THE PRACTICE OF INTERVENTIONAL RADIOLOGY
with Online Cases and Videos

THE PRACTICE OF INTERVENTIONAL RADIOLOGY
with Online Cases and Videos

KARIM VALJI, MD
Professor of Radiology
Chief of Interventional Radiology
University of Washington
Seattle, Washington

ELSEVIER
SAUNDERS

1600 John F. Kennedy Blvd.
Ste 1800
Philadelphia, PA 19103-2899

THE PRACTICE OF INTERVENTIONAL RADIOLOGY WITH ONLINE
CASES AND VIDEOS   ISBN: 978-1-4377-1719-8

Notices

Knowledge and best practice in this field are constantly changing. As new research and experience
broaden our understanding, changes in research methods, professional practices, or medical
treatment may become necessary.

Practitioners and researchers must always rely on their own experience and knowledge in
evaluating and using any information, methods, compounds, or experiments described herein.
In using such information or methods they should be mindful of their own safety and the safety
of others, including parties for whom they have a professional responsibility.

With respect to any drug or pharmaceutical products identified, readers are advised to check
the most current information provided (i) on procedures featured or (ii) by the manufacturer of
each product to be administered, to verify the recommended dose or formula, the method and
duration of administration, and contraindications. It is the responsibility of practitioners, relying
on their own experience and knowledge of their patients, to make diagnoses, to determine
dosages and the best treatment for each individual patient, and to take all appropriate safety
precautions.

To the fullest extent of the law, neither the Publisher nor the authors, contributors, or editors,
assume any liability for any injury and/or damage to persons or property as a matter of
products liability, negligence or otherwise, or from any use or operation of any methods,
products, instructions, or ideas contained in the material herein.

Library of Congress Cataloging-in-Publication Data

Valji, Karim.
  The practice of interventional radiology : with online cases and videos / Karim Valji.
      p. ; cm.
  Based on: Vascular and interventional radiology / Karim Valji. 2nd ed. c2006.
  Includes bibliographical references and index.
  ISBN 978-1-4377-1719-8 (hardcover : alk. paper)
  I. Valji, Karim. Vascular and interventional radiology. II. Title.
  [DNLM: 1. Radiography, interventional—methods—Atlases.
  2. Angiography—methods—Atlases. 3. Vascular Diseases—radiography—Atlases. WN 17]
LC classification not assigned
616.1'307572—dc23   2011041700

Acquisitions Editor: Pamela Hetherington
Developmental Editor: Joanie Milnes
Publishing Services Manager: Jeffrey Patterson
Senior Project Manager: Mary G. Stueck
Design Direction: Louis Forgione

Working together to grow
libraries in developing countries

www.elsevier.com | www.bookaid.org | www.sabre.org

ELSEVIER   BOOK AID International   Sabre Foundation

Printed in China

Last digit is the print number: 9 8 7 6 5 4 3 2 1

For Susanna

Contributors

Hamed Aryafar, MD
Assistant Clinical Professor of Radiology
Department of Radiology
University of California
San Diego, California
Chapter 4: Percutaneous Biopsy

Horacio R. D'Agostino, MD, FICS, FACR, FSIR
Professor of Radiology, Surgery, and Anesthesiology;
Chairman, Department of Radiology
Louisiana State University Health Sciences Center
Shreveport, Louisiana
Chapter 5: Transcatheter Fluid Drainage

Eric J. Hohenwalter, MD
Associate Professor of Radiology and Surgery
Division of Vascular and Interventional Radiology
Department of Radiology
Medical College of Wisconsin
Milwaukee, Wisconsin
Chapter 24: Interventional Oncology

Thomas B. Kinney, MD, MSME
Professor of Clinical Radiology
Director of HHT Clinic
Department of Radiology
University of California
San Diego, California
Chapter 4: Percutaneous Biopsy

Matthew Kogut, MD
Assistant Professor of Interventional Radiology
University of Washington
Seattle, Washington
Chapter 23: Urologic and Genital Systems

Todd L. Kooy, MD
Assistant Professor of Radiology
Department of Radiology
University of Washington
Seattle, Washington
Chapter 23: Urologic and Genital Systems

Gregory Lim
Mills-Peninsula Health Services
Burlingame, California
Chapter 21: Gastrointestinal Interventions

Ajit V. Nair
Associate Physician
Kaiser Permanente Medical Center
Modesto, California
Chapter 5: Transcatheter Fluid Drainage

Steven B. Oglevie, MD
Chief of Interventional Radiology
Hoag Memorial Hospital Presbyterian
Newport Beach, California
Chapter 23: Urologic and Genital Systems

Erik Ray, MD
Assistant Professor of Radiology
University of Washington
Seattle, Washington
Chapter 19: Hemodialysis Access

William Rilling, MD
Professor of Radiology and Surgery
Medical College of Wisconsin
Milwaukee, Wisconsin
Chapter 24: Interventional Oncology

Gerant Rivera-Sanfeliz
Associate Professor of Radiology
University of California
San Diego, California
Chapter 21: Gastrointestinal Interventions

Anne C. Roberts, MD
Professor of Radiology
Chief of Vascular and Interventional Radiology
Department of Radiology
University of California;
San Diego Medical Center
Thornton Hospital
La Jolla, California
Chapter 19: Hemodialysis Access

Steven C. Rose, MD
Professor of Radiology
University of California
San Diego Medical Center
San Diego, California
Chapter 22: Biliary System

David Sella
Department of Radiology
Mayo Clinic
Jacksonville, Florida
Chapter 24: Interventional Oncology

Tony P. Smith, MD
Professor of Radiology;
Division Chief of Peripheral and
    Neurological Interventional Radiology
Department of Radiology
Duke University Medical Center
Durham, North Carolina
Chapter 20: Neurointerventions

Sandeep Vaidya, MD
Assistant Professor of Radiology
Department of Radiology
University of Washington
Seattle, Washington
Chapter 21: Gastrointestinal Interventions

Preface

For centuries the design and function of medical textbooks remained largely unchanged. However, the ongoing revolution in digital technology affects almost every human endeavor and its influence on "book learning" is no exception. The rising generation of students and trainees has thoroughly embraced new interactive and dynamic educational tools. These materials emphasize visual elements, smaller "bites" of learning, and immediate access to cited primary sources. For a specialty such as interventional radiology (IR) that is so image-rich and procedure driven, the standard printed textbook is becoming an anachronism. There may be heated debate about the merits of the old and new ways, but change is unavoidable. The web-based features of this book were included to appeal to these new modes for learning IR.

The Practice of Interventional Radiology is largely based on the second edition of my previous text, *Vascular and Interventional Radiology,* which was published in 2006. Why the title change? Many hospital radiology divisions and even the American Board of Radiology still use the more traditional term. But almost all young trainees and an increasing number of patients around the world call our specialty (in their own native language), quite simply, "IR": interventional radiology. The appellation has stuck, and we should embrace it.

As before, my goal is to present the entire spectrum of vascular and nonvascular image-guided interventional procedures in a rigorous but practical, concise, and balanced fashion. Two new chapters have been added to fill noticeable gaps in the previous work—one covering neurointerventional procedures and a second devoted to interventional oncology. I doubt many readers will miss the one deleted chapter on lymphangiography. The introductory section of the book provides a foundation for the discipline, including chapters on the pathology of vascular diseases (the historic core of IR), the fundamentals of patient care, and basic interventional techniques. The bulk of the remaining chapters are clustered in sections and cover each of the major vascular beds. The final section contains material on nonvascular interventional procedures (organized by organ system) and a final chapter on oncologic interventions. Disease pathogenesis and natural history, relevant aspects of imaging studies, specific IR techniques and their expected outcomes, and the relative merits of various treatment modalities are emphasized throughout. For every procedure, I have summarized the best available evidence to support—or occasionally refute—the value of a particular therapy. The technical details of many procedures are described

in some depth. Still, the craft of our work can and should only be learned by extensive hands-on training from experienced practitioners.

The book includes over 1500 illustrations, many of them new. When appropriate, color has been added to radiographic images. All of the line drawings were redone in color to improve clarity. References were thoroughly updated. The citations are extensive but not exhaustive; they should direct the reader to the most important current—as well as classic or historic—publications covering each topic. For many of them, hyperlinks are included in the web-based version of the book that allow direct access to the actual journal articles.

The online book format has allowed several new features. The user can access a digital form of the text through the publisher's website for use on a computer (or, ultimately, an electronic reader). As an e-book, the reader will be able to highlight, dog-ear, and otherwise personalize the content to make it an enduring study guide. A major new element is the online library of over 100 unknown IR case studies that encompass the essential diseases and procedures that should be familiar to all imagers and interventionalists. The clinical cases and procedures are completely distinct from those found in the body of the text. The modules are interactive—questions are posed on each screen about the findings on the images presented, the differential diagnosis, characteristics of the particular disease, and possible treatment options. More advanced technical questions are aimed at actual IR practitioners. Each case is ultimately linked to the appropriate section of the main online text, giving the interested reader more detailed information about the subject under study. The other notable addition is a collection of short videos comprised of fluoroscopic sequences and/or movies taken at the interventional table. These subtitled clips illustrate many basic and some more complex interventional techniques. Some videos will be available with the launch of the book; others will be added over time.

The authorship is somewhat unusual for such a broad medical textbook. As with previous editions, I am the sole author for the introductory sections and most of the material concerned with vascular interventions. I leave it to the reader to decide whether that was hubris on my part. The nonvascular interventional chapters were originally written by IR faculty at the University of California, San Diego. All of them have been revised or largely rewritten by colleagues at my new home—the University of Washington in Seattle. Finally, I invited several noted authorities from outside institutions to write the two new chapters on neurointerventions and interventional oncology

As before, the book is aimed primarily at trainees in diagnostic radiology and interventional radiology. The IR fellow should master all of the material set forth in the text. The case library is geared to residents who do not intend to practice the specialty. These individuals still need to gain a basic understanding of the nature of and indications for IR procedures to become competent practicing diagnostic radiologists. For interventionalists finished with primary training, the book should serve as a comprehensive review of the current state of the field and also as a reference source for occasional consultation. Finally, it may be of value to physicians in other specialties who have an interest in performing selected IR procedures; however, it can only supplement (and certainly not replace) extensive formal training in these subjects.

Karim Valji

Acknowledgments

I am indebted to my publishing team at Elsevier/Saunders, led by Pam Hetherington, Joanie Milnes, and Mary Stueck. I am also grateful to David Wolbrecht of UW Creative at the University of Washington for a first-rate job in editing and producing the video and fluoroscopic clips included in the online version of this book.

I am privileged to work with an exceptional group of colleagues in interventional radiology and vascular surgery at the University of Washington and Harborview Medical Center in Seattle. Many of them enthusiastically contributed to this project with revised chapters for the book. In addition, a substantial number of the new figures come directly from interventional cases they performed as part of their daily practice.

For two decades, I have had the great pleasure of training interventional radiology fellows and diagnostic radiology residents at the University of California, San Diego and the University of Washington. I wrote all of my books specifically with them in mind. As I have said before, it is these trainees who keep me feeling young, fresh, and inspired.

Karim Valji

Contents

Core Cases in Interventional Radiology

1. Aberrant Right Subclavian Artery (6)
2. Blue Toe Syndrome from Aortic Plaque (8)
3. Normal Upper Extremity Arterial Anatomy (9)
4. Circumaortic Left Renal Vein (10)
5. Traumatic Leg Arteriovenous Fistula (8)
6. Normal Celiac Artery Anatomy (11)
7. Splenic Artery Aneurysm (12)
8. Acute Pulmonary Embolism with Thrombolytic Therapy (14)
9. Percutaneous Cholecystostomy (22)
10. Diverticular Abscess Drainage (5)
11. Normal Inferior Vena Cava Anatomy (16)
12. Superior Vena Cava Occlusion (17)
13. Aortic Dissection with Stent Placement (6)
14. Abdominal Aortic Aneurysm (AAA) Endovascular Repair with Type II Endoleak (7)
15. Postoperative Lymphocele Drainage and Sclerosis (5)
16. Biliary Stent Placement for Malignant Obstruction (22)
17. High Origin of Radial Artery, Variant (9)
18. Renal Artery Stent Placement with Rupture (10)
19. Separate Origins of Hepatic and Splenic Arteries (11)
20. Abdominal Drainage of GIST Tumor (5)
21. Uterine Artery Embolization for Fibroid Tumors (13)
22. Bronchial Artery Embolization for Hemoptysis from Tuberculosis (14)
23. Megacava with Filter Placement (16)
24. Percutaneous Treatment of Ureteral Leak (23)
25. Portal Vein Embolization Prior to Partial Liver Resection (24)
26. Retrieval of Retained Intravascular Foreign Body (18)
27. Aortic Coarctation (6)
28. Thrombosed Popliteal Artery Aneurysm (8)
29. Subclavian Steal Syndrome (9)
30. Retroperitoneal Biopsy of Sarcoma (4)
31. Retroaortic Left Renal Vein (10)
32. Post-biopsy Colonic Bleed with Embolotherapy (11)
33. Treatment of TIPS Dysfunction (12)
34. Pelvic Congestion Syndrome with Embolotherapy (13)
35. Renal Cyst Sclerosis (5)
36. Percutaneous Nephrostomy for Ureteral Obstruction by Stone (23)
37. Chronic Iliofemoral Vein Thrombosis with Stent Placement (15)
38. Retrieval of IVC Filter with Retained Thrombus (16)
39. Superior Vena Cava Syndrome with Stent Placement (17)
40. Percutaneous Thyroid Biopsy (4)
41. Biliary-Enteric Anastomotic Stricture with Stone Disease (22)
42. Leriche Syndrome of Abdominal Aorta (7)
43. Acute Femoropopliteal Artery Bypass Graft Occlusion (8)
44. Post-biopsy Renal AV Fistula with Embolotherapy (10)
45. Transtracheal Neck Mass Biopsy (4)
46. Celiac Compression (Median Arcuate Ligament) Syndrome (11)
47. Splenic Artery Pseudoaneurysm with Embolotherapy (12)
48. Pulmonary AVM with Embolotherapy (14)
49. Circumaortic Left Renal Vein with IVC Filter Placement (16)
50. Transgluteal Drainage with Ureteral Perforation (5)
51. Acute Secondary Axillosubclavian Vein Thrombosis with Lytic Therapy (17)
52. Aortic Dissection (Stanford A) (6)
53. Inflammatory Aortic Aneurysm (7)
54. Pelvic Trauma with Embolotherapy (8)
55. Post-transplant Portal Vein Stenosis (12)
56. Hypothenar Hammer Syndrome (9)
57. Renal Cell Carcinoma with IVC Invasion (10)
58. Liver Bleeding from Angiosarcoma with Embolotherapy (24)
59. Chronic Left Iliac Vein Occlusion (May Thurner Syndrome) (15)
60. Dialysis Access Balloon Angioplasty (19)
61. Port Catheter Tip in Azygous Vein (18)
62. Unusual Thoracic Aortic Aneurysm (MAGIC Syndrome) (6)
63. Percutaneous Treatment of Biliary Stones (22)
64. Subclavian and Brachial Artery Embolism with Lysis (9)
65. Type II Endoleak after Endovascular Aneurysm Repair (7)
66. Blunt Renal Artery Trauma with Embolotherapy (10)
67. Chronic Mesenteric Ischemia from SMA Occlusion (11)
68. Gastric Varices with Splenorenal Shunt (12)
69. Adrenal Biopsy (4)
70. Popliteal Artery Entrapment (8)
71. IVC Duplication with Filter Placement (16)
72. Cephalic Vein Stenosis with Angioplasty in Patient with Dialysis Graft (19)
73. Right Aortic Arch (6)
74. Buerger Disease of Lower Extremity (8)
75. Hepatic Amebic Abscess Drainage (5)
76. Renal Artery Fibromuscular Dysplasia with Angioplasty (10)

Online only at expertconsult.com
(associated chapters in parentheses).

BASIC PRINCIPLES AND TECHNIQUES

1

Pathogenesis of Vascular Diseases

Karim Valji

Historically, the cornerstone of interventional radiology (IR) is the vascular system, which since the 1950s was the province of angiographers. Modern IR practice now encompasses almost every part of the body. Although interventionalists must gain a strong foundation in the pathology of all organ systems that they treat, a substantial volume of work still happens within blood vessels. As such, all practitioners engaged in IR, regardless of background, must be particularly expert in the pathogenesis of diseases of the arteries and veins.

ARTERIES

Normal Structure

Human arteries are composed of three layers (Fig. 1-1). The *intima* consists of a sheet of endothelial cells lining the vessel lumen and a thin subendothelial matrix. The *endothelium* has a variety of critical functions.[1] It controls hemostasis largely by acting as a barrier between circulating blood and the thrombogenic subendothelial layer. Endothelial cells can indirectly alter vessel caliber when changes in blood oxygen tension, pressure, or flow are detected. The endothelium produces and responds to a variety of factors that are vital to arterial repair after injury.

The *media* is separated from the intima by the internal elastic lamina. This layer is primarily composed of collagen, elastin, and smooth muscle cells arranged in longitudinal and circumferential bundles. *Elastic (conduit) arteries* (i.e., aorta, aortic arch vessels, iliac artery, and pulmonary arteries) propel blood forward because dense bands of elastin let these vessels expand during systole and contract during diastole.[2] In the smaller-caliber *muscular arteries*, smooth muscle cells predominate, and the circumferential orientation of the cells allows the lumen to dilate or constrict in response to various stimuli.

The *adventitia* is composed of a fibrocellular matrix that includes fibroblasts, collagen, and elastin. In some vessels, an external elastic lamina separates the media from this outermost layer. Sympathetic nerves penetrate into the vessel wall and can alter smooth muscle tone in the media. A fine network of blood vessels, the *vasa vasorum,* supplies the adventitia of larger arteries and provides nutrients to this layer and the outer media. The intima and inner media are nourished by diffusion from the lumen.

Small arteries become *arterioles*, which are 40 to 200 micrometers (µm) in diameter. Arterioles lead into *capillaries.* Direct arteriovenous communications without interposed capillary networks exist in some vascular beds. These connections allow diversion of blood away from certain parts of the body in physiologic and pathologic states, such as shunting of blood from the skin and extremities in a hypotensive individual.

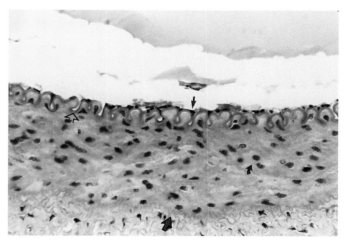

FIGURE 1-1 Photomicrograph of a normal artery (hematoxylin-eosin stain, original magnification ×40). A single layer of endothelial cells *(small arrow)* lines the internal elastic *lamina (open arrow).* The media is primarily made up of smooth muscle cells *(curved arrow).* The external elastic lamina *(large arrow)* separates the media from the adventitia.

Functional Disorders

Arterial tone and luminal diameter are regulated by several mechanisms[1]:

- Cells in the vascular wall release smooth muscle vasodilators (e.g., prostacyclin, nitric oxide) or vasoconstrictors (e.g., endothelin, thromboxane A_2) to regulate downstream blood flow.
- Vasomotor nerves act through neurotransmitters such as norepinephrine and acetylcholine.
- Circulating agents (e.g., angiotensin II and vasopressin) also affect vascular tone.

Vasodilation is seen primarily in low-resistance systems, such as arteriovenous fistulas, arteriovenous malformations, and hypervascular tumors, and in collateral circulations (Fig. 1-2). Vasoconstriction usually is the result of vascular trauma or low-flow conditions (Fig. 1-3). Ingestion or infusion of certain drugs (e.g., vasopressin, dopamine, epinephrine) also can lead to vasospasm (Fig. 1-4). *Raynaud disease* is a functional disorder primarily affecting the small arteries of the hands and feet in which intermittent vasospasm is caused by external stimuli[3] (see Chapter 9). The hallmarks of vasospasm are resolution over time or relief with vasodilators.

Arterial *"standing"* or *"stationary"* *waves* are an imaging curiosity that may be confused with functional vasospasm[4] (Fig. 1-5). Standing waves have been noted at both catheter

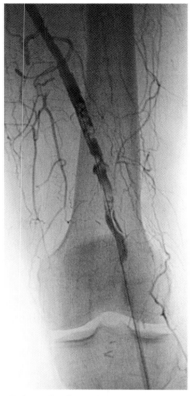

FIGURE 1-2   Enlarged collateral vessels bypass a popliteal artery occlusion.

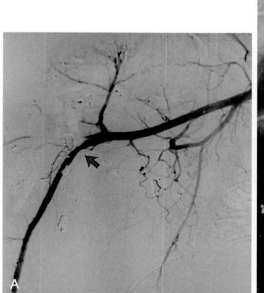

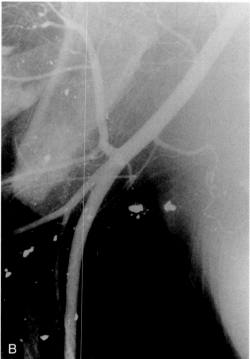

FIGURE 1-3   Post-traumatic arterial vasospasm. **A,** The *arrow* indicates focal narrowing of the upper right brachial artery. **B,** A follow-up arteriogram obtained 3 days later shows complete resolution of spasm.

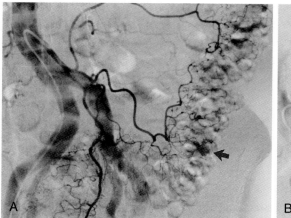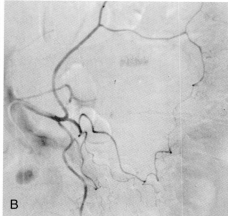

FIGURE 1-4 Vasopressin-induced vasospasm. **A,** Inferior mesenteric arteriogram shows extravasation in the left colon. **B,** After infusion of vasopressin, the vessels are diffusely constricted and the bleeding has stopped.

and magnetic resonance (MR) angiography. Their precise cause is unknown, but a leading hypothesis invokes secondary retrograde flow (typical in high resistance arteries) as the explanation for this temporary oscillating pattern.[5,6]

Atherosclerosis

Atherosclerosis is the most common disease affecting the vascular system and the leading cause of morbidity and mortality in the Western world. It develops as a result of an *inflammatory response* to lipid storage in the arterial wall.[7] Various provocative factors for disease may act as triggers for inflammation (see later discussion). The common inciting event is endothelial dysfunction mediated through the immune system. The damaged endothelium induces platelet activation, which in turn causes white blood cell adhesion to the vascular wall.[8] Lipoproteins and monocytes enter the subendothelial space and produce "fatty streaks" composed largely of foam cells.[9] A variety of factors are released in response to this pathologic process. These substances cause medial smooth muscle cells to migrate to and then proliferate in the intima. Overproduction of collagen, elastin, and proteoglycans gives the lesion a fibrotic character. Chronic inflammation ensues. With time, medial thinning, cellular necrosis, and plaque calcification and degeneration occur (Fig. 1-6). Ultimately, plaque fracture, ulceration, hemorrhage, or thrombosis may occur.

A number of risk factors for atherosclerosis have been identified (Box 1-1). However, these conditions do

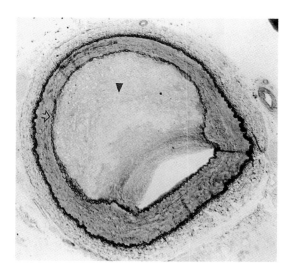

FIGURE 1-5 Standing (stationary) waves in the proximal right superficial femoral artery *(arrow)*. These appear as subtle periodic oscillations in the lumen contour.

FIGURE 1-6 Atherosclerosis in a human coronary artery (elastin stain, original magnification ×20). An advanced acellular intimal plaque markedly narrows the vessel lumen. Multiple cholesterol clefts *(arrowhead)* are seen. The internal elastic lamina *(open arrow)* is relatively intact. *(Specimen courtesy of Ahmed Shabaik, MD, San Diego, Calif.)*

not account for all cases of the disease. There are several other markers for the development of atherosclerosis.[10] *C-reactive protein (CRP)* is an acute phase reactant that accumulates in blood in the presence of an inflammatory state. Elevated serum CRP is strongly associated with progression of atherosclerotic lesions in asymptomatic patients and in those with established disease.[11] High levels of the amino acid *homocysteine* are also associated with a significant risk of arterial and venous thrombosis. Finally, increased *arterial stiffness* (i.e., diminished arterial distensibility) is now recognized as an important independent predictor for future cardiovascular disease.[12]

Atherosclerosis causes symptoms by blood flow reduction, thrombotic occlusion, plaque ulceration with distal embolization, and rarely by penetration into and

through the media. Plaques can produce mild to severe irregularity of the wall or smooth, concentric narrowing (Fig. 1-7). A protruding plaque can mimic a luminal filling defect (Fig. 1-8). Significant atherosclerosis is most commonly seen at branch points and at certain anatomic sites, including the coronary arteries, carotid artery bifurcation, infrarenal abdominal aorta, and lower extremity arteries. Most affected patients have diffuse disease at many sites. Arterial luminal narrowing has several causes, although atherosclerosis is the most common (Box 1-2).

Neointimal Hyperplasia and Restenosis

Neointimal hyperplasia is the "scar" produced by arteries (and veins) in response to significant injury or altered hemodynamics. Even though neointimal hyperplasia has features in common with atherosclerosis, it is a different pathophysiologic process. When caused by endovascular or surgical maneuvers (e.g., balloon angioplasty or stent placement), neointimal hyperplasia is triggered by clot formation and wall stretching at the site of injury.[13] Over several days, monocytes and lymphocytes infiltrate the thrombus, which is itself partially resorbed. Growth factors released from smooth muscle cells, macrophages, and platelets cause smooth muscle cell proliferation and migration to form a thickened intima (Figs. 1-9 and 1-10). This evolution is complete within 3 to 6 months after injury.[14] As with atherosclerosis, there is growing evidence that inflammation plays a central role in neointimal hyperplasia and restenosis.[15,16]

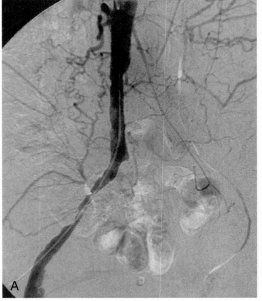 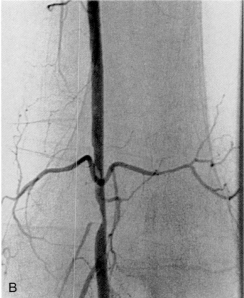

FIGURE 1-7 Atherosclerosis. **A,** Typical diffuse disease involving the abdominal aorta and right iliac artery. There is also thrombotic occlusion of the left iliac and right internal iliac arteries. **B,** Focal eccentric narrowing of the popliteal artery.

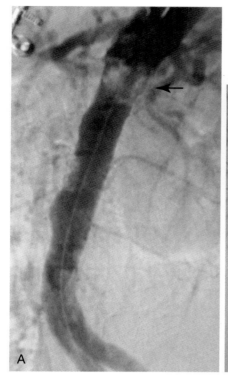
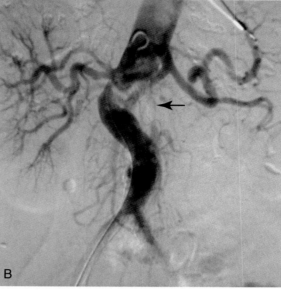

FIGURE 1-8 Plaque masquerading as thrombus. Lateral aortogram shows apparent embolus in the midabdominal aorta *(arrow).* **B,** Frontal image reveals that the defect is a large polypoid plaque arising from the left side of the aorta *(arrow).*

The degree of luminal narrowing *(restenosis)* after angioplasty or stent placement depends on the exuberance of the neointimal hyperplastic response and the extent of vascular remodeling. Negative remodeling, which may be caused by elastic recoil of the vessel or progressive thickening of the adventitia, can be partially controlled by placement of a stent.

Thrombosis

The ingredients for thrombosis are platelets and other cellular blood elements, coagulation proteins, and often an abnormal endothelium. Clot formation begins with platelet adhesion and aggregation on the subendothelial vascular surface.[17] Platelets release substances (e.g., adenosine diphosphate [ADP] and thromboxane A_2)

BOX 1-2

CAUSES OF ARTERIAL LUMINAL NARROWING

- Atherosclerosis
- Intimal hyperplasia
- Vasospasm
- Low-flow state
- Dissection
- Vasculitis
- Neoplastic or inflammatory encasement
- Fibromuscular dysplasia
- Extrinsic compression

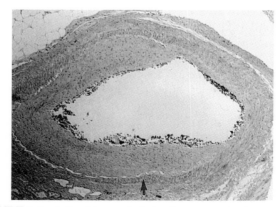

FIGURE 1-9 Intimal hyperplasia in a human renal artery (hematoxylin-eosin stain, original magnification ×40). The concentric thickening of the intima can be identified along with smooth muscle cells, fibroblasts, and matrix material. The internal elastic lamina *(arrow)* denotes the boundary between intima and media. *(Specimen courtesy of Ahmed Shabaik, MD, San Diego, Calif.)*

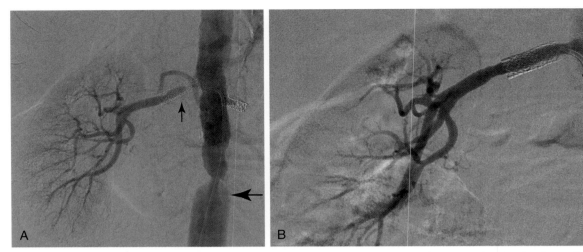

FIGURE 1-10   Intimal hyperplasia. **A,** Aortogram shows narrowing throughout the lumen of a previously placed right renal artery stent *(small arrow).* The neointimal hyperplasia is most severe proximally. Incidental note is made of an occluded left renal artery stent and infrarenal abdominal aortic stenosis *(large arrow).* **B,** Following balloon angioplasty, the narrowing of the right renal artery is markedly reduced.

that further accelerate platelet activation. Aggregation of platelets occur by cross-linking of fibrinogen and von Willebrand factor through *platelet surface* $\alpha_{IIb}\beta3$ *integrin receptors* (formerly designated as IIb/IIIa). Activation of the complex coagulation pathway (which begins with factor VII and tissue factor) leads to the formation of a "prothrombinase complex" (antiphospholipids bound to activated factors Va and Xa). Prothrombin is thus converted to *thrombin,* which is the critical enzyme responsible for transformation of *fibrinogen* to *fibrin.* A stable clot is formed from platelets, red blood cells, and white blood cells enmeshed within a fibrin matrix.

The coagulation cascade is regulated at almost every step to prevent uncontrolled thrombus formation at injured sites or remote locations. The primary "natural" anticoagulants are protein C, protein S, and antithrombin (AT). The former are vitamin K–dependent proteins activated by thrombomodulin-bound thrombin. Activated protein C (APC) binds with activated protein S to form the "APC complex," which degrades several procoagulant factors. Finally, intact endothelial cells produce heparin-like molecules, which promote AT-mediated inactivation of numerous coagulation enzymes.

Classically, thrombosis occurs in the presence of vessel injury, slow flow, or a thrombophilic (hypercoagulable) state (i.e., *Virchow triad*). However, recent experimental work suggests that underlying inherited or secondary thrombophilia is the primary instigator of pathologic clot formation. In most cases, thrombi form at sites of preexisting disease (e.g., atherosclerosis, intimal hyperplasia) or acute trauma (see Figs. 1-2 and 1-7).

In addition to thrombosis, arterial occlusion has several other causes (Box 1-3).

BOX 1-3

CAUSES OF ARTERIAL OCCLUSION

- Thrombosis
- Embolism
- Dissection
- Trauma
- Neoplastic invasion
- Extrinsic compression
- Vasculitis or vasculopathy
- Functional defect (e.g., drug-induced)

Thrombophilia

A variety of hereditary and acquired disorders predispose to venous or arterial thrombosis[17] (Boxes 1-4 and 1-5). Several inherited thrombophilias slightly to moderately increase the risk of pathologic thrombi. However, nontraumatic clot formation is much more likely in an individual when multiple congenital or secondary risk factors are present. *Arterial thrombosis* is particularly associated with antiphospholipid syndrome (APS), heparin-induced thrombocytopenia (HIT), protein C and S deficiencies, and myeloproliferative disorders (polycythemia vera and essential thrombocytosis.) Certain clinical situations should raise the suspicion for undiagnosed thrombophilia[17] (Box 1-6).

Factor V Leiden refers to a mutation at the 1691 position of the gene coding for factor V. The activated cofactor is made resistant to activated protein C, thereby

BOX 1-4

MAJOR INHERITED THROMBOPHILIAS

- Factor V gene mutation (G1691A) (factor V Leiden, activated protein C [APC] resistance)
- Prothrombin (factor II) gene mutation (G20210A)
- Hyperhomocysteinemia
- Antithrombin deficiency
- Protein S deficiency
- Protein C deficiency
- Elevated factor VIII
- Elevated factors IX or XI

BOX 1-5

SECONDARY THROMBOPHILIAS

- Antiphospholipid syndrome*
- Malignancy
  - Many antitumor and supportive medications (e.g., thalidomide, erythropoietin)
- Heparin-induced thrombocytopenia
- Myeloproliferative disorders
  - Polycythemia vera
  - Essential thrombocythemia
- Paroxysmal nocturnal hemoglobinuria
- Nephrotic syndrome
- Inflammatory bowel disease
- Advanced age
- Surgery
- Immobility
- Trauma
- Obesity
- Pregnancy/postpartum state
- Estrogen and hormonal therapies (e.g., contraceptives, replacement, selective estrogen receptor modulators)
- Central venous catheters

*APS may occur as a primary disorder without underlying systemic lupus erythematosus or other rheumatologic disorder.

BOX 1-6

CLINICAL AND LABORATORY FEATURES OF PRIMARY THROMBOPHILIAS

- Recurrent VTE or VTE in young patient without established risk factors
- Unprovoked thrombosis at unusual sites (e.g., mesenteric vessels, portal vein, renal veins)
- In situ arterial thrombosis
- Unexplained rethrombosis during thrombolysis or other recanalization procedures
- Resistance to heparin during interventions (i.e., unresponsive activated clotting time) related to antithrombin deficiency or consumption
- Unexplained elevation in baseline partial thromboplastin time related to lupus anticoagulant and possible antiphospholipid syndrome

VTE, venous thromboembolic disease.

Prothrombin gene mutation refers to a single point defect at the 20210 nucleotide position of the prothrombin gene that causes *elevated* levels of prothrombin in blood and renders the protein relatively resistant to APC. Like factor V Leiden, this inherited disorder only adds significantly to the risk of *recurrent* VTE when other hypercoagulable risk factors are also present.[18-20]

Antithrombin (AT) deficiency is a rare inherited autosomal dominant disorder expressed as lack of enzyme production (type I) or abnormal enzyme function (type II).[21] AT is a key protein in regulation of coagulation by inactivation of thrombin and a variety of other coagulation factors. Although AT deficiency is a rare thrombophilia, it carries a 10- to 30-fold increased lifetime relative risk of venous (and less often arterial) thrombosis.[18,19] An acquired form of AT deficiency is associated with liver disease and nephrotic syndrome.

Protein C and *protein S deficiencies* (as measured by activity or serum concentration) may be inherited or acquired. There is a 75% to 90% lifetime risk for VTE (and less often arterial thrombosis) in affected individuals with family members who have suffered a thrombotic event.[19,22] Acquired protein C or S deficiency can be seen with septic shock, advanced liver disease, vitamin K antagonists (e.g., warfarin), HIV infection, nephrotic syndrome, acute inflammation, pregnancy, or oral contraceptive therapy.

blunting its natural anticoagulant effect.[18] Factor V Leiden is the most common inherited thrombophilia in Caucasian populations (about 5%). The lifetime risk for venous thromboembolic disease (VTE) for heterozygotes is increased 3- to 8-fold.[19]

Elevated coagulation factor levels are being recognized as a relatively frequent cause for apparently idiopathic thrombophilia. In particular, excessive levels of factors VIII, IX, and XI are associated with increased risk for VTE, although specific genetic abnormalities have not yet been isolated.[23,24]

Hyperhomocysteinemia refers to elevated blood levels of homocysteine, its oxidative metabolite homocystine, and other disulfides.[17] A specific mutation in the gene for methylenetetrahydrofolate reductase (MTHFR) may cause mild hyperhomocysteinemia. When homocysteine levels are elevated, there is a significant added risk for venous or arterial thrombosis.[25] *Homocystinuria* is a rare autosomal recessive disorder caused by mutations of the cystathionine beta-synthase gene. The illness is marked by exceedingly high levels of homocysteine, arterial or venous thrombosis at an early age, premature atherosclerosis, Marfanoid features, and mental retardation.

Antiphospholipid syndrome (APS) is the most common acquired thrombophilia.[17,26] The hallmarks of these conditions are apparently unprovoked vascular thrombosis and persistent elevation of antiphospholipid (aPL) antibodies of the lupus anticoagulant, anticardiolipin, or anti-beta-2-glycoprotein I type.[27] The frequency of primary and secondary forms (the latter associated with connective tissue disorders such as systemic lupus erythematosus [SLE]) is about equal. The prototypical patient is a young to middle-aged woman with apparently idiopathic arterial or venous thrombosis. The risk for recurrent thrombotic events is significant. Because healthy people may transiently demonstrate aPL antibodies, positive clinical and laboratory criteria are needed for diagnosis.

Heparin-induced thrombocytopenia (HIT) is triggered by antibodies to heparin-platelet factor IV complexes in blood. These antibody complexes can precipitate platelet activation and degranulation, tissue factor and procoagulant release, and ultimately pathologic clot formation. About 3% of individuals who receive unfractionated heparin and 1.5% of those who receive low molecular weight heparin compounds will develop thrombocytopenia (<50% of baseline) within 4 to 10 days of the start of treatment in any form.[28] Up to 50% of these patients will suffer HIT-related thrombosis (HITT), manifested by new or worsening VTE, arterial thrombosis, skin necrosis, or catheter-related deep vein thrombosis (DVT).[29] When bleeding or thrombosis occurs, *all* heparin products must be stopped and replaced with a direct thrombin inhibitor.

Malignancy-associated hypercoagulability (once called *Trousseau syndrome*) is a multifactorial condition related to cellular release of procoagulants, tissue factors, cytokines, and platelet activators.[30] Cancer is associated with impaired fibrinolysis, production of aPL antibodies, and acquired resistance to APC (Fig. 1-11). Thrombophilia is

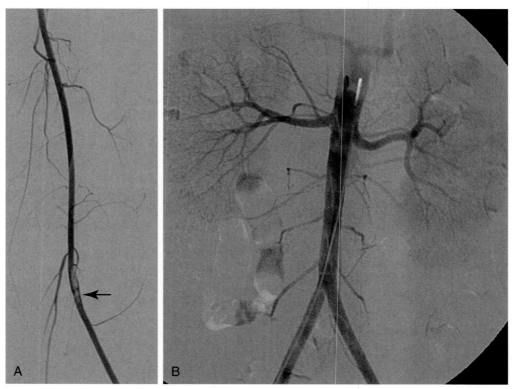

FIGURE 1-11   Thrombophilia-induced in situ thrombosis. **A,** Left leg arteriogram in a young woman with antiphospholipid syndrome shows an isolated thrombus *(arrow).* No other vascular disease was found in the legs or pelvis **(B).**

particularly common in several hematologic malignancies and in tumors of the pancreas, uterus, ovary, brain, stomach, lung, and prostate.[17]

Embolism

An embolus is any material that passes through the circulation and eventually lodges in a downstream vessel. Macroembolism and microembolism of the arterial circulation have numerous causes (Box 1-7).

Macroemboli usually are clots that originate from the heart or a central artery. Atherosclerotic plaque also can fragment and obstruct peripheral arteries. Emboli tend to lodge at arterial bifurcations or at sites of preexisting disease. After the embolic event occurs, the distal arteries constrict, and new thrombus propagates proximally and distally to the level of the next large collateral branches. It may be impossible to differentiate thrombotic from embolic occlusions by imaging, although an acute embolus has several classic angiographic features (Box 1-8 and Fig. 1-12). Real or apparent luminal filling defects are also observed with intimal flaps, protruding atherosclerotic plaques, inflow defects, and rarely with intraluminal tumor (Fig. 1-13; see also Fig. 1-8). An arterial *inflow defect* is caused by unopacified blood entering an artery beyond an obstruction through a collateral vessel.

Microemboli are seen in patients with ulcerated, protruding atherosclerotic plaques. Platelet-fibrin deposits can be released spontaneously into the distal circulation from a site of underlying disease. Cholesterol crystals (100 to 200 μ) also may shower into the distal circulation from a plaque.[31] Spontaneous release of small atheroemboli cause the *blue toe* (or *blue finger*) *syndrome*. However, the event may be associated with surgical manipulation, catheterization procedures, or treatment with anticoagulants or fibrinolytic agents.[32] Widespread embolization into the legs, kidneys, head, or intestinal tract can result in acute renal failure, stroke, profound lower extremity or intestinal ischemia, and even death[33] (see Chapter 2).

Aneurysms and Arterial Dilation

An aneurysm is defined as focal or diffuse dilation of an artery by more than 50% of its normal diameter.[34] In a *true aneurysm*, all three layers of the arterial wall are dilated but remain intact (Fig. 1-14). Degenerative (atherosclerosis-associated) aneurysms fall into this

---

BOX 1-8

ANGIOGRAPHIC SIGNS OF ACUTE ARTERIAL EMBOLISM

- Meniscus or filling defect
- Mild or absent diffuse vascular disease
- Lack of contralateral disease (in extremity arteries)
- Poorly developed collateral circulation
- Emboli or abrupt occlusions at other sites

BOX 1-7

SOURCES OF ARTERIAL EMBOLI

- Heart
  - Left atrial or ventricular thrombus
  - Endocardial vegetations
  - Atrial myxoma
- Thrombus superimposed on vascular disease (including aneurysms)
- Atherosclerotic plaque
- Catheterization procedures
  - Catheter-related thrombus
  - Plaque disruption
  - Gas bubbles
- Paradoxical emboli from the venous circulation
- Foreign bodies
  - Catheter or wire fragments
  - Gunshot pellets

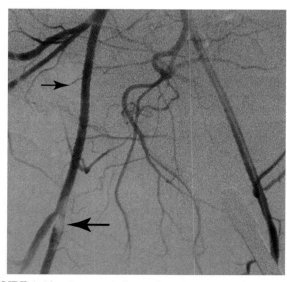

FIGURE 1-12   Acute embolus to the right common/superficial femoral artery *(large arrow)*. Note absence of other vascular disease, normal left common femoral artery, and lack of significant collateral circulation. Also note incidental finding of standing waves in the right external iliac artery *(small arrow)*.

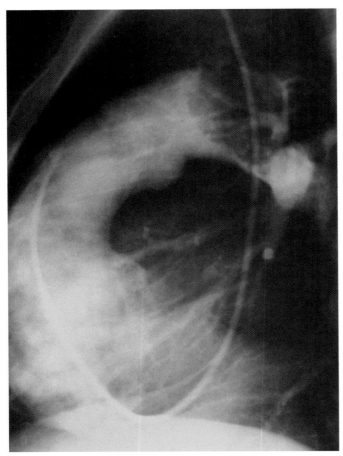

FIGURE 1-13   Main pulmonary artery sarcoma seen on a lateral pulmonary arteriogram.

category. In a *false aneurysm (pseudoaneurysm),* one or more layers of the arterial wall are disrupted (Fig. 1-15). Blood must be (temporarily) contained by the outer adventitia and surrounding supportive tissue. Trauma and infectious, neoplastic, or inflammatory masses typically produce pseudoaneurysms.[35] True aneurysms usually are *fusiform* with diffuse dilation involving the entire circumference of an artery. False aneurysms often are *saccular* with focal, eccentric dilation involving part of the circumference of the vessel. However, these morphologic features are not always reliable for pathologic distinction.

True and false aneurysms have a variety of causes (Box 1-9). *Degenerative aneurysms* are the most common. Although atherosclerosis and degenerative aneurysms are linked and often coexist in an individual, the two conditions are distinct disorders.[36] Degenerative aneurysms form because of inflammatory damage to the vessel wall and hemodynamic forces that produce remodeling.[37,38] The most common sites for degenerative aneurysms are the infrarenal abdominal aorta, descending thoracic aorta, and common iliac artery. Aneurysms of the popliteal, common femoral, internal iliac, brachiocephalic, and subclavian arteries are less common. Imaging features include diffuse arterial dilation, intimal calcification, and sometimes mural thrombus (see Fig. 1-14). The latter, which is common at most sites except the thoracic aorta, can obstruct branch vessels and give the lumen a smooth appearance.

Infectious (mycotic) aneurysms are caused by localized infection of the arterial wall.[39,40] They occur after inoculation of a preexisting aneurysm or from infection and progressive dilation of a previously normal artery. The infection can arise through seeding of the artery from the lumen or vasa vasorum, invasion from a neighboring

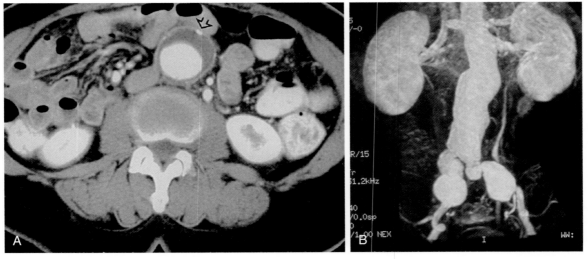

FIGURE 1-14   **A,** True degenerative aneurysm of the abdominal aorta with dilation of the entire aortic wall, luminal thrombus, and intimal calcification *(open arrow).* **B,** Maximum intensity projection gadolinium magnetic resonance angiogram shows large infrarenal true abdominal aortic aneurysm with extension to both iliac arteries.

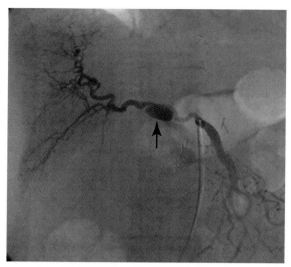

FIGURE 1-15   Pseudoaneurysm at anastomosis of liver transplant hepatic artery *(arrow)*.

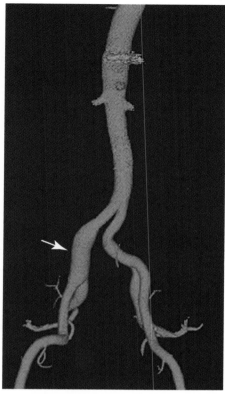

FIGURE 1-16   Ehlers-Danlos syndrome, type IV. Diffuse dilation of the right common iliac artery is noted *(arrow)* on shaded-surface display contrast-enhanced computed tomography angiography.

BOX 1-9

CAUSES OF ARTERIAL ANEURYSMS

- Atherosclerosis-associated degeneration
- Trauma
- Infection
- Inflammation
- Neoplastic invasion
- Vasculitis (see Box 1-10)
- Noninflammatory vasculopathy (see Box 1-10)
- Chronic dissection
- Congenital

---

infection, or from penetrating trauma. Infectious aneurysms are typically saccular, occur at unusual sites, and can be multiple (see Figs. 6-28 and 7-25). They are most commonly seen in the aorta, viscera, and lower extremity arteries. In addition to bacterial infections, tuberculous arteritis may cause an aneurysm to form.[41]

Traumatic pseudoaneurysms follow blunt trauma (e.g., deceleration injury), criminal penetrating trauma, and medical procedures (e.g., catheterization, surgical repair) (see Fig. 6-21). Like infectious aneurysms, they usually are saccular and eccentric and often occur in the absence of other vascular disease. Other causes of aneurysms are considered in the following sections (Fig. 1-16).

The potential complications of aneurysms and pseudoaneurysms are rupture, thrombosis, distal embolization of mural clot, compression of critical arteries (e.g., renal artery), and erosion of adjacent organs. The frequency of each of these complications varies with the type of aneurysm and its location. Aneurysm expansion is governed by *Laplace's law* (wall tension = pressure × radius). As a rule, the larger the aneurysm, the more rapid the rate of expansion and the greater the likelihood of rupture.

Several forms of arterial dilation may be confused with an aneurysm:

- Arterial *ectasia* is the age-related change that causes arteries to become dilated, tortuous, and lengthened (Fig. 1-17). Ectasia is particularly common in the thoracic aorta, abdominal aorta, and iliac and splenic arteries.
- *Arteriomegaly* is the diffuse enlargement of a long arterial segment (Fig. 1-18). It is typically seen in the iliac, carotid, and femoropopliteal vessels. The underlying pathology may be elastin deficiency within the media.[42]
- Compensatory dilation of inflow arteries occurs in high-flow states such as arteriovenous malformations and fistulas, hemodialysis grafts, and hypervascular tumors.
- Poststenotic dilation results from turbulence beyond a site of significant arterial narrowing (Fig. 1-19).

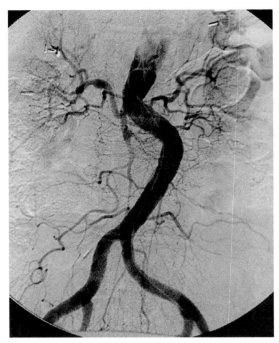

FIGURE 1-17   Ectasia of the aorta and iliac arteries in an elderly patient.

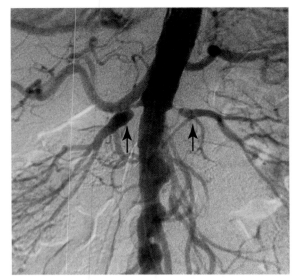

FIGURE 1-19   Poststenotic dilation of the right and left renal arteries beyond bilateral ostial stenoses *(arrows)*.

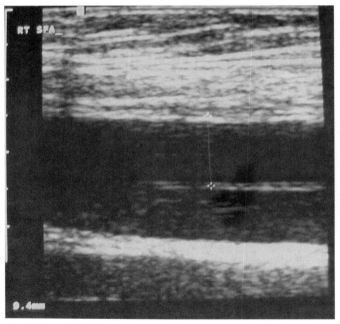

FIGURE 1-18   Diffuse arteriomegaly seen on longitudinal ultrasound. The right superficial femoral artery diameter (normally 5 to 6 mm) is 9 to 10 mm throughout its entire course.

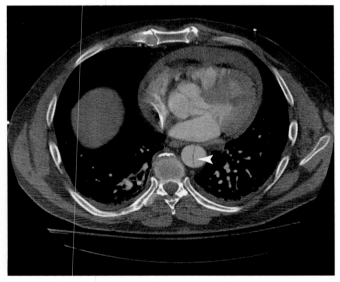

FIGURE 1-20   Acute aortic dissection on CT scan showing intimal flap *(arrowhead)* between the true and false lumen.

Dissection

Arterial dissection is a separation of layers of the vessel wall, usually between the intima and media or within the media. In most cases, an intimal tear initially connects the natural arterial lumen *(true lumen)* with the intramural space *(false lumen)*[43] (Fig. 1-20). An exit tear may later reconnect the false and true lumens and permit blood to flow freely through both channels. Branches along the course of the dissection can be fed by either lumen. Occasionally, the dissection is completely isolated from the lumen (i.e., *intramural hematoma;* see Fig. 6-30). The most common causes of aortic dissection are long-standing hypertension, chronic degeneration of the media, and trauma.

The major complications of dissection are rupture and end-organ ischemia. Rupture through the adventitia often occurs at the site of the intimal tear. Ischemia

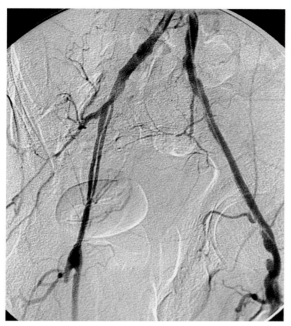

FIGURE 1-21   Chronic dissection of the right external iliac artery with a double-barrel lumen from a prior catheterization procedure.

results from obstruction of a branch vessel by the intimal flap or from slow flow in a branch fed by the nondominant lumen. In some cases, the false channel enlarges and compresses the true lumen. Left untreated, the false lumen can rupture, persist (*chronic dissection*), enlarge, or thrombose (Fig. 1-21).

Vasculitis

The hallmark of vasculitis is inflammation (and sometimes necrosis) of the blood vessel wall[44] (Box 1-10). The acute phase of these illnesses often is marked by constitutional symptoms and an elevated erythrocyte sedimentation rate (ESR) or CRP level. In the chronic phase, the effects of vascular damage, such as arterial narrowing, thrombosis, necrosis with aneurysm formation, or rupture become apparent.[45,46] Among the various disorders, the affected sites and severity of disease are wide ranging. Vasculitis should always be considered when obstructive or aneurysmal vascular disease occurs in strange circumstances (e.g., with a young patient or unusual location, distribution, or appearance). However, a number of purely infectious processes and noninflammatory vasculopathies can have an identical appearance on imaging studies (see Box 1-10).

Takayasu arteritis (TA) is a chronic, inflammatory vasculitis of large elastic arteries.[47,48] An autoimmune process has been implicated. In the acute stage, the adventitia and media are infiltrated with T cells, monocytes, and

---

BOX 1-10
MAJOR VASCULITIDES AND VASCULOPATHIES

Large Vessel (aorta and primary branches)

- Vasculitis
  - Takayasu arteritis
  - Giant cell arteritis
  - Connective tissue disorder
  - Radiation
  - Behçet syndrome
- Infections
  - Bacterial aneurysms
  - Syphilis
  - Tuberculosis
- Vasculopathies
  - Marfan syndrome
  - Ehlers-Danlos syndrome
  - Fibromuscular dysplasia
  - Human immunodeficiency virus (HIV) infection
  - Middle aortic syndrome
  - Neurofibromatosis
  - Loeys-Dietz syndrome

Medium and Small Vessel (first or second order aortic and distal branches)

- Vasculitis
  - Polyarteritis nodosa (PAN)
  - Buerger disease
  - Kawasaki disease
  - Behçet syndrome
  - Radiation arteritis
  - Connective tissue disorder
- Infections
  - Hepatitis B and C
  - Bacterial aneurysm
- Vasculopathies
  - Fibromuscular dysplasia
  - Marfan syndrome
  - Ehlers-Danlos syndrome
  - HIV infection
  - Drug-induced (e.g., cannabis, cocaine)
  - Grange syndrome

---

granulocytes entering through the vasa vasorum. Destruction and fibrosis progress inward through the entire vessel wall, leading to luminal narrowing or dilation.[49] If intimal thickening and associated calcification predominate, the lesion may be difficult to distinguish from atherosclerosis. TA primarily affects the aorta, its first order branches, and the pulmonary arteries. Several classification systems have been devised to categorize the distribution of disease.[50] In most patients, the thoracic and/or abdominal aorta and some of their principal branches (i.e., arch, renal, mesenteric, or iliac arteries) are involved. The pulmonary arteries are also affected in many cases.

TA is most commonly seen in Japan, China, Southeast Asia, India, and Latin America. However, it is being diagnosed more frequently in Western countries.[48] There is a strong female predilection, and most patients come to medical attention when they are teenagers or young adults. Clinical symptoms and signs in the chronic phase include upper extremity (and occasionally lower extremity) ischemia, arm blood pressure discrepancies, renovascular hypertension, cerebral ischemia, headaches, mesenteric ischemia, and angina. There is some controversy regarding the optimal clinical/imaging criteria required to make the diagnosis. However, most schemes involve some combination of appropriate demographic, clinical, and imaging features.[49]

Imaging is usually done with sonography, MR angiography, and positron emission tomography (PET).[51-53] However, the ability of MR to assess activity of disease is controversial.[54] In the acute or subacute stages, thickening and contrast enhancement of the arterial wall is evident.[55,56] The aorta itself may be dilated or narrowed[57,58] (Fig. 1-22). Long, smooth stenoses or complete occlusions of the proximal portions of the major aortic branches also are typical (see Fig. 6-25). Dilation or frank aneurysm of aortic branches is much less common (see Fig. 7-26). Arterial obstructions are treated when the patient has chronic end-organ ischemia, such as renovascular hypertension or arm "claudication." Aneurysm rupture is unusual, and operative treatment of asymptomatic aneurysms is rarely indicated. Involvement of the proximal subclavian and carotid arteries is more common with TA than giant cell arteritis.

Giant cell arteritis (GCA, formerly called *temporal arteritis)* is an immune-related large- and medium-vessel vasculitis similar to but distinct from TA.[47,59] The pathologic findings are analogous, with early T-lymphocyte, histiocyte, and giant cell vessel infiltration of the media and late luminal narrowing or thrombosis. The precise etiology is unknown, but autoimmune, genetic, and hormonal factors have been suggested. However, the chronic symptoms and vascular distribution are different from TA. Many of those afflicted are of Scandinavian descent. It is virtually never seen in patients younger than 50 years of age, and women are affected more commonly than men.[60] Acute symptoms include fever, headache, polymyalgia rheumatica, and scalp tenderness; rarely, visual loss follows. The ESR and CRP are elevated, and thrombocytosis may be present. Temporal artery biopsy still has a central role in diagnosis.

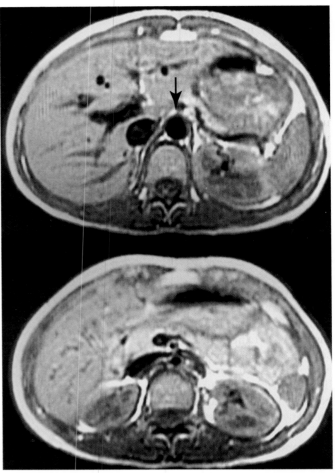

FIGURE 1-22   Takayasu arteritis of the abdominal aorta by magnetic resonance imaging. The caliber of the upper abdominal aorta *(arrow)* is normal *(top).* Narrowing of the aortic lumen and concentric thickening of the aortic wall are seen in the middle abdomen *(bottom).*

The characteristic imaging findings are long, smooth stenoses or occlusions, particularly in the external carotid artery and its branches (e.g., temporal artery). Extracranial GCA usually affects the distal subclavian or axillary artery.[61] Lesions are sometimes difficult to differentiate from atherosclerosis. Aortic aneurysms have been described also. PET imaging is valuable in diagnosis and assessment of GCA.[53,54]

Buerger disease (formerly *thromboangiitis obliterans*) is usually included in the list of vasculitides affecting small and medium-sized arteries and veins. However, the disease begins as an occlusive inflammatory thrombus with almost no involvement of the wall itself.[62] Serologic markers to suggest vasculitis are notably absent. With time, the clot becomes organized and the vessel wall fibrotic. Affected vascular segments are separated by essentially normal vessels. The cause of Buerger disease is unknown, although an immunologic abnormality has been postulated. Unlike most other vasculitides, the condition usually is confined to the extremities; involvement of mesenteric branches and other sites is rare.[63,64] Buerger disease attacks the lower and upper extremity arteries in 90% and 50% of cases, respectively. A superficial (or sometimes deep) thrombophlebitis occurs in up to 40% of patients.

All patients are smokers or have used tobacco products.[62] Although the disease is historically associated with young Jewish men of Ashkenazi descent, it is now recognized more widely within the general population. It is a common cause of severe chronic limb ischemia in smokers younger than 40 years of age. Involvement of more than one limb is the rule. On imaging studies, the arteries proximal to the elbow and the knee are relatively spared. Sources of emboli can be excluded. Abrupt occlusions of distal arteries with entirely normal skip areas are seen along with tortuous ("corkscrew") collateral vessels (see Figs. 8-20 and 9-31). These findings are inevitably present in asymptomatic limbs. Similar angiographic features have been reported in patients who use illicit drugs and in connective tissue disorders.[65] Diagnosis is important for prognostic reasons. The disease will remit if all tobacco exposure is avoided. Patients must be told emphatically about the likelihood of amputation with continued smoking. Novel therapeutic approaches have yet to accomplish the benefit of complete abstinence.[66]

Polyarteritis nodosa (PAN) is a necrotizing vasculitis of small and medium-sized arteries usually found in middle-aged patients.[67] Certain infections, such as hepatitis B, are clearly associated with the disease, but in most cases, the cause is unknown. An almost identical form of arteritis has been described in drug abusers.[68] PAN often begins with nonspecific constitutional symptoms. It can ultimately attack the kidneys, gastrointestinal tract, spleen, liver, skin, and peripheral nerves and muscles.[69,70] Symptoms are related to the vascular pathology of aneurysm rupture or arterial thrombosis.[70,71] Multiple small (<1 cm) saccular aneurysms *(microaneurysms)* and occlusions of distal arteries are very characteristic but not pathognomonic (Fig. 1-23). A similar appearance has been described for other diseases such as drug abuse, Sjögren syndrome, and Wegener granulomatosis.[72] CT scans may show renal or perirenal hematomas and focal thickening of the bowel wall.

Connective tissue disorders may lead to an arteritis.[73] With few exceptions, however, clinical vasculitis is not a prominent feature of these diseases. The affected sites vary widely. Rheumatoid arthritis and other related illnesses can cause inflammation in the aortic root with aortic regurgitation; aneurysm formation is rare. SLE can be complicated by symptomatic small vessel arteritis in the lung, kidneys, intestinal tract, or digits.

Behçet syndrome is a rare connective tissue disorder marked by oral and genital ulcers, uveitis, and skin lesions.[74,75] This unusual condition is primarily seen

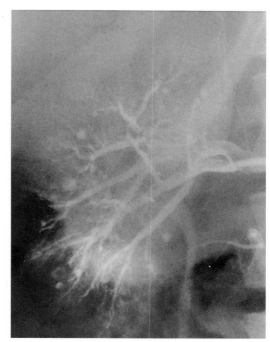

FIGURE 1-23   Polyarteritis nodosa of the right kidney with multiple microaneurysms of distal intrarenal vessels.

in young adults in a geographic swath from the Mediterranean (especially Turkey) to eastern Asia. Although most patients suffer from central nervous system involvement, a minority (particularly young men) are subject to panvasculitis (arterial and venous). The involved vessels show a severe cellular inflammatory reaction that ultimately scars the entire wall and may lead to aneurysm formation or vascular occlusion. Characteristic findings include superficial or deep venous thrombosis (about one third of cases), inferior vena cava (IVC) thrombosis with Budd-Chiari syndrome, aneurysms or pseudoaneurysms (characteristically of the *pulmonary artery*), and arterial obstructions.[76]

Kawasaki disease is a necrotizing vasculitis of medium-sized arteries that primarily afflicts young children.[77] The cause is unknown, but obscure infection has been postulated. Early signs are fever, lesions on the skin and oral mucosa, and cervical lymphadenopathy. Late sequelae (especially in untreated patients) include coronary artery aneurysms, myocarditis, and coronary artery stenoses.[78] Peripheral aneurysms (e.g., brachial, femoral, and renal arteries) also have been reported.

Radiation arteritis can develop in arteries of any size after high-dose radiotherapy (20 to 80 Gy).[79,80] In large- and medium-sized vessels, radiation causes myointimal fibrosis, ischemic necrosis, intimal atherosclerotic-like changes, thrombotic or fibrotic occlusion, and even rupture.[81,82] Radiation-induced arterial disease usually presents 5 or more years after therapy. The unique feature is localization of disease to the radiation portal.

Angiography shows smooth luminal narrowing, irregular mural plaques, or complete occlusion (Fig. 1-24). On the other hand, human veins are relatively resistant to the effects of radiotherapy.[82]

Noninflammatory Vasculopathies

Fibromuscular dysplasia (FMD) is a group of related noninflammatory disorders distinguished by arterial narrowing, small (and rarely large) aneurysms, and dissections.[83] The cause is poorly understood, but genetic, hormonal, and mechanical stress factors are suggested.

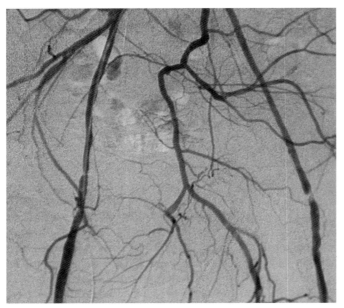

FIGURE 1-24   Radiation arteritis affecting both common femoral arteries in a patient who underwent radiation therapy for cervical cancer 7 years earlier. Note absence of other vascular disease.

FMD most often attacks the renal arteries. Less common sites include the carotid artery, external iliac, and mesenteric arteries.[84,85] Multiple beds are involved in about one fourth of cases.[86] Up to six distinct pathologic subtypes have been described (see Table 10-2). The *medial fibroplasia* type is the most common.[83] Medial smooth muscle cells are largely replaced by fibrous tissue and extracellular matrix. These thickened segments alternate with regions of severe thinning of the media. The effect on the lumen is alternating aneurysms (larger than the normal artery) and focal stenoses ("string of beads") (Fig. 1-25). The less common forms of fibromuscular dysplasia, such as perimedial fibroplasia and intimal fibroplasia, cause beading (beads smaller than the normal artery), smooth and tapered stenosis, focal bandlike narrowing, dissection, or aneurysms without stenoses (see Figs. 10-21 and 10-22).

Marfan syndrome is an autosomal dominant disorder that occurs in about 1 in 3000 to 5000 individuals.[87] Mutation in the *FBN1* gene that codes for fibrillin-1 results in structurally deficient microfibrils in the aortic media and activation of media-destroying matrix metalloproteinases (MMP) by upregulated transforming growth factor–beta (TGF-β) levels.[88] The cellular structure of the media becomes disorganized and weakened. Up to one third of affected individuals have de novo noninherited defects. The telltale thinning and elongation of the limbs may be accompanied by ocular abnormalities and cardiovascular complications. The latter are frequent and include aneurysm or dissection of the proximal ascending aorta ("sinotubular ectasia"), aortic insufficiency, mitral valve prolapse or calcification, and pulmonary artery dilation[89] (see Fig. 6-26).

Ehlers-Danlos syndromes are a set of rare genetic disorders of collagen production.[90] The Villefranche classification has six subtypes, but considerable clinical overlap

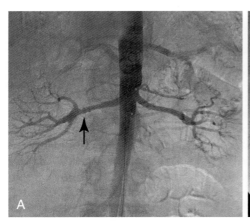
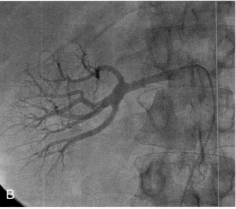
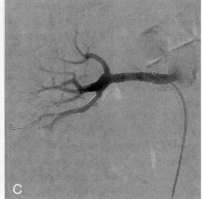

FIGURE 1-25   Medial fibroplasia type of fibromuscular dysplasia of the distal right renal artery. **A** and **B**, Aortogram and selective right renal arteriogram show typical "string of beads" appearance of distal artery *(arrow)*. Notably, the proximal renal artery and abdominal aorta look normal. **C**, Following balloon angioplasty, luminal patency is markedly improved.

exists.[91] The most common findings are skin hyperextensibility, delayed wound healing, joint hypermobility, and spontaneous ecchymoses. However, in the rare *type IV (vascular) subgroup,* the skin is remarkably thin but joints are not hyperextensible.[91,92] The underlying defect is a mutation in the gene coding for type III procollagen (COL3A1); as a consequence, this important structural protein is defective and deficient in the arterial media. Vascular events almost always occur before age 40 and include spontaneous arterial rupture, dissections, false aneurysms, carotid-cavernous fistula, and severe angiographic complications (Fig. 1-26 and see Fig. 9-29). Almost any artery can be affected. Intestinal and gravid uterine rupture are also encountered with this devastating condition.

Segmental arterial mediolysis (SAM) is a fascinating disease of unknown cause that leads to destruction of arterial medial smooth muscle cells and eventual replacement by fibrin and granulation tissue.[93] Over time, extension to the entire arterial wall can produce multiple spontaneous dissections, focal dilation, aneurysms, and arterial occlusions. It has been postulated that SAM is related to fibromuscular dysplasia.[94] The disorder primarily affects the mesenteric arteries and less frequently the cerebral, renal, and coronary circulations.[95,96] A classic presentation is intraabdominal bleeding from

aneurysm rupture. SAM may be difficult to distinguish from PAN by imaging alone; both entities can produce multiple bizarre aneurysms in medium-sized visceral arteries (see Fig. 11-39).

Loeys-Dietz syndrome is a recently identified autosomal dominant connective tissue disorder resulting from genetic defects in the genes coding for TGF-β receptors.[97] The characteristic features include arterial (especially aortic) aneurysms and dissections, global arterial tortuosity, hypertelorism, bifid uvula, cleft lip, and congenital heart disease. *Grange syndrome* is another newly described entity encompassing multifocal aneurysms and stenoses, bone fragility, brachysyndactyly, and cardiac abnormalities.[98]

Extrinsic Compression

The lumen of an artery can be narrowed by a variety of extrinsic sources, including inflammatory masses, tumors, hematomas or other fluid collections, musculoskeletal structures, and cutaneous compression.

ARTERIES AND VEINS

Neoplasms

Primary vascular tumors are exceedingly rare, and sarcomas of the aorta, pulmonary artery, or IVC account for most of them[99-102] (see Fig. 1-13). Most tumors of the aorta and pulmonary artery are *intimal angiosarcomas* that produce large luminal masses or emboli. *Mural angiosarcomas* (which typically invade contiguous structures) are less common. Most IVC tumors are *leiomyosarcomas* (see Fig. 16-27). Extravascular benign and malignant tumors have several possible effects on neighboring vessels. These patterns of hypervascularity, neovascularity, vascular displacement, and vascular invasion may be seen alone or in combination.

Hypervascularity occurs because neoplasms require abundant blood supply for significant growth. Tumors liberate several substances, including tumor angiogenesis factors, that induce formation of new blood vessels. These "tumor vessels" are blood channels and spaces devoid of smooth muscle cells.[103-105] The angiographic hallmark of these changes is *neovascularity,* which appears as bizarrely formed small arterial branches that have alternating dilated and narrowed segments and an angulated course (Fig. 1-27 and see Figs. 10-33 to 10-35). Other features of hypervascular tumors include enlargement of the feeding artery, an increased number of small arteries, dense contrast opacification of the mass ("tumor blush"), filling of enlarged vascular spaces (pools or lakes), and, occasionally, arteriovenous shunting. The classic hypervascular tumors are renal cell carcinoma, hepatocellular carcinoma, choriocarcinoma, endocrine tumors, and leiomyosarcoma.

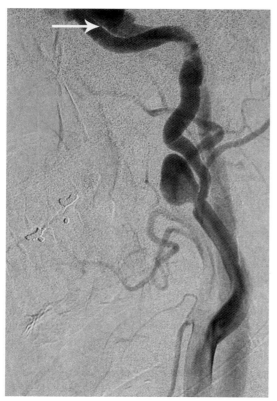

FIGURE 1-26 Saccular internal carotid artery aneurysm in a patient with Ehlers-Danlos syndrome. Also note a carotid-cavernous fistula *(arrow).*

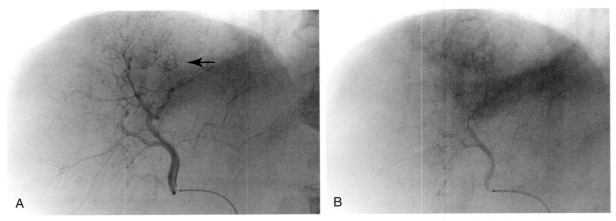

FIGURE 1-27   **A,** Hepatoma of the right lobe of the liver produces hypervascularity and neovascularity in the arterial phase of the hepatic angiogram *(arrow).* Note displacement of branches around the large mass. **B,** Later phase of the angiogram shows inhomogeneous tumor stain.

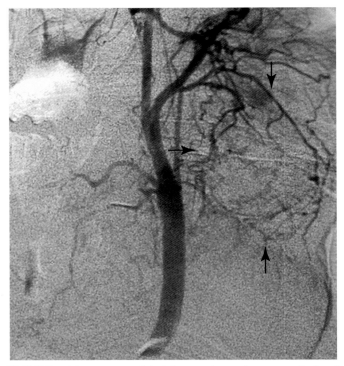

FIGURE 1-28   Branches of the left external carotid artery are displaced around a large metastatic mass from cutaneous melanoma *(arrows).*

Vascular invasion is another consequence of some tumors. Many solid neoplasms show little blood vessel proliferation. Instead, they are infiltrative or scirrhous and compress, encase, or completely occlude adjacent arteries or veins. Usually it is impossible to differentiate these changes from those caused by an inflammatory mass. Invasive tumors include adenocarcinomas of the intestinal tract, pancreatic adenocarcinoma, breast carcinoma, and most lung cancers. Vascular displacement occurs during malignant growth. Some tumors primarily

displace neighboring arteries or veins (Fig. 1-28). Mild hypervascularity or neovascularity may be seen in some of these cases.

Intravascular venous invasion is characteristic of a few malignancies, most notably hepatocellular carcinoma and renal cell carcinoma (Fig. 1-29; see also Fig. 12-17). At angiography, fine tumor vessels are occasionally identified within the thrombus.

Inflammatory Disorders

Every acute inflammatory process increases blood flow to the site and causes dilation of feeding arteries, hypervascularity, and parenchymal stain that can mimic a hypervascular tumor (Fig. 1-30). Chronic inflammatory masses, such as pancreatic pseudocysts, can displace, encase, occlude, or rupture into blood vessels (see Fig. 12-44).

Arteriovenous Communications

Development of the capillary system between arterioles and venules occurs through capillary network, retiform, and gross differentiation stages. Direct communications between arteries and veins without an interposed capillary network can be normal or pathologic. The distinction between vascular malformations and vascular tumors is often confusing. The modified Hamburg classification originally devised by John Mulliken and colleagues is most widely accepted and has been endorsed by the International Society for the Study of Vascular Anomalies[106,107] (Box 1-11).

Vascular malformations are congenital lesions composed of dilated, thin-walled venous, arterial, or lymphatic channels without proliferating cells.[108,109] They are always present at birth (although often detected later in life). They tend to grow slowly and continuously with the child but

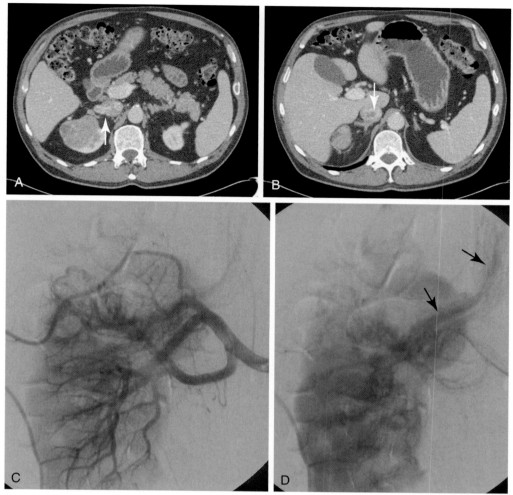

FIGURE 1-29 Right renal cell carcinoma with renal vein and inferior vena cava invasion. **A,** CT scan shows a heterogeneous enhancing mass in the right kidney, with extension to the renal vein *(arrow).* **B,** Inferior vena cava invasion is also noted *(arrow).* **C,** Early phase of right renal arteriogram shows the hypervascular mass in the upper pole of the kidney. **D,** Later phase shows linear "threads and streaks" in right renal vein and IVC related to tumor thrombus *(arrows).*

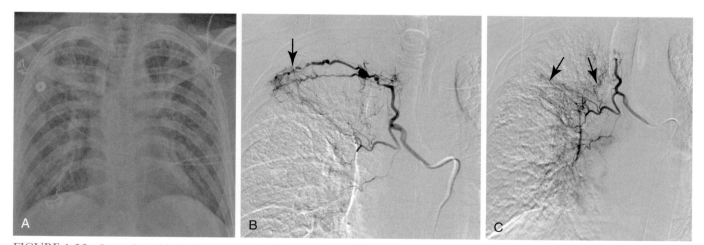

FIGURE 1-30 Severe bronchiectasis causes massive hemoptysis. **A,** Chest radiograph shows severe bilateral upper lobe airway disease. **B,** Arteriography of right intercostal-bronchial artery trunk shows marked hypervascularity in the lateral upper lobe from collateral intercostal vessels *(arrow).* **C,** Following microsphere embolization of the intercostal segment, the hypervascularity in the hilum from the bronchial branches themselves becomes evident *(arrows).*

are subject to rapid expansion with injury or hormonal stresses.[110] They never regress. Many are associated with an underlying clinical syndrome. Vascular malformations are most frequently located in the extremities, head, neck, and pelvis, but they may be found at almost any site in the body.

- *Venous malformations (VMs)* have slightly dilated or nondilated inflow arteries, variable flow patterns, and large spongy venous spaces. They are the most common type of vascular malformation and can occur almost anywhere on the body.[111] Multiple skin lesions on the trunk, soles, and palms are seen with *blue-rubber bleb nevus syndrome*. Certain VMs are sometimes mistakenly called hemangiomas (e.g., "adult liver hemangioma").
- *Capillary malformations* produce the so-called "port wine stain" skin lesion.
- *Arteriovenous malformations (AVMs)* result from failure of regression of the retiform plexus ("nidus") that directly connects arteries and veins in the fetus. They are distinguished by marked dilation of the feeding vessels, hypervascularity, numerous arteriovenous connections around the nidus, early venous filling, and rapid venous washout (Fig. 1-31). AVMs typically pass through several stages, from dormancy, to expansion with associated pulsation and thrill, to destruction with pain, bleeding or ulceration, to decompensation and possibly heart failure.[110] Trauma, hormonal changes, and ischemia seem to encourage growth; the latter response is one of several reasons to avoid proximal occlusion of feeding arteries.

BOX 1-11

VASCULAR ANOMALIES

- Vascular tumors
  - Hemangioma
  - Kaposiform hemangioendothelioma
  - Pyogenic granuloma
  - Hemangiopericytoma
  - Glomuvenous malformation
  - Cavernous angioma
- Vascular malformations
  - Venous malformation
  - Arteriovenous malformation
  - Arterial malformation
  - Lymphatic malformation
  - Capillary malformation
  - Combined types

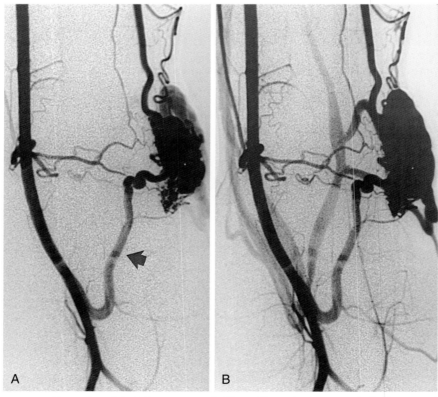

FIGURE 1-31   Arteriovenous malformation of the left upper arm. **A,** The malformation is primarily fed by the radial recurrent artery *(arrow)* and branches of the deep brachial artery. **B,** Early and rapid venous filling occurs during the arterial phase of the angiogram.

• *Lymphatic malformations (LMs)* are categorized as microcystic, macrocystic, or mixed. In the past, they were referred to as *lymphangiomas* or *cystic hygromas*. Most LMs are found in the head or neck, with the remainder occurring in the axilla, trunk, or extremities.[110] Many lesions have associated soft tissue or skeletal overgrowth; the overlying skin is often marked by a bluish tinge.

Benign vascular tumors undergo periods of cellular proliferation and usually involute over time. They may be cutaneous or found in internal organs, including the brain, liver, spleen, pancreas, and kidneys (see Fig. 12-41). *Capillary hemangiomas* are in a growth phase; *cavernous hemangiomas* are in a quiescent stage and marked by normal-caliber feeding vessels, large vascular channels, and early filling of vascular spaces that persists through the venous phase of a contrast imaging study (Fig. 1-32).

Telangiectasias are focal lesions composed of dilated arterioles, capillaries, and venules. They are typically found on the skin and mucous membranes but can be seen also in visceral organs. *Hereditary hemorrhagic telangiectasia (HHT,* once called *Osler-Weber-Rendu syndrome)* is an autosomal dominant disorder in which telangiectasias are present on the lips and mouth and in the intestinal tract, liver, spleen, lung, and brain[112,113] (Fig. 1-33; see Fig. 11-36).

Most patients are found to have mutations in the endoglin *(ENG)* or activin type-II-like receptor kinase *(ALK1)* genes that code for endothelial receptors of the TGF-β type. These proteins are intimately involved in maintaining overall vascular integrity. A definitive diagnosis requires the presence of three of the following conditions: recurrent spontaneous epistaxis, multiple telangiectasias, visceral vascular malformations, and autosomal dominant inheritance.[114]

Arteriovenous fistulas (AVFs) are almost always acquired direct connections between an artery and neighboring vein. Most arteriovenous fistulas are caused by trauma. Color Doppler sonography or MR angiography can often identify the site of communication along with the enlarged feeding artery and early and rapid filling of the draining vein (Fig. 1-34; see Figs. 7-12 and 10-31). AVFs can close spontaneously or enlarge over time. Patients often are asymptomatic but may present with local symptoms, distal ischemia (from a steal phenomenon), or high-output heart failure. Very rarely, fistulas are congenital.[115]

Arteriovenous shunts are normally present in many vascular beds. These *physiologic shunts* sometimes become quite prominent[116] (Fig. 1-35). They may be seen also in certain disease states, such as cirrhosis and in hypervascular tumors (Fig. 1-36).

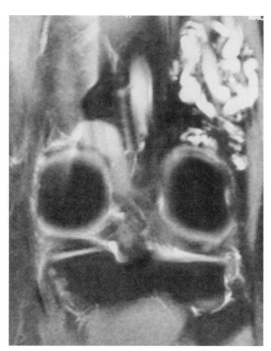

FIGURE 1-32   Hemangioma lateral to the distal left femur seen on gadolinium-enhanced magnetic resonance angiogram. Note enlarged, tortuous venous spaces.

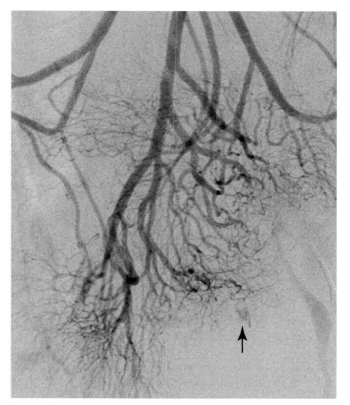

FIGURE 1-33   Telangiectasias of the jejunum *(arrow)* in a patient with hereditary hemorrhagic telangiectasia.

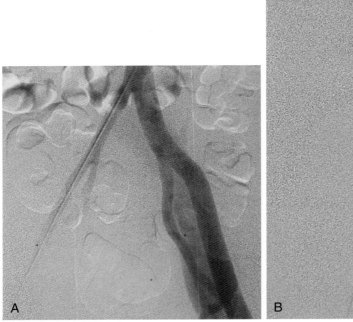

FIGURE 1-34   **A,** Arteriovenous fistula between the superficial femoral artery and vein after femoral artery catheterization. Note the marked enlargement of the left iliac arteries compared with the right side. **B,** Selective injection in the left common femoral artery in oblique projection identifies the site of communication.

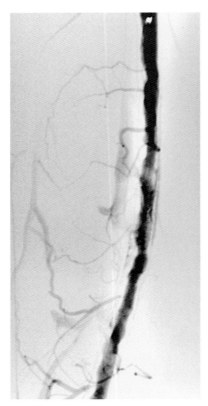

FIGURE 1-35   Prominent arteriovenous shunts after balloon angioplasty of the superficial femoral artery in a patient with peripheral vascular disease.

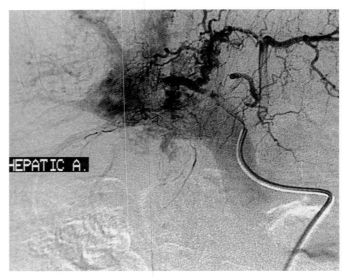

FIGURE 1-36   Profound hepatic arterioportal shunting in a patient with cirrhosis and hepatocellular carcinoma on hepatic arteriography.

Vascular Injury

Arteries and veins can be damaged in many ways.[117] Penetrating injuries may be caused by sharp objects, gunshot wounds, bone fragments, or medical procedures. Gunshot wounds produce vascular injury by

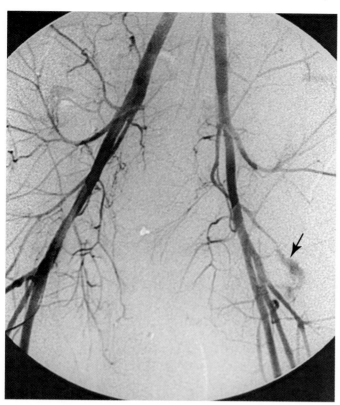

FIGURE 1-37   Extravasation from the left inferior gluteal artery *(arrow)* after pelvic trauma from a motor vehicle accident.

direct penetration or when a vessel is stretched by the temporary cavitation effect of a moving bullet.[118]

Blunt arterial trauma is typically caused by rapid deceleration, moving objects, crush injuries, or falls from a height. Deceleration injuries result from sudden compression of the vessel or from shearing or twisting forces. Bone fracture or joint dislocation also can cause blunt arterial damage (see Fig. 8-52). Hemorrhage or edema into a confined space, such as the anterior tibial compartment of the calf, sometimes results in a *compartment syndrome* that may compromise the arterial circulation in the extremity.[119]

The wide spectrum of traumatic arterial injuries includes intimal flaps, intraluminal thrombus, complete tear with extravasation or thrombosis, dissection, arteriovenous fistula, pseudoaneurysm formation, vasospasm, intramural hematoma, or extrinsic compression from hematoma (Fig. 1-37; see also Figs. 1-3 and 1-34). Rarely, bullets or gunshot pellets embolize within the arterial or venous circulation. Venous injuries are also common with penetrating injuries but rarely require imaging evaluation.

Invasion by neighboring inflammatory or neoplastic masses is another cause of vascular injury. Disruption of an artery causes frank extravasation or a pseudoaneurysm.

VEINS

Normal Structure and Function

Veins are composed of intima, media, and adventitia, but unlike arteries, there is less distinction among these layers. Veins are thinner, less elastic, and more compliant than arteries. *Venous valves* are bicuspid leaflets that direct blood flow toward the heart. They are typically located near venous tributaries, at which point a slight bulge above the valve attachments is seen (see Fig. 17-2). The numerous valves in medium-sized veins of the extremities become less frequent as the veins course centrally. With the exception of the *eustachian valve* below the right atrium, the superior and inferior vena cavae are valveless.

Because the aggregated veins of the body have tremendous capacitance, they serve a critical function in maintaining homeostasis with rapid changes in blood volume. Systemic venous blood is propelled centrally by several effects. Most important is extrinsic compression by the muscular "calf pump." Additional forces include the resting gradient between systemic venules (about 12 to 18 mm Hg) and the right atrium (4 to 7 mm Hg), cyclic changes in intrathoracic and intraabdominal pressure, and venous tone.[120] When a person is supine, the fall in intrathoracic pressure during inspiration increases blood flow from the IVC to the heart. The rise in intrathoracic or intraabdominal pressure during expiration or a Valsalva maneuver reduces blood flow from the abdomen into the thorax. Venous hemodynamics in the legs and arms are discussed further in Chapters 15 and 17.

Venospasm

Functional venous narrowing usually is caused by minor injury, including manipulation during angiographic procedures. The cardinal feature of venospasm is resolution with time. Spasm may also respond to vasodilating agents.

Acute Venous Thromboembolic Disease

Venous thrombosis occurs through a complex process involving cellular blood elements, coagulation proteins, and the vascular wall. Thrombophilic conditions are the most important factor in VTE[17,121] (see Boxes 1-4 and 1-5). Slow flow and vein injury are less important.

Fresh thrombus produces an intraluminal filling defect (Fig. 1-38). At sonography, the clot also alters normal vein compressibility and flow phasicity caused by reflected atrial or respiratory activity. Thrombus should not be confused with unopacified blood (inflow defect) or overlying bowel gas (Fig. 1-39).

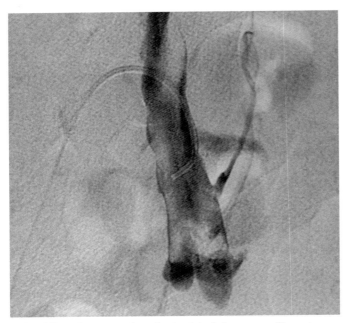

FIGURE 1-38   Acute thrombosis of the left common iliac vein seen with selective catheterization from the right common femoral vein.

Once venous clot forms, several outcomes are possible.

- **Progression.** A cascade of events may lead to extension of thrombosis. Upregulation of *selectins* (glycoproteins found on endothelial cells and platelets) is followed by creation of procoagulant *microparticles* (phospholipid cell membrane fragments).[121,122] In a particular individual, the fate of an acute venous clot depends on the site of thrombosis, any underlying thrombophilic factors, and anticoagulant or thrombolytic treatment.[123] Less than one third of untreated calf vein thrombi will progress centrally. Conversely, in excess of one third of patients with "proximal" (above the knee) DVT will demonstrate clot progression despite therapeutic anticoagulation.[124]
- **Resolution.** Acute leg vein thrombosis is *usually* followed by at least partial recanalization of the lumen.[125] Regression of clot (mediated primarily through monocyte activity) occurs by endogenous fibrinolysis, fragmentation, neovascularization, and ultimately clot retraction.[121] Clot dissolution is almost complete after about 6 to 12 weeks. In the superficial and deep veins of the leg, clot may lyse completely and leave vein walls and valves intact. At other sites (e.g., upper extremity veins, portal venous system, hepatic veins, IVC), complete resolution is less common. The affected

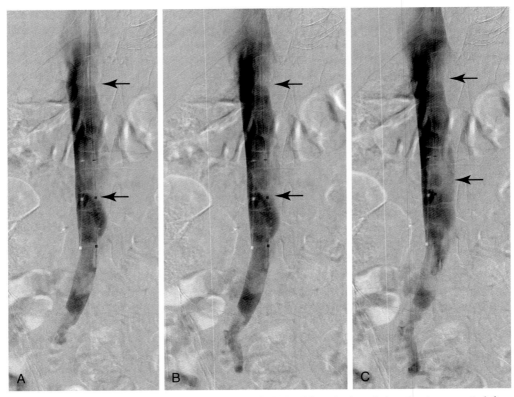

FIGURE 1-39   Venacavography reveals inflow defects from unopacified blood from both moieties of a circumaortic left renal vein *(arrows)*. The hallmark of this finding is change over the course of the injection **(B** and **C).**

vein wall remains thickened and scarred, minimally compliant, and associated with valve damage.

- **Pulmonary embolism** is the most feared complication of systemic DVT. The reported frequency is 10%.[126] Since the groundbreaking study of Barritt and Jordan in 1960,[127] numerous studies have proven that therapeutic anticoagulation of sufficient duration will reduce the risk significantly.

- **Chronic occlusion, vein/valve injury, and/or associated venous reflux** (Fig. 1-40). Even though most venous segments will recanalize after acute DVT, some valve damage is the rule. The major *late* sequelae from valvular damage with or without persistent obstruction is the *post-thrombotic syndrome*, which is characterized by limb swelling, hyperpigmentation, and "venous" ulcers. Although more than half of patients with VTE may suffer mild forms of this vexing problem, severe symptoms develop in fewer than one fourth of cases.[121] The major predictors of post-thrombotic syndrome are the rate of clot resolution, recurrence of thrombosis, and the extent and distribution of reflux and obstruction.

Rarely, malignancies invade neighboring veins and produce tumor thrombus that mimics bland clot (see Fig. 1-29). The most susceptible veins are the portal, renal, and hepatic veins and the IVC.

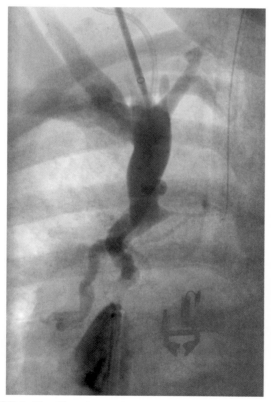

FIGURE 1-40 Chronic superior vena cava occlusion with well-developed collateral circulation.

Chronic Venous Diseases

Chronic disorders of the veins are typically divided into primary (no discernable reason for vein dysfunction) and secondary forms (which by definition follows some acute venous event.) Primary *chronic venous insufficiency (CVI)* is predicated on some type of valve dysfunction, often involves venous reflux but not venous obstruction. The spectrum ranges from telangiectasias and varicose veins (which afflict about 20% of the general population) to active ulceration (<1%). Despite centuries of study, the exact etiology of *varicose veins* is still obscure.[128,129] The unifying feature is valve dysfunction and incompetence which develops at multiple sites over a short time.[130] The pathologic abnormalities are well described (intimal thickening, mural fibrosis, elastic fiber atrophy, poor contractility and compliance.) Whether these findings are primary or secondary is not established.

Secondary CVI is characterized by venous hypertension with ambulation.[130] The disorder may be the result of reflux alone from valves damaged by prior thrombosis or reflux combined with chronic venous obstruction. The major determinants of venous pressure are reflux (caused by abnormal vein valves), venous obstruction, and failure of the calf pump (a function of central vein patency, abnormal joint or muscle activity, and valve failure). This secondary form of valve incompetence (about four times less common than the primary form) may occur after an episode of acute venous thrombosis. Malfunction of the *perforating veins* (from primary valve incompetence or reflux from deep vein occlusion) between the superficial and deep systems is critical. Elevated pressure is transmitted to superficial veins, which leads to distended skin capillaries and transfer of fluid, macromolecules, and red blood cells to the interstitium.[130] A cycle of chronic inflammation is set in motion.

In most countries, CVI is one of the most common chronic disabling conditions in the population. It is more often seen in women (especially after multiple births), in older or obese patients, and in individuals with family history. The American Venous Forum has created a classification system for chronic venous diseases (CEAP) that denotes *c*linical class, *e*tiology, *a*natomic location of obstruction and reflux, and *p*athology (reflux vs. obstruction).[131] From this scheme, disease is divided among seven grades (class 0, absent signs; class 1, telangiectasias; to class 6, active venous limb ulcers).

Neointimal Hyperplasia

Neointimal hyperplasia is the reaction of veins to acute injury or chronic hemodynamic changes. Clinically, the disease is seen most often in venous bypass grafts and

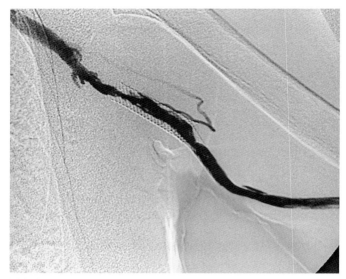

FIGURE 1-41 Intimal hyperplasia within a Wallstent placed in the outflow vein of a hemodialysis access graft.

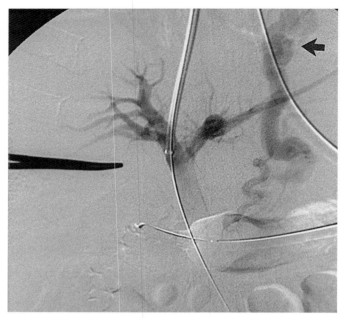

FIGURE 1-42 Gastroesophageal varices *(arrow)* fill from a direct portal vein injection in a patient with portal hypertension.

the outflow veins of hemodialysis grafts (Fig. 1-41). The thickened intima is composed almost entirely of smooth muscle cells with little connective tissue matrix.[132] For this reason, these lesions tend to be more elastic and more resistant to balloon dilation than comparable arterial stenoses.

Varices and Aneurysms

A *varix* is a dilated, tortuous vein. Varices occur at many sites in the body, including the legs and anorectal area (common) and associated with intestinal, gonadal, or renal veins (uncommon). They result from chronically elevated pressure in the venous circulation from any cause (see varicose veins above) (Fig. 1-42). The clinical sequelae include ulceration, bleeding, thrombosis, pain, and cosmetic deformity.

Venous aneurysms are quite rare[133] (see Fig. 15-20). Most are true aneurysms with an intact vein wall. Common sites are the internal jugular vein, popliteal, and portal veins and the superior and inferior vena cavae.[134,135] False aneurysms usually occur after trauma. Venous aneurysms of the neck and thorax are typically asymptomatic. Abdominal venous aneurysms may result in pain, bleeding, or thrombosis. Lower extremity venous aneurysms are complicated by thrombosis or pulmonary embolism.

Extrinsic Compression

The lumen of veins can be narrowed by inflammatory masses, tumors, hematomas or other fluid collections, fibromuscular bands, and external compression (Fig. 1-43).

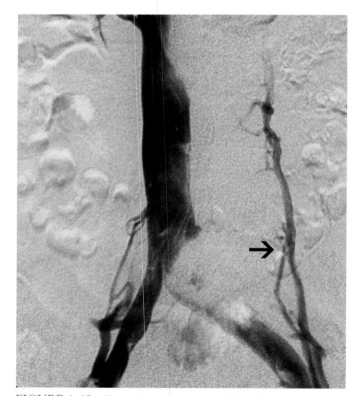

FIGURE 1-43 Extrinsic compression of the left common iliac vein and inferior vena cava proven by computed tomography. Note filling of collateral ascending lumbar veins *(arrow),* demonstrating the hemodynamic significance of this compression.

BOX 1-12

CAUSES OF VENOUS LUMINAL NARROWING

- True narrowing
  - Chronic venous thrombosis
  - Intimal hyperplasia
  - Venospasm
  - Extrinsic compression
- Apparent narrowing
  - Streaming blood or underfilling of veins
  - Hemodynamic forces (e.g., Valsalva maneuver)
  - Venturi effect

Real or apparent venous narrowing can have other causes (Box 1-12). Coaptation of vein walls during rapid contrast injection through an endhole catheter is caused by the Venturi effect (increased velocity of high-pressure contrast jet causing a reduction in neighboring pressure and associated coaptation of compliant vein walls).

References

1. Martins e Silva J, Saldanha C. Arterial endothelium and atherothrombogenesis. I—intact endothelium in vascular and blood hemostasis. *Rev Port Cardiol* 2006;**25**:1061.
2. Greenwald SE. Ageing of the conduit arteries. *J Pathol* 2007;**211**:157.
3. Bakst R, Merola JF, Franks Jr AG, et al. Raynaud's phenomenon: pathogenesis and management. *J Am Acad Dermatol* 2008;**59**:633.
4. Lehrer H. The physiology of angiographic arterial waves. *Radiology* 1967;**89**:11.
5. Peynircioglu B, Cil BE, Karcaaltincaba M. Standing or stationary arterial waves of the superior mesenteric artery at MR angiography and subsequent conventional arteriography. *J Vasc Interv Radiol* 2007;**18**:1329.
6. Norton PT, Hagspiel KD. Stationary arterial waves in magnetic resonance angiography. *J Vasc Interv Radiol* 2005;**16**:423.
7. Ross R. Atherosclerosis: an inflammatory disease. *N Engl J Med* 1999; **340**:115.
8. Insull Jr W. The pathology of atherosclerosis: plaque development and plaque responses to medical treatment. *Am J Med* 2009;**122**:S3.
9. Landmesser U, Hornig B, Drexler H. Endothelial function: a critical determinant in atherosclerosis? *Circulation* 2004;**109**(Suppl. 1):I127.
10. Hackam DG, Anand SS. Emerging risk factors for atherosclerotic vascular disease. A critical review of the evidence. *JAMA* 2003;**290**:932.
11. Liapis CD, Avgerinos ED, Kadoglou NP, et al. What a vascular surgeon should know and do about atherosclerotic risk factors. *J Vasc Surg* 2009;**49**:1348.
12. Maki-Petaja KM, Wilkinson IB. Antiinflammatory drugs and statins for arterial stiffness reduction. *Curr Pharm Des* 2009;**15**:290.
13. Weintraub WS. The pathophysiology and burden of restenosis. *Am J Cardiol* 2007;**100**:3K.
14. Rajagopal V, Rockson SG. Coronary restenosis: a review of mechanisms and management. *Am J Med* 2003;**115**:547.
15. McCowan TC, Eidt JF. Angioplasty, C-reactive protein, and the patient at risk. *Radiology* 2003;**227**:314.
16. Schillinger M, Exner M, Mlekusch W, et al. Endovascular revascularization below the knee: 6-month results and predictive value of C-reactive protein. *Radiology* 2003;**227**:419.
17. Valji K, Linenberger M. Chasing clot: thrombophilic states and the interventionalist. *J Vasc Interv Radiol* 2009;**20**:1403.
18. Dahlback B. Advances in understanding pathogenic mechanisms of thrombophilic disorders. *Blood* 2008;**112**:19.
19. Lijfering WM, Brouwer JL, Veeger NJ, et al. Selective testing for thrombophilia in patients with first venous thrombosis. Results from a retrospective family cohort study on absolute risk for currently known thrombophilic defects in 2479 relatives. *Blood* 2009;**113**:5314.
20. Ho WK, Hankey GJ, Quinlan DJ, et al. Risk of recurrent venous thromboembolism in patients with common thrombophilia. *Arch Intern Med* 2006;**166**:729.
21. Maclean PS, Tait RC. Hereditary and acquired antithrombin deficiency: epidemiology, pathogenesis, and treatment options. *Drugs* 2007;**67**:1429.
22. Brouwer JL, Lijfering WM, TenKate MK, et al. High long-term absolute risk of recurrent venous thromboembolism in patients with hereditary deficiencies of protein S, protein C, or antithrombin. *Thromb Haemost* 2009;**101**:93.
23. Doggen CJ, Rosendaal FR, Meijers JC. Levels of intrinsic coagulation factors and the risk of myocardial infarction among men: opposite and synergistic effects of factors XI and XII. *Blood* 2006;**108**:4045.
24. Bank I, Libourel EJ, Middeldorp S, et al. Elevated levels of FVIII:C within families are associated with an increased risk for venous and arterial thrombosis. *J Thromb Haemost* 2005;**3**:79.
25. Frederiksen J, Juul K, Grande P, et al. Methylenetetrahydrofolate reductase polymorphism (C677TT), hyperhomocysteinemia, and risk of ischemic cardiovascular disease and venous thromboembolism: prospective and case-control studies from the Copenhagen City Heart Study. *Blood* 2004;**104**:3046.
26. Lockshin MD, Erkan D. Treatment of the antiphospholipid syndrome. *N Engl J Med* 2003;**349**:1177.
27. Insko EK, Haskal ZJ. Antiphospholipid syndrome: patterns of life-threatening and severe recurrent vascular complications. *Radiology* 1997;**202**:319.
28. Baldwin ZK, Spitzer AL, Ng VL, et al. Contemporary standards for the diagnosis and treatment of heparin-induced thrombocytopenia (HIT). *Surgery* 2008;**143**:305.
29. Chong BH, Isaacs A. Heparin-induced thrombocytopenia: what clinicians need to know. *Thromb Haemost* 2009;**101**:279.
30. Linenberger ML, Wittkowsky AK. Thromboembolic complications of malignancy. Part 1: Risks. *Oncology* (Williston Park) 2005;**19**:853.
31. Meyrier A. Cholesterol crystal embolism: diagnosis and treatment. *Kidney Int* 2006;**69**:1308.
32. Fukumoto Y, Tsutsui H, Tsuchihasi M, et al. The incidence and risk factors of cholesterol embolization syndrome, a complication of cardiac catheterization: a prospective study. *J Am Coll Cardiol* 2003;**42**:211.
33. Kronzon I, Tunick PA. Aortic atherosclerotic disease and stroke. *Circulation* 2006;**114**:63.
34. Johnston KW, Rutherford RB, Tilson MD, et al. Suggested standards for reporting on arterial aneurysms. *J Vasc Surg* 1991;**13**:452.
35. Keeling AN, McGrath FP, Lee MJ. Interventional radiology in the diagnosis, management, and followup of pseudoaneurysms. *Cardiovasc Intervent Radiol* 2008;**32**:2.
36. Hirsch AT, Haskal ZJ, Hertzer NR, et al. ACC/AHA 2005 Practice Guidelines for the management of patients with peripheral arterial disease (lower extremity, renal, mesenteric, and abdominal aortic). *Circulation* 2006;**113**:e463.

37. Miller FJ. Aortic aneurysms. It's all about the stress. *Arterioscler Thromb Vasc Biol* 2002;**22**:1948.
38. Lindholt JS, Shi GP. Chronic inflammation, immune response, and infection in abdominal aortic aneurysms. *Eur J Vasc Endovasc Surg* 2006;**31**:453.
39. Lee WK, Mossop PJ, Little AF. Infected (mycotic) aneurysms: spectrum of imaging appearances and management. *Radiographics* 2008;**28**:1853.
40. Hsu RB, Lin FY. Infected aneurysm of the thoracic aorta. *J Vasc Surg* 2008;**47**:270.
41. Canaud L, Marzelle J, Bassinet L, et al. Tuberculous aneurysms of the abdominal aorta. *J Vasc Surg* 2008;**48**:1012.
42. Lawrence PF, Wallis C, Dobrin PB, et al. Peripheral aneurysms and arteriomegaly: is there a familial pattern? *J Vasc Surg* 1998;**28**:599.
43. Patel PD, Arora RR. Pathophysiology, diagnosis, and management of aortic dissection. *Ther Adv Cardiovasc Dis* 2008;**2**:439.
44. Gornik HL, Creager MA. Aortitis. *Circulation* 2008;**117**:3039.
45. Khasnis A, Langford CA. Update on vasculitis. *J Allergy Clin Immunol* 2009;**123**:1226.
46. Stone JH. Vasculitis: a collection of pearls and myths. *Rheum Dis Clin North Am* 2007;**33**:691.
47. Seko Y. Giant cell and Takayasu arteritis. *Curr Opin Rheumatol* 2007;**19**:39.
48. Maksimowicz-McKinnon K, Hoffman GS. Takayasu arteritis: what is the long term prognosis? *Rheum Dis Clin North Am* 2007;**33**:777.
49. Ogino H, Matsuda H, Minatoya K, et al. Overview of late outcome of medical and surgical treatment for Takayasu arteritis. *Circulation* 2008;**118**:2738.
50. Hata A, Noda M, Moriwaki R, et al. Angiographic findings of Takayasu arteritis: new classification. *Int J Cardiol* 1996;**54**(Suppl): S155.
51. Tso E, Flamm SD, White RD, et al. Takayasu arteritis: utility and limitations of magnetic resonance imaging in diagnosis and treatment. *Arthritis and Rheumatism* 2002;**46**:1634.
52. Pipitone N, Salvarani C. Role of imaging in vasculitis and connective tissue disease. *Best Pract Res Clin Rheumatol* 2008;**22**:1075.
53. Walter MA. [(18)F] fluorodeoxyglucose PET in large vessel vasculitis. *Radiol Clin North Am* 2007;**45**:735.
54. Blockmans D, Bley T, Schmidt W. Imaging for large-vessel vasculitis. *Curr Opin Rheumatol* 2009;**21**:19.
55. Chung JW, Kim HC, Choi YH, et al. Patterns of aortic involvement in Takayasu arteritis and its clinical implications: evaluation with spiral computed tomography angiography. *J Vasc Surg* 2007;**45**:906.
56. Sueyoshi E, Sakamoto I, Uetani M. MRI of Takayasu's arteritis: typical appearance and complications. *AJR Am J Roentgenol* 2006;**187**:W569.
57. Matsunaga N, Hayashi K, Sakamoto I, et al. Takayasu arteritis: protean radiologic manifestations and diagnosis. *Radiographics* 1997:**17**:579.
58. Canyigit M, Peynircioglu B, Hazirolan T, et al. Imaging characteristics of Takayasu arteritis. *Cardiovasc Intervent Radiol* 2007;**30**:711.
59. Cid MC, Garcia-Martinez A, Lozano E, et al. Five clinical conundrums in the management of giant cell arteritis. *Rheum Dis Clin North Am* 2007;**33**:819.
60. Wang X, Hu Z-P, Lu W, et al. Giant cell arteritis. *Rheumatol Int* 2008;**29**:1.
61. Schmidt WA, Seifert A, Gromnica-Ihle E, et al. Ultrasound of proximal upper extremity arteries to increase the diagnostic yield in large-vessel giant cell arteritis. *Rheumatology* 2008;**47**:96.
62. Olin JW, Shih A. Thromboangiitis obliterans (Buerger's disease). *Curr Opin Rheumatol* 2006;**18**:18.
63. Kobayashi M, Kurose K, Kobata T, et al. Ischemic intestinal involvement in a patient with Buerger disease: case report and literature review. *J Vasc Surg* 2003;**38**:170.
64. Leung DK, Haskal ZJ. SIR 2006 film panel case: mesenteric involvement and bowel infarction due to Buerger disease. *J Vasc Interv Radiol* 2006;**17**:1087.
65. Marder VJ, Mellinghoff IK. Cocaine and Buerger disease: is there a pathogenetic association? *Arch Intern Med* 2000;**160**:2057.
66. Paraskevas KI, Liapis CD, Briana DD, et al. Thromboangiitis obliterans (Buerger's disease): searching for a therapeutic strategy. *Angiology* 2007;**58**:75.
67. Saleh A, Stone JH. Classification and diagnostic criteria in systemic vasculitis. *Best Pract Res Clin Rheumatol* 2005;**19**:209.
68. Citron BP, Halpern M, McCarron M, et al. Necrotizing angiitis associated with drug abuse. *N Engl J Med* 1970;**283**:1003.
69. Jee KN, Ha HK, Lee IJ, et al. Radiologic findings of abdominal polyarteritis nodosa. *AJR Am J Roentgenol* 2000;**174**:1675.
70. Ebert ED, Hagspiel KD, Nagar M, et al. Gastrointestinal involvement in polyarteritis nodosa. *Clin Gastroenterol Hepatol* 2008;**6**:960.
71. Stanson AW, Friese JL, Johnson CM, et al. Polyarteritis nodosa: spectrum of angiographic findings. *Radiographics* 2001;**21**:151.
72. Hoffman GS, Kerr GS, Leavitt RY, et al. Wegener granulomatosis: an analysis of 158 patients. *Ann Intern Med* 1992;**116**:488.
73. Turesson C, Matteson EL. Vasculitis in rheumatoid arthritis. *Curr Opin Rheumatol* 2009;**21**:35.
74. Chae EJ, Do KH, Seo JB, et al. Radiologic and clinical findings of Behcet disease: comprehensive review of multisystemic involvement. *Radiographics* 2008;**28**:e31.
75. Yurdakul S, Yazici H. Behcet's syndrome. *Best Pract Res Clin Rheumat* 2008;**22**:793.
76. Park JH, Chung JW, Joh JH, et al. Aortic and arterial aneurysms in Behçet disease: management with stent-grafts—initial experience. *Radiology* 2001;**220**:745.
77. Harnden A, Takahashi M, Burgner D. Kawasaki disease. *BMJ* 2009;**338**:1133.
78. Newburger JW, Takahasi M, Gerber MA, et al. Diagnosis, treatment and long-term management of Kawasaki disease: a statement for health professionals from the committee on rheumatic fever, endocarditis, and Kawasaki disease, council on cardiovascular disease in the young, American Heart Association. *Pediatrics* 2004;**114**:1708.
79. Jurado JA, Bashir R, Burket MW. Radiation-induced peripheral artery disease. *Catheter Cardiovasc Interv* 2008;**72**:563.
80. Baerlocher MO, Rajan DK, Ing DJ, et al. Primary stenting of bilateral radiation induced external iliac stenoses. *J Vasc Surg* 2004;**40**:1028.
81. Modrall JG, Sadjadi J. Early and late presentations of radiation arteritis. *Semin Vasc Surg* 2003;**16**:209.
82. Fajardo LF. The pathology of ionizing radiation as defined by morphologic patterns. *Acta Oncologica* 2005;**44**:13.
83. Olin JW, Pierce M. Contemporary management of fibromuscular dysplasia. *Curr Opin Cardiol* 2008;**23**:527.
84. Furie DM, Tien RD. Fibromuscular dysplasia of arteries of the head and neck: imaging findings. *AJR Am J Roentgenol* 1994;**162**:1205.
85. Yamaguchi R, Yamaguchi A, Isogai M, et al. Fibromuscular dysplasia of the visceral arteries. *Am J Gastroenterol* 1996;**91**:1635.
86. Stokes JB, Bonsib SM, McBride JW. Diffuse intimal fibromuscular dysplasia with multiorgan failure. *Arch Intern Med* 1996;**156**:2611.
87. Keane MG, Pyeritz RE. Medical management of Marfan syndrome. *Circulation* 2008;**117**:2802.
88. Matt P, Habashi J, Carrel T, et al. Recent advances in understanding Marfan syndrome: should we now treat surgical patients with losartan? *J Thorac Cardiovasc Surg* 2008;**135**:389.
89. DePaepe AM, Devereux RB, Dietz HC, et al. Revised diagnostic criteria for the Marfan syndrome. *Am J Med Genet* 1996;**62**:417.
90. Pepin M, Schwarze U, Superti-Furga A, et al. Clinical and genetic features of Ehlers-Danlos syndrome type IV, the vascular type. *New Engl J Med* 2000;**342**:673.
91. Callewaert B, Malfait F, Loeys B, et al. Ehlers-Danlos syndromes and Marfan syndrome. *Best Pract Res Clin Rheum* 2008;**22**: 165.
92. Germain DP. Ehlers-Danlos syndrome type IV. *Orphanet J Rare Dis* 2007;**2**:32.

93. Slavin RE. Segmental arterial mediolysis: course, sequelae, prognosis, and pathologic-radiologic correlation. *Cardiovasc Pathol* 2009;**18**:352.

94. Slavin RE, Saeki K, Bhagavan B, et al. Segmental arterial mediolysis: a precursor to fibromuscular dysplasia? *Mod Pathol* 1995;**8**:287.

95. Soulen MC, Cohen DL, Itkin M, et al. Segmental arterial mediolysis: angioplasty of bilateral renal artery stenoses with 2-year imaging follow-up. *J Vasc Interv Radiol* 2004;**15**:763.

96. Ryan JM, Suhocki PV, Smith TP. Coil embolization of segmental arterial mediolysis of the hepatic artery. *J Vasc Interv Radiol* 2000;**11**:865.

97. Loeys BL, Schwarze U, Holm T, et al. Aneurysm syndromes caused by mutations in the TGF-beta receptor. *N Engl J Med* 2006;**355**:788.

98. Wallerstein R, Augustyn AM, Wallerstein D, et al. A new case of Grange syndrome without cardiac findings. *Am J Med Genet A* 2006;**140**:1316.

99. Chiche L, Mongredien B, Brocheriou I, et al. Primary tumors of the thoracoabdominal aorta: surgical treatment of 5 patients and review of the literature. *Ann Vasc Surg* 2003;**17**:354.

100. Abularrage CJ, Weiswasser JM, White PW, et al. Aortic angiosarcoma presenting as distal embolization. *Ann Vasc Surg* 2005;**19**:744.

101. Hagspiel KD, Hunter YR, Ahmed HK, et al. Primary sarcomas of the distal abdominal aorta: CT angiography findings. *Abdom Imaging* 2004;**29**:507.

102. Cho SW, Marsh JW, Geller DA, et al. Surgical management of leiomyosarcoma of the inferior vena cava. *J Gastrointest Surg* 2008;**12**:2141.

103. Ferrara N. Vascular endothelial growth factor. *Arterioscler Thromb Vasc Biol* 2009;**29**:789.

104. Folkman J. Role of angiogenesis in tumor growth and metastasis. *Semin Oncol* 2002;**29**(Suppl. 16):15.

105. Folkman J. Angiogenesis: an organizing principle for drug discovery? *Nat Rev Drug Discov* 2007;**6**:273.

106. Mulliken JB, Fishman SJ, Burrows PE. Vascular anomalies. *Curr Probl Surg* 2000;**37**:517.

107. Gloviczki P, Duncan A, Kalra M, et al. Vascular malformations: an update. *Perspect Vasc Surg Endovasc Ther* 2009;**21**:133.

108. Chiller KG, Frieden IJ, Arbiser JL. Molecular pathogenesis of vascular anomalies: classification into three categories based upon clinical and biochemical characteristics. *Lymphat Res Biol* 2003;**1**:267.

109. Fayad LM, Hazirolan T, Bluemke D, et al. Vascular malformations in the extremities: emphasis on MR imaging features that guide treatment options. *Skeletal Radiol* 2006;**35**:127.

110. Arneja JS, Gosain AK. Vascular malformations. *Plast Reconstr Surg* 2008;**121**:195e.

111. Marler JJ, Mulliken JB. Current management of hemangiomas and vascular malformations. *Clin Plast Surg* 2005;**32**:99.

112. Abdalla SA, Letarte M. Hereditary haemorrhagic telangiectasia: current views on genetics and mechanisms of disease. *J Med Genet* 2006;**43**:97.

113. Lacout A, Pelage JP, Lesur G, et al. Pancreatic involvement in hereditary hemorrhagic telangiectasia: assessment with multidetector helical CT. *Radiology* 2010;**254**:479.

114. Pollak JS, Saluja S, Thabet A, et al. Clinical and anatomic outcomes after embolotherapy of pulmonary arteriovenous malformations. *J Vasc Interv Radiol* 2006;**17**:35.

115. Doehlemann C, Hauser M, Nicolai T, et al. Innominate artery enlargement in congenital arteriovenous fistula with subsequent tracheal compression and stridor. *Pediatr Cardiol* 1995;**16**:287.

116. Vallance R, Quin RO, Forrest H. Arteriovenous shunting complicating occlusive atherosclerotic peripheral vascular disease. *Clin Radiol* 1986;**37**:389.

117. Scalea TM, Sclafani S. Interventional techniques in vascular trauma. *Surg Clin North Am* 2001;**81**:1281.

118. Hollerman JJ, Fackler ML, Coldwell DM, et al. Gunshot wounds: 1. Bullets, ballistics, and mechanisms of injury. *AJR Am J Roentgenol* 1990;**155**:685.

119. Kosir R, Moor FA, Selby JH, et al. Acute lower extremity compartment syndrome (ALECS) screening protocol in critically ill trauma patients. *J Trauma* 2007;**63**:268.

120. Meissner MH, Moneta G, Burnand K, et al. The hemodynamics and diagnosis of venous disease. *J Vasc Surg* 2007;**46**:4S.

121. Meissner MH, Wakefield TW, Ascher E, et al. Acute venous disease: venous thrombosis and venous trauma. *J Vasc Surg* 2007;**46**:25S.

122. Wakefield TW, Myers DD, Henke PK. Role of selectins and fibrinolysis in VTE. *Thromb Res* 2009;**123**:S35.

123. Kearon C. Natural history of venous thromboembolism. *Circulation* 2003;**107**(23 (Suppl. 1)):I22.

124. Caps MT, Meissner MH, Tullis MJ, et al. Venous thrombosis stability during acute phase of therapy. *Vasc Med* 1999;**4**:9.

125. van Ramshorst B, vanBemmelen PS, Honeveld H, et al. Thrombus regression in deep venous thrombosis. Quantification of spontaneous thrombolysis with duplex scanning. *Circulation* 1992;**86**:414.

126. Beyth RJ, Cohen AM, Landefeld CS. Long-term outcome of deep-vein thrombosis. *Arch Intern Med* 1995;**155**:1031.

127. Hirsh J, Bates SM. Clinical trials that have influenced the treatment of venous thromboembolism: a historical perspective. *Ann Intern Med* 2001;**134**:409.

128. Raju S, Neglen P. Clinical practice. Chronic venous insufficiency and varicose veins. *N Engl J Med* 2009;**360**:2319.

129. Kouri B. Current evaluation and treatment of lower extremity varicose veins. *Am J Med* 2009;**122**:513.

130. Meissner MH, Glovicki P, Bergan J, et al. Primary chronic venous disorders. *J Vasc Surg* 2007;**46**:54S.

131. Porter JM, Moneta GL. Reporting standards in venous disease: an update. International Consensus Committee on Chronic Venous Disease. *J Vasc Surg* 1995;**21**:635.

132. Allaire E, Clowes AW, Endothelial cell injury in cardiovascular surgery. the intimal hyperplastic response. *Ann Thorac Surg* 1997;**63**:582.

133. Calligaro KD, Ahmad S, Dandora R, et al. Venous aneurysms: surgical indications and review of the literature. *Surgery* 1995;**117**:1.

134. Davidovic L, Dragas M Bozic V, et al. Aneurysm of the inferior vena cava: a case report and review of the literature. *Phlebology* 2008;**23**:184.

135. Bergqvist D, Bjorck M, Ljungman C. Popliteal venous aneurysms—a systematic review. *World J Surg* 2006;**30**:273.

Patient Evaluation and Care

Karim Valji

In 1967, Dr. Alexander Margulis proposed a new subspecialty within the family of imaging sciences which he called "interventional radiology."[1] For some time thereafter, interventional radiologists (IRs) were consultants who performed minimally invasive angiographic procedures (at the request of clinicians) with little or no responsibility for patient care before or after. This practice model has been transformed over the past 40 years. Interventionalists (including the many subspecialists from other fields who also do this work) now assume full clinical responsibility for their patients—they are true "clinicians." As such, IRs are obligated to conduct the initial patient assessment, determine the best course of therapy, *and* provide long-term care and management after the procedure is completed. Experienced interventionalists will agree that a successful and safe technical outcome depends as much on preprocedure and postprocedure care as it does on performing the case itself. The concepts set down in this chapter form the cornerstone of modern interventional radiology practice. The details and nuances may vary among institutions, but the principles are universal.

PREPROCEDURE CARE

Patient Referral and Contact

For simple diagnostic and interventional procedures (e.g., vascular access placement), patient referral without direct contact between physicians is appropriate. For more complex or controversial clinical problems, a discussion between the interventionalist and the referring physician ensures that the appropriate procedure is done, the potential risks for the individual patient are appreciated by everyone involved, and the likely outcome is understood.

The interventionalist should review the medical history and all pertinent diagnostic tests and imaging studies *before* seeing the patient. With this approach, one can avoid raising the specter of an intervention that is ultimately not indicated. The initial conversation between patient and physician is vitally important and should occur as far away

(in time and space) from the interventional suite as possible. The goals of the interview and examination are to establish rapport, review the history firsthand, explain the procedure in detail (and thus obtain informed consent), and reduce anxiety. Family and significant others are encouraged to participate in the discussion. Ideally, inpatients are assessed the day before the case is scheduled. Outpatients are evaluated in a clinic or office dedicated to this work, where support staff (trainees, nurses, physician extenders, and administrative assistants) are fully engaged in IR.[2]

History and Physical Examination

The clinical evaluation includes several components (Box 2-1). The physician must be confident that there are appropriate indications for the proposed intervention based on "best practice" criteria established in the medical literature or endorsement by the Society of Interventional Radiology (SIR) and the Cardiovascular and Interventional Radiology Society of Europe (CIRSE).[3] Risk factors that may require a delay or modification of the proposed procedure or an alternative therapy are sought (Boxes 2-2 and 2-3). A focused physical examination is performed, but it is prudent to assess the airway, lungs, heart, and abdomen in almost all patients. For angiographic procedures, the interventionalist should evaluate and document the following parameters:

- Proposed puncture site (contraindications include, for example, groin infection, common femoral artery aneurysm, overlying hernia, fresh incision, recent injury)
- All extremity pulses, using a Doppler ultrasound probe when necessary
- Status of extremities (e.g., color, perfusion, presence of swelling, ulceration)

Thrombophilic (hypercoagulable) states are an important risk factor for vascular thrombosis and can be associated with significant complications from diagnostic and therapeutic vascular procedures.[4-6] The major hereditary and acquired disorders are listed in

---

BOX 2-1

EVALUATION OF THE PATIENT

- History of current problem
- Pertinent medical and surgical history
- Review of organ systems
  - Cardiac
  - Pulmonary
  - Renal
  - Hepatic
  - Hematologic (e.g., coagulopathy, thrombophilic state)
  - Endocrine (e.g., diabetes)
- History of allergies or adverse reactions to sedatives/anesthetics
- Current medications (including prescribed/illicit narcotics or sedatives)
- Directed physical examination
  - Weight
  - Airway
- Heart and lungs

BOX 2-2

PRIMARY RISK FACTORS FOR IODINATED CONTRAST MATERIAL REACTIONS

- Previous allergic reaction to iodinated contrast
- Other drug allergy
- Asthma
- Reaction to skin allergens

BOX 2-3

PRIMARY RISK FACTORS FOR CONTRAST-INDUCED NEPHROPATHY

- Preexisting renal dysfunction (serum creatinine >1.2-1.5 mg/dL, 106-132 mmol/L)
- Diabetes
- Dehydration
- Hypotension
- Congestive heart failure
- Large contrast dose
- Advanced age
- Anemia (hematocrit <40%)
- Nephrotoxic drugs

BOX 2-4

AMERICAN SOCIETY OF ANESTHESIOLOGY PHYSICAL STATUS CLASSIFICATION SCHEME

P1 A normal healthy patient
P2 A patient with mild systemic disease
P3 A patient with severe systemic disease
P4 A patient with severe systemic disease that is a constant threat to life
P5 A moribund patient who is not expected to survive without the operation

---

Chapter 1 (see Boxes 1-4 and 1-5). These conditions should be suspected when thrombosis occurs in young patients, at atypical sites, in the absence of underlying vascular disease, with familial tendency, or with apparent resistance to anticoagulants.

Sedation and Analgesia Requirements

Most procedures on adults are performed with moderate sedation under the supervision of the operating physician. It is wise (and often hospital policy) to have an anesthesiologist or nurse anesthetist handle sedation and analgesia for sicker patients (e.g., American Society of Anesthesiology physical status classification system categories 3 or above[7] [Box 2-4]). In certain circumstances, regional, monitored, or general anesthesia is preferable (Box 2-5).

Informed Consent

It is the obligation of the physician or physician extender performing any medical procedure to explain the proposed intervention to the patient, to the parent of a minor patient, or to the legal representative or the closest relative if the patient is not competent to give consent.[8,9] If the patient is not fluent in the native language of the health care team, a trained medical translator (*not* a relative or friend) should assist with consent. If telephone consent from a family member or legal representative is necessary, a witness must document the conversation. In

---

BOX 2-5

CONDITIONS THAT MAY REQUIRE MONITORED/ GENERAL ANESTHESIA

- Young age (children)
- Advanced age
- Morbid obesity
- Potential airway compromise (e.g., history of sleep apnea)
- Chronic narcotic use or abuse
- Severe heart, lung, or liver disease
- Increased risk of aspiration
- Very painful or prolonged procedures (e.g., biliary tract dilation)
- Patient inability to cooperate

---

the United States, the "implied consent" doctrine is considered to be in force with any medical procedure in which a delay could lead to severe disability, severe pain, or death. In this rare situation, consent is unnecessary if the patient cannot give his or her own approval *and* no legal representative is immediately available.[9]

To give informed consent, the patient must understand the need for undergoing the procedure, potential risks and expected immediate and long-term outcomes, the consequences of refusing the intervention, and the nature of alternative studies or therapies. To avoid "exceeding" consent, the discussion should include conceivable interventions (e.g., thrombolysis, angioplasty, or stent placement in a patient undergoing angiography for evaluation of peripheral vascular disease).

Informed consent is both a legal and medical concept. In the United States, some states have adopted a "prudent patient" standard that is based on the information an average patient needs to make a decision regarding medical care. Other states use a standard based on the information that a "prudent physician" in the community would have discussed for such a procedure. The interventionalist should explain the various elements of the intervention that could result in an untoward event:

- Access, including the possibility of local infection, bleeding, or hematoma formation (and pseudoaneurysm, arteriovenous fistula, thrombosis or dissection with arteriography)
- Needle, catheter, or guidewire manipulation en route to and at the intended site of angiography or intervention (e.g., risk of bleeding, organ injury, dissection, vessel perforation or thrombosis, nerve damage, arrhythmias, stroke)

- Administration of
  - Contrast agents, including allergic reactions and nephrotoxicity
  - Sedatives and analgesics (e.g., respiratory depression, hypotension)
  - Other medications that may be required during or after the procedure (e.g., allergic reaction, bleeding from anticoagulants)
- Radiation injury from prolonged fluoroscopic procedures

The particular risks for specific diagnostic and interventional procedures are discussed in later chapters. As a rough guide, the overall incidence of major complications (Box 2-6) should be no more than 1% to 2% for the more common interventions (e.g., vascular access placement, inferior vena cava filter placement, percutaneous biopsy and drainage procedures, dialysis access interventions).[10-12] However, older patients and those with established risk factors are more likely to suffer a bad outcome such as bleeding, infection, thrombosis, renal dysfunction, or allergic reactions to administered drugs.[13]

In addition to having the patient (or legal representative) sign a consent form, a preprocedure note stating that informed consent was obtained *must* be placed in the medical record before starting the case. Some practitioners list both common and serious (but rare) risks, but others prefer to be less specific. The thrust of the conversation and patient queries should be documented. The preprocedure note also includes a brief medical history, the specific indications for the procedure, directed physical examination, and results of relevant imaging and laboratory tests.

BOX 2-6

SOCIETY OF INTERVENTIONAL RADIOLOGY DEFINITIONS OF ADVERSE EVENTS

Minor Complications

- No therapy, no consequence
- Nominal therapy, no consequence; includes overnight admission for observation only

Major Complications

- Require therapy, minor hospitalization (≤48 hr)
- Require major therapy, unplanned increase in level of care, prolonged hospitalization (>48 hr)
- Permanent adverse sequelae
- Death

Laboratory Testing

The purpose of preprocedure laboratory testing is to minimize risk by detecting (and when feasible correcting) relevant abnormalities, altering the technique as needed, or canceling the case and choosing a safer treatment. Preprocedure studies may be *routine (screening)* or *selective (directed)*.[14] Indiscriminate testing has proved to be of little value in virtually every medical and surgical study ever published.[15-17] However, selective testing is warranted before vascular and interventional procedures. Screening is generally unnecessary in otherwise healthy patients younger than 40 years of age. Testing is certainly advisable in older adults and those with predisposing risk factors. The acceptable interval between test result and procedure varies among hospitals and clinical situations and cannot be generalized.

Renal Function

Serum creatinine is still widely used as a proxy for kidney function, but it is an imprecise measure of such. Estimated glomerular filtration rate (eGFR) is a more accurate indicator of renal insufficiency. Contrast-induced nephropathy (CIN) is marked by a significant rise in serum creatinine level (0.5 mg/dL or 25% of baseline) 1 to 3 days after intravascular administration and by resolution at 7 to 10 days. This (usually) transient dysfunction is related to direct toxic effects on the kidney by oxygen free radicals or ischemia of the renal medulla.[18] In the general population and in patients with eGFR greater than 60 mL/min (stage 1 or 2 chronic kidney disease), the overall risk of CIN after diagnostic angiography is low (<2%). The risk increases to about 5% in patients with preexisting mild renal dysfunction and 33% or greater in patients with diabetes *and* severe renal insufficiency (eGFR <30 mL/min, stage 4 or 5 chronic kidney disease).[19] Only a small fraction of patients who suffer this complication require long-term hemodialysis. However, some experts believe concerns about CIN are exaggerated and that use of iodinated contrast should not be avoided in patients with moderate renal dysfunction.[19]

The traditional approach to preventing CIN is hydration with intravenous (IV) saline (1 to 1.5 mL/kg/hr) for 6 to 12 hours before and at least several hours after intravascular contrast administration. In addition, several other measures should be considered when the risk is increased:

- The total volume of contrast agent is strictly limited. Contrast material is diluted as much as possible without compromising diagnostic quality.
- The lowest osmolality agent is used.
- Carbon dioxide may replace or supplement standard iodinated contrast in some situations (see Chapter 3).

Several pharmacologic regimens may reduce the likelihood of CIN (see discussion below).

Until recently, gadolinium-based contrast agents were favored as a safe alternative to iodinated materials during intravascular interventions in patients with baseline renal insufficiency. Some of these agents pose a risk (albeit very small) for causing *nephrogenic systemic fibrosis* in individuals with preexisting severe chronic or acute renal insufficiency (eGFR <30 mL/min.). This rare disorder is characterized by widespread and often debilitating dermal (and sometimes visceral organ) sclerosis.[20,21] As such, gadolinium-based agents are no longer used during vascular procedures unless renal function is essentially normal.

Coagulation Parameters

Significant bleeding from interventional procedures is uncommon. It is an axiom in interventional radiology (IR) that the individual risk is largely a function of the coagulation status of the patient (Box 2-7), the likelihood of traversing a major artery or vein, and the ability to detect and then manually control bleeding when it occurs. In fact, there are equivocal data regarding the value of coagulation screening tests in predicting the likelihood of bleeding from invasive procedures.[22,23] Nonetheless, routine screening for coagulopathy is the practice in many institutions based on tradition and sometimes stated policy. A more judicious approach is favored by some practitioners:

- For diagnostic and most therapeutic vascular procedures, individuals with known or suspected risk factors for bleeding should be tested (see Box 2-7).
- With thrombolytic therapy or endovascular interventions that may require parenteral antithrombin

---

BOX 2-7

RISK FACTORS FOR BLEEDING FROM VASCULAR AND INTERVENTIONAL PROCEDURES

- Thrombocytopenia
- Anticoagulant medications
- Liver disease
- History of bleeding diathesis
- Malignant hypertension
- Malnutrition
- Hematologic malignancy
- Splenomegaly
- Disseminated intravascular coagulation
- Selected chemotherapeutic agents

or antiplatelet agents, the substantial risk of local or remote bleeding supports routine testing.

- Many nonvascular interventional procedures (e.g., deep large-core biopsy or fluid drainage, nephrostomy, biliary drainage) can result in hemorrhage that is only apparent after substantial blood loss and is often difficult to control; thus, testing is done routinely. Other procedures (e.g., small-gauge superficial biopsy) do not require screening tests.

Commonly performed coagulation tests are outlined in Box 2-8. Thresholds for defining a coagulopathy and measures for correcting them[22-25] are outlined in Tables 2-1 and 2-2. Based on limited but promising experience using more relaxed parameters for tunneled central venous catheter placement, some practitioners insert such devices when the INR is less than 2.0 or the platelet count is greater than 25,000/dL.[26]

Patient Preparation

Diet and Hydration

When moderate sedation is planned, oral intake or gastrostomy feeding restrictions must comply with institutional guidelines. Typically, patients are limited to clear liquids within 6 hours and are given nothing by mouth (NPO) within 2 hours of the expected start time to prevent aspiration from vomiting caused by contrast agents, sedatives, or individual patient factors.[27] For inpatients who will receive significant volumes of intravascular contrast, overnight IV hydration should be considered when feasible. Outpatients are encouraged to drink plenty of fluids. IV fluids should be ordered in consultation with the referring physician for patients with cardiac or renal disease.

Medications

Patients are instructed to take their regular medications (particularly cardiac, respiratory, and antihypertensive drugs) with a few sips of water on the day of the procedure, with certain exceptions:

- Insulin-dependent diabetic patients may inject their usual insulin doses for early morning cases or reduce their morning dose by one half for midday cases to avoid hypoglycemia.
- Non–insulin-dependent diabetics may withhold drugs until after the procedure.[28] Blood glucose monitoring is advisable during the case.

BOX 2-8

COAGULATION SCREENING BEFORE INTERVENTIONAL RADIOLOGY PROCEDURES

Routine

- Platelet count
- International normalized ratio (INR). The INR standardizes the variability in responsiveness of different thromboplastin assays to warfarin anticoagulation. In most patients, the target therapeutic range for INR is 2.0 to 3.0.
- Prothrombin time (PT)
- Activated partial thromboplastin time (aPTT)

Selective

- Hemoglobin and hematocrit in patients who will undergo deep, large-bore biopsy, drainage, or thrombolysis procedures
- Bleeding time in patients with suspected qualitative platelet dysfunction or with minimal elevation of the PT or aPTT
- Fibrinogen before planned thrombolytic procedures (optional)

TABLE 2-1   Safety Thresholds for Coagulation Parameters

Parameter	Threshold
International normalized ratio (INR)	1.6-1.8
Prothrombin time (PT)	<3 sec from control
Partial thromboplastin time (PTT)	<6 sec from control
Platelet count (normal INR/PTT)	>50,000/mm³
Platelet count (abnormal INR/PTT)	>50-100,000/mm³
Bleeding time	<8 min

TABLE 2-2   Correction of Coagulation Abnormalities

Parameter	Response
International normalized ratio	Withhold warfarin, bridge with heparin or low molecular weight heparin (see Box 2-9)
	Fresh-frozen plasma (FFP), 2-4 bags or 10-15 mL/kg
	Vitamin K, 1-3 mg IV; may be repeated after 6-8 hr
Partial thromboplastin time	Withhold heparin 2-6 hr before procedure
	FFP, 2-4 bags or 10-15 mL/kg
Platelet count	Platelet transfusion (10 units to increase count by 50,000-100,000/mm³)
Bleeding time	Cryoprecipitate (0.2 bag/kg)
	Desmopressin (DDAVP), 0.4 µg/kg over 30 min
	Platelet transfusion
Fibrinogen	FFP, 10-15 mL/kg

IV, *intravenously.*

- Diabetic patients with preexisting renal dysfunction who take the oral hypoglycemic metformin (Glucophage) are at a very small risk for severe (and sometimes fatal) lactic acidosis resulting from metformin accumulation if CIN occurs after an angiographic procedure.[29] In these individuals, metformin is withheld for 48 hours before elective cases, at the time of the procedure for urgent cases, and 48 hours afterward.[30] The drug may be resumed after obtaining a new serum creatinine.
- Heparin is stopped 2 to 4 hours (depending on the most recent partial thromboplastin time [PTT] value) before most interventional procedures and restarted several hours later.
- Warfarin therapy complicates many IR procedures. The drug is usually withheld for 3 to 5 days before elective cases. Often, a low molecular weight (LMW) or unfractionated heparin bridge is necessary to protect the patient from a thrombotic or embolic event[31,32] (Box 2-9). If the PT or INR is mildly elevated on the day of the study, infusion of fresh frozen plasma should be considered.

BOX 2-9

INDICATIONS AND PROTOCOL FOR ANTICOAGULATION "BRIDGE" AFTER WITHHOLDING WARFARIN

- Prosthetic heart valve (most cases)
- VTE within 1 year
  - Severe thrombophilia
  - Active cancer
- Atrial fibrillation with history of stroke/TIA and additional risk factor
- Recurrent VTE

Day −5 Stop warfarin
Day −3 Start LMWH
Day −1 Check INR, hold LMWH after morning dose
Day 0 Stop unfractionated heparin 4 hours before (if prescribed)
Day +1 Restart LMWH and warfarin

Adapted from Vinik R, Wanner N, Pendleton RC: Periprocedural antithrombotic management: a review of the literature and practical approach for the hospitalist physician. *J Hosp Med* 2009;4:551.
INR, International Normalized Ratio; *LMWH*, low molecular weight heparin; *TIA*, transient ischemic attack; *VTE*, venous thromboembolic disease.

- LMW heparin compounds (e.g., enoxaparin [Lovenox]) will generally not alter standard coagulation tests. Studies in coronary interventions have failed to show a significant added risk of bleeding when these agents are administered.[33] However, there is a paucity of published data on their impact during noncoronary interventions. It is wise to hold doses for 24 hours before elective cases.
- Most practitioners favor discontinuation of aspirin or clopidogrel (Plavix) about 7 to 10 days before elective, high-risk procedures. This step is not necessary for lower risk procedures, such as tunneled central venous catheter insertion. However, if the agents were given in conjunction with bare or drug-eluting coronary stents, they should *not* be discontinued without the consent of a cardiologist.[31]
- Preprocedure sedation (e.g., lorazepam [Ativan], 0.5 to 2.0 mg orally) is favored by some interventionalists.

Contrast Reaction Pretreatment

Severe allergic reactions follow less than 1 in 10,000 doses of the most commonly used intravascular nonionic isosmolar contrast materials.[34,35] The value of universal pretreatment of patients with a history of a prior contrast material reaction is being questioned. Nonetheless, it remains accepted practice in many institutions to premedicate patients with a history of moderate to severe contrast allergy before giving these drugs. Even with pretreatment, so-called breakthrough reactions do occur.[36]

A variety of protocols are acceptable, but all include a corticosteroid taken at least 12 hours beforehand.[35,37] There is *no* evidence that oral or IV steroids are of any benefit when given immediately before contrast is injected.[37] Accepted regimens include:

- Corticosteroid: 32 mg methylprednisolone (Medrol) orally or 50 mg prednisone orally 12 hours, 7 hours (optional), and 2 hours before the procedure (mandatory)
- Histamine (H_1) receptor blocker: 25 to 50 mg diphenhydramine (Benadryl) orally 1 to 2 hours before the procedure (optional)

Prevention of Contrast-Induced Nephropathy

N-*acetylcysteine* (NAC, *Mucomyst*) is an antioxidant that behaves as a scavenger of oxygen free radicals and inhibitor of certain proteins implicated in kidney damage from iodine-based contrast media. Even though results of clinical trials have been mixed, the preponderance of evidence suggests that NAC is indeed more renal protective than IV hydration alone in patients with underlying renal insufficiency.[38-42] Dosing protocols vary, but typically patients receive 600 to 1200 mg orally twice on the day before, day of, and day after the procedure. Because of the low bioavailability of oral NAC, higher doses may be more effective.[43,44] Ascorbic acid is another antioxidant that has been studied for prevent of CIN. However, NAC appears to be the superior agent.[44]

IV sodium bicarbonate infusion results in alkalinization of the renal medulla and urine. Several randomized studies have shown that bicarbonate infusion (e.g., 154 mEq/L as 3 mL/kg/hr bolus for 1 hour before contrast administration, followed by 1 mL/kg/hr for 6 hours afterward) is more effective than saline hydration alone in preventing CIN in patients with some degree of renal dysfunction undergoing angiographic procedures.[45,46]

Finally, one trial found that the combination of NAC and bicarbonate infusion therapy was substantially more beneficial than either agent alone in this setting.[47] Although some experts dismiss the role of pharmacologic protection, many practitioners have adopted this combined approach.[48]

Prophylactic Antibiotics in Adults

Despite the widespread prescription of antimicrobial agents to prevent IR-related infections, there is almost no good evidence to support their routine use. One nonrandomized series of patients undergoing percutaneous gastrostomy indeed benefited from prophylactic antibiotics.[49] Still, experienced interventionists know that certain high-risk procedures (e.g., "virgin" biliary drainage, nephrostomy for stone disease) can directly lead to bacteremia or frank sepsis.

In principle, antibiotics are reserved for interventions that are:[50,51]

* "Clean-contaminated" (traverse a normally colonized viscus or lumen)
* Frankly "dirty" (active infection such as abscess)
* Intended to produce tissue necrosis (e.g., ablative procedures)

Surgical practice dictates that IV antibiotics be given within 20 to 60 minutes of skin incision/puncture.[52] Supplemental doses may be required for long cases. In some situations, antibiotics are continued for several days afterward (e.g., biliary drainage). The preferred antimicrobials vary widely among physicians and institutions, and new antibiotics appear almost every month. General guidelines have been described (Box 2-10), but each group should establish protocols in conjunction with infectious disease colleagues.[50,52]

Patients with prosthetic heart valves, history of bacterial endocarditis, or other valvular abnormalities are prone to serious infection from several bacteria species (most notably *Enterococcus*) during

---

BOX 2-10

ANTIBIOTIC PROPHYLAXIS IN INTERVENTIONAL RADIOLOGY

Recommended

Biliary procedures
Genitourinary procedures (with noted exceptions)
Drainage of suspected abscesses
Embolization intended to invoke target ischemia/ infarction (e.g., chemoembolization, uterine artery embolization)
Transjugular intrahepatic portosystemic shunt
Endograft (covered stent) placement (aorta, peripheral arteries, dialysis access)

Controversial

Gastrostomy and gastrojejunostomy
Vascular access device placement
Hemodialysis access treatment
Radiofrequency ablation of solid tumors
Intravascular stent placement
Transplant cholangiography

Not Recommended

Routine angiographic, angioplasty and thrombolysis procedures
Urinary tract tube changes and checks in patients without known infection
Clear fluid aspirations (e.g., renal cyst)
Endovenous laser ablation
Inferior vena cava filter placement
Biopsy (unless transrectal route)

---

invasive procedures. Appropriate antibiotic prophylaxis is warranted when a colonized or infected structure will be breached.[50]

Correction of Coagulopathies

Management of coagulation abnormalities is outlined in Table 2-2. PT/INR prolongation commonly results from warfarin therapy, liver disease, vitamin K deficiency, or disseminated intravascular coagulopathy. Prolongation of the PTT is most often seen with heparin therapy. Qualitative platelet defects often occur in patients with uremia or consumptive coagulopathies. Some agents, such as platelets, fresh frozen plasma, or desmopressin, should be given just before an intervention.

INTRAPROCEDURE CARE

"Time Out"

Immediately before starting any interventional or surgical procedure, and with the entire operating team present, The Joint Commission mandates a "time out" or "shout out."[53] Identity is established by announcing the name, medical record number, and birthdate on the patient's wrist band. The impending procedure is verbalized along with the site and side of intervention (e.g., "intraarterial embolization of the right kidney"). The signed consent form is reconciled with the clinically indicated intervention. The on-site existence of any specialized equipment necessary for the procedure is confirmed. Finally, any known drug allergies are stated.

Radiation Safety

The radiation dose to the patient can be minimized by limiting fluoroscopy time and the number of digital acquisitions, using the lowest imaging frame rates necessary to obtain diagnostic information during fluoroscopy, careful beam collimation, and use of lead shields (including gonadal protection when appropriate). Some complex or prolonged IR cases lead to significant radiation exposure and a real risk for radiation dermatitis.[54-57] Transient skin injury may occur after a dose of 2 Gy. Permanent damage usually requires doses greater than 5 Gy. The procedures with greatest overall risk include transjugular intrahepatic portosystemic shunt, embolization, and intravascular stent placement in the abdomen or pelvis.

Therefore, a measure of radiation exposure should be included in the dictated report for *all* IR procedures. Fluoroscopy time is a relatively poor proxy for dose and associated radiation risk. Peak skin dose (PSD), air kerma (in mGy), and dose area product (DAP, in Gycm²) are more accurate indicators.[58] Doses should be carefully monitored for the higher risk cases or when multiple sequential procedures are performed.

Interventionalists are at particular risk for excessive radiation exposure over their lifetimes.[59,60] The major complications of long-term radiation exposure in these providers include cataracts, certain solid organ cancers, and hematologic malignancies. Personal radiation monitoring badges must be worn at all times. Operators should protect themselves by wearing protective clothing, such as body aprons, thyroid wraps, and leaded glasses. Interventionalists should be diligent about using careful beam collimation, last image hold, and moveable leaded barriers during fluoroscopy and manual acquisition of digital images. Finally, appropriate tube angulation can greatly reduce radiation exposure to the arm during nonvascular procedures and dialysis access interventions.

Infectious Disease Precautions

The risk for transmission of blood-borne pathogens from physician to patient during interventional cases is vanishingly small. However, the risk for transmission from patient to operator is very real.[61-63] In particular, infection with hepatitis B or C virus and human immunodeficiency virus (HIV) is of particular concern to health care workers.

Because of the potentially grave consequences of these infections, Universal Precautions should be followed, as mandated in the United States by the Occupational Safety and Health Administration. These measures include use of surgical gowns, masks, protective eyewear, and two pairs of gloves. Gloves should be changed every few hours during long procedures and whenever glove integrity is breached.[64] A secure place for all sharp objects is kept on the interventional table (Online video 3-1). Needles are never recapped with a gloved hand alone. If a needle stick does occur, the occupational safety department should be consulted immediately.

Patient Monitoring

The interventionalist should note the baseline vital signs before the procedure begins. The patient undergoes continuous monitoring of electrocardiogram, respiratory rate, end tidal carbon dioxide, and oxygen saturation (by pulse oximetry). Automated cuff blood pressure measurement is obtained every 5 to 10 minutes, depending on the patient's condition. The nurse records these factors, the degree of sedation, and overall patient status every 5 to 10 minutes throughout the case. Oxygen is given by nasal cannula or face mask to maintain the oxygen saturation above 90% to 92%.

Fluid Management

The type and rate of IV fluid infusion are based on preexisting conditions (e.g., diabetes, renal failure, congestive heart failure) and the volume of intravascular contrast material being given. As a general rule, fluids are run at about 1 mL/kg/hr. One study found that the incidence of renal dysfunction after angiography was lower with vigorous saline hydration alone than with the use of mannitol or furosemide to induce diuresis after the procedure.[65] A Foley catheter is placed when angiographic imaging over the pelvis is required and for patient comfort and monitoring of urine output during long or complex interventions.

Sedation and Analgesia

Patients undergoing interventional radiologic procedures always experience some anxiety and pain, but the degree of discomfort may not reflect the invasiveness of the intervention. Perhaps the most important (and sometimes undervalued) measure to reduce anxiety and pain is reassurance. Patients can tolerate an invasive procedure more easily when the operator and other personnel show genuine concern for the patient's fears and discomfort and alert him or her to each sensation about to be felt as the case proceeds.

The goals of sedation during interventional procedures are relief of pain, anxiolysis, partial amnesia, and control of patient behavior. In most cases, these goals can be met with *moderate ("conscious") sedation,* in which the individual is calm, drowsy, and may even close his or her eyes but is responsive to verbal commands and able to protect his reflexes and airway.[66,67] *Deep sedation* (in which protective reflexes are lost) and *general anesthesia* are required for some cases but should be administered only by an anesthesiologist or other provider specially trained in these techniques.

The standard analgesic and sedative agents employed in IR are narcotics, benzodiazepines, and neuroleptic tranquilizers. A wide variety of drugs can be used to produce moderate sedation. One of the most popular combinations is midazolam and fentanyl.[67,68]

Midazolam (Versed) is a short-acting intravenous benzodiazepine that acts on GABA receptors to cause central nervous system depression (including anxiolysis and antegrade amnesia). It is metabolized by the liver. The onset of action is 2 to 4 minutes, and the duration of effect is about 45 to 60 minutes.[66] The standard initial dose is 0.5 to 1.0 mg IV. Additional boluses are given every 3 to 5 minutes to achieve the desired level of sedation. The optimal dose often is lower in patients with small body mass, advanced age, liver or cardiopulmonary disease, baseline hypotension, or a depressed level of consciousness. The major side effects of midazolam are respiratory depression and apnea.

Fentanyl (Sublimaze) is a short-acting narcotic opioid analgesic that also is metabolized by the liver. Its onset of intravenous action is 2 to 4 minutes, and the duration of effect is about 30 to 60 minutes.[66] The initial and incremental IV dose is 25 to 50 µg. Relatively large amounts may be required in patients with a history of chronic narcotic use or abuse. Major side effects include nausea, pruritus, dysphoria, and respiratory depression.

After the initial administration, additional doses are generally required every 3 to 10 minutes to maintain a continuous level of comfort. If an acceptable response to sedatives and analgesics is not observed *before* the case starts, the patient may not tolerate the more painful and prolonged interventions that may follow. In this unusual circumstance, it may be wise to request the assistance of an anesthetist or terminate the procedure. Sometimes a patient does not exhibit the expected response to standard dosages of these drugs. Addition of other synergistic IV agents (e.g., *hydromorphone [Dilaudid]* 1 to 2 mg IV and *diphenhydramine [Benadryl]* 25 to 50 mg) may be safer and more effective than relying on escalating amounts of fentanyl and midazolam. The interventional nurse must work closely with the interventionalist to achieve a steady but safe level of sedation and analgesia until the case is finished.

The chief signs of overmedication are a drop in oxygen saturation and respiratory depression. Some patients display a delayed or hypersensitive reaction to even small doses of these medications. Oxygen administered by nasal cannula or face mask is given if the oxygen saturation falls below 90%.

Pediatric sedation is the subject of numerous reviews.[69]

Treatment of Adverse Events and Reactions

Adverse events are relatively infrequent during interventional procedures. Successful management depends on recognizing problems quickly, acting promptly, and employing basic resuscitative efforts:

- Continuous patient monitoring
- Protecting the patient's airway
- Securing the intravenous line and administering fluids as needed
- Giving supplemental oxygen
- Calling for assistance early

Some of the more common clinical scenarios are outlined in Boxes 2-11 through 2-14.

Reaction to Sedatives and Analgesics

The most common symptoms of overdose are hypoxia, respiratory depression, and unresponsiveness. Less commonly, patients exhibit nausea, vomiting, hypotension, bradycardia, agitation, or confusion. Hypoxia alone usually resolves with supplemental oxygen, a neck tilt or jaw thrust to maintain the airway, and withholding additional sedatives. Nausea and vomiting respond to a variety of antiemetic agents, including 2.5 to 10 mg IV of the dopamine antagonist *prochlorperazine (Compazine)* or the serotonin 5-HT$_3$ blocker *ondansetron (Zofran)*, 4 mg IV.

BOX 2-11

CAUSES OF
INTRAPROCEDURAL
HYPOTENSION

- Overmedication with sedatives/analgesics
- Bleeding
- Sepsis
- Contrast or drug reaction
- Myocardial infarction
- Pulmonary embolism (including air embolism)

BOX 2-12

CAUSES OF INTRAPROCEDURAL HYPOXIA/RESPIRATORY DEPRESSION

- Overmedication with sedatives/analgesics
- Airway interference (e.g., morbid obesity, history of sleep apnea)
- Congestive heart failure
- Aspiration
- Pneumothorax
- Pulmonary embolism (including air embolism)

BOX 2-13

CAUSES OF INTRAPROCEDURAL ALTERED MENTAL STATUS

- Sedative/analgesic medication
- Hypoglycemia
- Anxiety
- Hypoxia
- Vasovagal reaction
- Bleeding/hypovolemia
- Myocardial infarction or dysrhythmia
- Stroke

BOX 2-14

CAUSES OF INTRAPROCEDURAL RIGORS

- Contrast or drug reaction
- Sepsis/bacteremia

Patients with profound or prolonged respiratory depression or hypotension should receive supplemental oxygen, airway maintenance, and antagonists to the offending drugs. *Naloxone (Narcan)* is an opiate antagonist. The initial dose of 0.2 to 0.4 mg given by IV push may be repeated every 1 to 2 minutes. *Flumazenil (Romazicon)* is a benzodiazepine antagonist. The initial dose of 0.2 mg given by IV push may be repeated every minute or so up to a total dose of 1 to 3 mg. Repeated injections of these agents may be needed to treat overmedication.

Vasovagal Reaction

Symptoms include hypotension with bradycardia, nausea, and diaphoresis. Immediate treatment includes elevation of the legs, rapid infusion of IV fluids, and administration of atropine. *Atropine* is a muscarinic, cholinergic blocking agent that affects the heart, bronchial and intestinal smooth muscle, central nervous system, secretory glands, and iris.[70] The initial dose is 0.5 to 1 mg IV, which may be repeated every 3 to 5 minutes up to a total dose of 2.5 mg. Major side effects include confusion, dry mouth, blurred vision, and bladder retention. The drug can be reversed with 1 to 4 mg IV of physostigmine.

Hypertension

The most common causes of hypertension during interventional procedures are uncontrolled baseline hypertension, failure to take routine antihypertensive medications, anxiety or pain, bladder distention, and hypoxia. Many patients become normotensive after sedatives and analgesics are given. The major risks of sustained hypertension are local bleeding after removal of an angiographic catheter or remote bleeding in patients undergoing treatment with anticoagulants or fibrinolytic agents. If severe hypertension persists, several drugs should be considered.[71,72]

Labetalol is a selective alpha-1 and nonselective beta adrenergic blocking agent and potent antihypertensive drug. A 20-mg IV dose is injected over 2 minutes. The dosage may be doubled again every 10 minutes to a total of 300 mg. The action is rapid (5 to 10 minutes) and prolonged (3 to 6 hours). Labetalol should be avoided in patients with asthma or congestive heart failure.

Enalaprilat is an angiotensin-converting enzyme (ACE) inhibitor that is quite effective for periprocedural hypertension. The usual dosage is 1.25 mg IV given over 5 minutes and again at 6 hours if necessary.

Sublingual *nifedipine* was once considered a first line agent in this setting. The drug has fallen out of favor because of scattered reports of life-threatening hypotension and dysrhythmias. The newer calcium channel blocker *clevidipine* (1 to 2 mg IV per hour) is a better alternative.

Hydralazine 5 to 10 mg by slow IV push (and repeated after 20 to 30 minutes) is a good backup antihypertensive drug.

Oral *clonidine* (initial dose 0.1 to 0.2 mg) may be useful in the postprocedure period.

Bleeding

When tachycardia and hypotension occur without other explanation or the patient complains of unexpectedly severe pain along the route of intervention, occult hemorrhage may be present. In this situation, bleeding will be undetectable by observation alone. Rapid infusion of fluid should be started; a blood count, coagulation screen, and type and cross should be obtained; and imaging assessment of potentially damaged structures should be considered.

Mild Contrast Agent Reaction

Patient reassurance is crucial in the management of all contrast reactions, regardless of severity.[73,74] Symptoms of a mild contrast reaction are myriad but commonly include urticaria, nausea and vomiting, cough, mild shaking, sweats, and anxiety.[37] Hives usually require no specific treatment. If itching is bothersome or the rash is widespread, treatment with *diphenhydramine (Benadryl)* (25 to 50 mg IV) is helpful. Persistent symptoms may be addressed with an intravenous antiemetic, such as prochlorperazine 2.5 to 10 mg or droperidol 0.625 to 1.25 mg.

Moderate Contrast Agent Reaction

Moderate reactions to contrast are manifested by mild bronchospasm or wheezing, mild facial or laryngeal edema, tachycardia (or bradycardia), and hypertension or hypotension.[37] Patients receiving beta-adrenergic blocking agents may not become tachycardiac. Bronchospasm is relieved with supplemental oxygen, an inhaled bronchodilator such as 2 or 3 puffs of *metaproterenol (Alupent)*, and *subcutaneous* administration of 0.1 mg (0.1 mL) of a *1:1000 concentration of epinephrine*, which may be repeated every 15 minutes. Isolated hypotension and tachycardia should respond to leg elevation, rapid infusion of IV fluids (normal saline or Ringer's lactate), and 10 to 20 μg/kg/min of dopamine (as needed).

Severe Contrast Agent Reaction

Life-threatening reactions to contrast (heralded by severe bronchospasm or laryngospasm, profound hypotension, convulsions, or cardiac dysrhythmias) are exceedingly rare. These events require immediate, aggressive treatment with supplemental oxygen, rapid IV fluid infusion, and *IV* administration of 0.1 mg (1 mL) of a *1:10,000 concentration of epinephrine*. The dose may be repeated every 2 to 3 minutes. Epinephrine must be given with care in patients with cardiac dysrhythmias, coronary artery disease, or those undergoing treatment with nonselective beta-adrenergic blocking agents. These reactions may progress to complete cardiovascular collapse.

Hypoglycemia

Patients with diabetes who receive insulin or oral hypoglycemic agents may become hypoglycemic during the procedure. Symptoms may include mental confusion, agitation, tremors, seizures, and cardiac arrest, which is rare. However, individuals with a profoundly low glucose level may be completely asymptomatic. If hypoglycemia is suspected or detected, an infusion of 5% to 10% dextrose is started and the blood glucose level checked or rechecked. If symptoms are severe or the serum glucose level is dangerously low, one ampule (50 mL) of 50% dextrose given by IV push is necessary.

Dysrhythmias

Cardiac dysrhythmias that occur during IR procedures often are caused by guidewire or catheter manipulation in the heart, by metabolic abnormalities (such as hypoxia, hypercarbia, or electrolyte imbalances), or by myocardial ischemia. Mechanically induced dysrhythmias usually revert after repositioning the guidewire. Sustained dysrhythmias should be treated in consultation with a cardiologist or physician with experience in such situations.

Supraventricular tachycardias (>150 beats/minute) appear as regular, narrow QRS (<0.12 sec) complexes on an electrocardiogram. Some resolve with a chest thump or vagal action (e.g., energetic cough or Valsalva maneuver). If not, the first line treatment in *asymptomatic* patients is an IV bolus of *adenosine*, which slows the sinus rate and atrioventricular node conduction velocity.[75,76] The initial dose is 6 mg given by rapid IV push; a 12-mg dose may be required if there is no response after several minutes. The onset of action is immediate, and transient asystole (about 5 seconds) should be anticipated. An alternative to adenosine is the calcium channel blocking agent *diltiazem*; a loading dose of 0.25 mg/kg is given by slow IV push. When these measures fail, a cardiologist should be promptly called. In symptomatic patients, immediate synchronized cardioversion is warranted.

Ventricular tachycardia (VT) has a regular wide complex QRS (>0.12 sec) on an electrocardiogram. When caused by guidewire manipulation in the heart, it is usually transient and reverts with a chest thump or having the patient cough vigorously. Symptomatic or hemodynamically unstable patients with this dangerous rhythm require immediate cardioversion with a synchronized shock (200 watt-sec). Asymptomatic sustained (>30 sec) monomorphic VT is treated with *amiodarone*.[77] The initial dose is 150 to 300 mg given IV over 5 to 10 minutes followed by an infusion of 1050 mg/day. The onset of action is almost immediate. Major side effects include confusion, seizures, and cardiopulmonary depression. Alternative agents in this situation include *procainamide* and *ajmaline*.

Sepsis

Bacteremia is a concern during nonvascular interventions, particularly those that involve manipulation of abscesses or the biliary and urinary systems.[78] Fever, chills, or rigors are common; frank septic shock occurs much less frequently. Broad spectrum antibiotics should be started immediately if they have not already been given. Rigors usually respond to 25 to 50 mg IV of *meperidine (Demerol)*. Hypotension from sepsis can be initially managed with IV saline boluses and a 10- to 20-μg/kg/min infusion of dopamine.

Seizures

Seizures may be idiopathic or a reaction to drugs given during the procedure (e.g., contrast agents). Treatment includes protection of the patient's airway and body, supplemental oxygen, and 5 to 10 mg IV of *diazepam (Valium)* or 1 mg IV of midazolam (Versed) as needed.

Air Embolism

This event is a rare occurrence during vascular access placement.[79] Most patients remain asymptomatic, but hypoxia and hypotension can occur. Some experts advocate placing the patient in a left lateral decubitus position to prevent air from entering the right ventricular outflow tract. Unfortunately, by the time the event is detected by fluoroscopy, air has usually migrated into the pulmonary arteries. Air embolism is rarely fatal. Treatment usually is supportive, including supplemental oxygen, IV fluids, and continuous patient monitoring.

Cardiopulmonary Arrest

Cardiorespiratory collapse may result from the patient's underlying condition (e.g., massive pulmonary embolus, multiorgan failure) or some aspect of the procedure itself (e.g., contrast agent reaction, oversedation). Regardless of the cause, basic life support maneuvers must be started immediately, including alerting a code team, establishing an airway, and beginning cardiopulmonary resuscitation.

POSTPROCEDURE CARE

Vascular Catheter Removal

Catheters are withdrawn immediately after vascular and interventional procedures unless ongoing intervention is necessary (e.g., overnight thrombolysis, abscess drainage). Additional lidocaine is given at the puncture site if sheath dwell time has been more than several hours. Especially prior to arterial catheter removal, blood pressure should be well controlled. The risk of hemorrhagic complications can be reduced in patients who have received heparin if catheter removal is delayed until the activated clotting time (ACT) falls into the high-normal range (typically less than 200 seconds).

Specific details of puncture site hemostasis and use of compressive dressings or arterial closure devices are considered in Chapter 3. For arterial punctures, manual compression is applied directly at, above, and below the puncture site to stop bleeding but maintain blood flow. Pressure is applied for 10 to 20 minutes or until bleeding has stopped. Femoral vein punctures usually need about 5 to 10 minutes of compression. Hemostasis at internal jugular

vein puncture sites is facilitated by elevating the patient's head. If a hematoma is present afterward, it should be marked on the skin and documented in the patient's chart.

Patient Monitoring

Initial postprocedure monitoring follows the same protocol as that used during the intervention. After arterial catheterization, the puncture site and distal pulses should be checked throughout the observation period: for example, every 15 minutes for 1 hour, every 30 minutes for the next hour, and every hour thereafter. The length of outpatient monitoring varies with the type of procedure and the method of hemostasis (manual compression or closure device). Generally, patients are observed for 30 to 90 minutes after the last dose of sedatives or analgesics is given and until institutional discharge criteria are met. After diagnostic femoral or brachial arteriography, a 4- to 6-hour observation period is routine (unless a closure device is used). After diagnostic femoral or jugular venography, a 2- to 4-hour observation period is common.

Orders

Patient orders should include the following directions:

- Vital signs and access site checks: Monitoring usually is done every 15 minutes for the first hour and then tapered over the observation period.
- Activity: The patient is kept at bed rest until near the end of the monitoring period.
- Pain control: Immediate postprocedure analgesia is primarily accomplished with oral and parenteral opioids.[80]
- Diet: After sedatives and analgesics wear off, patients can be given liquids or a soft solid meal.
- Hydration: IV hydration usually is continued throughout the postprocedure period if intravascular contrast was given. IV access should be maintained while the patient recovers from moderate sedation.

Management of Acute Complications

Identification and management of delayed complications of various vascular and interventional procedures are considered in detail in Chapter 3. The most common acute angiographic complications are described here.

Puncture site bleeding or hematoma in most cases produces localized firm swelling. Treatment includes prolonged local compression and correction of any precipitating factors (e.g., coagulopathy, hypertension). If the patient has received heparin and hemostasis cannot be achieved in a reasonable period, *protamine sulfate* can be used to reverse anticoagulation.[81] By itself, protamine is a weak anticoagulant; 10 mg of protamine neutralizes 1000 units of heparin. A typical IV dose of 20 to 40 mg is injected *slowly* over 10 minutes. Rapid injection can produce profound hypotension, bradycardia, flushing, and dyspnea. Individuals with a history of previous protamine therapy, treatment with protamine-containing insulin (e.g., isophane [NPH] insulin), or fish allergy are at increased risk for anaphylactic reactions and should not receive the drug.[82]

Patients with an enlarging hematoma or postprocedure hypotension are followed with serial hemoglobin/hematocrit measurement. Unexplained hypotension or a falling hematocrit may be the only signs of occult internal bleeding. In this case, CT scanning may be helpful to localize the bleeding site. A marked drop in hematocrit or massive hematoma may require blood transfusion, transcatheter embolization, or surgical evacuation. Arterial occlusion results from thrombosis or dissection at the puncture site. Femoral or brachial artery occlusion is suspected by a loss of distal pulses or the development of ischemic symptoms. Duplex sonography or catheter angiography of the affected limb should be performed.

Distal embolization can arise from a clot that formed on the catheter or punctured artery. These emboli often are silent. Some cases of asymptomatic embolization may be treated conservatively with observation and anticoagulation. A patient with a threatened limb should undergo diagnostic arteriography. Cholesterol embolization is a rare complication that follows disruption of an atherosclerotic plaque by manipulation of catheters or guidewires.[83] Cholesterol microemboli are showered into distal vascular beds, including those of the legs, kidneys, or bowel. Patients develop severe leg pain and a reddish, netlike pattern on the lower abdomen and legs ("livedo reticularis"), but the pedal pulses remain intact. Renal failure is common, and the mortality rate is high.

Discharge Instructions and Follow-up

Several criteria must be met before discharge of outpatients after IR procedures (Box 2-15). Patients should receive written instructions about care of the access or puncture site, catheter exit site, or external catheter. Postprocedure antibiotics or medications (if any), treatment of postprocedure pain, and warning signs of complications and how to deal with them (including a physician or nurse contact) are discussed with the patient. A responsible adult should accompany the patient home and preferably stay with him or her until the following day.

Performing an interventional procedure entails a commitment to follow-up and long-term care of the patient, including daily rounds for inpatients or periodic outpatient visits. A follow-up appointment should be scheduled to evaluate the results of therapy, identify complications, and determine the need for further interventions.

BOX 2-15

DISCHARGE CRITERIA AFTER OUTPATIENT INTERVENTIONAL PROCEDURES

- Stable vital signs with no respiratory depression
- Alert and oriented
- Able to drink, void, and ambulate
- Minimal residual pain
- Minimal nausea
- No bleeding at access site
- Discharge with competent adult

References

1. Margulis AR. Interventional diagnostic radiology: a new subspecialty. *AJR Am J Roentgenol* 1967;**99**:763.
2. Practice Guideline for Interventional Clinical Practice. American College of Radiology; American Society of Interventional and Therapeutic Neuroradiology; Society of Interventional Radiology. *J Vasc Interv Radiol* 2005;**16**:149.
3. Sacks D, McClenny TE, Cardella JF, et al. Society of Interventional Radiology clinical practice guidelines. *J Vasc Interv Radiol* 2003;**14** (9 (Pt. 2)):S199.
4. Dahlbäck B. Advances in understanding pathogenic mechanisms of thrombophilic disorders. *Blood* 2008;**112**:19.
5. Bick RL. Hereditary and acquired thrombophilic disorders. *Clin Appl Thromb Hemost* 2006;**12**:125.
6. Valji K, Linenberger M. Chasing clot: thrombophilic states and the interventionalist. *J Vasc Interv Radiol* 2009;**20**:1403.
7. American Society of Anesthesiologists (ASA). ASA physical status classification system. Available from: www.asahq.org/clinical/physicalstatus.htm.
8. Berlin L. Informed consent. *AJR Am J Roentgenol* 1997;**169**:15.
9. American College of Radiology (ACR). ACR practice guideline on informed consent for image-guided procedures, revised 2006 (Res. 32). Available from: www.acr.org/SecondaryMainMenuCategories/quality_safety/guidelines/iv/informed_consent_image_guided.aspx.
10. Egglin TKP, O'Moore PV, Feinstein AR, et al. Complications of peripheral arteriography: a new system to identify patients at increased risk. *J Vasc Surg* 1995;**22**:787.
11. Katzenschlager R, Ugurluoglu A, Ahmadi A, et al. Incidence of pseudoaneurysm after diagnostic and therapeutic angiography. *Radiology* 1995;**195**:463.
12. Arepally A, Oechsle D, Kirkwood S, et al. Safety of conscious sedation in interventional radiology. *Cardiovasc Intervent Radiol* 2001;**24**:185.
13. Fifi JT, Meyers PM, Lavine SD, et al. Complications of modern diagnostic cerebral angiography in an academic medical center. *J Vasc Interv Radiol* 2009;**20**:442.
14. Murphy TP, Dorfman GS, Becker J. Use of preprocedure tests by interventional radiologists. *Radiology* 1993;**186**:213.
15. Johnson H, Knee-Ioli S, Butler TA, et al. Are routine preoperative laboratory screening tests necessary to evaluate ambulatory surgical patients? *Surgery* 1988;**104**:639.
16. Mantha S, Roizen MF, Madduri J, et al. Usefulness of routine preoperative testing: a prospective single-observer study. *J Clin Anesth.* 2005;**17**:51.

17. Smetana GW, Macpherson DS. The case against routine preoperative laboratory testing. *Med Clin North Am* 2003;**87**:740.

18. Curhan GC. Prevention of contrast nephropathy. *JAMA* 2003;**289**:606.

19. Katzberg RW, Newhouse JH. Intravenous contrast medium-induced nephrotoxicity: is the medical risk really as great as we have come to believe? *Radiology* 2010;**256**:21.

20. Juluru K, Vogel-Claussen J, Macura KJ, et al. MR imaging in patients at risk for developing nephrogenic systemic fibrosis: protocols, practices, and imaging techniques to maximize patient safety. *Radiographics* 2009;**29**:9.

21. Shellock FG, Spinazzi A. MRI safety update 2008: part I. MRI contrast agents and nephrogenic systemic fibrosis. *AJR Am J Roentgenol* 2008;**191**:1129.

22. Segal JB, Dzik WH, Transfusion Medicine/Hemostasis Clinical Trials Network. Paucity of studies to support that abnormal coagulation test results predict bleeding in the setting of invasive procedures: an evidence-based review. *Transfusion* 2005;**45**:1413.

23. Dzik WH. Predicting hemorrhage using preoperative coagulation screening assays. *Curr Hematol Rep* 2004;**3**:324.

24. Iorio A, Basileo M, Marchesini E, et al. The good use of plasma. A critical analysis of five international guidelines. *Blood Transfus* 2008;**6**:18.

25. Stroncek DF, Rebulla P. Platelet transfusions. *Lancet* 2007;**370**:427.

26. Haas B, Chittams JL, Trerotola SO. Large-bore tunneled central venous catheter insertion in patients with coagulopathy. *J Vasc Interv Radiol* 2010;**21**:212.

27. Gross JB, Bailey PL, Caplan RA, et al. Practice guidelines for sedation and analgesia by non-anesthesiologists. *Anesthesiology* 1996;**84**:459.

28. Parra D, Legreid AM, Beckey NP, et al. Metformin monitoring and change in serum creatinine levels in patients undergoing radiologic procedures involving administration of intravenous contrast media. *Pharmacotherapy* 2004;**24**:987.

29. Nawaz S, Cleveland T, Gaines PA, et al. Clinical risk associated with contrast angiography in metformin treated patients: a clinical review. *Clin Radiol* 1998;**53**:342.

30. Glucophage (metformin) package insert. Princeton (NJ): Bristol-Myers Squibb Co.; 2009. Available from: http://packageinserts.bms.com/pi/pi_glucophage.pdf.

31. Vinik R, Wanner N, Pendleton RC. Periprocedural antithrombotic management: a review of the literature and practical approach for the hospitalist physician. *J Hosp Med* 2009;**4**:551.

32. Douketis JD, Berger PB, Dunn AS, et al. The perioperative management of antithrombotic therapy: American College of Chest Physicians evidence based clinical practice guidelines. 8th ed. *Chest* 2008;**133**:299S.

33. Bhatt DL, Lee BI, Castarella PJ, et al. Safety of concomitant therapy with eptifibatide and enoxaparin patients undergoing percutaneous coronary intervention: results of the Coronary Revascularization Using Integrilin and Single Bolus Enoxaparin Study. *J Am Coll Cardiol* 2003;**41**:20.

34. Tramer MR, von Elm E, Loubeyre P, et al. Pharmacologic prevention of serious anaphylactic reactions due to iodinated contrast media: systematic review. *BMJ* 2006;**333**:675.

35. Wang CL, Cohan RH, Ellis JH, et al. Frequency, outcome, and appropriateness of treatment of nonionic contrast media reactions. *AJR Am J Roentgenol* 2008;**191**:409.

36. Kim SH, Lee SH, Lee SM, et al. Outcomes of premedication for non-ionic radio-contrast media hypersensitivity reactions in Korea. *Eur J Radiol* 2010 [Epub ahead of print].

37. American College of Radiology. Manual on contrast media v7. Reston (VA): American College of Radiology; 2004–2011. Available from: www.acr.org/SecondaryMainMenuCategories/quality_safety/contrast_manual.aspx.

38. Shyu K-G, Cheng J-J, Kuan P. Acetylcysteine protects against acute renal damage in patients with abnormal renal function undergoing a coronary procedure. *J Am Coll Cardiol* 2002;**40**:1383.

39. Tepel M, van der Giet M, Schwarzfeld C, et al. Prevention of radiographic-contrast agent-induced reductions in renal function by acetylcysteine. *N Engl J Med* 2000;**343**:180.

40. Kay J, Chow WH, Chan TM, et al. Acetylcysteine for prevention of acute deterioration of renal function following elective coronary angiography and intervention. A randomized controlled trial. *JAMA* 2003;**289**:553.

41. Kelly AM, Dwamena B, Cronin P, et al. Meta-analysis: effectiveness of drugs for preventing contrast-induced nephropathy. *Ann Intern Med* 2008;**148**:284.

42. Diaz-Sandoval LJ, Kosowsky BD, Losordo DW. Acetylcysteine to prevent angiography-related renal tissue injury (the APART trial). *Am J Cardiol* 2002;**89**:356.

43. Stenstrom DA, Muldoon LL, Armijo-Medina H, et al. N-acetylcysteine use to prevent contrast medium-induced nephropathy: premature phase III trials. *J Vasc Interv Radiol* 2008;**19**:309.

44. Jo S-H, Koo B-K, Park J-S, et al. N-acetylcysteine versus ascorbic acid for preventing contrast-induced nephropathy in patients with renal insufficiency undergoing coronary angiography: NASPI study—a prospective controlled trial. *Am Heart J* 2009;**157**:576.

45. Merten GJ, Burgess WP, Gray LV, et al. Prevention of contrast-induced nephropathy with sodium bicarbonate: a randomized controlled trial. *JAMA* 2004;**291**:2328.

46. Navaneethan SD, Singh S, Appasamy S, et al. Sodium bicarbonate therapy for prevention of contrast-induced nephropathy: a systematic review and meta-analysis. *Am J Kid Dis* 2009;**53**:617.

47. Briguori C, Airoldi F, D'Andrea D, et al. Renal insufficiency following contrast media administration trial (REMEDIAL): a randomized comparison of 3 preventative strategies. *Circulation* 2007;**115**:1211.

48. Barrett BJ, Parfrey PS. Preventing nephropathy induced by contrast medium. *N Engl J Med* 2006;**354**:379.

49. Cantwell CP, Perumpillichira JJ, Maher MM, et al. Antibiotic prophylaxis for percutaneous radiologic gastrostomy and gastrojejunostomy insertion in outpatients with head and neck cancer. *J Vasc Interv Radiol* 2008;**19**:571.

50. Venkatesan AM, Kundu S, Sacks D, et al. Practice guidelines for adult antibiotic prophylaxis during vascular and interventional radiology procedures. *J Vasc Interv Radiol* 2010;**21**:1611.

51. Dravid VS, Gupta A, Zegel HG, et al. Investigation of antibiotic prophylaxis usage for vascular and non-vascular interventional procedures. *J Vasc Interv Radiol* 1998;**9**:401.

52. Beddy P, Ryan JM. Antibiotic prophylaxis in interventional radiology—anything new? *Tech Vasc Interv Radiol* 2006;**9**:69.

53. Angle JF, Nemcek Jr AA, Cohen AM, et al. Quality improvement guidelines for preventing wrong site, wrong procedure, and wrong person errors: application of the joint commission "Universal Protocol for Preventing Wrong Site, Wrong Procedure, Wrong Person Surgery" to the practice of interventional radiology. *J Vasc Interv Radiol* 2008;**19**:1145.

54. Wagner LK, McNeese MD, Marx MV, et al. Severe skin reactions from interventional fluoroscopy: case report and review of the literature. *Radiology* 1999;**213**:773.

55. Miller DL, Balter S, Cole PE, et al. Radiation doses in interventional radiology procedures: The RAD-IR study. Part I: overall measures of dose. *J Vasc Interv Radiol* 2003;**14**:711.

56. Miller DL, Balter S, Cole PE, et al. Radiation doses in interventional radiology procedures: The RAD-IR study. Part II: skin dose. *J Vasc Interv Radiol* 2003;**14**:977.

57. Marx MV. The radiation dose in interventional radiology: knowledge brings responsibility. *J Vasc Interv Radiol* 2003;**14**:947.

58. Miller DL, Balter S, Wagner LK, et al. Quality improvement guidelines for recording patient radiation dose in the medical record. *J Vasc Interv Radiol* 2004;**15**:423.

59. Stratakis J, Damilakis J, Hatzidakis A, et al. Occupational radiation exposure from fluoroscopically guided percutaneous transhepatic biliary procedures. *J Vasc Interv Radiol* 2006;**17**:863.

60. Klein LW, Miller DL, Balter S, et al. Occupational health hazards in the interventional laboratory: time for a safer environment. *J Vasc Interv Radiol* 2009;**20**:147.

61. Reddy P, Liebovitz D, Chrisman H, et al. Infection control practices among interventional radiologists: results of an online survey. *J Vasc Interv Radiol* 2009;**20**:1070.

62. Hansen ME, Miller III GL, Redman HC, et al. Needle-stick injuries and blood contacts during invasive radiologic procedures: frequency and risk factors. *AJR Am J Roentgenol* 1993;**160**:1119.

63. Baffoy-Fayard N, Maugat S, Sapoval M, et al. Potential exposure of hepatitis C virus through accidental blood contact in interventional radiology. *J Vasc Interv Radiol* 2003;**14**:173.

64. Hansen ME, McIntire DD, Miller III GL. Occult glove perforations: frequency during interventional radiologic procedures. *AJR Am J Roentgenol* 1992;**159**:131.

65. Solomon R, Werner C, Mann D, et al. Effects of saline, mannitol, and furosemide on acute decreases in renal function induced by radiocontrast agents. *N Engl J Med* 1994;**331**:1416.

66. Patatas K, Koukkoulli A. The use of sedation in the radiology department. *Clin Radiol* 2009;**64**:655.

67. Martin ML, Lennox PH. Sedation and analgesia in the interventional radiology department. *J Vasc Interv Radiol* 2003;**14**:1119.

68. American Society of Anesthesiologists Task Force on Sedation and Analgesia by Non-anesthesiologists. Practice guidelines for sedation and analgesia by non-anesthesiologists. *Anesthesiology* 2002;**96**:1004.

69. Gozal D, Gozal Y. Pediatric sedation/anesthesia outside the operating room. *Curr Opin Anesthesiol* 2008;**21**:494.

70. McEvoy GK, editor. *AHFS Drug Information 2002*. Bethesda (MD): American Society of Health-System Pharmacists; 2002.

71. Waybill MM, Waybill PN. A practical approach to hypertension in the 21st century. *J Vasc Interv Radiol* 2002;**14**:961.

72. Marik PE, Varon J. Perioperative hypertension: a review of current and emerging therapeutic agents. *J Clin Anesth* 2009;**21**:220.

73. Nayak KR, White AA, Cavendish JJ, et al. Anaphylactoid reactions to radiocontrast agents: prevention and treatment in the cardiac catheterization laboratory. *J Invasive Cardiol* 2009;**21**:548.

74. Davidson CJ, Erdogan AK. Contrast media: procedural capacities and potential risks. *Rev Cardiovasc Med* 2008;**9**:S24.

75. Patel A, Markowitz SM. Atrial tachycardia: mechanisms and management. *Expert Rev Cardiovasc Ther* 2008;**6**:811.

76. Holdgate A, Foo A. Adenosine versus intravenous calcium channel antagonists for the treatment of supraventricular tachycardia in adults. *Cochrane Database Syst Rev* 2006;**18**:CD005154.

77. Trappe HJ. Treating critical supraventricular and ventricular arrhythmias. *J Emerg Trauma Shock* 2010;**3**:143.

78. Smith TP, Ryan JM, Niklason LE. Sepsis in the interventional radiology patient. *J Vasc Interv Radiol* 2004;**15**:317.

79. Vesely T. Air embolism during insertion of central venous catheters. *J Vasc Interv Radiol* 2001;**12**:1291.

80. Hatsiopoulou O, Cohen RI, Lang EV. Postprocedure pain management of interventional radiology patients. *J Vasc Interv Radiol* 2003;**14**:1373.

81. McEvoy GK, editor. *AHFS Drug Information 2002*. Bethesda (MD): American Society of Health-System Pharmacists, 2002. p. 1453.

82. Levy JH, Adkinson Jr NF. Anaphylaxis during cardiac surgery: implications for clinicians. *Anesth Analg* 2008;**106**:392.

83. Bashore TM, Gehrig T. Cholesterol emboli after invasive cardiac procedures. *J Am Coll Cardiol* 2003;**42**:217.

3

Standard Angiographic and Interventional Techniques

Karim Valji

VASCULAR ACCESS

Anesthesia (Online Videos 3-1 and 3-2)

A local anesthetic is given at the start of every angiographic or interventional procedure. The preferred agent is 1% or 2% lidocaine (Xylocaine), which inhibits sodium channels involved in the conduction of nerve impulses. An intradermal skin wheal is made with a 25-gauge needle. The deeper subcutaneous tissues are anesthetized with a long 22- or 25-gauge needle. Intravascular injection must be avoided by intermittent aspiration. The pain from lidocaine injection is caused by the low pH of commercially available preparations. Discomfort is eased with "buffered lidocaine," which is prepared by admixing the drug with sodium bicarbonate (1 mL of 0.9% $NaHCO_3$ solution in 10 mL of 1% lidocaine).[1] Patients with a lidocaine allergy may receive an ester- rather than an amine-based anesthetic (e.g., 1% chloroprocaine).[2]

Retrograde Femoral Artery Catheterization (Online Video 3-2)

In 1953, Sven Ivar Seldinger first described the method for percutaneous arterial catheterization involving a needle, guidewire, and catheter.[3] The common femoral artery (CFA) is the safest and simplest arterial access route because it is large, superficial, usually disease free, and can be compressed against the femoral head to close the puncture. However, this approach should be avoided when the patient has a CFA aneurysm, local infection, overlying bowel, or a fresh incision. Within several weeks after placement, synthetic grafts in the groin also may be accessed safely using a single-wall needle.

When the skin is entered over the bottom of the femoral head and the needle is angled at 45 degrees, the needle usually enters the CFA at its midpoint[4] (Fig. 3-1). The inguinal crease is a poor landmark for skin puncture.[5] If the puncture is low (into the superficial femoral artery [SFA] or deep femoral artery [DFA]), the risk of thrombosis, pseudoaneurysm, or arteriovenous fistula formation is significantly increased.[6,7] If the puncture is too high (into the external iliac artery above the inguinal ligament), the risk of retroperitoneal or intraperitoneal bleeding is increased.[8] The bony landmarks for the inguinal ligament—a line running from the anterior superior iliac spine to the pubic tubercle—provide only a rough approximation.[9]

A small, superficial skin nick is made directly over the arterial pulse. A clamp is used to dissect the subcutaneous tissues. Although the advantages of real-time sonographic guidance for femoral artery puncture are obvious (Fig. 3-2), many practitioners continue to rely on the traditional method of manual palpation of the artery unless entry is difficult. A pulsatile artery may be surprisingly hard to puncture if the skin nick is malpositioned, the artery is unusually mobile, underlying disease exists, or vasospasm follows repeated attempts. In these situations, the operator should consider making a second skin nick directly over the arterial pulse or at a *slightly* higher location, waiting until a strong pulse has returned, or using the opposite groin. It is sometimes possible to catheterize the abdominal aorta even in the face of iliac artery occlusion if some flow can be detected by ultrasound in the CFA and an angled catheter and hydrophilic guidewire are used to traverse the occlusion.

The course of the artery is palpated while an 18-gauge needle is advanced at a 45-degree angle toward the femoral head (Fig. 3-3). It is safer to use a 21-gauge micropuncture needle set in coagulopathic patients (Fig. 3-4). If double-wall technique is used, the stylet is removed after bone is reached, and additional lidocaine is injected. The hub of the needle is depressed and then slowly withdrawn until pulsatile blood returns. Many interventionalists prefer a single-wall entry into the vessel. However, because single-wall needles have a beveled tip, the tip may be partially subintimal despite brisk pulsatile blood return. Slow return of dark blood usually

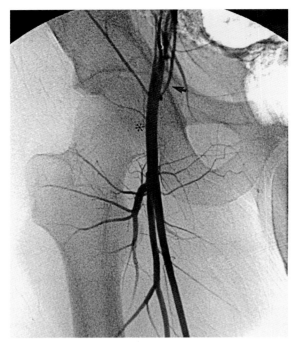

FIGURE 3-1   Common femoral artery puncture. The inguinal ligament is demarcated by the inferior epigastric artery *(arrow)*. The ideal arterial entry site is indicated by the *asterisk*.

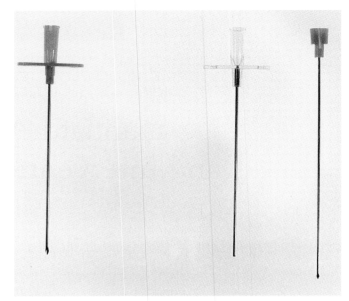

FIGURE 3-3   Needles for vascular catheterization. The single-wall needle *(left)* has a sharp beveled edge. The Seldinger-type needle with stylet *(right)* can also be used for most arterial catheterization procedures.

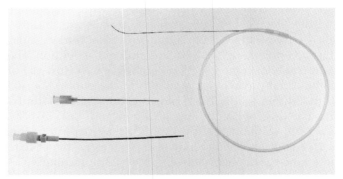

FIGURE 3-4   Micropuncture access set with a 21-gauge needle, a 0.018-inch steerable guidewire, and a 4-French transitional dilator.

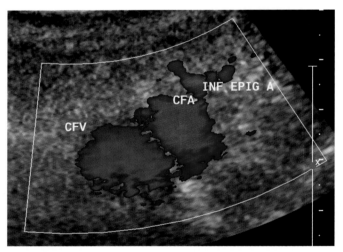

FIGURE 3-2   Color Doppler ultrasound of the left groin shows the relationship between left common femoral vein *(CFV)* and the left common femoral artery *(CFA)*. Note the inferior epigastric artery origin, which denotes the bottom of the inguinal ligament.

is a sign of venous entry; the site is then compressed and a more lateral puncture is made.

A 0.035- or 0.038-inch Bentson or floppy J-tipped guidewire is carefully inserted and advanced under fluoroscopy. Resistance to passage usually means that the tip of the needle is partially subintimal, up against the sidewall, or abutting common femoral or iliac artery

plaque. The wire should never be forced. A small change in needle position (e.g., medial to lateral, shallow to steep angle, slight withdrawal) usually allows the wire to pass; if not, contrast can be injected to identify the reason for resistance. If the guidewire still cannot be advanced, the needle is removed, compression is applied for a few minutes, and the artery is repunctured. Occasionally, the guidewire enters the deep iliac circumflex artery rather than the external iliac artery (Fig. 3-5). In this case, it is withdrawn and redirected.

After the guidewire is advanced to the abdominal aorta, a vascular sheath (or the bare angiographic catheter) is placed (Fig. 3-6). If the iliac arteries are severely diseased, it may be easier and safer to first place the sheath in the external iliac artery and then negotiate a

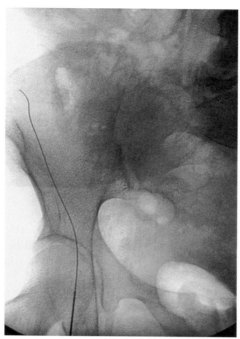

FIGURE 3-5   The guidewire has entered the deep iliac circumflex artery. Notice that the needle enters the common femoral artery over the middle of the femoral head.

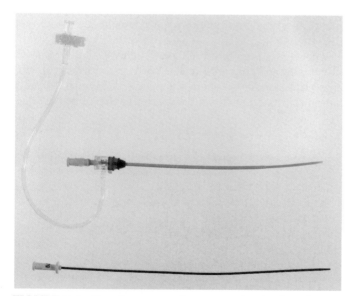

FIGURE 3-6   Vascular access catheters: vascular sheath with a sidearm and inner dilator *(top)* and a tapered dilator *(bottom)*.

hydrophilic guidewire into the aorta. Catheter advancement often is difficult in patients with marked obesity, heavily diseased arteries, or a scarred groin. In this case, placement of a stiff or super-stiff guidewire, overdilation of the access site by one French (Fr) size, or use of a stiff, tapered catheter (e.g., Coons dilator) may be helpful.

The puncture site is examined immediately after the catheter is inserted. Mild oozing usually stops after several minutes of gentle compression. A larger vascular sheath is placed if oozing persists or a hematoma starts to form. If the pulse has diminished, an angiogram of the iliac and common femoral artery is obtained immediately. If the catheter is occluding a critical stenosis, heparin is given, and the obstruction is treated with angioplasty.

Antegrade Femoral Artery Catheterization (Online Video 3-2)

Antegrade ("downhill") puncture of the CFA is sometimes required for infrainguinal procedures.[10] The skin puncture is made over the *top* of the femoral head to enter the middle of the CFA below the inguinal ligament[11] (see Fig. 3-1). In obese patients, it is helpful to tape the pannus onto the abdomen. A steep needle angle (>60 degrees) should be avoided because catheters and sheaths may be difficult to insert or may kink after placement. The guidewire often enters the DFA. Access into the SFA is accomplished in several ways[12-14]:

*   Replace the entry wire with an angled, steerable hydrophilic wire, which can often be manipulated into the SFA.
*   Place an angled catheter into the DFA, mark the skin entry site with a clamp, and then slowly withdraw the catheter while injecting the contrast medium. Once the catheter tip is at the bottom of the CFA, it is directed medially and a steerable guidewire is advanced into the SFA.
*   Withdraw the guidewire into the needle, redirect the needle toward the opposite arterial wall, and readvance the wire.

Brachial Artery Catheterization

Brachial artery catheterization is less desirable than CFA access because it is associated with a higher rate of adverse events. The neurologic complications that are the unfortunate hallmark of this technique are related to the particular anatomy of the brachial artery (see later discussion). From axilla to elbow, it runs within the *medial brachial fascial compartment*, a tight space bound by dense fibrous tissue.[15] The radial nerve exits this sheath in the distal axilla, the ulnar nerve in the lower third of the upper arm, and the median nerve continues throughout its course. This route may be necessary or advantageous for:

*   Patients with absent femoral pulses or known infrarenal abdominal aortic occlusion
*   Recanalization of steeply downgoing mesenteric or renal arteries

- Treatment of obstructions in upstream extremity arteries or downstream dialysis fistulae
- Patients with a history of cholesterol embolization during previous retrograde aortic catheterization

Decades ago, axillary artery puncture was abandoned for the high left brachial artery to diminish the complications associated with the former route.[16,17] Many experienced operators now choose a low (distal) brachial artery site for arterial catheterization.[18] Theoretically, right arm access exposes the patient to greater risk of embolic stroke with the catheter crossing all three arch vessels. The right arm is preferred if the brachial systolic blood pressure is significantly lower on the left (>20 mm Hg), suggesting significant left subclavian artery disease.

Real-time sonographic guidance greatly simplifies vessel puncture. With the arm abducted, a 21-gauge micropuncture or 18-gauge single-wall needle is advanced into the artery at a 45-degree angle. The guidewire often enters the ascending thoracic aorta. With an angled or pigtail catheter in the aortic arch, a hydrophilic guidewire can be negotiated into the descending thoracic aorta.

Alternative Arterial Access Routes

Retrograde popliteal artery access is becoming acceptable for certain femoral artery interventions.[19] However, it is premature to claim the safety of this novel route compared with more traditional access sites.

There are few reasons to perform direct *translumbar arteriography,* one being treatment of endoleak after endovascular graft placement (see Chapter 7). At first glance, the technique would appear unduly risky, but it is notable that generations ago, 5- to 7-Fr catheters were inserted directly into the aorta for diagnostic angiography with surprisingly few bad outcomes.[20]

Femoral Vein Catheterization (Online Video 3-4)

Before performing common femoral vein (CFV) catheterization, any existing lower extremity venous sonograms or computed tomography scans should be reviewed to confirm vessel patency. The CFV usually lies 0.5 to 1.5 cm medial to the CFA. Skin entry is made just medial to the arterial pulse and just below the bottom of the femoral head. In some patients, the vein is slightly medial and deep to the artery.[21] A single-wall needle is preferred to avoid unknowingly traversing the artery before entering the vein.

Most interventionalists use a 21-gauge micropuncture needle or ultrasound guidance to minimize the possibility of inadvertent arterial puncture, especially in coagulopathic patients. For "blind" entry, the neighboring CFA is palpated continuously. The needle is advanced with intermittent aspiration and is redirected if transmitted pulsations from the artery are felt at the hub. Sometimes, the tip coapts both sides of the vein and pierces the back wall without blood return on needle entry. The needle is then slowly withdrawn while aspiration is maintained. After blood returns freely, the guidewire is advanced into the inferior vena cava (IVC), and a sheath or diagnostic catheter is placed. Frequently, the wire tip meets resistance in a small ascending lumbar vein. If the guidewire is floppy, it may be advanced further until it buckles into the IVC. After several unsuccessful attempts at "blind" CFV puncture, sonography should be used. It might reveal venous thrombosis, chronic disease, or an abnormally positioned vein.

Internal Jugular Vein Catheterization (Online Video 3-5)

Internal jugular vein access is required for certain procedures (e.g., transjugular intrahepatic portosystemic shunt [TIPS] creation) and preferred for many others (e.g., vascular access placement, internal spermatic vein embolization, inferior vena cava filter placement). In most cases, the right internal jugular vein is chosen over the left.

The vessel is entered above the clavicle, always with direct sonographic guidance. With the transducer oriented in a transverse plane, the needle is advanced from a lateral approach or directly superior to the vein (Fig. 3-7).

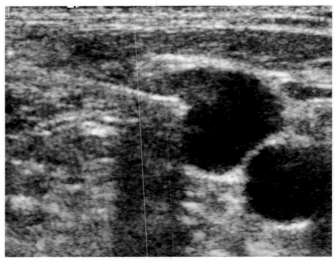

FIGURE 3-7   Right internal jugular vein entry under sonographic guidance in the transverse plane. Needle enters from lateral approach; carotid artery is medial to the vein.

A micropuncture set can be used to minimize trauma to the internal carotid artery if it is accidentally pierced. Entry into the venous system is confirmed by following the course of a guidewire advanced toward the right atrium.

Axillary/Subclavian Vein Catheterization

Subclavian vein access to the central venous system is discouraged for several reasons. Venous stenosis or occlusion is much more frequent after placement of subclavian vein catheters.[22] There is also a small risk of pneumothorax that is virtually nonexistent with internal jugular access. Finally, bleeding is more difficult to control if the subclavian artery is accidentally entered or venous access is lost. If this route must be used, puncture should always be made with sonographic guidance. The preferred point of entry is the central axillary vein at the level of the coracoid process. With the ultrasound transducer held in a longitudinal plane, the axillary/subclavian artery is identified first. A micropuncture needle is then advanced into the vein, which is situated just inferior to the artery (see Fig. 18-8).

Arterial Closure Devices (Online Video 3-6)

For more than 50 years, manual compression has been the standard approach for obtaining hemostasis of vascular catheterization puncture sites. However, this method requires additional operator time and rather prolonged patient bedrest afterward. Gaining hemostasis in anticoagulated patients or after large arterial sheaths (≥7 Fr) are removed can be problematic. Arterial closure devices are meant to reduce time to ambulation while allowing effective and safe vascular closure, even in the face of anticoagulation.[23-27] Three categories of devices are currently in use:

- Collagen material placed on the external surface of the punctured artery (e.g., AngioSeal device) (Fig. 3-8)
- Suture-mediated closure systems (e.g., Perclose Proglide and Starclose devices)
- External skin patches that accelerate coagulation (e.g., V-Pad, D-stat Dry Patch)

No one device is superior to the others, although patches and collagen-mediated products are not appropriate for larger holes (e.g., greater than 8 to 9 Fr). Device failure or need for conversion to manual compression is uncommon (<15% of cases) and rare for experienced operators. Some of these systems significantly reduce time to hemostasis and time to ambulation, particularly in anticoagulated patients.[23,28-33] Overall, the complication rate is comparable to manual compression. Still,

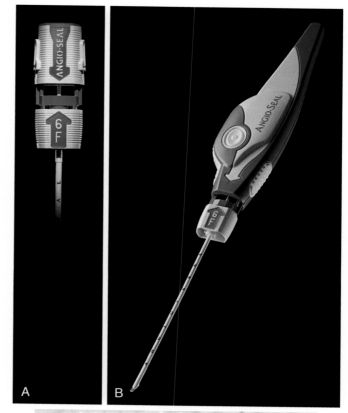

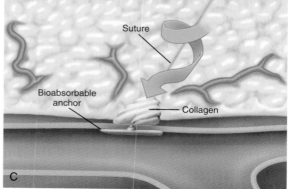

FIGURE 3-8 AngioSeal closure device. **A** and **B,** Two versions of the device. **C,** Illustration of footplate fixed to the inner wall of the artery, with collagen plug being deployed on the outer surface *(green arrow).* This mechanism is anchored to the skin with the white suture. *(Images courtesy of St. Jude Medical.)*

routine use of these devices is controversial for several reasons:

- The list of exclusionary criteria for many of these devices is long and includes uncontrolled hypertension, puncture outside the CFA, small caliber artery (<5 mm), existing hematoma, and double wall puncture. In addition, collagen-based systems should not be used if closure is delayed, repeat arterial puncture is anticipated, or groin operation is planned.

- Certain rare adverse events are specific to these devices. Local thrombosis or embolization of an AngioSeal anchor or part of a collagen plug has been reported, as has device failure requiring operative removal.[34] Most important, the presence of a foreign body adjacent to or in the artery increases the possibility (albeit remote) of local infection, which often requires surgical treatment and can be life-threatening.[35]

Certainly, a closure device should be considered when a large arterial sheath must be withdrawn or interruption of anticoagulation for sheath removal is inadvisable. Fresh sterile preparation of the access site is recommended; intravenous (IV) antibiotics may be indicated in some situations.

Complications

Specific complications of interventional procedures are considered in subsequent chapters. Complications after venous catheterization include bleeding or hematoma, thrombosis, and infection. Even when large sheaths are used, major events are seen in less than 5% of cases.

Table 3-1 outlines the most common adverse outcomes from femoral artery catheterization.[36-39] Minor bleeding or hematoma formation occurs in less than 10% of simple femoral artery catheterization procedures. Major bleeding requiring transfusion or surgical evacuation is relatively rare (<1%), but more likely when sheath size increases or anticoagulants and fibrinolytic agents are used. Blood may collect in the thigh, groin, retroperitoneum, or, rarely, the peritoneal space. Retroperitoneal hemorrhage should be suspected in a patient with an unexplained drop in hematocrit, hypotension, or flank pain (Fig. 3-9).

With proper technique, catheterization-related pseudoaneurysms are relatively uncommon (about 1% to 6%); arteriovenous fistulas are quite rare[39,40] (see Fig. 1-34). Most small (<2 cm) pseudoaneurysms close spontaneously. Large or persistent lesions require treatment (Fig. 3-10, see later discussion). Femoral artery thrombosis or occlusion usually is caused by dissection, spasm, or

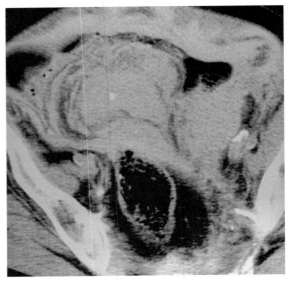

FIGURE 3-9   Massive hemorrhage after right femoral artery catheterization seen on axial computed tomography scan.

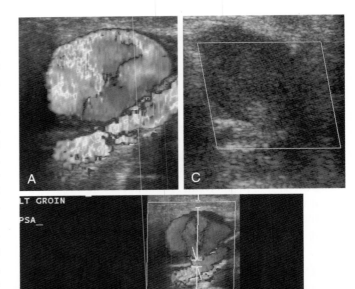

FIGURE 3-10   Postcatheterization femoral artery pseudoaneurysm treated with thrombin injection. **A,** Color Doppler ultrasound shows large pseudoaneurysm contiguous with superficial femoral artery. **B,** Waveform analysis reveals classic "to-and-fro" flow in the neck of the pseudoaneurysm. **C,** Following percutaneous thrombin injection, flow in the pseudoaneurysm has been abolished.

TABLE 3-1   Complications of Femoral Artery Catheterization

Type	Frequency (%)
Minor bleeding or hematoma	6–10
Major hemorrhage requiring therapy	<1
Pseudoaneurysm	1–6
Arteriovenous fistula	0.01
Occlusion (thrombosis or dissection)	<1
Perforation or extravasation	<1
Distal embolization	<0.10

pericatheter clot (Fig. 3-11). Cholesterol embolization from traumatic disruption of an atherosclerotic plaque is a rare but potentially devastating complication of arteriography[41] (see Chapter 2).

Other potential adverse events include nausea and vomiting, vasovagal reactions, and contrast media–related reaction or nephropathy. Cardiac events (e.g., arrhythmias, angina, heart failure) and neurologic events (e.g., seizures, femoral nerve injury, stroke) also can occur during vascular interventions.[42]

The reported frequency of complications from axillary or brachial artery access ranges from 2% to 24%.[16-18,20] In contemporary series, catheterization-related events with mid or low brachial artery puncture are less common but not negligible (0.44% [for diagnostic studies with 4-Fr catheters] to 6.5% [for interventional procedures with larger sheaths and anticoagulants]).[18,43] This vessel is more prone to thrombosis or pseudoaneurysm formation than the CFA (see Fig. 9-14). Distal neuropathy is a distinct but uncommon sequela of brachial artery puncture related to the tight anatomic space shared by the artery and several peripheral nerves (see earlier discussion). Thus even small hematomas can cause nerve compression. Sensory or motor neuropathy is reported in about 2% to 7% of patients who undergo this procedure.[16-18,43] The deficit is more likely to become permanent if early surgical decompression is not accomplished as soon as the problem is suspected. The other devastating neurologic complication of retrograde brachial artery catheterization is cerebral embolization of pericatheter clot, which has been reported in up to 4% of cases but is much less common in actual practice.[17]

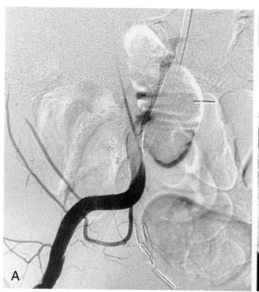
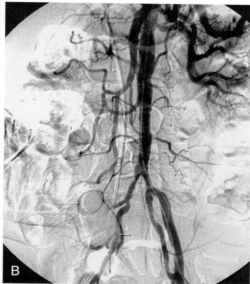
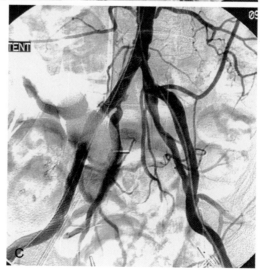

FIGURE 3-11 Right iliac artery and aortic dissection from retrograde femoral artery catheterization. **A,** Injection from the right external iliac artery shows a dissection with a thin channel of contrast in the false lumen. **B,** Aortogram from the left common femoral artery shows narrowing of the distal abdominal aorta and right common iliac artery and complete occlusion of the right external iliac artery. **C,** A guidewire was placed across the aortic bifurcation and through the true lumen into the right external iliac artery. The entire segment was reopened with a Wallstent.

Treatment of Postcatheterization Pseudoaneurysms and Arteriovenous Fistulas

Ultrasound-guided compression repair is effective in many cases of postcatheterization pseudoaneurysms.[44-46] In this technique, the ultrasound transducer is used to compress the neck of the pseudoaneurysm while flow is maintained in the SFA (Fig. 3-12). Patients are then kept at bedrest for 4 to 6 hours. Follow-up sonography is required to confirm permanent thrombosis. Pseudoaneurysm closure is successful in about 75% to 85% of cases. However, the method is painful (usually requiring moderate sedation), time-consuming, and sometimes ineffective, particularly in patients receiving anticoagulation.[47] Compression repair is not advised when flow in the neck cannot be obliterated or for lesions located above the inguinal ligament.

Ultrasound-guided percutaneous thrombin injection has become the first-line treatment for angiography-related pseudoaneurysms.[46-51] Thrombin injection also has been used to treat postcatheterization brachial artery pseudoaneurysms.[52] The procedure is quick, relatively painless, and highly effective. After excluding an arteriovenous fistula and using real-time ultrasound guidance, a 22- or 25-gauge needle is inserted into the body of the pseudoaneurysm away from the neck (see Fig. 3-10). Bovine thrombin (1000 units/mL) is injected into the lesion over 5 to 10 seconds. Most pseudoaneurysms require well under 1000 units for complete thrombosis. Clot formation is monitored with color Doppler imaging. The success rate is 90% or greater, even in the face of anticoagulation. Complete closure may be more problematic with complex pseudoaneurysms.[48] A failed first attempt should be repeated. However, the patient and operator should be aware that prior exposure to thrombin (topical or otherwise) can lead to antibody formation and the small risk of anaphylactic reaction. Although complications are rare, there are several reports of limb-threatening embolization or downstream thrombosis.[53-55] The presence of a wide or short aneurysm neck may predispose to this serious event.

Arteriovenous fistulas are much less common than pseudoaneurysms after femoral artery catheterization (Fig. 3-13 and see Fig. 1-34). Many fistulas close spontaneously. Repair is recommended if they persist for more than 2 months, increase twofold or more in size, or become symptomatic. As an alternative to operation, covered stents have been deployed to close fistulas. However, the published experience is too limited to endorse this approach as a routine measure.[56-58] In rare instances, embolization of a long track is feasible (see Fig. 8-53).

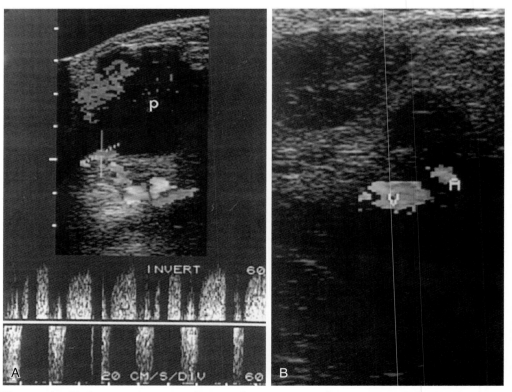

FIGURE 3-12   Ultrasound-guided compression repair of a postcatheterization pseudoaneurysm. **A,** Color Doppler sonogram shows a large pseudoaneurysm *(p)* arising from the left common femoral artery with classic "to-and-fro" flow at the aneurysm neck. **B,** After 30 minutes of compression of the neck, the pseudoaneurysm has thrombosed. Flow is maintained in the femoral artery *(A)* and vein *(V)*.

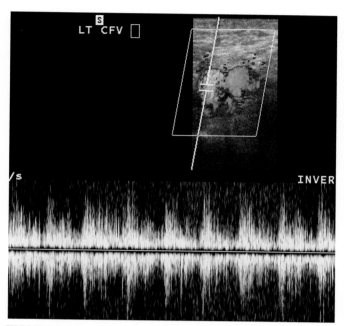

FIGURE 3-13 Postcatheterization femoral artery arteriovenous fistula. Transverse color Doppler sonography shows pulsatile flow in the left common femoral vein.

BASIC ANGIOGRAPHIC AND INTERVENTIONAL TOOLS

Catheters and Guidewires (Online Videos 3-1 and 3-7 to 3-9)

The interventionalist can choose from a vast assortment of commercially available guidewires and catheters. Proper selection of materials can be learned only through hands-on training and experience.

The primary characteristics of guidewires are listed in Box 3-1. All wires have a relatively soft, tapered segment of variable length at the working end. Standard guidewires are made of a stainless steel coil wrapped tightly around an inner mandril that narrows at the working end of the wire. A central safety wire filament is incorporated also to prevent complete separation if the wire breaks. Hydrophilic guidewires are extremely useful in diseased or tortuous vessels. Standard guidewire diameters are 0.035 and 0.038 inch. Finer-gauge wires (e.g., 0.014 and 0.018 inch) are available for use with microcatheters or small-caliber needles. Standard guidewire lengths are 145 cm and 175 cm. A long (260 to 300 cm) exchange wire may be needed for selective catheter changes. The more commonly used guidewires are outlined in Table 3-2.

Angiographic and interventional catheters are made of polyurethane, polyethylene, nylon, or Teflon. Many catheters are wire-braided for extra torqueability. Others are coated with a hydrophilic polymer to improve trackability. Catheters vary in length, diameter, and the presence of side holes. Outer catheter diameter is designated by French size (3 Fr = 1 mm). The standard angiographic catheter is 4 or 5 Fr.

Several types are available:

- *Straight catheters* come in many shapes (Fig. 3-14). Nonbraided catheters can be reshaped by heating them under a steam jet.
- *Reverse-curve catheters*, in which the tip is advanced into a vessel by catheter withdrawal at the groin, are available in many designs (Fig. 3-15).

BOX 3-1

CHARACTERISTICS OF INTERVENTIONAL GUIDEWIRES

- Composition and coating
- Diameter
- Total length
- Taper length
- Tip configuration
- Torqueability
- Stiffness
- Radiopacity

TABLE 3-2 Commonly Used Guidewires

Type	Function
STANDARD (0.035- or 0.038-inch)	
Bentson and floppy J tip wires	Standard access wire
Newton LT/LLT	Standard working wire
Hydrophilic wires (e.g., Terumo)	Use in tortuous or diseased vessels
Extra stiff wires (e.g., Amplatz)	Insertion of larger devices, resistant catheter passage
Exchange wires (e.g., Rosen)	Exchange of long angiographic catheters or devices or remote distance from access
Tapered wires (e.g., TAD wire)	Placement of devices into sensitive territories
Moveable core wires	Variable floppy working segment
MICROWIRES (0.012- to 0.018-inch)	
Cope mandril	Standard micropuncture access wire
Transcend Fathom	Floppy, steerable microwire
Syncro	Floppy, highly steerable and trackable microwire
V-18	Steerable, stiffer microwire
BMW	Steerable, stiffer microwire
Platinum plus	Steerable, stiffer microwire

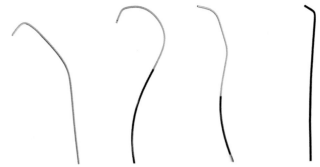

FIGURE 3-14　Basic straight angiographic catheters. *Left to right,* spinal, cobra, headhunter, and angled shapes.

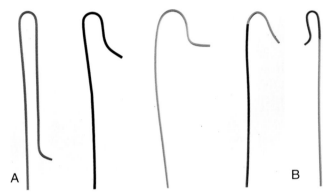

FIGURE 3-15　Basic reverse-curve catheters. **A,** *Left to right,* Roberts Uterine Catheter (RUC), Simmons (sidewinder), Shetty, and visceral hook. **B,** Sos selective catheter. *(Courtesy of Angiodynamics.)*

Although these catheters are versatile, they must first be reformed after insertion into the aorta or IVC[59] (Fig. 3-16 and Online Video 3-7). Some straight catheters can also be manipulated into a reverse-curve shape by formation of a "Waltman loop"[60] (Fig. 3-17). To eliminate the minute risk of cerebral embolization, some experienced interventionalists never re-form a catheter in the aortic arch if the region of interest is entirely below the diaphragm.

- *Pigtail-type catheters* are used for angiography in large vessels and for drainage procedures (urinary, biliary, fluid collections) (Fig. 3-18). Angiographic catheters have multiple side holes along the distal shaft that produce a tight bolus of contrast, which prevents subintimal dissection from a high-pressure contrast jet exiting the end-hole alone. Drainage catheters have side holes in the pigtail loop and sometimes the distal shaft. The loop is formed and secured by tightening a string attached to the tip, running within the lumen of the catheter, and exiting the catheter hub. The loop is designed to prevent catheter dislodgement.

- *Sheaths* are thin-walled valved catheters placed at the skin access site (see Fig. 3-6). In General, true outer sheath diameter is two sizes larger than the stated Fr size. They prevent oozing or hematoma around the puncture and minimize vessel trauma from multiple catheter exchanges. In addition, long sheaths can be advanced into a vessel undergoing treatment. Contrast medium can then be injected through sheath side arm while access to the intervention site is maintained with a guidewire or small catheter. Vascular and peel-away sheaths also are useful in nonvascular interventional procedures for maintaining access and placing multiple guidewires, among other reasons.

- *Guiding catheters* allow safer or more secure passage of devices into vessels (e.g., renal artery stent placement or coil embolization of pulmonary arteriovenous malformations [AVMs]). These catheters sometimes are inserted through larger sheaths placed at the vascular access site.

- *Microcatheters* pass through standard angiographic catheters and make angiography and intervention in small or tortuous arteries (e.g., mesenteric artery branches, infrapopliteal arteries) simple and safe. They are guided by small-caliber (e.g., 0.014 to 0.018-inch) steerable wires (Online Video 3-9 and see Table 3-2). Two commonly used microcatheters are the ProGreat and standard and high-flow Renegade devices. The Prowler microcatheter is constructed with preshaped tips. Only some catheters (e.g., Marathon) are appropriate for delivery of certain liquid embolic agents (e.g., Onyx). For embolotherapy, microcoils should not be delivered through high-flow microcatheters in which they can get stuck.

Pressure Measurements

Intravascular pressure monitoring is primarily used to determine the hemodynamic significance of stenoses, assess the results of revascularization procedures, and diagnose pulmonary artery or portal venous hypertension. A pressure gradient is far more accurate than multiple angiographic images for proving the significance of a vascular stenosis.[61] Hemodynamic measurements must be obtained with meticulous attention to detail to minimize artifacts.

The pressure gradient across a stenosis in a tube with flowing fluid is defined by *Poiseuille's law*:

$$\Delta P = \frac{8\eta QL}{\pi r^4}$$

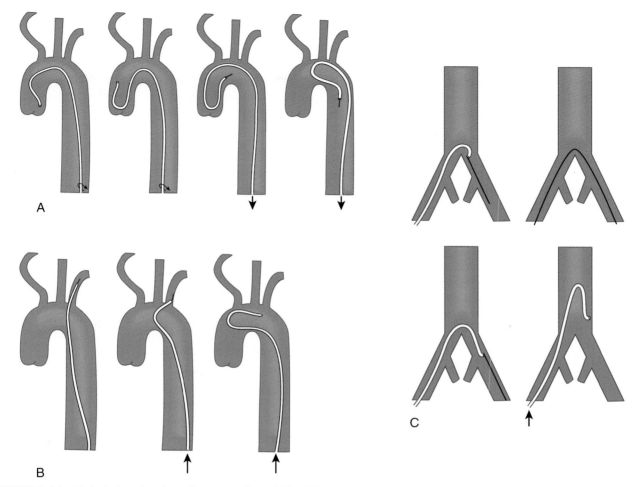

FIGURE 3-16   Methods for reforming a Simmons catheter. *(Adapted from Kadir S.* Diagnostic angiography. *Philadelphia: WB Saunders; 1986. p. 74.)*

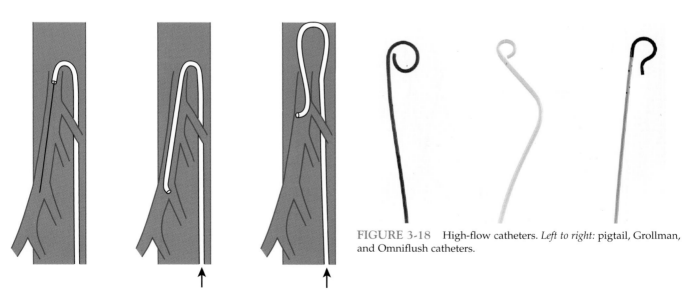

FIGURE 3-17   Method for forming a Waltman loop. *(From Kadir S.* The loop catheter technic. *Med Radiogr Photog 1981;57:22. Reprinted courtesy of Eastman Kodak Company.)*

FIGURE 3-18   High-flow catheters. *Left to right:* pigtail, Grollman, and Omniflush catheters.

In the equation, ΔP = pressure gradient, Q = blood flow, L = length of the stenosis, η = blood viscosity, and r = radius. In medium-sized arteries, blood flow is unchanged until the luminal diameter is reduced by 50%, which corresponds to a cross-sectional area reduction of 75% (Fig. 3-19). Blood flow falls precipitously as the diameter stenosis approaches 75% (about a 95% reduction in cross-sectional area). The relationship between flow reduction and luminal diameter becomes more complex with diffuse disease or tandem lesions. Pressure gradients are affected by blood flow. For example, as the peripheral arterial resistance in the legs drops with exercise, the magnitude (and therefore the clinical significance) of proximal pressure gradients increases.

The thresholds used to define a significant arterial pressure gradient are controversial. Resting systolic and mean gradients from 5 to 34 mm Hg have been suggested.[62-64] Absolute or relative gradients after flow augmentation (intraarterial injection of a vasodilator) are favored by some experts. As a general rule, a resting systolic gradient of *10 mm Hg or greater* is considered significant in the arterial system. In the central veins, a focal gradient of *3 to 6 mm Hg or greater* can be flow-limiting.

Pressure gradients are most accurate when simultaneous measurements are obtained from endhole catheters on either side of a stenosis. However, often it is more practical to use a single catheter to measure a "pullback pressure" across the lesion. With this method, however, the gradient may be spuriously elevated if the diameters of the catheter and vessel are similar (e.g., arteries ≤5 mm in diameter). A useful tool for determining hemodynamic significance of lesions in medium- and small-caliber arteries is a pressure guidewire (e.g., PrimeWire Prestige).[65,66]

Contrast Agents

Standard contrast materials used for vascular and interventional procedures are iodinated organic compounds.

- Ionic monomeric agents have a single triply iodinated benzene ring and form salts in plasma.
- Ionic dimeric agents (e.g., ioxaglate) contain twice the number of iodine atoms per molecule.
- Nonionic monomeric agents are less toxic because of lower osmolality, nondissociation in solution, and increased hydrophilicity.
- Nonionic dimeric agents are isosmolar (or nearly so) with plasma and are the least toxic of the available materials.

Iodinated contrast agents can produce numerous systemic effects after intravascular administration[67] (Box 3-2). The severity of these alterations depends largely on the osmolality of the preparation. At similar iodine concentrations, low osmolar contrast materials (LOCMs; ionic dimers and nonionic agents) have a significantly lower osmolality (600 to 800 mOsm/kg) than high osmolar contrast material (HOCMs; ionic monomers) with osmolality at 1400 to 2000 mOsm/kg. *Iodixanol (Visipaque)* is the only

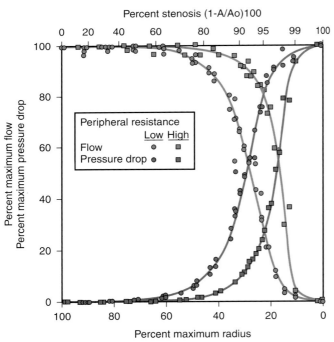

FIGURE 3-19   Relationship between arterial blood flow (y axis), cross-sectional area reduction (upper x axis), and luminal diameter (lower x axis). *(From Sumner DS. Hemodynamics and diagnosis of arterial disease: basic techniques and applications. In: Rutherford RB, editor.* Vascular surgery. *3rd ed. Philadelphia: WB Saunders; 1989. p. 24.)*

BOX 3-2

POSSIBLE SYSTEMIC EFFECTS OF INTRAVASCULAR CONTRAST AGENTS

- Hypervolemia
- Vasodilation
- Hemodilution
- Endothelial damage
- Altered heart rate, blood pressure, and respiration
- Constricted renal vessels
- Osmotic diuresis
- Damaged renal tubules
- Altered red cells
- Altered blood-brain barrier permeability
- Increased pulmonary artery resistance and pressure

isosmolar agent (290 mOsm/kg) currently available in the United States.

In most centers, nonionic agents are chosen for all intravascular applications. Minor side effects, such as nausea, vomiting, and local pain, are much less common with these drugs.[67] The overall incidence of adverse events with LOCM is less than 1%. The frequency of moderate to severe reactions is estimated at about 0.1% to 0.2% for HOCM and 0.01% to 0.02% for LOCM. The frequency of fatal reactions is less than 0.005% and not significantly different between the two classes of material.[68] There are only small differences in imaging quality among the various agents at the same iodine concentration,[69,70] The evidence is strong but not indisputable that contrast nephropathy is less likely in at-risk patients with use of iodixanol.[71-75] At centers in which cost issues are of particular concern, an argument can be made for selective use of nonionic material.

In patients with renal dysfunction or a history of life-threatening allergy, alternative contrast agents should be considered. Use of these media may limit or completely eliminate the need for iodinated material.

Carbon dioxide has been used extensively as a contrast agent for digital imaging in a variety of arterial and venous beds[76-80] (Fig. 3-20). The gas rapidly dissolves in blood and is eliminated from the lung less than 30 seconds after injection. There is no risk of allergic reaction or nephrotoxicity. An airtight system of reservoir bag, tubing, and syringes is constructed to purge a delivery syringe of room air and substitute instrument grade CO_2 (Online Video 3-10). For abdominal aortography or inferior venacavography, a 60-mL syringe is required. The catheter is then primed with the gas before rapid injection. Some patients experience discomfort with injection. The quality of images is generally inferior to those obtained with iodinated contrast. In addition, complications can arise from gas trapping and "vapor lock," especially in the pulmonary artery, abdominal aortic aneurysms, and the inferior mesenteric artery. *The agent cannot be used in arteries above the diaphragm because of the risk of intracerebral embolization.*

Gadolinium-based contrast materials can be used in individuals with a history of anaphylactic reaction to iodinated agents and normal renal function. However, they

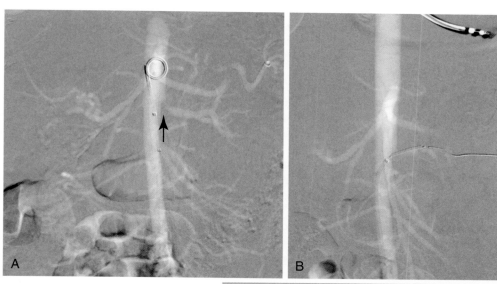

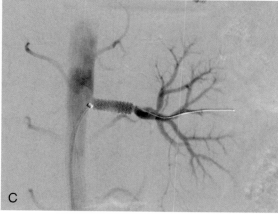

FIGURE 3-20 Carbon dioxide angiography for renal artery stent placement in a patient with underlying renal insufficiency. **A,** Abdominal aortogram shows proximal left renal artery stenosis *(arrow).* **B,** Carbon dioxide is used to confirm proper position of stent just before deployment. **C,** The single iodinated contrast arteriogram shows an excellent result with mild spasm at the distal end of the stent.

are not safe for intravascular use in patients with acute renal failure, chronic kidney disease (eGFR [estimated glomerular filtration rate] <30 mL/min), or dialysis dependence. In these populations, there is clear dose-related causation between some of these drugs and the highly debilitating disorder of nephrogenic systemic fibrosis[81-83] (NSF, see Chapter 2).

Pharmacologic Adjuncts

Antiplatelet Agents

Aspirin (acetylsalicylic acid, ASA) is a moderate inhibitor of platelet aggregation. It works by irreversibly inactivating cyclooxygenase (COX), a critical enzyme in the production of a key enzyme (thromboxane A_2) required for platelet function.[84,85] The drug is rapidly absorbed from the stomach; platelet function is inhibited within 1 hour of ingestion and continues for the lifetimes of existing platelets (about 7 to 10 days). Aspirin prolongs the bleeding time without significantly affecting other coagulation parameters. Patients often are maintained on a daily dose of 325 mg for at least several months after recanalization procedures.

Thienopyridines are more potent oral antiplatelet agents that irreversibly inhibit binding of adenosine diphosphate (ADP) to platelet receptors, thus preventing platelet-fibrinogen binding and $\alpha_{IIB}\beta3$ integrin (glycoprotein [GP] IIb/IIIa)–mediated platelet activation and aggregation.[86,87] The first-generation agent *ticlopidine (Ticlid)* is rarely prescribed because of certain relative drawbacks. The second-generation drug *clopidogrel (Plavix)* is in widespread use. The standard loading dose is 300 mg orally, with typical daily dosage of 75 mg. The new third-generation agent *prasugrel* may be useful in patients who are "nonresponders" to clopidogrel.[86] Combination therapy (aspirin + clopidogrel) is favored in many situations for patients with coronary artery disease. However, current recommendations favor monotherapy for primary prevention of cardiovascular events in the subset of individuals with peripheral arterial disease.[88,89] For interventionalists, clopidogrel (alone or in combination with aspirin) may be useful in some patients following arterial recanalization procedures. These agents also show promise in preventing restenosis after angioplasty, stent insertion, or bypass graft placement. The major downside to thienopyridines is bleeding. In patients requiring certain invasive procedures, clopidogrel must be withheld for 7 to 10 days to reverse the bleeding tendency.

Cilostazol (Pletal) is a phosphodiesterase III inhibitor that has antiplatelet, antithrombotic, smooth muscle antiproliferative, and vasodilatory effects.[90-92] There is abundant evidence that long-term therapy (50 to 100 mg orally twice daily) increases exercise ability and overall quality of life in patients with intermittent claudication.

There is also growing support for its additive benefit in preventing restenosis after some endovascular recanalization procedures.[93] Significant drug interactions can occur with certain cytochrome P450 inhibitors (e.g., diltiazem, erythromycin, and omeprazole).

$\alpha_{IIB}\beta3$ Integrin (GP IIb/IIIa) receptor inhibitors are a class of potent cell receptor antagonists that act on the final common pathway to platelet aggregation. Although interplatelet binding is inhibited, platelet attachment to subendothelial elements is maintained. Although these parenteral drugs have great potential for enhancing revascularization in acute coronary syndromes, the experience in peripheral arterial disease has been somewhat disappointing.[94-96] As such, these agents should not be used routinely but instead should be reserved for selected cases, such as slow response to thrombolytic agents, thrombophilic states, need for rapid revascularization, or infrageniculate interventions (Table 3-3). It is important to carefully monitor platelet levels, which can fall precipitously during treatment.

Antithrombin Agents

Heparin is a polyanionic protein that binds with antithrombin (AT), among other plasma proteins and cells.[97] The resulting complex inhibits clot formation by inactivating thrombin and factor Xa. This effect is dependent on a specific pentasaccharide sequence present on unfractionated heparin and other synthetic drugs (see later discussion). Because thrombin is the critical enzyme in clot formation, heparin is a potent antithrombotic agent. The drug is cleared from the body in two phases. Rapid initial clearance by fairly indiscriminate binding to plasma proteins and endothelial cells is followed by slower clearance by the kidneys. The biologic half-life varies widely among individuals, but it is roughly 1 hour at typical therapeutic doses (5000 units IV bolus followed by 500 to 1500 units/hr infusion). *Protamine*, a

TABLE 3-3 $\alpha_{IIB}\beta3$ Integrin (GP IIB/IIIA) Platelet Inhibitor Agents

Generic (Trade Name)	Structure	Half-Life	Dosage
Abciximab (ReoPro)	Monoclonal antibody	8-12 hr	Bolus 0.25 mg/kg Infuse 0.125 µg/kg/min over 12 hr
Eptifibatide (Integrilin)	Synthetic peptide	2.5 hr	Bolus 180 µg/kg t = 0,10 min Infuse 2.0 µg/kg/min over 18-24 hr
Tirofiban (Aggrastat)	Nonpeptide tyrosine	2 hr	Bolus 0.10 µg/kg Infuse 0.15 µg/min over 18-24 hr

cationic protein derived from salmon sperm, completely reverses the anticoagulant effect (see Chapter 2).

Because heparin pharmacokinetics are unpredictable, its effect must be measured. During vascular procedures, the antithrombotic response can be followed with the activated clotting time (ACT), which reflects whole blood clotting.[98] Normal and therapeutic ranges are specific to each manufacturer's device. The activated partial thromboplastin time (PTT) is used to monitor long-term anticoagulation. The therapeutic range is 1.5 to 3.5 times the control value.[99] One protocol for adjusting heparin doses based on the PTT obtained every 4 to 6 hours was recently proposed by a panel of experts.[100] Patients who are extremely resistant to heparin may require titration by direct heparin assay or a switch to a low molecular weight heparin (LMWH) agent (see later discussion).

The major complications of heparin therapy are bleeding, *heparin-induced thrombocytopenia (HIT)* (see Chapter 1), and osteopenia (with long-term use). The risk of bleeding is a function of drug dose, concomitant use of thrombolytic agents, recent surgery or trauma, baseline coagulation status, kidney function, and age. To screen for HIT, platelet levels should be monitored two or three times a week.

LMWH has more predictable and persistent anticoagulant activity than unfractionated heparin.[97,101,102] This class of drugs includes *enoxaparin (Lovenox), dalteparin (Fragmin), reviparin,* and *tinzaparin (Innohep).* The primary mechanism of action is inhibition of factor Xa and thrombin mediated through antithrombin. Unlike unfractionated heparin, LMWH exhibits almost no indiscriminate cellular or protein binding. As such, clearance is dose-independent, and the half-life (about 4 hours) is much longer. The dose must be reduced in patients with renal disease; the drug is avoided altogether in severe renal insufficiency (eGFR <30 mL/min).

LMWH is becoming the standard prophylactic regimen in prevention of deep venous thrombosis (e.g., before major orthopedic or abdominal surgery) and often replaces the heparin/warfarin sequence for treatment of acute deep venous thrombosis.[102,103] Major advantages over unfractionated heparin include ease of administration (once or twice daily by subcutaneous injection), no need for monitoring, and a low (<2%) frequency of HIT.[97] Bleeding is still a major concern with long-term use.

Fondaparinux (Arixtra) is a synthetic pentasaccharide that corresponds to the critical portions of the heparin molecule responsible for binding to antithrombin.[97] It only targets factor Xa and has a much longer half-life (about 17 hours) than heparin-related agents. One drawback of this drug is the lack of an available reversing agent. On the other hand, it may be prescribed in patients with a history of HIT.[104]

Direct thrombin inhibitors (bivalirudin [Angiomax], argatroban, and *lepirudin [Refludan])* are recombinant or synthetic agents that inhibit both free and circulating thrombin. Unlike heparin-related compounds, they do not require antithrombin for activity.[103,105,106] The anticoagulative effect is much more predictable than with unfractionated heparin. Whereas they are used widely during coronary interventions, experience in other vascular beds is limited.[107,108] However, these drugs play a crucial role in patients with a history of HIT.[109]

Warfarin (Coumadin) is an oral antithrombotic agent that inhibits vitamin K–dependent liver synthesis of the proenzymes for coagulation factors II, VII, IX, and X.[110] Despite many drawbacks (including inconsistent dose-response, need for frequent monitoring, and nontrivial bleeding complications), warfarin is still widely used to prevent and treat arterial and venous thrombotic events. It has a half-life of 36 to 42 hours. A full anticoagulative effect is not achieved until 3 to 7 days after therapy is started. Drug monitoring and reversal are discussed in Chapter 2. A wide variety of foods and medications can potentiate or inhibit the anticoagulant effect of warfarin.

Antispasmodic Agents

Vasodilators are used during vascular procedures to prevent or relieve vasospasm and occasionally to augment arterial flow.[111] One of the more commonly used agents is the direct smooth muscle relaxant *nitroglycerin* (100 to 200 µg IA or IV), which has a half-life of 1 to 4 minutes. Calcium channel blockers, including *verapamil,* can be used also. This drug class is contraindicated in patients with elevated intracranial pressure and certain cardiac conditions. Adverse effects include hypotension, tachycardia, and nausea. However, these reactions are uncommon with standard dosages.

VASCULAR INTERVENTIONAL TECHNIQUES

Balloon Angioplasty

Percutaneous transluminal balloon angioplasty (PTA) remains the first line minimally invasive technique for treatment of stenoses in the vascular, biliary, and urinary systems (Fig. 3-21). PTA was conceived by Dotter and Judkins,[112] who first used sequential dilators to open an occluded SFA. Gruentzig[113] is credited with the development of balloon angioplasty catheters that are the basis of the current method. In many situations, PTA is performed in conjunction with stent placement to obtain optimal results (see later discussion).

Mechanism of Action

Inflation of an angioplasty balloon in a stenotic artery causes desquamation of endothelial cells, splitting or dissection of the atherosclerotic plaque and adjacent intima,

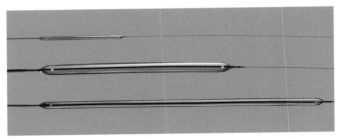

FIGURE 3-21   Balloon angioplasty catheters. *(Image provided courtesy of Boston Scientific. © 2010 Boston Scientific Corporation or its affiliates. All rights reserved.)*

and stretching of the media and adventitia.[114,115] There is virtually no compression of the plaque itself. This controlled stretch injury increases the cross-sectional area of the vascular lumen. Platelets and fibrin cover the denuded surface immediately. Over the next several weeks, reendothelialization of the intima occurs, and the artery remodels. Clinically significant *restenosis* is the consequence of vascular remodeling (e.g., recoil) and prolific neointimal hyperplasia that reflects an inflammatory response to the injury. On the other hand, PTA of venous stenoses stretches the entire vein wall, usually without causing a frank tear.

Patient Selection

The specific indications for PTA are considered in later chapters. Vascular angioplasty should only be performed when all of the following conditions are met: the obstruction is hemodynamically significant, reopening the vessel is likely to improve the patient's symptoms or clinical condition, and other treatment options are less attractive.

As a rule, balloon angioplasty alone is less effective or relatively unsafe in the following situations:

- Stenosis adjoining an aneurysm (owing to higher risk for rupture)
- Bulky, polypoid atherosclerotic plaque (owing to higher risk for distal embolization)
- Diffuse disease (Fig. 3-22)
- Long-segment stenosis or occlusion

Technique (Online Video 3-11)

The important factors in device selection are balloon diameter, balloon length, catheter profile (a function of shaft size and balloon material), peak inflation pressure, and trackability.

- The shortest balloon that will span the lesion is chosen. However, if the balloon is too short and not centered precisely, it may be squeezed away from the stenosis during inflation ("watermelon seed effect").
- Low-profile balloon systems that accommodate microwires are now popular for treatment of

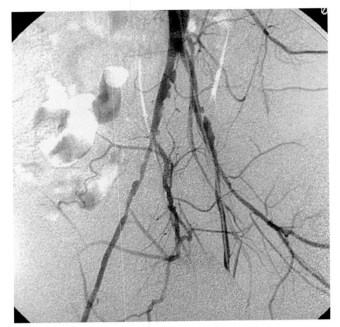

FIGURE 3-22   Balloon angioplasty alone is unlikely to be effective for diffuse disease in the right common and external iliac arteries.

medium- and small-caliber arteries (e.g., renal, hepatic, small peripheral arteries).
- For most arteries and veins, better results are obtained with slight overdilation (about 10% to 15%). However, it is sometimes prudent to start with smaller diameter balloons and upsize as needed.
- Atherosclerotic plaques yield with inflation pressures of 5 to 10 atm. Venous and graft stenoses may require much higher pressures (18 to >24 atm).
- Vessel rupture may occur if the balloon is too big or the rated balloon inflation pressure is exceeded (Fig. 3-23). The mechanism behind angioplasty-induced vascular rupture may be related to sudden overdistention of the balloon or a high-pressure fluid jet created when the balloon bursts.[116] In some instances, the balloon breaks after the artery has torn.[117]

Cutting balloons with microthin longitudinal blades running along the balloon surface are used to treat stenoses that fail to efface even high-pressure balloons.[118-120] The primary applications of these devices are resistant lesions in hemodialysis grafts and arterial bypass grafts.

Three drug classes should always be considered as possible adjuncts to any vascular recanalization procedure, including angioplasty.

- *Anti-platelet:* In some vascular beds, aspirin or a thienopyridine platelet inhibitor (e.g., clopidogrel) is given beforehand to prevent postangioplasty thrombosis and for several months thereafter to limit restenosis.

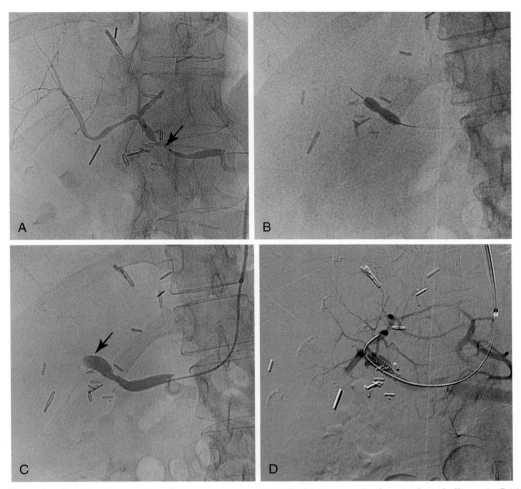

FIGURE 3-23 Transplant hepatic artery rupture from excess pressure applied to an oversized angioplasty balloon. **A,** Critical stenosis of liver transplant arterial stenosis *(arrow)* on celiac arteriogram. **B,** First balloon treatment failed to break the stenosis. A second balloon that was 2 mm larger than the calculated vessel diameter was inflated above the recommended pressure. The balloon ruptured. **C,** Arteriography shows contained rupture beyond the anastomosis *(arrow).* **D,** After successful passage of a guidewire, treatment with intravenous heparin and intraarterial nitroglycerin, stent placement reestablished flow in the artery.

- *Antithrombin:* Heparin (or a direct thrombin inhibitor) is administered immediately before crossing the obstruction, continued for the duration of the procedure, and, in some cases, continued afterward to prevent thrombosis (e.g., with small vessels, poor runoff, or slow flow). Heparin is not always necessary in large, high-flow veins.
- *Antispasm:* Vasodilators are used to prevent or relieve angioplasty-induced vasospasm, which is especially problematic in the renal, mesenteric, infrapopliteal, and upper extremity arteries (see Fig. 12-37).

Initial placement of a preshaped guiding sheath or catheter up to the target vessel can simplify post-PTA angiograms and allow a guidewire to remain across the treatment site. With an angiographic catheter or the balloon catheter itself near the stenosis, the lesion is crossed with a guidewire (Fig. 3-24). Stenoses in veins and large arteries can be crossed safely with a variety of guidewires. Microwires or steerable, tapered wires with very floppy tips may be needed to traverse critical lesions in small vessels or those more prone to dissection. Roadmapping often is helpful. Forceful guidewire manipulation during any arterial intervention can quickly result in a dissection or occlusion (Fig. 3-25).

Over the guidewire, the balloon is advanced across the stenosis. A stiff guidewire with a soft flexible tip or a lower-profile device may be tried if the catheter will not pass easily. With the balloon centered over the obstruction, it is inflated with dilute contrast material using an inflation device to control the balloon pressure. Manual inflation with a 10 cc polycarbonate syringe interposed with a flow switch is a cheaper alternative in lower-risk situations. Smaller syringes generate higher pressures within a somewhat predictable range.[121] A guidewire must exit the endhole for at least several centimeters to

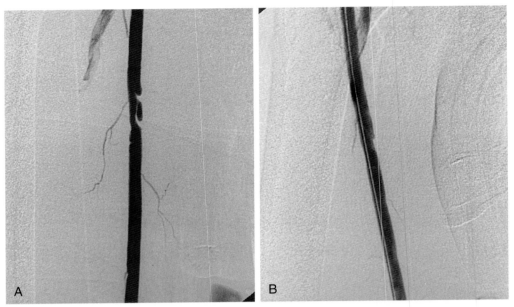

FIGURE 3-24   Balloon angioplasty of eccentric right superficial femoral artery stenosis **(A)** produces a widely patent vessel **(B).**

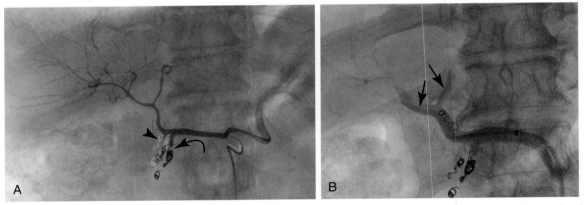

FIGURE 3-25   Hepatic artery dissection from guidewire manipulation. **A,** Celiac arteriogram after embolization of the gastroduodenal artery *(curved arrow)* and retroduodenal artery *(arrowhead)* in preparation for radiotherapy for hepatocellular carcinoma. Coils were placed in the presumed right gastric artery. The coils migrated to the proper hepatic artery (PHA). **B,** Attempts to snare and remove them caused formation of an occlusive dissection of the PHA that extended into the right and left hepatic arteries *(arrows).*

prevent the rigid catheter tip from injuring the vessel as the balloon expands. The "waist" produced by an atherosclerotic stenosis yields suddenly as the plaque cracks. Venous stenoses sometimes open more gradually. Optimal inflation parameters (number, duration, and pressure) are not firmly established outside the coronary circulation. Venous stenoses sometimes require two to three inflations of 30 to 120 seconds to achieve a good result.

Patients may express mild discomfort during balloon inflation. If the patient complains of severe pain, the balloon should be immediately deflated unless the operator is confident that the balloon is not significantly oversized.

If pain persists after deflation, vessel rupture must be excluded with angiography while maintaining guidewire access. If the vessel has ruptured, the balloon is immediately reinflated across the site for 5 to 10 minutes to prevent bleeding. By itself, this maneuver may seal the tear. If not, a stent (uncovered or covered depending on the vessel) can be inserted[122] (see Fig. 19-13). Urgent operative repair is hardly ever necessary.

It is standard teaching that a guidewire remain across the lesion while the deflated balloon is withdrawn and postangioplasty angiography is done. However, many interventionalists "abandon" stenoses in large arteries and veins. If a sheath or guiding catheter is being used, contrast injections are made around a standard 0.035-inch guidewire. A technically successful result is typically defined as a residual luminal diameter stenosis of less than 30%. Sometimes it is imperative to obtain a pressure gradient across the angioplasty site. The optimal goal is an arterial systolic gradient less than 5 to 10 mm Hg or mean venous gradient less than 3 to 5 mm Hg. An inadequate PTA result may occur for several reasons:

- *Large dissection.* Minor dissection is an expected result of balloon angioplasty. However, large, flow-limiting dissections can threaten the outcome of the procedure. If repeated prolonged balloon inflation fails to tack down the flap, stent placement should be considered.
- *Elastic recoil.* Some stenoses (particularly in veins) may fully dilate with balloon inflation but return to their stenotic caliber after deflation. Treatment with a slightly larger balloon (or even a cutting balloon) may be effective. In some cases, however, stent placement is required to maintain patency.
- *Resistant stenoses.* Some lesions will not yield even with multiple, prolonged, high-pressure inflations (>24 atm). In this case, use of a slightly larger balloon or a cutting balloon should be considered.

If the results of PTA are suboptimal or the risk of rethrombosis is significant (e.g., transplant artery stenosis), heparin infusion is often continued at least overnight.

Results and Complications

The efficacy of PTA depends on many factors. In general, the best results are obtained with short, solitary, concentric, noncalcified stenoses with good downstream outflow. For arterial stenoses, the procedure is technically successful in greater than 90% of patients.[123-126] Long-term results vary widely for different vascular beds (see later chapters). The overall complication rate is about 10% (Box 3-3). Major complications that require specific therapy occur in about 2% to 3% of cases.

Vessel occlusion (1% to 7% of procedures) can result from acute thrombosis, dissection, or vasospasm. An IV bolus of heparin and an intraarterial vasodilator should be given immediately. Repeat angioplasty or stent placement is performed to tack down a dissection. Local infusion of a fibrinolytic agent dissolves most acute thrombi.

Distal embolization occurs after 2% to 5% of arterial angioplasty procedures. Emboli are typically composed of fresh lysable thrombus, old organized clot, or unlysable atherosclerotic plaque. Treatment options include anticoagulation alone (for insignificant emboli), local thrombolytic infusion, mechanical thrombectomy, percutaneous aspiration, or surgical embolectomy.

BOX 3-3

COMPLICATIONS OF VASCULAR BALLOON ANGIOPLASTY

- Access site complications (see Table 3-1)
- Thrombosis
- Vessel rupture
- Distal embolization
- Flow-limiting dissection
- Pseudoaneurysm
- Guidewire perforation
- Acute kidney injury

Atherectomy Devices

Unlike balloon angioplasty catheters, atherectomy devices actually remove excess tissue from the walls of stenotic arteries or veins. Their early popularity in the 1990s waned because long-term results were no better and in some cases worse than with PTA or stent placement.[127,128] Significantly higher complication rates with certain atherectomy devices have been reported in some series. Despite these discouraging results, several atherectomy catheters are still on the market and others are in development, largely to handle failures of angioplasty.[129-131]

Bare and Covered Metallic Stents

Mechanism of Action

Stents maintain luminal patency by providing a rigid lattice that compresses atherosclerotic disease, neointimal hyperplasia, or dissection flaps and limits or prevents remodeling and elastic recoil. In addition, alterations in wall shear stress imposed by the stent may retard the process of neointimal hyperplasia (see Chapter 1). Thinning of the media is a consistent feature of stented arteries.[132]

Immediately after vascular stent insertion, fibrin coats the luminal surface. Intraprocedural anticoagulation or rapid blood flow prevents immediate thrombosis of the device. Over several weeks, this thin layer of clot is replaced by fibromuscular tissue. Eventual reendothelialization of the stented vessel largely protects it from late thrombosis.

Patient and Stent Selection

Stents are used in a host of vascular and nonvascular disorders (Box 3-4). The product variety is wide, and new stents come on the market every year (Box 3-5).

BOX 3-4

INDICATIONS FOR STENT PLACEMENT

- Primary treatment of coronary, renal, mesenteric, and transplant arterial obstructions
- Primary treatment or secondary salvage of peripheral arterial obstructions
- Endovascular repair of thoracic and abdominal aortic diseases
- Central venous obstructions not responsive to percutaneous transluminal balloon angioplasty alone
- Hemodialysis access related obstructions
- Immediate or long-term failures of balloon angioplasty (arterial and venous)
- Complications of angioplasty or catheterization procedures (e.g., dissection)
- Malignant biliary strictures
- Creation of endovascular portosystemic shunts

BOX 3-6

ADVANTAGES OF STENT DESIGNS

Uncovered Balloon Expandable

- Greater radial force and hoop strength
- More precise placement

Uncovered Self-Expanding

- Minimal plastic deformation from external forces
- More flexible and trackable
- Conform to changing vessel diameters

Covered

- Vessel sealing (ruptures, aneurysms, arteriovenous fistulas)
- Prevent in-stent restenosis

BOX 3-5

PROPERTIES OF STENTS

- Longitudinal flexibility
- Elastic deformation (tendency to return to nominal diameter)
- Plastic deformation (tendency to maintain diameter imposed by external forces)
- Radial and hoop strength
- Composition
- Metallic surface area
- Radiopacity
- Shortening with deployment
- MR imaging compatibility

TABLE 3-4   Stent Selection

Balloon Expandable	Self-Expanding
Uncovered Stent	
Precise arterial placement (e.g., renal, mesenteric, proximal iliac arteries)	Long-segment arterial disease (e.g., iliac artery)
	At sites of motion (e.g., CFA, popliteal artery)
Arterial dissection flap	Site of extrinsic compression (e.g., left iliac vein)
	Biliary obstructions
Covered Stent	
Arterial rupture (e.g., postangioplasty)	Long-segment arterial disease (e.g., femoropopliteal artery)
Pseudoaneurysm and AVF exclusion	Hemodialysis access–related obstruction
	Portosystemic shunts (TIPS)
	Biliary obstructions
	Intestinal obstructions

AVF, *arteriovenous fistula;* CFA, *common femoral artery;* TIPS, *transjugular intrahepatic portosystemic shunt.*

Stents may have U.S. Food and Drug Administration approval or European CE mark for use in particular vascular beds. If a physician chooses to use a device "off-label," the patient should consent to this decision. Stent selection is based on a variety of factors (Box 3-6); a very simplified algorithm is outlined in Table 3-4.

Self-expanding stents are compressed onto a catheter and deployed by uncovering a constraining sheath or membrane (Figs. 3-26 and 3-27). Most are composed of nitinol (a nickel/titanium alloy) or the metallic alloy Elgiloy. The final diameter of the stent is a function of the outward elastic load of the stent and the inward forces of elastic wall recoil or extrinsic compression. For vascular use, nominal diameters are 4 to 24 mm for placement through 5- to 12-Fr sheaths. Stents are oversized by 1 to 2 mm (and even more in large veins) to ensure firm vessel apposition and prevent migration. When the path to the lesion is tortuous or steeply angled (e.g., over the aortic bifurcation), these stents

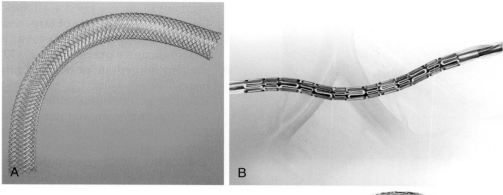

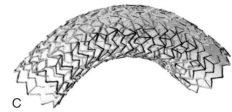

FIGURE 3-26   Bare metal stent designs. **A,** Wallstent. **B,** Compressed balloon expandable Express stent. **C,** Expanded Express stent. *(Images provided courtesy of Boston Scientific. © 2010 Boston Scientific Corporation or its affiliates. All rights reserved.)*

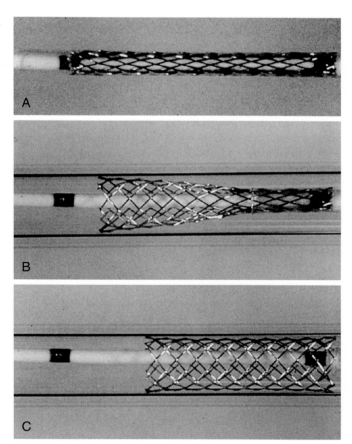

FIGURE 3-27   Deployment of Wallstent. **A,** The constraining membrane covers the compressed stent. **B,** The membrane is partially withdrawn. If necessary, the stent can be pulled back in the vessel, or the stent can be recovered by the constraining membrane. **C,** The stent is completely deployed. *(Courtesy of Schneider USA Inc., Minneapolis, Minn.)*

may be easier to use than some balloon-expandable ones. Finally, they are suitable for target vessel segments that change diameter (e.g., common to external iliac artery) because they are more likely to appose the entire arterial wall.

Balloon-expandable stents are premounted on angioplasty balloons in a compressed state and then deployed by balloon inflation (see Fig. 3-26). They have somewhat greater hoop strength than self-expanding designs and thus initially retain the diameter of the balloon. Placement is somewhat more precise than with even new self-expanding models, and longitudinal shortening is essentially zero. They have almost no elastic deformity but considerable plastic deformity.[133] Therefore balloon-expandable stents should generally not be used at sites that are subject to external compression (e.g., superficial arm veins, subclavian vein at the costoclavicular ligament, adductor canal in the leg, around joints).[134] For vascular use, stent diameters range from 4 to 12 mm placed through 5- to 10-Fr introducers. Early versions of balloon- and self-expandable nitinol stents had some problems with late stent fracture.[135]

Covered stents are metallic devices lined on the luminal and/or abluminal surface with a thin layer of synthetic graft material (Fig. 3-28). The metal lattice is made of nitinol or Elgiloy. The most popular fabric is expanded polytetrafluoroethylene (ePTFE). The presence of this relatively impermeable material seals the lumen and prevents neointimal proliferation in the stented segment.[136-138]

Drug-eluting stents are designed to prevent restenosis after recanalization.[139-141] Compounds that inhibit

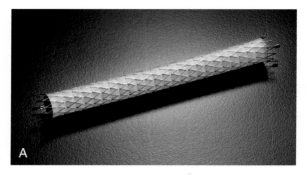

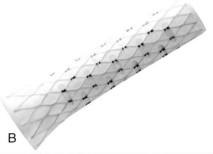

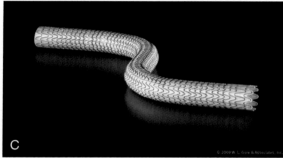

FIGURE 3-28   Covered stents. **A,** Fluency stent graft. **B,** Flair stent graft. **C,** Viabahn stent graft. *(Images courtesy of Bard Peripheral Vascular and W.L. Gore and Associates.)*

smooth muscle cell proliferation are introduced into a polymer that is bonded to the stent and slowly released into the arterial wall. Despite the theoretical benefits of these devices, there is no substantial evidence to date that they are more effective in peripheral arteries than uncovered stents.

Common Technical Points (Online Video 3-12)

Anticoagulants and antiplatelet agents are often given during vascular stent placement. Postprocedure anticoagulation is used selectively.

The following general principles apply to vascular stent placement:

- Select a guiding catheter or sheath that will accommodate the largest stent device anticipated.
- Choose a stent slightly larger in diameter than the normal vessel and longer than the diseased

segment to ensure good wall apposition (see Fig. 17-23). In the case of large veins (e.g., brachiocephalic veins or vena cava), stents should be significantly oversized (e.g., 30% to 50%) to prevent immediate or delayed migration to the heart.

- If precise placement is critical (e.g., renal artery stents), perform angiograms in several projections through the guiding catheter to confirm the location just before deployment.
- Some self-expanding stent designs tend to move during release. Follow the manufacturer's recommendations closely and perform this step with great care.
- Avoid covering vascular branches (unless intentional) or extending a stent into a branch that is clearly too small for the balloon inflating the stent.
- Use one or more stents to cover the entire obstruction. Residual disease at the mouth of a stent can promote acute thrombosis or restenosis.
- Be certain tandem stents are well overlapped. Gaps that develop between stents predispose to restenosis.
- If it becomes necessary to recross a freshly placed stent, be certain the guidewire does not pass through the interstices of the stent before entering the central lumen. A J-tipped guidewire is helpful for this purpose.

Enzymatic Thrombolysis

Patient Selection

Thrombolysis refers to any procedure that removes clot from a blood vessel including enzymatic fibrinolysis, mechanical thrombectomy, and thromboaspiration. Thrombolysis is primarily indicated for treatment of acute occlusion of hemodialysis grafts, iliac and infrainguinal arteries, bypass grafts, central venous catheters, upper extremity arteries, central upper or lower veins unresponsive to anticoagulation, and central pulmonary arteries. Thrombolysis is an acceptable therapy when the anticipated technical and long-term outcome is comparable to surgical treatment, revascularization can be accomplished quickly enough to avoid irreversible ischemia, and the risks of the procedure are reasonable. Contraindications to enzymatic fibrinolysis are outlined in Box 3-7.

Thrombolytic Agents

Enzymatic thrombolysis is accomplished with one of several fibrinolytic agents.[142,143] The key enzyme in clot dissolution is *plasmin*, a nonspecific serine protease that cleaves fibrin and circulating fibrinogen into a variety of fibrin degradation products. Plasmin is inhibited by several circulating antiplasmins. The precursor of plasmin is plasminogen, which is converted by naturally occurring or exogenous *plasminogen activators (PAs)*. These agents are the basis for thrombolytic therapy.[144,145] The various drugs are characterized by differences in half-life, *fibrin affinity* (ability to bind fibrin), and *fibrin specificity* (preferential activation of fibrin [clot]-bound plasminogen). Plasminogen activators are inactivated by inhibitors such as PAI-1.

Streptokinase (SK) is a naturally occurring polypeptide derived from group C streptococci. A streptokinase-plasminogen complex converts a second molecule of plasminogen to plasmin. The biologic half-life of streptokinase is about 23 minutes.[146] Antibodies present from prior streptococcal infection or streptokinase treatment may preclude use of the drug. For this reason, among others, SK is rarely used in clinical practice.

Recombinant tissue–type plasminogen activator (t-PA, alteplase, Activase) is a naturally occurring serine protease produced by endothelial cells. The drug is manufactured by recombinant DNA techniques. Its biologic half-life is about 4 to 6 minutes. t-PA is a weak plasminogen activator in the absence of fibrin. Its activity is enhanced about 1000-fold in the presence of fibrin. However, fibrin specificity is dose-dependent. Currently, t-PA is the principal fibrinolytic agent for noncoronary interventions.

Reteplase (r-PA, Retavase) is a recombinant mutant form of t-PA in which the finger domain of the molecule is removed (decreasing fibrin affinity and possibly enhancing diffusion into thrombus) along with epidermal growth factor and kringle 1 domains (increasing half-life to about 13 to 16 minutes). Unlike t-PA, reteplase has not been the subject of multiple large clinical trials to establish its relative efficacy and safety in noncoronary

vessels.[95] *Tenecteplase (TNK)* is a relatively new variant of t-PA formed by removal of the T, N, and K domains. The agent has markedly enhanced fibrin specificity and increased resistance to PAI-1. Its half-life is about 20 to 24 minutes.

Alfimeprase is a direct plasminogen activator that is being touted as a valuable alternative to the existing indirect PAs.[147,148] At this time, it remains an investigational drug.

Following current dosing regimens, the safety and efficacy of these agents is similar. No one drug has been proven superior to the others. With regard to limiting systemic effects and associated bleeding complications, the theoretical advantages of these fibrinolytics have not entirely borne out in clinical practice.

Technique

Systemic administration is only used for acute coronary thrombosis, acute ischemic stroke, and pulmonary embolism. *Catheter-directed thrombolysis* is done by one of the following methods[149-152]:

- Intraarterial infusion
- Stepwise infusion (gradual advancement of end-hole catheter into lysing clot)
- Graded infusion (start with high dose, continue with lower dose)
- Continuous intrathrombic infusion
- Clot "lacing" with a bolus dose followed by continuous intrathrombic infusion

The concept of high-dose intrathrombic infusion thrombolysis is based on the technique described by McNamara and Fischer.[150] Pulse-spray pharmacomechanical thrombolysis (PSPMT) is a method for accelerated clot dissolution developed by Bookstein and colleagues in which concentrated fibrinolytic agent is injected directly into clot as a high-pressure spray through a catheter with many side holes[151,153] (Fig. 3-29). Direct intrathrombic infusion seems to shorten the time for lysis and may limit systemic effects of the drug.

Oral antiplatelet agents are administered before and after thrombolysis to help prevent acute rethrombosis. Heparin (or bivalirudin) is given during and occasionally after the procedure to limit pericatheter thrombus, acute thrombosis, or post-PTA occlusion. With t-PA and its derivatives, the standard heparin dose is a 5000-unit IV bolus followed by infusion at about 500 units/hr. However, some practitioners prefer to administer only low-dose heparin (50 to 100 units/hr) through the indwelling access sheath. A standard dose of bivalirudin for peripheral interventions is 0.75 mg/kg IV bolus followed by 1.75 mg/kg/hr infusion. The safety of long-duration infusions is unknown.

Following diagnostic arteriography, the occlusion is engaged with a guidewire from an antegrade or retro-

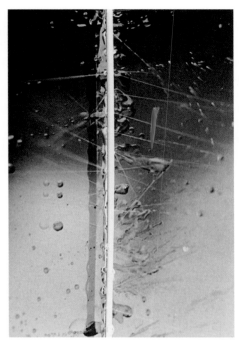

FIGURE 3-29   Pulse-spray thrombolysis catheter with high-pressure fluid spray.

grade approach (Fig. 3-30). Hydrophilic wires are especially useful for this purpose. If the occlusion cannot be crossed ("guidewire traversal test"), thrombolysis is much less likely to be successful.[154] However, a short trial of fibrinolytic agent infusion to "soften" the clot may be warranted. The drug is delivered through a multiside hole catheter with tip-occluding wire (e.g., Unifuse catheter) or through a coaxial infusion microcatheter (microMewi system) residing within the diagnostic catheter (Online Video 3-13). Ideally, the entire thrombus is bathed in the thrombolytic solution. Table 3-5 provides rough dosing guidelines for peripheral arteries and veins.[143-145,155]

The patient is monitored for bleeding complications and reperfusion in an intensive care or intermediate care unit. The heparin drip is then adjusted by monitoring the PTT every 4 to 6 hours during infusion to maintain at 60 to 80 seconds. Fibrinogen levels can be checked periodically; the risk of hemorrhage may increase when the serum level falls below 100 to 150 mg/dL, in which case the infusion usually is stopped or slowed.[156,157] Angiograms are repeated at 4- to 12-hour intervals to assess the degree of lysis and to adjust doses and catheter position. When lysis is complete or near complete (>90% to 95%), underlying disease is treated with angioplasty, stents, or both. Arterial thrombolysis usually is accomplished in less than 24 hours. Venous lysis may require much more time.

If clot dissolution is unusually sluggish or rethrombosis occurs, several possibilities should be considered. Inadequate anticoagulation is corrected by increasing the heparin dose or substituting a direct thrombin inhibitor. In small vessels, vasospasm may be present and is aggressively treated with vasodilators. Consideration should be given to loading the patient with clopidogrel or starting an IV $\alpha_{IIB}\beta3$ integrin inhibitor infusion to inactivate platelets.

After thrombolysis, residual disease often is found in the vessel wall (atherosclerotic plaque, intimal hyperplasia) or the lumen (organized clot, fibrin- and platelet-rich clot, embolus composed of one or more of these elements). Mural plaque or intimal hyperplasia is treated with angioplasty and sometimes stent placement. Percutaneous aspiration, mechanical thrombectomy, or operative removal may be required for residual luminal disease resistant to thrombolytics (see later). Angioplasty of such material can cause fragmentation and embolization. At the end of the procedure, a completion angiogram is obtained to document vessel patency and search for occult downstream emboli, which should be treated by local fibrinolytic infusion through a microcatheter.

Results and Complications

Immediate and long-term results of enzymatic thrombolysis are discussed in later chapters.[142-145,158-161] Hemorrhage may occur at the access site, regions of altered vascular integrity (e.g., recent vascular punctures, fresh graft anastomoses), or remote sites (e.g., retroperitoneum, brain, gastrointestinal tract). Bleeding can happen for several reasons. Circulating plasminogen activator will deplete plasminogen activator inhibitors and generate unbound plasmin. As antiplasmins are exhausted, a systemic "lytic state" results. t-PA and its derivatives are less likely to degrade unbound fibrinogen than older fibrinolytic agents. But because they are fibrin-specific, they may preferentially dissolve hemostatic plugs at remote sites of minor trauma and cause major bleeding (e.g., intracranial hemorrhage).

Total thrombolytic dose and overall infusion time have some bearing on bleeding risk, but the relationship is hardly linear. In some studies, significant fibrinogen depletion is strongly associated with increased risk for major hemorrhage, but in other studies it is not.[145,156,157] In many cases, bleeding is the result of excessive anticoagulation, not the fibrinolytic agent itself.

Distal embolization is detected in about 10% of peripheral arterial revascularization procedures and does not seem to a function of the thrombolytic method. An attempt should be made to lyse distal clot by advancing a small-caliber infusion microcatheter directly to the embolus. Unlysable clot may be left in place or removed

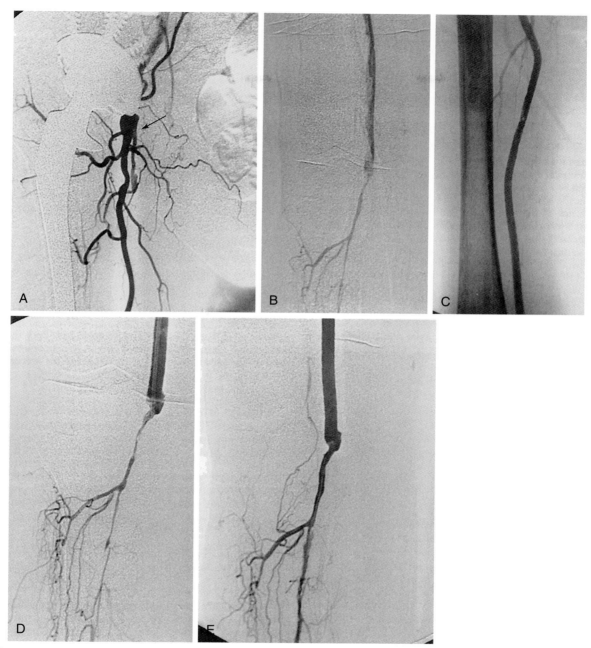

FIGURE 3-30 Combined pulse-spray and infusion thrombolysis of an occluded femoropopliteal bypass graft. **A,** The graft is occluded at its origin *(arrow).* **B,** After pulse-spray thrombolysis with bolus dose of fibrolytic agent, significant clot lysis has occurred. **C,** After overnight infusion of the drug, the body of the graft is almost entirely free of clot. **D,** A long stenosis in the distal popliteal artery and tibioperoneal trunk is revealed. **E,** After balloon angioplasty, the graft outflow is significantly improved.

TABLE 3-5 Fibrinolytic Agent Dosing Regimens

Agent	Infusion Dose	Maximum Bolus	Maximum Dose
t-PA	0.5-1.0 mg/hr 0.001-0.02 mg/kg/hr	10 mg	40 mg
Reteplase	0.25-1.0 U/hr	2-5 U	20 U

surgically, depending on the nature of the occlusion and the condition of the patient.

Complications directly related to revascularization of the extremities include *reperfusion syndrome* and *compartment syndrome.* Revascularization of a nonsalvageable necrotic limb can release lactic acid, myoglobin, and other substances that may lead to acute kidney injury and cardiovascular instability. Bleeding into a treated (or even untreated) limb may significantly elevate muscular compartment pressures and require fasciotomy (Table 3-6).

Mechanical Thrombectomy

Percutaneous thrombectomy devices are emerging as an attractive alternative or adjunct to enzymatic thrombolysis or aspiration thrombectomy.[162-165] Existing thrombectomy catheters can be classified by their mechanism of action as (1) clot maceration and aspiration or (2) clot pulverization into microparticles. However, none of the available models has entirely lived up to expectations to replace enzymatic thrombolysis by improving technical efficacy of clot removal and lowering the risk for adverse events. Adjunctive enzymatic lysis often is needed to complete thrombus removal. Bleeding complications are not completely eliminated (up to 10% to 15% in some series). The rate of distal embolization ranges from 5% to 15%. Vessel perforation or dissection is reported in 5% to

12% of cases. Finally, device failure is an occasional problem with some catheters. However, these catheters play a critical role in patients at undue risk for bleeding from fibrinolytic agents who are otherwise appropriate candidates for endovascular thrombectomy.

There are a variety of devices available around the world. Three of the more popular catheters are considered as follows:

- The *Arrow-Trerotola percutaneous thrombectomy device (PTD)* is composed of a nitinol basket that acts like an egg-beater on relatively fresh thrombus (Fig. 3-31). The device is placed over a guidewire into the thrombus. The activated device spins at 3000 rpm. The macerated clot is then aspirated through the sideport of a sheath. The PTD is primarily used in treatment of thrombosed hemodialysis access and iliofemoral deep vein thrombosis.[166-168] It may also have applications in other vascular territories (e.g., mesenteric veins, pulmonary artery).
- The *AngioJet thrombectomy catheter* is a flexible device that is inserted directly into the thrombus (Fig. 3-32). Based on the Bernouilli principle, high-speed saline jets exit the end of the catheter, producing a low pressure space that sucks clot into the catheter for maceration. The clot fragments are propelled back through the catheter and evacuated from the body. The principal indications for use are iliofemoral deep vein thrombosis and dialysis access thrombosis.[169] However, it is widely used in other vascular beds.[170] It has two main drawbacks: the occasional occurrence of bradyarrythmias

TABLE 3-6   Complications of Enzymatic Thrombolysis

Complication	Frequency (%)
Minor puncture site bleeding	5-25
Major bleeding requiring transfusion or surgery	3-7
Distal embolization	2-15
Pericatheter thrombosis	—
Reperfusion syndrome	—
Compartment syndrome	—
Drug reactions	—
Vessel or graft extravasation	—

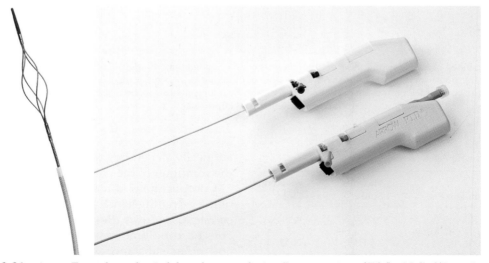

FIGURE 3-31   Arrow-Trerotola mechanical thrombectomy device. *(Images courtesy of Teleflex Medical/Arrow International.)*

FIGURE 3-32 AngioJet thrombectomy device. **A,** Drawing shows high pressure saline jets *(arrows)* that are propelled backwards within the catheter lumen, creating a pressure drop that draws clot into the catheter. **B,** Drawing illustrates mechanism of clot pulverization. *(Images courtesy of MEDRAD International.)*

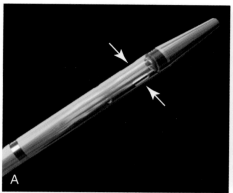
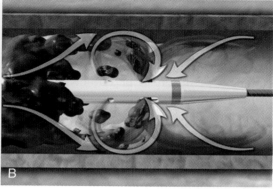

(which are sometimes life-threatening) or hyperkalemia and renal failure related to profound intravascular hemolysis.[171,172]

- The *Trellis peripheral infusion system* is comprised of a delivery catheter with a 10 or 20 cm length of multiple side holes surrounded by two balloons that isolate the occluded treatment segment (Fig. 3-33). An oscillating dispersion wire between the balloons admixes clot and fibrinolytic agent. The highly macerated clot is then aspirated out of the vessel. In theory, this arrangement prevents distal embolization and escape of thrombolytic agent into the systemic circulation. Again, it is used primarily (but not solely) in treatment of acute iliofemoral deep vein thrombosis.[173-175]

Embolotherapy (Online Videos 3-14 through 3-18)

Patient Selection

Transcatheter embolization is done for the following reasons[176]:

- To stop or prevent bleeding
- To destroy tissue (e.g., neoplasms)
- To occlude vascular abnormalities (e.g., aneurysms, AVMs, varicoceles)
- To redistribute blood flow (e.g., portal vein embolization to induce contralateral liver lobe hypertrophy)
- To treat endoleak after stent graft placement

FIGURE 3-33 Trellis-8 peripheral infusion system. **A,** Access to a popliteal vein for iliofemoral deep vein thrombolysis. **B,** The Trellis catheter has been advanced into the thrombus over a guidewire, and the upper balloon inflated. **C,** With both balloons inflated and the occlusion isolated, fibrinolytic agent is infused through the side holes of the sinusoidal wire. **D,** The device is activated, spinning the infusion wire to macerate clot and admix the lytic agent. *(© Covidien. Used with permission.)*

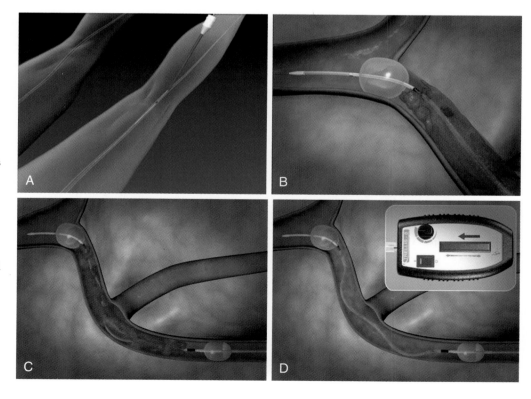

For the treatment of hemorrhage, the goal of embolotherapy is to reduce flow to the bleeding site and allow endogenous clotting but still maintain collateral perfusion to neighboring tissue (Fig. 3-34). For tissue obliteration or vascular malformation occlusion, the goal is to completely eliminate perfusion to or outflow from the target site (including potential collaterals) while preserving nearby tissue (see Fig. 10-34). Embolization has several advantages over surgery.[176,177] Vital structures are not damaged en route to the bleeding site or organ, tissue loss is minimized by limiting occlusion to target vessels, and the risks associated with an operation are avoided. With currently available materials, superselective embolization is possible almost anywhere in the body.

The decision to perform embolotherapy is based on several factors, including the risks of embolization, the feasibility and efficacy of alternative procedures, and the experience of the operator. Beforehand, a thorough angiographic evaluation is needed to define the bleeding site or abnormality, the path to the target, and the state of existing and potential collateral vessels.

Materials and Technique

A vascular sheath is placed to maintain access in case the delivery catheter becomes occluded with embolic material. Delivery catheters must not have side holes through which embolic material can escape. In some cases, the diagnostic catheter can be advanced without difficulty. Otherwise, a coaxial microcatheter is inserted and directed to the target site using a steerable guidewire. Coils may get stuck in the lumen of some high-flow microcatheters, so an appropriate device must be chosen. The outer catheter should be secured in a stable position. In some cases (e.g., pulmonary AVM occlusion), a larger guiding catheter or sheath is advanced close to the proposed site of device placement.

In vascular systems with extensive collateral circulation (e.g., mesenteric and peripheral arteries), the operator must be cognizant of potential routes of blood flow. In this situation, it may be imperative to "close the back door" to prevent rebleeding (see Figs. 8-54 and 11-32).

A wide assortment of embolic agents are available for vascular occlusion (Table 3-7).

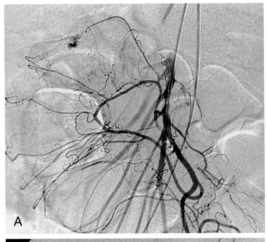
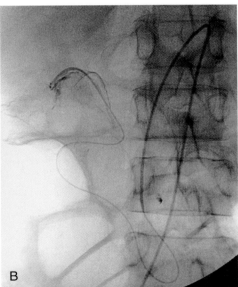
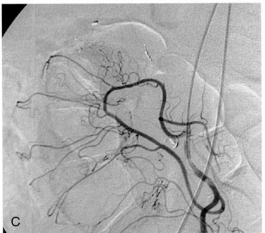

FIGURE 3-34 Embolization of a bleeding site in the hepatic flexure of the colon. **A,** Extravasation from a vasa recta arising from the middle colic branch of the superior mesenteric artery. **B,** A 3-Fr microcatheter was placed through the long RUC catheter directly into the branch feeding the bleeding site. **C,** After placement of two microcoils, extravasation has stopped. Perfusion to adjacent bowel has been maintained.

TABLE 3-7   Commonly Used Embolic Agents

Material	Vascular Occlusion
PERMANENT	
Macrocoils	P
Microcoils	P
Amplatzer plug	P
Polyvinyl alcohol (PVA) particles	D
Microspheres	D
Alcohol	P, D
Sodium tetradecyl sulfate (SDS, 3%)	P, D
Glue	P, D
Onyx	P, D
"TEMPORARY"	
Gelfoam pieces	P
Occlusion balloon catheter	P
Thrombin	P

D, *distal;* P, *proximal.*

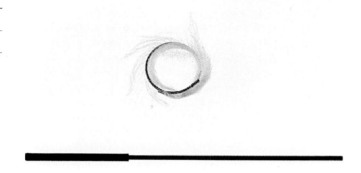

FIGURE 3-35   Macrocoil with loader.

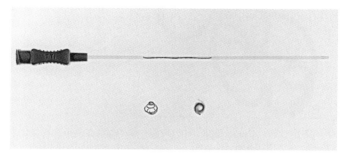

FIGURE 3-36   Microcoils with unwound coil in a plastic loader.

The selection of an agent for embolotherapy is based on the particular goals of treatment:

- *Temporary or permanent occlusion.* Permanent occlusion is generally required for progressive diseases (e.g., tumors, inflammatory processes). Temporary occlusion is appropriate for most self-limited pathology (e.g., traumatic lesions).
- *Proximal or distal embolization.* Embolization into or around small arteries or beyond venules is used to stop flow through a vessel when remaining collateral vessels will not compromise the result (e.g., pseudoaneurysms, traumatic extravasation). Distal embolization at the arteriolar or capillary level is needed to destroy tissue or stop flow through a vessel when new collateral vessels could lead to recurrence of the problem (e.g., tumors, bronchial artery bleeding, AVMs).

Coils are used for permanent vascular occlusion. (Online video 3-14) Macrocoils are made of guidewire material with polyester threads attached to promote thrombosis (Fig. 3-35). They are available in a variety of lengths, diameters (2 to 15 mm), and shapes for use with standard 5-Fr (0.035- or 0.038-inch) nonhydrophilic catheters. The unwound coil preloaded in a metal tube is pushed into the catheter and then deployed with a guidewire or a brisk fluid pulse. Before inserting the coil, it is prudent to test whether the catheter tip will back away when the guidewire is advanced alone or saline pulse is made.

Microcoils are made for passage through microcatheters. They come preloaded in a plastic or metal delivery loader (Fig. 3-36 and Online Video 3-15). Most are composed of platinum, and they are manufactured in a wide variety of shapes and sizes. Some microcoils are less thrombogenic than macrocoils and should generally be used with Gelfoam (see later discussion).

Coil selection is primarily based on the diameter and length of the vessel to be occluded. The nominal coil diameter should be slightly larger than the target vessel. If the coil is too small, it can migrate distally or proximally into a sidebranch, with sometimes disastrous results (e.g., through a pulmonary AVM into the brain; see Fig. 3-25). If the coil is too large, it may unravel proximally and obstruct nontarget branches (e.g., intracranial aneurysms) or even embolize to a distant site. Although more costly and complicated to use, *detachable coils* permit complete coil formation within the target vessel before release to ensure optimal sizing. Release from the deployment wire is achieved by mechanical (Interlock coils) or electrolytic (Guglielmi detachable coils [GDC]) means (Fig. 3-37). Once a large coil is secured in the vessel, additional coils of the same or smaller size are densely packed in front of it to make a "nest." Gelatin sponge sometimes is used along with coils to promote rapid thrombosis.

Amplatzer vascular plugs are relatively new devices that are extremely useful for occlusion of large and medium vessels (Fig. 3-38). There are several forms on the market. The occluder is preattached to a wire and passed through a guiding catheter or sheath. It conforms to the target vessel when exposed by withdrawing the

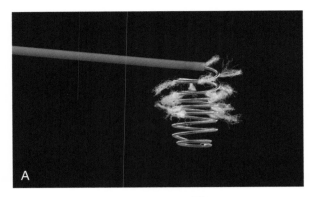

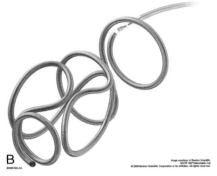

FIGURE 3-37   Detachable coils. *(Images provided courtesy of Boston Scientific. © 2010 Boston Scientific Corporation or its affiliates. All rights reserved.)*

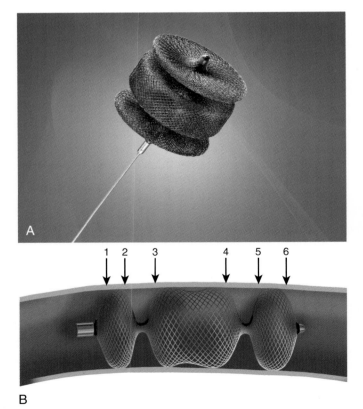

FIGURE 3-38   Amplatzer II vascular plug. **A,** Plug connected to delivery catheter. **B,** Expanded plug in place in vessel. *(© AGA Medical. Reprinted with permission.)*

sheath (see Fig. 7-15). If the plug is unstable, it may be removed. It is deployed by simple counterclockwise rotation of the delivery wire. Although Amplatzer plugs are extremely popular among interventionalists, their long-term behavior is not established.[178,179]

Gelfoam is water-insoluble surgical hemostatic sponge that expands on contact with fluids.[180] Gelfoam incites a foreign body reaction in blood vessels within 2 to 3 weeks of insertion. This process resolves over time, such that the material is not present several months afterward.[181] Depending on the embolic needs and catheter size, Gelfoam sheets are cut into individual small pledgets ("torpedoes") or scored into very small cubes (Fig. 3-39). Larger pieces are delivered individually with a tuberculin syringe in dilute contrast material. Smaller pieces may be suspended in contrast material and injected as a slurry in small increments until the blood column is static (Online Videos 3-16 and 3-17). Overzealous injection can cause reflux of material. Ischemic complications are rare but have been reported.[182,183] Gelfoam powder may be particular hazardous in this regard.

Polyvinyl alcohol (PVA) particles occlude small arteries and arterioles (50 to 2500 μm) (Fig. 3-40). PVA causes an inflammatory reaction in the vessel wall. These particles tend to aggregate within the vessel lumen and occasionally do not provide complete or permanent vascular occlusion. The agent, which expands on contact with fluid, is commercially available in narrow size ranges (e.g., from 100 to 300 μm, 900 to 1200 μm). In practice, most applications require 300 to 500 μm or 500 to 700 μm sizes. For delivery, one vial of particles is suspended in about 10 mL of dilute contrast material, mixed immediately before injection in a three-way stopcock system, and infused slowly under fluoroscopic guidance. After each aliquot is given, contrast is injected to assess flow. Dilute suspensions of small particles (<500 to 700 μm) pass easily through most microcatheters.

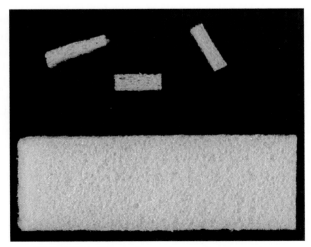

FIGURE 3-39   Gelfoam sheet and cut torpedoes.

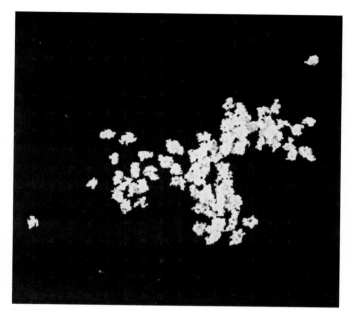

FIGURE 3-40   Polyvinyl alcohol particles (1000 to 1500 μm) in a dry state.

Tris-acryl gelatin microspheres (Embospheres) and *PVA microspheres (Contour SE Microspheres* and *Bead Block)* are spherical particles that cause relatively permanent occlusion.[184] Owing to their uniform size and inability to clump, they are easier to deliver through microcatheters than PVA (Fig. 3-41 and Online Video 3-18). In addition, there is more precise correlation between particle size and diameter of occluded vessels.[185] Unlike with PVA particles, a substantial fraction of this material migrates out of the vessel lumen over time. These agents have been used in a variety of vascular beds with good clinical results. However, there may be more risk of ischemia or infarction with microspheres than with PVA particles of comparable size because of more distal vascular occlusion or escape through arteriovenous shunts.[186,187] There is some evidence that Contour particles are especially compressible,

resulting in more distal (and somewhat less predictable level of) occlusion than comparably sized Embospheres. Thus the various microspheric agents are not interchangeable.[185]

Absolute ethanol is an extremely toxic liquid that causes permanent vascular occlusion forward from the point of contact. It is a particularly dangerous agent and should be handled with great care. Alcohol completely denatures proteins in the vessel wall, causing a painful inflammatory reaction that can extend into the perivascular spaces and injure adjacent tissues, vessels, and nerves. The alcohol volume is estimated by first injecting contrast until the desired level of vascular filling is achieved. In the arterial system, the liquid may be delivered through the lumen of an inflated occlusion balloon to prevent reflux (Fig. 3-42). Patients should be warned that moderate to intense pain may follow embolization. In many cases, general or epidural anesthesia is required for the procedure and aggressive analgesia used afterward.

Sodium tetradecyl sulfate 3% (*SDS, Sotradecol*) is a mild detergent that causes immediate and intense injury to vascular endothelium, followed quickly by separation of the intima and media along with thrombus formation.[188] In clinical practice, it is often delivered as a foam created by agitating the solution with air in a syringe system. SDS is an extremely versatile embolic agent used primarily in obliterating pathologic veins (e.g., venous malformations, male varicocele).[189] Complications are rare and usually self-limited.[190]

Ethylene vinyl alcohol copolymer (*Onyx*) is a nonadhesive liquid that is gaining popularity particularly in neurovascular and peripheral vascular interventions.[191] Catheters are prefilled with a small volume of dimethyl sulfoxide (DMSO) to prevent precipitation of the drug. The delivery system must be compatible with DMSO, which can dissolve many plastic catheters. Onyx, which is radiopaque, is then slowly injected to endpoint. Outside the brain, it has been used in treating AVMs and endoleaks after endovascular aneurysm repair.[192,193]

FIGURE 3-41   Magnified image of hydrated polyvinyl alcohol particles (**A**) and tris-acryl gelatin microspheres (**B**). (*From Andrews RT, Binkert CA. Relative rates of blood flow reduction during transcatheter arterial embolization with tris-acryl gelatin microspheres or polyvinyl alcohol: quantitative comparison in a swine model. J Vasc Interv Radiol 2003;14:1311. Reprinted with permission.*)

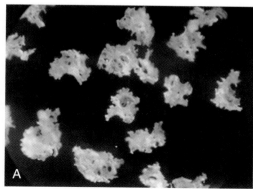

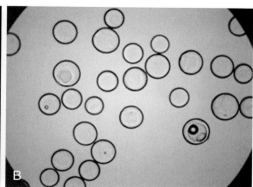

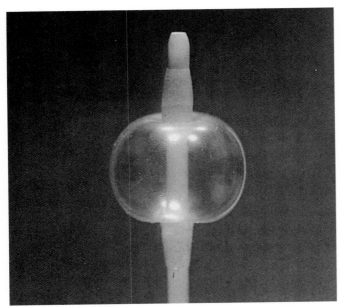

FIGURE 3-42   The balloon occlusion catheter can be used as a temporary occlusive device or to avoid reflux during delivery of certain embolic agents.

Cyanoacrylates (glues) are liquid adhesives and versatile embolic agents.[194] Glues cause acute inflammatory changes in treated vessels and provide effectively permanent occlusion. Their liquid nature allows them to penetrate directly into the nidus of AVMs. Several derivatives exist; in the United States, *n*-butyl cyanoacrylate (*n*-BCA, Trufill) is currently approved for use in cranial AVMs. The primary noncranial application is also for AVMs, but glues have been used in a variety of other settings, including aneurysms and pseudoaneurysms, aortobronchial fistulas, varicocele treatment, and gastrointestinal bleeding.[194-198]

Cyanoacrylates solidify on contact with ionic surfaces (e.g., blood). Therefore, the delivery system is purged with dextrose before and after injection; great care must be taken to avoid any contact with blood or saline before injection. The glue is admixed with Ethiodol to provide radiopacity and to control the time for polymerization (cyanoacrylate-to-oil ratio of 1:1 to 1:4 corresponding to solidification interval of about 1 to 4 seconds, respectively). The volume of agent (usually 0.1 to 0.5 mL) is estimated by several test injections of contrast through the microcatheter placed just proximal to the AVM nidus. The complexity of the technique (estimating injection volume and rate, preparation of the mixture, avoidance of contact with blood, saline, or polycarbonate syringes, proper purging of the entire system with dextrose, agent delivery and dextrose flush, and immediate withdrawal of the microcatheter to avoid gluing the tip to the vessel) demands considerable expertise and experience.

Ethanolamine oleate and *sodium morrhuate* are fatty acid–based sclerosing agents used primarily for endoscopic treatment of gastroesophageal varices and transcatheter embolization of gastric varices.[199] Sodium morrhuate also is indicated for sclerotherapy of varicose veins. They cause a mild inflammatory reaction that ultimately leads to vessel fibrosis and occlusion. Both agents have been used for transvenous treatment of intestinal varices in portal hypertension and for venous malformations.

Results and Complications

With available microcatheter systems, embolotherapy is technically successful in more than 90% of attempts.[176] Immediate and long-term results for specific applications are considered in later chapters.

The major risks of transcatheter embolization are ischemia of adjacent tissue and nontarget embolization. Ischemia can be minimized by careful placement of embolic material. Nontarget embolization is avoided by patience and meticulous technique during the procedure.

Postembolization syndrome is a frequent occurrence after embolization. The symptoms usually begin immediately or within 24 hours of embolization, and consist of fever, nausea and vomiting, and localized pain. Supportive care usually is sufficient, including antipyretics, antiemetics, and analgesia (sometimes requiring patient-controlled anesthesia). Patients should be carefully evaluated for infection or evidence of infarction.

References

1. Ruegg TA, Curran CR, Lamb T. Use of buffered lidocaine in bone marrow biopsies: a randomized, controlled trial. *Oncol Nurs Forum* 2009;**36**:52.
2. McEvoy GK, editor. Chloroprocaine Hydrochloride. AHFS Drug Information 98. Bethesda (MD): American Society of Health-System Pharmacists; 1998. p. 2661.
3. Seldinger SI. Catheter replacement of the needle in percutaneous arteriography. *Acta Radiol* 1953;**39**:368.
4. Irani F, Kumar S, Colyer Jr WR. Common femoral artery access techniques: a review. *J Cardiovasc Med* (Hagerstown) 2009;**10**:517.
5. Garrett PD, Eckart RE, Bauch TD, et al. Fluoroscopic localization of the femoral head as a landmark for common femoral artery cannulation. *Catheter Cardiovasc Interv* 2005;**65**:205.
6. Illescas FF, Baker ME, McCann R, et al. CT evaluation of retroperitoneal hemorrhage associated with femoral arteriography. *AJR Am J Roentgenol* 1986;**146**:1289.
7. Altin RS, Flicker S, Naidech HJ. Pseudoaneurysm and arteriovenous fistula after femoral artery catheterization: association with low femoral punctures. *AJR Am J Roentgenol* 1989;**152**:629.
8. Chan YC, Morales JP, Reidy JF, et al. Management of spontaneous and iatrogenic retroperitoneal haemorrhage: conservative management, endovascular intervention or open surgery? *Int J Clin Pract* 2008;**62**:1604.
9. Rupp SB, Vogelzang RL, Nemcek Jr AA, et al. Relationship of the inguinal ligament to pelvic radiographic landmarks: anatomic correlation and its role in femoral arteriography. *J Vasc Interv Radiol* 1993;**4**:409.

10. Nice C, Timmons G, Bartholemew P, et al. Retrograde vs. antegrade puncture for infra-inguinal angioplasty. *Cardiovasc Intervent Radiol* 2003;**26**:370.

11. Spijkerboer AM, Scholten FG, Mali WP, et al. Antegrade puncture of the femoral artery: morphologic study. *Radiology* 1990;**176**:57.

12. Sacks D, Summers TA. Antegrade selective catheterization of femoral vessels with a 4- or 5-F catheter and safety wire. *J Vasc Interv Radiol* 1991;**2**:325.

13. Saddekni S, Srur M, Cohn DJ, et al. Antegrade catheterization of the superficial femoral artery. *Radiology* 1985;**157**:531.

14. Bishop AF, Berkman WA, Palagallo GL. Antegrade selective catheterization of the superficial femoral artery using a moveable core guide wire. *Radiology* 1985;**157**:548.

15. Smith DC, Mitchell DA, Peterson GW, et al. Medial brachial fascial compartment syndrome: anatomic basis of neuropathy after transaxillary arteriography. *Radiology* 1989;**173**:149.

16. Lipchik EO, Sugimoto H. Percutaneous brachial artery catheterization. *Radiology* 1986;**160**:842.

17. Chitwood RW, Shepard AD, Shetty PC, et al. Surgical complications of transaxillary arteriography: a case-control study. *J Vasc Surg* 1996;**23**:844.

18. Chatziioannou A, Ladopoulos C, Mourikis D, et al. Complications of lower-extremity outpatient arteriography via low brachial artery. *Cardiovasc Intervent Radiol* 2004;**27**:31.

19. Evans C, Peter N, Gibson M, et al. Five-year retrograde transpopliteal angioplasty results compared with antegrade angioplasty. *Ann R Coll Surg Engl* 2010;**92**:347.

20. Gaines PA, Reidy JF. Percutaneous high brachial aortography: a safe alternative to the translumbar approach. *Clin Radiol* 1986;**37**:595.

21. Baum PA, Matsumoto AH, Teitelbaum GP, et al. Anatomic relationship between the common femoral artery and vein: CT evaluation and clinical significance. *Radiology* 1989;**173**:775.

22. Trerotola SO, Kuhn-Fulton J, Johnson MS, et al. Tunneled infusion catheters: increased incidence of symptomatic venous thrombosis after subclavian versus internal jugular venous access. *Radiology* 2000;**217**:89.

23. Hoffer EK, Bloch RD. Percutaneous arterial closure devices. *J Vasc Interv Radiol* 2003;**14**:865.

24. Balzer JO, Scheinert D, Diebold T, et al. Postinterventional transcutaneous suture of femoral artery access sites in patients with peripheral arterial occlusive disease: a study of 930 patients. *Catheter Cardiovasc Interv* 2001;**53**:174.

25. Das R, Ahmed K, Athanasiou T, et al. Arterial closure devices versus manual compression for femoral haemostasis in interventional radiological procedures: a systemic review and meta-analysis. *Cardiovasc Intervent Radiol* 2010 [Epub ahead of print].

26. Koreny M, Riedmuller E, Nikfardjam M, et al. Arterial puncture closing devices compared with standard manual compression after cardiac catheterization: systematic review and meta-analysis. *JAMA* 2004;**291**:350.

27. Hon LQ, Ganeshan A, Thomas SM, et al. An overview of vascular closure devices: what every radiologist should know. *Eur J Radiol* 2010;**73**:181.

28. Martin JL, Pratsos A, Magargee E, et al. A randomized trial comparing compression, Perclose Proglide and Angio-Seal VIP for arterial closure following percutaneous coronary intervention: the CAP trial. *Catheter Cardiovasc Interv* 2008;**71**:1.

29. Wong SC, Bachinsky W, Cambier P, et al. A randomized comparison of a novel bioabsorbable vascular closure device versus manual compression in the achievement of hemostasis after percutaneous femoral procedures: the ECLIPSE (Ensure's Vascular Closure Device Speeds Hemostasis) trial. *JACC Cardiovasc Interv* 2009;**2**:785.

30. Deuling JH, Wermeulen RP, Anthonio RA, et al. Closure of the femoral artery after cardiac catheterization: a comparison of Angio-Seal, StarClose and manual compression. *Catheter Cardiovasc Interv* 2008; **71**:518.

31. Jaff MR, Hadley G, Hermiller JB, et al. The safety and efficacy of the StarClose Vascular Closure System: the ultrasound substudy of the CLIP study. *Catheter Cardiovasc Interv* 2006;**68**:684.

32. Hermiller JB, Simonton C, Hinoshara T, et al. The StarClose Vascular Closure System: interventional results from the CLIP study. *Catheter Cardiovasc Interv* 2006;**68**:677.

33. Gray BH, Miller R, Langan III EM, et al. The utility of the StarClose arterial closure device in patients with peripheral arterial disease. *Ann Vasc Surg* 2009;**23**:341.

34. Biancari F, D'Andrea V, DiMarco C, et al. Meta-analysis of randomized trials on the efficacy of vascular closure devices after diagnostic angiography and angioplasty. *Am Heart J* 2010;**159**:518

35. Azmoon S, Pucillo AL, Aronow WS, et al. Vascular complications after percutaneous coronary intervention following hemostasis with the Mynx vascular closure device versus the AngioSeal vascular closure device. *J Invasive Cardiol* 2010;**22**:175.

36. Singh H, Cardella JF, Cole PE, et al. Quality improvement guidelines for diagnostic arteriography. *J Vasc Interv Radiol* 2003;**14** (9 (Pt. 2)):S283.

37. Egglin TK, O'Moore PV, Feinstein AR, et al. Complications of peripheral arteriography: a new system to identify patients at increased risk. *J Vasc Surg* 1995;**22**:787.

38. Darcy MD, Kanterman RY, Kleinhoffer MA, et al. Evaluation of coagulation tests as predictors of angiographic bleeding complications. *Radiology* 1996;**198**:741.

39. Katzenschlager R, Ugurluoglu A, Ahmadi A, et al. Incidence of pseudoaneurysm after diagnostic and therapeutic angiography. *Radiology* 1995;**195**:463.

40. Toursarkissian B, Allen BT, Petrinec D, et al. Spontaneous closure of selected iatrogenic pseudoaneurysms and arteriovenous fistulae. *J Vasc Surg* 1997;**25**:803.

41. Fukumoto Y, Tsutsui H, Tsuchihasi M, et al. The incidence and risk factors of cholesterol embolization syndrome, a complication of cardiac catheterization: a prospective study. *J Am Coll Cardiol* 2003;**42**:211.

42. Jarosz JM, McKeown B, Reidy JF. Short-term femoral nerve complications following percutaneous transfemoral procedures. *J Vasc Interv Radiol* 1995;**6**:351.

43. Alvarez-Tostado JA, Moise MA, Bena JF, et al. The brachial artery: a critical access for endovascular procedures. *J Vasc Surg* 2009; **49**:378.

44. Coley BD, Roberts AC, Fellmeth BD, et al. Postangiographic femoral artery pseudoaneurysms: further experience with US guided compression repair. *Radiology* 1995;**194**:307.

45. Tisi PV, Callam MJ. Treatment for femoral pseudoaneurysms. *Cochrane Database Syst Rev* 2009;CD004981.

46. Ahamad F, Turner SA, Torrie P, et al. Iatrogenic femoral artery pseudoaneurysms—a review of current methods of diagnosis and treatment. *Clin Radiol* 2008;**63**:1310.

47. Morgan R, Belli A-M. Current treatment methods for postcatheterization pseudoaneurysms. *J Vasc Interv Radiol* 2003;**14**:697.

48. Krueger K, Zaehringer M, Soehngen F-D, et al. Femoral pseudoaneurysms: management with percutaneous thrombin injections—success rates and effects on systemic coagulation. *Radiology* 2003; **226**:452.

49. Schneider C, Malisius R, Kuechler R, et al. A prospective study on ultrasound-guided percutaneous thrombin injection for treatment of iatrogenic post-catheterisation femoral pseudoaneurysms. *Int J Cardiol* 2009;**131**:356.

50. Krueger K, Zaehringer M, Strohe D, et al. Postcatheterization pseudoaneurysm: results of US-guided percutaneous thrombin injection in 240 patients. *Radiology* 2005;**236**:1104 .

51. Hofmann I, Wunderlich N, Robertson G, et al. Percutaneous injection of thrombin for the treatment of pseudoaneurysms: the German multicentre registry. *EuroIntervention* 2007;**3**:321.

52. Sheiman RG, Brophy DP, Perry LJ, et al. Thrombin injection for the repair of brachial artery pseudoaneurysms. *AJR Am J Roentgenol* 1999;**173**:1029.

53. Sadiq S, Ibrahim W. Thromboembolism complicating thrombin injection of femoral artery pseudoaneurysm: management with intraarterial thrombolysis. *J Vasc Interv Radiol* 2001;**12**:633.

54. D'Ayala M, Smith R, Zanieski G, et al. Acute arterial occlusion after ultrasound-guided thrombin injection of a common femoral artery pseudoaneurysm with a wide, short neck. *Ann Vasc Surg* 2008;**22**:473.

55. Ohlow MA, Secknus MA, von Korn H, et al. Percutaneous thrombin injection for treatment of iatrogenic femoral artery pseudoaneurysms: a case for caution. *Angiology* 2008;**59**:372.

56. Tsetis D. Endovascular treatment of complications of femoral arterial access. *Cardiovasc Intervent Radiol* 2010;**33**:457.

57. Onal B, Kosar S, Gumus T, et al. Postcatheterization femoral arteriovenous fistulas: endovascular treatment with stent-grafts. *Cardiovasc Intervent Radiol* 2004;**27**:453.

58. Thalhammer C, Kirchherr AS, Uhlich F, et al. Postcatheterization pseudoaneurysms and arteriovenous fistulas: repair with percutaneous implantation of endovascular covered stents. *Radiology* 2000;**214**:127.

59. Silberstein M, Tress BM, Hennessy O. Selecting the right technique to reform a reverse curve catheter (Simmons style): critical review. *Cardiovasc Intervent Radiol* 1992;**15**:171.

60. Waltman AC, Courey WR, Athanasoulis C, et al. Technique for left gastric artery catheterization. *Radiology* 1973;**109**:732.

61. Tetteroo E, van Engelen AD, Spithoven JH, et al. Stent placement after iliac angioplasty. Comparison of hemodynamic and angiographic criteria. *Radiology* 1996;**201**:155.

62. Bonn J. Percutaneous vascular intervention: value of hemodynamic measurements. *Radiology* 1996;**201**:18.

63. Kinney TB, Rose SC. Intraarterial pressure measurements during angiographic evaluation of peripheral vascular disease: techniques, interpretation, applications, and limitations. *AJR Am J Roentgenol* 1996;**166**:277.

64. Archie Jr JP. Analysis and comparison of pressure gradients and ratios for predicting iliac stenosis. *Ann Vasc Surg* 1994;**8**:271.

65. Cavendish JJ, Carter LI, Tsimikas S. Recent advances in hemodynamics: noncoronary applications of a pressure sensor angioplasty guidewire. *Catheter Cardiovasc Interv* 2008;**71**:748.

66. Garcia LA, Carrozza Jr JP. Physiologic evaluation of translesion pressure gradients in peripheral arteries: comparison of pressure wire and catheter-derived measurements. *J Interv Cardiol* 2007;**20**:63.

67. American College of Radiology. Manual on contrast media, V7. Reston, Va., American College of Radiology. Available at www.acr.org/SecondaryMainMenuCategories/quality_safety/contrast_manual.aspx.

68. Cochran ST. Anaphylactoid reactions to radiocontrast media. *Curr Allergy Asthma Rep* 2005;**5**:28.

69. Lawrence V, Matthai W, Hartmaier S. Comparative safety of high-osmolality and low-osmolality radiographic contrast agents: report of a multidisciplinary working group. *Invest Radiol* 1992;**27**:2.

70. Druy EM, Bettmann MA, Jeans W. A double-blind study of iopromide 300 for peripheral arteriography. Results of a multi-institutional comparison of iopromide with iohexol and iopamidol. *Invest Radiol* 1994;**29**(Suppl. 1):S102.

71. Solomon RJ, Natarajan MK, Doucet S, et al. Cardiac angiography in renally impaired patients (CARE) study: a randomized double-blind trial of contrast-induced nephropathy in patients with chronic kidney disease. *Circulation* 2007;**115**:3189.

72. Laskey W, Aspelin P, Davidson C, et al. Nephrotoxicity of iodixanol versus iopamidol in patients with chronic kidney disease and diabetes mellitus undergoing coronary angiographic procedures. *Am Heart J* 2009;**158**:822.

73. Mehran R, Nikolsky E, Kirtane AJ, et al. Ionic low osmolar versus nonionic iso-osmolar contrast media to obviate worsening nephropathy after angioplasty in chronic renal failure patients: the ICON (Ionic versus non-ionic Contrast to Obviate worsening Nephropathy after angioplasty in chronic renal failure patients) study. *JACC Cardiovasc Interv* 2009;**2**:415.

74. Nie B, Cheng WJ, Li YF, et al. A prospective, double-blind, randomized, controlled trial on the efficacy and cardiorenal safety of iodixanol vs. iopromide in patients with chronic kidney disease undergoing coronary angiography with or without percutaneous coronary intervention. *Catheter Cardiovasc Interv* 2008;**72**:958.

75. Jo SH, Youn TJ, Koo BH, et al. Renal toxicity evaluation and comparison between Visipaque (iodixanol) and Hexabrix (ioxaglate) in patients with renal insufficiency undergoing coronary angiography: the RECOVER study: a randomized controlled trial. *J Am Coll Cardiol* 2006;**48**:924.

76. Shaw DR, Kessel DO. The current status of the use of carbon dioxide in diagnostic and interventional angiographic procedures. *Cardiovasc Intervent Radiol* 2006;**29**:323.

77. Caridi JG, Hawkins Jr IF, Klioze SD, et al. Carbon dioxide digital subtraction angiography: the practical approach. *Tech Vasc Interv Radiol* 2001;**4**:57.

78. Heye S, Maleux G, Marchal GJ. Upper extremity venography: CO_2 versus iodinated contrast material. *Radiology* 2006;**241**:291.

79. Maleux G, Nevens F, Heye S, et al. The use of carbon dioxide wedged hepatic venography to identify the portal vein: comparison with direct catheter portography with iodinated contrast medium and analysis of predictive factors influencing level of opacification. *J Vasc Interv Radiol* 2006;**17**:1771.

80. Hawkins IF, Cho KJ, Caridi JG. Carbon dioxide in angiography to reduce the risk of contrast-induced nephropathy. *Radiol Clin North Am* 2009;**47**:813.

81. Prince MR, Zhang HL, Prowda JC, et al. Nephrogenic systemic fibrosis and its impact on abdominal imaging. *Radiographics* 2009;**29**:1565.

82. Altun E, Martin DR, Wertman R, et al. Nephrogenic systemic fibrosis: change in incidence following a switch in gadolinium agents and adoption of a gadolinium policy—report from two U.S. universities. *Radiology* 2009;**253**:689.

83. Abujudeh HH, Kaewlai R, Kagan A, et al. Nephrogenic systemic fibrosis after gadopentetate dimeglumine exposure; case series of 36 patients. *Radiology* 2009;**253**:81.

84. Kereiakes DJ. Adjunctive pharmacotherapy before percutaneous coronary intervention in non-ST-elevation acute coronary syndromes: the role of modulating inflammation. *Circulation* 2003;**108**(16 (Suppl. 1)):III22.

85. Mohler III ER. Combination antiplatelet therapy in patients with peripheral arterial disease: is the best therapy aspirin, clopidogrel, or both? *Cath Cardiovasc Intervent* 2009;**74**:S1.

86. Wiviott SD, Antman EM, Braunwald E. Prasugrel. *Circulation* 2010;**122**:394.

87. Cannon CP, CAPRIE investigators. Effectiveness of clopidogrel versus aspirin in preventing acute myocardial infarction in patients with symptomatic atherothrombosis (CAPRIE trial). *Am J Cardiol* 2002;**90**:760.

88. Bhatt DL, Fox KA, Hacke W, et al. Clopidogrel and aspirin versus aspirin alone for the prevention of atheroembolic events. *N Engl J Med* 2006;**354**:1706.

89. Tran H, Anand SS. Oral antiplatelet therapy in cerebrovascular disease, coronary artery disease, and peripheral arterial disease. *JAMA* 2004;**292**:1867.

90. Chapman TM, Goa KL. Cilostazol: a review of its use in intermittent claudication. *Am J Cardiovasc Drugs* 2003;**3**:117.

91. Kambayashi J, Liu Y, Sun B, et al. Cilostazol as a unique antithrombotic agent. *Curr Pharm Des* 2003;**9**:2289.

92. Olin JW, Sealove BA. Peripheral artery disease: current insight into the disease and its diagnosis and management. *Mayo Clin Proc* 2010;**85**:678.

93. Lee SW, Park SW, Kim YH, et al. Drug-eluting stenting followed by cilostazol treatment reduces late restenosis in patients with diabetes mellitus—the DECLARE-DIABETES trial. *J Am Coll Cardiol* 2008;**51**:1181.

94. Duda, Tepe G, Luz O, et al. Peripheral artery occlusion: treatment with abciximab plus urokinase versus urokinase alone—a randomized pilot trial (the PROMPT study). *Radiology* 2001;**221**:689.

95. Ouriel K, Castaneda F, McNamara T, et al. Reteplase monotherapy and reteplase/abciximab combination therapy in peripheral arterial occlusive disease: results from the RELAX trial. *J Vasc Interv Radiol* 2004;**15**:229.

96. Tepe G, Hopfenzitz C, Dietz K, et al. Peripheral arteries: treatment with antibodies of platelet receptors and reteplase for thrombolysis—APART trial. *Radiology* 2006;**239**:892.

97. Weitz DS, Weitz JI. Update on heparin: what do we need to know? *J Thromb Thrombolysis* 2010;**29**:199.

98. Simko RJ, Tsung FF, Stanek EJ. Activated clotting time versus activated partial thromboplastin time for therapeutic monitoring of heparin. *Ann Pharmacother* 1995;**29**:1015.

99. Bates SM, Weitz JI, Johnston M, et al. Use of a fixed activated partial thromboplastin time ratio to establish a therapeutic range for unfractionated heparin. *Arch Intern Med* 2001;**161**:385.

100. Kearon C, Ginsberg JS, Julian JA, et al. Comparison of fixed dose weight adjusted unfractionated heparin and low molecular weight heparin for acute treatment of venous thromboembolism. *JAMA* 2006;**296**:935.

101. Raskob GE, Hirsch J. Controversies in timing of the first dose of anticoagulant prophylaxis against venous thromboembolism after major orthopedic surgery. *Chest* 2003;**124**(Suppl. 6):379S.

102. Louzada ML, Majeed H, Wells PS. Efficacy of low-molecular-weight heparin versus vitamin K antagonists for long term treatment of cancer-associated venous thromboembolism in adults: a systemic review of randomized controlled trials. *Thromb Res* 2009;**123**:837.

103. Fareed J, Hoppensteadt DA, Bick RL. Management of thrombotic and cardiovascular disorders in the new millennium. *Clin Appl Thromb Hemost* 2003;**9**:101.

104. Lobo B, Finch C, Howard A, et al. Fondaparinux for the treatment of patients with acute heparin-induced thrombocytopenia. *Thromb Haemost* 2008;**99**:208.

105. Shammas NW. Complications in peripheral vascular interventions: emerging role of direct thrombin inhibitors. *J Vasc Interv Radiol* 2005;**16**(2 (Pt. 1)):165.

106. Allie DE, Lirtzman MD, Wyatt CH, et al. Bivalirudin as a foundation anticoagulant in peripheral vascular disease: a safe and feasible alternative for renal and iliac interventions. *J Invasive Cardiol* 2003;**15**:334.

107. Katzen BT, Ardid MI, MacLean AA, et al. Bivalirudin as an anticoagulant agent: safety and efficacy in peripheral interventions. *J Vasc Interv Radiol* 2005;**16**:1183.

108. De Luca G, Marino P. Antithrombotic therapies in primary angioplasty: rationale, results, and future directions. *Drugs* 2008;**68**:2325.

109. Hong MS, Amanullah AM. Heparin induced thrombocytopenia: a practical review. *Rev Cardiovasc Med* 2010;**11**:13.

110. Hirsh J, Fuster V. Guide to anticoagulant therapy. Part 2: oral anticoagulants. *Circulation* 1994;**89**:1469.

111. Stoeckelhuber BM, Suttmann I, Stoeckelhuber M, et al. Comparison of the vasodilating effects of nitroglycerin, verapamil, and tolazoline in hand angiography. *J Vasc Interv Radiol* 2003;**14**:749.

112. Dotter CT, Judkins MP. Transluminal treatment of arteriosclerotic obstruction. *Circulation* 1964;**30**:654.

113. Gruentzig A, Hopff H. Perkutane Rekanalisation chronischer arterieller Verschluesse mit einem neuen Dilatationskatheter. *Dtsch Med Wochenschr* 1974;**99**:2502.

114. Castaneda-Zuniga WR, Formanek A, Tadavarthy M, et al. The mechanism of balloon angioplasty. *Radiology* 1980;**135**:565.

115. Block PC, Baughman KL, Pasternak RC, et al. Transluminal angioplasty: correlation of morphologic and angiographic findings in an experimental model. *Circulation* 1980;**61**:778.

116. Duebel HP, Gliech V, Bunk G, et al. Rupture of PTCA balloons—an in vitro study. *Z Kardiol* 1997;**86**:968.

117. Zollikofer CL, Salomonowitz E, Castaneda-Zuniga WR, et al. The relation between arterial and balloon rupture in experimental angioplasty. *AJR Am J Roentgenol* 1985;**144**:777.

118. Engelke C, Morgan RA, Belli AM. Cutting balloon percutaneous transluminal angioplasty for salvage of lower limb arterial bypass grafts: feasibility. *Radiology* 2002;**223**:106.

119. Engelke C, Sandhu C, Morgan RA, et al. Using 6-mm cutting balloon angioplasty in patients with resistant peripheral artery stenosis: preliminary results. *AJR Am J Roentgenol* 2002;**179**:619.

120. Vorwerk D, Adam G, Muller-Leisse C, et al. Hemodialysis fistulas and grafts: use of cutting balloons to dilate venous stenoses. *Radiology* 1996;**201**:864.

121. Foering K, Chittams JL, Trerotola SO. Percutaneous transluminal angioplasty balloon inflation with syringes: who needs an inflator? *J Vasc Interv Radiol* 2009;**20**:629.

122. Bittl JA. Venous rupture during percutaneous treatment of hemodialysis fistulas and grafts. *Catheter Cardiovasc Interv* 2009;**74**:1097.

123. Rosenfield K, Schainfeld R, Isner JM. Percutaneous revascularization in peripheral arterial disease. *Curr Prob Cardiol* 1996;**21**:7.

124. Johnston KW, Rae M, Hogg-Johnston SA, et al. Five-year results of a prospective study of percutaneous transluminal angioplasty. *Ann Surg* 1987;**206**:403.

125. Anand S, Creager M. Peripheral arterial disease. *Clin Evid* 2002;**7**:79.

126. Society of Interventional Radiology Standards of Practice Committee. Guidelines for percutaneous transluminal angioplasty. *J Vasc Interv Radiol* 2003;**14**(9 (Pt. 2)):S209.

127. Tielbeek AV, Vroegindeweij D, Buth J, et al. Comparison of balloon angioplasty and Simpson atherectomy for lesions in the femoropopliteal artery: angiographic and clinical results of a prospective randomized trial. *J Vasc Interv Radiol* 1996;**7**:837.

128. McLean GK. Percutaneous peripheral atherectomy. *J Vasc Interv Radiol* 1993;**4**:465.

129. Shrikhande GV, McKinsey JF. Use and abuse of atherectomy: where should it be used? *Semin Vasc Surg* 2008;**21**:204.

130. Biskup NI, Ihnat DM, Leon LR, et al. Infrainguinal atherectomy: a retrospective review of a single-center experience. *Ann Vasc Surg* 2008;**22**:776.

131. Schwarzwaelder U, Zeller T. Debulking procedure: potential device specific indications. *Tech Vasc Interv Radiol* 2010;**13**:43.

132. Palmaz JC. Intravascular stents: tissue-stent interactions and design considerations. *AJR Am J Roentgenol* 1993;**160**:613.

133. Lossef SV, Lutz RL, Mundorf J, et al. Comparison of mechanical deformation properties of metallic stents with use of stress-strain analysis. *J Vasc Interv Radiol* 1994;**5**:341.

134. Karnabatidis D, Katsanos K, Spilliopoulos S, et al. Incidence, anatomical location, and clinical significance of compressions and fractures in infrapopliteal balloon expandable metal stents. *J Endovasc Ther* 2009;**16**:15.

135. Schillinger M, Minar E. Past, present, and future of femoropopliteal stenting. *J Endovasc Ther* 2009;**16**:I147.

136. Haskal ZJ, Trerotola S, Dolmatch B, et al. Stent graft versus balloon angioplasty for failing dialysis access grafts. *N Engl J Med* 2010;**362**:494.

137. Saad WE, Darwish WM, Davies MG, et al. Stent-grafts for transjugular intrahepatic portosystemic shunt creation: specialized TIPS stent-graft versus generic stent-graft/bare stent combination. *J Vasc Interv Radiol* 2010;**21**:1512.

138. McQuade K, Gable D, Pearl G, et al. Four-year randomized prospective comparison of percutaneous ePTFE/nitinol self-expanding

stent graft versus prosthetic femoral-popliteal bypass in the treatment of superficial femoral artery occlusive disease. *J Vasc Surg* 2010;**52**:584.

139. Ansel GM, Lumsden AB. Evolving modalities for femoropopliteal interventions. *J Endovasc Ther* 2009;**16**:II82.

140. Bosiers M, Deloose K, Keirse K, et al. Are drug-eluting stents the future of SFA treatment? *J Cardiovasc Surg* (Torino) 2010;**51**:115.

141. Duda SH, Bosiers M, Lammer J. Sirolimus-eluting versus Bare Nitinol stent for obstructive superficial femoral artery disease: the SIROCCO II trial. *J Vasc Interv Radiol* 2005;**16**:331.

142. Marder VJ, Novokhatny V. Direct fibrinolytic agents: biochemical attributes, preclinical foundation, and clinical potential. *J Thromb Haemost* 2009;**8**:433.

143. Razavi MK, Lee DS, Hofmann LV. Catheter-directed thrombolytic therapy for limb ischemia: current status and controversies. *J Vasc Interv Radiol* 2004;**15**:13.

144. Semba CP, Bakal CW, Calis KA, et al. Alteplase as an alternative to urokinase. *J Vasc Interv Radiol* 2000;**11**:279.

145. Valji K. Evolving strategies for thrombolytic therapy of peripheral vascular occlusion. *J Vasc Interv Radiol* 2000;**11**:411.

146. Margaglione M, Grandone E, DiMinno G. Mechanisms of fibrinolysis and clinical use of thrombolytic agents. *Prog Drug Res* 1992;**39**:197.

147. Ouriel K, Cynamon J, Weaver FA, et al. A phase I trial of alfimeprase for peripheral arterial thrombolysis. *J Vasc Interv Radiol* 2005;**16**:1075.

148. Moise MA, Kashyap VS. Alfimeprase for the treatment of acute peripheral arterial occlusion. *Expert Opin Biol Ther* 2008;**8**:683.

149. Ouriel K, Shortell CK, DeWeese JA, et al. A comparison of thrombolytic therapy with operative revascularization in the initial treatment of acute peripheral arterial ischemia. *J Vasc Surg* 1994;**19**:1021.

150. McNamara TO, Fischer JR. Thrombolysis of peripheral arteries and bypass grafts: improved results using high dose urokinase. *AJR Am J Roentgenol* 1985;**144**:769.

151. Bookstein JJ, Fellmeth B, Roberts A, et al. Pulsed-spray pharmacomechanical thrombolysis: preliminary clinical results. *AJR Am J Roentgenol* 1989;**152**:1097.

152. Valji K, Bookstein JJ, Roberts AC, et al. Pulse-spray pharmacomechanical thrombolysis of thrombosed hemodialysis grafts: long-term experience and comparison of original and current techniques. *AJR Am J Roentgenol* 1995;**164**:1495.

153. Valji K, Roberts AC, Davis GB, et al. Pulsed spray thrombolysis of arterial and bypass graft occlusions. *AJR Am J Roentgenol* 1991;**156**:617.

154. Ouriel K, Shortell CK, Azodo MV, et al. Acute peripheral arterial occlusion: predictors of success in catheter-directed thrombolytic therapy. *Radiology* 1994;**193**:561.

155. Benenati J, Shlansky-Goldberg R, Meglin A, et al. Thrombolytic and antiplatelet therapy in peripheral vascular disease with use of reteplase and/or abciximab. *J Vasc Interv Radiol* 2001;**12**:796.

156. The STILE investigators. Results of a prospective randomized trial evaluating surgery versus thrombolysis for ischemia of the lower extremity. The STILE trial. *Ann Surg* 1994;**220**:251.

157. Earnshaw JJ, Westby JC, Gregson RHS, et al. Local thrombolytic therapy of acute peripheral arterial ischaemia with tissue plasminogen activator: a dose ranging study. *Br J Surg* 1988;**75**:1196.

158. Semba CP, Murphy TP, Bakal CW, et al. Thrombolytic therapy with use of alteplase (rt-PA) in peripheral arterial occlusive disease: review of the clinical literature. *J Vasc Interv Radiol* 2000;**11**:149.

159. van den Berg JC. Thrombolysis for acute arterial occlusion. *J Vasc Surg* 2010;**52**:512.

160. Kessel DO, Berridge DC, Roberston I. Infusion techniques for peripheral arterial thrombolysis. *Cochrane Database Syst Rev* 2004; CD000985.

161. Working party on thrombolysis in the management of limb ischemia. Thrombolysis in the management of lower limb peripheral arterial occlusion—a consensus document. *J Vasc Interv Radiol* 2003;**14**(9 (Pt. 2)):S337.

162. Walker TG. Acute limb ischemia. *Tech Vasc Interv Radiol* 2009;**12**:117.

163. Nazir SA, Ganeshan A, Uberoi R. Endovascular treatment options in the management of lower limb deep venous thrombosis. *Cardiovasc Intervent Radiol* 2009;**32**:861.

164. Turmel-Rodrigues L, Sapoval M, Pengloan J, et al. Manual thromboaspiration and dilation of thrombosed dialysis access: mid-term results of a simple concept. *J Vasc Interv Radiol* 1997;**8**:813.

165. Beyssen B, Sapoval M, Emmerich J, et al. Acute femoro-popliteal ischemia—new therapeutic approach: respective role of thromboaspiration and in situ thrombolysis. *Chirurgie* 1996;**121**:127.

166. Shatsky JB, Berns JS, Clark TW, et al. Single-center experience with the Arrow-Trerotola percutaneous thrombectomy device in the management of thrombosed native dialysis fistulas. *J Vasc Interv Radiol* 2005;**16**:1605.

167. Vashchenko N, Korzets A, Neiman C, et al. Retrospective comparison of mechanical percutaneous thrombectomy of hemodialysis arteriovenous grafts with the Arrow-Trerotola device and the lyse and wait technique. *AJR Am J Roentgenol* 2010;**194**:1626.

168. Rao AS, Konig G, Leers SA, et al. Pharmacomechanical thrombectomy for iliofemoral deep vein thrombosis: an alternative in patients with contraindications to thrombolysis. *J Vasc Surg* 2009;**50**:1092.

169. Littler P, Cullen N, Gould D, et al. AngioJet thrombectomy for occluded dialysis fistulae: outcome data. *Cardiovasc Intervent Radiol* 2009;**32**:265.

170. Dosluoglu HH, Chen GS, Harris LM, et al. Rheolytic thrombectomy, angioplasty, and selective stenting for subacute isolated popliteal artery occlusions. *J Vasc Surg* 2007;**46**:717.

171. Dwarka D, Schwartz SA, Smyth SH, et al. Bradyarrhythmias during use of the AngioJet system. *J Vasc Interv Radiol* 2006;**17**:1693.

172. Dukkipati R, Yang EH, Adler S, et al. Acute kidney injury caused by intravascular hemolysis after mechanical thrombectomy. *Nat Clin Pract Nephrol* 2009;**5**:112.

173. Sarac TP, Hilleman D, Arko FR, et al. Clinical and economic evaluation of the Trellis thrombectomy device for arterial occlusions: preliminary analysis. *J Vasc Surg* 2004;**39**:556.

174. O'Sullivan GJ, Mhuircheartaigh JN, Ferguson D, et al. Isolated pharmacomechanical thrombolysis plus primary stenting in a single procedure to treat acute thrombotic superior vena cava syndrome. *J Endovasc Ther* 2010;**17**:115.

175. Hilleman DE, Razavi MK. Clinical and economic evaluation of the Trellis-8 infusion catheter for deep vein thrombosis. *J Vasc Interv Radiol* 2008;**19**:377.

176. Angle JF, Siddiqi NH, Wallace MJ, et al. Quality improvement guidelines for percutaneous transcatheter embolization: Society of Interventional Radiology Standards of Practice Committee. *J Vasc Interv Radiol* 2010;**21**:1479.

177. Lee BB, Do YS, Yakes W, et al. Management of arteriovenous malformations: a multidisciplinary approach. *J Vasc Surg* 2004;**39**:590.

178. Pech M, Kraetsch A, Wieners G, et al. Embolization of the gastroduodenal artery before selective internal radiotherapy: a prospectively randomized trial comparing platinum-fibered microcoils with the Amplatzer Vascular Plug II. *Cardiovasc Intervent Radiol* 2009;**32**:455.

179. Trerotola SO, Pyeritz RE. Does use of coils in addition to Amplatzer vascular plugs prevent recanalization? *AJR Am J Roentgenol* 2010;**195**:766.

180. Abada HT, Golzarian J. Gelatin sponge particles: handling characteristics for endovascular use. *Tech Vasc Interventional Rad* 2007;**10**:257.

181. Barth KH, Strandberg JD, White RI. Long-term follow-up of transcatheter embolization with autologous clot, Oxycel and Gelfoam in domestic swine. *Invest Radiol* 1977;**3**:273.

182. Collier JP, Fignon A, Tranquart F, et al. Uterine necrosis after arterial embolization for postpartum hemorrhage. *Obstet Gynecol* 2002;**100**:1074.

183. Hare WS, Holland CJ. Paresis following internal iliac artery embolization. *Radiology* 1983;**146**:47.

184. Siskin GP, Dowling K, Virmani R, et al. Pathologic evaluation of a spherical polyvinyl alcohol embolic agent in a porcine renal model. *J Vasc Interv Radiol* 2003;**14**:89.

185. Laurent A. Microspheres and nonspherical particles for embolization. *Tech Vasc Interventional Rad* 2007;**10**:248.

186. Pelage J-P, LeDref O, Beregi J-P, et al. Limited uterine artery embolization with tris-acryl gelatin microspheres for uterine fibroids. *J Vasc Interv Radiol* 2003;**14**:15.

187. Brown KT. Fatal pulmonary complication after arterial embolization with 40-120 μm tris-acryl gelatin microspheres. *J Vasc Interv Radiol* 2004;**15**:197.

188. Orsini C, Brotto M. Immediate pathologic effects on the vein wall of foam sclerotherapy. *Dermatol Surg* 2007;**33**:1250.

189. Reiner E, Pollak JS, Henderson KJ, et al. Initial experience with 3% sodium tetradecyl sulfate foam and fibered coils for management of adolescent varicocele. *J Vasc Interv Radiol* 2008;**19**:207.

190. Guex JJ. Complications and side effects of foam sclerotherapy. *Phlebology* 2009;**24**:270.

191. Ayad M, Eskioglu E, Mericle RA. Onyx: a unique neuroembolic agent. *Expert Rev Med Devices* 2006;**3**:705.

192. Martin ML, Dolmatch BL, Fry PD, et al. Treatment of type II endoleak with Onyx. *J Vasc Interv Radiol* 2001;**12**:629.

193. Castaneda F, Goodwin SC, Swischuk JL, et al. Treatment of pelvic arteriovenous malformations with ethylene vinyl alcohol copolymer (Onyx). *J Vasc Interv Radiol* 2002;**13**:513.

194. Pollak JS, White RI. The use of cyanoacrylate adhesives in peripheral embolization. *J Vasc Interv Radiol* 2001;**12**:907.

195. Yamakado K, Nakatsuka A, Tanaka N, et al. Transcatheter arterial embolization of ruptured pseudoaneurysms with coils and n-butyl cyanoacrylate. *J Vasc Interv Radiol* 2000;**11**:66.

196. Hiraki T, Mimura H, Kanazawa S, et al. Transcatheter embolization of an aortobronchial fistula with n-butyl cyanoacrylate. *J Vasc Interv Radiol* 2002;**13**:743.

197. Kim BS, Do HM, Razavi M. N-butyl cyanoacrylate glue embolization of splenic artery aneurysms. *J Vasc Interv Radiol* 2004;**15**:91.

198. Frodsham A, Berkmen T, Ananian C, et al. Initial experience using n-butyl cyanoacrylate for embolization of lower gastrointestinal hemorrhage. *J Vasc Interv Radiol* 2009;**20**:1312.

199. Kiyosue H, Mori H, Matsumoto S, et al. Transcatheter obliteration of gastric varices: Part 2. Strategy and techniques based on hemodynamic features. *Radiographics* 2003;**23**:921.

Percutaneous Biopsy

Hamed Aryafar, Thomas B. Kinney

Percutaneous biopsy is a widely used interventional technique for obtaining tissue samples.[1,2] The crucial element of the procedure is image guidance, which facilitates accurate and safe needle passage. Percutaneous biopsy with image guidance is less invasive and less expensive than most surgical methods. The procedure has become safer and more effective with advances in imaging, specialized cytologic analyses, and small-gauge, thin-walled needles. Cross-sectional imaging with computed tomography (CT), ultrasound, and magnetic resonance imaging (MRI) permits safe diagnosis of small, remote lesions that once were completely inaccessible in this way. The accuracy of percutaneous biopsy for the diagnosis of malignancy in the chest and abdomen is about 85% to 95%.[3] Definitive diagnosis of benign lesions is less accurate, however. Further advances in biopsy and cytopathologic methods should improve these results.

The most common indication for percutaneous biopsy is the diagnosis of malignancy, including primary neoplasms, metastatic disease, tumor staging, and recurrent disease after treatment. The procedure also is used for diagnosis of inflammatory or infectious processes, abnormal fluid collections, and diffuse organ disease. Relative contraindications include uncorrectable coagulation abnormalities, lack of a safe percutaneous pathway to the lesion, and an uncooperative patient in whom motion may increase the risk of bleeding.[4] Biopsy usually is not indicated in a patient who will undergo surgery regardless of the biopsy results or if the results will not change the management of the patient (e.g., the patient is already in hospice care).

TECHNIQUE

Patient Preparation

The patient's history, clinical status, and imaging studies should be reviewed and discussed with the referring physicians. Routinely performed coagulation studies include hematocrit, platelet count, prothrombin time, partial thromboplastin time, and international normalized ratio[5] (INR) (see Chapter 2). Coagulopathies should be corrected with appropriate transfusions of platelets, fresh-frozen plasma, vitamin K, or packed red blood cells. Although institutional thresholds vary, transfusions should be considered when the INR is greater than 1.5 or when platelet count is less than $50,000/mm^3$. However, numerous studies have shown the relatively low predictive value of abnormal screening parameters in predicting bleeding.[5,6] Surgical series also have indicated that preoperative coagulation studies correlate poorly with postoperative bleeding.[6] Recent Society of Interventional Radiology practice guidelines offer useful coagulation and transfusion parameters for percutaneous biopsy depending on whether the lesions are superficial (minimal risk); deeper intraabdominal, thoracic, or retroperitoneal (moderate risk); or renal (significant risk).[7] Interventionalists must be careful to screen their patients for use of potent antiplatelet agents such as clopidogrel (Plavix). These agents should be discontinued at least 5 days before moderate or significant risk biopsies. Care should be taken before discontinuing Plavix if it is prescribed to maintain patency of a coronary artery stent. A cardiology consult may be necessary to avoid stent complications based on type of stent used (drug-eluting vs. bare metal) and timing of stent placement.[8,9]

Materials

A wide array of needles are available for percutaneous biopsy procedures.[10] Needles can be classified by caliber or gauge, tip configuration, and mechanism of sample acquisition. Needle sizes are divided broadly into smaller gauge (20 to 25 gauge) and larger gauge (14 to 19 gauge).[3] Thinner-gauge needles often provide adequate cytologic material and often histologic material as well. Smaller-caliber needles also minimize bleeding, providing a margin of safety when multiple passes are required. Traversing bowel may at times be necessary, and complications can be minimized by using thin-gauge needles.[4] However, they can be somewhat difficult to direct into lesions because they tend to deflect significantly, particularly in deep-seated lesions. Larger needles are easier to direct and provide better samples for cytology and histology, often with fewer needle passes. The risk for hemorrhage may increase as needle size increases.[5] Needles also are classified by tip configuration[10] (Fig. 4-1). Needles vary in the angle and bevel of the tip. The Chiba and spinal needles have bevel angles of 25 and 30 degrees, respectively. Greene, Madayag, and Franseen (or Crown) needles have 90-degree tips. Needle tips are classified also into noncutting (aspiration needles such as the Chiba or spinal) and cutting (end-cut or side-cut) types. Needles can be manual, spring-loaded, or automated.

The wide selection of needle types suggests that no design is clearly optimal and that needle selection should be based on physician preference in conjunction with consideration of the specific biopsy task at hand. In general, initial samples are obtained for cytologic analysis with fine-gauge (22-gauge) Chiba or spinal needles. If these needles do not yield satisfactory samples, a Franseen needle often yields cells for cytologic study. Superficial lesions are easier to reach; deep-seated ones may require larger-gauge needles to provide sufficient stiffness to direct the needle accurately.

The vulnerability of organs along the anticipated path of the biopsy needle (e.g., pleura, bowel) may dictate needle selection, because smaller-gauge needles (>19 gauge) are relatively safe.

Preprocedure imaging characteristics also may guide needle selection. For example, smaller-gauge needles are used for metastatic disease and in patients with a known primary malignancy. In patients with no known primary malignancy at the time of biopsy or in patients with suspected lymphoma, multiple passes with fine-gauge needles or several passes with a large-gauge needle often are required to obtain adequate tissue for diagnosis. Physician experience is an important factor; automated devices yield better results when the operator is less experienced at obtaining core material by manual aspiration.

Imaging Guidance

The important factors in choosing an imaging modality for biopsy are lesion characteristics (e.g., size, location, depth), ability to visualize the abnormality, and operator experience and preference. Generally, the shortest path to the lesion is considered when planning the imaging approach, with the possible exception of peripherally located hypervascular hepatic lesions and when preprocedure imaging demonstrates better tissue yield from a different axis (e.g., elongated but thin lesion).

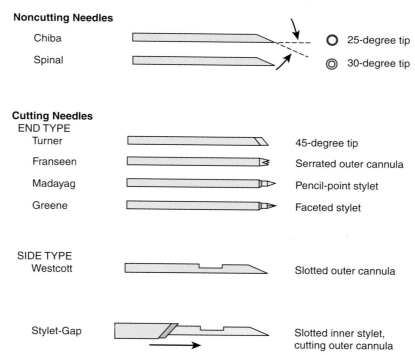

FIGURE 4-1 Standard needles used for percutaneous biopsy. All of the needles come with stylets. The spinal needle has a thicker wall than the Chiba needle. Unlike an 18-gauge spinal needle, an 18-gauge Chiba needle can accommodate a 0.035-inch guidewire. This feature is useful when aspiration yields infected fluid that requires drainage.

Fluoroscopy

Fluoroscopy is a common technique for biopsy of lung and pleural masses (Fig. 4-2). In the abdomen, fluoroscopy can be used for fine-needle biopsy of obstructing lesions of the biliary and urinary systems outlined by contrast material from percutaneously placed catheters. Disadvantages of this method include added radiation exposure to the operator and inability to visualize adjacent structures as the needle is advanced. Cross-sectional imaging studies (e.g., CT, ultrasound, MRI) can be helpful in planning an approach when fluoroscopy is used.

Sonography

Ultrasound is very useful for biopsy of intraabdominal lesions, including masses in the liver, pancreas, or kidney; bulky adenopathy in the retroperitoneum or root of the mesentery; and large adrenal masses.[11] In the chest, ultrasound is used for aspiration of pleural-based masses and fluid collections and occasionally can be used in the biopsy of peripheral pulmonary parenchymal lesions.

A complete diagnostic ultrasound study is obtained first to determine the conspicuity of the lesion, its depth, and a safe angle of approach. Ultrasound-guided biopsy can be performed with a free-hand technique or with the use of ultrasound guides. Sterilized probes or sterile probe covers allow real-time imaging while the biopsy is performed. Advantages of ultrasound include the lack of ionizing radiation, real-time imaging of needle position, and the multiplanar imaging capability that facilitates complex angled approaches often required to biopsy upper quadrant abdominal masses. Disadvantages include impaired visualization of deep lesions and obscuration by overlying bowel gas or bone. Additionally,

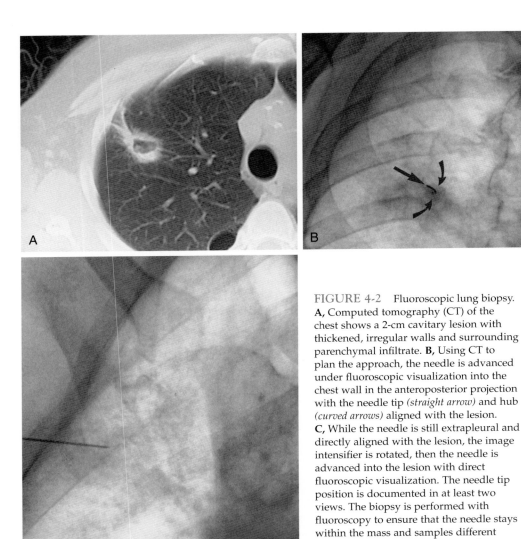

FIGURE 4-2 Fluoroscopic lung biopsy. **A,** Computed tomography (CT) of the chest shows a 2-cm cavitary lesion with thickened, irregular walls and surrounding parenchymal infiltrate. **B,** Using CT to plan the approach, the needle is advanced under fluoroscopic visualization into the chest wall in the anteroposterior projection with the needle tip *(straight arrow)* and hub *(curved arrows)* aligned with the lesion. **C,** While the needle is still extrapleural and directly aligned with the lesion, the image intensifier is rotated, then the needle is advanced into the lesion with direct fluoroscopic visualization. The needle tip position is documented in at least two views. The biopsy is performed with fluoroscopy to ensure that the needle stays within the mass and samples different regions of the lesion. In this case, the diagnosis was coccidioidomycosis.

operator variability in experience and technique can play a part in sonographically guided biopsies.

Specifically designed and somewhat costly reflective needles are available. However, standard biopsy needles are visualized adequately at real-time sonography, particularly with gentle motion of the needle tip. Low-frequency transducers (e.g., 3.5-MHz sector probe) are needed for deeper lesions. Higher-frequency transducers (e.g., 7-MHz linear or phased-array probe) are used for biopsy of superficial masses such as thyroid nodules. Specifically designed probes for transvaginal and transrectal imaging have needle guides to facilitate biopsy of pelvic lesions.

The needle can be inserted perpendicular to the transducer, which may facilitate visualization by improved reflections from the needle shaft[11] (Fig. 4-3). Alternatively, the needle can be inserted in close to the ultrasound transducer. Ideally, the entire needle should be visualized during passage through the tissues into the mass (Fig. 4-4). If the needle is not visible, misalignment between the needle path and ultrasound beam is occurring. A slight rocking motion (or panning) back and forth of the ultrasound transducer may help visualize the needle. A gentle in-out motion of the needle or stylet may increase conspicuity of the needle tip as well. In every case, the needle tip should be documented as a discrete echogenic focus within the lesion in at least two views before biopsy (Fig. 4-5).

The advent of three-dimensional sonography has aided percutaneous biopsy by precise delineation of mass lesions and adjacent structures (e.g., blood vessels and bile ducts) in the anticipated needle pathway.[12] It also has been useful in guiding transjugular liver procedures and regional tumor ablation procedures because orthogonal images can be obtained in planes that are anatomically useful to the interventionalist performing the procedure. Three-dimensional sonography, however, has not gained significant popularity in most practices.

Computed Tomography

CT is used for biopsy of smaller intraabdominal and thoracic lesions not well visualized by ultrasound or fluoroscopy. The patient is first scanned in the anticipated biopsy position (e.g., prone, supine, oblique) with images obtained through the target area (Fig. 4-6). Intravenous contrast may be helpful in delineating vascular structures, in determining the vascularity of the target lesion, and for biopsy of lesions not well seen on unenhanced images (Fig. 4-7). A variety of devices is available to mark the skin during scanning and to determine the needle insertion site and angle.

A vertical needle pathway is preferable because it avoids the need for triangulation or accurate angle measurements. The needle should be visualized in the axial plane during the biopsy. Occasionally, gantry angulation

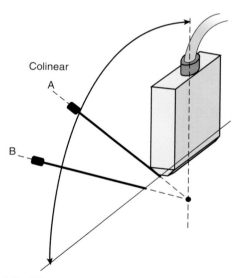

FIGURE 4-3   Ultrasound-guided percutaneous biopsy. Using freehand technique, the needle is placed at one end of the longitudinal face of the ultrasound probe (A). The shaft is aligned parallel to the transducer as the needle is advanced to keep it within the sonographic field of view. If the needle is poorly seen, a more perpendicular angle (B) with the transducer may improve ultrasonographic reflections and make the needle more conspicuous. Needle guides are available on some ultrasound machines to simplify the biopsy.

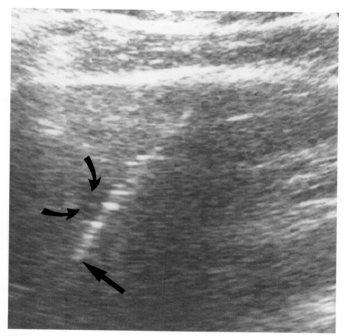

FIGURE 4-4   Ultrasound-guided percutaneous biopsy with visualization of the entire needle shaft (straight arrow) as it passes beyond a focal liver mass (curved arrows).

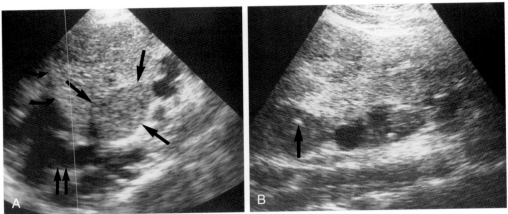

FIGURE 4-5 Ultrasound-guided percutaneous biopsy of a hepatic mass. The patient had cryptogenic cirrhosis and an incidental hypoechoic, 6-cm lesion in the medial segment of the left lobe. **A,** The sagittal image shows the lesion *(straight arrows)*, pericardium *(curved arrows)*, and inferior vena cava *(double arrows)*. **B,** Real-time imaging shows the brightly echogenic needle tip within the lesion *(arrow)*.

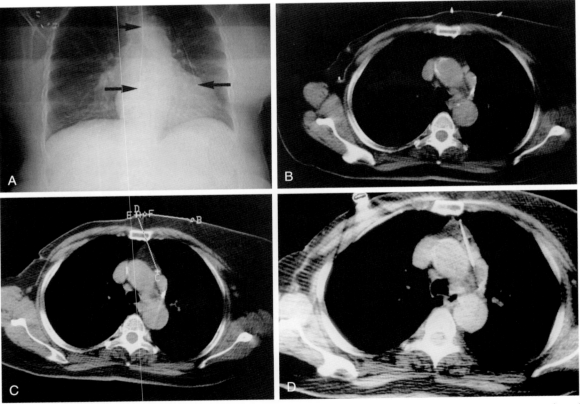

FIGURE 4-6 Technique for computed tomography (CT)-guided percutaneous biopsy. The patient had undergone resection for colon carcinoma. Rising carcinoembryonic antigen titers were found later along with mediastinal lymphadenopathy on a CT scan. **A,** Using the initial diagnostic CT scan as a guide, the patient is positioned in the scanner with a grid marker taped to the skin *(arrows)* near the anticipated needle entry site. **B,** Scans are obtained through the lesion, and the table position that best shows the lesion is identified. Note the grid bars on the skin overlying the mass. **C,** Cursors measure the distance between grid bars *(F-B)*, which allows determination of the cephalocaudal location of the lesion. The planned skin entry site is labeled *A,* and the depth of lesion is the distance from *A* to *C.* **D,** The needle is advanced in stages as serial scans follow its progress into the lesion. The needle tip is seen as a beam-hardening artifact. In this case, no malignant tissue was recovered.

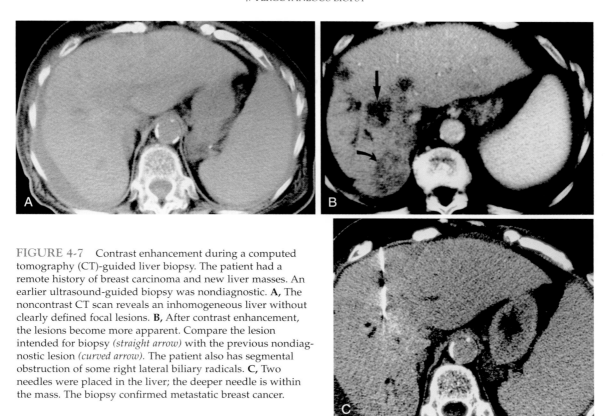

FIGURE 4-7   Contrast enhancement during a computed tomography (CT)-guided liver biopsy. The patient had a remote history of breast carcinoma and new liver masses. An earlier ultrasound-guided biopsy was nondiagnostic. **A,** The noncontrast CT scan reveals an inhomogeneous liver without clearly defined focal lesions. **B,** After contrast enhancement, the lesions become more apparent. Compare the lesion intended for biopsy *(straight arrow)* with the previous nondiagnostic lesion *(curved arrow)*. The patient also has segmental obstruction of some right lateral biliary radicals. **C,** Two needles were placed in the liver; the deeper needle is within the mass. The biopsy confirmed metastatic breast cancer.

may be helpful to visualize cranial-caudal angled approaches (e.g., adrenal biopsy, transthoracic biopsy with overlying ribs).

The advantages of CT include high-resolution image quality and the ability to visualize all structures in the path of the lesion including bowel. Disadvantages include additional radiation exposure for the patient, lack of real-time feedback during needle advancement and biopsy, and difficulty in using angled approaches required for targeting abdominal masses high under the diaphragm. Spiral CT improves needle tip localization because of minimal respiratory motion artifact and fast scanning times.

CT fluoroscopy allows real-time monitoring of needle positioning during percutaneous biopsy. Since its introduction in 1996, various studies have outlined advantages and disadvantages of this technique for biopsy of various targets.[13] Advantages of CT fluoroscopy over conventional CT include the ability to time a patient's breathing to access moving lesions or to avoid ribs and other overlying structures. CT fluoroscopy allows the needle and lesion to be visualized during sampling to be sure the needle tip is properly located within the lesion. Using CT fluoroscopy in near real-time imaging requires either that the operator's hands be in the radiation beam

or that special needle holders be used. The technique also is useful to perform peripheral lesional biopsy when central necrosis is present. CT fluoroscopy is not used universally, because some investigators are concerned about added radiation exposure and conflicting studies about reduced procedure times. CT fluoroscopy has been used most often for transthoracic biopsy, for which high rates of technical success have been reported with sensitivity ranging from 89% to 95% and specificity of 100%.[14] Several recent studies have shown that using intermittent "quick check" CT fluoroscopy between needle advancements instead of continuous (near real-time) fluoroscopy can reduce radiation doses significantly.[15,16]

Magnetic Resonance Imaging

Several investigators have described initial experiences with MR-guided percutaneous biopsies. Potential advantages include the ability to image lesions not readily seen by other modalities, multiplanar imaging capability, near real-time imaging during needle insertion, lack of ionizing radiation, and potential use of MR-guided tumor ablation in conjunction with biopsy.[17] Disadvantages include the need for specially designed needles compatible with MR scanners, higher imaging costs, and special magnet configurations (i.e., open designs) to facilitate needle insertion.

Magnetic field–based electronic guidance systems are a special class of equipment that uses a low magnetic field with position sensors on the patient fused with previously obtained cross-sectional imaging to provide near real-time targeting.[18,19]

Using a computer-calculated map, the operator can position the needle based solely on the prior imaging or can be coupled with real-time ultrasound or CT for true concordance. These systems can be useful in targeting lesions that are only visible on contrast-enhanced CT images.

Sampling Technique (Online Case 45)

Most biopsies are performed with the patient in a supine position, although prone and oblique positions can be used when necessary. With a few exceptions, the shortest path to the lesion is preferred. Hypervascular hepatic lesions should be approached through a sizable parenchymal track to reduce hemorrhagic complications[20] (Fig. 4-8). The likelihood of pneumothorax is reduced by minimizing the number of pleural surfaces crossed during chest and some abdominal biopsies. It is optimal to avoid traversing lung, pleura, pancreas, gallbladder, dilated or obstructed biliary ducts, and bowel during biopsy procedures. Small and large bowel can be crossed safely with small-gauge needles if no other pathway is available. However, sampling of intraabdominal fluid collections through bowel loops is not advisable.

Usually it is best to start with smaller needles (e.g., 22-gauge) that can serve as localizers for subsequent needle placement. Sampling can be performed with or without suction. Suctioning sample is obtained by small

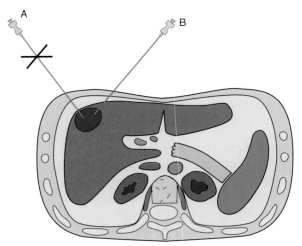

FIGURE 4-8   Biopsy of suspected hypervascular peripheral hepatic lesions. Bleeding is more likely if the parenchymal track is short *(A)*, With a tangential approach *(B)*, a long parenchymal track should tamponade bleeding.

oscillating and rotating motions of the needle hub while 5 to 10 mL of continuous suction is applied with a 10-mL syringe connected by extension tubing. During needle advancement and biopsy, the patient should suspend respiration to minimize inadvertent motion of the needle or target. With ultrasound, fluoroscopy, and CT fluoroscopy, the position of the needle tip can be observed continuously during biopsy so that different sectors of the lesion are sampled to increase the diagnostic yield. Before the needle is removed, the suction is released to prevent the entire sample from being aspirated into the tubing or syringe. Ideally, the biopsy is performed with a cytopathologist present.

If the sample is predominantly composed of red blood cells, a better sample may be obtained with a smaller-gauge needle (e.g., 25-gauge). A nonaspiration technique also can be used in which the needle is advanced and retracted through the lesion without suction.[21] Large lesions with necrotic centers may require biopsy of peripheral tissue to make a diagnosis (Fig. 4-9).

Single-Needle Technique

With the single-needle method, the needle is advanced into position, and its location is confirmed (Fig. 4-10). If the needle location is unsatisfactory, it is left in place to guide placement of a second needle. Each biopsy sample that is obtained requires a new needle be placed into the lesion, adding to the complexity of the case and increasing risks for complications such as bleeding. This technique allows sampling of different regions of a mass, which may improve biopsy yield. This technique is very useful for biopsy of superficial lesions such as thyroid nodules.

Two-Needle Technique

With the two-needle method, a needle is placed initially just superficial to the lesion to serve as a guide for subsequent needle passage and biopsy with a tandem or coaxial technique (see Fig. 4-10). Precise needle placement needs to be done only once. The coaxial method is particularly useful with smaller or deep lesions that are difficult to localize. It has the further advantage that a single puncture of the visceral organ capsule (or pleura) is made, regardless of the number of biopsy needle passes that are made. A disadvantage of this method is that the sampling path of the biopsy needle is limited by the direction of the outer guiding needle. Several different commercially available coaxial sets are now available and are particularly useful for biopsy of thoracic and deep abdominal lesions. Care should be maintained when using different needles from different vendors as slight size/length incompatibilities may arise, making biopsy difficult or impossible.

Additional special equipment is available, such as a modified coaxial system (e.g., 23-gauge needle with

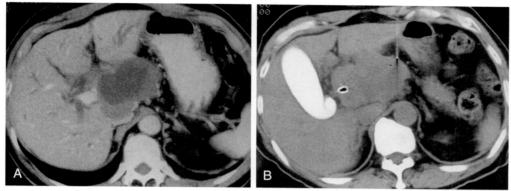

FIGURE 4-9   Value of sampling multiple regions of a lesion during percutaneous biopsy. The patient had an epigastric mass, obstructive jaundice, and ascending cholangitis. **A,** Computed tomography (CT) demonstrates a large pancreatic mass encasing the hepatic artery and displacing the portal vein, with extension of the mass into the porta hepatis. The patient had undergone biliary stenting with nondiagnostic bile duct brushings. Initial samples from a CT-guided biopsy (not shown) from the center of the lesion revealed only necrotic cells. **B,** Sampling the periphery of the lesion revealed adenocarcinoma. The gallbladder contrast is residual from a recent endoscopic retrograde cholangiopancreatography.

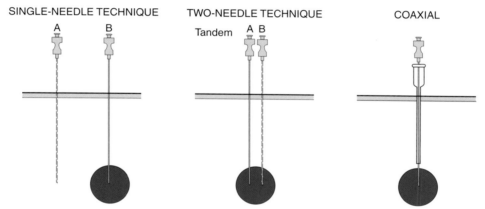

FIGURE 4-10   Single- and double-needle techniques for percutaneous biopsy. *Left,* Single-needle technique. If the initial pass misses the lesion, the needle *(A)* is used to redirect a second needle *(B)* into the lesion. With each attempt, a new needle is reinserted with imaging guidance. *Center,* Two-needle technique. With the tandem method, a second needle *(A)* is slid alongside the landmark needle *(B)* and then used to perform the biopsy. The original needle is left in place to guide subsequent needle insertions. *Right,* With the coaxial method, a larger needle (18- or 19-gauge) is inserted just up to the mass. The biopsy is performed with a longer, smaller-gauge needle (22-gauge) inside the outer guiding needle.

removable hub is used to guide a 19-gauge biopsy needle), for additional cost.

Specimen Handling

An optimal cytologic specimen consists of a small amount of soft or semiliquid material with minimal bloody contamination.[22] Smears should be composed of a thin layer of cells and fragments; blood dilutes and obscures the diagnostic material. Clotting of the specimen can be minimized by expeditious sample preparation and prerinsing the aspiration syringe and needle with a small amount of heparinized saline. Small-gauge needles (e.g., 25-gauge) also limit the blood content of the aspirate.

A small amount of aspirated material first is placed on a slide. The material is spread and then air-dried or fixed in alcohol. Air-dried samples are stained with Diff-Quik (Baxter Healthcare, McGraw Park, Ill.) for prompt diagnosis. Larger tissue fragments or material are placed in a tube or container of 10% neutral buffered formalin for processing as a cell block. This step is particularly important when immunohistochemical staining is required for diagnosis. Occasionally, the core sample can be used to perform a "touch preparation" in which the core sample is smeared across a slide or multiple slides and then the core is placed in formalin, the touch preparations are then processed similarly as other cytologic samples.[23] The remaining core sample is processed for histologic examination. "Touch prep" or "core roll preparation" has been shown to improve the diagnostic yield during the biopsy when compared with fine-needle aspiration (FNA) alone.[23-25] In combination with FNA, this allows for fewer passes to obtain a diagnostic sample without significantly altering the histologic sample.

Care After Biopsy

After the biopsy sample is obtained, imaging is performed to exclude potential complications (e.g., upright chest radiographs 1 and 4 hours after percutaneous chest biopsy or sonography of perihepatic spaces, paracolic gutters, and pelvis after percutaneous liver biopsy). The patient is monitored for 2 to 4 hours after the procedure while intravenous access is maintained, and vital signs are obtained frequently. If the patient has remained stable and no new clinical symptoms develop (e.g., chest pain, shortness of breath, abdominal pain, distention), the patient is discharged home with a family member after the patient assessment of procedure and anesthesia scoring system exceeds the threshold level. If vital signs are abnormal or symptoms develop, additional imaging may be required to exclude a complication.

SPECIFIC APPLICATIONS

Chest

Patient Selection

Percutaneous chest biopsy is performed for evaluation of nodules or masses in the lung, hilum, mediastinum, pleura, and chest wall.[26-28] In general, masses that involve lobar or segmental bronchi on chest radiography or CT suggest the presence of an endobronchial lesion, and these are best approached with bronchoscopy. On the other hand, peripherally located lesions are not that accessible with bronchoscopy and are easily reached with percutaneous biopsy. The most common indication for percutaneous chest biopsy is the diagnosis of a solitary pulmonary nodule (SPN), which is a rounded, well-defined mass of less than 3 cm that is largely surrounded by lung. Percutaneous biopsy, particularly core biopsy in conjunction with FNA, has been advocated for diagnosing pneumonia and diseases that mimic pneumonia (i.e., bronchiolitis obliterans organizing pneumonia, neoplasms [lymphoma, bronchoalveolar cell carcinoma], eosinophilic pneumonia, vasculitis [Wegener's granulomatosis]).[27] Percutaneous biopsy should be strictly avoided

with suspected vascular lesions (e.g., arteriovenous malformation, pulmonary varix) and *Echinococcus* cysts. Relative contraindications to lung biopsy include severe obstructive pulmonary disease, moderate to severe pulmonary hypertension, contralateral pneumonectomy, ventilator dependence, and inability to cooperate with breathing instructions. These patients are at increased risk of or are less able to tolerate pneumothorax after biopsy.

The workup of pulmonary lesions varies significantly among institutions with regard to the use of percutaneous needle biopsy or surgical resection for an SPN. The probability that an SPN represents a primary lung tumor rather than a metastasis from a known malignancy depends largely on the primary tumor type (e.g., 1:1.2 for colon cancer, 3.3:1 for breast cancer, 3.3:1 for bladder cancer, and 8.3:1 for head and neck cancers).[26] The false-negative rate for needle biopsy in patients with malignancy is relatively high (up to one third of procedures).[28,29] The cases in which clinical suspicion of malignancy is high require repeat biopsy or close follow-up. In some centers, a potentially malignant SPN in a low-risk operative patient often is resected without prior needle biopsy.

Technique

CT is helpful in planning all chest biopsies. CT can identify the most accessible lung lesion or an extrapulmonary mass that can be biopsied more safely (e.g., liver or adrenal gland). CT also outlines bullae that should be avoided to reduce the likelihood of postbiopsy pneumothorax.

Sonography can be used for some pleural or pleural-based masses. Fluoroscopy-guided chest biopsies are greatly facilitated with the use of a C-arm (see Fig. 4-2). The needle and hub are aligned with the lesion in one view while the needle is placed initially through the skin. The tube is then rotated into the orthogonal projection as the needle is advanced to the proper depth within the lesion. Aspiration of material is performed under direct fluoroscopic visualization, with spot images documenting needle position in various projections. The technique for CT biopsy is described above in the CT section. Anterior mediastinal masses can be approached through the sternum[30] (see Fig. 4-6). With very large mediastinal masses a parasternal approach can be used, keeping in mind the course of the internal mammary arteries (Fig. 4-11). Artificial widening of the extrapleural (paravertebral or substernal) space by injection of saline has been used to facilitate biopsy of lesions located in the posterior or anterior mediastinum.[31] An alternative approach to mediastinal lesions avoids visceral pleural traversal by using an existing pleural effusion or an iatrogenically created pneumothorax.[32]

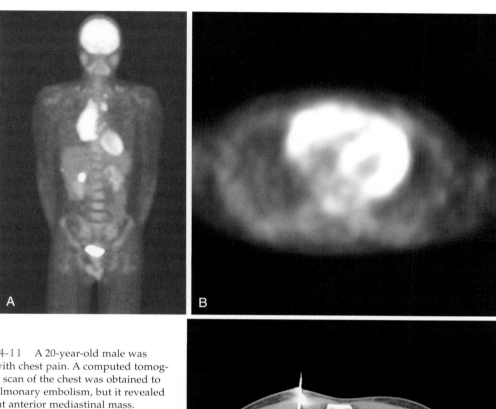

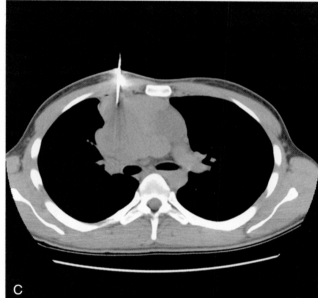

FIGURE 4-11   A 20-year-old male was admitted with chest pain. A computed tomography (CT) scan of the chest was obtained to exclude pulmonary embolism, but it revealed a large right anterior mediastinal mass. **A,** A whole-body positron emission tomography (PET) scan in coronal projection shows intense uptake along the right mediastinal border. **B,** Axial PET scan confirms the intense uptake of the right anterior mediastinal mass. Also note uptake in cardiac structures. **C,** CT image of biopsy procedure that was performed with coaxial 22- and 20-gauge needles for cytology and several passes with an 18-gauge coring needle. It is imperative to identify the location of the internal mammary artery using this approach so that it is not compromised. The final diagnosis was Hodgkin lymphoma.

If a significant pneumothorax occurs, a chest tube can be placed and the biopsy procedure continued or postponed (see later). Upright chest radiographs are obtained after the procedure (e.g., immediately and 4 hours after) to exclude a pneumothorax.

Results

Percutaneous needle biopsy of the chest is 80% to 95% accurate in the diagnosis of malignant lesions with a lower yield for benign lesions.[27-29,33] The probability of malignancy is partly a function of size[34] (Table 4-1). Patients with a nonspecific biopsy result need close

TABLE 4-1   Relationship Between Pulmonary Nodule Size and Malignancy

Diameter of Solitary Pulmonary Nodule (cm)	Malignant (%)
0-1	36
1-2	51
2-3	82
>3	97

follow-up, with repeat imaging and possible repeat percutaneous biopsy.

Complications

The most common complication of lung biopsy is pneumothorax, which occurs in 10% to 35% of cases.[28] The risk of pneumothorax is increased with preexisting lung disease (smoking), smaller lesion size, no history of prior thoracic surgery, and advanced age.[35] Nearly all pneumothoraces appear on the 1-hour postbiopsy chest film, and essentially all are detected on radiographs obtained 4 hours after biopsy.[36]

Most cases can be managed conservatively; repeat films are obtained to document stability, reduction, or resolution of the pneumothorax. Treatment is required for about 5% to 15% of patients, based on development of symptoms, an enlarging pneumothorax, or pneumothorax that occupies more than 25% of the hemithorax. Some pneumothoraces respond to simple aspiration with a plastic cannula.[37,38] In a minority of cases, however, a chest drainage tube is required.

For chest tube placement, anterior access is gained through the second intercostal space in the midclavicular line. A direct trocar technique is used to place an 8- to 10-French (Fr) chest tube if a large pneumothorax is present to expedite treatment. Smaller pneumothoraces can be treated using the Seldinger method as well. Air is removed by aspiration, Pleur-Evac device, or Heimlich valve. Some operators clamp the tube (or place to water seal) soon after placement and remove it if the pneumothorax does not recur soon thereafter. Otherwise, patients are admitted overnight.

Additional complications include pulmonary hemorrhage, hemothorax (Fig. 4-12), hemoptysis, malignant needle tract seeding, and systemic air embolism[39,40] (Fig. 4-13). If significant pulmonary hemorrhage occurs, the patient should be turned so that the biopsied side is down, keeping the hemorrhage outside of the unaffected healthy lung. Systemic air embolism is a rare (<0.07%), potentially fatal complication. The formation of a communication between an airway and a pulmonary vein is one assumed mechanism of air embolism

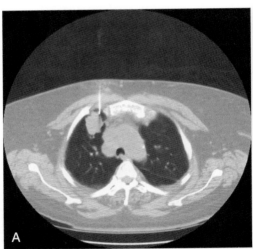
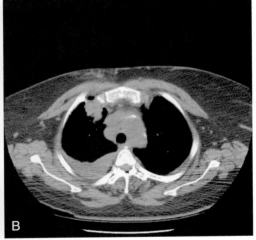
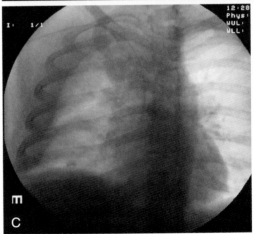

FIGURE 4-12 A 54-year-old female patient with a 20 pack-year history of smoking was admitted with a right upper lobe lung mass and right hilar and mediastinal lymphadenopathy. She was sent for percutaneous lung biopsy. She had thrombocytopenia and was given platelet transfusions. **A,** Computed tomography (CT) image shows the course of the needle, which is right parasternal and into the right upper lobe lesion. **B,** A postbiopsy CT image of the chest showed no pneumothorax, but there was interval development of pleural effusion with attenuation similar to that of muscle consistent with hemothorax. **C,** Plain chest radiograph confirms the hemothorax, which was evacuated with chest tube insertion. Treatment options at this point may include angiography to attempt to identify the bleeding site, such as an intercostal or internal mammary artery, which could be embolized. She was found to have small cell lung cancer.

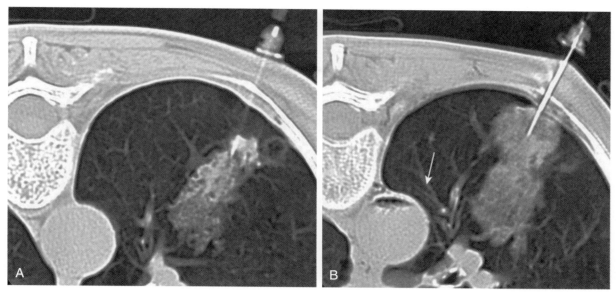

FIGURE 4-13   A 77-year-old woman with a long history of cigarette smoking and emphysema and on home oxygen use was found
to have a left lower lobe pulmonary nodule. She was referred for percutaneous lung biopsy. **A,** Computed tomography (CT) image during
the biopsy, performed with the patient in a prone position, shows the needle in the lesion with pulmonary hemorrhage extending
anteriorly from the lesion. **B,** The patient had an uncontrolled episode of coughing during which air was aspirated into the needle. She had
a grand mal seizure. A repeat CT scan of the chest demonstrates air within the thoracic aorta *(arrow),* intercostal, and spinal arteries. She
responded to supportive measures and was found to have a lung adenocarcinoma, which was treated with radiation therapy (she was not
a surgical candidate).

during biopsy. An uncooperative patient who coughs
during the biopsy procedure may contribute to pulmonary venous air by increasing air pressure in the
bronchial tree. Another source of air emboli is transient
position of the needle tip in a pulmonary vein. Finally,
it is conceivable that air introduced into the pulmonary arterial circulation may pass through the lung
microcirculation and into the pulmonary veins. Embolized air bubbles can cause stroke, transient ischemic
attack, myocardial ischemia, or even cardiac arrest.
Hyperbaric oxygen is one possible treatment modality
for such cases.[41]

Liver

Patient Selection

Liver biopsy may be performed by an operative, percutaneous, or transvenous route. Surgical biopsy is
indicated when an abdominal operation is planned regardless of the biopsy results. Percutaneous techniques
are used to obtain fine-needle aspirates for cytology
and core biopsy; the latter is required when architec-
tural detail is needed for diagnosis and staging of diffuse liver diseases. Transvenous liver biopsy is used for
nonfocal biopsies (e.g., staging cirrhosis) in patients
with coagulation disorders, massive ascites, portal hypertension, morbid obesity, or large vascular tumors
(see Chapter 12). Reports differ about the relative
safety of percutaneous biopsy in patients with massive
ascites.[42]

Technique

The primary indication for percutaneous liver biopsy is
the diagnosis of focal liver lesions (Box 4-1). Liver biopsy
is performed with image guidance to evaluate diffuse liver
disease such as hepatitis and cirrhosis. Hepatic masses
can be approached with ultrasound or CT, including CT
fluoroscopy (see Fig. 4-7). Real-time imaging with sonography greatly facilitates the procedure (see Figs. 4-4 and
4-5). CT is necessary for lesions that are not well seen by
ultrasound. CT of small liver lesions is affected by respiratory motion, although this problem is minimized with
spiral techniques. Many hepatic masses that require
biopsy lie deep to the lower ribs and the pleural space.
When possible, a subcostal approach should be chosen to
avoid traversing the pleura and producing a pneumothorax. A steep subcostal approach combined with deep
inspiration often is required to reach lesions high on the
dome of the liver. Ultrasound is preferred in this case, because sufficient gantry angulation with CT usually is not
possible. An intercostal, transpleural approach avoiding
aerated lung can be done with CT with a small risk of
pneumothorax.[43] Recognition of colonic interposition (i.e.,
Chilaiditi syndrome) also is important when planning a
liver biopsy (Fig. 4-14).

Aspiration biopsy for cytologic analysis is sufficient
for many focal hepatic lesions. However, core biopsy is
required for the diagnosis of certain liver tumors and
generalized liver disease.[44]

Care should be taken to traverse at least 1 to 2 cm
of normal liver parenchyma to reach any pathologic

BOX 4-1

FOCAL LESIONS
OF THE LIVER

Benign Lesions

- Simple cyst*
- Cavernous hemangioma*
- Focal nodular hyperplasia*
- Regenerating nodule
- Adenoma*
- Focal fatty replacement*
- Amebic abscess†
- Pyogenic abscess
- Echinococcal cyst*†
- Hematoma*
- Infarct
- Pseudoaneurysm*

Malignant Lesions

- Hepatocellular carcinoma*†
- Cholangiocarcinoma
- Metastases
- Lymphoma
- Angiosarcoma

*Imaging alone may provide a diagnosis.
†Laboratory studies (e.g., serology) may aid the diagnosis.

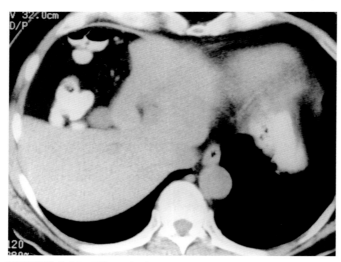

FIGURE 4-14 Effect of colonic position on percutaneous liver biopsy. The initial biopsy to exclude hemochromatosis was performed without imaging guidance and was nondiagnostic. The proximal portion of the right colon is interposed between the right lobe of the liver and the hemidiaphragm. Biopsy through this route is relatively unsafe.

liver lesion to decrease the likelihood of extracapsular hemorrhage. [20]

Results

A retrospective study of 510 percutaneous liver biopsies using cytology alone showed a 1% frequency of nondiagnostic biopsies and a 94% sensitivity and a 93% specificity for tumor.[45] False-positive results occurred in 18 cases (7% of all benign lesions), and false-negative results occurred in 14 cases (5% of all malignant lesions). Cytologic liver biopsy may be limited for the following reasons:

- Inherent pathologic similarity of hemangioma, focal nodular hyperplasia, and hepatic adenoma to well-differentiated hepatocellular carcinoma
- Reactive changes in hepatocytes related to acute and chronic inflammation or infection mimicking malignant cells
- Liver cirrhosis and parasitic infections failing to yield a cytologic diagnosis

Most hemangiomas can be diagnosed with scintigraphy, MRI, or CT scanning. Suspected hemangiomas can be biopsied safely when small needles are used (e.g., 20 to 25 gauge) and the needle passes through a normal parenchymal track en route to the lesion.[20,46] Biopsy of hemangiomas most often yields blood. The presence of endothelial cells suggests hemangioma; the finding of capillary vessels in conjunction with blood and endothelial cells is diagnostic (Fig. 4-15).

Ultrasound-guided biopsy of portal venous thrombi is safe and effective.[47] The procedure is aided by color flow imaging.

Complications

The major complications of percutaneous liver biopsy are bleeding, pneumothorax, malignant needle track seeding, and infection. Although rare, fatal hemorrhage can result, particularly after biopsy of a hemangioma or hypervascular neoplasm. Hemorrhagic complications from liver biopsy of diffuse liver diseases are less common than with biopsy of malignant lesions. Bleeding usually occurs within several hours of the procedure and often can be managed conservatively.[48] Hemorrhage may occur into the peritoneum or into the biliary system (i.e., hemobilia). Less than 5% of outpatient liver biopsy patients requires admission. At Doppler sonography, a "patent track" sign after liver biopsy (particularly if persistent for more than 5 minutes) strongly predicts postbiopsy bleeding.[49]

The most common signs of significant bleeding are abdominal or shoulder pain and hemodynamic instability. When clinical suspicion arises, serial hematocrits and CT or ultrasound imaging should be obtained. Suspicion for hemobilia should be raised if clinical

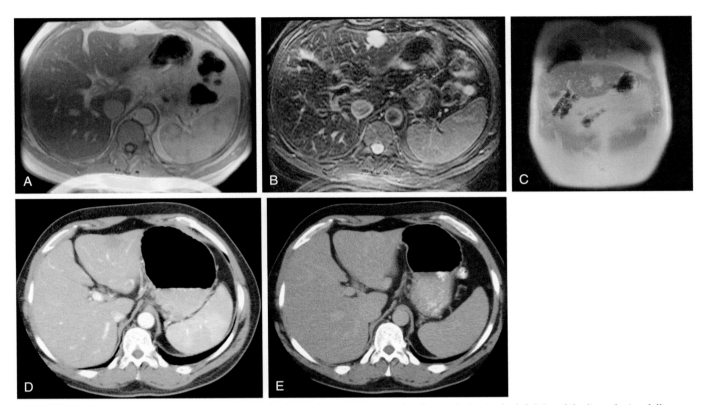

FIGURE 4-15 A 67-year-old man with a history of colorectal cancer was found to have a lesion in the left lobe of the liver during follow-up imaging. Axial T1- and T2-weighted and coronal T1 MR images of the liver (**A, B,** and **C**) were thought to be atypical for hemangioma, and biopsy was suggested. Computed tomography (CT) images in arterial and delayed phases confirm the CT findings (**D** and **E**). A biopsy was performed with ultrasound and the diagnosis was hemangioma. There was no postbiopsy bleeding.

symptoms are present, but no definite hemorrhage is noted on imaging. Subtle findings such as high attenuating material in the gallbladder on CT is also important for diagnosis. In patients who continue to bleed, angiography and transcatheter embolization may be required to control bleeding. Needle track seeding is less frequent than with biopsy of the pancreas. Fatal carcinoid crisis has been reported after biopsy of liver metastases.[50]

Adrenal Gland (Online Case 69)

Patient Selection

Percutaneous biopsy is used for diagnosing focal lesions of the adrenal gland. The most common adrenal masses are nonfunctioning adenomas and metastases[51] (Box 4-2). Adrenal adenomas are seen in as many as 5% of patients undergoing CT for unrelated reasons. In an asymptomatic patient with an adrenal mass, the size of the mass and the presence or absence of a primary malignancy must be considered in determining the need for biopsy. When adrenal lesions are larger than 3 cm, the likelihood of malignancy is significant. Even in patients with a known primary and an adrenal lesion, the likelihood of a positive biopsy is only about 50%. In some cases, nonfunctioning adenomas can be diagnosed confidently by CT (noncontrast CT with threshold values to detect low attenuation or contrast washout methods) or chemical shift MRI without the need for tissue sampling. Application of these cross-sectional methods has reduced the number of adrenal biopsies yielding benign diagnoses to less than 12% in patients with extraadrenal malignancies.[52] When adrenal masses larger than 1 cm are detected in patients undergoing imaging procedures for nonadrenal problems, these lesions are called adrenal *incidentalomas*.[53] Guidelines have been published to help in workup of these lesions.[54,55] Functioning cortical adenomas and pheochromocytomas are best characterized by means of biochemical assays. All hormonally active tumors causing Conn syndrome (aldosterone hypersecretion) are resected after confirmation by adrenal vein sampling (see Chapter 13). Inactive tumors are resected based on size, imaging characteristics, and interval growth. Percutaneous biopsy of these incidentalomas is generally not warranted.

Technique

Adrenal masses often are best approached from the back, respecting the location of pleural reflections. Other routes include a transhepatic approach for right-sided

---

BOX 4-2

FOCAL LESIONS OF THE ADRENAL GLANDS

Unilateral Lesions

- Metastases
- Primary adenocarcinoma
- Benign adenoma*†
  - Functional
  - Nonfunctional
- Pheochromocytoma†
- Neuroblastoma
- Myelolipoma*
- Adrenal cyst*

Bilateral Lesions

- Metastases
- Hemorrhage*
- Tuberculosis or histoplasmosis
- Bilateral pheochromocytoma†

*Imaging alone may provide a diagnosis.
†Laboratory studies may aid the diagnosis.

BOX 4-3

FOCAL LESIONS OF THE PANCREAS

Neoplastic Lesions

- Ductal adenocarcinoma
- Islet cell (neuroendocrine) tumor
- Cystic neoplasm
- Papilloma (intraductal)
- Lymphoma
- Sarcoma or other mesenchymal tumor

Nonneoplastic Lesions

- Focal pancreatitis
- Abscess
- Hemorrhage (including pseudoaneurysms)
- Pseudocyst
- Fluid collection
- Hydatid cysts

---

lesions and an anterior approach for left-sided lesions; the latter route is associated with a 6% incidence of pancreatitis.[56]

Results and Complications

In a large study of percutaneous biopsy of adrenal masses, the reported sensitivity was 93%, accuracy was 96%, and the negative predictive value was 91%.[57] Repeat biopsy was recommended in cases in which the sample did not contain benign adrenal tissue or malignant cells. Adrenal adenoma and adrenocortical carcinoma may be difficult to distinguish histopathologically. If a discrepancy exists between the imaging and pathology results, surgical intervention may be advocated.

The complication rate after adrenal biopsy is 1% to 11%. The most common complication is pneumothorax. Postprocedure chest radiographs may be obtained to exclude this possibility. Other adverse events include bleeding, pancreatitis, hemothorax, and, rarely, precipitation of a hypertensive crisis from biopsy of an unsuspected pheochromocytoma.[58] Reported complications from biopsy of pheochromocytomas have included transient headaches, labile blood pressures, abdominal pain, hemodynamic instability, uncontrolled hemorrhage, and death. Because pheochromocytoma has no specific imaging features, the diagnosis is based on clinical suspicion with confirmatory testing via a 24-hour urine collection for catecholamines (and their breakdown products) or serum catecholamines.

Pancreas

The differential diagnosis of pancreatic masses is wide (Box 4-3). Pancreatic biopsies are often safely and easily performed by endoscopic ultrasound. Operative candidates undergo biopsy at that time. Percutaneous pancreatic biopsy is performed for diagnosis of suspected pancreatic neoplasm in nonoperable patients or when endoscopic biopsy is unsuccessful.

Pancreatic biopsy is performed with CT or ultrasound guidance. If the stomach or small bowel lies along the anticipated needle pathway, small-caliber needles (e.g., 20 to 22 gauge) should be used. A posterior transcaval approach to pancreatic biopsy of lesions in or near the head of the pancreas has recently been described.[14]

Historically, the overall yield for percutaneous biopsy diagnosis of pancreatic malignancy is about 80%.[10] These modest results are related to the scirrhous nature of the tumor and the surrounding desmoplastic, inflammatory reaction. More recent series have reported accuracies of 86% and 95% for CT and ultrasound-guided biopsy, respectively.[59] The higher success with ultrasound guidance may relate to the better lesional conspicuity of pancreatic lesions with ultrasound. CT with contrast may improve the accuracy of pancreatic biopsy findings. Results are better for larger lesions (>3 cm) with larger needles (16- to

19-gauge) and when the lesion is located in the body or tail of the gland.[59] In addition to standard cytologic evaluation of tissue, fluid analysis for viscosity, enzymes, and tumor markers may be valuable for cystic lesions.[60]

Complications develop after approximately 3% of procedures and include hemorrhage, pancreatitis, and pancreatic duct fistulas. Pancreatitis may be more common after biopsy of a normal gland.[61] Because rapid intraabdominal spread of disease has been described after intraoperative biopsy of pancreatic tumors, some surgeons believe that percutaneous biopsy should be avoided if curative resection is planned. Track seeding from needle biopsy has been reported, but it is rare.[62]

Kidney

Patient Selection

Renal disorders may be divided into diffuse processes that produce chronic kidney disease (CKD) and focal mass lesions.[63] Large-core biopsy for CKD often is performed by a nephrologist, with limited imaging guidance. Occasionally, a radiologist is asked to perform such a biopsy when the nephrologist is unable to obtain adequate material. Percutaneous kidney biopsy by an interventional radiologist has several established indications (Box 4-4).

The expanded role of percutaneous biopsy of small renal masses has been influenced by advances in cytology, immunocytochemistry, and cytogenetics and by refinement of local ablative techniques and nephron sparing surgery.[64]

Technique

Biopsy of focal renal masses is usually performed with ultrasound guidance.[63] CT is required when the mass is difficult to visualize with sonography (Fig. 4-16). A posterior approach is used.

Biopsy for CKD and transplantation complications usually is performed with ultrasound guidance. Biopsy of the lower pole is preferred to avoid vessels in the renal hilum or possible injury to the liver or spleen. Large-core samples (with 16- to 18-gauge usually automated devices) are required to obtain the 5 to 10 glomeruli needed for diagnosis.[65-67] Transjugular renal biopsy can be applied in patients at high risk for bleeding complications.[68]

Results and Complications

Using 18-gauge needles, a diagnosis is established in 85% to 95% of patients with chronic kidney disease.[63]

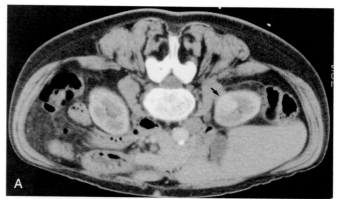
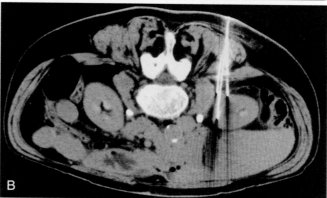

FIGURE 4-16 Computed tomography (CT)-guided kidney biopsy. **A,** CT in the prone position shows a hyperdense right renal mass *(arrow)* in a patient with cutaneous melanoma. Grid bars are taped to the skin over the lesion. **B,** Three passes were made with 22-gauge Chiba needles. The outer needles missed the lesion but were left in place to assist with accurate placement of the third needle just beyond the mass.

BOX 4-4

INDICATIONS FOR KIDNEY BIOPSY

Established

- Chronic kidney disease when imaging is difficult (e.g., obese patients, atrophic kidneys) or initial biopsy is inadequate
- Focal renal mass in a patient with underlying malignancy
- Focal renal mass in a nonoperative patient
- Focal renal mass in a patient with fever of unknown origin

Emerging

- Small (≤3 cm) solid renal mass
- Renal mass being considered for percutaneous ablation
- Indeterminant cystic renal mass

Complications follow about 1% to 6% of percutaneous renal biopsies.[65,69] After biopsy, small arteriovenous fistulas and pseudoaneurysms are relatively common. Many of these close spontaneously without the need for treatment. Significant hematomas with falling hematocrit levels and persistent gross hematuria are uncommon. A prospective study of biopsies for chronic kidney disease in 471 patients found that 161 patients (34.1%) experienced postbiopsy bleeding (33.3% hematomas, 0.4% gross hematuria, 0.4% arteriovenous fistula).[70] Major complications occurred in six patients (1.2%), with two requiring blood transfusions, three requiring angiograms, and one requiring nephrectomy. There were no deaths. Angiographic evaluation and transcatheter embolization are required occasionally for treatment of bleeding that does not stop with conservative measures.

Other Abdominal and Pelvic Sites (Online Case 30)

Splenic biopsy is rarely performed because focal masses are uncommon. Although there is particular concern about splenic hemorrhage, biopsy with 20- to 22-gauge Chiba or spinal needles is relatively safe.[71] Biopsy may be performed with CT or ultrasound guidance. The largest, most superficial lesion usually is chosen; the splenic hilum, colon, kidney, lung, and pleura should be avoided. Hemorrhage is the most common complication (typically 0 to 1.5% but as high as 10% of patients); other complications include pneumothorax, pleural effusion, and colonic injury.

Retroperitoneal masses can be approached from an anterior or posterior route. The major disadvantage of the anterior approach is that bowel may be traversed. However, this route is reasonable if cytologic analysis using small-caliber needles is sufficient. If lymphoma is suspected, core biopsy may be required for immunocytochemical studies, flow cytometry, cytogenetic analysis, or molecular studies, and a posterior route is preferable. Biopsies of almost all retroperitoneal masses are conducted under CT or ultrasound guidance.

Metastatic lymphadenopathy from tumors of the gastrointestinal and genitourinary tracts can be diagnosed in about 65% to 90% of cases.[72] Historically, the diagnostic accuracy of percutaneous biopsy in patients with lymphoma is about 20% lower than for nonlymphomatous retroperitoneal lesions. Later series reported higher success rates.[73] A negative percutaneous biopsy cannot entirely exclude a malignant process. If several properly performed biopsy attempts fail to provide a cytologic or histologic diagnosis, an excisional biopsy may be required. The yield for rare malignant forms of retroperitoneal fibrosis is relatively low, and surgical biopsy often is needed to identify the diffusely dispersed malignant cells that are characteristic of this condition.[74]

Peritoneal soft tissue masses and mesenteric lymphadenopathy are amenable to percutaneous biopsy techniques. Ultrasound guidance greatly facilitates biopsy of these entities.[75] Such lesions often are better visualized by external compression with the ultrasound transducer to displace bowel loops overlying the mass. Deeper lesions can be approached with CT (Fig. 4-17). Biopsy of peritoneal masses poses a small risk of ileus or peritonitis (<1%).

Pelvic lymphadenopathy or soft tissue masses can be approached through transperitoneal (anterior or transgluteal), extraperitoneal, transvaginal, or transrectal routes. The transvaginal approach is useful especially for biopsy of primary or recurrent adnexal or ovarian masses.[76] For diagnosis of metastatic prostate cancer, CT-guided biopsy with thin section CT is accurate in up to 97% of cases.[77]

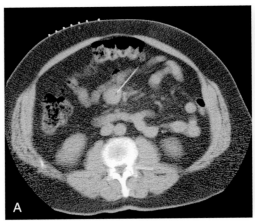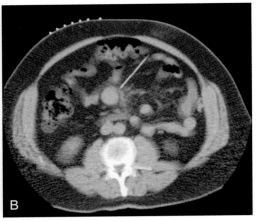

FIGURE 4-17   An 80-year-old man with abdominal pain was found to have lymphadenopathy that slowly enlarged on serial computed tomography (CT) scans of the abdomen. **A** and **B,** CT-guided biopsy shows percutaneous biopsy performed around surrounding adjacent bowel loops.

Presacral masses in patients who have undergone abdominoperineal resection can be evaluated with percutaneous biopsy. Although such masses are not uncommon in postoperative patients, a rising carcinoembryonic antigen level or asymmetric thickening of the presacral space may indicate recurrence. These lesions are accessed easily through a transgluteal approach, taking care to avoid the sciatic nerve running in the anterior third of the greater sciatic notch.

Percutaneous biopsy techniques also can be applied to a variety of uncommon intraabdominal or intrapelvic lesions, including omental cakes, mesenteric root masses, and mucosal lesions of the stomach, bile ducts, or urinary tract (Fig. 4-18).

Thyroid (Online Case 40)

Patient Selection

Thyroid nodules are the most common pathologic finding in the thyroid gland.[78] In general, about 4% to 7% of the population of the United States has clinically palpable thyroid nodules. The incidence of thyroid nodules increases with age and is more prevalent in females of all ages. Autopsy studies indicate that clinical examination has limited ability to detect nodules, particularly smaller nodules and nodules situated deeper within the thyroid gland. Several studies also have shown that ultrasound reveals occult nodules in about 50% patients who have a normal thyroid gland on physical examination.[78] Many nodules come to attention as a result of other diagnostic imaging studies, such as chest CT, carotid sonography, and cervical spine MRI. Less than 5% of thyroid nodules are malignant.

Thyroid cancer is the most common malignancy of the endocrine system, with more than 80% representing papillary thyroid carcinoma. More than 37,000 new cases of thyroid cancer were expected to be diagnosed in the United States in 2009, with 163 deaths expected to be attributable to thyroid cancer.[79] Risk factors for thyroid cancer include family history of thyroid malignancy, a history of prior head and neck radiation, age younger than 30 years or older than 60 years, and patients with multiple endocrine neoplasia type 2.[80]

Clearly, there is a need to differentiate the uncommon but important thyroid carcinoma from the common, insignificant thyroid nodule (Table 4-2). However, there is much overlap in the ultrasonographic appearance of benign and malignant nodules[81] (Fig. 4-19). Ultrasonographic features suggesting malignancy include a solid, hypoechoic nodule; punctate calcifications; a poorly defined, indistinct, or blurred lesional margin; direct invasion of the nodule through the thyroid capsule; and central rather than peripheral vascularity within the lesion.[78,82] Hyperechoic nodules, cystic nodules, and nodules with complete halos are typically benign. Size of a nodule is not a reliable indicator of the benign or malignant nature of thyroid nodules. In most cases, FNA biopsy of the thyroid can differentiate benign nodules from thyroid neoplasms, which has reduced the number of patients undergoing surgical excision of benign nodules. Several criteria are available for determining

TABLE 4-2   Differential Diagnosis of Thyroid Nodules

Benign	Malignant
Hyperplastic nodule; adenomatous nodule	Primary (papillary, follicular, Hürthle, medullary, anaplastic)
Follicular or Hürthle cell adenoma	Metastases (renal, breast, melanoma)
Lymphocytic thyroiditis	Lymphoma
Cyst (pure cyst is rare: <3%)	

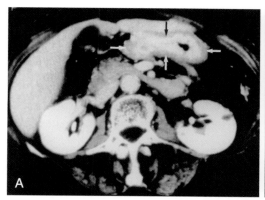
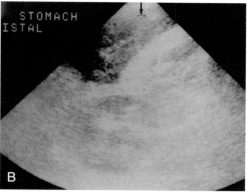

FIGURE 4-18   Percutaneous gastric wall biopsy. The patient had multiple negative endoscopic gastric biopsies. The upper gastrointestinal series had a linitis plastica appearance. **A,** Computed tomography scan shows diffuse gastric wall thickening *(arrows)*. **B,** The biopsy under sonographic guidance *(arrow)* revealed signet cell–positive gastric carcinoma.

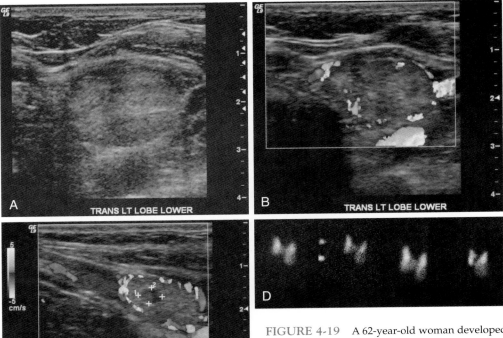

FIGURE 4-19   A 62-year-old woman developed hoarseness and had a thyroid ultrasound demonstrating a left lower pole thyroid nodule (**A, B,** and **C**). **D,** A nuclear medicine thyroid scan performed 6 hours after oral administration of 232 μCi I[123] demonstrated a cold nodule in the lower left pole. A percutaneous aspiration of the left lower pole nodule with several passes with 25-gauge needles revealed a follicular neoplasm.

whether a nodule should be biopsied. The three most popular ones are the Kim criteria, American Association of Clinical Endocrinologists criteria, and the Society of Radiologists in Ultrasound criteria.[80,83,84] One recent study suggests that the former two protocols are more accurate than the latter one.[85]

Technique

The patient lies supine on a stretcher. Neck extension aids in visualizing the thyroid gland, which is obtained by placing a rolled towel behind the patient's lower neck. Sonography is performed with a high-frequency (8 to 15 MHz) linear array transducer to localize the nodule to be biopsied. A sterile ultrasound probe is set up and sterile gel placed on the patient's neck. After local anesthesia is applied, a 3-cm, 25-gauge needle is then placed into the lesion with continuous sonographic visualization. Specimens may be obtained by either a nonaspiration or an aspiration technique. The patient is instructed to refrain from talking, breathing, or swallowing while the biopsy is being performed. With the nonaspiration technique, cells are pulled into the needle by capillary effect. With this technique, the biopsy is performed by moving the needle back and forth vigorously through the nodule until bloody material is seen at the hub of the needle. The suction aspiration technique

is performed by connecting a 10-mL syringe to the 25-gauge needle with connecting tubing. A similar biopsy motion is used while suction is applied with 1- to 2-mL aspiration of the syringe. The samples are placed onto a slide. If the gross appearance of the smear appears scant, additional passes (up to 6 or 8) should be made, assessing different parts of the nodule to increase the biopsy yield. Some investigators have used 20- and 22-gauge cutting-needle biopsy guns for lesions that are hypocellular, particularly if the lesion is larger than 1 cm.

Results and Complications

Reported rates of diagnostic accuracy range from 85% to 95%.[78,86] The use of thyroid FNA biopsy has been shown to reduce the number of thyroidectomies by approximately 50%, roughly double the surgical yield of carcinoma, and reduce the overall cost of medical care in these patients by 25%. The yield from biopsy of cystic thyroid nodules is lower, with about 39% of cases yielding unsatisfactory cytologic results.[87] The appropriate action following a nondiagnostic biopsy is controversial. Follow-up is at the discretion of the referring physician. Management options include repeat biopsy, surgery, or close imaging surveillance. One study found that repeat biopsy of such cases revealed malignant lesions in about half of the cases.[88] These authors suggested that operators wait at least 3 months before repeating the biopsy because needle-induced reparative cellular atypia complicates subsequent cytologic diagnosis. The complication rate from thyroid biopsy is less than 1% and most relate to small hematomas.[80]

METHODS TO REACH INACCESSIBLE LESIONS

In general, the shortest path between skin and lesion is chosen for percutaneous biopsy, but occasionally this may not be possible because of interposed bowel, bone, lung, pleura, or major vessels. Techniques to overcome these problems are described earlier, including transsternal biopsies, displacement of structures by injected fluid or carbon dioxide, and manual compression with an ultrasound transducer. The "triangulation method" was described by vanSonnenberg in 1981 as a method to solve cranial or caudal angled approaches to lesions.[89] This technique uses the Pythagorean theorem or lengths of triangles to calculate the proper cranial or caudal angles. In certain cases, angling the gantry may solve these cranial-caudal angulation problems, which is particularly helpful when the ribs cover subpleural pulmonary masses.

A few studies have described use of custom-made curved needles to access lesions with interposed structures[72,90] (Fig. 4-20). In one method, a 20- to 23-gauge needle is introduced with fluoroscopic guidance in a direction away from the lesion to avoid the interposed structure, and gradual change is made in direction of the needle insertion when the curved part of the needle has been inserted so that the lesion is accessed. Repeat biopsies with this technique require additional needles because this approach is coaxial. A second method employs a coaxial technique with custom bent thin-walled 19-gauge needles that are then inserted with CT or MR fluoroscopy. A 21-gauge needle is advanced through the arc-shaped, outer 19-gauge needle to perform the biopsy. A variation is to use a straight 18-gauge needle through which a curved 22-gauge needle is advanced.[14]

References

1. Bret PM, Fond A, Casola G, et al. Abdominal lesions: a prospective study of clinical efficacy of percutaneous fine-needle biopsy. *Radiology* 1986;**159**(2):345.
2. Hopper KD. Percutaneous, radiographically guided biopsy: a history. *Radiology* 1995;**196**(2):329.
3. Reading CC, Charboneau JW, James EM, Hurt MR. Sonographically guided percutaneous biopsy of small (3 cm or less) masses. *AJR Am J Roentgenol* 1988;**151**(1):189.
4. Charboneau JW, Reading CC, Welch TJ. CT and sonographically guided needle biopsy: current techniques and new innovations. *AJR Am J Roentgenol* 1990;**154**(1):1.
5. Silverman SG, Mueller PR, Pfister RC. Hemostatic evaluation before abdominal interventions: an overview and proposal. *AJR Am J Roentgenol* 1990;**154**(2):233.
6. Shapiro M. Approach to the patient with a coagulopathy. *J Vasc Interv Radiol* 1996;**7**:73.
7. Malloy PC, Grassi CJ, Kundu S, Gervais DA, Miller DL, Osnis RB, et al. Consensus guidelines for periprocedural management of coagulation status and hemostasis risk in percutaneous image-guided interventions. *J Vasc Interv Radiol* 2009;**20**(Suppl. 7): S240.
8. Fleisher LA, Beckman JA, Brown KA, Calkins H, Chaikof E, Fleischmann KE, et al. ACC/AHA 2007 Guidelines on perioperative cardiovascular evaluation and care for noncardiac surgery: executive summary. *Circulation* 2007;**116**(17):1971.
9. Brilakis ES, Banerjee S, Berger PB. Perioperative management of patients with coronary stents. *J Am Coll Cardiol* 2007;**49**(22): 2145.
10. Gazelle GS, Haaga JR. Guided percutaneous biopsy of intraabdominal lesions: *AJR Am J Roentgenol* 1989;**153**(5):929.
11. Matalon TA, Silver B. US guidance of interventional procedures. *Radiology* 1990;**174**(1):43.
12. Rose SC, Roberts AC, Kinney TB, Pretorius DH, Nelson TR. Three-dimensional ultrasonography for planning percutaneous drainage of complex abdominal fluid collections. *J Vasc Interv Radiol* 2003;**14**(4):451.
13. Katada K, Kato R, Anno H, Ogura Y, Koga S, Ida Y, et al. Guidance with real-time CT fluoroscopy: early clinical experience. *Radiology* 1996;**200**(3):851.
14. Gupta S. New techniques in image-guided percutaneous biopsy. *Cardiovasc Intervent Radiol* 2004;**27**(2):91.
15. Silverman SG, Tuncali K, Adams DF, Nawfel RD, Zou KH, Judy PF. CT fluoroscopy-guided abdominal interventions: techniques, results, and radiation exposure. *Radiology* 1999;**212**(3):673.
16. Carlson SK, Bender CE, Classic KL, Zink FE, Quam JP, Ward EM, et al. Benefits and safety of CT fluoroscopy in interventional radiologic procedures. *Radiology* 2001;**219**(2):515.
17. Silverman SG. Percutaneous abdominal biopsy: recent advances and future directions. *Semin Interv Radiol* 1996;**13**(01):3.
18. Wallace MJ, Gupta S, Hicks ME. Out-of-plane computed-tomography-guided biopsy using a magnetic-field-based navigation system. *Cardiovasc Intervent Radiol* 2006;**29**(1):108.

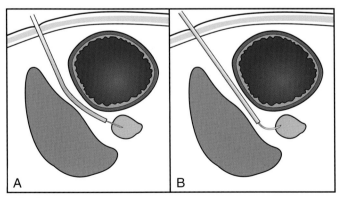

FIGURE 4-20 The use of curved needles to biopsy difficult to access lesions. A soft tissue mass is located medial to the iliac wing and posterior to the cecum. **A,** A thin-walled, curved, outer, 19-gauge needle is used to direct a thinner 21-gauge needle into the mass for biopsy. **B,** A straight 18- or 19-gauge needle is advanced proximal to the lesion. A 22-gauge needle with a bent tip is advanced through the straight needle into the lesion for biopsy. It is not possible to use a coring needle in this type of setup.

19. Wood BJ, Zhang H, Durrani A, Glossop N, Ranjan S, Lindisch D, et al. Navigation with electromagnetic tracking for interventional radiology procedures: a feasibility study. *J Vasc Interv Radiol* 2005;**16**(4):493.

20. Solbiati L, Livraghi T, Pra LD, Ierace T, Masciadri N, Ravetto C. Fine-needle biopsy of hepatic hemangioma with sonographic guidance. *AJR Am J Roentgenol* 1985;**144**(3):471.

21. Kinney TB, Lee MJ, Filomena CA, Krebs TL, Dawson SL, Smith PL, et al. Fine-needle biopsy: prospective comparison of aspiration versus nonaspiration techniques in the abdomen. *Radiology* 1993;**186**(2):549.

22. Dodd LG, Mooney EE, Layfield LJ, Nelson RC. Fine-needle aspiration of the liver and pancreas: a cytology primer for radiologists. *Radiology* 1997;**203**(1):1.

23. Hahn PF, Eisenberg PJ, Pitman MB, Gazelle GS, Mueller PR. Cytopathologic touch preparations (imprints) from core needle biopsies: accuracy compared with that of fine-needle aspirates. *AJR Am J Roentgenol* 1995;**165**(5):1277.

24. Chandan VS, Zimmerman K, Baker P, Scalzetti E, Khurana KK. Usefulness of core roll preparations in immediate assessment of neoplastic lung lesions: comparison to conventional CT scan-guided lung fine-needle aspiration cytology. *Chest* 2004;**126**(3): 739.

25. Liao WY, Jerng JS, Chen KY, Chang YL, Yang PC, Kuo SH. Value of imprint cytology for ultrasound-guided transthoracic core biopsy. *Eur Respir J* 2004;**24**(6):905.

26. Quint LE, Park CH, Iannettoni MD. Solitary pulmonary nodules in patients with extrapulmonary neoplasms. *Radiology* 2000;**217**(1): 257.

27. Thanos L, Galani P, Mylona S, Pomoni M, Mpatakis N. Percutaneous CT-guided core needle biopsy versus fine needle aspiration in diagnosing pneumonia and mimics of pneumonia. *Cardiovasc Intervent Radiol* 2004;**27**(4):329.

28. Perlmutt LM, Johnston WW, Dunnick NR. Percutaneous transthoracic needle aspiration: a review. *AJR Am J Roentgenol* 1989; **152**(3):451.

29. Calhoun P, Feldman PS, Armstrong P, Black WC, Pope TL, Minor GR, et al. The clinical outcome of needle aspirations of the lung when cancer is not diagnosed. *Ann Thorac Surg* 1986;**41**(6):592.

30. D'Agostino HB, Sanchez RB, Laoide RM, Oglevie S, Donaldson JS, Russack V, et al. Anterior mediastinal lesions: transsternal biopsy with CT guidance. Work in progress. *Radiology* 1993; **189**(3):703.

31. Langen HJ, Klose KC, Keulers P, Adam G, Jochims M, Günther RW. Artificial widening of the mediastinum to gain access for extrapleural biopsy: clinical results. *Radiology* 1995;**196**(3): 703.

32. Bressler EL, Kirkham JA. Mediastinal masses: alternative approaches to CT-guided needle biopsy. *Radiology* 1994;**191**(2):391.

33. Johnston WW. Percutaneous fine needle aspiration biopsy of the lung. A study of 1,015 patients. *Acta Cytol* 1984;**28**(3):218.

34. Zerhouni EA, Stitik FP, Siegelman SS, Naidich DP, Sagel SS, Proto AV, et al. CT of the pulmonary nodule: a cooperative study. *Radiology* 1986;**160**(2):319.

35. Covey AM, Gandhi R, Brody LA, Getrajdman G, Thaler HT, Brown KT. Factors associated with pneumothorax and pneumothorax requiring treatment after percutaneous lung biopsy in 443 consecutive patients. *J Vasc Interv Radiol* 2004; **15**(5):479.

36. Perlmutt LM, Braun SD, Newman GE, Oke EJ, Dunnick NR. Timing of chest film follow-up after transthoracic needle aspiration. *AJR* 1986;**146**:1049.

37. Yankelevitz DF, Davis SD, Henschke CI. Aspiration of a large pneumothorax resulting from transthoracic needle biopsy. *Radiology* 1996;**200**(3):695.

38. Yamagami T, Kato T, Iida S, Hirota T, Yoshimatsu R, Nishimura T. Efficacy of manual aspiration immediately after complicated pneumothorax in CT-guided lung biopsy. *J Vasc Interv Radiol* 2005;**16**(4):477.

39. Arnold BW, Zwiebel WJ. Percutaneous transthoracic needle biopsy complicated by air embolism. *AJR Am J Roentgenol* 2002;**178** (6):1400.

40. Cardella JF, Bakal CW, Bertino RE, Burke DR, Drooz A, Haskal Z, et al. Quality improvement guidelines for image-guided percutaneous biopsy in adults. *J Vasc Interv Radiol* 2003;**14**(9 (Pt. 2)):S227.

41. Ashizawa K, Watanabe H, Morooka H, Hayashi K. Hyperbaric oxygen therapy for air embolism complicating CT-guided needle biopsy of the lung. *AJR Am J Roentgenol* 2004;**182**(6):1606.

42. Murphy FB, Barefield KP, Steinberg HV, Bernardino ME. CT- or sonography-guided biopsy of the liver in the presence of ascites: frequency of complications. *AJR Am J Roentgenol* 1988;**151**(3): 485.

43. Gervais DA, Gazelle GS, Lu DS, Han PF, Mueller PR. Percutaneous transpulmonary CT-guided liver biopsy: a safe and technically easy approach for lesions located near the diaphragm. *AJR Am J Roentgenol* 1996;**167**(2):482.

44. Rivera-Sanfeliz G, Kinney TB, Rose SC, Agha AKM, Valji K, Miller FJ, et al. Single-pass percutaneous liver biopsy for diffuse liver disease using an automated device: experience in 154 procedures. *Cardiovasc Intervent Radiol* 2005;**28**(5):584.

45. Lüning M, Schröder K, Wolff H, Kranz D, Hoppe E. Percutaneous biopsy of the liver. *Cardiovasc Intervent Radiol* 1991;**14** (1):40.

46. Cronan JJ, Esparza AR, Dorfman GS, Ridlen MS, Paolella LP. Cavernous hemangioma of the liver: role of percutaneous biopsy. *Radiology* 1988;**166**(1 (Pt. 1)):135.

47. Withers CE, Casola G, Herba MJ, Viloria J. Intravascular tumors: transvenous biopsy. *Radiology* 1988;**167**(3):713.

48. Janes CH, Lindor KD. Outcome of patients hospitalized for complications after outpatient liver biopsy. *Ann Intern Med* 1993;**118**(2):96.

49. Kim KW, Kim MJ, Kim HC, Park SH, Kim SY, Park MS, et al. Value of "patent track" sign on Doppler sonography after percutaneous liver biopsy in detection of postbiopsy bleeding: a prospective study in 352 patients. *AJR Am J Roentgenol* 2007;**189** (1):109.

50. Bissonnette RT, Gibney RG, Berry BR, Buckley AR. Fatal carcinoid crisis after percutaneous fine-needle biopsy of hepatic metastasis: case report and literature review. *Radiology* 1990;**174**(3 (Pt. 1)): 751.

51. Dunnick NR, Korobkin M, Francis I. Adrenal radiology: distinguishing benign from malignant adrenal masses. *AJR Am J Roentgenol* 1996;**167**(4):861.

52. Paulsen SD, Nghiem HV, Korobkin M, Caoili EM, Higgins EJ. Changing role of imaging-guided percutaneous biopsy of adrenal masses: evaluation of 50 adrenal biopsies. *AJR Am J Roentgenol* 2004;**182**(4):1033.

53. Thompson GB, Young WF. Adrenal incidentaloma. *Curr Opin Oncol* 2003;**15**(1):84.

54. Berland LL, Silverman SG, Gore RM, et al. Managing incidental findings on abdominal CT: white paper on the ACR incidental findings committee. *J Am Coll Radiol* 2010;**7**:754.

55. Boland GW, Blake MA, Hahn PR, Mayo-Smity WW. Incidental adrenal lesions: principles, technique, and algorithms for imaging characterization. *Radiology* 2008;**249**:756.

56. Kane NM, Korobkin M, Francis IR, Quint LE, Cascade PN. Percutaneous biopsy of left adrenal masses: prevalence of pancreatitis after anterior approach. *AJR Am J Roentgenol* 1991;**157**(4):777.

57. Silverman SG, Mueller PR, Pinkney LP, Koenker RM, Seltzer SE. Predictive value of image-guided adrenal biopsy: analysis of results of 101 biopsies. *Radiology* 1993;**187**(3):715.

58. Casola G, Nicolet V, vanSonnenberg E, Withers C, Bretagnolle M, Saba RM, et al. Unsuspected pheochromocytoma: risk of blood-pressure alterations during percutaneous adrenal biopsy. *Radiology* 1986;**159**(3):733.

59. Brandt KR, Charboneau JW, Stephens DH, Welch TJ, Goellner JR. CT- and US-guided biopsy of the pancreas. *Radiology* 1993;**187**(1):99.

60. Lewandrowski K, Lee J, Southern J, Centeno B, Warshaw A. Cyst fluid analysis in the differential diagnosis of pancreatic cysts: a new approach to the preoperative assessment of pancreatic cystic lesions. *AJR Am J Roentgenol* 1995;**164**(4):815.

61. Smith EH. Complications of percutaneous abdominal fine-needle biopsy. Review. *Radiology* 1991;**178**(1):253.

62. Ferrucci JT, Wittenberg J, Margolies MN, Carey RW. Malignant seeding of the tract after thin-needle aspiration biopsy. *Radiology* 1979;**130**(2):345.

63. Vassiliades V, Bernardino M. Percutaneous renal and adrenal biopsies. *Cardiovasc Interv Radiol* 1991;**14**:50.

64. Silverman SG, Gan YU, Mortele KJ, Tuncali K, Cibas ES. Renal masses in the adult patient: the role of percutaneous biopsy. *Radiology* 2006;**240**(1):6.

65. Mostbeck GH, Wittich GR, Derfler K, Ulrich W, Walter RM, Herold C, et al. Optimal needle size for renal biopsy: in vitro and in vivo evaluation. *Radiology* 1989;**173**(3):819.

66. Cozens NJ, Murchison JT, Allan PL, Winney RJ. Conventional 15 G needle technique for renal biopsy compared with ultrasound-guided spring-loaded 18 G needle biopsy. *Br J Radiol* 1992;**65**(775):594.

67. Nyman RS, Cappelen-Smith J, al Suhaibani H, Alfurayh O, Shakweer W, Akhtar M. Yield and complications in percutaneous renal biopsy. A comparison between ultrasound-guided gun-biopsy and manual techniques in native and transplant kidneys. *Acta Radiol* 1997;**38**(3):431.

68. Misra S, Gyamlani G, Swaminathan S, et al. Safety and diagnostic yield of transjugular renal biopsy. *J Vasc Interv Radiol* 2008;**19**:546.

69. Sateriale M, Cronan JJ, Savadler LD. A 5-year experience with 307 CT-guided renal biopsies: results and complications. *J Vasc Interv Radiol* 1991;**2**(3):401.

70. Manno C, Strippoli GFM, Arnesano L, Bonifati C, Campobasso N, Gesualdo L, et al. Predictors of bleeding complications in percutaneous ultrasound-guided renal biopsy. *Kidney Int* 2004;**66**(4):1570.

71. Quinn SF, vanSonnenberg E, Casola G, Wittich GR, Neff CC. Interventional radiology in the spleen. *Radiology* 1986;**161**(2):289.

72. Lawrence DD, Carrasco CH, Fornage B, Sneige N, Wallace S. Percutaneous lymph node biopsy. *Cardiovasc Intervent Radiol* 1991;**14**(1):55.

73. Silverman SG, Lee BY, Mueller PR, Cibas ES, Seltzer SE. Impact of positive findings at image-guided biopsy of lymphoma on patient care: evaluation of clinical history, needle size, and pathologic findings on biopsy performance. *Radiology* 1994;**190**(3):759.

74. Amis ES. Retroperitoneal fibrosis. *AJR Am J Roentgenol* 1991;**157**(2):321.

75. Memel DS, Dodd GD, Esola CC. Efficacy of sonography as a guidance technique for biopsy of abdominal, pelvic, and retroperitoneal lymph nodes. *AJR Am J Roentgenol* 1996;**167**(4):957.

76. Bret PM, Guibaud L, Atri M, Gillett P, Seymour RJ, Senterman MK. Transvaginal US-guided aspiration of ovarian cysts and solid pelvic masses. *Radiology* 1992;**185**(2):377.

77. Oyen RH, Poppel HPV, Ameye FE, de Voorde WAV, Baert AL, Baert LV. Lymph node staging of localized prostatic carcinoma with CT and CT-guided fine-needle aspiration biopsy: prospective study of 285 patients. *Radiology* 1994;**190**(2):315.

78. Lewis BD, Charboneau JW, Reading CC. Ultrasound-guided biopsy and ablation in the neck. *Ultrasound Q* 2002;**18**(1):3.

79. Jemal A, Siegel R, Ward E, Hao Y, Xu J, Thun MJ. Cancer Statistics, 2009. *CA Cancer J Clin* 2009;**59**(4):225.

80. Frates MC, Benson CB, Charboneau JW, Cibas ES, Clark OH, Coleman BG, et al. Management of thyroid nodules detected at US: Society of Radiologists in Ultrasound consensus conference statement. *Radiology* 2005;**237**(3):794.

81. Ahuja AT, Metreweli C. Ultrasound of thyroid nodules. *Ultrasound Q* 2000;**16**(3):111.

82. Papini E, Guglielmi R, Bianchini A, Crescenzi A, Taccogna S, Nardi F, et al. Risk of malignancy in nonpalpable thyroid nodules: predictive value of ultrasound and color-Doppler features. *J Clin Endocrinol Metab* 2002;**87**(5):1941.

83. Gharib H, Papini E, Valcavi R, Baskin HJ, Crescenzi A, Dottorini ME, et al. American Association of Clinical Endocrinologists and Associazione Medici Endocrinologi medical guidelines for clinical practice for the diagnosis and management of thyroid nodules. *Endocr Pract* 2006;**12**(1):63.

84. Kim EK, Park CS, Chung WY, Oh KK, Kim DI, Lee JT, et al. New sonographic criteria for recommending fine-needle aspiration biopsy of nonpalpable solid nodules of the thyroid. *AJR Am J Roentgenol* 2002;**178**(3):687.

85. Ahn SS, Kim EK, Kang DR, Lim SK, Kwak JY, Kim MJ. Biopsy of thyroid nodules: comparison of three sets of guidelines. *AJR Am J Roentgenol* 2010;**194**(1):31.

86. Hegedüs L, Bonnema SJ, Bennedbaek FN. Management of simple nodular goiter: current status and future perspectives. *Endocr Rev* 2003;**24**(1):102.

87. O'Malley ME, Weir MM, Hahn PF, Misdraji J, Wood BJ, Mueller PR. US-guided fine-needle aspiration biopsy of thyroid nodules: adequacy of cytologic material and procedure time with and without immediate cytologic analysis. *Radiology* 2002;**222**(2):383.

88. Baloch Z, LiVolsi VA, Jain P, Jain R, Aljada I, Mandel S, et al. Role of repeat fine-needle aspiration biopsy (FNAB) in the management of thyroid nodules. *Diagn Cytopathol* 2003;**29**(4):203. doi.org/10.1002/dc.10361.

89. vanSonnenberg E, Wittenberg J, Ferrucci JT, Mueller PR, Simeone JF. Triangulation method for percutaneous needle guidance: the angled approach to upper abdominal masses. *AJR Am J Roentgenol* 1981;**137**(4):757.

90. Sze DY. Use of curved needles to perform biopsies and drainages of inaccessible targets. *J Vasc Interv Radiol* 2001;**12**(12):1441.

5

Transcatheter Fluid Drainage

Ajit V. Nair, Horacio R. D'Agostino

TECHNIQUE

Although no longer novel, percutaneous fluid drainage (PFD) represents a paradigm shift in the treatment of sterile and infected fluid collections throughout the body, largely replacing traditional surgical incision and drainage and washout operations, which have been relegated to second-line therapies behind image-guided drainage. They are amongst the most common procedures performed in interventional radiology, and are frequently amongst the most satisfying, in that the effects of these procedures can often be immediate and provide significant relief of a patient's suffering.[1-5]

Patient Selection

Almost any fluid collection found in the chest, abdomen or pelvis, as well as much of the musculoskeletal system, may be amenable to percutaneous fluid drainage, whether by simple needle aspiration or placement of a drainage catheter, as long as a safe pathway for needle insertion is available and any underlying coagulopathy is corrected.[6]

Patient Preparation

As with all interventional procedures, coagulopathies must be corrected before intervention (see Chapter 2). Study of previous cross-sectional imaging and plain radiography is crucial in proper patient positioning and sterile preparation. Often, patients with suspected infected fluid collections are already receiving antibiotics at the time of drainage. If not, the decision to provide prophylactic coverage is left to the discretion of the interventional radiologist and should be based on the patient's current clinical condition. Although there is no consensus regarding first-line antibiotic coverage, commonly a second- or third-generation cephalosporin may be administered within 1 hour of the procedure, with a combination of clindamycin and gentamicin

reserved for patients with penicillin allergy.[7] This prophylaxis does not interfere with cultures of fluid aspirated from the collection. Many of these procedures may be performed with local anesthesia alone; conscious sedation may be provided intravenously for more anxious patients. General anesthesia is indicated for children and uncooperative patients. Proper informed consent must be obtained.

Imaging Guidance and Access

Of critical importance to the safe performance of drainage procedures is the proper selection of needle access and image guidance. Sonography is preferred because of its low cost, lack of ionizing radiation, and real-time needle localization in multiple planes. Collections located deep within the body or poorly visualized with sonography are drained using intermittent computed tomography (CT) guidance. Fluoroscopy may be used in the drainage of gas-filled collections that can be visualized, although care must be taken to study cross-sectional imaging to ensure safe needle access without traversal of interposed vital organs or structures. In the deep pelvis, transrectal and transvaginal sonography may provide a safe and effective access route to collections that would be otherwise inaccessible.

The route offering the shortest distance from skin to collection is often the preferred access window for needle and catheter placement. This is not always possible, however, because of the interposition of organs or vessels along the access route. Transpleural drainage of high abdominal fluid collections (i.e., perisplenic abscesses or liver abscesses), while often providing the shortest route, is less preferable and should be avoided if a safe subphrenic pathway is available to avoid potential empyema. Prior imaging studies are used in the selection of the access route, as well as in the positional preparation of the patient and choice of imaging modality for drainage guidance. The area to be drained is then examined with the imaging modality of choice to confirm the viability of the chosen access route. The patient is then prepped and draped in a sterile fashion, and local anesthetic is administered to the access site. Local anesthesia should be generously applied to both the skin surface and the deep tissues, particularly at innervated surfaces such as the peritoneum, pleura, or organ capsule (i.e., liver, kidney). Good local anesthesia maximizes patient comfort and minimizes the need for intravenous conscious sedation.

Needle selection is based on the objective of the procedure (i.e., aspiration vs. drainage catheter placement) and location of the collection to be drained. Generally, small-caliber needles (18- to 22-gauge) are chosen with a length sufficient to reach the collection. Eighteen-gauge Chiba and Hawkins needles have thinner walls than comparable spinal needles and are preferable when drain placement is desired, because they accept a 0.035-inch guidewire.

After the application of local anesthesia, a scalpel is used to puncture the skin and underlying fascia to allow for ease of needle and possible catheter insertion. This maneuver is particularly useful when using a sonographic needle guide for real-time imaging.

Sonography and fluoroscopy allow for needle localization under direct imaging guidance (Fig. 5-1). Imaging under CT is performed intermittently during needle insertion, advancing the needle before acquiring a limited CT slice to determine needle location and trajectory. Successful puncture of the collection, wire localization, and drainage placement are all confirmed by CT (Fig. 5-2).

DIAGNOSTIC ASPIRATION

Diagnostic aspiration of fluid collections is a useful tool for both diagnosis and treatment. It can be used to obtain a sample to determine the transudative or exudative nature of a collection, can assist in the tailoring of the appropriate antibiotic regimen, and helps determine the appropriate drainage catheter. Aspiration may be performed as a stand-alone procedure or may precede drain placement, because aspiration is the first step in the placement of a percutaneous drain.

As noted in the previous section, small-caliber needles (18- to 22-gauge) are typically selected for aspiration. Alternatively, an over-the-needle catheter system may be employed, such as the Yueh or OneStep catheter systems. These are 4- and 5-French (Fr) catheters that slide into position over the introducer needle, much like a peripheral intravenous catheter. Such systems are useful for aspiration of simple fluid collections of some volume, in which a drainage catheter placement is not indicated, such as a therapeutic thoracentesis or paracentesis (Fig. 5-3).

Aspiration of fluid confirms needle location in the collection. Fluid characteristics are assessed qualitatively (e.g., color, viscosity, turbidity, odor), and the sample is sent for Gram stain, culture, sensitivity, cytology (if there is concern for malignancy), and other tests as necessary. If catheter placement is to follow, only a small fluid sample (<5 mL) is removed initially, because decompression of the collection may complicate or preclude tube insertion. Conversely, complete aspiration should be performed if imaging shows the collection to be too small for drainage catheter placement, thus assisting in its resolution. Dry aspiration from an 18-gauge needle well positioned within the collection may indicate that the lesion is either very viscous or not drainable. Often, the ability to pass a guidewire, and ultimately a catheter, into the collection determines whether drainage is possible. If not, the tissue may then be biopsied with specimens sent for cytology and microbiology.

Conversion of an aspiration procedure to drainage catheter placement is based on multiple factors. One small, retrospective study found that more than half of all sterile pancreatic fluid collections found in acute pancreatitis treated with long-term catheter drainage underwent bacterial colonization.[8] Thus, by convention, sterile pleural effusions or ascites are often treated with therapeutic aspiration alone, because placement of an indwelling drainage catheter can promote infection of these collections. The same is true for fluid collections elsewhere, such as joint effusions. Infected collections often require placement of a drainage catheter; however, aspiration may be performed on collections that are too small for placement of a drainage catheter. Drains are placed for symptomatic collections that recur after therapeutic aspiration, such as cysts and pseudocysts. One-step needle aspiration without catheter insertion may be performed in certain locations without expected communication with the gastrointestinal, biliary, or urinary tracts. This approach has reported success rates up to 90% in selected cases.[6,9-12]

CATHETER INSERTION

Choice of catheter size and type is determined by the type and character of the fluid to be drained. Air and thin fluids are drained with 8- and 10-Fr catheters. Viscous fluids and fluids containing particulates require larger drainage catheters ranging from 12- to 26-Fr. Most drainage catheters have an inner retention mechanism, such as the locking pigtail (Cope loop) or Malecot drains (Fig. 5-4).

Drainage catheters may be placed using different techniques: direct trocar, tandem-trocar, and Seldinger.

The *direct trocar technique* can be safely performed on large superficial collections. After application of local anesthesia, the skin is incised with a scalpel and the

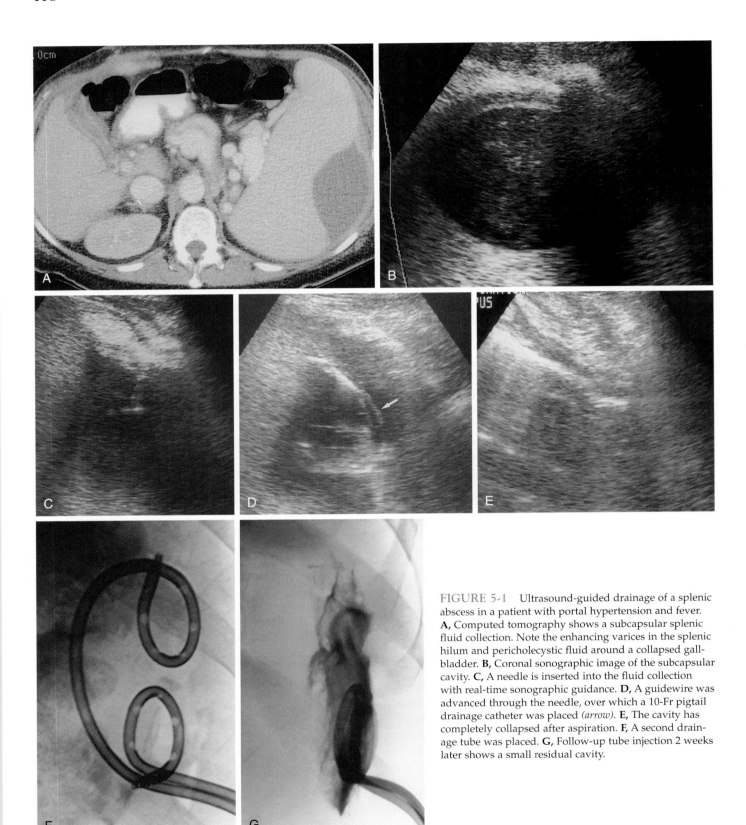

FIGURE 5-1 Ultrasound-guided drainage of a splenic abscess in a patient with portal hypertension and fever. **A,** Computed tomography shows a subcapsular splenic fluid collection. Note the enhancing varices in the splenic hilum and pericholecystic fluid around a collapsed gallbladder. **B,** Coronal sonographic image of the subcapsular cavity. **C,** A needle is inserted into the fluid collection with real-time sonographic guidance. **D,** A guidewire was advanced through the needle, over which a 10-Fr pigtail drainage catheter was placed *(arrow)*. **E,** The cavity has completely collapsed after aspiration. **F,** A second drainage tube was placed. **G,** Follow-up tube injection 2 weeks later shows a small residual cavity.

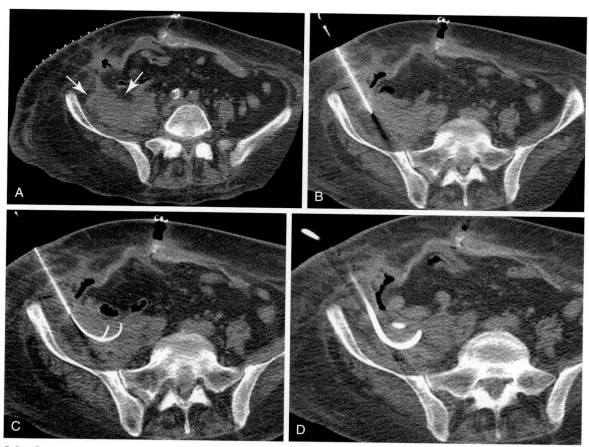

FIGURE 5-2 Computed tomography (CT)-guided drainage of right lower quadrant abscess. **A,** CT shows collection of fluid and gas in the right lower quadrant consistent with abscess *(arrows)*. Note radiopaque marking grid overlying the anterior surface of the right lower quadrant. **B,** Access needle is directed into the collection under intermittent CT guidance. **C,** A guidewire is advanced and curled in the collection. **D,** Using Seldinger technique, a pigtail drainage catheter is placed over the wire.

FIGURE 5-3 Over-the-needle catheter system for aspiration. **A,** Yueh catheter with introducer needle in place. **B,** The catheter is advanced over the needle, allowing for removal of the needle and Luer-lock attachment of an aspiration system, such as a vacuum-container.

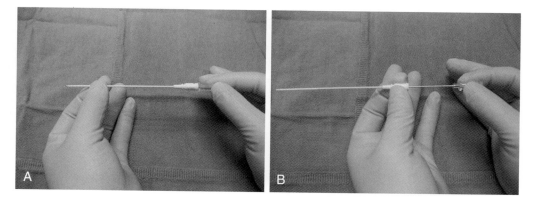

incision spread with a Kelly clamp. The catheter is directly inserted into the collection with the inner cannula and stylet. The stylet is then removed and the cannula is aspirated. The catheter is then inserted over the cannula or guidewire.

The *tandem-trocar technique* is a variation of the trocar technique, in which the distance between the skin and collection is measured by imaging and marked on the catheter shaft. The catheter, with the metal cannula and stylet, is placed in the skin hole next to the previously inserted needle and advanced into the collection under imaging guidance. The stylet is removed, and material can be aspirated. A 0.035-inch guidewire is then advanced through the cannula, and the catheter is inserted over the cannula and guidewire into the collection. Use of the guidewire decreases the risk of perforation of the

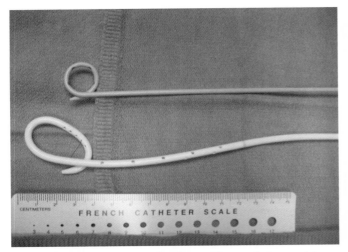

FIGURE 5-4 Locking pigtail catheters. These catheters contain a Cope loop retention system with side holes within the loop for drainage. Note the lower catheter, commonly used for biliary drainage, contains larger side holes that extend along the shaft.

back wall of the cavity, disrupts septations allowing for better drainage, and assists in the coiling of the pigtail catheter.

The *Seldinger technique* is the most common method of catheter placement and is suitable for drainage of all collections, particularly those that are small or difficult to access. After access has been achieved with an 18-gauge needle, a 0.035-inch guidewire is inserted through the needle and coiled in the collection (see Fig. 5-2). The tract is serially dilated and the catheter is inserted over the guidewire using the metal cannula without the stylet. The catheter is then advanced over the cannula and wire and coiled in the collection.

After catheter insertion, postplacement imaging is performed to document proper catheter location. The collection is then evacuated. Fluid levels determined by specific gravity are not uncommon, and one can often find a collection that initially yields thin fluid, followed by viscous aspirate and finally serosanguineous fluid. The fluid can become blood tinged when the cavity is nearly empty and suction is applied to the dry walls of the former collection (Fig. 5-5).

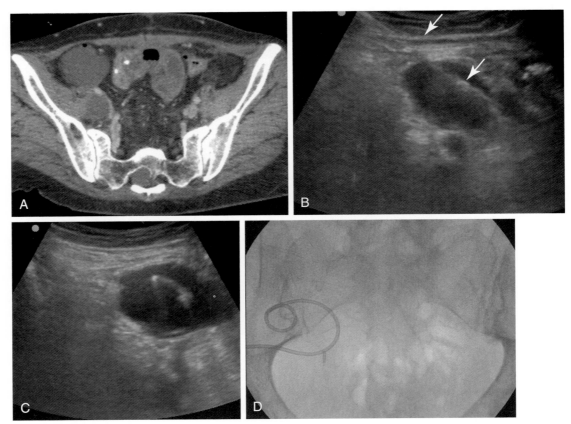

FIGURE 5-5 Ultrasound-guided placement of a drainage catheter in a right lower quadrant abscess using Seldinger technique. **A,** Computed tomography demonstrates right lower quadrant fluid collection. **B,** Ultrasound-guided access into the collection. The guidewire has been placed through the needle into the collection *(arrows).* **C,** Ultrasound shows the pigtail drain inside the collection. **D,** Fluoroscopic image demonstrates the location of the catheter within the right lower quadrant.

Catheter Care

A large-bore, three-way stopcock is attached to the catheter hub. The cavity is irrigated with 10- to 20-mL aliquots of normal saline until the aspirated fluid is clear. To prevent bacteremia and sepsis, avoid overdistention of the collection.

The catheter is then secured to the skin such that it does not kink or pull with patient movement. Catheters are often secured to the skin with 2-0 nonabsorbable suture. Alternatively, an adhesive retention device may be used. Adhesive tape wrapped around the catheter and applied to the skin may provide added security.

Gravity drainage to a collection bag is typical in most cases, particularly when the fluid being drained is nonviscous. Thicker material may require a suction drainage bag or application of low intermittent wall suction, as well as frequent irrigation to break up viscous material and prevent catheter clogging. Continuous low wall suction is used for thoracic collections. Drains placed in the pleural space are connected to a Pleur-evac water-seal device, which contains a fluid collection chamber and a safety mechanism to prevent excessive suction. The Pleur-evac is then attached to wall suction (Fig. 5-6). High-output collections, which often involve gastrointestinal and urinary fistulas, may require continuous low wall suction to keep the cavity dry and promote healing.

Postprocedure Care

Postplacement, drainage catheters require routine maintenance to ensure proper function and complete resolution of the collection. The catheter, its connections, and its fixation devices are checked daily for all inpatients and during clinic visits for outpatients. Dressings should be changed daily, and the drain site must be kept clean and dry.

All drainage catheters require regular irrigation to maintain patency. Without regular irrigation, all drainage catheters will occlude, regardless of their size. Proper irrigation involves the following steps:

- Place a syringe in the stopcock and aspirate residual fluid
- Inject 10 to 20 mL of normal saline
- Aspirate the irrigant
- Reflush the catheter with 5 mL of normal saline

Routine irrigation is performed two to three times each day. This maneuver may be performed by the floor nurses on inpatients, and by the patient or caretaker for outpatients. Viscous collections may require more frequent irrigation (e.g., every 4 to 6 hours). Daily catheter output is recorded, with the amount of irrigant solution subtracted to obtain the true drainage output.

A 2- to 4-mg dose of tissue plasminogen activator (t-PA) in 10 to 20 mL or more of normal saline may be instilled in drains that are properly positioned in viscous collections that are refractory to drainage after normal routine irrigation. Typically, such collections are loculated (e.g., infected hematomas). In such cases, t-PA is infused through the catheter, which is then capped for 1 to 2 hours to allow the t-PA to liquefy the collection. The catheter is then reopened to drainage. Several prospective studies suggest that routine catheter flushing using fibrinolytics instead of saline decreases the total time to abscess resolution, length of hospital stay, and therefore total cost of care.[13,14] In general, the patient's acute condition resolves within 24 to 48 hours after drain placement.

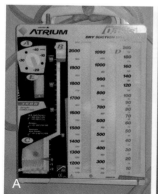
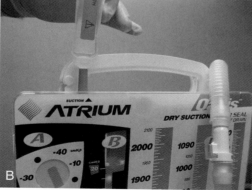
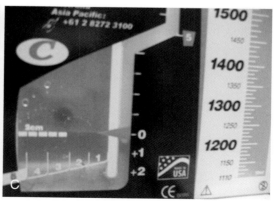

FIGURE 5-6   Dry-suction water-seal chest drain. **A,** This drainage system contains a graduated chamber for collecting fluid, a water seal chamber to evaluate for air leak, and a pressure regulator. **B,** The water-seal chamber is filled with saline. This connection is then attached to suction. Tubing to the right is attached to the chest tube. **C,** Water-seal chamber. Air bubbles in this chamber indicate an air leak within the chest tube system.

Clinical Management: Postprocedure Imaging, Catheter Manipulation and Removal

Management of drainage catheters is based on the patient's clinical course and the output of the drainage catheter (Table 5-1):

1. If the patient's clinical status significantly improves or resolves, and the catheter output has decreased to an immeasurable amount (<10 mL/day), the catheter may be removed, unless a fistula is suspected or present.

2. If the patient's condition fails to improve or worsens after drain placement, and catheter output has decreased, cross-sectional imaging may be obtained for further evaluation. These patients may require repositioning or exchange of the drain, upsizing of the catheter, a more frequent irrigation regimen (or supplementation with fibrinolytics), or placement of a new drain in a different collection.[15] CT is the preferred imaging modality, because it provides a complete survey of the anatomic compartment and allows for assessment of the drain in relation to the fluid collection as well as visualization of any other undrained collections. Chest radiographs are useful to assess diffuse thoracic collections after drain placement. Chest CT is helpful in the case of a loculated thoracic fluid collection.

3. If the patient's condition fails to improve or worsens, and the catheter output has remained stable or increased, the drainage catheter is left in place and routine maintenance continued. In such cases, further investigation may be required to look for another source of the patient's condition.

4. If the patient's condition has improved, but drainage output has remained stable or increased, a catheter sinogram is indicated to evaluate for a fistula or to evaluate the size of the cavity before possible cyst or lymphocele sclerosis.

A drainage catheter may require repositioning if it has become dislodged from the collection, or if the collection is loculated and the drain has only evacuated a portion of it. Such findings are often determined by CT. In these cases, the patient returns to the fluoroscopy suite, where a catheter sinogram is performed to outline the extent of the collection relative to the end of the catheter. The size of the cavity is assessed as well; when the size of the collection does not resolve despite proper drainage, a necrotic or cystic tumor should be suspected.

A stiff 0.035-inch guidewire is inserted into the tube after the hub is cut off to release the internal locking mechanism. Under fluoroscopy, the wire is manipulated into the collection outlined by contrast from the sinogram. The catheter is then removed over the wire and replaced with a new one; the size of the catheter may be increased if the collection is particularly viscous (Fig. 5-7).

Fistulas pose a special problem when dealing with percutaneous drainage catheters. Fistulas close with proper drainage, unless:

- The system (e.g., respiratory, gastrointestinal, urinary, biliary) is obstructed distally.
- Infection or tumor resides in the fistula tract.
- The patient has impaired healing (e.g., poor nutrition, steroid therapy).

Fluid collections recur if the fistula has not healed by the time the drainage catheter is removed. Sometimes a fistula is seen on catheter sinogram despite minimal drainage from the catheter because fluid can escape through another route. In this situation, the catheter is clamped for 1 to 3 days to allow reaccumulation of fluid. If no collection is identified by imaging, the catheter can be removed. Fluid collections associated with fistulas may require prolonged drainage (sometimes up to months). Persistent low-output drainage can be managed by downsizing the drainage tube and gradually removing it over 3 to 5 days. Presumably, this technique allows collapse and closure of the tract as the catheter is pulled out.

Ultimately, the catheter is removed if:

- The patient's clinical condition has improved
- Laboratory tests have normalized
- Catheter output has decreased to an immeasurable amount (<10 mL/day)
- The fluid cavity has resolved
- There is absence of fistula

RESULTS AND COMPLICATIONS

The success rate of PFD combined with antibiotics and nutritional support is about 90% for simple collections (cysts, unilocular abscesses). The cure rate drops to 70% for complex collections such as infected hematomas, multilocular abscesses, abscesses complicated by bowel fistula, pancreatic abscesses, and infected necrotic pancreatic collections.[15,16] Drainage failures often are attributed to residual undrained collections, premature tube removal, or inadequate position (or number) of catheters. However, even when PFD is not completely curative, it

TABLE 5-1   Algorithm for Percutaneous Fluid Drain Management

	CLINICAL STATUS	
	Improved	Stable/Declined
Decreased drainage output	Remove catheter	Reimage and reassess
Increased or stable output	Sinogram to evaluate for fistula	Leave catheter in place and continue maintenance

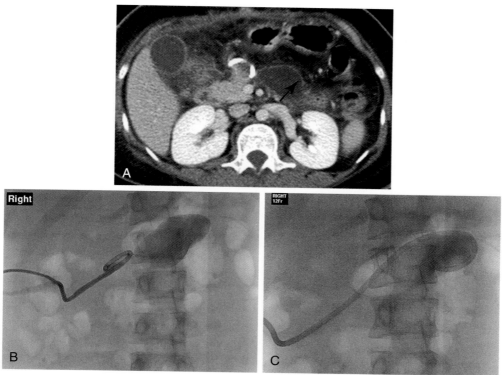

FIGURE 5-7 Drain catheter reposition after drain output decreased. **A,** Computed tomography (CT) scan shows drainage catheter pigtail no longer in the largest portion of the collection *(arrow)*, after having successfully drained the material surrounding the tube. **B,** Catheter sinogram under fluoroscopy shows main portion of the abscess cavity beyond the pigtail loop. The contrast-filled sac provides a target for repositioning the tube. **C,** Catheter repositioned into the remaining collection. The former catheter was removed over a stiff guidewire, which was advanced into the larger collection for drain replacement.

often converts an emergent operation (with its attendant risks) to an elective procedure or obviates the need for a two-stage operation (e.g., diverting colostomy).

The major complications of PFD are bleeding, bowel or bladder perforation, and sepsis. Hemorrhage is more likely to occur in a patient with an uncorrected coagulopathy or when a suboptimal access route was used for catheter insertion. Inadvertent bowel perforation may take place when bowel motility is impaired by adhesions or ileus. If a loop of bowel is traversed en route to a fluid collection, a second catheter is placed in the collection. The first catheter is withdrawn until its tip is in the bowel lumen. This enterostomy catheter is removed when a mature track has formed. If an abnormally distended loop of bowel is mistaken for an abscess, aspiration yields yellow-green fluid that contains bubbles and is not foul smelling. In this situation, the catheter should not be removed but rather kept in place for 10 to 15 days until a track has formed. The catheter then can be removed safely, and the track closes spontaneously.

Perforation of the bladder may occur while draining lower abdomen fluid collections, regardless of the access route. Foley catheter insertion in the bladder before the procedure may avoid this complication. On recognition of bladder perforation by a drainage catheter, the catheter is removed. A Foley catheter is placed (if not already present) to ensure good bladder drainage. The Foley catheter is left in place for 5 to 7 days to allow healing of the perforation. The catheter then is clamped for 4 hours and removed if no urine leak is evident.

SPECIFIC APPLICATIONS

Chest

PFD is indicated for treatment of pneumothorax, empyema, malignant pleural effusion, pericardial effusion, lung abscess and mediastinal abscess.[17] Imaging guidance may be provided by sonography, fluoroscopy, or CT, with sonographic guidance being the most common. Typically, catheters placed in the chest cavity are connected to a water-seal drainage device.

Bleeding risk is posed by the intercostal and internal mammary arteries. Transection of the intercostal vessels is largely avoided by inserting needles and catheters over the upper border of the ribs. The internal mammary vessels are avoided by placement of needles and catheters at least 5 cm lateral to the sternal margins, or by direct visualization of these vessels during placement under CT or sonography.

Pneumothorax has been treated traditionally by surgical large-bore chest tube placement, but is very amenable to small-bore catheter placement by the interventionalist. Additionally, pneumothorax is a common complication of percutaneous lung biopsy and should be managed by the interventionalist, as its treatment has many aspects in common with abscess drainage.[18] Indications for chest tube placement include large-volume pneumothorax (>30% of the hemithorax), the appearance of symptoms (e.g., dyspnea, decrease in blood-oxygen saturation), or need to re-expand the lung to continue with lung biopsy.

In free-flowing pneumothoraces, catheter insertion is performed using anatomic landmarks or under fluoroscopic guidance. With the patient supine, the anterior chest wall is sterilized. Local anesthesia is provided at the skin level as well as at the pleural surface; if adequate local anesthesia at the pleural interface is attained, catheter insertion can be virtually painless for the patient. An 18-gauge needle is inserted between the second and third anterior ribs in the midclavicular line with suction applied through a syringe until air is aspirated. An alternative site in women and in men with bulky pectoralis muscles is the fourth or fifth intercostal space at the anterior axillary line. A stiff 0.035-inch guidewire is inserted and angled toward the apex of the hemithorax. An 8-Fr catheter is then inserted over the wire with the pigtail formed at the apex of the pleural space. The tube is then connected to a Heimlich valve or a waterseal drainage device immediately after placement and is left connected to drainage for at least 12 hours. The catheter can be removed when the lung remains expanded on a follow-up chest radiograph obtained 2 hours after clamping the tube (Fig. 5-8).

Loculated pneumothoraces may require placement of a chest tube using CT guidance. Loculations may prevent complete evacuation of the pneumothorax, in that sections of the lesion may be walled off from the compartment containing the chest tube. Under CT guidance, these loculations can be identified and a chest tube placed through the septation; alternatively, individual catheters may be placed in each loculated compartment. Needle, wire, and catheter placement is similar to that of free-flowing pneumothoraces, except intermittent CT imaging is performed to guide needle and tube placement.

Empyema is an infected pleural collection usually caused by pneumonia, bronchiectasis, or trauma. Empyemas evolve in the following three stages[19]:

- Acute (exudative) phase, indicated by the presence of a nonviscous, nonloculated effusion
- Subacute phase, in which the fluid is fibrinous or purulent and the cavity may have loculations
- Chronic (organizing) phase, when there is organization of the exudate with adhesion of the visceral and parietal pleurae (i.e., "pleural peel")

The diagnosis is made at the time of aspiration by the presence of gross pus, fluid pH 7.2 or lower, bacteria identified by Gram stain, or a fluid glucose less than 40 mg/dL.[20,21] CT diagnosis may be made by identification of the "split pleura sign," in which the visceral and parietal pleura are thickened on contrast-enhanced CT and divided by pleural fluid.[22] Acute and subacute empyema is treated successfully by PFD in greater than 80% of cases; chronic empyemas respond much less well.[23,24] Catheters are typically placed using ultrasound and fluoroscopy after diagnostic aspiration; CT may be used to access loculated collections, which may require multiple tubes. Fluid viscosity is used to determine the size of the catheter placed, usually ranging from 12 to 24 Fr. The catheter is connected to a water-seal drainage

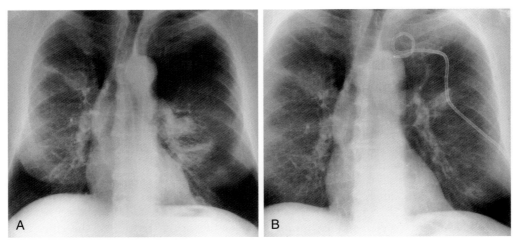

FIGURE 5-8   Postbiopsy pneumothorax tube placement. **A,** The patient developed a large, symptomatic left pneumothorax after percutaneous biopsy of a lung mass with a 22-gauge Chiba needle. **B,** The pneumothorax was treated by evacuation through a pigtail catheter placed in the second intercostal space.

device and continuous low wall suction after insertion. Intrapleural t-PA instillation is necessary to improve drainage, particularly in fibrinous collections.[25] A 2- to 4-mg dose of t-PA in 10 to 20 mL of saline, depending on the size of the tube and collection, is administered and the tube is clamped for several hours before drainage is resumed. This step can be performed every 8 hours and may be done for several days to ensure resolution of the collection. Empyema catheters are removed when there is improvement in clinical and laboratory parameters, no sign of air leak to indicate a bronchocutaneous fistula, and drainage of less than 10 mL/day.

Malignant pleural effusions tend to recur rapidly after therapeutic thoracentesis. Closure of the pleural cavity (pleurodesis) with a sclerosing agent (e.g., tetracycline, doxycycline, talc, diluted sodium hydroxide, bleomycin) is an effective way to prevent recurrent effusions in more than 80% of patients.[26] Before sclerosis, the pleural fluid is drained completely. Usually, several sessions of sclerosis are needed to achieve fusion of the pleural surfaces. More recently, placement of tunneled pleural drains (Pleur X catheters) has gained favor in the treatment of malignant pleural effusions in terminal patients, particularly those who failed pleurodesis.[27] Such catheters allow for intermittent drainage to be performed by the patient or caretaker, with a theoretical decrease in the risk of infection or pneumothorax formation in the outpatient setting.

Placement of these catheters involves traditional percutaneous access of the fluid in the pleural space, typically caudally within the chest. The catheter is then tunneled under the skin between the ribs near the midclavicular line to the access site, where it is placed into the pleural space through a peel-away sheath. The catheter is accessible to the patient for periodic drainage, with the exposed portion distal to the site where it enters the pleural space. Infrequently, these catheters are complicated by leakage, migration, loculation of the effusion, or infection.

Lung abscess is an infected collection of the lung parenchyma. Primary abscesses usually are the consequence of aspiration and are caused by anaerobic bacteria. Secondary abscesses arise from an adjacent infection or hematogenous spread (e.g., pneumonia, lung cyst, septic emboli). About 90% of lung abscesses respond to antibiotics, postural drainage, and bronchoscopic lavage. Those that do not resolve with more conservative measures require percutaneous drainage.[28-31] The procedure is performed with fluoroscopic or CT guidance (Fig. 5-9). A catheter pathway through abnormal lung is preferred to avoid pneumothorax and collapse of the healthy lung. Rarely, this is not possible and normal lung must be traversed by the drainage catheter. The patient is positioned to keep the opposite hemithorax nondependent to avoid aspiration of the abscess fluid into the normal lung. Catheter insertion in a lung abscess establishes a controlled

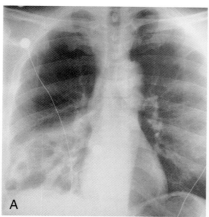
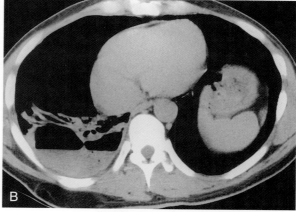
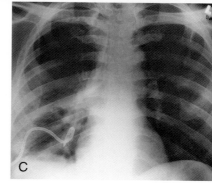

FIGURE 5-9   Lung abscess drainage in a patient with acquired immunodeficiency syndrome and Salmonella pneumonia. **A** and **B,** A complex cavity with air-fluid levels is seen in the right lower lobe. **C,** The abscess was drained with a 12-Fr drainage catheter placed by tandem trocar technique under computed tomography guidance.

bronchocutaneous fistula that can be detected by air leak in the water-seal chamber of the Pleur-evac. A large air leak from a bronchocutaneous fistula can cause respiratory insufficiency in a critically ill patient. To avoid this problem, the catheter used to drain a lung abscess should be no larger than 12 to 14 Fr.

Mediastinal abscess is an emergent, life-threatening infection that usually occurs after thoracic surgery or endoscopy.[32] CT or sonography combined with fluoroscopy is used for image-guided tube placement with a parasternal or paraspinous approach to avoid the lung (Fig. 5-10).

Pericardial effusions require drainage when there is impairment of diastolic filling of the ventricles. The causes of large symptomatic pericardial effusions include renal insufficiency, metabolic or immunologic diseases, infection, trauma (such as biopsy) and malignancy.[33] Pericardial catheter drainage is performed under sonographic guidance with or without fluoroscopy. Malignant pericardial effusions have a high recurrence rate. Septic pericardial effusions are rare and are successfully drained percutaneously.

Liver (Online Case 75)

Pyogenic (bacterial) liver abscess may result from cholangitis, iatrogenic or criminal trauma, hematogenous septic emboli from enteric abscesses (e.g., appendicitis, diverticulitis), or tumor.[34] Percutaneous drainage has largely replaced operative treatment.[35] Acute cholangitis typically develops in patients with partial or total biliary obstruction caused by gallstones or tumor. PFD is well accepted as first-line therapy for these abscesses.[36-38] Tube insertion is done with sonographic or CT guidance. Care should be taken to avoid traversing the pleura, which may lead to empyema. Percutaneous drainage can treat

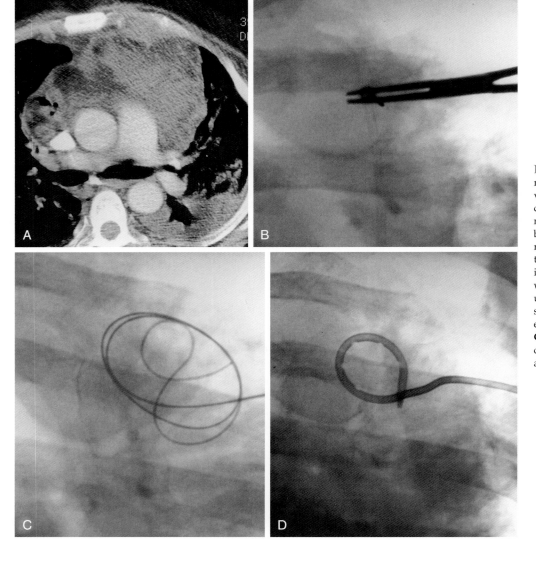

FIGURE 5-10 Suspected mediastinal abscess after extravascular placement of a left subclavian central line. **A,** Inhomogeneous soft tissue density with air bubbles is present in the anterior mediastinum. Note the pleural thickening and left lower lobe infiltrate. **B,** A 16-gauge Angiocath was inserted into the collection under sonographic and fluoroscopic guidance, and serosanguineous material was aspirated. **C,** A guidewire was coiled in the cavity, over which a 10-Fr drainage catheter was inserted **(D).**

the abscess and may decompress the biliary tree if there is distal biliary obstruction. However, additional biliary drainage may be required to control sepsis. PFD is not feasible for widespread microabscesses, but may still provide benefit in complex or multiloculated collections.[39] Single-step needle aspiration without tube placement had gained some popularity for noncholangitic pyogenic liver abscesses, but later studies questioned this approach.[40-42] Percutaneous needle aspiration without catheter placement may have a role to play in the management of collections that are too small to allow for catheter placement (generally less than 5 cm in size), with catheter placement showing greater benefit in larger lesions.[43]

Hydatid cyst disease is caused by the parasite *Echinococcus granulosus*. The characteristic CT finding is multiloculated hepatic cysts with daughter collections. Medical therapy is the standard treatment.[44] Invasive procedures (PFD or surgery) are reserved for failures of drug therapy.[45-47] In the past, PFD was avoided strictly because of the fear of leakage of scolices with ensuing anaphylactic shock or peritoneal spread. However, published series describe favorable results in controlling the disease with a combination of oral albendazole and percutaneous drainage.[48,49] Albendazole therapy begins 2 weeks before drainage and is continued until the catheter is removed. Puncture, aspiration, injection, and reaspiration (PAIR) technique is typically performed. To avoid seeding the abdominal cavity at the time of drainage, aliquots of hydatid-fluid aspirate should be replaced with hypertonic (33%) saline solution. When the entire cyst is filled with saline solution, a catheter is inserted and left to gravity drainage. A catheter sinogram is performed later to assess communication with the bile ducts. If no communication is found, absolute alcohol is injected to assist in removal of the germinative layer of the cyst. Bile staining or pus in the hydatid cyst cavity is a sign that the parasites are dead.

Amebic abscess is diagnosed with serologic tests and is almost always eradicated with drug therapy such as metronidazole. Indications for amebic abscess drainage include failure of medical therapy, perforated abscess, and large collections in a peripheral location or the left lobe of the liver.[50-52] Abscesses at these sites are prone especially to rupture into the peritoneum, pericardium, or pleural space. Percutaneous drainage effectively controls symptoms from amebic abscess (Fig. 5-11). The usual duration of catheterization is less than 1 week. An alternative approach is simple aspiration with a large-bore needle or single-step catheter drainage and removal.

Congenital liver cysts usually are multiple and fall along the spectrum of polycystic kidney disease. Infrequently, symptomatic dominant cysts require drainage and sclerosis.[53] However, solitary cystic liver lesions may be malignant (e.g., primary cystadenocarcinoma, metastatic disease) and are treated by surgical resection. *Metastatic cystic tumors* may benefit from palliative drainage to alleviate mass effect–caused discomfort. The method of cyst and lymphocele sclerotherapy are described later in this chapter.

Post-traumatic biloma results from liver injury from blunt or penetrating trauma, or abdominal surgery.[54,55] Bile accumulation from disrupted bile ducts may not require drainage if it is small, sterile, and asymptomatic. Usually, though, bilomas become infected and require percutaneous drainage (Fig. 5-12). The presence of a biliary fistula may prolong the duration of catheterization. Biliary fistulas usually close unless there is total transection of a bile duct or distal biliary obstruction.

Ischemic fluid collections are complex bilomas caused by focal liver infarction. Liver infarcts result from severe compromise of the hepatic circulation and are seen in patients with portal vein thrombosis, occlusion of branches of the hepatic artery, or profound hypotension. Infarcts may become infected and require drainage.

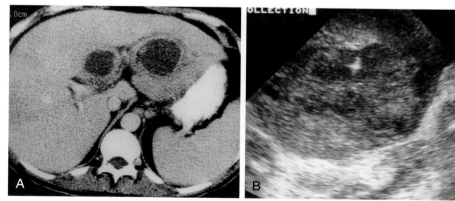

FIGURE 5-11 Amebic liver abscess drainage. **A,** Computed tomography scan shows two large, low-density masses with enhancing rims and surrounding edema in the left lobe and caudate lobe. Numerous small satellite lesions were seen throughout the liver on other images. **B,** A 22-gauge spinal needle was advanced into the left lobe cavity with sonographic guidance; frank pus was aspirated. A 12-Fr drainage catheter was placed by tandem trocar technique. The caudate lobe lesion was drained in a similar fashion.

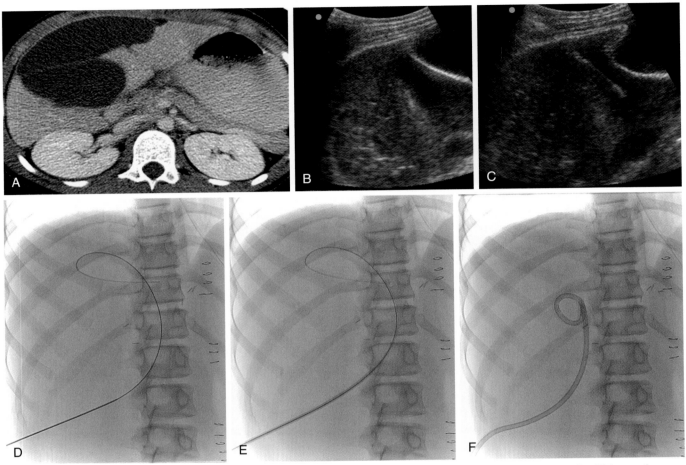

FIGURE 5-12   Biloma drainage after iatrogenic trauma during laparoscopic cholecystectomy. **A,** Computed tomography (CT) scan shows large, low-attenuation hepatic fluid collection consistent with biloma. **B** and **C,** Ultrasound demonstrates the mixed echogenicity collection and needle access. **D,** Fluoroscopy after ultrasound-guided needle access demonstrates wire placement. **E** and **F,** The track is dilated, followed by pigtail drainage catheter placement.

These collections are filled with necrotic liver parenchyma and bile. A biliary fistula is the rule after percutaneous drainage. Catheter sinograms reveal necrotic material in the bile ducts, which can cause biliary obstruction and maintain the fistula. Resolution of ischemic bilomas depends on adequate drainage, unobstructed bile ducts, and appropriate nutrition and vascular supply to allow for liver regeneration and healing of the collection cavity.

Spleen

Percutaneous drainage of splenic fluid collections is done for abscesses, liquefied infarcts, and symptomatic cysts.[56-59] Although splenic fluid collections are relatively rare, these can be safely approached by percutaneous means.[60,61] Drainage may be performed as a temporizing measure before splenectomy, or even as a curative measure with antibiotic therapy and without need for subsequent surgery.[62]

Splenic abscesses are caused by hematogenous seeding (as in intravenous drug abusers) or trauma or are spread from adjacent tissue. Tube insertion is done with sonographic or CT guidance[63] (see Fig. 5-1). Care should be taken to avoid transgressing bowel, kidney, or pancreas. Transpleural drainage is not recommended but can be done safely.[64] To prevent splenic hemorrhage, the catheter is inserted by traversing the least amount of splenic parenchyma possible.

Pancreas

Basic management of all pancreatic fluid collections includes bowel rest, parenteral antibiotics, and parenteral or enteral nutrition. PFD is indicated for *pancreatic pseudocysts* that become infected or cause symptoms such as continued pain or bowel or biliary obstruction[65,66] (Fig. 5-13). Percutaneous drainage also plays a major role in the management of necrotic collections and *pancreatic abscesses*[67-69] (Fig. 5-14).

Abscesses and pseudocysts may spread to the lesser sac, paracolic gutter or pararenal space, pelvis, and occasionally the thorax. Pancreatic phlegmon does not

FIGURE 5-13 Pancreatic pseudocyst drainage in a patient with an elevated white blood cell count and a history of pancreatitis. **A,** A large cystic mass is centered on the pancreatic tail. **B,** Using sonography, a 22-gauge Chiba needle was inserted into the collection. With the tandem trocar technique, a 10-Fr drainage catheter was placed. **C,** Because of persistent pain and white blood cell count elevation, a second catheter was inserted 3 days later to improve drainage. **D,** Two weeks later (with interval removal of one catheter), computed tomography shows resolution of the pseudocyst with a persistent, strandy soft tissue density consistent with ongoing peripancreatic inflammation.

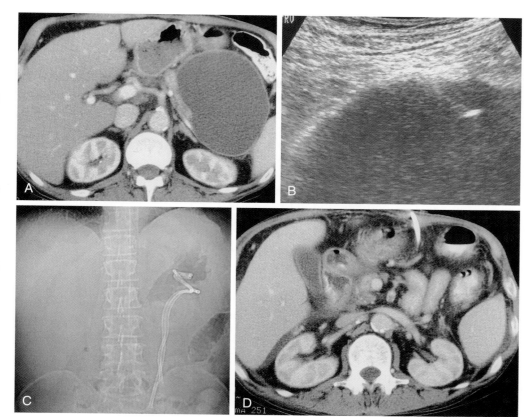

FIGURE 5-14 Pancreatic abscess after a Whipple procedure for pancreatic carcinoma. **A and B,** Two large cystic collections with rim enhancement are found in the operative bed and the porta hepatis. An efferent bowel loop from the diversion procedure is wrapped around the lateral aspect of one cavity. The pancreatic duct is dilated. Diffuse inflammatory changes have occurred in the peripancreatic region. **C and D,** Computed tomography scans 10 days after drainage show resolution of the collections.

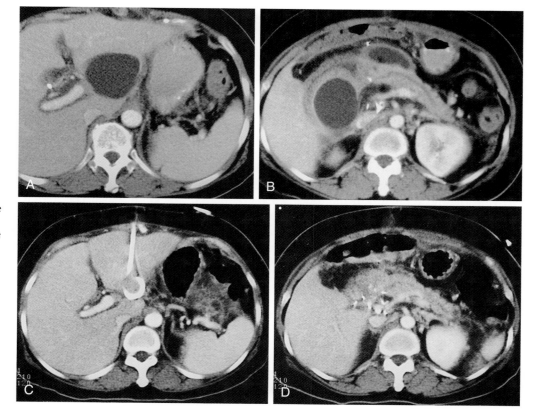

respond to PFD. Because of the complex nature of pancreatic abscesses and the frequency of associated fistulas, PFD (often with multiple tubes) usually is necessary for cure. Postoperative drainage of residual infected necrosis or abscess is highly effective and used instead of reoperation. A pancreatic fluid collection in a patient without risk factors or history of pancreatitis should raise the possibility of malignancy. Drainage of pancreatic fluid collections usually is accomplished through a direct transabdominal or retroperitoneal approach. However, transhepatic, transsplenic, and transgastric drainage often can be done safely.[70,71] Complications of PFD in the pancreas occur in about 10% of cases and usually involve bleeding, infection, pneumothorax, or empyema.

A *pancreatocutaneous fistula* establishes when a catheter is inserted to drain a pancreatic fluid collection. With the exception of chronic pancreatic pseudocysts, most pancreatic collections have purulent brownish or grayish fluid drainage. When the collection has resolved and debris evacuated, clear pancreatic fluid may continue to drain, causing prolonged duration of catheterization. Drainage of clear pancreatic fluid for more than 4 weeks is diagnostic of a persistent pancreatic fistula.[72] High-output pancreatic fistulas produce at least 300 mL/day. After acute inflammation has subsided, such fistulas can be reduced effectively by the administration of octreotide (50 to 150 mg, given subcutaneously three times daily). *Octreotide* (Sandostatin, Novartis Pharmaceuticals, East Hanover, N.J.) is a synthetic somatostatin analogue that inhibits pancreatic fluid and enzyme secretion.[73] Octreotide has no effect while there is active pancreatitis or infection. The compound may reduce the drainage volume of pancreatic fistulas even in presence of transection or occlusion of the pancreatic duct.[74]

Recently, there has been increased enthusiasm for percutaneous drainage of infected necrotic pancreatic collections.[75-77] In one study, large retroperitoneal drainage catheters were placed into pancreatic collections in patients admitted for acute pancreatitis or necrotizing pancreatitis complicated by infected acute postnecrotic collection or known infected pancreatic walled-off necrosis as diagnosed by CT. If there was a 75% reduction of the collection in 10 days, the collection was managed by drains alone; otherwise, video-assisted retroperitoneal debridement was performed through the drainage tract, thus avoiding open pancreatic debridement and its complications.[78]

Lower Abdomen and Pelvis (Online Cases 10, 20, and 50)

A variety of disorders can produce fluid collections in the lower abdomen and pelvis (Box 5-1). PFD, along with antibiotics and bowel resection in some cases, is the

---

BOX 5-1

LOWER ABDOMINAL AND PELVIC FLUID COLLECTIONS

- Perforated bowel abscess
- Appendicitis
- Diverticulitis
- Crohn disease
- Bowel tumor
- Cystic tumor
- Postoperative collections
- Pelvic inflammatory disease
- Tubo-ovarian abscess
- Lymphocele
- Urinoma
- Hematoma
- Prostatic abscess

---

primary treatment for many of these collections when they are infected, symptomatic, or produce obstruction. Percutaneous drainage often achieves a cure without surgery. After the abscess resolves, the indication for surgery depends on the nature and extent of underlying disease. PFD permits elective definitive surgery, allowing bowel resection, primary anastomosis, and wound closure. A colostomy or an open wound is therefore avoided. Patients with perforated tumors undergo surgery with the catheter in place for removal of the drainage tract en bloc with the specimen. PFD is effective for large, well-circumscribed *periappendiceal abscesses* without extension and for postappendectomy abscesses[79-81] (Fig. 5-15). *Diverticular abscesses* localized to the pelvis or mesentery without fecal spillage respond best to PFD.[82-85] Patients with perforated bowel abscess from Crohn disease may avoid emergent bowel resection with tube drainage.[86,87]

Fluid collections in the lower pelvis can be drained in several ways. The *transabdominal approach* usually is the simplest but may not be feasible because of interposed bowel. CT guidance normally is required, except for large superficial collections that can be visualized with sonography.

The *transgluteal approach* is common but can be complicated by catheter-associated pain. Catheters must be inserted close to the sacral and coccygeal margins to avoid the large gluteal vessels and the sciatic nerve running through the greater sciatic foramen.[88] Pain is often associated with placement through the piriformis muscle at the lateral margin of the sacrum. Placement below this muscle is recommended.

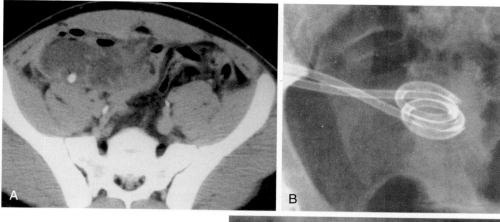

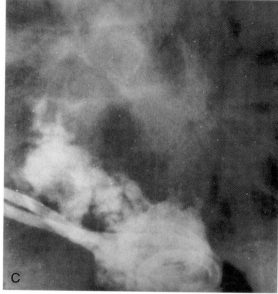

FIGURE 5-15 Periappendiceal abscess drainage. **A,** A large, complex collection with gas bubbles is seen in the right lower quadrant. Note the appendicolith in the posterior aspect of the collection. **B,** Ultrasound guidance was used to place two 12-Fr drainage catheters. **C,** Follow-up tube injection 5 days later shows a small residual cavity but no definite communication with bowel.

The *transrectal approach* is useful for infected collections adjacent to the rectum.[89-91] Sterile collections may become infected if drained in this fashion. Access is gained using an endocavitary sonographic probe (with biopsy guide) and fluoroscopy or CT guidance with the patient in a lateral decubitus position (Fig. 5-16). A Foley catheter is inserted into the bladder prior to transrectal and transvaginal drainage to allow better visualization of the collection and to minimize the risk of bladder puncture.

The *transvaginal approach* is exceedingly useful in women with fluid collections in contact with the vaginal wall.[92,93] It is performed with a vaginal sonographic probe (with a biopsy guide) and fluoroscopic guidance (Fig. 5-17). Catheter insertion through the muscular vaginal wall may be difficult.

Catheters placed transvaginally or transrectally benefit from having a locking pigtail loop (Cope) to prevent dislodgment when the patient is upright. The catheter is secured to the skin of the medial aspect of the thigh.

Patients tolerate transvaginal and transrectal catheters surprisingly well.

Sclerotherapy of Lymphoceles and Cysts (Online Case 15)

Lymphoceles usually are secondary to pelvic operations, particularly kidney transplantation and lymph node dissection. PFD is the procedure of choice but may require protracted tube placement (>1 month).

Management of true cysts and lymphoceles often requires intracavitary injection of a sclerosing agent.[94-96] Before sclerosis is performed, a catheter sinogram is performed to exclude communication of the drained cavity with vital structures such as vessels, ductal structures, or bowel. The amount of contrast injected for the sinogram allows for a measurement of the volume of sclerosant to be used. Sclerosis is successfully achieved by multiple injections of absolute alcohol, tetracycline, or iodine solutions.

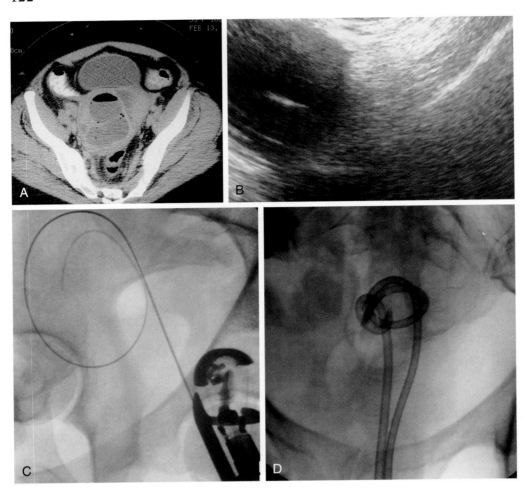

FIGURE 5-16   Transrectal drainage of a tubo-ovarian abscess. **A,** A complex cystic collection with rim enhancement is seen anterior to the rectum. **B,** With the patient in the right lateral decubitus position, a sonographic probe is inserted into the rectum. The needle is advanced into the collection through a needle guide. **C,** A guidewire is coiled in the cavity. **D,** After 10- and 12-Fr drainage catheters were placed, 200 mL of foul-smelling exudate was aspirated.

Barring the discovery of a fistula during sinography, the cavity is injected with the sclerosing agent until there is complete filling of the space without excessive pressure. The catheter is then clamped. The patient is allowed to move about for approximately one hour, with a variety of maneuvers employed to ensure contact of the sclerosing agent with all walls of the cavity. The catheter is then reopened to gravity drainage. Patients are instructed to record drainage output daily, with the expectation that output should diminish after each sclerotherapy procedure. The procedure is repeated within one week, again starting with a sinogram to document the size of the cavity prior to sclerosis. The catheter is removed when output has decreased to less than 10 mL/day and sinography demonstrates near complete collapse of the cavity.

Kidney and Retroperitoneum (Online Case 35)

Retroperitoneal collections include urinomas, perinephric abscess, renal abscess, renal cysts, iliopsoas muscle abscess, and necrotic tumors (most commonly cervical carcinoma metastases).[97] Most of these collections can be managed successfully with PFD (see Chapter 23). *Urinoma drainage* usually is done after percutaneous nephrostomy to divert the urine flow that maintains the collection. *Renal abscesses* usually have a phlegmonous component that may not respond to percutaneous drainage. Symptomatic *simple renal cysts* are treated with catheter drainage and sclerosis.

Musculoskeletal System

Muscular abscesses, hematomas, and lymphoceles are successfully drained percutaneously. Abscess recurrence caused by osteomyelitis depends on control of the bone infection. Hip effusions also have been drained percutaneously. Few data are available on the success rate of percutaneous drainage for joint effusions.

Iliopsoas muscle abscesses usually originate from an axial skeletal infection or other adjacent process (e.g., diverticulitis, appendicitis, infected lymph nodes).[98] Bilateral iliopsoas abscesses are usually caused by spondylitis. The offending organism is often *Mycobacterium tuberculosis* (Fig. 5-18).

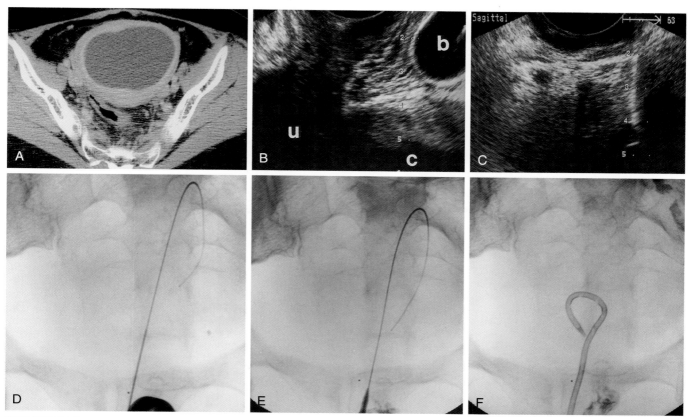

FIGURE 5-17 Transvaginal drainage of pyometrium caused by cervical obstruction from carcinoma. **A,** The uterus is dilated and fluid filled. **B,** Sagittal transvaginal sonography identifies the dilated uterus *(u)*, cervix *(c)*, and bladder with indwelling Foley catheter *(b)*. **C,** The transvaginal needle is advanced into the uterus. **D,** A guidewire is inserted through the needle. **E,** A 10-Fr drainage catheter is advanced over the guidewire. **F,** Final catheter placement in the uterine cavity.

FIGURE 5-18 Computed tomography (CT)-guided percutaneous drain placement in left psoas muscle abscess secondary to diverticulitis. **A,** CT scan shows gas and fluid collection within the left psoas muscle *(arrows).* **B,** Access needle is inserted under intermittent CT guidance. **C** and **D,** Wire and drainage catheter placement.

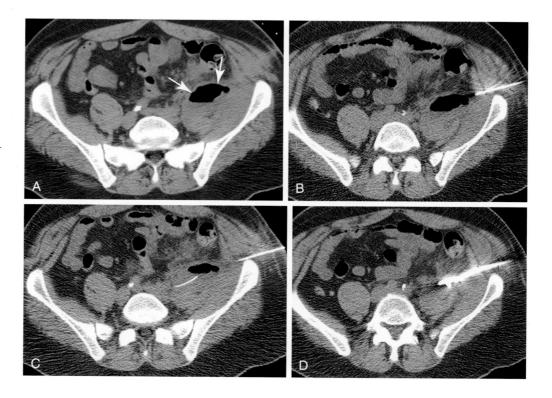

References

1. Mueller PR, vanSonnenberg E. Interventional radiology in the chest and abdomen. *N Engl J Med* 1990;**322**:1364.

2. vanSonnenberg E, D'Agostino HB, Casola G, et al. Percutaneous abscess drainage: current concepts. *Radiology* 1991;**181**:617.

3. Bakal CW, Sacks D, Burke DR, et al. Quality improvement guidelines for adult percutaneous abscess and fluid drainage. *J Vasc Interv Radiol* 1995;**6**:68.

4. Mueller PR, vanSonnenberg E, Ferrucci Jr JT. Percutaneous drainage of 250 abdominal abscesses and fluid collections. Part II: current procedural concepts. *Radiology* 1984;**151**:343.

5. vanSonnenberg E, Mueller PR, Ferrucci Jr JT. Percutaneous drainage of 250 abdominal abscesses and fluid collections. Part I: results, failures, and complications. *Radiology* 1984;**151**:337.

6. Wroblicka JT, Kuligowska E. One-step needle aspiration and lavage for the treatment of abdominal and pelvic abscesses. *AJR Am J Roentgenol* 1998;**170**:1197.

7. Venkatesan AM, Kundu S, Sacks D, et al. Practice guideline for adult antibiotic prophylaxis during vascular and interventional radiology procedures. *J Vasc Interv Radiol* 2010;**21**:1611.

8. Walser EM, Nealon WH, Marroquin S, et al. Sterile fluid collections in acute pancreatitis: catheter drainage versus simple aspiration. *Cardiovasc Intervent Radiol* 2006;**29**:102.

9. Kuligowska E, Keller E, Ferruci JT. Treatment of pelvic abscesses: value of one-step sonographically guided transrectal needle aspiration and lavage. *AJR Am J Roentgenol* 1995;**164**:201.

10. Miller FJ, Ahola DT, Bretzman PA, et al. Percutaneous management of hepatic abscess: a perspective by interventional radiologists. *J Vasc Interv Radiol* 1997;**8**:241.

11. Seeto RK, Rockey DC. Pyogenic liver abscess. Changes in etiology, management and outcome. *Medicine (Baltimore)* 1996;**75**:99.

12. Nielsen MB, Torp-Pedersen S. Sonographically guided transrectal or transvaginal one-step catheter placement in deep pelvic and perirectal abscesses. *AJR Am J Roentgenol* 2004;**183**:1035.

13. Laborda A, De Gregorio MA, Miguelena JM, et al. Percutaneous treatment of intraabdominal abscess: urokinase versus saline serum in 100 cases using two surgical scoring systems in a randomized trial. *Eur Radiol* 2009;**19**:1772.

14. Cheng D, Nagata KT, Yoon HC. Randomized prospective comparison of alteplase versus saline solution for the percutaneous treatment of loculated abdominopelvic abscesses. *J Vasc Interv Radiol* 2008;**19**:906.

15. Gee MS, Kim JY, Gervais DA, et al. Management of abdominal and pelvic abscesses that persist despite satisfactory percutaneous drainage catheter placement. *AJR Am J Roentgenol* 2010;**194**:815.

16. vanSonnenberg E, Wittich GR, Goodacre BW, et al. Percutaneous abscess drainage: update. *World J Surg* 2001;**25**:362.

17. Klein JS, Schultz S, Heffner JE. Interventional radiology of the chest: image-guided percutaneous drainage of pleural effusions, lung abscess and pneumothorax. *AJR Am J Roentgenol* 1995;**164**:581.

18. Cantin L, Chartrand-Lefebvre C, Lepanto L, et al. Chest tube drainage under radiological guidance for pleural effusion and pneumothorax in a tertiary care university teaching hospital: review of 51 cases. *Can Respir J* 2005;**12**:29.

19. Light RW. Parapneumonic effusions and empyema. *Clin Chest Med* 1985;**6**:55.

20. Christie NA. Management of pleural space: effusions and empyema. *Surg Clin North Am* 2010;**90**:919.

21. Porcel JM. Pleural fluid tests to identify complicated parapneumonic effusions. *Curr Opin Pulm Med* 2010;**16**:357.

22. Kraus GJ. The split pleura sign. *Radiology* 2007;**243**:297.

23. Lee MJ, Saini S, Brink JA, et al. Interventional radiology of the pleural space: management of thoracic empyema with image guided catheter drainage. *Semin Intervent Radiol* 1991;**8**:29.

24. Merriam MA, Cronin JJ, Dorfman GS, et al. Radiographically guided percutaneous catheter drainage of pleural fluid collections. *AJR Am J Roentgenol* 1988;**151**:1113.

25. Lee KS, Im J-G, Kim YH, et al. Treatment of thoracic multiloculated empyemas with intracavitary urokinase: a prospective study. *Radiology* 1991;**179**:771.

26. Loutsidis A, Bellenis I, Argiriou M, et al. Tetracycline compared with mechlorethamine in the treatment of malignant pleural effusions: a randomized trial. *Respir Med* 1994;**88**:523.

27. Thornton RH, Miller A, Covey AM, et al. Tunneled pleural catheters for treatment of recurrent malignant pleural effusion following failed pleurodesis. *J Vasc Interv Radiol* 2010;**21**:696.

28. vanSonnenberg E, D'Agostino HB, Casola G, et al. Lung abscess: CT guided drainage. *Radiology* 1991;**178**:347.

29. Moore AV, Zuger JH, Kelly MJ. Lung abscess: an interventional radiology perspective. *Semin Intervent Radiol* 1991;**8**:36.

30. Rice TW, Ginsberg RJ, Todd TR. Tube drainage of lung abscesses. *Ann Thorac Surg* 1987;**44**:356.

31. Wali SO, Shugaeri A, Samman YS, Abdelaziz M. Percutaneous drainage of pyogenic lung abscess. *Scand J Infect Dis* 2002;**34**:673.

32. Stavas J, vanSonnenberg E, Casola G, et al. Percutaneous drainage of infected and noninfected thoracic fluid collections. *J Thorac Imaging* 1987;**2**:80.

33. Kabukcu M, Demircioglu F, Yanik E, et al. Pericardial tamponade and large pericardial effusions: causal factors and efficacy of percutaneous catheter drainage in 50 patients. *Tex Heart Inst J* 2004;**31**:398.

34. Tazawa J, Sakai Y, Maekawa S, et al. Solitary and multiple pyogenic liver abscesses: characteristics of the patients and efficacy of percutaneous drainage. *Am J Gastroenterol* 1997;**92**:271.

35. Mezhir JJ, Fong Y, Jacks LM, et al. Current management of pyogenic liver abscess: surgery is now second-line treatment. *J Am Coll Surg* 2010;**210**:975.

36. Johnson RD, Mueller PF, Ferruci Jr JT, et al. Percutaneous drainage of pyogenic liver abscesses. *AJR Am J Roentgenol* 1985;**144**:463.

37. Do H, Lambiase RE, Deyoe L, et al. Percutaneous drainage of hepatic abscesses: comparison of results in abscesses with and without intrahepatic biliary communication. *AJR Am J Roentgenol* 1991;**157**:1209.

38. Gerzof SG, Johnson WC, Robbins AH, et al. Intrahepatic pyogenic abscesses: treatment by percutaneous drainage. *Am J Surg* 1985;**149**:487.

39. Liu CH, Gervais DA, Hahn PF, et al. Percutaneous hepatic abscess drainage: do multiple abscesses or multiloculated abscesses preclude drainage or affect outcome? *J Vasc Interv Radiol* 2009;**20**:1059.

40. Rajak CL, Gupta S, Jain S, et al. Percutaneous treatment of liver abscesses: needle aspiration versus catheter drainage. *AJR Am J Roentgenol* 1998;**170**:1035.

41. Yu SC, Ho SS, Lau WY, et al. Treatment of pyogenic liver abscess: prospective randomized comparison of catheter drainage and needle aspiration. *Hepatology* 2004;**39**:932.

42. Zerem E, Hadzic A. Sonographically guided percutaneous catheter drainage versus needle aspiration in the management of pyogenic liver abscess. *AJR Am J Roentgenol* 2007;**189**:W138.

43. Singh O, Gupta S, Moses S, et al. Comparative study of catheter drainage and needle aspiration in management of large liver abscesses. *Indian J Gastroenterol* 2009;**3**:88.

44. Smego RA Jr, Sebanego P. Treatment options for hepatic cystic echinococcosis. *Int J Infect Dis* 2005;**9**:69.

45. Saremi F, McNamara TO. Hydatid cysts of the liver: long-term results of percutaneous treatment using a cutting instrument. *AJR Am J Roentgenol* 1995;**165**:1163.

46. Bret PM, Fond A, Bretagnolle M, et al. Percutaneous aspiration and drainage of hydatid cysts of the liver. *Radiology* 1988;**168**:617.

47. Mueller PR, Dawson SL, Ferruci JT Jr, et al. Hepatic echinococcal cyst: successful percutaneous drainage. *Radiology* 1985;**155**:627.

48. Dziri C, Haouet K, Fingerhut A. Treatment of hydatid cyst of the liver: where is the evidence? *World J Surg* 2004;**28**:731.

49. Etlik O, Arslan H, Bay A, et al. Abdominal hydatid disease: long-term results of percutaneous treatment. *Acta Radiol* 2004;**45**:383.

50. Baijal SS, Agarwal DK, Roy S, et al. Complex ruptured amebic liver abscesses: the role of percutaneous catheter drainage. *Eur J Radiol* 1995;**20**:65.

51. vanSonnenberg E, Mueller PR, Schiffman HR, et al. Intrahepatic amebic abscesses: indications for and results of percutaneous catheter drainage. *Radiology* 1985;**156**:631.

52. Ken JG, vanSonnenberg E, Casola G, et al. Perforated amebic liver abscesses: successful percutaneous treatment. *Radiology* 1989;**170**:195.

53. vanSonnenberg E, Wroblicka JT, D'Agostino HB, et al. Symptomatic hepatic cysts: percutaneous drainage and sclerosis. *Radiology* 1994;**190**:387.

54. Pachter HL, Knudson MM, Esrig B, et al. Status of nonoperative management of blunt hepatic injuries in 1995: a multicenter experience with 404 patients. *J Trauma* 1996;**40**:31.

55. Faust TW, Reddy KR. Postoperative jaundice. *Clin Liver Dis* 2004;**8**:151.

56. Quinn SF, vanSonnenberg E, Casola G, et al. Interventional radiology in the spleen. *Radiology* 1986;**161**:289.

57. Ng KK, Lee TY, Wan YL, et al. Splenic abscess: diagnosis and management. *Hepatogastroenterology* 2002;**49**:567.

58. Thanos L, Dailiana T, Papaioannou G, et al. Percutaneous CT-guided drainage of splenic abscess. *AJR Am J Roentgenol* 2002;**179**:629.

59. Tasar M, Ugurel MS, Kocaoglu M, et al. Computed tomography-guided percutaneous drainage of splenic abscesses. *Clin Imaging* 2004;**28**:44.

60. Kang M, Kalra N, Gulati M, et al. Image guided percutaneous splenic interventions. *Eur J Radiol* 2007;**64**:140.

61. Ferraioli G, Bruneti E, Gulizia R, et al. Management of splenic abscess: report on 16 cases from a single center. *Int J Infect Dis* 2009;**13**:524.

62. Choudhury SR, Debnath PR, Jain P, et al. Conservative management of isolated splenic abscess in children. *J Ped Surg* 2009;**45**:372.

63. Chou YH, Hsu CC, Tiu CM, et al. Splenic abscess: sonographic diagnosis and percutaneous drainage or aspiration. *Gastrointest Radiol* 1992;**17**:262.

64. McNicholas MM, Mueller PR, Lee MJ, et al. Percutaneous drainage of subphrenic fluid collections that occur after splenectomy: efficacy and safety of transpleural versus extrapleural approach. *AJR Am J Roentgenol* 1995;**165**:355.

65. Torres WE, Evert MB, Baumgartner BR, et al. Percutaneous aspiration and drainage of pancreatic pseudocysts. *AJR Am J Roentgenol* 1986;**147**:1007.

66. vanSonnenberg E, Wittich GR, Casola G, et al. Percutaneous drainage of infected and noninfected pancreatic pseudocysts: experience in 101 cases. *Radiology* 1989;**170**:757.

67. vanSonnenberg E, Wittich GR, Chon KS, et al. Percutaneous radiologic drainage of pancreatic abscesses. *AJR Am J Roentgenol* 1997;**168**:979.

68. D'Agostino HB, Fotoohi M, Aspron MM, et al. Percutaneous drainage of pancreatic fluid collections. *Semin Intervent Radiol* 1996;**13**:101.

69. Steiner E, Mueller PR, Hahn PF, et al. Complicated pancreatic abscesses: problems in interventional management. *Radiology* 1988;**167**:443.

70. Matzinger FR, Ho CS, Yee AC, Gray RR. Pancreatic pseudocysts drained through a percutaneous transgastric approach: further experience. *Radiology* 1988;**167**:431.

71. Mueller PF, Ferrucci Jr JT, Simeone JF, et al. Lesser sac abscesses and fluid collections: drainage by transhepatic approach. *Radiology* 1985;**155**:615.

72. Fotoohi M, D'Agostino HB, Wollman B, et al. Persistent pancreatocutaneous fistula after percutaneous drainage of pancreatic fluid collections: role of cause and severity of pancreatitis. *Radiology* 1999;**213**:573.

73. Gyr KE, Meier R. Pharmacodynamic effects of Sandostatin in the gastrointestinal tract. *Digestion* 1993;**54**(Suppl. 1):14.

74. D'Agostino HB, vanSonnenberg E, Sanchez RB, et al. Treatment of pancreatic pseudocysts with percutaneous drainage and octreotide. Work in progress. *Radiology* 1993;**187**:685.

75. Echenique AM, Sleeman D, and Yrizarry J. Percutaneous catheter-directed debridement of infected pancreatic necrosis: results in 20 patients. *J Vasc Interv Radiol* 1998;**9**:565.

76. D'Agostino HB, Venable D, Gimenez M, et al. Percutaneous video-endoscopy-assisted removal of necrotic debris from pancreatic fluid collections. Baltimore (MD): SCVIR 27th Annual Scientific Meeting, April 6–April 11, 2002. *J Vasc Interv Radiol Supplement* 2002;**13**:S104.

77. Mui LM, Wong SK, Ng EK, et al. Combined sinus tract endoscopy and endoscopic retrograde cholangiopancreatography in management of pancreatic necrosis and abscess. *Surg Endosc* 2005;**19**:393.

78. Horvath K, Freeny P, Escallon J, et al. Safety and efficacy of video-assisted retroperitoneal debridement for infected pancreatic collections. *Arch Surg* 2010;**145**:817.

79. vanSonnenberg E, Wittich GR, Casola G, et al. Periappendiceal abscesses: percutaneous drainage. *Radiology* 1987;**163**:23.

80. Jamieson DH, Chait PG, Filler R. Interventional drainage of appendiceal abscesses in children. *AJR Am J Roentgenol* 1997;**169**:1619.

81. Jeffrey RB Jr, Federle MP, Tolentino CS. Periappendiceal inflammatory masses: CT directed management and clinical outcome in 70 patients. *Radiology* 1988;**167**:13.

82. Neff CC, vanSonnenberg E, Casola G, et al. Diverticular abscesses: percutaneous drainage. *Radiology* 1987;**163**:15.

83. Mueller PR, Saini S, Wittenberg J, et al. Sigmoid diverticular abscesses: percutaneous drainage as an adjunct to surgical resection in 24 cases. *Radiology* 1987;**164**:321.

84. Ambrosetti P, Chautems R, Soravia C, et al. Long-term outcome of mesocolic and pelvic diverticular abscesses of the left colon: a prospective study of 73 cases. *Dis Colon Rectum* 2005;**48**:787.

85. Gervais DA, Ho CH, O'Neill MJ, et al. Recurrent abdominal and pelvic abscesses: incidence, results of repeated percutaneous drainage, and underlying causes in 956 drainages. *AJR Am J Roentgenol* 2004;**182**:463.

86. Casola G, vanSonnenberg E, Neff CC, et al. Abscesses in Crohn disease: percutaneous drainage. *Radiology* 1987;**163**:19.

87. Doemeny JM, Burke DR, Meranze SG. Percutaneous drainage of abscesses in patients with Crohn's disease. *Gastrointest Radiol* 1988;**13**:237.

88. Ryan JM, Murphy BL, Boland GW. Use of the transgluteal route for percutaneous abscess drainage in acute diverticulitis to facilitate delayed surgical repair. *AJR Am J Roentgenol* 1998;**170**:1189.

89. Pereira JK, Chait PG, Miller SF. Deep pelvic abscesses in children: transrectal drainage under radiologic guidance. *Radiology* 1996;**198**:393.

90. Lomas DJ, Dixon AK, Thomson HJ, et al. CT guided drainage of pelvic abscesses: the peranal transrectal approach. *Clin Radiol* 1992;**45**:246.

91. Gazelle GS, Haaga JR, Stellato TA, et al. Pelvic abscesses: CT guided transrectal drainage. *Radiology* 1991;**181**:49.

92. vanSonnenberg E, D'Agostino HB, Casola G, et al. US-guided transvaginal drainage of pelvic abscesses and fluid collections. *Radiology* 1991;**181**:53.

93. Nosher JL, Winchman HK, Needell GS. Transvaginal pelvic abscess drainage with US guidance. *Radiology* 1987;**165**:872.

94. Gilliland JD, Spies JB, Brown SB, et al. Lymphoceles: percutaneous treatment with povidone-iodine sclerosis. *Radiology* 1989;**171**:227.

95. Sawhney R, D'Agostino HB, Zinck S, et al. Treatment of postoperative lymphoceles with percutaneous drainage and alcohol sclerotherapy. *J Vasc Interv Radiol* 1996;**7**:241.

96. Tasar M, Gulec B, Saglam M, et al. Posttransplant symptomatic lymphocele treatment with percutaneous drainage and ethanol sclerosis. Long-term follow-up. *Clin Imaging* 2005;**29**:109.

97. Paley M, Sidhu PS, Evans RA, et al. Retroperitoneal collections—aetiology and radiological implications. *Clin Radiol* 1997;**52**:290.

98. Gupta S, Suri S, Gulati M, et al. Ilio-psoas abscesses: percutaneous drainage under image guidance. *Clin Radiol* 1997;**52**:704.

SECTION II

AORTA AND PERIPHERAL ARTERIES

6

Thoracic Aorta

Karim Valji

ARTERIOGRAPHY

Thoracic aortography usually is done through a femoral artery approach. In individuals with a history of catheterization-related cholesterol embolization, angiography is sometimes performed via the proximal left brachial artery to avoid recurrent showering of plaque fragments. Although catheter angiography is rarely required in patients with suspected traumatic aortic injury, in that situation the arch should be traversed with a guidewire. Advancing a formed pigtail catheter into a traumatic pseudoaneurysm can be lethal.[1] A pigtail or similarly shaped catheter is placed about 2 cm above the aortic valve to avoid catheter recoil into the left ventricle during rapid contrast injection. A steep right posterior oblique projection is standard. Additional projections are obtained as needed.

ANATOMY

Development

In the fetus, two paired blood vessels (dorsal and ventral aortae) form in the chest.[2] The ventral aortae merge into the aortic sac, which forms parts of the ascending aorta, aortic arch, and pulmonary trunk. The left dorsal aorta becomes the descending thoracic aorta. Six pairs of *branchial arches*

connect these two major vascular channels (Fig. 6-1 and Table 6-1). The normal left aortic arch persists while the right arch involutes beyond the origin of the right subclavian artery. The remaining portion of the right arch becomes the brachiocephalic (innominate) artery.

Normal Anatomy

The *aortic valve* is composed of three leaflets that form the three *sinuses of Valsalva*: right, left, and posterior or noncoronary[3] (Fig. 6-2). The *right* and *left coronary arteries* arise from their respective sinuses. Beyond the sinus segment, the ascending aorta courses anteriorly and superiorly. This region is enclosed within the fibrous pericardium. In adults, its mean diameter at end diastole is 2.8 cm.[4] The aorta then passes over the main pulmonary artery and left main stem bronchus. The *brachiocephalic, left common carotid,* and *left subclavian arteries* take off in turn from the upper surface of the aortic arch.

Just beyond the origin of the left subclavian artery, the aorta narrows at the *aortic isthmus*. It then widens slightly beyond this point at the *aortic spindle*. The *ligamentum arteriosum,* a remnant of the ductus arteriosus, tethers the aorta to the left pulmonary artery at the isthmus. In some cases, a shallow, smooth, symmetric outpouching persists: the *ductus diverticulum,* or "ductus bump" (Fig. 6-3).

The descending thoracic aorta runs in front of the spine. In adults, its mean diameter at end diastole is

FIGURE 6-1 Embryologic development of the thoracic aorta. The numbers in the first panel refer to the branchial arches. *CCA,* common carotid artery; *DAo,* dorsal aortae; *DA,* ductus arteriosus; *ECA,* external carotid artery; *ICA,* internal carotid artery; *PA,* pulmonary artery; *RSCA,* right subclavian artery; *TA,* thoracic aorta; *VA,* ventral aortae. (*Adapted from: Langman J.* Medical Embryology. *3rd ed. Baltimore: Williams & Wilkins; 1975:235.*)

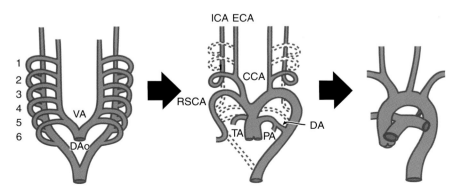

TABLE 6-1   Fate of Embryologic Aortic and Branchial Vessels

Embryologic Vessel	Neonatal Vessel
Ventral aorta (upper)	External carotid artery
Dorsal aorta (upper)	Internal carotid artery
Branchial arch 1	Maxillary artery
Branchial arch 2	Hyoid and stapedial arteries
Branchial arch 3	Carotid arteries
Branchial arch 4	Aortic arch
Branchial arch 5	Involutes
Branchial arch 6	Pulmonary artery, ductus arteriosus
7th intersegmental artery	Subclavian artery

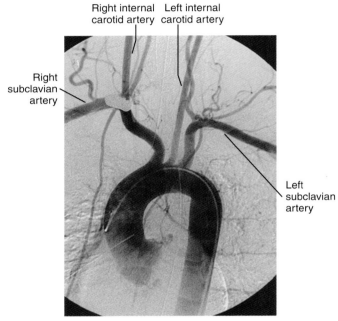

FIGURE 6-2   Normal thoracic aortogram in right posterior oblique projection.

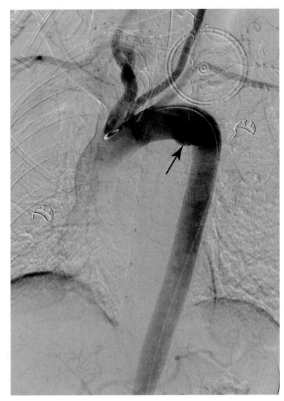

FIGURE 6-3   Normal thoracic aortogram in left posterior oblique projection demonstrates a prominent ductus diverticulum *(arrow)*.

about 2.2 cm.[4] Nine pairs of *posterior intercostal arteries* (levels 3 through 11) exit the descending aorta. The first and second posterior intercostal arteries are branches of the *superior intercostal artery*, which arises from the costo-cervical branch of the subclavian artery (see Chapter 9). The *subcostal arteries* take off at the level of the 12th ribs. One or more *bronchial arteries* supply each lung and originate as separate branches or bronchointercostal trunks typically at the fourth to sixth thoracic level (see Chapter 14). Numerous small vessels that supply the chest wall, mediastinum, esophagus, spinal cord, and pericardium are rarely seen during aortography.

Variant Anatomy (Online Cases 1 and 73)

Congenital anomalies of the thoracic aorta can be explained by abnormal evolution of the dorsal and ventral aortae and the branchial arches using the hypothetical double aortic arch system proposed by Edwards[5] (Box 6-1). The aorta, pulmonary artery, and anomalous branches may form vascular rings that compress the trachea or esophagus. Aortic arch variants often are associated with congenital cardiac anomalies.[6]

A common origin of the brachiocephalic and left common carotid arteries or origin of the left common carotid

---

BOX 6-1

CONGENITAL ANOMALIES OF THE THORACIC AORTA

- Aberrant right subclavian artery
- Right aortic arch
  - Aberrant left subclavian artery
  - Mirror-image branching
- Coarctation of the aorta
- Double aortic arch
- Cervical aortic arch
- Aberrant left brachiocephalic artery
- Isolated left subclavian artery
- Circumflex aorta
- Persistence of the fifth aortic arch

artery from the root of the brachiocephalic artery (bovine arch) is reported in 3% to 29% of the population based on autopsy and imaging studies; the true figure is probably closer to 10% to 15%[7,8] (Fig. 6-4). The origin of the term *bovine arch* is disputed. It may reflect the configuration of the vessels (like a bull's horn); this anatomy is not typical in cattle. Takeoff of the left vertebral artery directly from the arch is an uncommon variant (see Fig. 6-4). Separate origin of the right subclavian and common carotid arteries from the arch is rare.

An *aberrant right subclavian artery* is the most common aortic arch malformation of clinical significance, with a reported frequency of 0.4% to 2.3%.[9] This anomaly results from involution of the embryonic aortic segment between the right subclavian and right common carotid arteries. The right subclavian artery becomes the last branch of the aortic arch (Fig. 6-5). It usually passes behind the trachea and esophagus to reach the right side of the chest. The vessel may indent the posterior surface of the esophagus, but patients rarely have symptoms.[10] The aberrant artery often originates from a dilated portion of the most distal remnant of the right aortic arch, the so-called diverticulum of Kommerell.

Right aortic arch with aberrant left subclavian artery is the most common of the several types of right aortic arch, occurring in about 0.1% of the population.[11] The root cause is involution of the left aortic arch between the left common and left subclavian arteries with persistence of the embryologic right arch. The order of aortic arch branching is therefore left carotid artery, right carotid artery, right subclavian artery, and left subclavian artery. The arch passes over the right main stem bronchus and descends on either side of the spine (Fig. 6-6). Despite the presence of a vascular ring, respiratory and esophageal symptoms are infrequent. Few of these individuals have associated congenital heart disease.

Right aortic arch with mirror-image branching imposes a branch order of left brachiocephalic artery, right common carotid artery, and right subclavian artery.[12] The descending thoracic aorta is virtually always to the right of the

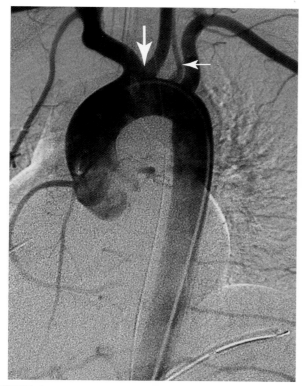

FIGURE 6-4 Bovine aortic arch *(large arrow)* with anomalous origin of left vertebral artery from the aortic arch *(small arrow).*

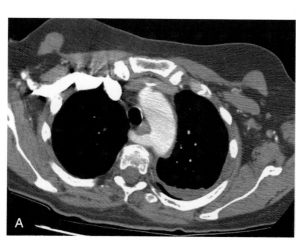
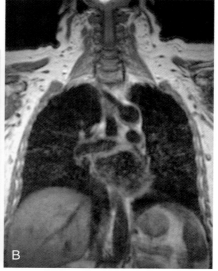

FIGURE 6-5 Aberrant right subclavian artery. **A,** The artery runs posterior to the trachea and esophagus on computed tomography angiography. **B,** Aberrant vessel arises as the last branch of the aortic arch on black-blood magnetic resonance image. *(Courtesy of Eric Goodman, MD, San Diego.)*

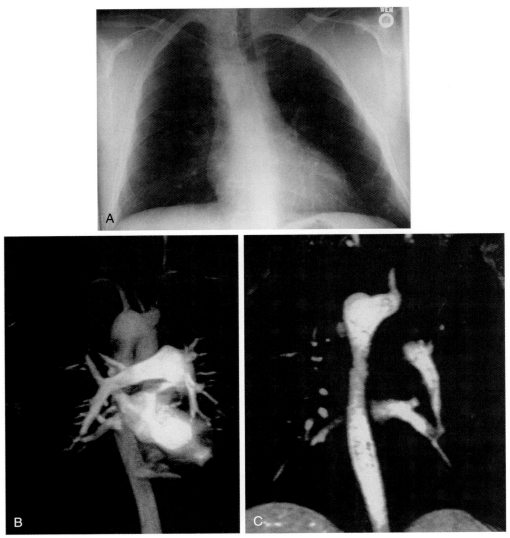

FIGURE 6-6 Right aortic arch with aberrant left subclavian artery. **A,** Chest radiograph shows right-sided aorta displacing the trachea to the left. **B,** Coronal three-dimensional MR angiography with cine breath-hold technique shows the right aortic arch. **C,** The left subclavian artery is the final branch of the aortic arch and arises from a large diverticulum.

spine. Some form of congenital heart disease is found in 90% to 95% of patients, including tetralogy of Fallot, truncus arteriosus, double-outlet right ventricle, and transposition of the great vessels. About one third of patients with tetralogy of Fallot have a right aortic arch, usually of this type. Although the vascular ring created by the right arch and ligamentum arteriosum produces tracheal or esophageal compression, patients usually have no symptoms.

MAJOR DISORDERS

Atherosclerosis

Atherosclerosis is the most common disease affecting the thoracic aorta, but usually it is silent. Plaques cause symptoms when fragments embolize into the brain or peripheral circulation. Emboli usually are released from "protruding" plaques with a mobile component that is probably overlying thrombus.[13] Most of these symptomatic lesions are found in the aortic arch and descending thoracic aorta. About one third of patients with such atheromas suffer distal embolization within 1 year of detection. Cholesterol crystals may shower into the distal circulation (spontaneously or after aortic manipulation) and result in renal insufficiency, bowel ischemia, or *blue toe syndrome.*[14]

Suspected thoracic aortic atherosclerosis in patients with unexplained stroke or peripheral embolization is studied by transesophageal echocardiography (TEE), computed tomography (CT), magnetic resonance imaging (MRI), or positron emission tomography (PET) imaging.[13,15] The disease produces an irregular contour to the aortic lumen, typically in the arch or distal aorta

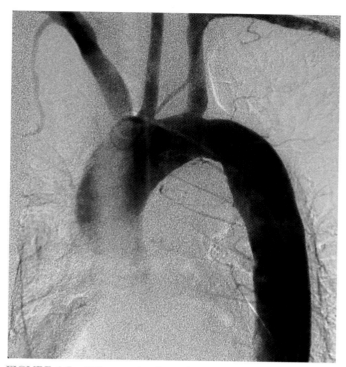

FIGURE 6-7   Diffuse aortic atherosclerosis seen on arch aortography.

CAUSES OF THORACIC AORTIC ANEURYSMS

- Degenerative ("atherosclerotic")
- Bicuspid aortic valve
- Trauma
  - Blunt or penetrating
  - Postoperative
- Chronic dissection
- Noninflammatory vasculopathy
  - Marfan syndrome
  - Ehlers-Danlos syndromes
  - Loeys-Dietz syndrome
- Infection (bacterial, syphilitic, tuberculous)
- Vasculitis (see Box 6-5)
- Congenital (sinus of Valsalva aneurysm)

TABLE 6-2   Classic Appearance of Thoracic Aortic Aneurysms

Type	Features
Degenerative	Fusiform aneurysm of the descending aorta with atherosclerotic changes
Post-traumatic	Saccular pseudoaneurysm at the aortic isthmus
Postoperative	Saccular aneurysm at stent-graft termination, suture line, or cannulation site
Bacterial	Saccular, eccentric aneurysm at an unusual site
Marfan syndrome	Aneurysm of aortic root and tubular segment (sinotubular or annuloaortic ectasia)
Syphilitic	Saccular ascending aortic or arch aneurysm sparing the aortic root
Takayasu arteritis	Wall thickening and enhancement (early) Diffuse fusiform dilation of the aorta with branch stenoses or occlusions (late)
Post-stenotic	Dilation beyond an obstruction (e.g., aortic stenosis, coarctation)

(Fig. 6-7). Rarely, ulcerated plaque penetrates into the aortic wall (see later discussion). Other causes for narrowing of the aortic lumen include dissection (with encroachment by the false lumen), arteritis, and noninflammatory vasculopathies (see Box 1-10).

Degenerative Aneurysms (Online Case 96)

Etiology and Natural History

Thoracic aortic aneurysms (TAAs) and pseudoaneurysms have many causes[16-18] (Box 6-2). The classic features of several types are summarized in Table 6-2. The pathologic and imaging features of the uncommon forms are considered in later sections of this chapter.

About 75% of TAAs are *degenerative ("atherosclerotic") aneurysms* that form because of weakening of the aortic wall by enhanced proteolytic activity or hemodynamic forces that cause pathologic remodeling.[16-18] Most degenerative thoracic aneurysms involve the descending segment; about 5% are thoracoabdominal.[19] The most common cause of **isolated** ascending aortic aneurysm is intrinsic medial degeneration[20] (e.g., Marfan syndrome, see Chapter 1).

Compared with abdominal aortic aneurysms, the natural history of thoracic aneurysms is less well understood. The most feared complication is rupture. Based on Laplace's law (wall stress = pressure × radius), the strongest predictor of rupture is *aneurysm size*. Less important risk factors for TAA rupture are advanced age, hypertension, chronic lung disease, and renal failure.[21] The likelihood of rupture is low if the aneurysm is less than 5 cm in diameter, unless the rate of expansion exceeds about 1 cm/yr. After a TAA reaches *5 to 6 cm in diameter,* the risk of subsequent rupture increases substantially (i.e., 5-year mortality between 38% and 64%).[22-25] As a rule, such patients should undergo elective aneurysm repair.

Clinical Features

Most affected patients are older and asymptomatic at the time the aneurysm is discovered on a routine chest radiograph or CT scan obtained for unrelated reasons. Unusual complaints related to compression of adjacent organs include dysphagia, respiratory distress, superior vena cava syndrome, and hoarseness from impingement of the recurrent laryngeal nerve. Some individuals with intact aneurysms do complain of chest or back pain. However, symptoms are expected when the aneurysm ruptures. They include chest pain, hypotension, massive hemoptysis (from *aortobronchial fistula*), hematemesis (from the even rarer *aortoesophageal fistula*), and dyspnea from leakage into the pleural space.

Imaging

CHEST RADIOGRAPHY

Plain chest radiographs show enlargement of the ascending aorta, descending aorta, or both. A massive aneurysm can erode the vertebral bodies or sternum. Atelectasis can result from compression of the airways. A left pleural effusion suggests the possibility of rupture.

TRANSESOPHAGEAL ECHOCARDIOGRAPHY

TEE can both detect and size TAA.[26] However, TEE is less valuable for aneurysm staging, evaluation of adjacent structures, or postoperative surveillance.

COMPUTED TOMOGRAPHY

CT is the standard tool for the diagnosis of suspected TAA, surveillance of known aneurysms, and detection of sac rupture.[27] Aneurysm diameter and length, presence of mural thrombus, and associated atherosclerotic disease are well depicted by CT (Fig. 6-8). A high-density "crescent" in the mural thrombus may be a harbinger of contained or imminent rupture. Multiplanar reformatted and shaded-surface display images provide exquisite views of the aneurysm, its relationship to adjacent structures (e.g., compression of the pulmonary artery), and involvement of arch vessels.[16,28]

MAGNETIC RESONANCE IMAGING

MRI is probably the best modality for studying TAA in patients in stable condition, although it is not effective after endograft repair. Gadolinium-enhanced MR angiography characterizes the entire extent of the aneurysm, its effect on neighboring organs, branch vessel involvement, the aortic valve, and the heart.[6,29] Several features can sometimes differentiate degenerative aneurysms from other types (see Table 6-2).

Treatment

SURGICAL THERAPY

The traditional treatment for TAAs is operative.[30] As a rule, they are repaired when the diameter exceeds 5 to 6 cm or the patient is symptomatic (see earlier discussion).

An *interposition graft* is placed by end-to-end anastomosis of a synthetic conduit between the excised ends of the aorta. Alternatively, the diseased portion of the aorta is wrapped around the graft material sewn to the aorta at both ends as an *inclusion graft*. With proximal aortic disease, an *elephant trunk* technique may be employed.[31] The ascending aortic and arch segments are replaced with graft material and branch vessels connected into it; the distal free end of the graft floats in the descending thoracic aorta. At a later stage, the surgeon creates a permanent anastomosis to the normal lower descending thoracic aorta.

Major complications of operative TAA repair include stroke, myocardial infarction, and renal failure. Paraplegia is a rather unique and devastating event caused by exclusion of branches to the spinal artery. It is more frequent with repair of thoracoabdominal aneurysms. The frequency of spinal cord injury is well under 10% with the use of intraoperative maneuvers such as distal perfusion, hypothermia, and monitoring of evoked potentials.[32,33] Preoperative spinal arteriography may be useful in this setting to allow reimplantation of major spinal artery branches.[34] In contemporary series, the overall mortality rate for elective repair is still substantial but far better than for operation with rupture (3% to 8% vs. 22%).[32,33]

ENDOVASCULAR THERAPY

Thoracic endovascular aneurysm repair (TEVAR) with stent grafts is an attractive alternative to open surgery for selected patients with stable or ruptured degenerative TAAs.[35-37] Several devices are approved by the U.S. Food and Drug Administration for treatment of this particular disorder (Table 6-3 and Fig. 6-9). The choice of stent graft is based on patient factors, aneurysm characteristics, and operator preference. The *TAG device* can be inserted rapidly but with somewhat less precision than other endografts. The *Talent device* (and the newer iteration *Valiant stent*) allows accurate deployment and is easier to use with severe aortic angulation or iliac artery access tortuosity. Finally, the *Zenith device* has the lowest profile (at present) and permits the most accurate deployment.

Technical success and immediate aneurysm thrombosis is noted in more than 90% of cases with very low mortality rates[38] (see Fig. 6-8). Unlike endograft treatment of abdominal aortic aneurysms (see Chapter 7), the most common type of endoleak with TAA (up to 30% of cases) is a type I defect at an attachment site.[39,40] In this situation, additional interventions (further balloon treatment, insertion of additional stents or stent grafts) are usually necessary. Uncommon early complications include stroke and paraplegia from exclusion of side branches feeding the spinal cord.[41] Late complications involve proximal

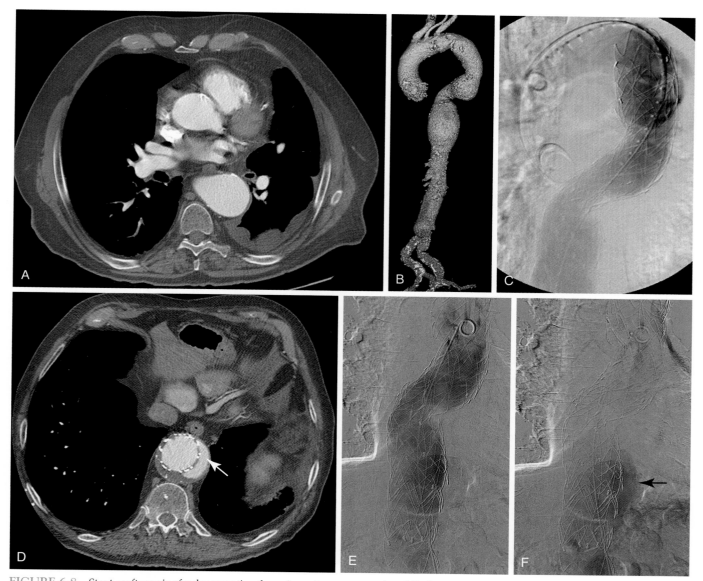

FIGURE 6-8   Stent graft repair of a degenerative thoracic aortic aneurysm. **A** and **B,** On contrast-enhanced computed tomography (CT) scans, two regions of saccular dilation of the descending thoracic aorta (almost extending to the abdominal segment) are evident. **C,** The stent graft is in place and is widely patent. **D,** On follow-up CT, a crescentic region of contrast appears outside the graft but within the aneurysm sac *(arrow).* **E** and **F,** Catheter aortography demonstrates the leak that occurs at a graft attachment site *(arrow).*

and distal endoleaks, aneurysm growth at the edges of the device, stent graft movement, kinking or fracture, and aneurysm rupture.

The choice between open and endovascular repair of TAA is made difficult by the almost complete lack of randomized, controlled trials comparing the two approaches.[36,37] Two large, prospective, single-arm trials with historical controls noted significantly lower early morbidity and mortality and paraplegia rates with TEVAR.[38,42] Reported outcomes were technical success 96%, major adverse events 41%, 30-day mortality 2.1%, paraplegia 1.5%, stroke 3.6%, aneurysm rupture at 1 year 0.5%, migration 4%, and endoleak 12.2%. One study observed

better 1-year mortality with TEVAR, whereas the other showed no difference at 2 years. A recent metaanalysis calculated a significantly lower incidence of neurologic injury and perioperative mortality with TEVAR.

Dissection (Online Cases 13 and 52)

Etiology

A dissection is a longitudinal split in the media of the aortic wall. In most cases, an intimal tear connects this medial channel with the aortic lumen. Dissections confined to the aortic wall are *intramural hematomas*[43] (see later discussion).

TABLE 6-3   FDA-Approved Stent Grafts for Thoracic Aortic Disease

Type	Talent	Zenith	TAG
Manufacturer	Medtronic	Cook, Inc	W.L. Gore Associates
Components	Single	Two part	Single
Construction	Nitinol/ polyester	Stainless steel/ Dacron	Nitinol/ePTFE
Bare segment	Available	Available	
Delivery system	22-25 Fr	20-22 Fr	"Large"
Device diameter	22-46 mm	22-42 mm	26-40 mm
Device length		10.8-21.6 cm	10, 15, 20 cm
Features	Very flexible Very trackable Wide size range	Low profile Precise placement	Easy deployment

ePTFE, *expanded polytetrafluoroethylene.*

The pathogenesis of aortic dissection is not entirely understood.[44] Dissection is usually attributed to hemodynamic stresses such as long-standing hypertension or to abnormalities of the media (some of which are congenital)[45] (Box 6-3). In the former group, the pathologic basis for dissection is unclear; only mild medial degeneration is seen histologically. In the latter group, degeneration of medial smooth muscle, elastin, or collagen matrix can be identified. The reason that pregnant women are at greater risk for dissection is unknown, although hemodynamic factors and hormonal effects have been implicated. Illicit drug use (particularly cocaine and methamphetamines) is being recognized as an increasingly frequent cause of acute dissection.[46] Occasionally, aortic dissection is caused by trauma (e.g., deceleration injury, catheterization procedures).[47]

Regardless of the underlying pathology, the inciting event usually is an intimal tear. Sometimes, the dissection begins spontaneously within the aortic wall, possibly from rupture of the vasa vasorum. The intimal tear connects the lumen in direct continuity with the aortic valve *(true lumen)* with the channel of blood in the media *(false lumen).* The dissection propagates distally, proximally, or in both directions as blood under high pressure expands the false channel. Blood flow in the false lumen usually is slower than in the true lumen. The false channel, however, can become large and compress the true lumen. The dissection usually stops at an aortic branch or atherosclerotic plaque. In many cases, it extends to the aortic bifurcation or beyond.

The location and extent of the dissection has important implications for treatment and prognosis. The DeBakey and Stanford classifications are illustrated in Figure 6-10. Stanford *type A dissections,* which usually begin with a tear just above the aortic valve and always involve the ascending aorta, account for about two thirds of cases.[48] *Type B dissections,* which usually begin with a tear just beyond the origin of the left subclavian artery and only involve the descending aorta, account for the remaining cases. Sometimes, a dissection that

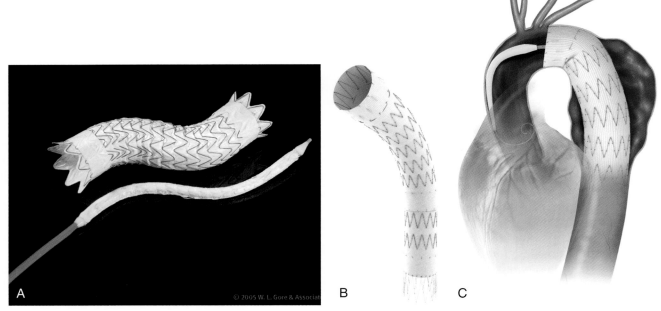

FIGURE 6-9   Stent graft devices for thoracic aortic disease. **A,** TAG graft. **B,** Zenith graft. **C,** Schematic of Zenith graft for exclusion of a descending thoracic aortic aneurysm. (**A,** *Courtesy of W.L. Gore Associates;* **B,** *Courtesy of Cook, Inc.)*

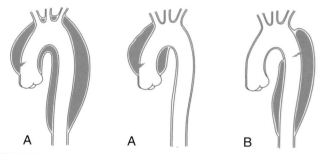

FIGURE 6-10 Classification for aortic dissection. Figures *(from left to right)* correspond to DeBakey types I, II, and III, and the Stanford classification *(A or B)* is stated for each. *(Adapted from: Kadir S. Diagnostic Angiography. Philadelphia: WB Saunders; 1986:141.)*

begins at this site extends distally and proximally toward the aortic valve.

Natural History

Early complications of aortic dissection are the result of complete rupture (often at the site of the intimal tear) or ischemia. Advances in diagnosis and treatment have improved outcomes, but even in the best of hands the mortality rate still exceeds 18% to 25%.[49,50] Rupture, which often is fatal, can occur from the ascending aorta into the pericardium, from the aortic arch into the mediastinum, or from the descending aorta into the mediastinum or left pleural space. In about half of patients with type A dissection, aortic regurgitation follows damage to the aortic root.

If the intimal flap obstructs a major aortic branch or flow is diminished in the true or false channel supplying an organ, ischemia can result (so-called *malperfusion syndrome*). In most of these cases, the obstruction is "dynamic" (prolapse of flap into vessel orifice or inadequate flow in the lumen feeding the tissue).[49] In this situation, some type of fenestration to increase blood pressure in the stagnant lumen is indicated (see later discussion). Less often, "static" obstruction from extension of the flap into a major branch is responsible for target organ ischemia. In this event, direct recanalization by stent insertion or operative bypass is necessary.

Over time, untreated dissections can persist (i.e., *chronic dissection*), enlarge, thrombose, or rupture. A dissection is consider chronic if it is present for more than 2 weeks. Late complications of untreated chronic dissections include aneurysm formation and delayed ischemic events. Even with appropriate medical therapy, 25% to 40% of surviving patients will go on to aneurysm formation.[44]

Clinical Features

Aortic dissection is one of several diseases included in the *acute aortic syndromes* which feature the constellation of chest pain and chronic hypertension[51] (see later discussion). These disorders are easily confused with the *acute coronary syndromes*. In modern series, men suffer aortic dissections about four or five times as frequently as women. Most patients are older than 50 years and have one or more risk factors for dissection (see Box 6-3). Hypertension is present in about three fourths of patients and is even more common in patients with type B dissection. The classic presentation is the sudden onset of searing chest or back pain. Patients also may present with a stroke, renal failure or renovascular hypertension, mesenteric ischemia, lower extremity ischemia, or even paraplegia from obstruction of spinal artery branches of the descending aorta.

Imaging

CHEST RADIOGRAPHY

Plain radiographs of the chest may point to the diagnosis of aortic dissection. The most common findings are an increase in size of the thoracic aorta, a double aortic arch contour, widening of the mediastinal silhouette, pleural effusion, and tracheal shift.[52] A completely normal chest radiograph does not exclude the diagnosis.

COMPUTED TOMOGRAPHY

CT is widely used for evaluation of acute aortic dissection.[16,52,53] CT is readily available, relatively noninvasive, and accommodates critically ill patients.

Scans reveal an intimal flap separating the two lumens, often with different enhancement patterns (Fig. 6-11).

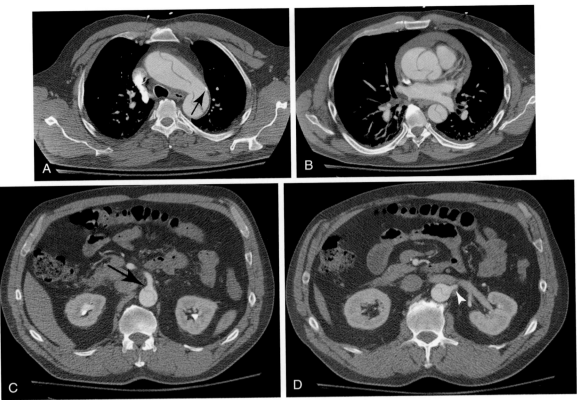

FIGURE 6-11   Stanford type A aortic dissection. **A** and **B,** Contrast-enhanced chest computed tomography shows a complex dissection flap passing through the entire aortic arch. Spot of calcification on lateral wall of arch denotes the intima *(arrow),* indicating that the true lumen is lateral and false lumen more medial at that level. **C,** The compressed true lumen *(arrow)* supplies the superior mesenteric artery. **D,** The true lumen also supplies the left renal artery *(arrowhead).*

Other possible findings are dilation of the aorta, compression of the true lumen by the false lumen, thrombosis of the false lumen, mediastinal hematoma, and pleural or pericardial effusion. A localized dissection must be differentiated from an intramural hematoma or a penetrating aortic ulcer (see later discussion).

It is important to distinguish the true lumen from the false lumen and the relationship of all major aortic branches to them. The true lumen is the one in continuity with the aortic valve. The most reliable features of the true lumen are outer wall calcification and eccentric flap calcification[53] (see Fig. 6-11). The false lumen usually has a larger cross-sectional area and an acute angle between the flap and the outer aortic wall (Fig. 6-12). In most type B aortic dissections, the false lumen is posterior and lateral to the true lumen in the chest and then spirals down the aorta in a somewhat unpredictable fashion.

MAGNETIC RESONANCE IMAGING

Gadolinium-enhanced MR angiography also is extremely accurate for diagnosing and staging aortic dissection.[29,54,55] The risks of iodinated contrast material are avoided. Aortic branch vessels, the aortic valve, and the heart can be evaluated with MRI. Its major limitations are longer scanning times and difficulties with monitoring critically ill patients. Cine imaging will help detect aortic insufficiency. MR images can identify an intimal flap and different signal intensities in the true and false lumens caused by variations in blood flow or by clot (Fig. 6-13). Noncommunicating dissection (i.e., intramural hematoma) can usually be differentiated from a communicating dissection with slow flow.

TRANSESOPHAGEAL ECHOCARDIOGRAPHY

TEE is performed with multiplanar color flow Doppler techniques.[26] The procedure can be performed at the bedside in less than 30 minutes with the patient under moderate sedation. TEE is favored by cardiologists because it is fast and convenient. Besides identifying an intimal flap, echocardiography also can detect aortic insufficiency and extension of dissection into the coronary arteries. It is extremely sensitive but somewhat less specific than CT and MRI. The aortic arch is a relative blind-spot for this modality.

CATHETER ANGIOGRAPHY

Aortography was once the primary method for preoperative diagnosis of aortic dissection but is now only necessary prior to TEVAR or other endovascular interventions.

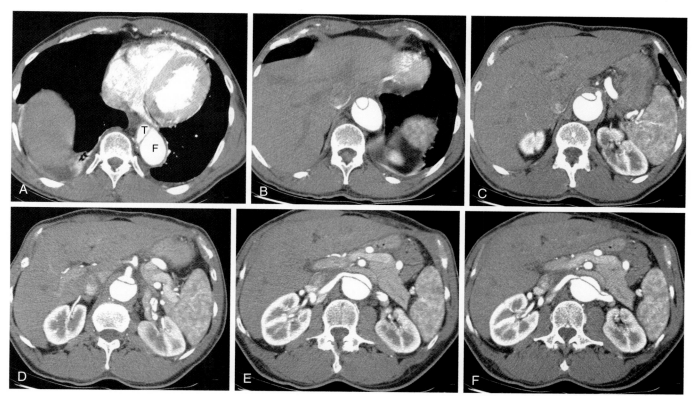

FIGURE 6-12   Stanford type B dissection **(A and B)** with extension into the abdominal aorta seen with computed tomography angiography (*T*, true lumen; *F*, false lumen). Note relationship of lumens to celiac **(C)**, superior mesenteric **(D)**, right renal **(E)**, and left renal arteries into which the dissection flap extends **(F)**. The dissection continued down both iliac arteries to the groin (not shown).

Aortography is more risky and less sensitive than cross-sectional techniques in the detection of acute dissection. The imager can entirely miss the diagnosis of intramural hematoma or chronic dissection with thrombosis of the false lumen.

CT or MR images guide catheterization of the true and/or false lumens from a common femoral or brachial artery approach. Special care should be taken to avoid extending or overinjecting the false lumen if it is catheterized. Abdominal or pelvic arteriography usually is needed to follow the dissection to the level of reentry. A lucent flap between the true and false lumens is diagnostic (Fig. 6-14). Delayed filling and slow washout of the false lumen are characteristic. The true lumen may be narrowed by an expanding false channel. The relationship of branch vessels to the two lumens should be established.

CHOICE OF IMAGING MODALITY

Multidetector CT and MR angiography have similar accuracy in the diagnosis of aortic dissection.[29,56] The optimal approach to the patient with suspected or known dissection depends on the relative availability of equipment, condition of the patient, and capability of operators.

Treatment

SURGICAL THERAPY

Management of patients with acute aortic dissection depends on the location and extent of the dissection, existence of complications, and the general health of the patient. Patients with type B dissection are first treated medically with blood pressure control. There is a consensus that most patients with Stanford type A dissection should undergo repair with graft insertion or primary obliteration of the false lumen.[44,50] The aortic valve is replaced when necessary. Repair is performed if there is a complication (e.g., renal failure, mesenteric ischemia), rapid expansion, or impending rupture signaled by continuing pain or hypotension. Notably, mortality rates are substantially reduced if mesenteric ischemia (when present) is treated before attending to the aortic pathology itself.[57] Chronic dissections usually are treated when the aortic diameter exceeds 6 cm or the patient has symptoms.

ENDOVASCULAR THERAPY

Endovascular methods have been devised to treat both acute and late complications of aortic dissection. These techniques include uncovered stent placement, balloon fenestration, and stent graft insertion.

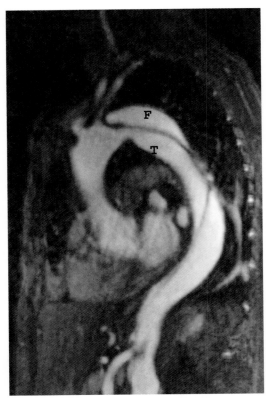

FIGURE 6-13   Type B aortic dissection seen on three-dimensional magnetic resonance angiography in oblique sagittal plane (*T*, true lumen; *F*, false lumen). The dissection spirals down into the abdominal aorta.

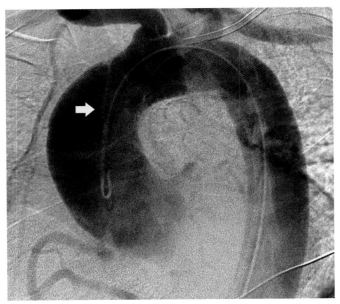

FIGURE 6-14   Stanford type A dissection on arch aortography in the right posterior oblique projection. An intimal tear is seen in the proximal ascending aorta *(arrow)*.

When "static obstruction" causes malperfusion to an organ, an uncovered stent can tack down an intimal flap extending into a branch vessel and reopen the artery. With "dynamic obstruction," equalization of pressure in both lumens often relieves end organ ischemia. This condition is accomplished by *aortic flap balloon fenestration*.[58,59] Both the true and false lumens are engaged through separate arterial access sites. In some cases it is necessary to puncture the proximal right brachial artery to enter the true lumen. Careful catheter arteriography is done to delineate the precise position of the flaps and relationship to all major primary branches. A large-caliber needle within a protective cannula (e.g., Roesch-Uchida TIPS) is used to pierce the intimal flap and connect one lumen with the other. Typically, the puncture is made from the constricted true lumen into the expanded false lumen. Some interventionalists use intravascular ultrasound (IVUS) to facilitate the needle pass. Alternatively, an occlusion balloon inflated in the apposing lumen may serve as a target. Once the flap is transgressed and a stiff guidewire advanced, the hole is then widened with a 15- to 20-mm–diameter angioplasty balloon (Fig. 6-15). Several fenestrations should be made.

Finally, stent grafts are now favored to permanently correct many early complications of malperfusion syndrome and to prevent (or later treat) aneurysm formation.[36,37,49,60] The primary goals are to seal the entry tear and eliminate flow in the false lumen. Treatment of chronic dissections can be more difficult because of the development of multiple entry flaps or predominance of the false lumen. Choosing appropriate cases requires careful analysis of high-quality CT arteriograms. A proximal landing zone of 2 cm is generally required; covering the left subclavian artery is often necessary but may not be as safe as often thought.[41] Ideally, the graft is extended at least 10 cm beyond the entry tear. Sometimes, commercially available devices will not accommodate a markedly dilated aorta. The diameter, tortuosity, or heavy calcification of the femoral and iliac arteries may preclude endovascular treatment without an open iliac conduit.[49]

Both the true and false lumens are accessed; brachial artery puncture may be necessary. Placement of the device is guided by catheter angiography and often IVUS. Great care is taken when inflating compliant balloons used to mold the device to the aortic wall. A recent report from the EUROSTAR aortic stent graft registry noted 89% technical success, 8.4% 30-day mortality, and 90% 1-year survival among 131 treated patients, most of whom had type B dissections.[41] However, in a recent large multicenter trial comparing TEVAR with optimal medical therapy in patients with uncomplicated type B dissection, no benefit was found in 2-year survival or frequency of adverse events.[61]

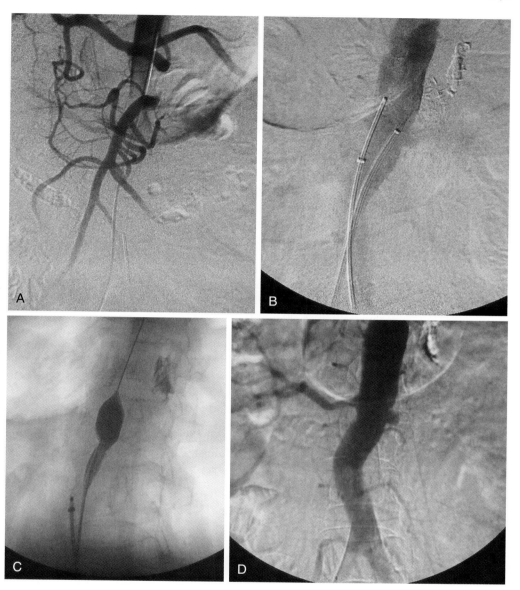

FIGURE 6-15 Balloon fenestration of a type B aortic dissection. **A,** Abdominal aortography shows right and left common femoral artery (CFA) catheters lying in the true lumen, which feeds the celiac and superior mesenteric arteries with poor flow to the right renal artery and none to the left. **B,** Intravascular ultrasound introduced from the left CFA, Rosch-Uchida TIPS set introduced from the right CFA. Puncture was made posterolaterally and proven to be intraluminal. **C,** Angioplasty with 18-mm balloon is performed. **D,** Repeat angiography shows improved flow to the right renal artery and equivalent flow in both aortic lumens.

Follow-up Imaging

All patients with aortic dissection, whether treated medically or surgically, need routine follow-up examinations to evaluate the dissection (or graft) and to detect complications.[62,63] The surgeon or interventionalist is concerned about several issues:

- Patency, fixation, and stability of the graft or endograft
- Presence of endoleak after endograft placement
- Status of the false lumen (e.g., persistent flow, extension, expansion, thrombosis)
- Degree of aortic insufficiency

The most common late sequelae are progressive expansion of the false lumen, aneurysm or pseudoaneurysm formation at graft anastomoses or stent graft edges, endograft migration, and endoleak (see Chapter 7).

Aortic Trauma (Online Case 91)

Etiology and Natural History

Motor vehicle accidents are responsible for most thoracic aortic injuries by rapid deceleration of a passenger or pedestrian. Other causes include falls from a height, crush injuries, and penetrating wounds. Deceleration trauma usually result in an intimal or transmural tear (rupture), which is almost immediately fatal in about 80% to 90% of cases.[64,65] Dissection is less common.[47] Rarely, the injury produces an aortic intramural hematoma or complete transection with thrombosis.

Immediate survival of an aortic tear is possible if the rupture is contained by periadventitial tissues to form a fragile pseudoaneurysm. One widely held explanation for these injuries is that relatively fixed and mobile parts of the aorta experience unequal forces at the moment of impact. These forces, which may be caused by traction, torsion, shearing, or compression, lacerate the aortic wall.[66] The actual mechanisms are unknown.

Aortic injury can occur at any site or at multiple sites. In up to 75% to 90% of accident scene survivors, the tear is located at the aortic isthmus just beyond the left subclavian artery. Less commonly, a defect is found at the aortic root, origins of the arch vessels, or lower descending aorta. The mortality rate for blunt aortic trauma is extremely high if left untreated, and many of these patients die within the first 24 hours after injury.[67] However, mortality has dropped with contemporary management protocols[68] (see later discussion). Without repair, a chronic pseudoaneurysm may develop and remain silent for decades. These cases may come to medical attention as incidental findings on chest radiographs or CT scans.

Clinical Features

The violence of the event may not correlate with the likelihood of aortic injury. Clinical symptoms and signs are not particularly helpful in screening patients. For these reasons, every patient with the appropriate "mechanism of injury" is suspect. Because the consequence of missing an aortic injury is so grave, imaging studies are used liberally.

Imaging

CHEST RADIOGRAPHY

A plain radiograph is obtained for every patient with significant chest trauma. Radiographs are most useful with the patient in an upright position, although this is rarely feasible. A ruptured aorta produces a host of findings[69] (Box 6-4). The most sensitive signs are widening of the superior mediastinum (ultimately a subjective call), indistinctness of the aortic arch contour, and loss of the descending aortic shadow (Fig. 6-16). Fewer than 1% to 2% of patients with normal chest radiographs are subsequently found to have an aortic laceration. In practice, most stable patients with a mechanism for injury proceed to CT scanning.

COMPUTED TOMOGRAPHY

Multidetector thoracic CT angiography can detect and characterize significant aortic injury with very close to 100% accuracy.[69-72] In addition to indirect signs of bleeding, direct signs include intraluminal flaps, pseudoaneurysm, irregular contour, dissection, or intramural hematoma (Figs. 6-17 through 6-19). Particular care

---

> ### BOX 6-4
>
> ## CHEST RADIOGRAPHIC SIGNS ASSOCIATED WITH AORTIC INJURY
>
> - Abnormal contour of the arch or descending aorta
> - Mediastinal widening
> - Loss of the aorticopulmonary window
> - Tracheal shift to the right
> - Depressed left main stem bronchus
> - Nasogastric tube displacement to the right
> - Widened paraspinal lines
> - Left apical cap
> - Upper rib fractures
> - Lung contusion or opacification
> - Left hemothorax or pneumothorax

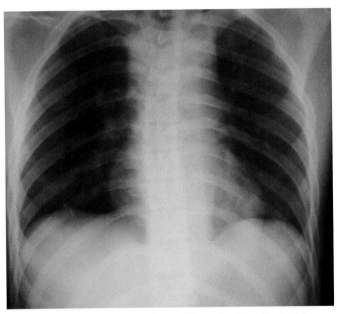

FIGURE 6-16   The supine chest radiograph of a patient with a traumatic aortic tear shows marked widening of the mediastinum and loss of the normal aortic knob.

---

must be taken to identify abnormalities at the origins of the arch vessels.

CATHETER AORTOGRAPHY

Catheter arteriography is only employed when CT is uninterpretable or inconclusive, angiography is being done urgently for possible embolization of other arterial injuries, and prior to stent graft placement. Guidewire hangup, particularly near the aortic isthmus, may be the first indication of an aortic tear. Aortography is then

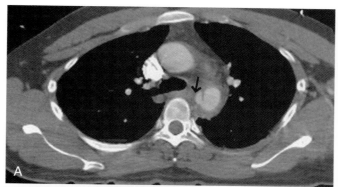

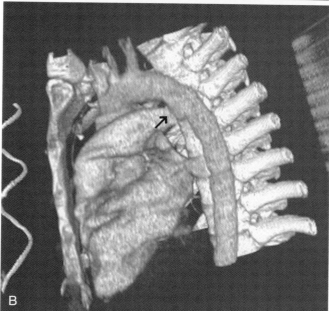

FIGURE 6-17 **A,** Aortic tear with typical appearance of a pseudoaneurysm *(arrow)* just beyond the left subclavian artery on axial computed tomography angiogram. Also note increased paraaortic density from mediastinal blood. **B,** Shaded-surface display reformatted image demonstrates pseudoaneurysm.

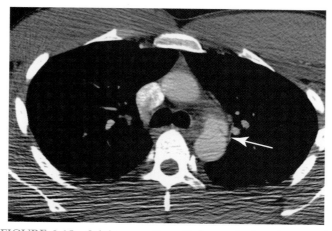

FIGURE 6-18 Subtle traumatic aortic flap on the lateral aspect of the aorta *(arrow)* identified with CT angiography.

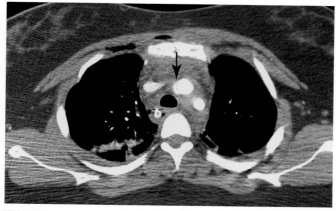

FIGURE 6-19 Computed tomography angiography shows an isolated traumatic pseudoaneurysm of the origin of the brachiocephalic/left common carotid artery (bovine arch, *arrow*) following a motor vehicle accident. A sternal fracture is present.

performed below this level with a small contrast injection to avoid further damage to the vessel.[1] The entire thoracic aorta, from the aortic valve to the diaphragmatic hiatus and including the arch vessels must be imaged. Aortography is always done in *at least two views* to exclude the diagnosis, typically a steep right posterior oblique projection and an orthogonal left posterior oblique or frontal projection. Subtle tears or intimal flaps can easily be missed on a single view (Fig. 6-20).

The usual aortographic finding is an irregular outpouching of the aorta just beyond the left subclavian artery (Fig. 6-21). These contained pseudoaneurysms can take on a variety of shapes and sizes. Less often, injury produces an intimal flap, arch vessel pseudoaneurysm or intimal flap, dissection, or (rarely) complete transection[73] (Fig. 6-22). *Novices sometimes mistake traumatic aortic rupture for a dissection, which is the wrong term for the typical abnormality.* Chronic traumatic pseudoaneurysms can be saccular or fusiform, and the wall often is heavily calcified.

Several entities can mimic an acute aortic injury[74]:

- The *ductus diverticulum* occurs at the usual site for deceleration injury. However, this normal variant usually has smooth, continuous edges with the aorta, no associated intimal flap, and rapid washout of contrast (see Fig. 6-3).
- An *infundibulum* of an aortic branch (usually left subclavian or bronchointercostal artery) can be mistaken for an injured segment. This error is avoided by noting its smooth, symmetric, conical margins and association with a normal vessel (Fig. 6-23).
- In older patients, ulcerated atherosclerotic plaque or a focal degenerative aneurysm may be impossible to differentiate from an acute traumatic injury.
- The normal widening of the *aortic spindle* should not be confused with a traumatic pseudoaneurysm.

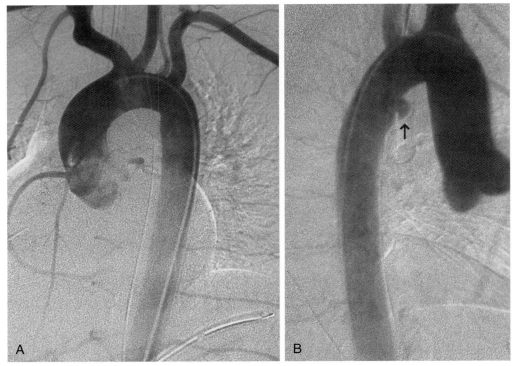

FIGURE 6-20   **A,** Standard right posterior oblique projection shows no evidence of blunt aortic injury. **B,** Shallow left posterior oblique projection shows abnormal outpouching from the proximal descending thoracic aorta *(arrow).*

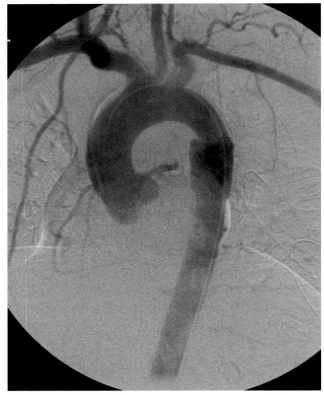

FIGURE 6-21   Traumatic rupture at the aortic isthmus on right posterior oblique arch aortography.

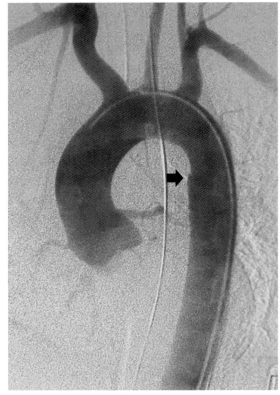

FIGURE 6-22   Subtle intimal flap in the upper descending thoracic aorta *(arrow)* from a deceleration injury (confirmed at operation).

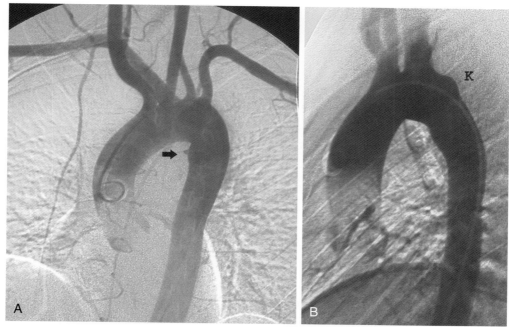

FIGURE 6-23   **A,** Bronchial artery diverticulum *(arrow)* and aberrant right subclavian artery on arch aortography. **B,** In steep right posterior oblique projection, a diverticulum of Kommerell *(K)* is evident.

OTHER MODALITIES

In general, TEE and MRI are not favored for the evaluation of blunt aortic trauma except to confirm other equivocal studies.[75] IVUS detects many of the typical findings of acute aortic injury.[76,77] Although its accuracy is debated, it can be a valuable adjunct during endograft placement.

Treatment

SURGICAL THERAPY

Traditionally, all acute traumatic aortic injuries were repaired immediately with primary resection or graft placement.[78] Recent trends in trauma care favor a slight delay in repair (open or endovascular), particularly in patients with severe intracranial injury or at high risk for thoracic surgery.[47,79,80] Beta-blocking agents are used liberally to lower blood pressure and heart rate and thus avoid free rupture before definitive treatment. Small intimal flaps may be managed medically with vigorous imaging follow-up. Chronic pseudoaneurysms usually require surgical treatment.

ENDOVASCULAR THERAPY

Recently, endovascular stent grafts have become the first line treatment for blunt aortic injury at many major trauma centers[79,81] (Fig. 6-24). To date, no randomized trials have compared stent graft and open treatment. The most convincing evidence comes from an American Society for the Surgery of Trauma multicenter prospective nonrandomized trial.[47] About two thirds of 193 patients underwent endograft insertion, and the remainder were treated with open operation. Mortality and paraplegia rates were significantly lower in the endograft group (7.2% vs. 23.5% and 0.8% vs. 2.9%, respectively). There were comparable rates of adverse events in the two cohorts. Endoleak was detected in 14.4% of the former group; most required additional device placement or conversion to open surgery. Notably, the mean interval between injury and definitive treatment was slightly more than 2 days. These conclusions are further supported by a recent meta-analysis of the published reports on the subject.[79]

Criteria for selection of patients is both device- and operator-dependent. The most important factors are:

- Length of the proximal landing zone (10 to 15 mm) beyond the left subclavian artery (or left common carotid artery if necessary)
- Aortic diameter (measured at several sites 1 to 2 cm from landing zones) compatible with current devices
- Femoral/iliac access artery that will accommodate device sheaths (typically 6 to 7 mm)
- Aortic arch angulation

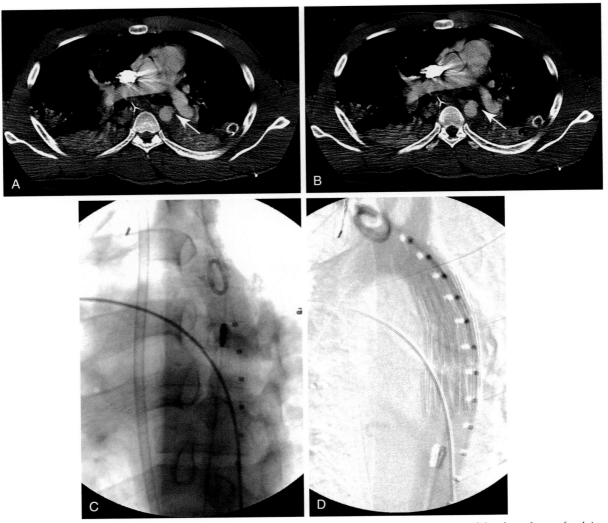

FIGURE 6-24 Traumatic aortic injury. **A** and **B,** Axial contrast-enhanced computed tomography scans of the chest show a focal, irregular outpouching of the proximal descending thoracic aorta *(arrow)*. Fluid density is present around the aorta at this level. A left chest tube is in place. There is bilateral lung consolidation. **C** and **D,** A stent graft is placed to repair the injury and avoid surgery.

OTHER DISORDERS

Vasculitis

Several types of vasculitis affect the thoracic aorta and its primary branches[82,83] (Box 6-5; see also Chapter 1). The consequence is arterial dilation, arterial narrowing, or both.

Takayasu arteritis (TA) is a chronic, inflammatory vasculitis of large elastic arteries[84,85] (see Chapter 1). It primarily affects the aorta, its major branches, and the pulmonary arteries. CT and MRI demonstrate variable patterns of enhancement in the early phase of the disease.[86-88] In the chronic stages, typical imaging findings include aortic dilation or irregularity, narrowing of the descending aorta, long stenoses or occlusions of arch vessels, wall thickening, calcifications, mural

---

BOX 6-5

VASCULITIDES AFFECTING THE THORACIC AORTA OR PRIMARY BRANCHES

- Takayasu arteritis
- Giant cell (temporal) arteritis
- Connective tissue disorders (e.g., rheumatoid arthritis)
- Behçet disease
- Kawasaki disease
- Radiation arteritis

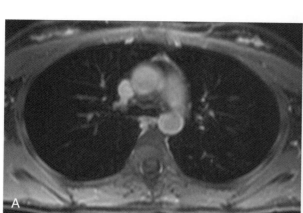
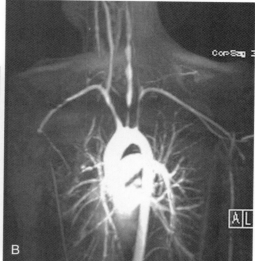

FIGURE 6-25   Takayasu arteritis. **A,** Gadolinium-enhanced magnetic resonance angiogram shows aortic wall thickening and enhancement. **B,** Maximum intensity projection image shows long, smooth left common carotid artery (CCA) and left subclavian and right subclavian artery stenoses with dilation of the upper left CCA.

thrombi, and, rarely, aortic insufficiency or dissection (Fig. 6-25).

In the quiescent phase of TA, branch obstructions are treated if there is end-organ ischemia (e.g., arm "claudication"). Balloon angioplasty is an attractive alternative to open surgery. Angioplasty is initially effective and safe for descending thoracic, abdominal aortic, and pulmonary artery stenoses. Early series suggested that restenosis was uncommon.[89-91] However, one recent series found an unacceptably high rate of late failure of angioplasty alone in a cohort of U.S. patients with symptomatic TA.[92] Intravascular stents have been used as an adjunct to angioplasty, but should only be employed when absolutely necessary.[93] It is advisable to delay surgery or percutaneous therapy until the acute constitutional symptoms have subsided.[94] Expanding aneurysms often require operative repair, although stent grafts have been used in this setting.[95]

Giant cell (temporal) arteritis is a vasculitis of large- and medium-sized arteries.[82,83,96] The disease has some features in common with Takayasu arteritis but is a distinct entity (see Chapter 1). Significant aortic disease, such as aneurysm, annular dilation, or aortic insufficiency, is relatively uncommon. Involved aortic branches have long, smooth stenoses alternating with normal segments. These findings, along with the distribution of disease, sometimes distinguish giant cell arteritis from atherosclerosis.

Collagen-vascular disorders, particularly those linked to the HLA-B27 antigen, occasionally produce aortitis.[97] Acute inflammation followed by fibrotic scarring occurs in the sinotubular portion of the ascending aorta and may extend into the ventricular septum and mitral valve apparatus. Aortic regurgitation can result; dilation of the aortic root is unusual.

Noninflammatory Vasculopathies (Online Case 62)

Marfan syndrome is an autosomal dominant disorder that affects the eyes, skeleton, muscles, and cardiovascular system[98] (see Chapter 1). The disease mutation in the FBN1 gene that codes for fibrillin-1 results in structurally deficient microfibrils in the aortic media and activation of media-destroying matrix metalloproteinases by upregulated transforming growth factor–beta (TGF-β) levels.[20,99] The cellular structure of the media becomes disorganized and weakened. However, up to one third of patients have a de novo noninherited defect. Affected individuals have characteristic thinning and elongation of the limbs along with other outward features. Cardiovascular complications are frequent and include aneurysm or dissection of the proximal ascending aorta, aortic insufficiency, mitral valve prolapse or calcification, and pulmonary artery dilation.[100] Aortic dilation in Marfan syndrome usually is confined to the aortic root, producing *sinotubular ectasia* with a characteristic "tulip bulb" appearance[101] (Fig. 6-26). The risk for type A dissection increases substantially when the aortic diameter exceeds 5 cm, growth rate accelerates (>0.5 cm/year), a family member suffered dissection, or a woman becomes pregnant.[98] In such cases, operative aortic replacement is indicated.

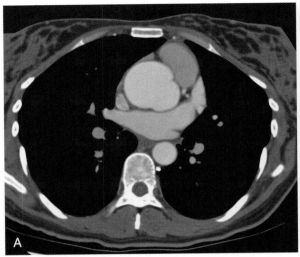
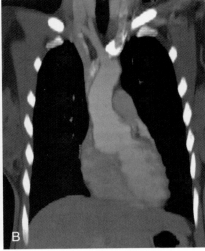

FIGURE 6-26   Marfan syndrome. **A,** Axial computed tomography angiogram demonstrates diffuse dilation of the aortic root involving the aortic sinuses. **B,** Coronal maximum-intensity projection shows fusiform aortic root dilation with characteristic "tulip bulb" appearance. *(Courtesy of Eric Goodman, MD, San Diego.)*

Ehlers-Danlos syndromes are a set of distinct genetic disorders of collagen production[102] (see Chapter 1). The rare vascular subtype (type IV) results from a genetic defect in type III procollagen. Translucent skin, easy bruising, and pneumothorax are present. The vascular manifestations are spontaneous arterial ruptures, aneurysms, occlusions, and arteriovenous or carotid-cavernous fistula. Historically, angiographers were warned to avoid catheterization in this population because of fears of severe complications.[103] In fact, arteriography and endovascular treatment can be done safely in many patients.[104]

Loeys-Dietz syndrome is a recently identified autosomal dominant connective tissue disorder resulting from genetic defects in the genes coding for TGF-β receptors.[105,106] The characteristic features include arterial (especially aortic) aneurysms and dissections, global arterial tortuosity, hypertelorism, bifid uvula, cleft lip, and congenital heart disease.

HIV-related vasculopathy is well known to affect medium- and small-caliber vessels. However, a rarer form of large vessel disease can cause solitary or multiple aneurysms in the aorta and its major branches.[107,108] The disease produces a leukocytoclastic reaction in the vasa vasorum and periadventitial tissues along with chronic inflammation. The aneurysms often are saccular in appearance (Fig. 6-27).

Infectious Aortitis and Aerodigestive Fistulas

Bacterial aortitis is caused by seeding of an aortic lesion such as atherosclerotic plaque or a preexisting aneurysm, septic embolization into the aortic vasa vasorum, transmural spread from an adjacent infection, or penetrating trauma. The inflamed wall can form an infected *(mycotic)* aneurysm or pseudoaneurysm.[109] Although infectious aneurysms are rare, the aorta and femoral artery are the most commonly affected sites. The usual pathogens are *Salmonella* species and *Staphylococcus aureus.*[110]

Some patients have localized pain, fever, and positive blood cultures. With this clinical picture, the presence of an uncalcified, smooth, eccentric saccular aneurysm is highly worrisome for mycotic aneurysm (Fig. 6-28). *Tuberculous aortitis* may develop from lymphangitic spread or contiguous extension of disease in the chest. *Syphilitic aortitis* has been largely eradicated in most parts of the world. About 10% of patients with long-standing, untreated tertiary syphilis develop cardiovascular disease including aortic aneurysms.[111] The proximal portion of the aorta is the most extensively involved, leading to aortic dilation with mural calcification, aortic insufficiency, coronary artery stenosis, or frank aneurysm formation. Aneurysms usually are saccular and typically spare the aortic sinuses.

Infected aortic pseudoaneurysms can erode into the respiratory or digestive system; likewise, inflammatory or malignant mediastinal processes can destroy the adjacent aortic wall. The end result may be an *aortoenteric* (e.g., *aortoesophageal*) *fistula* or *aortobronchial fistula.* These devastating lesions classically present with massive hematemesis or hemoptysis, respectively.

Despite the general prohibition of placing stent grafts at sites of known infection, these devices have been used in this setting to manage acute complications of infectious aortic aneurysms. However, covered stent insertion should only be considered a temporizing measure.[112,113]

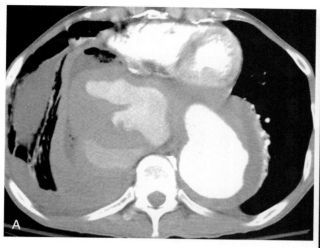

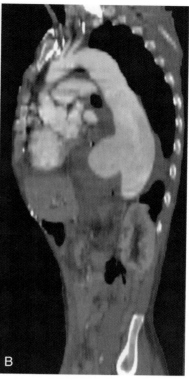

FIGURE 6-27 Human immunodeficiency virus–related vasculopathy. **A,** The disease causes diffuse dilation of the descending thoracic aorta along with a large saccular aneurysm with recent leak of high-density blood on transverse computed tomography angiography and oblique sagittal reformatted image **(B).**

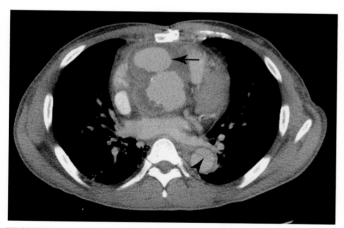

FIGURE 6-28 Infected pseudoaneurysm of the ascending thoracic aorta *(arrow)* with surrounding inflammatory tissue following surgical repair of an aortic dissection. Intimal flap is still evident in the descending thoracic aorta *(arrowhead).*

Penetrating Aortic Ulcer (Online Case 95)

Rarely, an ulcerated atherosclerotic aortic plaque penetrates into the media and forms a longitudinal hematoma in the vessel wall.[114] With time, a pseudoaneurysm may develop, or frank rupture may occur. *Penetrating aortic ulcers (PAUs)* often are found in the lower descending thoracic or upper abdominal aorta but may occur anywhere. As with aortic dissection, the patient is typically older and hypertensive. Most patients are asymptomatic, but some present with "acute aortic syndrome" (see earlier discussion). The lesion must be distinguished from true aortic dissection or intramural hematoma.[16,55]

The diagnosis is made by CT, MRI, or TEE.[115-117] The descending thoracic aorta often is diffusely dilated. Displaced intimal calcification and a focal ulcerated plaque with underlying mural hematoma are seen (Fig. 6-29). Intraluminal thrombus with neighboring intimal plaque can mimic PAU. Pleural or mediastinal fluid may be present.

The natural history of PAU is debated.[114] Many asymptomatic lesions fail to enlarge, but some lead to progressive aortic dilation, pseudoaneurysm formation, distal embolization, and—uncommonly—fatal rupture. Some clinical series have reported high rates of rupture (up to one third of cases) whereas others note a more benign course with no significant difference in outcomes from medical or surgical treatment.[118,119] Clearly, type A PAU is more malignant than type B. Most patients receive antihypertensive medications. Surgery or stent graft placement is performed in selected cases, including ascending aortic involvement, large ulcer diameter or depth, persistent pain, expansion, or rupture.[120-122] Percutaneous coil embolization of the ulcer has been described.[123]

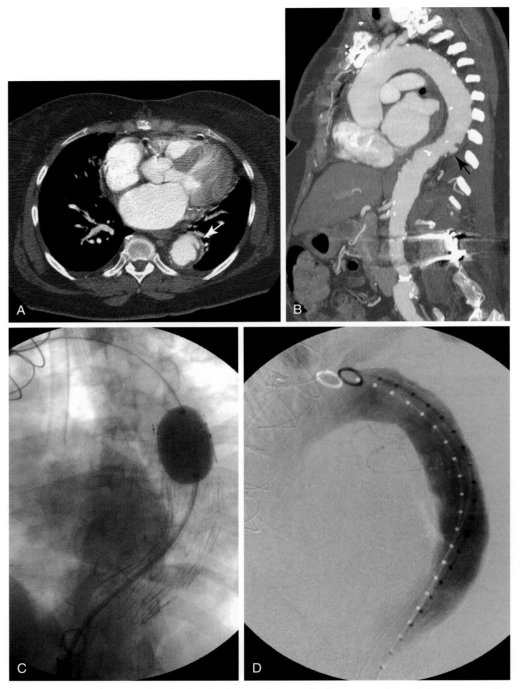

FIGURE 6-29   Penetrating aortic ulcer. **A** and **B,** Axial and reformatted parasagittal contrast-enhanced chest computed tomography scans show a very focal extension of contrast from the lumen into the wall of the mid-descending thoracic aorta *(arrow)*. There is diffuse atherosclerotic disease throughout the aorta. No frank dissection is seen. **C,** Patient underwent stent graft placement, which shows inflation of a large balloon used to tack the device down to the aortic wall. **D,** Final aortogram shows exclusion of the ulcer with a widely patent lumen.

Intramural Hematoma

In intramural hematoma (IMH), a localized hematoma develops spontaneously in the wall of the aorta without an intimal tear or overlying atherosclerotic plaque.[43,51,124,125] The postulated cause is rupture of aortic vasa vasorum; there is no proof for this premise.[114] Intramural hematoma is effectively a noncommunicating aortic dissection. It can progress to frank dissection or rupture but fortunately is much less likely to result in the *malperfusion syndrome* seen with aortic dissection. IMH is being diagnosed more frequently with the widespread use of cross-sectional imaging in patients with suspected aortic disease. The clinical picture is similar to that of aortic dissection, with sudden onset of chest or back pain in a middle-aged to elderly hypertensive individual. Classic teaching holds that intramural hematoma is a disease of the descending thoracic aorta (type B). Some reports show a significant distribution in the ascending aorta (type A).[124]

IMH usually is detected by CT or MRI, which shows a crescentic mural hematoma of medium to high density or signal intensity (depending on clot age) extending over a length of the thoracic aorta[115-117] (Fig. 6-30). There is no intimal flap nor flow within the collection. Intramural hematoma must be differentiated from other diseases that cause wall thickening, such as aortitis, atherosclerotic plaque, PAU, and mural thrombus.

IMH usually is treated by blood pressure and heart rate control with beta-adrenergic blockers unless the ascending aorta is involved.[125] The natural history is more benign than with aortic dissection, but the mortality rate is still substantial (related to aneurysm rupture or evolution to frank dissection, particularly with type A lesions).[114,126] Characteristics that favor complete resolution include type B lesion, younger age, diameter less than 4 cm, and thickness less than 1 cm.[43,125,127] Many interventionalists advocate stent graft insertion for the typical patient with type A IMH. Surgery or stent graft insertion usually is reserved for patients with type B IMH and persistent symptoms, expansion of the hematoma, aortic diameter greater than 6 cm, or progression to frank dissection or rupture.[49,128]

Coarctation of the Aorta (Online Case 27)

Congenital thoracic *aortic coarctation* occurs in 0.02% to 0.06% of individuals.[129] The obstruction takes the form of a discrete bandlike narrowing at or beyond the attachment of the ligamentum arteriosum (*postductal* form).[130] This anomaly should not be confused with *fetal coarctation*, which produces diffuse narrowing of the aortic arch and hypoplasia of left heart chambers (*preductal* form). Coarctation is associated with bicuspid aortic valve, patent ductus arteriosus, ventricular septal defect, and Turner syndrome. It usually is discovered in a child or young adult with upper extremity hypertension, diminished lower extremity pulses, or heart failure. To bypass the stenosis, blood flows from the anterior intercostal branches of the internal thoracic arteries retrograde into the posterior intercostal branches of the descending aorta. Enlargement and tortuosity of the intercostal arteries cause pressure erosion on the undersurface of the third through ninth ribs ("rib notching").

The characteristic findings of coarctation are severe discrete narrowing around the aortic isthmus, dilation of the ascending aorta, and enlarged internal thoracic and intercostal arteries (Fig. 6-31). Operative treatment of aortic coarctation is by direct resection with end-to-end anastomosis or by patch aortoplasty.[131] Balloon angioplasty and stent placement are attractive alternatives to surgery.[132,133] Long-term results are generally good, but restenosis or aneurysm formation at the treatment site occurs in about 20% of patients.

Pseudocoarctation of the aorta is a congenital elongation of the thoracic aorta with a discrete kink at the aortic isthmus.[5] Although it looks superficially similar to true coarctation, pseudocoarctation produces no pressure gradient across the kink and has no collateral circulation (Fig. 6-32). Occasionally, aneurysms form adjacent to the aortic twist.

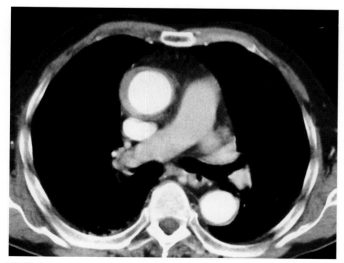

FIGURE 6-30 Intramural hematoma of the right lateral wall of the ascending aorta on computed tomography angiogram.

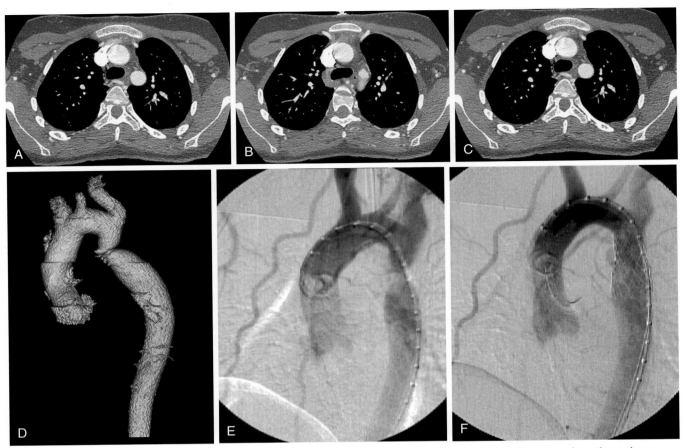

FIGURE 6-31   Coarctation of the aorta. **A** through **C,** Axial contrast-enhanced chest computed tomography images show that a short segment of the proximal descending thoracic aorta is narrowed. The remainder of the visualized aorta looks normal. The internal thoracic (mammary) arteries are prominent, as are multiple small posterior mediastinal vascular structures. **D,** The reformatted shaded-surface display image confirms the diagnosis. **E** and **F,** A stent graft is placed with excellent cosmetic result.

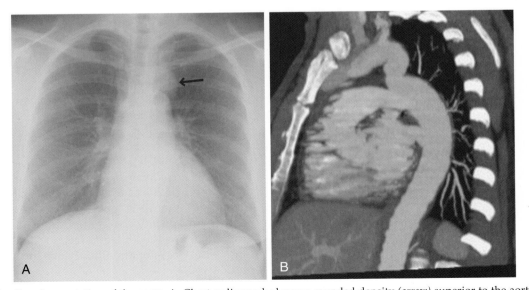

FIGURE 6-32   Pseudocoarctation of the aorta. **A,** Chest radiograph shows a rounded density *(arrow)* superior to the aortic knob. **B,** Oblique parasagittal reformatted computed tomography angiogram shows marked kinking of the descending thoracic aorta but no discrete stenosis. *(Courtesy of Eric Goodman, MD, San Diego.)*

References

1. LaBerge JM, Jeffrey RB. Aortic lacerations: fatal complications of thoracic aortography. *Radiology* 1987;**165**:367.

2. Collins P, editor. Embryology and development. In: Williams PL, Bannister LH, Berry MM, et al, editors. *Gray's anatomy*. 38th ed. New York: Churchill Livingstone; 1995, p. 312.

3. Gabella G, editor. Cardiovascular system. In: Williams PL, Bannister LH, Berry MM, et al, editors. *Gray's anatomy*. 38th ed. New York: Churchill Livingstone; 1995, p. 1505.

4. Lin FY, Devereux RB, Roman MJ, et al. Assessment of the thoracic aorta by multidetector computed tomography: age- and sex-specific reference values in adults without evident cardiovascular disease. *J Cardiovasc Comput Tomogr* 2008;**2**:298.

5. Edwards JE. Anomalies of derivatives of aortic arch systems. *Med Clin North Am* 1948;**91**:925.

6. Francois CJ, Carr JC. MR of the thoracic aorta. *Magn Reson Imaging Clin N Am* 2007;**15**:639.

7. Katz JC, Chakravarti S, Ko H, et al. Common origin of the innominate and carotid arteries: prevalence, nomenclature, and surgical implications. *J Am Soc Echocardiogr* 2006;**19**:1446.

8. Reppert MK, Lundgren EC, Dibos LA, et al. Variations in aortic arch branch vessel anatomy as seen by aortography. *Vasc Endovasc Surg* 1993;**27**:89.

9. Atkin GK, Grieve PP, Vattipally VR, et al. The surgical management of aortic root vessel anomalies presenting in adults. *Ann Vasc Surg* 2007;**21**:525.

10. Hara M, Satake M, Itoh M, et al. Radiographic findings of aberrant right subclavian artery initially depicted on CT. *Radiat Med* 2003;**21**:161.

11. Russo V, Renzulli M, LaPalombara C, et al. Congenital diseases of the thoracic aorta. Role of MRI and MRA. *Eur Radiol* 2006;**16**:676.

12. McElhinney DB, Hoydu AK, Gaynolr JW, et al. Patterns of right aortic arch and mirror imaging branching of the brachiocephalic vessels without associated anomalies. *Pediatr Cardiol* 2001;**22**:285.

13. Krozon I, Tunick PA. Aortic atherosclerotic disease and stroke. *Circulation* 2006;**114**:63.

14. Bashore TM, Gehrig T. Cholesterol emboli after invasive cardiac procedures. *J Am Coll Cardiol* 2003;**42**:217.

15. Gottsegen JM, Coplan NL. The atherosclerotic aortic arch: considerations in diagnostic imaging. *Prev Cardiol* 2008;**11**:162.

16. Chung JH, Ghoshhajra BB, Rojas CA, et al. CT angiography of the thoracic aorta. *Radiol Clin North Am* 2010;**48**:249.

17. Guo DC, Papke CL, He R, et al. Pathogenesis of thoracic and abdominal aortic aneurysms. *Ann N Y Acad Sci* 2006;**1085**:339.

18. Ruddy JM, Jones JA, Spinale FG, et al. Regional heterogeneity within the aorta: relevance to aneurysm disease. *J Thorac Cardiovasc Surg* 2008;**136**:1123.

19. Svensjö S, Bengtsson H, Bergqvist D. Thoracic and thoracoabdominal aortic aneurysm and dissection: an investigation based on autopsy. *Br J Surg* 1996;**83**:68.

20. Loeys B, DePaepe A. New insights into the pathogenesis of aortic aneurysms. *Verh K Acad Geneeskd Belg* 2008;**70**:69.

21. Griepp RB, Ergin MA, Galla JD, et al. Natural history of descending thoracic and thoracoabdominal aneurysms. *Ann Thoracic Surg* 1999;**67**:1927.

22. Elefteriades JA, Botta Jr DM. Indications for the treatment of thoracic aortic aneurysms. *Surg Clin North Am* 2009;**89**:845.

23. Perko MJ, Norgaard M, Herzog TM, et al. Unoperated aortic aneurysms: a survey of 170 patients. *Ann Thoracic Surg* 1995;**59**:1204.

24. Dapunt OE, Galla JD, Sadeghi AM, et al. The natural history of thoracic aortic aneurysms. *J Thorac Cardiovasc Surg* 1994;**107**:1323.

25. Cambria RA, Gloviczki P, Stanson AW, et al. Outcome and expansion rate of 57 thoracoabdominal aortic aneurysms managed nonoperatively. *Am J Surg* 1995;**170**:213.

26. Rousseau H, Chabbert V, Maracher MA, et al. The importance of imaging assessment before endovascular repair of thoracic aorta. *Eur J Vasc Endovasc Surg* 2009;**38**:408.

27. Agarwal PP, Chughtai A, Matzinger FRK, et al. Multidetector CT of thoracic aortic aneurysms. *Radiographics* 2009;**29**:537.

28. Castaner E, Andreu M, Gallardo X, et al. CT in nontraumatic acute thoracic aortic disease: typical and atypical features and complications. *Radiographics* 2003;**23**:S93.

29. Tatli S, Lipton MJ, Davison BD, et al. MR imaging of aortic and peripheral vascular disease. *Radiographics* 2003;**23**:S59.

30. Lawrie GM, Earle N, DeBakey ME. Evolution of surgical techniques for aneurysms of the descending thoracic aorta: twenty-nine years experience with 659 patients. *J Cardiac Surg* 1994; **9**:648.

31. Etz CD, Plestis KA, Kari FA, et al. Staged repair of thoracic and thoracoabdominal aortic aneurysms using the elephant trunk technique: a consecutive series of 215 first stage and 120 complete repairs. *Eur J Cardiothorac Surg* 2008;**34**:605.

32. Estrera AL, Miller CC, Chen EP, et al. Descending thoracic aortic aneurysm repair: 12-year experience using distal aortic perfusion and cerebrospinal fluid drainage. *Ann Thorac Surg* 2005;**80**:1290.

33. Yamauchi T, Takano H, Nishimura N, et al. Paraplegia and paraparesis after descending thoracic aortic aneurysm repair: a risk factor analysis. *Ann Thorac Cardiovasc Surg* 2006;**12**:179.

34. Savader SJ, Williams GM, Trerotola SO, et al. Preoperative spinal artery localization and its relationship to postoperative neurologic complications. *Radiology* 1993;**189**:165.

35. Jonker FH, Trimarchi S, Verhagen HJ, et al. Meta-analysis of open versus endovascular repair for ruptured descending thoracic aortic aneurysm. *J Vasc Surg* 2010;**51**:1026.

36. Abraha I, Romagnoli C, Montedori A, et al. Thoracic stent graft versus surgery for thoracic aneurysm. *Cochrane Database Syst Rev* 2009;CD006796.

37. Matsumura JS, Cambria RP, Dake MD, et al. International controlled clinical trial of thoracic endovascular aneurysm repair with the Zenith TX2 endovascular graft: 1-year results. *J Vasc Surg* 2008; **47**:247.

38. Fairman RM, Criado F, Farber M, et al. Pivotal results of the Medtronic Vascular Talent Thoracic Stent-Graft System: the VALOR trial. *J Vasc Surg* 2008;**48**:546.

39. Neuhauser B, Czermak BV, Fish J, et al. Type A dissection following endovascular thoracic aortic stent-graft repair. *J Endovasc Ther* 2005;**12**:74.

40. Stavropoulos SW, Charagundla SR. Imaging techniques for detection and management of endoleaks after endovascular aortic aneurysm repair. *Radiology* 2007;**243**:641.

41. Buth J, Harris PL, Hobo R, et al. Neurologic complications associated with endovascular repair of thoracic aortic pathology: incidence and risk factors. A study from the European Collaborators on Stent/Graft Techniques for Aortic Aneurysm Repair (EUROSTAR) registry. *J Vasc Surg* 2007;**46**:1103.

42. Bavaria JE, Appoo JJ, Makaroun MS, et al. Endovascular stent grafting versus open surgical repair of descending thoracic aortic aneurysms in low risk patients: a multicenter comparative trial. *J Thorac Cardiovasc Surg* 2007;**133**:369.

43. Evangelista A, Mukherjee D, Mehta R, et al. Acute intramural hematoma of the aorta: a mystery in evolution. *Circulation* 2005; **111**:1063.

44. Atkins MD, Black JH III, Cambria RP. Aortic dissection: perspectives in the era of stent-graft repair. *J Vasc Surg* 2006;**43**:30A.

45. Larson EW, Edwards WD. Risk factors for aortic dissection: a necropsy study of 161 cases. *Am J Cardiol* 1984;**53**:849.

46. Afonso L, Mohammed T, Thatai D. Crack whips the heart: a review of the cardiovascular toxicity of cocaine. *Am J Cardiol* 2007;**100**: 1040.

47. Demetriades D, Velhamos GC, Scalea TM, et al. Operative repair or endovascular stent graft in blunt traumatic thoracic aortic injuries:

results of an American Association for the Surgery of Trauma multicenter study. *J Trauma* 2008;**64**:561.

48. Cambria RP, Brewster DC, Gertler J, et al. Vascular complications associated with spontaneous aortic dissection. *J Vasc Surg* 1988;**7**:199.

49. Hagan PG, Nienaber CA, Isselbacher EM, et al. The international registry of acute aortic dissection (IRAD): new insights into an old disease. *JAMA* 2000;**283**:897.

50. Lauterbach SR, Cambria RP, Brewster DC, et al. Contemporary management of aortic branch compromise resulting from acute aortic dissection. *J Vasc Surg* 2001;**33**:1185.

51. Vilacosta I, Roman JA. Acute aortic syndrome. *Heart* 2001;**85**:365.

52. Fisher ER, Stern EJ, Godwin JD II, et al. Acute aortic dissection: typical and atypical imaging features. *Radiographics* 1994;**14**:1263.

53. LePage MA, Quint LE, Sonnad SS, et al. Aortic dissection: CT features that distinguish true lumen from false lumen. *Am J Roentgenol* 2001;**177**:207.

54. Liu Q, Lu JP, Wang F, et al. Three-dimensional contrast-enhanced MR angiography of aortic dissection: a pictorial essay. *Radiographics* 2007;**27**:1311.

55. Lohan DG, Krishnam M, Saleh R, et al. MR imaging of the thoracic aorta. *Magn Reson Imaging Clin N Am* 2008;**16**:213.

56. Sommer T, Fehske W, Holzknecht N, et al. Aortic dissection: a comparative study of diagnosis with spiral CT, multiplanar transesophageal echocardiography, and MR imaging. *Radiology* 1996;**199**:347.

57. Deeb GM, Williams DM, Bolling SF, et al. Surgical delay for acute type A dissection with malperfusion. *Ann Thorac Surg* 1997;**64**:1669.

58. Pradhan S, Elefteriades JA, Sumpio BE. Utility of the aortic fenestration technique in the management of acute aortic dissections. *Ann Thorac Cardiovasc Surg* 2007;**13**:296.

59. Barnes DM, Williams DM, Dasika NL, et al. A single-center experience treating renal malperfusion after aortic dissection with central aortic fenestration and renal artery stenting. *J Vasc Surg* 2008;**47**:903.

60. Karmy-Jones R, Simeone A, Meissner M, et al. Descending thoracic aortic dissections. *Surg Clin North Am* 2007;**87**:1047.

61. Nienaber CA, Rousseau H, Eggebrecht H, et al. Randomized comparison of strategies for type B aortic dissection: the INvestigation of STEnt Grafts in Aortic Dissection (INSTEAD) trial. *Circulation* 2009;**120**:2519.

62. Kusagawa H, Shimono T, Ishida M, et al. Changes in false lumen after transluminal stent-graft placement in aortic dissection: six years' experience. *Circulation* 2005;**111**:2951.

63. Blount KJ, Hagspiel KD. Aortic diameter, true lumen, and false lumen growth rates in chronic type B aortic dissection. *AJR Am J Roentgenol* 2009;**192**:W222.

64. Parmley LF, Mattingly TW, Manion WC, et al. Non-penetrating traumatic injury of the aorta. *Circulation* 1958;**17**:1086.

65. Cowley RA, Turney SZ, Hankins JR, et al. Rupture of the thoracic aorta cause by blunt trauma. *J Thorac Cardiovasc Surg* 1990;**100**:652.

66. Schmoker JD, Lee CH, Taylor RG, et al. A novel model of blunt thoracic aortic injury: a mechanism confirmed? *J Trauma* 2008;**64**:923.

67. Feczko JD, Lynch L, Pless JE, et al. An autopsy case review of 142 non-penetrating (blunt) injuries of the aorta. *J Trauma* 1992;**33**:846.

68. Fabian TC. Roger T. Sherman lecture. Advances in the management of blunt thoracic aortic injury: Parmley to the present. *Am Surg* 2009;**75**:273.

69. Steenburg SD, Ravenel JG, Ikonomidis JS, et al. Acute traumatic aortic injury: imaging evaluation and management. *Radiology* 2008;**248**:748.

70. Bruckner BA, DiBardino DJ, Cumbie TC, et al. Critical evaluation of chest computed tomography scans for blunt descending thoracic aortic injury. *Ann Thorac Surg* 2006;**81**:1339.

71. Ellis JD, Mayo JR. Computed tomography evaluation of traumatic rupture of the thoracic aorta: an outcome study. *Can Assoc Radiol J* 2007;**58**:22.

72. Demetriades D, Velmahos GC, Scalea TM, et al. Diagnosis and treatment of blunt thoracic aortic injuries: changing perspectives. *J Trauma* 2008;**64**:1415.

73. Fisher RG, Sanchez-Torres M, Thomas JW, et al. Subtle or atypical injuries of the thoracic aorta and brachiocephalic vessels in blunt thoracic trauma. *Radiographics* 1997;**17**:835.

74. Fisher RG, Sanchez-Torres M, Whigham CJ, et al. "Lumps" and "bumps" that mimic acute aortic and brachiocephalic vessel injury. *Radiographics* 1997;**17**:825.

75. Smith MD, Cassidy JM, Souther S, et al. Transesophageal echocardiography in the diagnosis of traumatic rupture of the aorta. *N Engl J Med* 1995;**332**:356.

76. Uflacker R, Horn J, Phillips G, et al. Intravascular sonography in the assessment of traumatic injury of the thoracic aorta. *AJR Am J Roentgenol* 1999;**173**:665.

77. Lee DE, Arslan B, Quieroz R, et al. Assessment of inter- and intraobserver agreement between intravascular US and aortic angiography of thoracic aortic injury. *Radiology* 2003;**227**:434.

78. Fabian TC, Richardson JD, Croce MA, et al. Prospective study of blunt aortic injury: Multicenter Trial of the American Association for the Surgery of Trauma. *J Trauma* 1997;**42**:374.

79. Xenos ES, Abedi NN, Davenport DL, et al. Meta-analysis of endovascular vs. open repair for traumatic descending thoracic aortic rupture. *J Vasc Surg* 2008;**48**:1343.

80. Cambria RP, Crawford RS, Cho JS, et al. A multicenter clinical trial of endovascular stent graft repair of acute catastrophe of the descending thoracic aorta. *J Vasc Surg* 2009;**50**:1255.

81. Alsac JM, Boura B, Desgranges P, et al. Immediate endovascular repair for acute traumatic injuries of the thoracic aorta: a multicenter analysis of 28 cases. *J Vasc Surg* 2008;**48**:1369.

82. Gornik HL, Creager MA. Aortitis. *Circulation* 2008;**117**:3039.

83. Khasnis A, Langford CA. Update on vasculitis. *J Allergy Clin Immunol* 2009;**123**:1226.

84. Seko Y. Giant cell and Takayasu arteritis. *Curr Opin Rheumatol* 2007;**19**:39.

85. Sueyoshi E, Sakamoto I, Uetani M. MRI of Takayasu's arteritis: typical appearance and complications. *AJR Am J Roentgenol* 2006;**187**:W569.

86. Chung JW, Kim HC, Choi YH, et al. Patterns of aortic involvement in Takayasu arteritis and its clinical implications: evaluation with spiral computed tomography angiography. *J Vasc Surg* 2007;**45**:906.

87. Matsunaga N, Hayashi K, Sakamoto I, et al. Takayasu arteritis: protean radiologic manifestations and diagnosis. *Radiographics* 1997;**17**:579.

88. Canyigit M, Peynircioglu B, Hazirolan T, et al. Imaging characteristics of Takayasu arteritis. *Cardiovasc Intervent Radiol* 2007;**30**:711.

89. Tyagi S, Kaul UA, Nair M, et al. Balloon angioplasty of the aorta in Takayasu's arteritis: initial and long-term results. *Am Heart J* 1992;**124**:876.

90. Rao SA, Mandalam KR, Rao VR, et al. Takayasu arteritis: initial and long term follow-up in 16 patients after percutaneous transluminal angioplasty of the descending thoracic and abdominal aorta. *Radiology* 1993;**189**:173.

91. Ogino H, Matsuda H, Minatoya K, et al. Overview of late outcome of medical and surgical treatment for Takayasu arteritis. *Circulation* 2008;**118**:2738.

92. Maksimowicz-McKinnon K, Clark TM, Hoffman GS. Limitations of therapy and a guarded prognosis in an American cohort of Takayasu arteritis patients. *Arthritis Rheum* 2007;**56**:1000.

93. Bali HK, Bhargava M, Jain AK, et al. De novo stenting of descending thoracic aorta in Takayasu arteritis: intermediate-term follow-up results. *J Invasive Cardiol* 2000;**12**:612.

94. Giordano JM, Leavitt RY, Hoffman G, et al. Experience with surgical treatment of Takayasu's disease. *Surgery* 1991;109:252.

95. Baril DT, Carroccio A, Palchik E, et al. Endovascular treatment of complicated aortic aneurysms in patients with underlying arteriopathies. *Ann Vasc Surg* 2006;**20**:464.

96. Nordborg E, Nordborg C. Giant cell arteritis: epidemiological clues to its pathogenesis and an update on its treatment. *Rheumatology* 2003;**42**:413.

97. Turesson C, Matteson EL. Vasculitis in rheumatoid arthritis. *Curr Opin Rheumatol* 2009;**21**:35.

98. Keane MG, Pyeritz RE. Medical management of Marfan syndrome. *Circulation* 2008;**117**:2802.

99. Dietz HC, Loeys BL, Carta L, et al. Recent progress towards a molecular understanding of Marfan syndrome. *Am J Med Genet* 2005;**139C**:4.

100. DePaepe AM, Devereux RB, Dietz HC, et al. Revised diagnostic criteria for the Marfan syndrome. *Am J Med Genet* 1996;**62**:417.

101. Ha HI, Seo JB, Lee SH, et al. Imaging of Marfan syndrome: multisystemic manifestations. *RadioGraphics* 2007;**27**:989.

102. Callewaert B, Malfait F, Loeys B, et al. Ehlers-Danlos syndromes and Marfan syndrome. *Best Prac Res Clin Rheum* 2008;**22**:165.

103. Zilocchi M, Macedo TA, Oderich GS, et al. Vascular Ehlers-Danlos syndrome: imaging findings. *AJR Am J Roentgenol* 2007;**189**:712.

104. Brooke BS, Arnaoutakis G, McDonnell NB, et al. Contemporary management of vascular complications associated with Ehlers Danlos syndrome. *J Vasc Surg* 2010;**51**:131.

105. Maleszewski JJ, Miller DV, Lu J, et al. Histopathologic findings in ascending aortas from individuals with Loeys-Dietz syndrome (LDS). *Am J Surg Pathol* 2009;**33**:194.

106. Williams JA, Loeys BL, Nwakanma LU, et al. Early surgical experience with Loeys-Dietz: a new syndrome of aggressive thoracic aortic aneurysm disease. *Ann Thorac Surg* 2007;**83**:S757.

107. Woolgar JD, Ray R, Maharaj K, et al. Colour Doppler and grey scale ultrasound features of HIV-related vascular aneurysms. *Br J Radiol* 2002;**75**:884.

108. Chetty R, Batitang S, Nair R. Large artery vasculopathy in HIV positive patients: another vasculitic enigma. *Hum Pathol* 2000;**31**:374.

109. Malouf JF, Chandrasekaran K, Orszulak TA. Mycotic aneurysms of the thoracic aorta: a diagnostic challenge. *Am J Med* 2003;**115**:489.

110. Oz MC, McNicholas KW, Serra AJ, et al. Review of Salmonella mycotic aneurysms of the thoracic aorta. *J Cardiovasc Surg* 1989;**30**:99.

111. Jackman Jr JD, Radolf JD. Cardiovascular syphilis. *Am J Med* 1989;**87**:425.

112. Lew WK, Rowe VL, Cunningham MJ, et al. Endovascular management of mycotic aortic aneurysms and associated aortoaerodigestive fistulas. *Ann Vasc Surg* 2009;**23**:81.

113. Kan CD, Lee HL, Yang YJ. Outcome after endovascular stent graft treatment for mycotic aortic aneurysm: a systematic review. *J Vasc Surg* 2007;**46**:906.

114. Sundt TM. Intramural hematoma and penetrating aortic ulcer. *Curr Opin Cardiol* 2007;**22**:504.

115. Krishnam MS, Tomasian A, Malik S, et al. Image quality and diagnostic accuracy of unenhanced SSFP MR angiography compared with conventional contrast-enhanced MR angiography for the assessment of thoracic aortic diseases. *Eur Radiol* 2010;**20**:1311.

116. Litmanovich D, Bankier AA, Cantin L, et al. CT and MRI in diseases of the aorta. AJR Am J Roentgenol 2009;**193**:928.

117. Yoo SM, Lee HY, White CS. MDCT evaluation of acute aortic syndrome. *Radiol Clin North Am* 2010;**48**:67.

118. Cho KR, Stanson AW, Potter DD, et al. Penetrating atherosclerotic ulcer of the descending thoracic aorta and arch. *J Thorac Cardiovasc Surg* 2004;**127**:1393.

119. Tittle SL, Lynch RJ, Cole PE, et al. Midterm followup of penetrating ulcer and intramural hematoma of the aorta. *J Thorac Cardiovasc Surg* 2002;**123**:1051.

120. Stone DH, Brewster DC, Kwolek CJ, et al. Stent graft versus open surgical repair of the thoracic aorta: mid term results. *J Vasc Surg* 2006;**44**:1188.

121. Brinster DR, Wheatley GH 3d, Williams J, et al. Are penetrating aortic ulcers best treated using an endovascular approach? *Ann Thorac Surg* 2006;**82**:1688.

122. Eggebrecht H, Herold U, Schmermund A, et al. Endovascular stent graft treatment of penetrating aortic ulcer: results over a median followup of 27 months. *Am Heart J* 2006;**151**:530.

123. Williams DM, Kirsh MM, Abrams GD. Penetrating atherosclerotic aortic ulcer with dissecting hematoma: control of bleeding with percutaneous embolization. *Radiology* 1991;**181**:85.

124. Ganaha F, Miller DC, Sugimoto K, et al. Prognosis of aortic intramural hematoma with and without penetrating aortic ulcer: a clinical and radiological analysis. *Circulation* 2002;**106**:342.

125. Sueyoshi E, Imada T, Sakamoto I, et al. Analysis of predictive factors for progression of type B aortic intramural hematoma with computed tomography. *J Vasc Surg* 2002;**35**:1179.

126. Maraj R, Rerkpattanapipat P, Jacobs LE, et al. Meta-analysis of 143 reported cases of aortic intramural hematoma. *Am J Cardiol* 2000;**86**:664.

127. Kaji S, Akasaka T, Katayama M, et al. Long term prognosis of patients with type B aortic intramural hematoma. *Circulation* 2003;**108**:9.

128. Kaji S, Akasaka T, Horibata Y, et al. Long-term prognosis of patients with Type A aortic intramural hematoma. *Circulation* 2002;**106**(Suppl I):248.

129. Mack G, Burch GH, Sahn DJ. Coarctation of the aorta. *Curr Treat Options Cardiovasc Med* 1999;**1**:347.

130. Tanous D, Benson LN, Horlick EM. Coarctation of the aorta: evaluation and management. *Curr Opin Cardiol* 2009;**24**:509.

131. Kaushal S, Backer CL, Patel JN, et al. Coarctation of the aorta: midterm outcomes of resection with extended end-to-end anastomosis. *Ann Thorac Surg* 2009;**88**:1932.

132. Egan M, Holzer RJ. Comparing balloon angioplasty, stenting, and surgery in the treatment of aortic coarctation. *Expert Rev Cardiovasc Ther* 2009;**7**:1401.

133. Kische S, Schneider H, Akin I, et al. Technique of interventional repair in adult aortic coarctation. *J Vasc Surg* 2010;**51**:1550.

CHAPTER

7

Abdominal Aorta

Karim Valji

AORTOGRAPHY

Abdominal aortography is performed using a 4- or 5-French (Fr) catheter with a pigtail or similar configuration. To properly evaluate the renal artery origins, the side holes of the catheter are positioned at the L1-L2 level. When visualization of the celiac and superior mesenteric arteries is necessary, higher catheter placement (above the T12 level) is required. Lateral projections are sometimes used to supplement frontal images in order to study the orifices of the mesenteric arteries. Particular care should be taken when catheterizing the abdominal aorta in patients known to have aneurysms or severe atherosclerotic disease to avoid dislodging mural thrombus or plaque.

ANATOMY

Development

In the embryo, the abdominal aorta is formed from the right and left dorsal aortae.[1] Numerous ventral splanchnic branches of the aorta supply the primitive digestive tract. These channels are eventually reduced to the celiac, superior mesenteric, and inferior mesenteric arteries. Lateral splanchnic branches supply organs arising from the mesonephric ridge, giving rise to the inferior phrenic, adrenal, renal, and gonadal arteries. Four sets of somatic arterial branches evolve into the intersegmental lumbar arteries.

Normal Anatomy

The *abdominal aorta* begins at the diaphragmatic hiatus.[2] The vessel runs in front of the spine and to the left of the inferior vena cava (IVC) until it bifurcates into the *common iliac arteries* at about the L4 vertebra. The normal caliber of the abdominal aorta increases with age; at the renal hila, its mean diameter varies from about 1.5 cm in women in the fourth decade of life to about 2 cm in men in the eighth decade.[3,4]

The abdominal aorta has three ventral branches (Figs. 7-1 and 7-2). The *celiac artery* arises at the T12-L1 level. It can initially take a forward, upward, or dowward course. The *superior mesenteric artery (SMA)* takes off at the L1-L2 level about 1 cm below the celiac axis. The *inferior mesenteric artery (IMA)* originates at the L3-L4 level, typically on the left anterolateral surface of the aorta.

The paired *inferior phrenic arteries* classically originate at or just above the celiac artery. They course superolaterally toward the central tendon of the hemidiaphragms, where they bifurcate. Paired *middle adrenal arteries* take off from the aorta adjacent to the SMA to provide partial blood supply to the adrenal glands. The *renal arteries* originate just

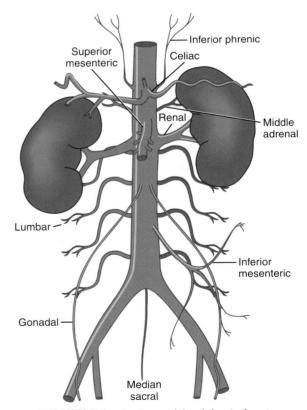

FIGURE 7-1   Anatomy of the abdominal aorta.

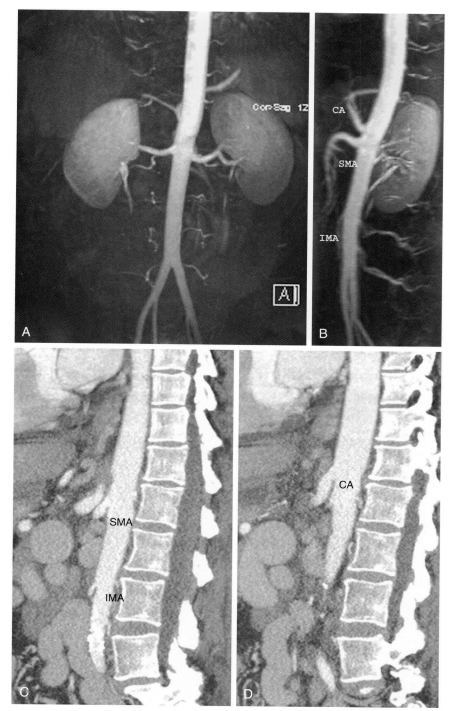

FIGURE 7-2 Normal MR angiogram of the abdominal aorta in frontal **(A)** and lateral **(B)** reformations. **C** and **D,** Computed tomography angiogram of the aorta in sagittal reformation. Ventral branches: *CA,* celiac artery; *IMA,* inferior mesenteric artery; *SMA,* superior mesenteric artery.

below or at the level of the SMA. The *gonadal (testicular or ovarian) arteries* are paired vessels off the anterolateral surface of the aorta just below the main renal arteries.

Four pairs of *lumbar arteries* exit the posterolateral aspect of the aorta. There are extensive anastomoses between these vessels, the lower intercostal arteries (superiorly), and the iliolumbar, deep iliac circumflex, and gluteal vessels (inferiorly). The *median sacral artery* takes off posteriorly just above the aortic bifurcation and descends toward the coccyx.

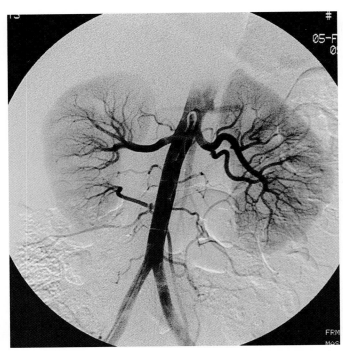

FIGURE 7-3   Multiple renal arteries. Two renal arteries supply the right kidney.

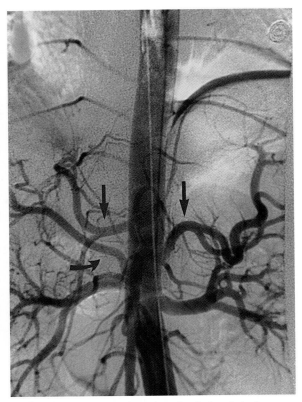

FIGURE 7-4   The common hepatic and splenic arteries have separate origins from the abdominal aorta *(straight arrows)*. Notice the right hepatic artery replaced to the superior mesenteric artery *(curved arrow)*.

The smaller somatic and splanchnic vessels (i.e., inferior phrenic, middle adrenal, gonadal, and median sacral arteries) are not always seen on routine abdominal aortograms. In a patient with an enlarged aorta or sluggish flow, the IMA may not opacify with a midabdominal aortic injection because of layering of contrast in the posterior (dependent) portion of the distal aortic lumen.

Variant Anatomy

Congenital anomalies of the abdominal aorta are rare. However, anomalies of the primary branches are common (see Chapters 10 and 11). Multiple renal arteries are present in about 25% to 35% of the population.[5-7] Although most accessory arteries are found just below the main renal artery, they may arise above the main trunk or as far distally as the iliac artery (Fig. 7-3).

Persistence of the embryonic ventral connection between the celiac artery and SMA with regression of the origin of one of these vessels leads to the rare *celiomesenteric artery*[8] (see Fig. 11-10). The hepatic, left gastric, or splenic arteries may have a separate origin from the aorta (Fig. 7-4). The inferior phrenic arteries can exit the top of the celiac (or rarely a renal) artery or form a common trunk from the aorta.[9,10] Rarely, a pair of lumbar arteries arise as a single branch from the posterior aspect of the aorta.

Collateral Circulation

With severe narrowing or complete occlusion of the abdominal aorta, several parietal and visceral collateral pathways divert blood flow around the obstructed segment. The chief parietal collateral routes are from the intercostal, subcostal, and lumbar arteries to the iliolumbar, lateral sacral, and superior gluteal branches of the internal iliac artery and to the deep and superficial iliac circumflex branches of the external iliac artery (Fig. 7-5). With the latter system, blood flows through the internal iliac artery to feed the external iliac artery in a retrograde direction. Interconnections between the lumbar arteries help to support this collateral network. A pathway also exists from the superior epigastric artery (terminal branch of the internal thoracic artery) to the inferior epigastric artery, which joins the common femoral artery.

The SMA and IMA are critical visceral conduits when the abdominal aorta is obstructed. With occlusion of the aorta *above* the level of the IMA, the SMA feeds the IMA through the middle colic and marginal arteries, which then connect with branches of the internal iliac artery through the rectal network (see Fig. 11-15). With occlusion of the abdominal aorta *below* the IMA origin, the

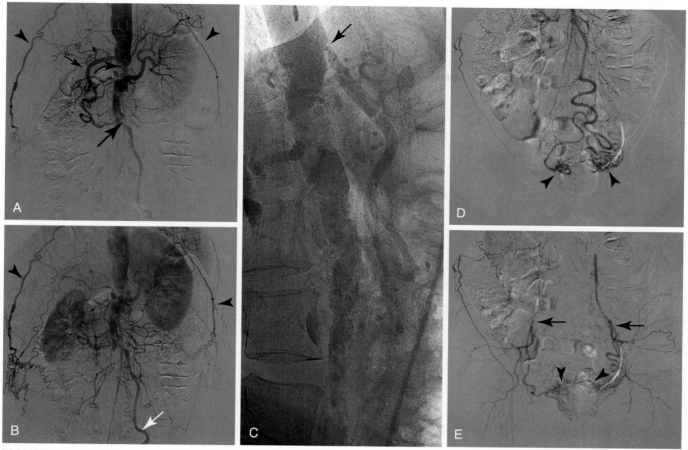

FIGURE 7-5   Distal aortic occlusion encompassing the superior mesenteric artery (SMA). **A** and **B,** Early and late phase frontal aortography show complete occlusion below the IMA *(large arrow).* A huge plaque obstructs the SMA origin *(curved arrow),* which is fed largely through celiac artery collaterals *(small arrow).* The IMA *(white arrow)* is huge, as are subcostal arteries headed toward the pelvis *(arrowheads).* The left renal artery is patent, but the right renal artery is severely diseased and feeds a small kidney. **C,** Lateral aortography also shows a tight celiac artery stenosis *(arrow)* and SMA occlusion. **D** and **E,** Pelvic imaging shows reconstitution of the internal iliac arteries *(arrows)* through the rectal network from the distal IMA *(arrowheads).* Parietal arteries also assist in diverting blood around the occlusion.

rectal collateral network (between the superior rectal branch of the IMA and the middle and inferior rectal branches of the internal iliac artery) may be an important communication (see Fig 7-5). In cases of short-segment aortic stenosis involving the SMA, the so-called *meandering mesenteric artery* can fill the SMA from the IMA circulation[11] (see Fig. 11-16).

MAJOR DISORDERS

Atherosclerosis

Atherosclerosis is the most common disease affecting the abdominal aorta (Fig. 7-6). This condition is considered as part of lower extremity peripheral vascular disease in Chapter 8.

Degenerative Abdominal Aortic Aneurysms (Online Cases 14 and 65)

Etiology

An arterial aneurysm is defined as a localized dilation of the vessel by 50% or more of its normal diameter.[12,13] By general agreement, an abdominal aortic aneurysm (AAA) is present in an adult when the wall-to-wall diameter of the infrarenal aorta exceeds 3 cm.[14] Most AAAs are infrarenal; in large series, up to 15% are suprarenal or juxtarenal (extending ≤1 cm from the renal arteries).[15-17] More than 20% of abdominal aneurysms extend into one or both common iliac arteries. The incidence of AAA has risen significantly during the last half century, and this phenomenon cannot be attributed entirely to earlier detection through screening or aging of the population.[18,19]

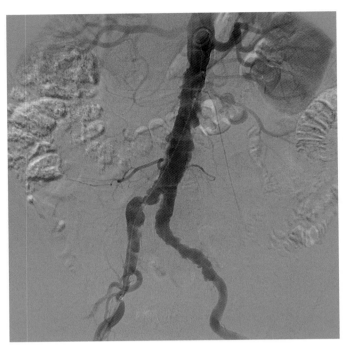

FIGURE 7-6   Atherosclerosis of the infrarenal abdominal aorta and both iliac arteries.

The vast majority of AAA are *degenerative* in nature. Although the strong association between abdominal aneurysms and atherosclerosis is well recognized, causation has not been proven.[20-22] Degenerative AAAs form because of genetic predisposition, immune-related inflammatory damage to the vessel wall, weakening of components of the media, and hemodynamic forces that produce remodeling.[20,23-25] The predilection for the infrarenal segment is possibly a consequence of reduced elastin content (relative to the suprarenal aorta) and a variety of hemodynamic factors. Although most AAAs are degenerative, a small percentage of patients develop aortic aneurysms for other reasons[26-28] (Box 7-1).

Natural History

The most common and feared complication of AAA is rupture, the likelihood of which is governed by *Laplace's law* (wall stress = pressure × radius). Rupture is thus mainly a function of aneurysm size.[29] Although the diameter of a typical AAA will grow by 1 to 4 mm per year, the rate of expansion is unpredictable in a particular patient, and the growth rate is not completely linear.[30,31] Expansion accelerates as the aneurysm gets bigger, even though periods of quiescence may occur. The rupture rate for AAAs that are 4 to 5.5 cm in diameter is about 0.7% to 1% per year.[32] Elective repair (open or endovascular) of smaller asymptomatic aneurysms (<5.5 cm in diameter) does not appear to be beneficial relative to the attendant risks if strict imaging surveillance is maintained[32-37] (see later discussion). The risk of AAA rupture increases substantially when the diameter is greater than 5 cm; for example, the 5-year risk of rupture of untreated AAAs of 5.5 cm or larger is 25% to 50%.[31,32,34]

Before the advent of endovascular therapy, AAA rupture was fatal in up to 90% of individuals.[38] More than 60% of such patients did not survive to reach medical care, and the mortality rate with emergent open surgery can exceed 75%.[38-40] When rupture occurs, the tear usually starts in the posterior or lateral wall of the aorta, with bleeding into the retroperitoneal space. Less often, the rupture occurs on the anterior wall, sometimes leading to hemorrhage into the peritoneal cavity.

Other sequelae of AAA include distal embolization, thrombosis, and aortocaval fistula. The latter complication occurs in fewer than 1% of untreated patients with AAA.[41]

Clinical Features

AAA is largely a disease of older adults and is strikingly more common in men than in women (approximately 6:1).[39,42] The other strong risk factors for AAA are smoking and family history. Additional associations include hypertension, coronary and peripheral arterial disease, and chronic obstructive pulmonary disease.

Most patients are asymptomatic at the time the aneurysm is detected, usually by imaging studies obtained for screening or unrelated problems. A rapidly expanding aneurysm may produce abdominal or back pain. Less than one fourth of affected individuals present with aneurysm rupture, which is suggested by the triad of abdominal or back pain, a pulsatile abdominal mass, and hypotension. Occasionally, patients have symptoms caused by extrinsic compression of adjacent

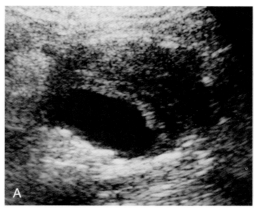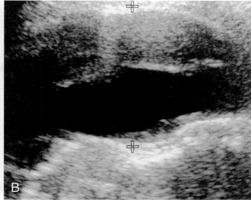

FIGURE 7-7   Abdominal aortic aneurysm. Transverse **(A)** and longitudinal **(B)** sonographic images document the size of the aneurysm and show extensive eccentric luminal thrombus.

organs, aneurysm thrombosis, distal embolization, or dissection. The rare patient with an aortocaval fistula may exhibit pain, a pulsatile abdominal mass, continuous abdominal bruit or thrill, congestive heart failure, lower extremity edema, or hematuria.

Imaging

Before considering invasive treatment, imaging studies are necessary for AAA detection and staging, surveillance of small aneurysms, and diagnosis of rupture or other complications.

SONOGRAPHY

Ultrasound (US) is the chief tool for detecting, sizing, and monitoring AAAs[35] (Fig. 7-7). The technique is almost 100% sensitive for aneurysm diagnosis. Body habitus or overlying structures (e.g., bowel gas) makes the test useless in some individuals. There is strong evidence that US screening programs in populations at risk will reduce overall mortality attributable to this lethal disease.[35,37] Sonography also is highly accurate in determining aneurysm size, the presence of mural thrombus, and associated abdominal pathology. US is less accurate in assessment of the cranial and caudal extent of the aneurysm, the relationship to and number of renal arteries, and the presence of iliofemoral arterial disease.

COMPUTED TOMOGRAPHY

Computed tomography angiography (CTA) is the principal modality for preprocedure and postprocedure assessment of patients with AAA[43-46] (Box 7-2). CT also is useful in following aneurysm growth in patients who cannot be imaged adequately with sonography. In those with underlying renal dysfunction, the need for iodinated contrast material is a major drawback of CTA.

The typical AAA is a fusiform dilation of the infrarenal abdominal aorta (Fig. 7-8). Intimal calcification and mural thrombus are common. If the aneurysm is saccular or eccentric without calcification or adjacent aortic disease, or is present in a young patient, uncommon causes should be considered (see Box 7-1).

CTA is the best means for evaluating patients with suspected AAA rupture.[45,47-49] Acute aneurysm rupture produces strandlike soft tissue density with high attenuation in the retroperitoneum adjacent to the aneurysm (often posteriorly) (Fig. 7-9). It may be difficult to pinpoint the exact site of leak. Several CT findings have been described as suggestive of impending aortic rupture, including a high-attenuation crescent sign within or between the luminal thrombus and the aortic wall.

Other entities can mimic acute aneurysm leak, including chronic rupture, perianeurysmal fibrosis from an inflammatory aneurysm (see later), lymphadenopathy, unopacified duodenum, and spontaneous retroperitoneal hemorrhage (Fig. 7-10).

BOX 7-2

IMAGING OF ABDOMINAL AORTIC ANEURYSMS BEFORE REPAIR

- Proximal and distal extent of aneurysm (including extension to iliac arteries)
- Number, location, and patency of renal arteries
- Presence of obstructive iliofemoral arterial disease
- Patency of mesenteric arteries
- Presence of associated anomalies or pathology (e.g., horseshoe kidney)
- Presence of inflammatory aneurysm
- Evidence of rupture
- Presence of inferior vena cava or renal vein anomalies

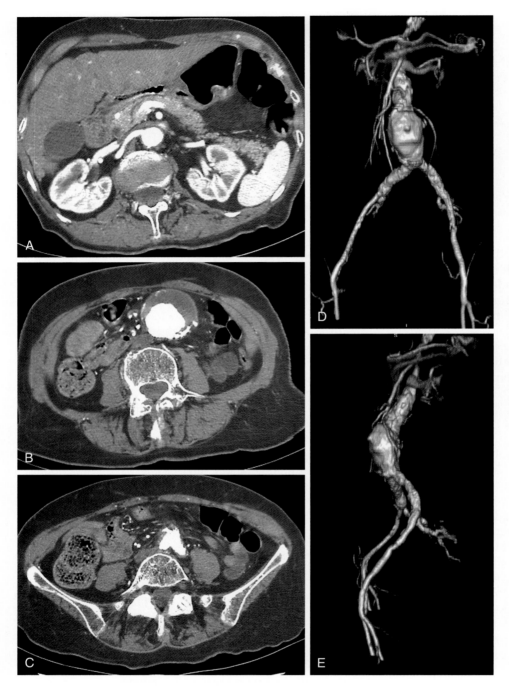

FIGURE 7-8 Infrarenal abdominal aortic aneurysm on computed tomography angiography. Axial images show aneurysm beginning below the renal arteries **(A)**, with large volume of mural thrombus and intimal calcification **(B)** and no involvement of the common iliac artery origins **(C).** Shaded surface display reconstructions in frontal **(D)** and lateral **(E)** projections nicely demonstrate the aneurysm, relationship to branch vessels, and status of the iliac arteries.

MAGNETIC RESONANCE IMAGING

Magnetic resonance imaging (MRI) is used in preprocedure and postprocedure assessment of some individuals with AAA[50-52] (Fig. 7-11). The diagnosis of *aortocaval fistula* is usually made by CT or MR angiography (Fig. 7-12). The communication most frequently develops between the distal aorta and IVC. In the absence of AAA, aortocaval fistula is either spontaneous or secondary to infection or trauma.[53,54] Stent grafts have been used to manage these rare lesions.[55]

Treatment

All patients with small AAAs should undergo routine imaging surveillance to follow growth. There is modest evidence that doxycycline (perhaps acting as an antiinflammatory agent) and coenzyme A reductase

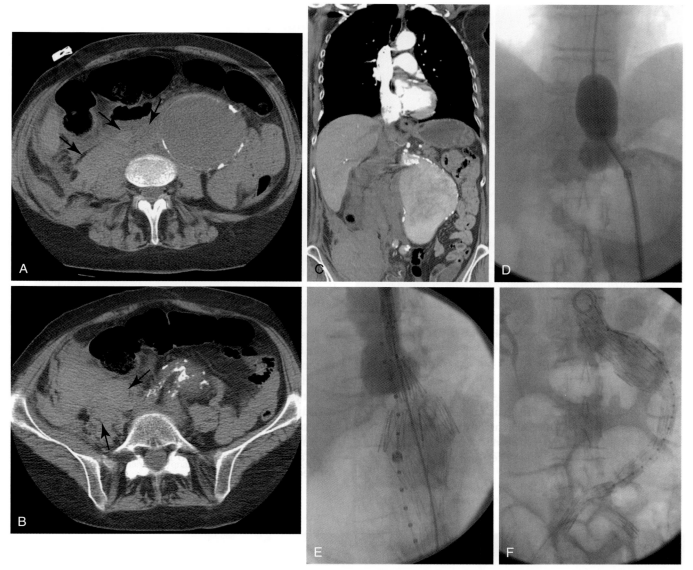

FIGURE 7-9   Acute rupture of an abdominal aortic aneurysm (AAA). Unenhanced axial (**A** and **B**) and contrast-enhanced reformatted coronal (**C**) CT images show a huge AAA that ends above the aortic bifurcation. There is high-density, heterogeneous soft tissue to the right of the aneurysm that represents recent leak *(arrows)*. **D, E,** and **F,** A stent-graft is being inserted emergently to treat the ruptured aneurysm.

inhibitors (statins) will slow the progression of AAA expansion.[56] The sole purpose of invasive AAA intervention is to prevent rupture.

PATIENT SELECTION

There is general agreement among vascular interventionalists that all AAA larger than 5 cm in transverse wall-to-wall diameter should be repaired electively and that smaller asymptomatic aneurysms be routinely followed by imaging studies.[33-37] Smaller AAAs are considered for repair if they are symptomatic (causing pain, tenderness, or distal embolization) or enlarging rapidly (>5 mm/6 months).

Of course, the benefits of watchful waiting with imaging surveillance in a particular individual must be weighed against the operative mortality rate for elective open or endovascular AAA repair (≤5%) and the high mortality rate associated with ruptured AAAs (50% to 75%).[36,39] Risk factors for rupture include female gender, advanced age, and continued smoking. The indications for open versus endovascular repair are evolving but are based primarily on anatomic factors, comorbid conditions, and patient/physician preference. Endovascular AAA repair (EVAR) with a stent graft should certainly be considered in patients with advanced age, significant operative risk, or

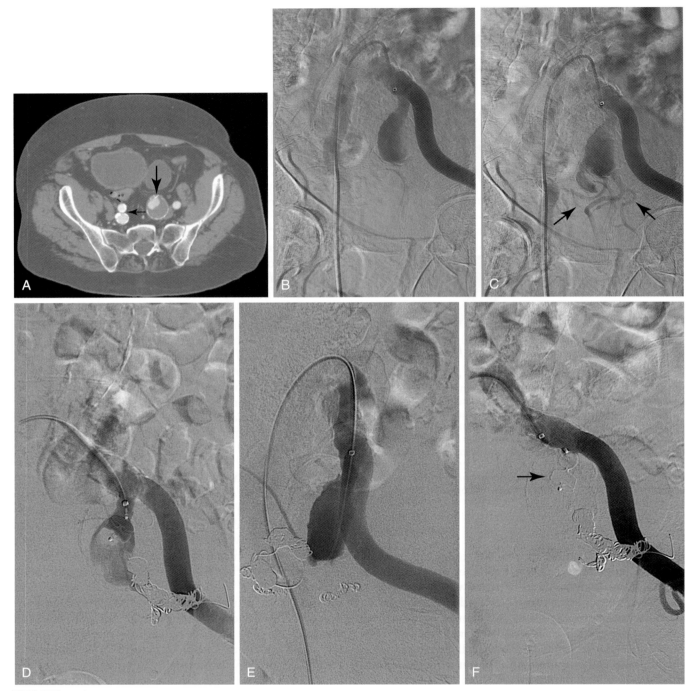

FIGURE 7-15   Internal iliac artery embolization prior to EVAR. **A,** Contrast-enhanced CT scan shows a large internal iliac artery aneurysm with extensive mural thrombus and intimal calcification *(large arrow)*. Right internal iliac artery is dilated and calcified *(small arrow)*. **B** and **C,** Catheter angiography outlines the aneurysm and branches beyond *(arrows)*. These distal branches must be excluded first with multiple coils **(D** and **E)** to prevent backfilling of the aneurysm before more proximal embolization with an Amplatzer plug **(F,** *arrow)*. Lesion is now completely excluded from the circulation.

TABLE 7-1   FDA-Approved Stent Grafts for Abdominal Aortic Aneurysms

Factor	AneuRx	Excluder	Zenith	TALENT	POWERLINK
Material	Nitinol, polyester	Nitinol, ePTFE	SS, polyester	Nitinol, polyester	Co-Ch, ePTFE
Design	2-piece, bifurcated	2-piece, modular	3-piece, modular	2-piece, bifurcated	Unibody, bifurcated
Proximal fixation	Infrarenal	Infrarenal	Suprarenal	Suprarenal	Infrarenal
Diameters	20-28 mm	22-31 mm	22-36 mm	22-36 mm	25-34 mm
Lengths	13.5-16.5 cm	12-18 cm	8.2-14 cm	15.5-18.5 cm	12-17.5 cm
Iliac limb diameter	12-20 mm	12-20 mm	8-24 mm	10-22 mm	16 mm
Aortic sheath	19, 21 Fr	18 Fr	18-22 Fr		21 Fr
Iliac sheath	16-19 Fr	12 Fr	14, 16 Fr		9 Fr

Co-Ch, *cobalt chromium alloy;* ePTFE, *expanded polytetrafluoroethylene;* Fr, *French;* SS, *stainless steel.*

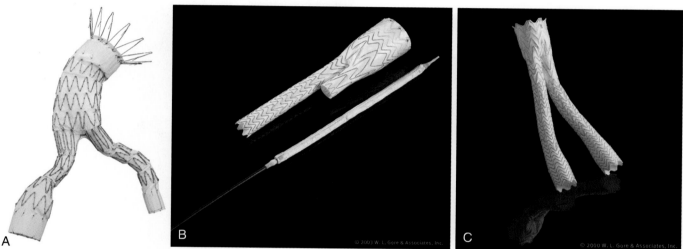

FIGURE 7-16   Endografts for abdominal aortic aneurysms. **A,** Zenith endograft. **B,** Excluder device, main module expanded *(top)* and wrapped *(bottom)* on deployment catheter. **C,** Excluder device with iliac limb extension in place. (**A,** *Courtesy of Cook, Inc;* **B** *and* **C,** *Courtesy of W. L. Gore and Associates.*)

Type I endoleak is defined as failure at the proximal or distal component attachment sites, most often inferior migration of the proximal stent and/or neck dilation[101] (Fig. 7-18). Neck dilation is known to progress over time after open aneurysm repair, but the surgical construction precludes leak. The behavior of the neck after EVAR depends to some extent on the self-expanding or balloon-expandable nature of the proximal component.[79] CT scans show hyperdense blood in the sac before contrast injection and focal extravasation contiguous with an attachment site after contrast.[102] Duplex ultrasound may depict the flow stream at this site.

Type III endoleak refers to delayed loss of integrity of an individual component stent or fabric. On CT images, the focal contrast collection does not correspond to attachment sites. In a summary of published series, mean frequency of delayed type I and III endoleaks were 6% and 1%, respectively. All type I and type III endoleaks require treatment upon detection (Fig. 7-19 and see Fig. 7-18). Grafts are salvaged by transarterial balloon dilation of leaky attachment sites or insertion of an additional stent graft cuff. Sometimes, the leak is sealed with glue or coils.[75] Conversion to open repair is rarely necessary.

Type II endoleak is by far the most common late event after EVAR. In this situation, blood flows in a retrograde direction through an aortic sac side branch and then must exit the aneurysm sac through the same vessel (simple) or another branch (complex). The *lumbar arteries, IMA,* or *internal iliac artery* (typically the iliolumbar branch) are the usual culprits. Rarely, an accessory renal or median sacral artery is responsible (Figs. 7-20 and 7-21). Contrast-enhanced CT shows focal extravasation in the sac away from the graft itself and usually remote from the device attachment points.[102] The leak may not be evident on the aortogram or selective arteriogram; superselective studies (e.g., microcatheterization of the marginal artery or the iliolumbar arterial collateral into a lumbar artery) are sometimes required[75] (see Fig. 7-20). Many type II endoleaks resolve spontaneously, so observation and imaging follow-up is often sufficient. If the aneurysm sac does not grow, most others have a benign course. However, aneurysm rupture in patients with this type of endoleak has been reported, and new endoleak has been discovered many years after the procedure.

Therefore the following subset of patients should be considered for treatment.[35,76,103-105]

- Persistent type II endoleak (>6 months)
- Type II endoleak with aneurysm expansion

There is still controversy regarding endoleak closure with persistent leak without sac expansion.[106,107]

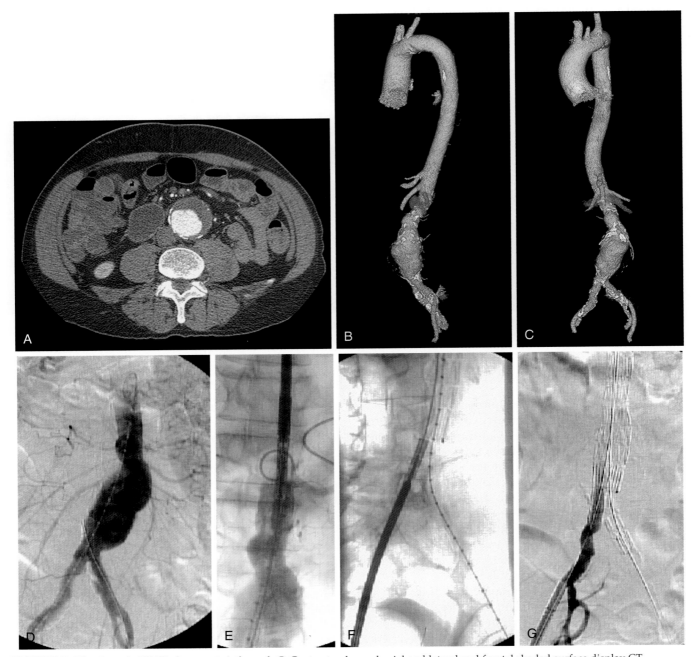

FIGURE 7-17   Steps in EVAR placement. **A** through **C**, Contrast-enhanced axial and lateral and frontal shaded surface display CT angiograms demonstrates a large infrarenal abdominal aortic aneurysm (AAA). **D**, Diagnostic aortography following bilateral femoral artery access. **E**, The main stent graft module is in place. **F**, Main module is deployed. **G**, Left iliac component in place.

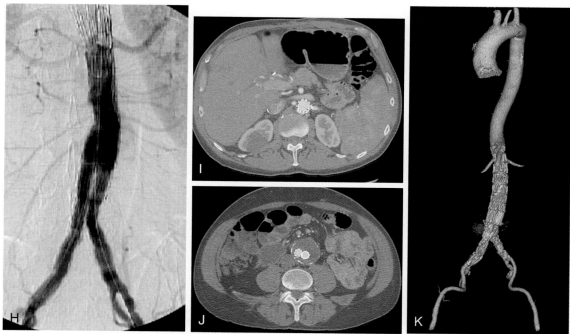

FIGURE 7-17, cont'd **H,** Final aortogram shows exclusion of the aneurysm. **I** through **K,** Follow-up axial and shaded surface display reformatted images show complete exclusion of AAA afterward with no evidence for endoleak. A postprocedure right renal infarct is identified.

TABLE 7-2   Outcomes of Endovascular Abdominal Aortic Aneurysm Repair

Technical success	95%
Access complications	
Hematoma	1%-5%
Infection	0%-11%
Arterial rupture/dissection	1%-4%
Other major early adverse events	
Acute renal failure	0%-17%
Lymphocele	0%-5%
Graft thrombosis	0%-7%
Stroke	0%-1%
Mesenteric ischemia	0%-2%
Paraplegia	0%-1%
30-day overall mortality	1%-4%
Endoleak rate at 2 yr	10%-20%
Device migration	2%
Limb occlusion/kink	3%-11%
Secondary procedures	2%-31%
Aneurysm expansion	1%-11%
Aneurysm shrinkage (1 yr)	15%-67%
Conversions (early and late)	<5%
Aneurysm rupture	0%-2%
2-yr survival	>85%

Several nonoperative methods are used to eliminate endoleak.[35,76]

- *Transarterial embolization* (see Fig. 7-20). Proximal occlusion of the feeding vessel alone has an unacceptable rate of failure or endoleak recurrence.[108] The optimal goal is superselective catheterization

BOX 7-4

POST-EVAR IMAGE ANALYSIS

- Morphology of aorta and endograft (changes in shape or structure)
- Aneurysm size
- Graft patency
- Endoleak (see text)
- Proximal or distal dilation
- Atherosclerosis
- Evidence for end organ ischemia (renal, mesenteric)

back into the aneurysm sac to allow obliteration of this space (with glue, coils, or Onyx) along with the culprit feeding and draining vessels. However, complex lesions treated in this fashion may still recur.[109] The procedure is generally quite safe, although aortoenteric fistula, colonic ischemia, and transient paraplegia have been reported.[76,110,111]

- *Translumbar sac and branch obliteration.*[76,112] Many experts think this approach provides a more durable result than transarterial treatment.[109,113,114] With the patient prone and following analysis of the CT angiogram, a 19-gauge sheath-needle

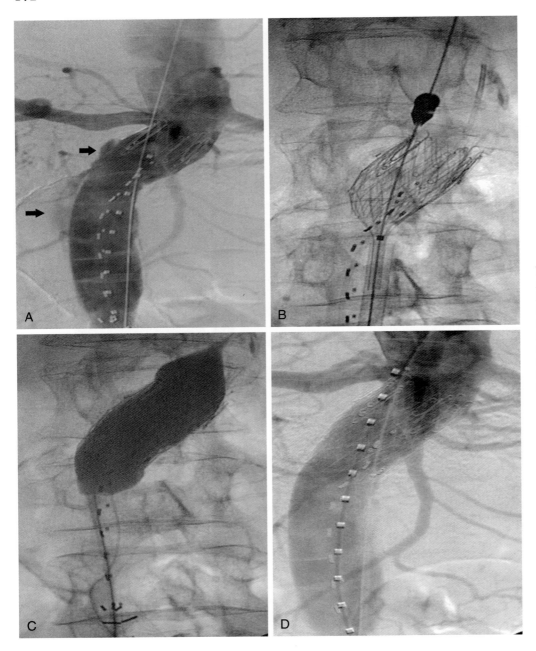

FIGURE 7-18   Type I endoleak. **A,** Catheter angiogram shows leak from the proximal attachment site *(arrows).* **B,** An aortic cuff is placed at this location. **C,** The leak is sealed by balloon dilation of the cuff. **D,** Final angiogram shows no evidence for residual leak. *(Courtesy of Gerant Rivera-Sanfeliz, San Diego, Calif.)*

or micropuncture system is inserted about one hand breadth from the midline toward the left lateral border of the spine from the left flank (or right flank if a transcaval approach is deemed necessary).[115] Once the aneurysm sac is entered, the pressure is measured and the sac is embolized with cyanoacrylate and/or coils (Fig. 7-22). Great care should be taken to prevent glue from backfilling into the IMA circulation. Thrombin has been used is this setting, but serious visceral injury has occurred.[116]

- *Laparoscopic branch ligation.*

Type IV endoleak was a transient feature of older devices with more porous fabric material that allowed early seepage of blood. They never required treatment.

Type V endoleak ("*endotension*") refers to aneurysm growth after EVAR with persistent pressurization of the sac without a detectable endoleak.[117] The etiology for this phenomenon is somewhat obscure, but is perhaps caused by a leak below the threshold for current imaging detection or persistent transgraft pressure (rather than flow) on the native aortic wall. Aneurysm rupture is theoretically possible. Endovascular methods may be used to treat this condition, and open

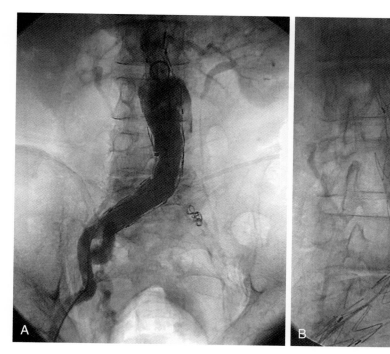

FIGURE 7-19 Type III endoleak. **A,** Catheter angiogram shows leak in proximal device material. **B,** Plain radiograph demonstrates stent graft separation. *(Courtesy of William Stavropoulos, Philadelphia, Pa.)*

TABLE 7-3 Endoleak Classification

Type		Definition
I		Attachment leak or failure
	IA	Proximal end
	IB	Distal end
	IC	Iliac component
II		Retrograde branch flow into aneurysm sac
	IIA	Simple (single inflow/outflow vessel)
	IIB	Complex (multiple inflow/outflow vessels)
III		Device deterioration or dehiscence
	IIIA	Disruption of modular stent components
	IIIB	Fabric defect
	IIIC	Other defect
IV		Graft porosity
V		Endotension

repair is rarely necessary. Future modifications in graft material may ultimately prevent this perplexing, uncommon problem.

Aortic Occlusive Disease (Online Case 42)

Etiology

Complete occlusion of the abdominal aorta can present as an acute or chronic event. The most common cause of *chronic* occlusion is thrombosis superimposed on severe atherosclerosis of the distal abdominal aorta and common iliac arteries. The *Leriche syndrome* describes such patients with buttock and thigh claudication, impotence, thigh muscle atrophy, and diminished femoral pulses.[118]

Thrombosis also may occur in the setting of less common entities that narrow the aorta.

Box 7-5 outlines the major causes for *acute* abdominal aortic occlusion.[119,120] About 50% to 65% of cases result from embolism.[121] Thrombosis of AAAs often follows disruption of mural thrombus followed by distal embolization.[122] In many cases, distal aortic occlusion propagates back toward the level of the renal arteries or SMA. The ultimate level of the occlusion is distributed about evenly above and below the origin of the IMA.

Clinical Features

Most patients with chronic aortic occlusion have a long history of smoking. Symptoms and signs depend largely on whether the occlusion is acute or chronic. Patients with acute occlusion may have sudden onset of bilateral lower extremity rest pain, absent pulses, cool and mottled skin, and neurologic deficits. Prior episodes of myocardial infarction or cardiac dysrhythmias are common. Patients with chronic occlusion usually complain of severe, progressive, bilateral leg claudication, along with impotence in some men. Distal leg pulses often are diminished or absent. However, with good collateral circulation, weak femoral pulses may be palpable in patients with complete long-standing occlusion.

Imaging

Acute and chronic occlusions are imaged with CT or MR angiography. When catheter arteriography is performed (usually because endovascular treatment is

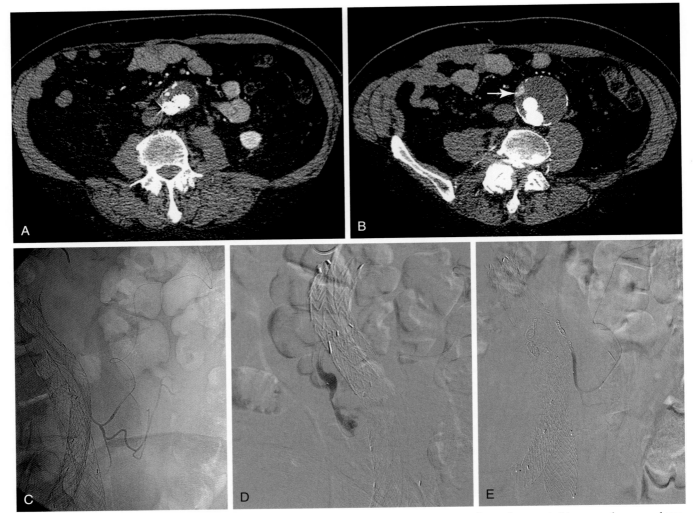

FIGURE 7-20   Type II endoleak following endovascular aneurysm repair. **A** and **B**, Contrast-enhanced computed tomography scans show filling of both iliac limbs of the aortic graft. Extravasation of contrast into the anterior portion of mural thrombus *(arrow)* indicates endoleak, probably from the inferior mesenteric artery (IMA). **C**, The superior mesenteric artery was catheterized. A coaxial microcatheter was negotiated into the middle colic artery, then the marginal artery and finally the left colic branch of the IMA. **D**, The microcatheter was advanced further through the IMA root and directly into the aneurysm sac, into which contrast spills. **E**, Coils were deposited back from the sac into the proximal IMA, closing the endoleak.

contemplated), a left brachial artery approach is recommended. However, it may be possible to enter the femoral artery using ultrasound guidance and traverse the occlusion with a hydrophilic guidewire, even with faint or absent pulses. The catheter should be advanced carefully into the abdominal aorta to within several centimeters of the site of occlusion.

Chronic occlusion invokes an extensive collateral circulation (see Fig. 7-5). A filling defect in the aorta indicates acute embolism or in situ thrombosis. Involvement of the renal or mesenteric arteries should be sought. Rarely, extension of a thoracic aortic dissection causes acute abdominal aortic occlusion.

Treatment

SURGICAL THERAPY

Historically, the mortality for patients with acute abdominal aortic occlusion was greater than 50%.[121] Patients with embolic aortic obstruction are treated with embolectomy in many cases.[120,121] For acute or chronic thrombotic occlusion, aortobifemoral bypass grafting is the procedure of choice.

ENDOVASCULAR THERAPY

Interventional radiology has a role in the management of chronic aortic occlusion, particularly when disease is isolated to the distal portion of the abdominal aorta.[123-125] Thrombolysis (to lyse fresh clot), angioplasty, and intra-

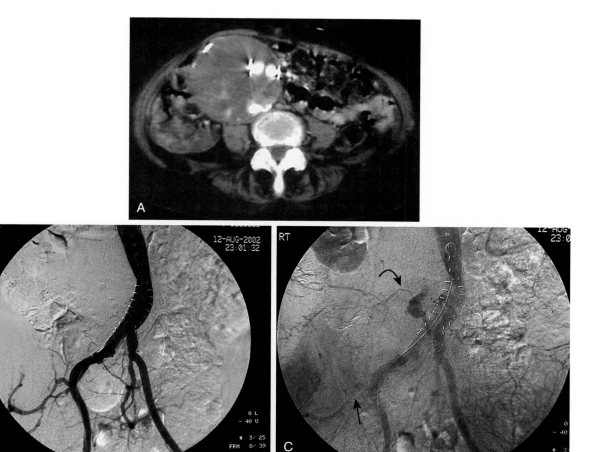

FIGURE 7-21   Type II endoleak in a patient lost to follow-up years after stent-graft placement. **A,** Computed tomography angiogram shows huge abdominal aortic aneurysm displaced to the right with patent endograft and contrast extravasation into clot, indicating endoleak. **B,** Early phase of catheter aortogram reveals a widely patent device. **C,** Late phase shows leak into aneurysm sac through internal iliac artery branches *(arrow)* feeding a right lumbar artery in a retrograde direction *(curved arrow). (Courtesy of Anne C. Roberts, MD, San Diego, Calif.)*

vascular stent placement have been used successfully in selected cases (see Chapter 8). However, long-term patency in large series of patients has not been established.

Dissection

Dissection of the abdominal aorta usually follows extension of a thoracic aortic dissection (see Chapter 6). Causes of *isolated abdominal aortic dissection* include trauma, catheterization, preexisting aneurysm, and a spontaneous event.[126,127] With cross-sectional imaging, an intimal flap is seen with differential flow signal or density in the true and false lumens. The true aortic lumen may appear tapered or narrowed because of expansion of the false lumen (Box 7-6 and Fig. 7-23). Progressive enlargement of the false lumen of a chronic aortic dissection can produce an aneurysm. Whereas many afflicted patients are handled with conservative management, extensive surveillance is important if endovascular or open repair is rejected.[128]

OTHER DISORDERS

Inflammatory Aortic Aneurysms (Online Case 53)

Inflammatory AAAs fall within the spectrum of the generalized disorder of *chronic periaortitis*, which includes this disease and idiopathic *retroperitoneal fibrosis (RPF)*.[40] RPF is distinguished from the former disorder by the absence of aortic aneurysm. Both entities are marked by cellular infiltration of the adventitia of the abdominal aorta and sometimes other retroperitoneal structures (including duodenum, ureters, IVC, and even left renal vein). The consequence is marked thickening of the aortic wall and a dense, periadventitial fibrotic reaction, which draws other organs toward the aorta and sometimes obstructs them. The precise cause is unknown, but the condition may involve an immune-related reaction to material within the aortic

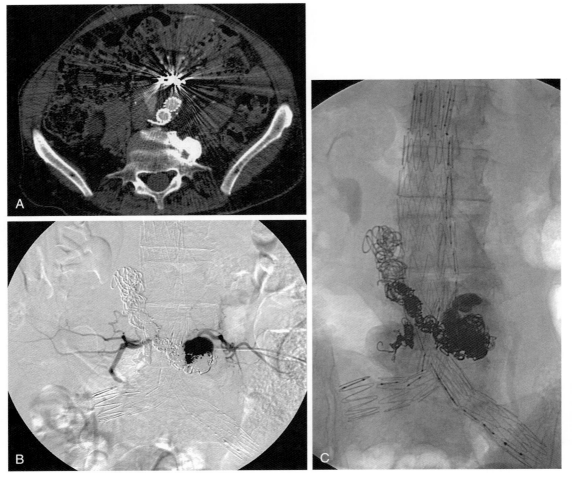

FIGURE 7-22   Recurrent type II endoleak treatment by translumbar embolization. Patient had type II endoleak treated 2 years earlier. **A,** Computed tomography angiogram shows persistent leak into aneurysm sac. **B,** Following translumbar catheter placement, there is antegrade filling of bilateral lumbar arteries. **C,** Multiple coils and *x*-butyl cyanoacrylate were used to fill the sac. *(Courtesy of William Stavropoulos, Philadelphia, Pa.)*

BOX 7-5

CAUSES OF ACUTE OCCLUSION OF THE ABDOMINAL AORTA

- Embolism (usually cardiac source)
- Thrombosis superimposed on atherosclerotic disease
- Thrombosis of abdominal aortic aneurysm
- Trauma
- Iatrogenic injury (e.g., catheterization)
- Thrombophilic state
- Dissection
- Extrinsic compression

BOX 7-6

CAUSES OF ABDOMINAL AORTIC NARROWING

- Atherosclerosis
- Dissection
- Aneurysm with mural thrombus
- Vasculitis
  - Takayasu arteritis
- Congenital coarctation syndromes
  - Neurofibromatosis
  - Williams syndrome
  - Congenital rubella
  - Tuberous sclerosis
  - Middle aortic syndrome
- Radiation aortitis

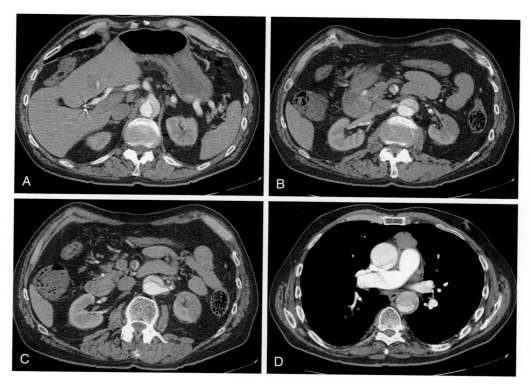

FIGURE 7-23 Extension of thoracic aortic dissection into the abdominal aorta as seen on contrast-enhanced computed tomography angiograms.

wall.[129,130] Genetic factors also have been implicated, including an association with the human leukocyte antigen molecule and autoimmune diseases.[131]

Inflammatory aneurysms account for about 3% to 10% of all AAAs.[40,132,133] Compared with patients with degenerative aortic aneurysms, this subgroup is somewhat younger, more likely to be male, and more often symptomatic at presentation, but much less likely to rupture (lifetime risk <5%).[40] Patients may have fever, weight loss, and an elevated erythrocyte sedimentation rate or C-reactive protein during the acute phase of the illness. Abdominal or back pain is much more common in patients with inflammatory aneurysms than in those with degenerative ones.

On CT or MRI, the diagnosis is suggested by a smooth, confluent rind of enhancing soft tissue around the anterior and lateral margins of the aorta[134,135] (Fig. 7-24). The posterior border of the aorta often is spared. Involvement of the small bowel, ureters, or IVC in the fibrotic process is characteristic. These features usually allow distinction from aortic rupture, metastatic disease, or lymphadenopathy (see Figs. 7-9 and 7-10). Identification of disease in adjacent organs is important before invasive treatment.

Most practitioners opt for a course of corticosteroids in the acute phase of the illness.[40] However, aneurysm repair appears to halt (and even reverse) the inflammatory process. Recently, EVAR has been used in this condition with perioperative mortality (about 2%) and regression of periaortic inflammation (65%) comparable to open repair.[136]

Infectious Aortic Aneurysms

Infectious (mycotic) aneurysms or *pseudoaneurysms* are caused by local seeding of diseased vessel wall (usually atherosclerotic plaque), seeding through the vasa vasorum, direct invasion from an adjacent infection, or penetrating trauma. Mycotic aneurysms account for about 1% to 2% of all AAA.[137] They are especially lethal, with a substantial risk for rapid growth, rupture, and postoperative mortality[138] Among the more common offending organisms are *Staphylococcus aureus* and *Salmonella* species.[137,139] Mycobacterial AAA are also described.[140] The thoracoabdominal and abdominal aorta are more commonly affected than the thoracic aorta. Most patients are intravenous drug abusers or alcoholics, or are immunocompromised.

Abdominal or back pain, fever, a pulsatile mass, elevated inflammatory markers (such as C-reactive protein and white blood cell count), and positive blood cultures may be present. The diagnosis is confirmed by cross-sectional imaging. The typical finding is a saccular, eccentric aneurysm, usually with little or no adjacent aortic disease[141] (Fig. 7-25). Enhancing periaortic soft tissue may be evident. Multiple aneurysms are common.

Patients are treated vigorously with intravenous antibiotics. If the patient does not undergo surgical

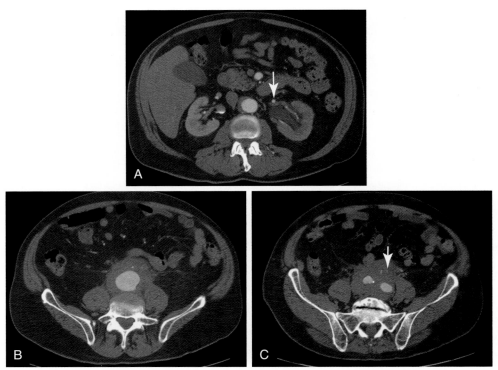

FIGURE 7-24 Inflammatory abdominal aortic aneurysm. **A** through **C,** Contrast-enhanced computed tomography scan shows the aortic aneurysm with a large rind of soft tissue around the anterolateral portion of the aorta. The inflammatory mass entirely surrounds the common iliac arteries. The inferior vena cava is obliterated by the mass, and a bowel loop has become enmeshed within it *(short arrow).* Left hydronephrosis *(long arrow)* indicates that at least the left ureter is involved.

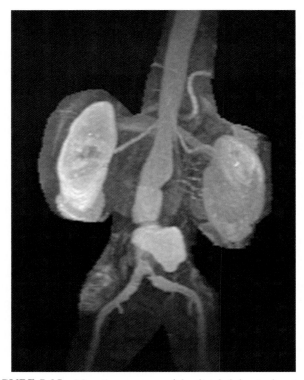

FIGURE 7-25 Mycotic aneurysm of the distal abdominal aorta on gadolinium-enhanced magnetic resonance angiogram.

repair, then long-term (sometimes lifelong) antimicrobial coverage along with aneurysm surveillance is mandatory. Early operation is recommended in most cases, usually with prosthetic graft placement or ligation and extraanatomic bypass grafting.[142,143] In many reports, 1-year mortality is substantial (>20%).[137,138,144] Intuitively, EVAR seems a mistake due to the risk for persistent infection, the inability to obtain tissue for culture, and the possibility for graft seeding. Somewhat surprisingly, stent graft placement may be both effective and safe as a bridge to definitive open surgical management, particularly in initially high-risk patients.[137,145-147] On occasion, EVAR is curative.

Penetrating Aortic Ulcer and Intramural Hematoma

See Chapter 6 for a full consideration of these two uncommon but important entities.[148]

Trauma

Injury to the abdominal aorta occurs from accidental, criminal, or iatrogenic penetrating trauma and, less commonly, from blunt trauma.[149-151] Penetrating injuries occur more frequently to the abdominal aorta than to the thoracic aorta. The most common causes of blunt trauma are motor vehicle crashes and crush injuries. Few patients survive to reach medical care. When the vascular disruption is minor (e.g., an intimal flap), patients may have no symptoms. Signs of major abdominal aortic injury include diminished pulses or a reduction in ankle-brachial indices. There is a classic association with lumbar spine fractures.

Unstable patients may go immediately to exploratory laparotomy without imaging studies. Those with abdominal trauma who are hemodynamically stable usually undergo CT scanning. The abnormalities range from a discrete intimal flap to dissection, intramural hematoma, penetrating tear, pseudoaneurysm, complete transection with acute thrombosis, or aortocaval fistula.[149-155] In the absence of AAA, *aortocaval fistula* usually is a complication of blunt or penetrating injury or lumbar disc surgery.[154]

The mortality rate from abdominal aortic injury is greater than 75% and is higher for suprarenal injuries.[150,151] The usual treatment is operation with aortic reconstruction or bypass graft placement. Endovascular stent grafts have also been used in this situation.[149,156,157]

Injury to abdominal aortic branches is considered in the related chapters. Injury to lumbar arteries should be suspected in any patient with blunt abdominal or pelvic trauma and evidence of significant retroperitoneal bleeding (see Chapter 8).

Vasculitis and Vasculopathy

Takayasu arteritis is an inflammatory vasculitis affecting large- and medium-sized elastic arteries. Details of this unusual entity are considered in Chapters 1 and 6. The typical patient is young and female, often of Asian descent. The abdominal aorta and its branches are involved in about two thirds of cases[158-160] (see Fig. 1-22). The most common imaging finding is smooth narrowing of the abdominal aorta, which may be focal, segmental, or diffuse; rarely, complete obstruction occurs (Fig. 7-26A and see Box 7-6). Associated narrowing of the proximal portions of the renal, mesenteric, or iliac arteries is common. Conversely, fusiform aneurysms of the aorta (usually suprarenal) and branch vessels are occasionally seen (see Fig. 7-26B). Most lesions remain stable after the disease becomes chronic.

Radiation arteritis may develop in large or small blood vessels. In large- and medium-sized arteries, high-dose radiotherapy can induce periarterial fibrosis, intimal atherosclerotic-like changes with mural thrombus formation, or frank fibrotic occlusion.[161] Radiation-induced arterial disease usually becomes apparent 5 or more years after therapy. Imaging reveals smooth narrowing of the affected vessels, irregular atherosclerotic-like lesions, or complete occlusion.[162,163]

HIV-related arteriopathy is well known to affect medium- and small-caliber vessels. However, a rarer

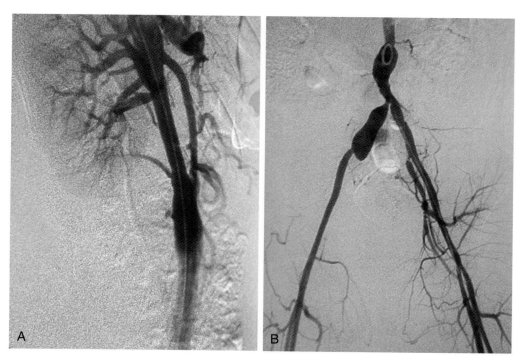

FIGURE 7-26   Takayasu arteritis. **A,** Typical smooth long-segment infrarenal aortic narrowing in a 7-year-old girl (lateral projection of abdominal aortogram). **B,** Atypical aortic and iliac artery aneurysms in another young girl.

large vessel vasculopathy can produce solitary or multiple aneurysms in the aorta and its major branches.[164] The disease provokes a leukocytoclastic reaction in the vasa vasorum and periadventitial tissues along with chronic inflammation. The aneurysms often are saccular in appearance (see Fig. 6-27).

Coarctation Syndromes (Online Case 88)

Several disorders associated with congenital coarctation syndromes can affect the abdominal aorta and its major branches[165-168] (see Box 7-6 and Chapter 1). In many patients, the etiology is obscure; it is postulated that overfusion of the paired dorsal aortas in the fetus is responsible for some cases.[166] Vascular involvement in *neurofibromatosis-1 (NF-1)* is common; when present, stenoses of the aorta and branch vessels (particularly the renal arteries) or arterial aneurysms are found. Narrowing of large- and medium-caliber vessels results from proliferation of neurofibromas or ganglioneuromatous tissue within the vascular wall.[165,166] *Williams syndrome* is a congenital disorder that includes infantile hypercalcemia, supravalvular aortic stenosis, elfin facies, and developmental delays.

This rare and diverse group of diseases is often the underlying cause of hypertension in children or young adults.[166] For operative staging, the coarctation syndromes are classified by the more cephalic site of disease: suprarenal, intrarenal, or infrarenal (most to least common). Imaging findings include smooth narrowing of the proximal or midabdominal aorta, narrowing of the proximal renal arteries in almost all cases, and stenoses or occlusions of the superior mesenteric or celiac artery with enlarged collateral vessels (Fig. 7-27; see Box 7-6 and see Fig. 10-20). Standard treatment is a thoracoabdominal bypass graft or patch aortoplasty along with renal and mesenteric artery reconstruction.[166]

Middle aortic syndrome (or atypical coarctation) produces narrowing of abdominal aorta, characteristically in its midportion and including major visceral branches.[169] Despite extensive research, there is still controversy about the relationships between middle aortic syndrome, Takayasu arteritis, and the congenital coarctation syndromes.[167] Some experts believe that middle aortic syndrome is simply a subtype of Takayasu arteritis and that the features in this subgroup of patients are found in the spectrum of patients with nonspecific aortoarteritis. Other investigators believe that these entities are distinct, although perhaps related, diseases. Middle aortic syndrome differs from Takayasu arteritis in the lack of geographic predilection, younger age at presentation (first and second decades of life), noninflammatory pathology, and absence of an acute febrile phase. Surgical revascularization is the standard treatment.[170] Stents have been used in this setting, but the durability of such an approach in this young population is unknown.[166,171-173]

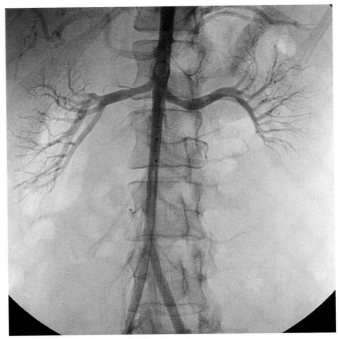

FIGURE 7-27   Aortic hypoplasia in Williams syndrome. Abdominal aortography shows diffuse narrowing of the infrarenal aorta. The central portions of both renal arteries are moderately dilated.

References

1. Collins P, editor. Embryology and development. In: Williams PL, Bannister LH, Berry MM, et al., editors. *Gray's anatomy.* 38th ed. New York: Churchill Livingstone; 1995. p. 318.
2. Gabella G, editor. Cardiovascular system. In: Williams PL, Bannister LH, Berry MM, et al., editors. *Gray's anatomy.* 38th ed. New York: Churchill Livingstone; 1995. p. 1547.
3. da Silva ES, Rodrigues Jr AJ, Castro de Tolosa EM, et al. Variation of infrarenal aortic diameter: a necropsy study. *J Vasc Surg* 1999; **29**:920.
4. Horejs D, Gilbert PM, Burstein S, et al. Normal aortoiliac diameters by CT. *J Comput Assist Tomogr* 1988;**12**:602.
5. Shokeir AA, el-Diasty TA, Nabeeh A, et al. Digital subtraction angiography in potential live-kidney donors: a study of 1000 cases. *Abdom Imaging* 1994;**19**:461.
6. Rankin SC, Jan W, Koffman CG. Noninvasive imaging of living related kidney donors: evaluation of CT angiography and gadolinium enhanced MR angiography. *AJR Am J Roentgenol* 2001; **177**:349.
7. Raman SS, Pojchamarnwiputh S, Muangsomboon K, et al. Surgically relevant normal and variant renal parenchymal and vascular anatomy in preoperative 16-MDCT evaluation of potential laparoscopic renal donors. *AJR Am J Roentgenol* 2007;**188**:105.
8. Kalra M, Panneton JM, Hofer JM, et al. Aneurysm and stenosis of the celiomesenteric trunk: a rare anomaly. *J Vasc Surg* 2003; **37**:679.
9. Gwon DI, Ko GY, Yoon HK, et al. Inferior phrenic artery: anatomy, variations, pathologic conditions, and interventional management. *Radiographics* 2007;**27**:687.
10. So YH, Chung JW, Yin Y, et al. The right inferior phrenic artery: origin and proximal anatomy on digital subtraction angiography and thin-section helical computed tomography. *J Vasc Interv Radiol* 2009;**20**:1164.
11. Inoue Y, Iwai T, Endo M. Determining variations in colonic circulation during aortic surgery. *Cardiovasc Surg* 1997;**5**:626.
12. Johnston KW, Rutherford RB, Tilson MD, et al. Suggested standards for reporting on arterial aneurysms. *J Vasc Surg* 1991;**13**:452.

13. Sakalihasan N, Limet R, Defawe OD. Abdominal aortic aneurysm. *Lancet* 2005;**365**:1577.

14. Wanhainen A. How to define an abdominal aortic aneurysm-influence on epidemiology and clinical practice. *Scand J Surg* 2008;**97**:105.

15. Johnston KW, Scobie TK. Multicenter prospective study of nonruptured abdominal aortic aneurysms. I. Population and operative management. *J Vasc Surg* 1988;**7**:69.

16. Nypaver TJ, Shepard AD, Reddy DJ, et al. Repair of pararenal abdominal aortic aneurysms: an analysis of operative management. *Arch Surg* 1993;**128**:803.

17. Jongkind V, Yeung KK, Akkersdijk GJ, et al. Juxtarenal aortic aneurysm repair: a systematic review. *J Vasc Surg* 2010;**52**:760.

18. Melton III LJ, Bickerstaff LK, Hollier LH, et al. Changing incidence of abdominal aortic aneurysms: a population-based study. *Am J Epidemiol* 1984;**120**:379.

19. Reitsma JB, Pleumeekers HJ, Hoes AW, et al. Increasing incidence of aneurysms of the abdominal aorta in The Netherlands. *Eur J Vasc Endovasc Surg* 1996;**12**:446.

20. Guo DC, Papke CL, He R, et al. Pathogenesis of thoracic and abdominal aortic aneurysms. *Ann N Y Acad Sci* 2006;**1085**:339.

21. Golledge J, Norman PE. Atherosclerosis and abdominal aortic aneurysm: cause, response, or common risk factors. *Arterioscler Thromb Vasc Biol* 2010;**30**:1075.

22. Abdul-Hussien H, Hanemaaijer R, Kleemann R, et al. The pathophysiology of abdominal aortic aneurysm growth: corresponding and discordant inflammatory and proteolytic processes in abdominal aortic and popliteal artery aneurysms. *J Vasc Surg* 2010;**51**:1479.

23. Miller FJ. Aortic aneurysms. It's all about the stress. *Arterioscler Thromb Vasc Biol* 2002;**22**:1948.

24. Ruddy JM, Jones JA, Spinale FG, et al. Regional heterogeneity within the aorta: relevance to aneurysm disease. *J Thorac Cardiovasc Surg* 2008;**136**:1123.

25. Rizas KD, Ippagunta N, Tilson III ND. Immune cells and molecular mediators in the pathogenesis of the abdominal aortic aneurysm. *Cardiol Rev* 2009;**17**:201.

26. Jost CJ, Gloviczki P, Edwards WD, et al. Aortic aneurysms in children and young adults with tuberous sclerosis: report of two cases and review of the literature. *J Vasc Surg* 2001;**33**:639.

27. Alpagut U, Ugurlucan M, Dayioglu E. Major arterial involvement and review of Behcet's disease. *Ann Vasc Surg* 2007;**21**:232.

28. Tucker Jr S, Rowe VL, Rao R, et al. Treatment options for traumatic pseudoaneurysms of the paravisceral abdominal aorta. *Ann Vasc Surg* 2005;**19**:613.

29. Powell JT, Brown LC. The natural history of abdominal aortic aneurysms and their risk of rupture. *Acta Chir Belg* 2001;**101**:11.

30. Kurvers H, Veith FJ, Lipsitz EC, et al. Discontinuous, staccato growth of abdominal aortic aneurysms. *J Am Coll Surg* 2004;**199**:709.

31. Brady AR, Thompson SG, Fowkes FG, et al. Abdominal aortic aneurysm expansion: risk factors and time intervals for surveillance. *Circulation* 2004;**110**:16.

32. Lederle FA. The natural history of abdominal aortic aneurysm. *Acta Chir Belg* 2009;109:7.

33. Ouriel K, Clair DG, Kent KC, et al. Endovascular repair compared with surveillance for patients with small abdominal aortic aneurysms. *J Vasc Surg* 2010;**51**:1081.

34. Powell JT, Brown LC, Forbes JF, et al. Final 12-year follow-up of surgery versus surveillance in the UK Small Aneurysm Trial. *Br J Surg* 2007;**94**:702.

35. Chaikof EL, Brewster DC, Dalman RL, et al. SVS practice guidelines for the care of patients with an abdominal aortic aneurysm: executive summary. *J Vasc Surg* 2009;**50**:880.

36. Lederle FA, Wilson SE, Johnson GR, et al. Immediate repair compared with surveillance of small abdominal aortic aneurysms. *N Engl J Med* 2002;**346**:1437.

37. Kim LG, Scott RA, Ashton HA, et al. A sustained mortality benefit from screening for abdominal aortic aneurysm. *Ann Intern Med* 2007;**146**:699.

38. Bengtsson H, Bergqvist D. Ruptured abdominal aortic aneurysm: a population-based study. *J Vasc Surg* 1993;**18**:74.

39. Singh K, Bonaa KH, Jacobsen BK, et al. Prevalence of and risk factors for abdominal aortic aneurysms in a population-based study: The Tromso Study. *Am J Epidemiol* 2001;**154**:236.

40. Hellmann DB, Grand DJ, Freischlag JA. Inflammatory abdominal aortic aneurysm. *JAMA* 2007;**297**:395.

41. Guzzardi G, Fossaceca R, Divenuto I, et al. Endovascular treatment of ruptured abdominal aortic aneurysm with aortocaval fistula. *Cardiovasc Intervent Radiol* 2010;**33**:853.

42. Ricotta II JJ, Malgor RD, Oderich GS. Endovascular abdominal aortic aneurysm repair: Part 1. *Ann Vasc Surg* 2009;**23**:799.

43. Budovec JJ, Pollema M, Grogan M. Update on multidetector computed tomography angiography of the abdominal aorta. *Radiol Clin North Am* 2010;**48**:283.

44. Bromley PJ, Kaufman JA. Abdominal aortic aneurysms before and after endograft implantation: evaluation by computed tomography. *Tech Vasc Interv Radiol* 2001;**4**:15.

45. Rakita D, Newatia A, Hines JJ, et al. Spectrum of CT findings in rupture and impending rupture of abdominal aortic aneurysms. *Radiographics* 2007;**27**:497.

46. Nyman R, Eriksson MO. The future of imaging in the management of abdominal aortic aneurysm. *Scand J Surg* 2008;**97**:110.

47. Fillinger MF, Racusin J, Baker RK, et al. Anatomic characteristics of ruptured abdominal aortic aneurysm on conventional CT scans: implications for rupture risk. *J Vasc Surg* 2004;**39**:1243.

48. Lederle FA, Johnson GR, Wilson SE, et al. Rupture rate of large abdominal aortic aneurysms in patients refusing or unfit for elective repair. *JAMA* 2002;**287**:2968.

49. Bhalla S, Menias CO, Heiken JP. CT of acute abdominal aortic disorders. *Radiol Clin North Am* 2003;**41**:1153.

50. Persson A, Dahlstrom N, Engellau L, et al. Volume rendering compared with maximum intensity projection for magnetic resonance angiography measurements of the abdominal aorta. *Acta Radiol* 2004;**45**:453.

51. Lookstein RA, Goldman J, Pukin L, et al. Time-resolved magnetic resonance angiography as a noninvasive method to characterize endoleaks: initial results compared with conventional angiography. *J Vasc Surg* 2004;**39**:27.

52. Atar E, Belenky A, Hadad M, et al. MR angiography for abdominal and thoracic aortic aneurysms: assessment before endovascular repair in patients with impaired renal function. *AJR Am J Roentgenol* 2006;**186**:386.

53. Torigian DA, Carpenter JP, Roberts DA. Mycotic aortocaval fistula: efficient evaluation by bolus-chase MR angiography. *J Magn Reson Imaging* 2002;**15**:195.

54. Rajmohan B. Spontaneous aortocaval fistula. *J Postgrad Med* 2002;**48**:203.

55. Lau LL, O'Reilly MJ, Johnston LC, et al. Endovascular stent-graft repair of primary aortocaval fistula with an abdominal aortoiliac aneurysm. *J Vasc Surg* 2001;**33**:425.

56. Baxter BT, Terrin MC, Dalman RL. Medical management of small abdominal aortic aneurysms. *Circulation* 2008;**117**:1883.

57. Brewster DC, Cronenwett JL, Hallett Jr JW, et al. Guidelines for the treatment of abdominal aortic aneurysms. Report of a subcommittee of the Joint Council of the American Association for Vascular Surgery and Society for Vascular Surgery. *J Vasc Surg* 2003;**37**:1106.

58. Towne JB. Endovascular treatment of abdominal aortic aneurysms. *Am J Surg* 2005;**189**:140.

59. Giles KA, Pomposelli FB, Hamdan AD, et al. Comparison of open and endovascular repair of ruptured abdominal aortic aneurysms from the ACS-NSQIP 2005–07. *J Endovasc Ther* 2009;**16**:365.

60. Cambria RP, Brewster DC, Abbott WM, et al. Transperitoneal versus retroperitoneal approach for aortic reconstruction: a randomized, prospective study. *J Vasc Surg* 1990;**11**:314.

61. Vu QD, Menias CO, Bhalia S, et al. Aortoenteric fistulas: CT features and potential mimics. *Radiographics* 2009;**29**:197.

62. Calligaro KD, Veith FJ, Yuan JG, et al. Intra-abdominal aortic graft infection: complete or partial graft preservation in patients at very high risk. *J Vasc Surg* 2003;**38**:1199.

63. Noel AA, Gloviczki P, Cherry Jr KJ, et al. Abdominal aortic reconstruction in infected fields: early results of the United States cryopreserved aortic allograft registry. *J Vasc Surg* 2002;**35**:847.

64. Mii S, Mori A, Sakata H, et al. Para-anastomotic aneurysms: incidence, risk factors, treatment, and prognosis. *J Cardiovasc Surg (Torino)* 1998;**39**:259.

65. Cendan JC, Thomas IV JB, Seeger JM. Twenty-one cases of aortoenteric fistula: lessons for the general surgeon. *Am Surg* 2004;**70**:583.

66. Busuttil SJ, Goldstone J. Diagnosis and management of aortoenteric fistulas. *Semin Vasc Surg* 2001;**14**:302.

67. Lew WK, Rowe VL, Cunningham MJ, et al. Endovascular management of mycotic aortic aneurysms and associated aortoaerodigestive fistulas. *Ann Vasc Surg* 2009;**23**:81.

68. Parodi JC, Palmaz JC, Barone HD. Transfemoral intraluminal graft implantation for abdominal aortic aneurysms. *Ann Vasc Surg* 1991;**5**:491.

69. Rydberg J, Kopecky KK, Johnson MS, et al. Endovascular repair of abdominal aortic aneurysms: assessment with multislice CT. *AJR Am J Roentgenol* 2001;**177**:607.

70. Geller SC. Imaging guidelines for abdominal aortic aneurysm repair with endovascular stent grafts. *J Vasc Interv Radiol* 2003;**14**:S263.

71. Lee CW, Kaufman JA, Fan C-M, et al. Clinical outcome of internal iliac artery occlusions during endovascular treatment of aorto-iliac aneurysmal disease. *J Vasc Interv Radiol* 2000;**11**:567.

72. Razavi MK, DeGroot M, Olcott C, et al. Internal iliac artery embolization in the stent graft treatment of aortoiliac aneurysms: analysis of outcomes and complications. *J Vasc Interv Radiol* 2000;**11**:561.

73. Soulen MC, Fairman RM, Baum RA. Embolization of the internal iliac artery: still more to learn. *J Vasc Interv Radiol* 2000;**11**:543.

74. Engelke C, Elford J, Morgan RA, et al. Internal iliac artery embolization with bilateral occlusion before endovascular aortoiliac aneurysm repair—clinical outcome of simultaneous and sequential intervention. *J Vasc Interv Radiol* 2002;**13**:667.

75. Rosen RJ, Green RM. Endoleak management following endovascular aneurysm repair. *J Vasc Interv Radiol* 2008;**19**:S37.

76. Jonker FHW, Aruny J, Muhs BE. Management of type II endoleaks: preoperative versus postoperative versus expectant management. *Semin Vasc Surg* 2009;**22**:165.

77. Heye S, Nevelsteen A, Maleux G. Internal iliac artery coil embolization in the prevention of potential type 2 endoleak after endovascular repair of abdominal aortoiliac and iliac artery aneurysms: effect of total occlusion versus residual flow. *J Vasc Interv Radiol* 2005;**16**:235.

78. Tan JWC, Yeo KK, Laird JR. Food and Drug Administration approved endovascular repair devices for abdominal aortic aneurysms: a review. *J Vasc Interv Radiol* 2007;**19**:S9.

79. Chuter TAM. Durability of endovascular infrarenal aneurysm repair: when does late failure occur and why? *Semin Vasc Surg* 2009;**22**:102.

80. Greenberg RK, Sternbergh III WC, Makaroun M, et al. Intermediate results of a United States multicenter trial of fenestrated endograft repair for juxtarenal abdominal aortic aneurysms. *J Vasc Surg* 2009;**50**:730.

81. Diehm N, Baum S, Benenati JF. Fenestrated and branched endografts: why we need them now. *J Vasc Interv Radiol* 2009;**19**:S63.

82. Zarins CK, AneuRx Clinical Investigators. The US AneuRx Clinical Trial: 6-year clinical update 2002. *J Vasc Surg* 2003;**37**:904.

83. Turnbull IC, Criado FJ, Sanchez L, et al. Five-year results for the Talent enhanced Low Profile System abdominal stent graft pivotal trial including early and long-term safety and efficacy. *J Vasc Surg* 2010;**51**:537.

84. Greenberg RK, Chuter TA, Sternbergh III WC, et al. Zenith AAA endovascular graft: intermediate-term results of the US multicenter trial. *J Vasc Surg* 2004;**39**:1209.

85. Kibbe MR, Matsumura JS. Excluder Investigators: The Gore Excluder US multi-center trial: analysis of adverse events at 2 years. *Semin Vasc Surg* 2003;**16**:144.

86. Criado FJ, Fairman RM, Becker GJ, et al. Talent LPS AAA stent graft: results of a pivotal clinical trial. *J Vasc Surg* 2003;**37**:709.

87. Prinssen M, Verhoeven EL, Buth J, et al. A randomized trial comparing conventional and endovascular repair of abdominal aortic aneurysms. *N Engl J Med* 2004;**351**:1607.

88. Schermerhorn ML, O'Malley AJ, Jhaveri A, et al. Endovascular vs. open repair of abdominal aortic aneurysms in the Medicare population. *N Engl J Med* 2008;**358**:464.

89. EVAR Trial Participants. Endovascular aneurysm repair versus open repair in patients with abdominal aortic aneurysm (EVAR trial 1): randomized, controlled trial. *Lancet* 2005;**365**:2179.

90. Matsumoto AH. What randomized controlled trials tell us about endovascular repair of abdominal aortic aneurysms. *J Vasc Interv Radiol* 2007;**19**:S18.

91. Brooks MJ, Brown LC, Greenhalgh RM. Defining the role of endovascular therapy in the treatment of abdominal aortic aneurysm: results of a prospective randomized trial. *Adv Surg* 2006;**44**:229.

92. The United Kingdom EVAR Trial Investigators. Endovascular versus open repair of abdominal aortic aneurysms. *N Engl J Med* 2010;**362**:1863.

93. deBruin JL, Baas AF, Buth J, et al. Long-term outcome of open or endovascular repair of abdominal aortic aneurysm. *N Engl J Med* 2010;**362**:1881.

94. Lederle FA, Freischlag JA, Kyriakides TC, et al. Outcomes following endovascular vs. open repair of abdominal aortic aneurysm: a randomized trial. *JAMA* 2009;**302**:1535.

95. Dillon M, Cardwell C, Blair PH, et al. Endovascular treatment of ruptured abdominal aortic aneurysm. *Cochrane Database Syst Rev* 2007:CD005261.

96. Ricotta II JJ, Malgor RD, Oderich GS. Ruptured endovascular abdominal aortic aneurysm repair: part II. *Ann Vasc Surg* 2010;**24**:269.

97. Monge M, Eskandari MK. Strategies for ruptured abdominal aortic aneurysms. *J Vasc Interv Radiol* 2007;**19**:S44.

98. Erzurum VZ, Sampram ES, Sarac TP, et al. Initial management and outcome of aortic endograft limb occlusion. *J Vasc Surg* 2004;**40**:419.

99. Kranokpiraksa P, Kaufman JA. Follow-up of endovascular aneurysm repair: plain radiography, ultrasound, CT/CT angiography, MR imaging/MR angiography, or what? *J Vasc Interv Radiol* 2008;**19**:S27.

100. Manning BJ, O'Neill SM, Haider SN, et al. Duplex ultrasound in aneurysm surveillance following endovascular aneurysm repair: a comparison with computed tomography aortography. *J Vasc Surg* 2009;**49**:60.

101. Stavropoulos SW, Baum RA. Imaging modalities for the detection and management of endoleaks. *Semin Vasc Surg* 2004;**17**:154.

102. Bashir MR, Ferral H, Jacobs C, et al. Endoleaks after endovascular abdominal aortic aneurysm repair: management strategies according to CT findings. *AJR Am J Roentgenol* 2009;**192**:W178.

103. Veith FJ, Baum RA, Ohki T, et al. Nature and significance of endoleaks and endotension: summary of opinions expressed at an international conference. *J Vasc Surg* 2002;**35**:1029.

104. Baum RA, Stavropoulos SW, Fairman RM, et al. Endoleaks after endovascular repair of abdominal aortic aneurysms. *J Vasc Interv Radiol* 2003;**14**(Pt. 1):1111.

105. Faries PL, Cadot H, Agarwal G, et al. Management of endoleak after endovascular aneurysm repair: cuffs, coils, and conversion. *J Vasc Surg* 2003;**37**:1155.

106. Jones JE, Atkins MD, Brewster DC, et al. Persistent type 2 endoleak after endovascular repair of abdominal aortic aneurysms is associated with late adverse outcomes. *J Vasc Surg* 2007;**46**:1.

107. Bernhard VM, Mitchell RS, Matsumura JS, et al. Ruptured abdominal aortic aneurysm after endovascular repair. *J Vasc Surg* 2002;**35**:1155.

108. Silverberg D, Baril DT, Ellozy S, et al. An 8-year experience with type II endoleaks: natural history suggest selective intervention is a safe approach. *J Vasc Surg* 2006;**44**:453.

109. Baum RA, Carpenter JP, Stavropoulos SW, et al. Treatment of type 2 endoleaks after endovascular repair of abdominal aortic aneurysms: comparison of transarterial and translumbar techniques. *J Vasc Surg* 2002;**35**:23.

110. Bush RL, Lin PH, Ronson RS, et al. Colonic necrosis subsequent to catheter-directed thrombin embolization of the inferior mesenteric artery via the superior mesenteric artery: a complication in the management of a type II endoleak. *J Vasc Surg* 2001;**34**:1119.

111. Bertges DJ, Villella ER, Makaroun MS. Aortoenteric fistula due to endoleak coil embolization after endovascular AAA repair. *J Endovasc Ther* 2003;**10**:130.

112. Baum RA, Cope C, Fairman RM, et al. Translumbar embolization of type 2 endoleaks after endovascular repair of abdominal aortic aneurysms. *J Vasc Interv Radiol* 2001;**12**:111.

113. Gorlitzer M, Mertikian G, Trnka H, et al. Translumbar treatment of type II endoleaks after endovascular repair of abdominal aortic aneurysm. *Interact Cardiovasc Thorac Surg* 2008;**7**:781.

114. Binkert CA, Alencar H, Singh J, et al. Translumbar type II endoleak repair using angiographic CT. *J Vasc Interv Radiol* 2006;**17**:1349.

115. Stavropoulos SW, Carpenter JP, Fairman RM, et al. Inferior vena cava traversal for translumbar endoleak embolization after endovascular abdominal aortic aneurysm repair. *J Vasc Interv Radiol* 2003;**14**:1191.

116. Gambaro E, Abou-Zamzam AM, Teruya TH, et al. Ischemic colitis following translumbar thrombin injection for treatment of endoleak. *Ann Vasc Surg* 2004;**18**:74.

117. Schwartz LB, Baldwin ZK, Curi MA. The changing face of abdominal aortic aneurysm management. *Ann Surg* 2003;**238**:S56.

118. Leriche R, Morel A. The syndrome of thrombotic obliteration of the aortic bifurcation. *Ann Surg* 1948;**127**:193.

119. Hirose H, Takagi M, Hashiyada H, et al. Acute occlusion of an abdominal aortic aneurysm—case report and review of the literature. *Angiology* 2000;**51**:515.

120. Tapper SS, Jenkins JM, Edwards WH, et al. Juxtarenal aortic occlusion. *Ann Surg* 1992;**215**:443.

121. Dossa CD, Shepard AD, Reddy DJ, et al. Acute aortic occlusion: a 40-year experience. *Arch Surg* 1994;**129**:603.

122. Patel H, Krishnamoorthy M, Dorazio RA, et al. Thrombosis of abdominal aortic aneurysms. *Am Surgeon* 1994;**60**:801.

123. Klonaris C, Katsargyris A, Tsekouras N, et al. Primary stenting for aortic lesions: from single stenoses to total aortoiliac occlusions. *J Vasc Surg* 2008;**47**:310.

124. Krankenberg H, Schlueter M, Schwencke C, et al. Endovascular reconstruction of the aortic bifurcation in patients with Leriche syndrome. *Clin Res Cardiol* 2009;**98**:657.

125. Moise MA, Alvarez-Tostado JA, Clair DG, et al. Endovascular management of chronic infrarenal aortic occlusion. *J Endovasc Ther* 2009;**16**:84.

126. Farber A, Wagner WH, Cossman DV, et al. Isolated dissection of the abdominal aorta: clinical presentation and therapeutic options. *J Vasc Surg* 2002;**36**:205.

127. Jonker FH, Schloesser FJ, Moll FL, et al. Dissection of the abdominal aorta. Current evidence and implications for treatment strategies: a review and meta-analysis of 92 patients. *J Endovasc Ther* 2009;**16**:71.

128. Trimarchi S, Tsai T, Eagle KA, et al. Acute abdominal aortic dissection: insight from the International Registry of Acute Aortic Dissection (IRAD). *J Vasc Surg* 2007;**46**:913.

129. Rasmussen TE, Hallett Jr JW. Inflammatory aortic aneurysms. A clinical review with new perspectives in pathogenesis. *Ann Surg* 1997;**225**:155.

130. Vaglio A, Corradi D, Manenti L, et al. Evidence of autoimmunity in chronic periaortitis: a prospective study. *Am J Med* 2003;**114**:454.

131. Haug ES, Skomsvoll JF, Jacobsen G, et al. Inflammatory aortic aneurysm is associated with increased incidence of autoimmune disease. *J Vasc Surg* 2003;**38**:492.

132. Leseche G, Schaetz A, Arrive L, et al. Diagnosis and management of 17 consecutive patients with inflammatory abdominal aortic aneurysm. *Am J Surg* 1992;**164**:39.

133. Di Marzo L, Sapienza P, Bernucci P, et al. Inflammatory aneurysm of the abdominal aorta. A prospective clinical study. *J Cardiovasc Surg (Torino)* 1999;**40**:407.

134. Iino M, Kuribayashi S, Imakita S, et al. Sensitivity and specificity of CT in the diagnosis of inflammatory abdominal aortic aneurysms. *J Comput Assist Tomogr* 2002;**26**:1006.

135. Wallis F, Roditi GH, Redpath TW, et al. Inflammatory abdominal aortic aneurysms: diagnosis with gadolinium enhanced T1-weighted imaging. *Clin Radiol* 2000;**55**:136.

136. Paravastu SC, Ghosh J, Murray D, et al. A systematic review of open versus endovascular repair of inflammatory abdominal aortic aneurysms. *Eur J Vasc Endovasc Surg* 2009;**38**:291.

137. Soerelius K, Mani K, Bjorck M, et al. Endovascular repair of mycotic aortic aneurysms. *J Vasc Surg* 2009;**50**:269.

138. Muller BT, Wegener OR, Grabitz K, et al. Mycotic aneurysms of the thoracic and abdominal aorta and iliac arteries: experience with anatomic and extra-anatomic repair in 33 cases. *J Vasc Surg* 2001;**33**:106.

139. Chan FY, Crawford ES, Coselli JS, et al. In situ prosthetic graft replacement for mycotic aneurysm of the aorta. *Ann Thorac Surg* 1989;**47**:193.

140. Canaud L, Marzelle J, Bassinet L, et al. Tuberculous aneurysms of the abdominal aorta. *J Vasc Surg* 2008;**48**:1012.

141. Macedo TA, Stanson AW, Oderich GS, et al. Infected aortic aneurysms: imaging findings. *Radiology* 2004;**231**:250.

142. Muller BT, Wegener OR, Grabitz K, et al. Mycotic aneurysms of the thoracic and abdominal aorta and iliac arteries: experience with anatomic and extra-anatomic repair in 33 cases. *J Vasc Surg* 2001;**33**:106.

143. Woon CY, Sebastian MG, Tay KH, et al. Extra-anatomic revascularization and aortic exclusion for mycotic aneurysms of the infrarenal aorta and iliac arteries in an Asian population. *Am J Surg* 2008;**195**:66.

144. Fillmore AJ, Valentine RJ. Surgical mortality in patients with infected aortic aneurysms. *J Am Coll Surg* 2003;**196**:435.

145. Tiesenhausen K, Hessinger M, Tomka M, et al. Endovascular treatment of mycotic aortic pseudoaneurysms with stent-grafts. *Cardiovasc Intervent Radiol* 2008;**31**:509.

146. Kan CD, Lee HL, Yang YJ. Outcome after endovascular stent graft treatment for mycotic aortic aneurysms: a systematic review. *J Vasc Surg* 2007;**46**:906.

147. Razavi MK, Razavi MD. Stent-graft treatment of mycotic aneurysms: a review of the current literature. *J Vasc Interv Radiol* 2008;**19**:S51.

148. Chao CP, Walker TG, Kalva SP. Natural history and CT appearances of aortic intramural hematoma. *Radiographics* 2009;**29**:791.

149. Yeh MW, Horn JK, Schecter WP, et al. Endovascular repair of an actively hemorrhaging gunshot wound to the abdominal aorta. *J Vasc Surg* 2005;**42**:1007.

150. Demetriades D, Theodorou D, Murray J, et al. Mortality and prognostic factors in penetrating injuries of the aorta. *J Trauma* 1996;**40**:761.

151. Michaels AJ, Gerndt SJ, Taheri PA, et al. Blunt force injury of the abdominal aorta. *J Trauma* 1996;**41**:105.

152. Nucifora G, Hysko F, Vasciaveo A. Blunt traumatic abdominal aortic rupture: CT imaging. *Emerg Radiol* 2008;**15**:211.

153. Aladham F, Sundaram B, Williams DM, et al. Traumatic aortic injury: computerized tomographic findings at presentation and after conservative therapy. *J Comput Assist Tomogr* 2010;**34**:388.

154. Davidovic LB, Kostic DM, Cvetkovic SD, et al. Aorto-caval fistulas. *Cardiovasc Surg* 2002;**10**:555.

155. Berthet JP, Marty-Ane CH, Veerapen R, et al. Dissection of the abdominal aorta in blunt trauma: endovascular or conventional surgical management? *J Vasc Surg* 2003;**38**:997.

156. Gunn M, Campbell M, Hoffer EK. Traumatic abdominal aortic injury treated by endovascular stent placement. *Emerg Radiol* 2007;**13**:329.

157. Hussain Q, Maleux G, Heye S, et al. Endovascular repair of an actively hemorrhaging stab wound injury to the abdominal aorta. *Cardiovasc Intervent Radiol* 2008;**31**:1023.

158. Khandelwal N, Kalra N, Gard MK, et al. Multidetector CT angiography in Takayasu arteritis. *Eur J Radiol* 2009;Aug [Epub ahead of print].

159. Choe YH, Han B-K, Koh E-M, et al. Takayasu's arteritis: assessment of disease activity with contrast-enhanced MR imaging. *AJR Am J Roentgenol* 2000;**175**:505.

160. Maksimowicz-McKinnon K, Clark TM, Hoffman GS. Limitations of therapy and a guarded prognosis in an American cohort of Takayasu arteritis patients. *Arthritis Rheum* 2007;**56**:1000.

161. Chuang VP. Radiation-induced arteritis. *Semin Roentgenol* 1994;**29**:64.

162. Israel G, Krinsky G, Lee V. The "skinny aorta." *Clin Imaging* 2002;**26**:116.

163. Luehr M, Siepe M, Beyersdorf F, et al. Extra-anatomic bypass for recurrent abdominal aortic and renal in-stent stenoses following radiotherapy for neuroblastoma. *Interact Cardiovasc Thorac Surg* 2009;**8**:488.

164. Chetty R, Batitang S, Nair R. Large artery vasculopathy in HIV-positive patients: another vasculitic enigma. *Hum Pathol* 2000;**31**:374.

165. Criado E, Izquierdo L, Lujan S, et al. Abdominal aortic coarctation, renovascular, hypertension, and neurofibromatosis. *Ann Vasc Surg* 2002;**16**:363.

166. Stanley JC, Criado E, Eliason JL, et al. Abdominal aortic coarctation: surgical treatment of 53 patients with a thoracoabdominal bypass, patch aortoplasty, or interposition aortoaortic graft. *J Vasc Surg* 2008;**48**:1073.

167. Connolly JE, Wilson SE, Lawrence PL, et al. Middle aortic syndrome: distal thoracic and abdominal coarctation, a disorder with multiple etiologies. *J Am Coll Surg* 2002;**194**:774.

168. Flynn PM, Robinson MB, Stapleton FB, et al. Coarctation of the aorta and renal artery stenosis in tuberous sclerosis. *Pediatric Radiol* 1984;**14**:337.

169. Delis KT, Gloviczki P. Middle aortic syndrome: from presentation to contemporary open surgical and endovascular treatment. *Perspect Vasc Surg Endovasc Ther* 2005;**17**:187.

170. Stanley JC, Criado E, Upchurch Jr GR, et al. Pediatric renovascular hypertension: 132 primary and 30 secondary operations in 97 children. *J Vasc Surg* 2006;**44**:1219.

171. Siwik ES, Perry SB, Lock JE. Endovascular stent implantation in patients with stenotic aortoarteriopathies: early and medium-term results. *Catheter Cardiovasc Interv* 2003;**59**:380.

172. Forbes TJ, Garekar S, Amin Z, et al. Procedural results and acute complications in stenting native and recurrent coarctation of the aorta in patients over 4 years of age. A multi-institutional study. *Catheter Cardiovasc Interv* 2007;**70**:276.

173. Brzezinska-Rajszys G, Qureshi SA, Ksiazyk J, et al. Middle aortic syndrome treated by stent implantation. *Heart* 1999;**81**:166.

Pelvic and Lower Extremity Arteries

Karim Valji

ARTERIOGRAPHY

Pelvic arteriography is performed with common femoral artery access using a pigtail or similarly shaped catheter placed at the aortic bifurcation. Even with diminished or absent femoral pulses, catheterization is sometimes possible using real-time ultrasound guidance and a steerable hydrophilic guidewire. A retrograde brachial artery puncture is made when femoral access is not possible. Some interventionalists prefer the brachial route in patients who have suffered cholesterol embolization during prior retrograde femoral artery catheterization procedures.

When an iliac artery is occluded, multiple ipsilateral lumbar arteries can serve as major collaterals into the pelvis; in this situation, the catheter side holes are positioned slightly below the renal arteries to opacify these vessels. In patients with peripheral arterial disease, bilateral, 25- to 30-degree oblique pelvic arteriograms often are needed to thoroughly assess iliac artery disease and to lay out the iliac and femoral artery bifurcations. The left posterior oblique projection opens the left iliac and right femoral bifurcations; the right posterior oblique projection opens the opposite bifurcations.

Bilateral lower extremity arteriography ("run-off" study) is done with the pigtail just above the aortic bifurcation. Serial images are obtained down to the feet. If only one leg needs to be examined, it is usual practice to catheterize the contralateral groin and direct a cobra or similarly shaped catheter over the aortic bifurcation (see Chapter 3). If a pigtail catheter is already in place, it can be gently unwound on the bifurcation and replaced with a straight catheter (see Fig. 3-16). A long, reverse-curve catheter simplifies entry into internal iliac artery branches (see Fig. 3-15).

When the tibial or pedal arteries are poorly visualized on the initial angiogram, they often are better seen by advancing a catheter into the common or superficial femoral artery and first injecting an intraarterial vasodilator (e.g., 100 to 200 μg of nitroglycerin). In patients with a history of severe contrast allergy or renal insufficiency, alternative noninvasive imaging should be attempted. If catheter angiography is required before treatment, carbon dioxide can be used exclusively or supplemented with small volumes of iodinated contrast[1-4] (see Chapter 3).

ANATOMY

Development

In the embryo, the lower extremities are supplied by the axial artery, which arises from the sciatic branch of the internal iliac artery.[5] This vessel ends in a plantar network in the developing foot. The femoral artery, which runs along the ventral aspect of the limb, is the continuation of the external iliac artery; it joins the axial artery at the knee to form the popliteal artery. The posterior tibial and peroneal arteries originate from the axial artery below the knee and run along the dorsal aspect of the calf. The anterior tibial artery takes off from the lower popliteal artery and courses along the ventral aspect of the calf. The superficial femoral artery eventually becomes the dominant vessel to the lower leg. The deep femoral artery arises near the bottom of the femoral head. Most of the axial artery regresses before birth; normally, the only remnants are portions of the inferior gluteal, popliteal, and peroneal arteries.

Normal Anatomy

The abdominal aorta divides into the common iliac arteries at the L4-L5 level[6] (Figs. 8-1A and 8-2). The *common iliac arteries* lie in front of the iliac veins and the inferior vena cava. They usually have no major branches; rarely, they give off aberrant iliolumbar or accessory renal arteries. The common iliac artery divides near the lumbosacral junction. The *external iliac artery* continues directly to the groin behind the inguinal ligament. This vessel also has no major branches. The *internal iliac artery* takes off medially and posteriorly. At the superior edge of the greater sciatic foramen, it usually divides into anterior and posterior trunks. The branching pattern of

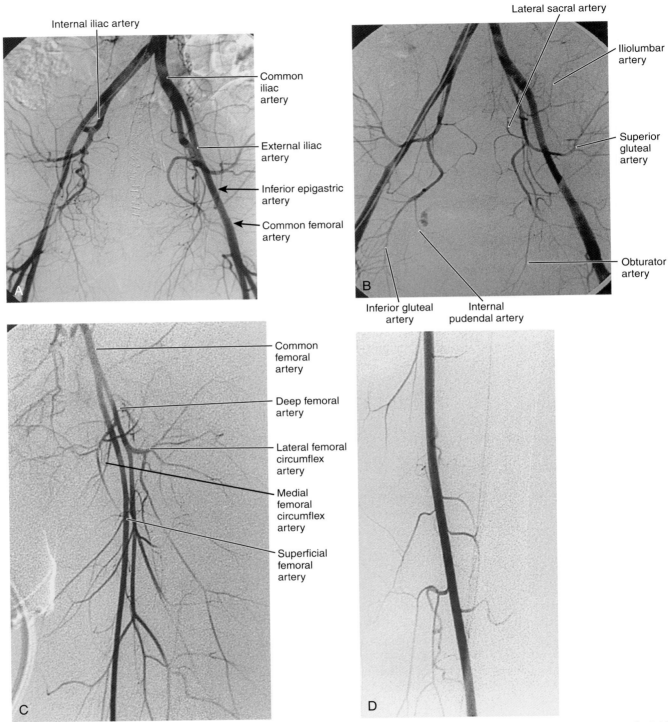

FIGURE 8-1   Normal pelvic and left lower extremity arteriograms. **A,** The abdominal aorta divides into the common iliac arteries at the L4-L5 level. **B,** The branching pattern of the internal iliac artery varies. **C,** The common femoral artery divides into the superficial femoral artery (SFA) and deep femoral artery near the bottom of the femoral head. **D,** The SFA passes down the anteromedial aspect of the thigh, dives into the flexor muscle compartment, and runs through the adductor (Hunter) canal.

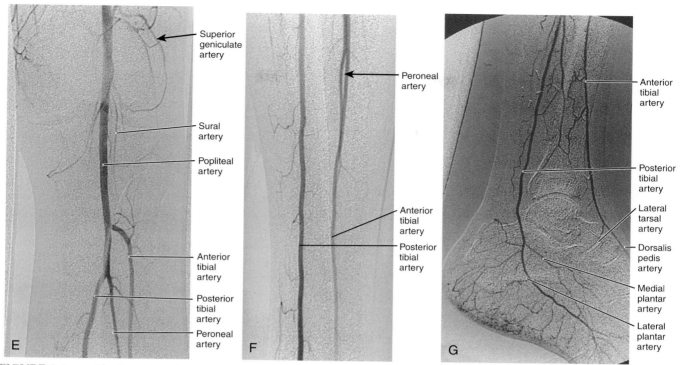

FIGURE 8-1, cont'd   **E** and **F,** At the distal border of the popliteus muscle, the popliteal artery divides. **G,** The dorsalis pedis artery gives off medial and lateral tarsal branches. The posterior tibial artery gives off medial and lateral plantar branches.

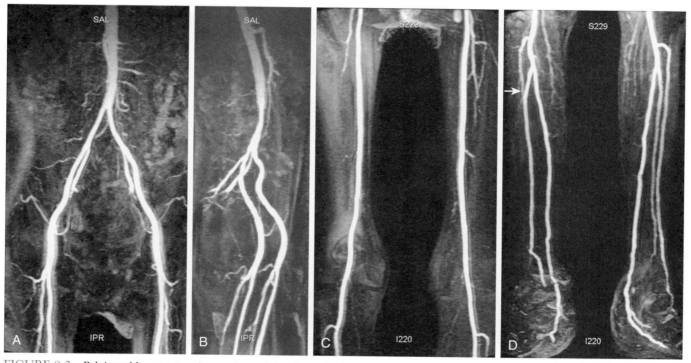

FIGURE 8-2   Pelvic and lower extremity maximum intensity projection magnetic resonance angiogram. Pelvis in frontal **(A)** and near lateral **(B)** views. Thigh **(C)** and calf **(D)** in frontal view. The right anterior tibial artery is occluded in the upper calf *(arrow).*

the internal iliac artery is quite variable (see Fig. 8-1B). Classically, the major branches of the *anterior* division are as follows:

- Obturator artery
- Internal pudendal artery, which supplies the external genitalia and rectum (see Fig. 13-11)
- Inferior gluteal artery, which nourishes muscles of the thigh and buttocks and the sciatic nerve
- Visceral arteries, which supply the bladder, rectum, and uterus or prostate through the superior and inferior vesicular, middle rectal, and uterine or prostatic arteries, respectively (see Fig. 13-16). They may be hard to identify on a routine pelvic arteriogram.

The major branches of the *posterior* division of the internal iliac artery are:

- Iliolumbar artery, which takes off laterally to supply the lumbar muscles
- Lateral sacral artery, which takes off medially toward the sacral foramina
- Superior gluteal artery, which is the largest branch of the division and feeds the gluteal muscles

At the junction of the external iliac and common femoral arteries (which corresponds to the inguinal ligament), the *inferior epigastric artery* exits medially (see Fig. 3-1). It runs alongside the rectus abdominis muscle before communicating with the superior epigastric branch of the internal thoracic (mammary) artery. The *deep iliac circumflex artery* takes off laterally and superiorly (see Fig. 3-5).

The *common femoral artery (CFA)* courses over the femoral head encased in the femoral sheath along with the femoral vein (medial or posteromedial) and the femoral nerve (lateral). Branches of the CFA include the superficial epigastric artery, superficial circumflex iliac artery (laterally), and external pudendal artery (medially); all of these are inconsistently seen at angiography. The CFA divides into the *superficial femoral artery (SFA)* and *deep femoral artery (DFA)* or *profunda femoris artery (PFA)* near the bottom of the femoral head (see Fig. 8-1C). A "high" bifurcation is occasionally seen. The DFA takes off laterally and posteriorly. Its major branches are the lateral femoral circumflex, medial femoral circumflex, and four or so pairs of perforating arteries.

The SFA passes down the anteromedial aspect of the thigh, dives into the flexor muscle compartment, and runs through the adductor (Hunter) canal (see Fig. 8-1D). The SFA then becomes the *popliteal artery*, which is posterior to the femur (surrounded by the heads of the gastrocnemius muscle) and deep to the popliteal vein. Its major muscular branches are the sural arteries and paired superior, middle, and inferior geniculate arteries, all of which form an anastomotic network around the knee.

At the distal border of the popliteus muscle, the popliteal artery divides.[7] The *anterior tibial artery* arises laterally, pierces the interosseous membrane, and then runs in front of the lower tibia (see Fig. 8-1E and F). It passes over the ankle onto the dorsum of the foot to become the *dorsalis pedis artery*. The *tibioperoneal trunk* is the direct continuation of the popliteal artery and bifurcates just beyond its origin into the posterior tibial and peroneal arteries. The *posterior tibial artery* runs posteriorly and medially in the flexor compartment. The *peroneal artery* runs between the posterior and anterior tibial arteries near the fibula. It is a small-caliber vessel unless functioning as a collateral in the face of tibial artery obstruction. In the distal calf, its perforating and communicating branches may join the anterior and posterior tibial arteries, respectively. Above the ankle, the artery divides into two calcaneal branches ("fish tail") that have anastomoses with the distal tibial arteries.

A network of malleolar arteries interconnect the tibial arteries above the ankle.[7] The dorsalis pedis artery gives off medial and lateral tarsal branches (see Fig. 8-1G). The posterior tibial artery passes behind the medial malleolus, where it divides into medial and lateral plantar arteries. The *plantar arch* is formed by the dominant lateral plantar branch of the posterior tibial artery and the distal dorsalis pedis artery. Smaller secondary arches are created by other branches of the distal tibial arteries. Metatarsal arteries arise primarily from the plantar arch.

Variant Anatomy (Online Case 102)

The most common variations in branching of the internal iliac artery involve anomalous origin of a named artery (e.g., obturator, inferior gluteal, or superior gluteal) from another major branch of either division.

The *persistent sciatic artery* is a rare anomaly (about 0.1% of the population) in which the embryologic sciatic artery remains the dominant inflow vessel to the leg.[8,9] The aberrant vessel arises from the internal iliac artery, passes through the greater sciatic foramen, and lies deep to the gluteus maximus muscle (Fig. 8-3). Above the knee, it joins the popliteal artery. The SFA is hypoplastic or absent. The anomaly is occasionally bilateral. Because of its relatively superficial position in the ischial region, the sciatic artery is prone to intimal injury or aneurysm formation.

Very rare femoral artery variants include the *saphenous artery* and *duplication of the SFA*.[10] Anomalies of the DFA are common, including a posterior or even medial origin of the main DFA trunk and separate origins of the medial and lateral circumflex femoral branches.

Tibial artery anomalies are present in about 3% to 10% of the population.[11-13] The variants often are bilateral. The

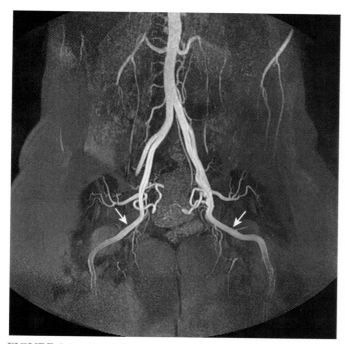

FIGURE 8-3   Bilateral persistent sciatic arteries. Maximum intensity projection MR angiogram shows a large vessel arising from each internal iliac artery (arrows) passing laterally over the femoral heads and running down the legs lateral to the expected position of the femoral arteries.

most frequent are "high" bifurcation or true trifurcation of the popliteal artery, common origin of the anterior tibial and peroneal arteries, and hypoplasia or absence of the anterior or posterior tibial artery (Fig. 8-4). In the latter case, the affected vessel is normal at its origin but gradually tapers in the mid to distal calf without discrete termination. A major branch of the peroneal artery often reforms the absent vessel above the ankle, resulting in normal pedal pulses.

Collateral Circulation

The pelvis and lower extremities have rich and complex systems of collateral circulation that maintain blood flow to the leg when proximal arteries are obstructed. The major routes are formed by branches of the internal iliac, deep femoral, and popliteal arteries (Fig. 8-5 and see Fig. 7-5):

- Common iliac artery obstruction: ipsilateral lumbar or contralateral lateral sacral branches to the deep iliac circumflex or the internal iliac artery (allowing retrograde or antegrade flow, respectively, into the external iliac artery)
- Internal iliac artery obstruction: inferior mesenteric artery to the inferior gluteal branches through the rectal network, lumbar to the

iliolumbar arteries, DFA to the gluteal arteries through femoral circumflex branches
- External iliac artery obstruction: posterior division of the internal iliac artery branches to the CFA through the deep iliac circumflex artery, anterior division of the internal iliac artery branches to circumflex femoral branches of DFA, transpelvic collaterals
- SFA obstruction: collaterals depend on the site and length of the obstruction; the DFA becomes the dominant route to the lower leg, with lateral femoral circumflex and perforating vessels supplying branches of the distal SFA and popliteal arteries
- DFA obstruction: internal iliac artery branches to medial and lateral circumflex femoral branches of the DFA
- Popliteal artery obstruction: geniculate and sural collateral networks
- Tibial artery obstruction: the peroneal artery is the principal collateral channel with anterior or posterior tibial artery obstruction

MAJOR DISORDERS

Chronic Peripheral Arterial Disease (Online Case 2)

Etiology

Obstructive disease of the pelvic and lower extremity arteries is one of the most frequent clinical problems encountered by interventionalists. In the United States, the overall prevalence is 3% to 10% of the general population; up to 20% of individuals older than age 70 suffer from this disorder.[14,15] The cardinal feature is diminished blood flow to the pelvis or legs with exercise or at rest.

Peripheral arterial disease (PAD) encompasses the following three clinical scenarios:

- Asymptomatic obstructive disease
- Intermittent claudication
- Chronic limb ischemia (CLI)

There are a variety of causes for lower extremity PAD (Box 8-1). However, the vast majority of cases result from atherosclerotic stenoses, superimposed thrombosis, or embolism. By a wide margin, atherosclerosis is the most common disease affecting the lower extremity arteries. Most of the established risk factors are well known[14,16] (Box 8-2). The pathophysiology of atherosclerosis and the emerging significance of certain inflammatory markers (e.g., C-reactive protein) in progression of disease and response to treatment are discussed in Chapter 1. In certain situations, the interventionalist should keep in mind the less common causes of PAD (Box 8-3).

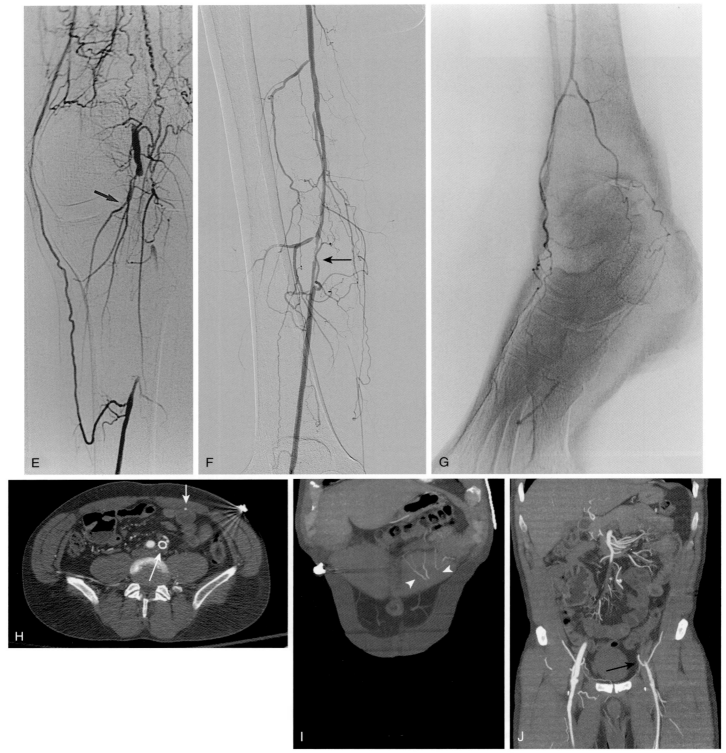

FIGURE 8-5, cont'd   **E,** Left femoropopliteal and proximal tibial artery occlusions. Deep femoral branches reconstitute a short segment of the midpopliteal artery, which supplies sural collaterals *(arrow)* into the calf. The posterior tibial artery is reconstituted in the midcalf. **F,** Critical stenosis of distal right superficial femoral artery *(arrow)* with multiple collateral channels. **G,** Posterior and anterior tibial artery occlusion, with the peroneal artery reconstituting the distal vessels in the foot. **H through J,** Thrombosis of left limb *(long white arrow)* of aortobifemoral bypass graft on axial and reformatted coronal contrast enhanced computed tomography images. The left leg is partially fed through superficial epigastric branches *(arrowheads)* of the distal left internal thoracic (mammary) artery. These vessels communicate with branches of the inferior epigastric artery *(black arrow)* which then fill the left common femoral artery.

BOX 8-1

CAUSES OF LOWER EXTREMITY PERIPHERAL ARTERIAL DISEASE

- Atherosclerosis
  - Thrombotic occlusion of underlying stenosis
- Embolism
  - Thromboembolism
  - Microembolization
- Trauma
  - Catheterization
- Aneurysm
  - Thrombosis (e.g., popliteal artery)
  - Distal embolization
- Neointimal hyperplasia
- Dissection
- Vasculitis
  - Buerger disease
  - HIV arteriopathy
  - Radiation therapy
  - Collagen vascular diseases
- Extrinsic compression
- Vasospastic drugs (e.g., vasopressin, ergots, methysergide)
- Raynaud disease
- Popliteal artery disorders
  - Popliteal artery entrapment
  - Cystic adventitial disease
- Fibromuscular dysplasia
- Iliac artery endofibrosis

BOX 8-2

RISK FACTORS FOR PERIPHERAL ARTERIAL DISEASE

- Diabetes
  - Insulin resistance without diabetes
- Smoking
- Hypertension
- Dyslipidemia (especially elevated total/high density lipoprotein cholesterol)
- Thrombophilic states (see Boxes 1-4 and 1-5)
- Age
- Non-white race

BOX 8-3

CLUES TO UNUSUAL CAUSES FOR PERIPHERAL ARTERIAL DISEASE

- Age <40 years
- No risk factors for atherosclerosis or thromboembolism
- Isolated, unilateral disease
- Disease at unusual sites (e.g., common femoral artery)

Atherosclerosis is a systemic disease. As such, it is typically diffuse and bilateral. However, there is a clear predilection for clinically significant disease in the distal aorta, common and external iliac arteries, distal SFA, and tibial arteries. The propensity for obstructions in the distal SFA as it passes through the adductor canal is related to turbulent flow and altered wall shear stress. These hemodynamic disturbances result from changes in curvature and tortuosity of this mobile vessel along with compression on the vessel by the adductor magnus muscle and fascia at the adductor canal.[17,18] Atherosclerotic plaques cause symptoms by impeding blood flow to the leg, inducing thrombotic occlusion, or through embolization of clot or plaque fragments. In CLI, obstructions are accompanied by abnormalities of skin microcirculation that further exacerbate ischemia.

Diabetes is a strong risk factor for PAD. Extensive tibial and pedal artery disease is characteristic; the aortoiliac and femoropopliteal segments are relatively spared. Medial calcification is distinctive of diabetic arterial disease and chronic end-stage renal disease. Arterial obstructions tend to be more severe than in patients with atherosclerosis, and the collateral circulation often is less effective. For these reasons, nonhealing ulcers, gangrene, and amputation are much more common in this population.

Macroemboli usually are thrombi that originate from the heart. Less often, clot or plaque fragments break off from aneurysms or atherosclerotic surfaces in the proximal arteries. Emboli usually lodge at branch points or sites of underlying disease. *Microemboli* are composed of platelet-fibrin deposits or cholesterol crystals arising from atherosclerotic plaques or aneurysms. These particles may be released spontaneously or during operative manipulation or catheterization. Microemboli can lead to *blue toe syndrome* or an *acute cholesterol embolization* event (see Chapter 1).

Clinical Features

By definition, the diagnosis of *chronic* PAD requires symptoms lasting more than 2 weeks. The severity of PAD often is graded according to the scale of Rutherford and Becker[19] (Table 8-1). At least 50% of patients with PAD are asymptomatic or have atypical symptoms; in some cases, limited physical activity prevents the onset of leg pain. Only 10% or so will ultimately develop CLI.[14] Chronic PAD is unusual before age 40. Men are affected more frequently than women, as are nonwhite individuals.[14] Most patients have one or more risk factors for disease (see Box 8-2). These patients usually suffer from associated coronary artery disease, cerebrovascular disease, or chronic renal insufficiency. PAD is an important marker of these conditions.

Intermittent claudication (IC) is the first symptom in some patients. IC is characterized by predictable and reproducible calf, thigh, or buttock muscle pain or fatigue with exercise (especially walking on an incline) that is invariably relieved by rest. The pain does not resolve with continued leg exercise. It rarely occurs in the foot. Unfortunately, a variety of unrelated conditions are often confused with true claudication, including spinal stenosis, nerve root compression, arthritis, chronic compartment syndrome, and venous claudication.[14,20] Still, a careful history will usually distinguish among these entities. In a minority of afflicted patients, the collateral circulation eventually becomes insufficient to prevent muscle ischemia at rest despite maximum peripheral vasodilation. *Chronic limb ischemia* is present when symptoms of rest pain or ischemic skin changes are combined with an ankle-brachial index less than 0.50 (see later discussion).

Rest pain is usually localized to the (distal) foot, is made worse with leg elevation (while sleeping), and is relieved with dependency (e.g., dangling the limb off the bed). The pain is often excruciating and unremitting and may require opiate analgesics for relief. Many of these patients also have peripheral neuropathic pain. Rest pain can be mistaken for isolated diabetic (or nondiabetic) peripheral neuropathy, complex regional pain syndrome, nerve root compression, or "night cramps."

However, these disorders are not associated with a low ankle blood pressure (see later).

Ischemic skin changes may follow if the obstructions worsen or revascularization is not done. *Ischemic ulcers* often start with trivial skin injury, which is particularly dangerous in patients with diabetes with peripheral neuropathy and altered sensation. The toes are most affected, although arterial heel and malleolar ulcers do occur. Again, ischemic ulcers must be distinguished from traumatic, venous, or neuropathic lesions.[14] Their appearance is sometimes distinctive: located on the toes (or heel), dry with a pale base, sharply marginated, and associated with severe pain. Ulcers about the malleoli or above the ankle are usually venous in origin (see Chapter 15). *Gangrene* is the feared sequela of CLI. Amputation may then be necessary. Diabetic patients suffer a major amputation rate that is 5- to 10-fold greater than the general PAD population.[14]

Physical signs of long-standing PAD include dependent rubor, leg coolness, delayed capillary refill (>1 second), and trophic changes (e.g., hair loss over the lower legs, thin shiny skin, nail thickening). With advanced PAD, ulcers and gangrenous changes occur. The interventionalist should document the status of the bilateral femoral, popliteal, dorsal pedis, and posterior tibial artery pulses. The peripheral pulses are evaluated on a 2-point scale (2 = full, 1 = diminished, 0 = absent). However, the pulse examination is notoriously nonspecific for the degree and location of PAD. Nonpalpable peripheral pulses should be examined with a Doppler probe. A venous signal may be pulsatile but vanishes with compression by the transducer.

Patients with blue toe syndrome complain of relatively acute onset of painful, bluish-colored toes on one or both feet.[21,22] The symptoms often resolve but may recur and occasionally lead to tissue loss. The peripheral pulses often are intact.

Natural History

Usually, the clinical progression of PAD is remarkably slow. Only 25% of individuals with IC note worsening of initial symptoms. In most patients, development of robust collateral circulation, adaptation of leg muscles, and self-imposed changes in activity or gait are responsible for the oftentimes benign course of the condition. No more than 10% of those diagnosed with PAD require revascularization for CLI within 5 years of presentation.[14]

However, once CLI is present, the overall prognosis is dismal. Within 1 year, 25% of such patients will require major amputation and another 25% will be dead. These disturbing figures reflect the nature of PAD: a systemic vascular disease with a very high mortality rate, largely from associated coronary artery disease or

TABLE 8-1   Rutherford-Becker Classification of Peripheral Arterial Disease

Grade	Category	Symptoms
0	0	None
I	1	Mild claudication
I	2	Moderate claudication
I	3	Severe (lifestyle-limiting) claudication
II	4	Rest pain
III	5	Nonhealing ulcers, focal gangrene
III	6	Major tissue loss

stroke (i.e., 30% at 5 years, 50% at 10 years).[14,15] Almost every patient who suffers from CLI is dead within a decade.

Noninvasive Testing

Noninvasive vascular studies identify at-risk patients with asymptomatic disease, confirm the diagnosis of PAD in those with an equivocal history or physical findings, determine the severity and level of obstructions, follow the progression of disease, and assess response to endovascular and surgical therapy. The most commonly used tests are the ankle-brachial and toe indexes, segmental blood pressure measurements, and plethysmography (pulse-volume recording).

The *ankle-brachial index (ABI)* is extremely sensitive (95%) and specific (almost 100%) for the diagnosis of PAD.[14,23] It is an absolutely essential part of the evaluation of all patients with known or suspected PAD. The systolic blood pressure at the ankle is divided by the systolic brachial arterial pressure to yield an index (Table 8-2). Rest pain usually requires an ABI less than 0.5 or an absolute ankle pressure less than 50 mm Hg. Ischemic ulcers can develop below a pressure of 50 to 70 mm Hg. However, calcified or noncompressible arteries (as found in patients with diabetes or chronic renal failure) falsely elevate pressure measurements and can lead to underestimation of disease severity. In this situation, *toe pressure measurements* are more useful. The toe index is normally greater than 0.60. An absolute toe pressure of greater than 30 mm Hg is generally required for wound healing.

Segmental blood pressures are obtained by sequentially inflating blood pressure cuffs around the upper thigh, lower thigh, calf, ankle, and toe. Several sets of guidelines have been established to interpret these values.[14,23] A drop of 20 to 30 mm Hg between levels (or comparing legs at the same level) suggests a significant stenosis or occlusion (Fig. 8-6A). Abnormal values at the upper thigh, lower thigh, calf, and ankle reflect obstructions in the aortoiliac segments, SFA, femoropopliteal segment, and tibial arteries, respectively (see Fig. 8-6B). However, the correlation is not always precise; for example, proximal femoral artery disease can mimic aortoiliac disease. Segmental pressure measurements after exercise can detect occult disease in

patients with suspicious symptoms and a normal study at rest (see Fig. 8-6C). While walking on an inclined treadmill, ankle and brachial pressure measurements are periodically recorded. A fall in ankle pressure is diagnostic of significant PAD.

Plethysmography (pulse volume recordings, PVR) utilizes changes in leg volume to reflect overall perfusion of the limb.[23] With mild or moderate PAD, digital or segmental pulse volume tracings are dampened; with severe occlusive disease, the waveform is almost flat. This technique is particularly useful when segmental pressure measurements are inaccurate, as in patients with noncompliant arteries.

Imaging

A correct diagnosis of chronic lower extremity PAD can almost always be made through a combination of clinical findings and noninvasive testing. Direct imaging is used almost solely to identify the nature, sites, and extent of disease in patients whose symptoms warrant endovascular or surgical treatment.

Atherosclerosis is typically diffuse, bilateral, and often strikingly symmetric. Patients with claudication usually have *single-level disease*. With the notable exception of diabetic patients, patients with CLI almost always have *multilevel disease*. Clinically relevant lesions include hemodynamically significant stenoses (as measured by pressure gradients or luminal diameter reduction of more than 50%), diffuse long-segment atherosclerosis, thrombotic occlusions, and ulcerated or exophytic plaques. Plaques may be characterized as focal or long, calcified or noncalcified, concentric or eccentric, and smooth or ulcerated.

COLOR DOPPLER SONOGRAPHY

Color Doppler ("duplex") sonography is favored in some laboratories for arterial mapping to depict and grade arterial stenoses and occlusions. The technique is sensitive (~80% to 90%) and quite specific (~95%).[23,24] The normal Doppler spectral pattern in these high-resistance arteries is triphasic, with rapid forward flow in systole followed by brief reversal of flow in early diastole. Direct and indirect indicators of significant PAD are listed in Box 8-4.

MAGNETIC RESONANCE ANGIOGRAPHY

Magnetic resonance (MR) angiography has revolutionized the evaluation of patients with PAD.[25-28] When properly performed, MR angiography provides images almost comparable in quality and form to conventional catheter angiography with none of the associated risks (see Fig. 8-2). The sensitivity and specificity of state-of-the-art MR angiography approaches or exceeds 95%[26-30] (Figs. 8-7 and 8-8).

MR angiography is contraindicated in certain patients (e.g., those with pacemakers, intracranial clips, severe

TABLE 8-2 Ankle-Brachial Index Classifications

Range	Rutherford Grade	Disease
<0.5	II or III	Chronic limb ischemia
0.51 to 0.90	I	Intermittent claudication
0.91 to 1.3	0	No significant PAD
>1.4	—	Noncompressible vessels, likely to have PAD

PAD, *peripheral artery disease.*

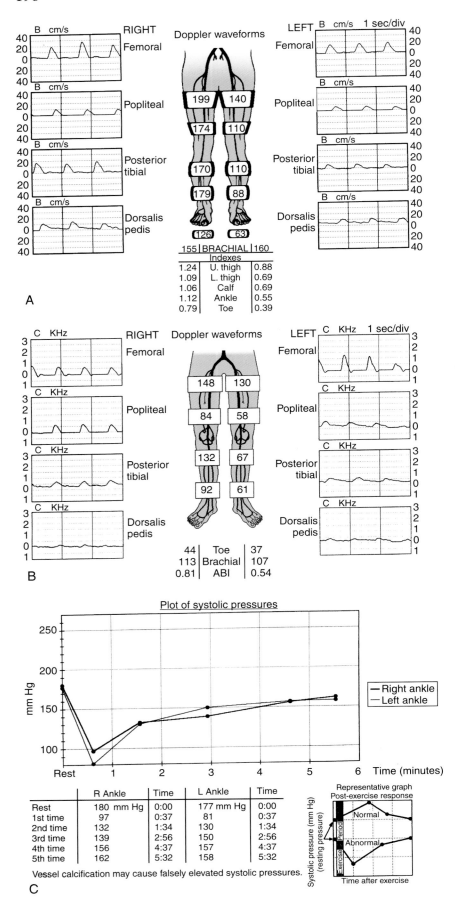

FIGURE 8-6   Segmental blood pressure measurements. **A,** Abnormal left upper thigh index (0.88) in a patient with left leg claudication. The angiogram showed a tight left common iliac artery stenosis. **B,** Bilateral drop in lower thigh pressures in a patient with bilateral leg claudication. Notice dampening of the normal waveform at this level. Angiography showed bilateral occlusions of the superficial femoral arteries. **C,** After exercise, the ankle pressures dropped abnormally in a patient with bilateral calf claudication and normal resting segmental pressures. The angiogram demonstrated bilateral tibial artery disease.

SONOGRAPHIC INDICATORS OF SIGNIFICANT PERIPHERAL ARTERIAL DISEASE

Direct Signs (Femoropopliteal System)

- Turbulent color flow pattern
- PSV >180 cm/sec
- PSV ratio at site .2

Indirect Signs (Aortoiliac System)

- Dampened waveform (from triphasic to monophasic)
- Decreased pulsatility
- Delayed systolic rise (acceleration)
- PSV <80 cm/sec

PSV, peak systolic velocity.

claustrophobia). Each institution must develop its own protocol for routine imaging of patients with PAD, and software and hardware are constantly evolving. The gadolinium injections and imaging acquisitions are coordinated such that the imaging interval is centered around the time of peak gadolinium concentration. Initial unenhanced two-dimensional time-of-flight acquisitions can be helpful in evaluating the calf and pedal vessels, but add substantial time to the examination. In addition to inspecting the maximum intensity projections in multiple planes, it is crucial to review source data to confirm findings.

COMPUTED TOMOGRAPHY ANGIOGRAPHY

The widespread availability of multidetector computed tomography (CT) scanners has made CT angiography an important tool in evaluation of a wide variety of vascular diseases, including PAD[31] (Fig. 8-9). The sensitivity and specificity with current technology is about 92% to 96% compared with catheter digital angiography.[32-35] The major pitfalls of CT angiography for PAD include pulsation artifacts (which are minimized with cardiac gating), contrast bolus mistiming, calcified vessels, and the presence of metallic objects (e.g., stents, coils) (Fig. 8-10).

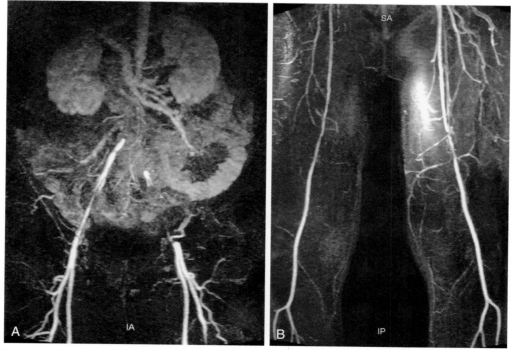

FIGURE 8-7   Chronic aortoiliac occlusion on maximum intensity projection magnetic resonance angiogram of the pelvis **(A)** and thigh **(B)**. There is complete occlusion of the distal aorta, proximal right common iliac artery, and left common and external iliac arteries. The right external iliac artery is diseased. Diffuse right superficial femoral artery (SFA) disease with a tight mid left SFA stenosis is present.

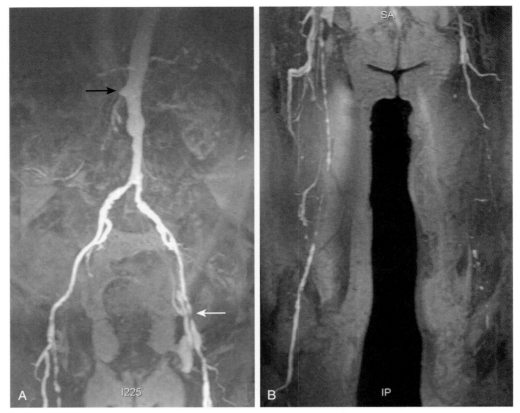

FIGURE 8-8   Acute occlusion of left deep femoral to below-knee popliteal artery bypass graft. History of a right nephrectomy and left renal artery stent **(A).** Magnetic resonance angiogram shows a small infrarenal abdominal aortic aneurism. The right renal artery is occluded *(black arrow).* The proximal left renal artery is obscured by the stent. Proximal portions of both common iliac arteries are stenotic. A stenosis is evident in the left common femoral artery *(white arrow).* **B,** The bypass graft is thrombosed. The right superficial femoral artery (SFA) is diffusely diseased, and the left SFA is occluded.

CATHETER ANGIOGRAPHY

Catheter arteriography remains the gold standard for evaluation of patients with symptomatic PAD. In practice, however, it is only requested when endovascular revascularization is being contemplated or high-quality CT or MR angiography cannot be obtained before planned surgery. A complete procedure includes the following components:

- Abdominal aortography
- Bilateral oblique pelvic arteriography
- Bilateral lower extremity run-off study (Fig. 8-11)
- Selective arteriography (sometimes in multiple projections or after intraarterial vasodilator injection) to evaluate equivocal findings
- Measurement of pressure gradients in the aorta and iliac arteries to determine the significance of moderate or suspicious stenoses (>5 to 10 mm Hg systolic)

However, a more tailored study is appropriate if MR or CT angiography is available or preexisting renal insufficiency makes contrast load a concern. When the angiogram is performed through the CFA on the less symptomatic leg, groin complications do not interfere with surgical bypass procedures, catheter occlusion of a stenotic iliac artery is less likely, and antegrade puncture for infrainguinal treatment of the affected leg can be performed in the same setting. On the other hand, direct access to iliac artery stenoses is available if the angiogram is performed on the side with diminished femoral pulses.

Visualization of the entire arterial circulation to the foot is mandatory because vascular surgical techniques allow bypass to the pedal arteries. Measurement of aortoiliac pressure gradients after vasodilator injection is particularly important in patients with claudication or before infrainguinal bypass graft placement (Fig. 8-12). The drop in peripheral vascular resistance and resulting increase in flow that occurs with exercise or after graft placement increase the significance of proximal stenoses (see Chapter 3).

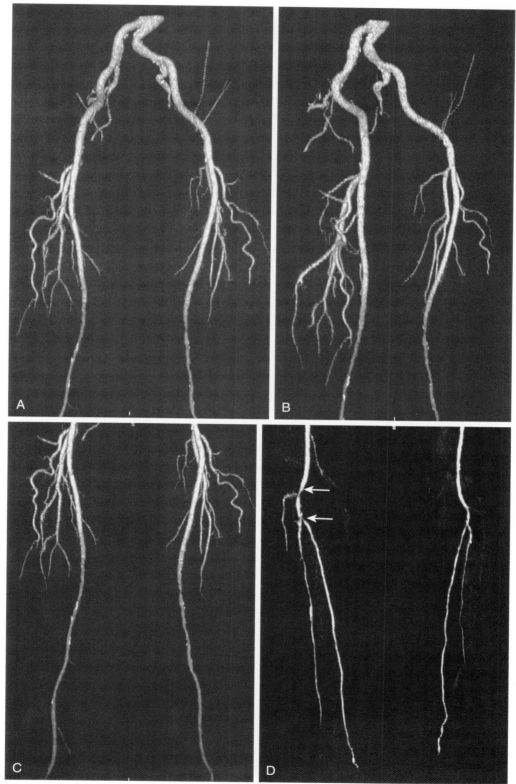

FIGURE 8-9 Pelvic and extremity arteries at computed tomography angiography, including the pelvis (**A** and **B**), thigh (**C**), and calf (**D**). Diffuse bilateral mid superficial femoral artery (SFA) disease is present. There are right distal popliteal and tibioperoneal trunk stenoses *(white arrows)*. Neither anterior tibial artery is opacified.

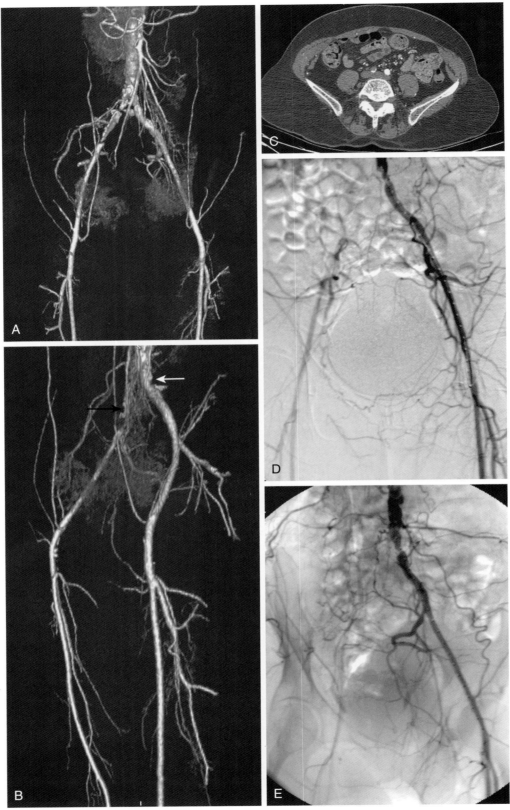

FIGURE 8-10   Correlation of computed tomography and catheter angiography for peripheral vascular disease. Frontal **(A)** and oblique **(B)** shaded-surface display computed tomography reconstructions suggest complete right common iliac artery occlusion *(black arrow)*, and moderate left common iliac artery stenosis *(white arrow)*. The former is confirmed on review of axial images **(C)**. Note that significant calcification partially obscures the occlusion on reformatted images. The findings were confirmed on a catheter angiogram in frontal **(D)** and left posterior oblique **(E)** projections.

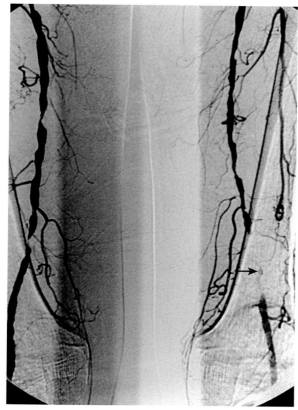

FIGURE 8-11   Diffuse bilateral atherosclerosis of superficial femoral arteries and short occlusion of the distal left superficial femoral artery *(black arrow)*.

Certain points in the interpretation of lower extremity run-off studies are worth comment:

- The only sign of an eccentric plaque along the posterior or anterior wall of an artery may be a relative dilution of the contrast column. Multiple projections or pressure gradients often are required to outline such lesions in profile (Fig. 8-13).
- Noncalcified aneurysms may go undetected if the lumen is lined with thrombus or the aneurysm is completely thrombosed (Fig. 8-14).
- In addition to thrombotic occlusion, nonopacification of arteries can result from inadequate filling (especially the tibial and pedal arteries) or congenital absence (see Fig. 8-4). Visualization of distal tibial vessels may be improved with selective studies after intraarterial vasodilator injection (Fig. 8-15).
- Luminal filling defects may be caused by emboli, in situ thrombosis, inflow defects (unopacified blood entering the contrast column), plaques seen en face, or dissection flaps (Fig. 8-16).
- Luminal narrowing has other causes than atherosclerosis (Figs. 8-17 through 8-20; see Box 8-1). The presence of atypical clinical or angiographic features should raise this possibility (see Box 8-3).
- Diabetic patients are prone to severe disease of the infrapopliteal arteries with relative sparing of proximal vessels (Fig. 8-21).

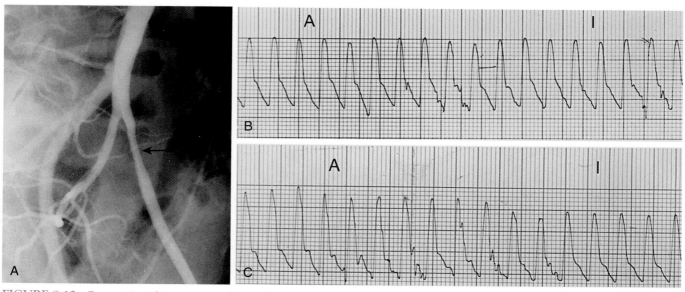

FIGURE 8-12   Provocation of a pressure gradient with vasodilators. **A,** This patient with left superficial femoral artery occlusion and a moderate left external iliac artery stenosis *(black arrow)* is about to undergo infrainguinal bypass graft placement. **B,** No pressure gradient was found between the aorta *(A)* and external iliac artery *(I)* with the initial pullback method. **C,** After intraarterial injection of 25 mg of tolazoline, the repeat pullback pressure measurement showed a systolic gradient of 20 mm Hg that warranted treatment.

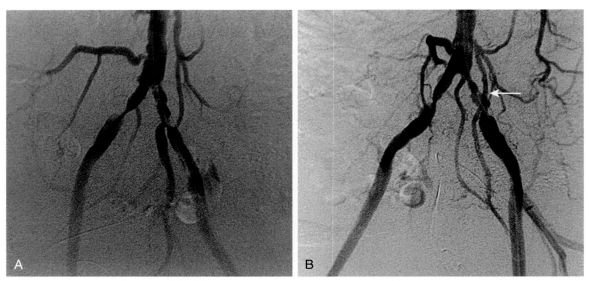

FIGURE 8-13   Eccentric atherosclerotic plaque. **A,** The left posterior oblique pelvic arteriogram shows right iliac stenosis and only moderate disease of the left common iliac artery. Note the enlarged right lumbar artery indicating the significance of the right-sided disease. **B,** The right posterior oblique projection shows the true severity of the left-sided disease *(white arrow).*

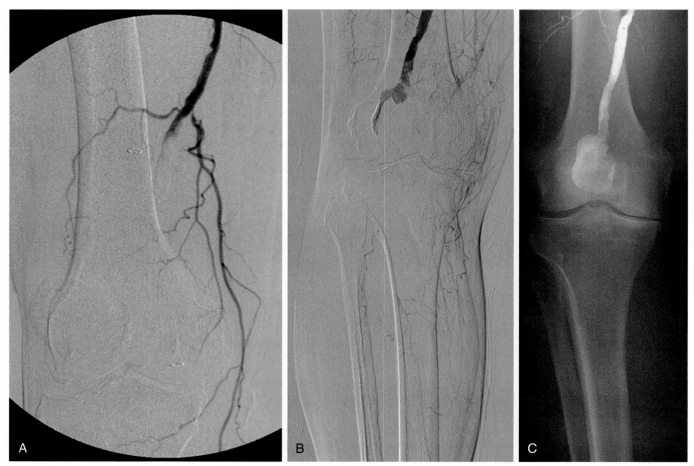

FIGURE 8-14   Right popliteal artery aneurysm. **A,** Initial right leg arteriogram shows complete occlusion of the upper popliteal artery. An aneurysm was not initially suspected. **B** and **C,** After partial thrombolysis, the aneurysm becomes apparent.

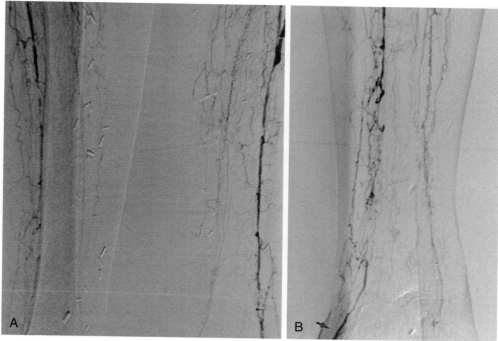

FIGURE 8-15 Enhanced opacification of tibial arteries after vasodilator injection. **A,** The initial run-off study fails to identify a target vessel for bypass graft placement in a patient with right leg rest pain. **B,** After a catheter was advanced into the right external iliac artery and 12.5 mg of tolazoline was injected, the repeat arteriogram showed a patent dorsal pedis artery at the ankle *(arrow).*

Medical Therapy

Many patients with asymptomatic PAD or intermittent claudication respond to medical therapy without the need for any type of imaging or intervention. The treatment goals are to stabilize or reduce lower extremity symptoms and prevent other cardiovascular events (e.g., myocardial infarction or stroke). The interventionalist must work aggressively with the patient to accomplish these goals[14,36] (Box 8-5). Drug therapy, risk factor modification, and a supervised exercise program remain the cornerstones of treatment for mild to moderate IC. Endovascular interventions should serve an adjunctive role.[37,38]

A host of pharmacologic agents have been tried for specific treatment of PAD. Most are not effective, including pentoxifylline, aspirin, vasodilators, and L-arginine.[14] Two drugs are valuable in patients with IC. *Cilostazol* is a phosphodiesterase-III inhibitor with several properties of direct benefit to claudicants.[39,40] There is strong evidence that long-term use will significantly increase walking distance and improve overall quality of life in this population. Side effects include diarrhea, headaches and palpitations. Cilostazol is contraindicated in patients with congestive heart failure. *Naftidrofuryl* is a 5-hydroxytryptamine antagonist the inhibits red cell and platelet aggregation and enhances striated muscle metabolism. Daily therapy affords similar benefits to cilostazol.[41-43]

For patients with CLI, the goals of therapy are relief of pain, healing of ulcers, avoidance of major amputation, and improvement in quality of life. Narcotic analgesics are appropriate before revascularization or for palliation. Along with aggressive antibiotic therapy for infections, local would care is essential.

Endovascular Therapy
PATIENT SELECTION

The mere presence of a peripheral arterial lesion (even an apparently significant one) in the absence of associated symptoms is not a license to intervene. An invasive procedure may convert a stenosis with a fairly benign natural history into a lesion that becomes rapidly and severely progressive and quite symptomatic.

The primary goals of intervention are improved quality of life, limb salvage, and prolonged survival. Revascularization should be considered for patients with the following:

- Moderate or severe intermittent claudication that does not respond adequately to medical measures (see Box 8-5). However, one rigorous analysis suggested that angioplasty is more cost-effective than exercise therapy in patients with IC.[44]
- Chronic limb ischemia

Selection of patients for endovascular versus open surgical therapy depends on a variety of patient factors and the site and nature of disease. For almost all arterial segments, results are better in groups suffering from claudication than those with CLI. The guidelines of the TransAtlantic Inter-Society Consensus on Peripheral Arterial Disease (TASC) working group are widely recognized[14] (Fig. 8-22).

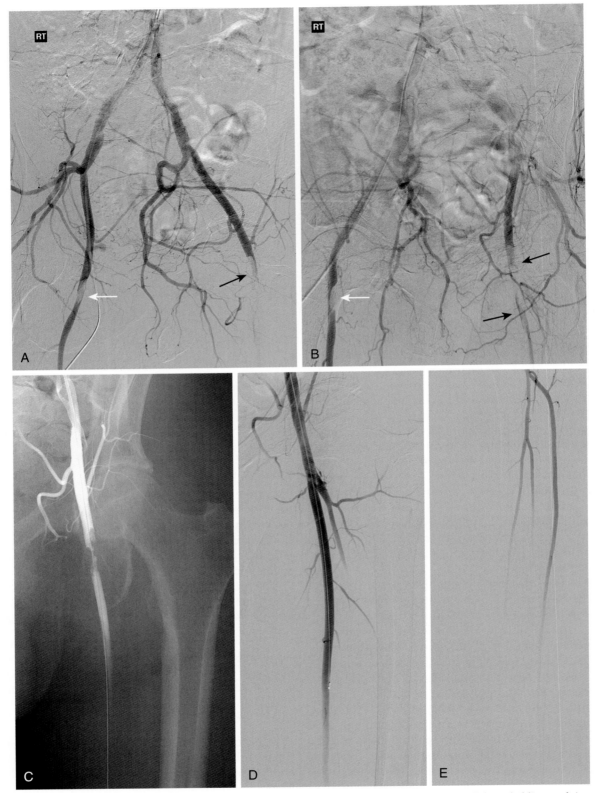

FIGURE 8-16 Embolism to both common femoral arteries (CFA) with severe left leg ischemia. **A** and **B,** Bilateral oblique pelvic arteriography shows a near occlusive embolus to the right CFA *(white arrow).* The right deep femoral artery is blocked. A left CFA embolus is almost completely obstructive and extends into the superficial and deep femoral arteries *(black arrow).* Blood flows from internal iliac artery collaterals into deep femoral artery branches. **C,** Following initial treatment with 12 mg of t-PA, there is some lysis of clot. **D** and **E,** Following additional thrombolytic therapy, the embolus is completely resolved with three vessel run-off in the calf.

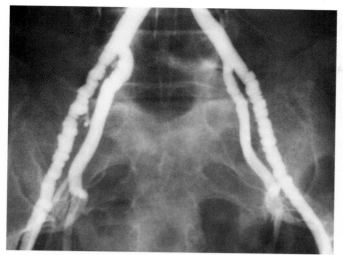

FIGURE 8-17   Fibromuscular dysplasia of both external iliac arteries.

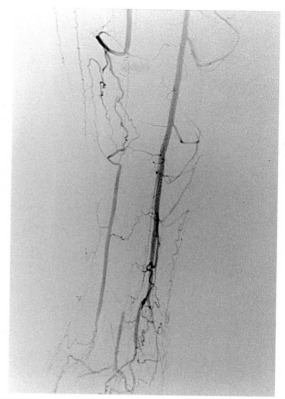

FIGURE 8-19   Buerger disease in a 45-year-old smoker. An arteriogram of the right calf shows abrupt occlusions of the tibial arteries with relatively normal intervening segments and tortuous corkscrew collaterals.

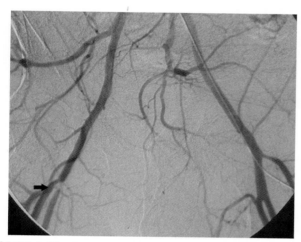

FIGURE 8-18   Puncture site neointimal hyperplasia at the origin of the right superficial femoral artery after cardiac catheterization (arrow). Notably, no other vascular disease is seen.

- Category A disease: endovascular treatment preferred
- Category B disease: endovascular treatment preferred, unless an operation is planned for other PAD
- Category C disease: surgical treatment preferred unless patient is at high risk for operation
- Category D disease: surgical treatment is much preferred, endovascular therapy is inferior

The technical details of percutaneous arterial revascularization are considered in detail in Chapter 3. Selection criteria, specific technical features, and outcomes at various sites are discussed herein. Perhaps in no other area of interventional radiology are reports of the efficacy of a procedure more disparate and confusing. Older radiologic

---

BOX 8-5

CONSERVATIVE MANAGEMENT OF PERIPHERAL ARTERIAL DISEASE

- (Supervised) exercise program
- Smoking cessation
- Dietary modifications (for weight and cholesterol control)
- Blood glucose control in diabetic patients (hemoglobin A1c < 7%)
- Blood pressure control (<140/90 mm Hg, <130/80 mm Hg if diabetic or renal failure, favor thiazides and ACE inhibitors)
- Statin therapy for dyslipidemia (to LDL cholesterol <100 mg/dL)
- Daily antiplatelet therapy (aspirin or clopidogrel) for associated CAD and CVD rather than PAD

ACE, angiotensin converting enzyme; CAD, coronary artery disease; CVD, cerebrovascular disease; LDL, low density lipoprotein.

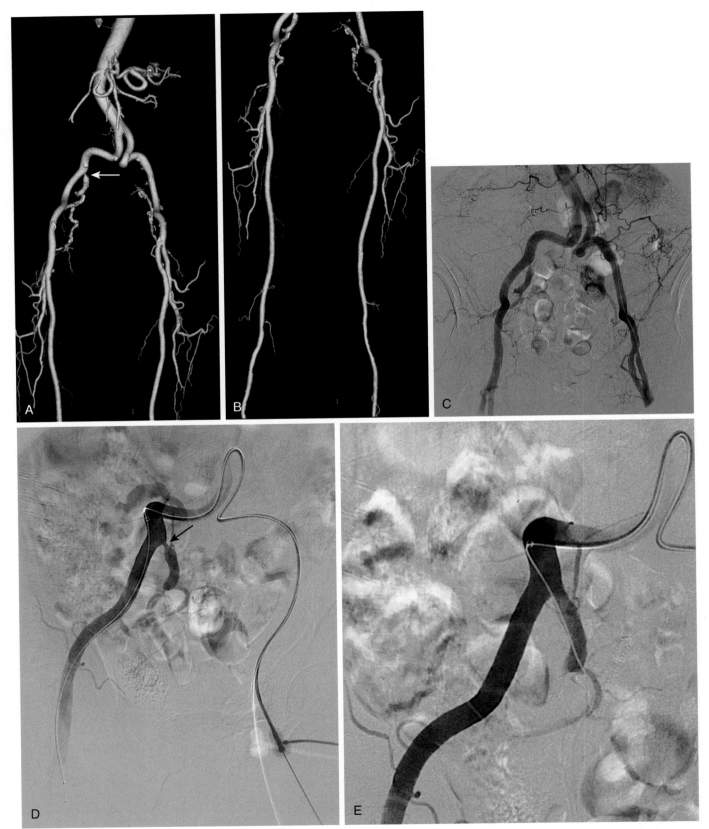

FIGURE 8-20   Radiation arteritis in a woman with a remote history of radiation therapy for cervical cancer and new right buttock claudication. **A** and **B,** Shaded-surface display reformatted CT angiography shows entirely normal lower extremity arteries except left internal iliac artery (IIA) occlusion and a moderate origin stenosis of the right internal iliac artery *(arrow)*. Pelvic arteriogram **(C)** and selective right common iliac arteriogram in left anterior oblique projection **(D)** confirm these findings and show enlarged lumbar arteries providing collateral circulation into the pelvis. **E,** Angioplasty of the right IIA gave a good technical result but did not improve symptoms, probably due to radiation-induced small vessel arteritis.

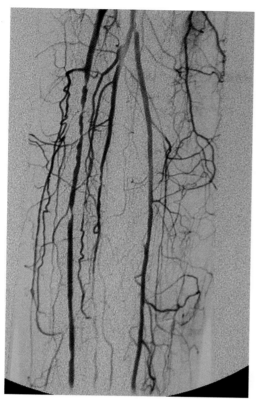

FIGURE 8-21   Peripheral vascular disease in a diabetic patient. Severe diffuse right tibial artery lesions with relatively mild disease proximally (not shown).

series focused primarily on technical success and patency rates. The outcomes summarized in Table 8-3 are rough estimates intended only to help educate patients and referring physicians. To properly compare endovascular procedures with surgical treatment, these modalities must be evaluated in terms of durable clinical improvement in ischemic symptoms, limb salvage, and survival.

It is interesting to note that arterial angioplasty and stent placement provoke an inflammatory reaction at the treated site. The response is marked by elevations of serum C-reactive protein and fibrinogen (among other factors) and is more intense after femoropopliteal percutaneous transluminal balloon angioplasty (PTA) than carotid or iliac artery PTA. This phenomenon may partly explain the increased frequency of clinical restenosis at this site.[45] The risk of restenosis also may be associated with higher preprocedure and postprocedure levels of C-reactive protein.[46,47]

INFRARENAL AORTIC STENOSIS (TASC B LESIONS)

Isolated, severe atherosclerotic abdominal aortic stenoses are relatively uncommon. They occur mostly frequently in middle-aged or elderly women who smoke and in patients with *hypoplastic aortic syndrome* (small aorta and hypoplastic iliofemoral arteries).[48] The traditional therapy

was surgical endarterectomy or bypass grafting. For endovascular repair, these lesions cause some trepidation for interventionalists because the theoretical risk of rupture is greater than at other sites due to the large diameter of the aorta. In reality, angioplasty is remarkably safe, effective, and durable at this location[49] (Fig. 8-23 and see Table 8-3). Primary hemodynamic patency at 10 years with PTA alone is close to 50%. Stents are certainly justified for failures of angioplasty and for large exophytic lesions that are more likely to shower emboli with balloon dilation.[50] In actual practice, and despite the lack of solid evidence, most interventionalists opt for primary stent placement for all infrarenal aortic stenoses.[51-55] In one small series, 3-year primary patency was 83% with primary stent insertion.[53]

AORTIC OCCLUSION AND SEVERE AORTOILIAC OCCLUSIVE DISEASE (TASC C AND D LESIONS)

This relatively uncommon form of PAD is typically seen in a somewhat younger population, most of whom smoke.[56] Symptoms of bilateral claudication (and impotence in men) are common *(Leriche syndrome)* (see Fig. 7-5). The singular risk of an untreated infrarenal aortic occlusion is proximal propagation of clot leading to renal or mesenteric artery thrombosis. For these TASC C and D lesions, first-line treatment is still aortobifemoral bypass (AFB) grafting. Inferior alternatives include endarterectomy, axillobifemoral grafting, or thoracoaortic femoral grafting. Recently, some aggressive interventionalists have tackled these difficult cases by endovascular reconstruction with (limited) thrombolysis, angioplasty, and stent insertion (bare or covered). Long-term patency is still inferior to AFB grafting, but is perhaps acceptable given the reduced risk of perioperative complications, similar amputation rates, and comparable 30-day mortality.[57-62] The reported primary patency rates at 3 and 5 years are 66% and 60% to 86%, respectively, with secondary patency rates of 90% and 80% to 98%, respectively. Hybrid interventions are becoming increasingly popular, whereby suprainguinal endovascular treatment is done in concert with CFA endarterectomy and/or infrainguinal bypass grafting [63]

ILIAC ARTERY STENOSIS (TASC A-D LESIONS)

Primary stent placement is now standard of care for all TASC type B and C iliac lesions.[57,64] Although formally considered operative territory, many interventionalists now handle type D iliac lesions. Balloon angioplasty is effective and durable for many simple iliac artery stenoses (Table 8-4). The oft-quoted Dutch Iliac Stent Trial and some other reports found no particular benefit to primary stent placement over selective stenting for type A and B lesions.[65,66] Even so, many experienced operators still prefer primary stent placement for all iliac artery stenoses. Primary stent placement is certainly justified in the following situations[67] (Fig. 8-24).

- Immediate failures of iliac angioplasty (e.g., residual pressure gradient [>5 to 10 mm Hg systolic], residual luminal stenosis [>30%], flow-limiting dissection flap)
- External iliac artery stenoses
- Subacute restenosis after balloon angioplasty

Predilation with a balloon catheter ensures that the lumen can be fully expanded and that the appropriate balloon and stent size is chosen to avoid vessel rupture. In reality, unless the lesion is heavily calcified, most interventionalists perform primary stent placement to expedite the procedure and theoretically decrease the risk of distal embolization of plaque fragments.

Stents must cover all of the diseased segment and ideally end at a relatively normal point on the artery. Notably, the internal iliac artery often remains patent even with a bare stent placed across its origin. Either self-expanding (SE) or balloon-expandable (BE) stents may be used[60,67,68] (see Chapter 3). When precise placement is critical (e.g., at the aortic bifurcation), BE stents are advantageous. When long arterial segments must be covered, SE stents are a wise choice. Although no single device has proven most effective or durable, there is good evidence that nitinol stents yield better long-term results than other materials.

For iliac disease at or just adjacent to the aortic bifurcation, so-called "kissing stents" are often placed. In this technique, bare stents are deployed simultaneously from both groins in both iliac arteries with the superior ends

Type A lesions
- Unilateral or bilateral stenoses of CIA
- Unilateral or bilateral single, short (≤3 cm) stenosis of EIA

Type B lesions
- Short (≤3 cm) stenosis of infrarenal aorta
- Unilateral CIA occlusion
- Single or multiple stenosis totaling 3-10 cm involving the EIA, not extending into the CFA
- Unilateral EIA occlusion not involving the origins of internal iliac or CFA

Type C lesions
- Bilateral CIA occlusions
- Bilateral EIA stenoses 3-10 cm long, not extending into the CFA
- Unilateral EIA stenosis extending into the CFA
- Unilateral EIA occlusion that involves the origins of internal iliac and/or CFA
- Heavily calcified unilateral EIA occlusion with or without involvement of origins of internal iliac and/or CFA

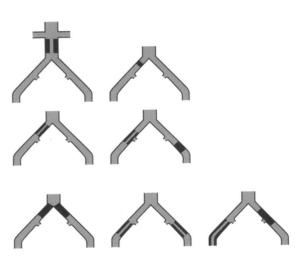

Type D lesions
- Infrarenal aortoiliac occlusion
- Diffuse disease involving the aorta and both iliac arteries, requiring treatment
- Diffuse multiple stenoses involving the unilateral CIA, EIA, and CFA
- Unilateral occlusions of both CIA and EIA
- Bilateral occlusions of EIA
- Iliac stenoses in patients with AAA requiring treatment and not amenable to endograft placement or other lesions requiring open aortic or iliac surgery

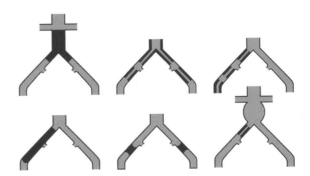

A

FIGURE 8-22   **A,** TASC II classification of aortoiliac lesions. (*Adapted from Norgren L, Hiatt WR, Dormandy JA, et al: Inter-society consensus for the management of peripheral arterial disease [TASC II]. Eur J Vasc Endovasc Surg 2007;33:S1.*)

Type A lesions
- Single stenosis ≤10 cm long
- Single occlusion ≤5 cm long

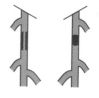

Type B lesions
- Multiple lesions (stenoses or occlusions), each ≤5 cm
- Single stenosis or occlusion ≤15 cm, not involving the infrageniculate popliteal artery
- Single or multiple lesions in the absence of continuous tibial vessels to improve inflow for a distal bypass
- Heavily calcified occlusion ≤5 cm long
- Single popliteal stenosis

Type C lesions
- Multiple stenoses or occlusions totaling >15 cm with or without heavy calcification
- Recurrent stenoses or occlusions that need treatment after two endovascular interventions

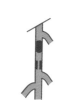

Type D lesions
- Chronic total occlusions of CFA or SFA (>20 cm, involving the popliteal artery)
- Chronic total occlusion of popliteal artery and proximal trifurcation vessels

B

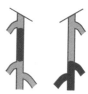

FIGURE 8-22, cont'd   **B,** TASC II classification of femoropopliteal lesions. *(Adapted from Norgren L, Hiatt WR, Dormandy JA, et al: Intersociety consensus for the management of peripheral arterial disease [TASC II]. Eur J Vasc Endovasc Surg 2007;**33**:S1.)*

TABLE 8-3   Results of Transcatheter Therapy for Chronic Peripheral Arterial Disease

Site and Disease	Therapy	Technical Success (%)	1-Yr Patency (%)	3-Yr Patency (%)	5-Yr Patency (%)
Abdominal aortic stenosis	Stent	70	60	50-80	50
Severe aortoiliac disease	Stent	90	66	60-86	
Iliac stenosis	Angioplasty	95	75-85	65-80	70
Iliac stenosis	Stent	98	90	75-80	70-80
Iliac occlusion	Stent	80-85	70-90	60	50-60
Femoropopliteal stenosis	Angioplasty	95	70-80	50-70	50-60
Femoropopliteal occlusion	Angioplasty	80-85	50-70	40-55	35-50
Femoropopliteal lesions	Stent (older)	98	50-60	40	—
Femoropopliteal lesions	Stent (nitinol)	98	75-85	60-75	—
Tibial obstruction*	Angioplasty	60-90	50-80	—	—

Two-year limb salvage of 60% to 80%.

touching in the very distal aorta[60,68] (see Fig. 8-24). In this way, overhanging aortic disease is covered and a unilateral stent extending into the aortic lumen will not infringe on the contralateral common iliac artery. However, this common practice may be unnecessary if the opposing iliac vessel is normal and the stent is deposited just up to the bifurcation.[69]

Table 8-3 summarizes the primary patency rates for endovascular iliac artery treatment.* Eight- to 10-year primary patency rates of iliac artery stents (including occlusions) have been reported at 46% to 74%.[70,71] Secondary patency rates at 3 years approach 90% to 95% with most devices. The most commonly reported predictors of long-term durability are male gender, abstinence from smoking, common iliac artery location, large arterial (stent) diameter, patent outflow arteries,

*See references 14, 58-60, 64, 65, 70-73.

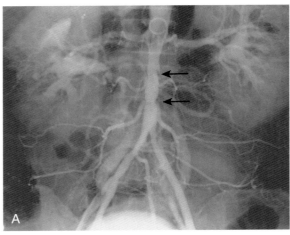

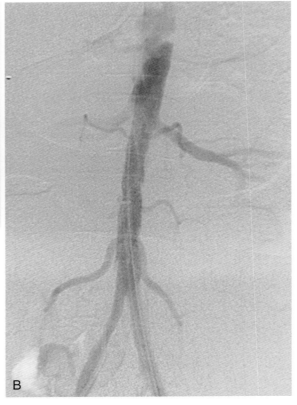

FIGURE 8-23 Abdominal aortic stenosis in an older woman with bilateral leg claudication. **A,** Tandem stenoses of the infrarenal aorta *(arrows)* are associated with a systolic pressure gradient of 30 mm Hg. **B,** The pressure gradient dropped to 5 mm Hg after balloon angioplasty.

TABLE 8-4 Ideal Conditions for Balloon Angioplasty of Lower Extremity Arteries

Lesion Characteristics	Patient Characteristics
Short	Nondiabetic
Concentric	Milder degrees of ischemia
Noncalcified	
Solitary	
Nonocclusive	
Large vessel	
Continuous in-line run-off	

short lesion length, and complete covering of the diseased segment.[14,70] For example, patency rates for common versus external iliac artery stent placement at 5 years in one study were 76% and 56%, respectively.[74] This response may be related to the smaller size of the vessel and the fact that hip flexion causes arterial angulation in this region (not just around the CFA as commonly believed).[75]

Complications (most of which are minor) occur in about 10% of cases and include puncture site injury or hematoma, acute stent thrombosis, distal embolization, stent dislodgment, pseudoaneurysm formation, and vessel rupture.

ILIAC ARTERY OCCLUSION (TASC TYPE B-D)

Endovascular therapy is an attractive alternative to surgery for some common or external iliac artery occlusions. Balloon angioplasty alone is not sufficient; all of these obstructions require a stent. It is also accepted practice to skip thrombolysis or mechanical thrombectomy and proceed directly to primary uncovered stent insertion once the obstruction is crossed.[76]

An ipsilateral groin approach provides the most direct pathway to the obstruction. It is also preferable when stents must be deployed up into the aorta. However, many devices can be advanced from the opposite groin over the bifurcation, through a guiding catheter or sheath, and then deployed in the main iliac artery trunks. Rarely, a brachial artery approach is necessary. The occlusion is crossed with a steerable hydrophilic guidewire. If the guidewire will only traverse the occlusion from the contralateral groin, the tip can be snared from the ipsilateral CFA and pulled through the sheath. An angiographic catheter is then placed in a retrograde direction for stent placement. Stents may be inserted even when guidewire passage is partially subintimal, as long as the wire reenters the lumen before reaching the aorta. Stents are deposited along the entire length of the occlusion, incorporating adjacent segments of significant atherosclerotic disease. Placement of stents well into the CFA is controversial (see later discussion).

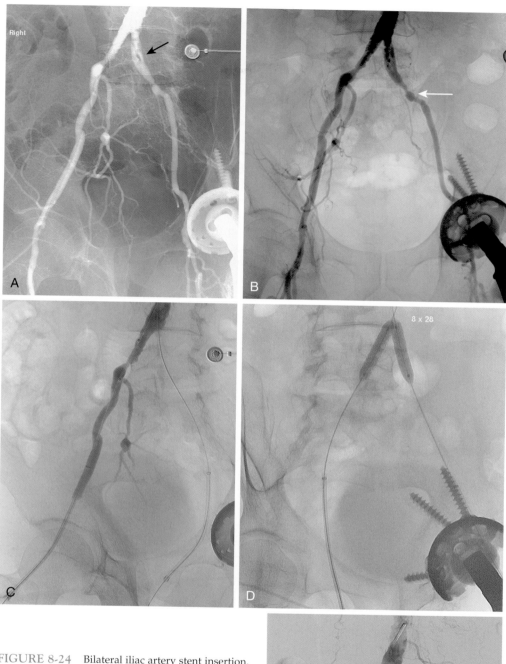

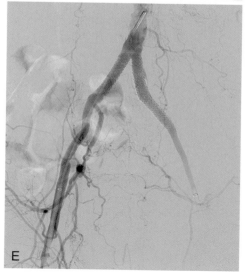

FIGURE 8-24   Bilateral iliac artery stent insertion.
A and **B,** Right posterior oblique and frontal pelvic
arteriography show a right common iliac artery
stenosis, weblike left common iliac artery stenosis
(black arrow), and proximal left external iliac artery
stenosis *(white arrow).* **C,** Retrograde access was
obtained at both groins and sheaths placed. The left
groin sheath totally occludes the left external iliac
artery. **D,** Balloon expandable stents were positioned
with proximal ends "kissing" and balloons inflated
simultaneously to deploy the stents. A second overlapping stent was inserted in the proximal left
external iliac artery. **E,** Final angiogram shows
widely patent vessels after stent insertion.

Revascularization of TASC B and C iliac artery occlusions is somewhat less successful than TASC A iliac stenoses[14] (see Table 8-3). However, the difference is largely attributable to cases in which the occlusion cannot be traversed with a guidewire. Thus, following a technically successful procedure, long-term patency rates are about 15% higher than published figures.[76-79] The overall complication rate is about 10%. The frequency of distal embolization is about 2% to 5% whether or not thrombolysis is performed.

INTERNAL ILIAC ARTERY STENOSIS

Occasionally, proximal internal iliac artery stenoses cause isolated buttock claudication.[80-82] Balloon angioplasty and stents have been used successfully to relieve such lesions.

COMMON FEMORAL ARTERY OBSTRUCTION

Often, isolated CFA stenoses and occlusions are best treated surgically (e.g., endarterectomy or patch angioplasty), because the operation is relatively simple and is more lasting than angioplasty.[83-85] Also, the long-term behavior of metallic stents near this site of constant motion has not been established.

DEEP FEMORAL ARTERY STENOSIS

Given the ease and durability of endarterectomy for focal proximal DFA disease, angioplasty or stenting is a second line treatment at this critical site (Fig. 8-25). Reports of long-term clinical success have been sporadic.[86-88]

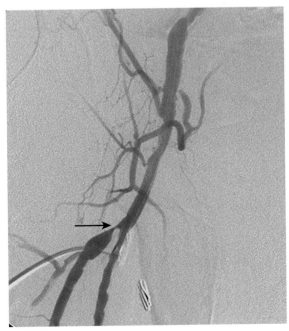

FIGURE 8-25   Tight proximal right deep femoral artery origin stenosis with post-stenotic dilation.

FEMOROPOPLITEAL ARTERY STENOSIS (TASC TYPES A AND B)

Endovascular therapy is first-line treatment for many femoropopliteal lesions in patients with appropriate symptoms[14,89,90] (Figs. 8-26 and 8-27). Unlike the iliac artery, the best endovascular approach is often controversial. The outcomes of "plain old" balloon angioplasty and bare stent placement in the femoropopliteal artery have been disappointing compared with applications in the iliac artery (Fig. 8-28). Leading explanations for this disparity invoke (1) the larger atherosclerotic burden of the long femoropopliteal segment, (2) constant extrinsic compression of the SFA at the adductor canal, and (3) hemodynamic stresses related to frequent and significant bending and shortening of the vessel with leg motion. Numerous strategies have been pursued to improve on early modest results.

- *Cutting balloons* have microtomes mounted on the balloon to incise plaque or fibrotic tissue. They may be valuable for lesions resistant to standard balloon dilation. However, patency and restenosis rates are inferior to those for conventional balloon angioplasty of de novo lesions or in-stent restenosis.[91-94]
- *Cryoplasty* entails balloon dilation of plaque combined with delivery of cold thermal energy.[95] Liquid nitrous oxide (rather than diluted contrast material) is used to inflate the balloon. As the agent rapidly assumes a gaseous state, a local $-10°$ C heat sink is created. The consequences are smooth muscle cell apoptosis (programmed cell death) to inhibit neointimal hyperplasia and restriction of arterial elasticity by thermal effects on collagen and elastin. Although the method has some proponents, it offers no significant benefit over (and is perhaps worse than) standard angioplasty.[96,97]
- *Drug-eluting balloons* deliver drug to the vascular wall that is believed to prevent restenosis of the artery (see later). The randomized FemPac and THUNDER trials in patients with femoropopliteal lesions showed proof of concept. Both reported significantly decreased late lumen loss and target lesion revascularization at 6 months in the group treated with *paclitaxel*-coated balloons.[98,99] However, the studies suffered from inadequate sample size and flawed clinical endpoints.[100] These devices are also undergoing investigation for management of in-stent restenosis.[101]
- *Brachytherapy* (endovascular radiation therapy) also has been touted as a means to limit the restenotic process in femoropopliteal obstructions, but most results have been discouraging.[102-104]

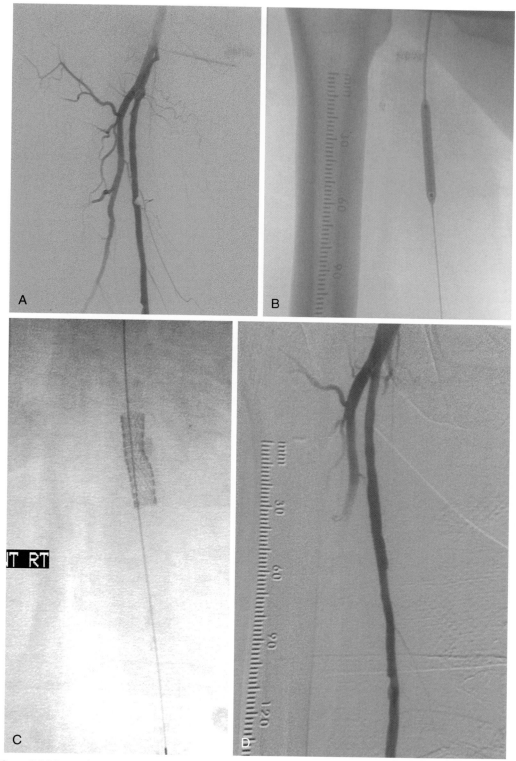

FIGURE 8-26   Superficial femoral artery angioplasty and stent placement. **A,** Arteriogram reveals an ideal lesion for angioplasty. **B,** Although the balloon inflated completely, follow-up angiogram showed elastic recoil (not shown). **C,** Nitinol SMART stent inserted to limit remodeling. **D,** Widely patent artery afterwards.

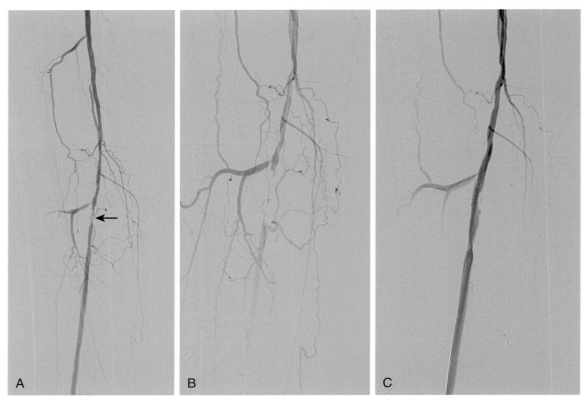

FIGURE 8-27   Superficial femoral artery (SFA) balloon angioplasty. **A,** Right leg arteriogram shows a critical mid-SFA stenosis *(arrow).*
B, A microwire and catheter were used to cross the site. The catheter is occlusive in the lesion. **C,** Following angioplasty with a 5-mm × 2-cm
balloon, there is marked improvement in patency and collateral circulation is diminished.

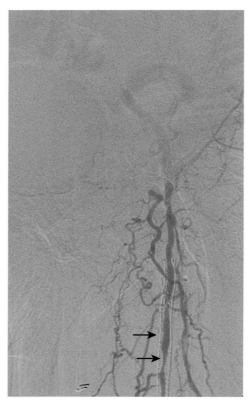

FIGURE 8-28   Exuberant diffuse restenosis 6 months after left
superficial femoral artery stent placement *(arrows).*

- *Atherectomy devices* have a long history in peripheral arterial interventions. However, the theoretical notion that removing plaque is preferable to remodeling it has not worked in practice. Outcomes with almost every atherectomy catheter that has been tried have been poor. The Silverhawk catheter (Fox Hollow) is currently approved by the U.S. Food and Drug Administration for peripheral arterial use. A joint on the working end of the catheter presses an open metallic container onto the vessel wall. A rotating blade shaves plaque (or neointimal hyperplasia) from the artery and deposits it into the container for removal. Again, although these devices have some enthusiasts, they have largely been abandoned by most interventionalists because of very mixed results.[105-110]

- *Self-expanding bare nitinol stents* have yielded lower angiographic restenosis rates and higher primary patency rates at 1 year than balloon angioplasty for the femoropopliteal arteries in some studies.[111,112] Metaanalyses of the literature have failed to show consistent benefit across angiographic and clinical parameters.[113,114] The controlled and randomized FAST, RESILIENT, Vienna ABSOLUTE, and ASTRON trials collectively provide modest support for use of these devices in complex or longer femoropopliteal lesions (e.g., >5 to 10 cm).[115-118] On the other hand, stents composed of other materials or of the balloon-expandable variety should be avoided. The advantages of nitinol include greater radial force and flexibility, minimal plastic deformity, and more predictable lesion coverage due to minimal shortening at deployment. Two vexing and persistent problems with some current devices are in-stent restenosis and stent fracture, both of which can reduce overall patency.[112,119]

- *Drug-eluting bare stents (DES)* are currently the subject of intense research for infrainguinal revascularization. They have shown dramatic results in the coronary circulation, where clinically significant restenosis has been markedly reduced. A polymer matrix is bonded to the bare metal stent. The matrix affords controlled release of an agent chosen to retard the process of neointimal hyperplasia. The principal drugs under study are *sirolimus* and *everolimus* (lipophilic macrocyclic drugs with immunosuppressive and antibiotic activity) and *paclitaxel* (a lipophilic diterpenoid that inhibits cell function by microtubule stabilization, thus preventing smooth muscle cell proliferation and migration).[120] To date, results of DES in femoropopliteal artery obstructions have been mixed. The SIROCCO (sirolimus-based) and STRIDES (everolimus-based) trials did not support use of these devices.[121,122] However, preliminary unpublished work from the Zilver PTX (paclitaxel-based) trial is quite promising.[123]

- *ePTFE covered stent grafts* show great promise for femoropopliteal obstructions that do not respond to balloon angioplasty.[124,125] A randomized, multicenter trial conducted more than 10 years ago (largely in claudicants) found significantly improved target vessel patency and limb ischemia status in the Viabahn stent graft group compared with angioplasty alone, particularly for lesions greater than 3 to 13 cm in length.[124] The ongoing VIASTAR trial will compare a bare nitinol stent with the Viabahn Propaten (heparin-bonded coating) platform. Most patients receive aspirin or clopidogrel before and for at least several months after covered stent placement.[126,127]

Table 8-5 summarizes current recommendations for treatment of femoropopliteal lesions. Methods must be tailored to the availability and local advisory board approval of the various devices.

FEMOROPOPLITEAL ARTERY OCCLUSION (TASC C AND D LESIONS)

At present, three endovascular options are considered. (see Table 8-5). For short (<3 to 5 cm) total femoropopliteal occlusions, bare nitinol stents are appropriate (Fig. 8-29).

TABLE 8-5 Endovascular Options for Femoropopliteal Arterial Obstructions

Lesion	Options
Short, simple FP stenosis	PTA
Resistant stenosis	Cutting balloon
Elastic recoil stenosis	Bare nitinol stent
Post PTA dissection	Bare nitinol stent
Complex >5-10 cm FP stenosis	Bare nitinol stent
Multiple FP stenoses	PTA or bare nitinol stent
Angioplasty failure	Bare nitinol stent
Short FP occlusion	Bare nitinol stent (or ePTFE stent graft)
Long segment FP occlusion	ePTFE stent graft or subintimal recanalization

ePTFE, *expanded polytetrafluoroethylene;* FP, *femoropopliteal;* PTA, *conventional balloon angioplasty.*

For longer femoropopliteal occlusions in patients who are not candidates for surgical bypass (due to lack of vein conduit or operative risks), recanalization of the entire occluded vessel with ePTFE-covered stents is perhaps the best choice (Fig. 8-30).

Subintimal angioplasty is advocated by some experts for treating long-segment femoropopliteal artery occlusions.[128-132] Again, this technique is usually reserved for patients with high operative risk or no suitable vein for bypass. A distal target vessel that will ultimately provide in-line run-off to the foot must be present. Access is gained through the contralateral or ipsilateral CFA, or retrograde from the popliteal artery. The optimal entry (diseased) and exit (nondiseased) points are determined. With an angled angiographic catheter wedged at the diseased upper (or lower) arterial segment, a 0.035-inch angled hydrophilic guidewire is directed subintimally. A small loop is formed with the wire; a reinforced, hydrophilic catheter is then advanced to the loop, and the entire unit is run down (or up) the subintimal space until the planned exit site is reached. The lumen is then reentered with the wire tip. Alternatively, the Outback reentry catheter accomplishes the same thing.[133-135] The entire channel is widened with an angioplasty balloon; stents are used selectively as needed. The reported technical success (in experienced hands) is 80% to 90%, and 1-year limb salvage rates are 75% to 90%. In one report, these salvage rates persisted at 3 years.[136]

There are two major risks from subintimal angioplasty: bleeding and worsening of ischemia. To prevent bleeding in case transmural perforation occurs, full anticoagulation is delayed until the channel is created. Rarely, coil embolization of the tract is necessary. In addition, worsening of ischemia may result from occlusion of important collateral branches if the procedure is not successful.

Mechanical revascularization devices (e.g., Amplatz thrombectomy catheter) have excellent technical success

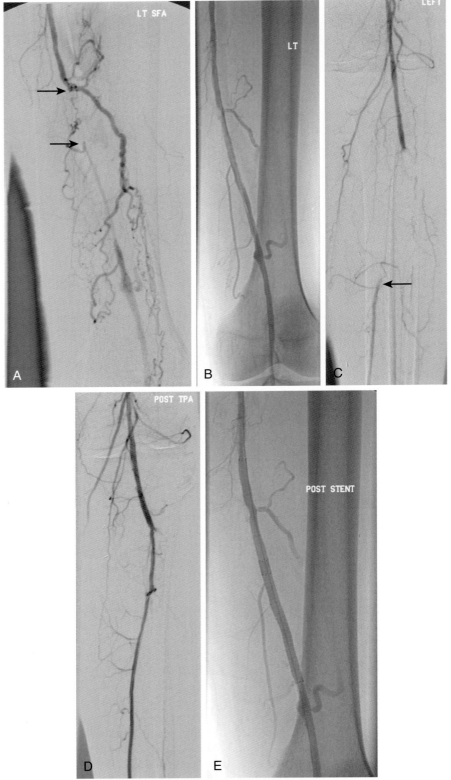

FIGURE 8-29 Angioplasty and stent placement for a left superficial femoral artery (SFA) occlusion. **A,** Distal SFA occlusion. Note that the actual length of the obstruction *(between arrows)* is relatively short because of backfilling from the collateral circulation. **B,** After 5-mm balloon angioplasty, a long dissection flap is seen. **C,** Embolic occlusion of the tibioperoneal trunk and anterior tibial artery *(arrow)* has occurred. **D,** After angioplasty, flow in the peroneal artery has been reestablished. **E,** Following placement of two overlapping SMART Control stents, the SFA is widely patent. *(Courtesy of David Lopresti, MD, San Diego, Calif.)*

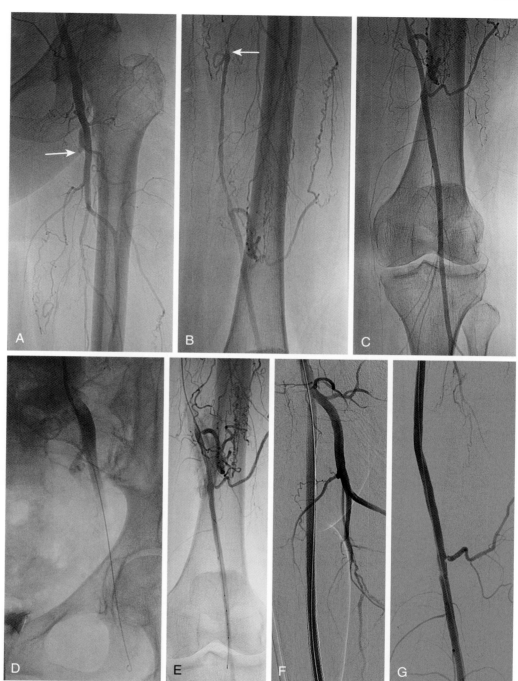

FIGURE 8-30 Superficial femoral artery (SFA) stent graft insertion for occlusive disease. A through C, Left leg arteriography shows an SFA occlusion beginning just beyond its origin *(arrow in A)* and extending to the mid thigh. A diseased SFA then reconstitutes *(arrow in B)*. The distal SFA and left popliteal arteries are normal. D, From the right groin, a curved vascular sheath is advanced into the left external iliac artery. A Rosen wire is advanced through the SFA occlusion. E, The entire obstruction was traversed and a guidewire has entered the above knee popliteal artery. F and G, Viabahn stent grafts were inserted in overlapping fashion to reconstruct the entire left SFA, which is now widely patent.

in some series, but long-term patency and limb salvage rates have not been substantiated.

TIBIAL ARTERY OBSTRUCTION

Infrapopliteal endovascular interventions are almost always performed for limb salvage (Fig. 8-31). Although durability of angioplasty is inferior to distal vein bypass grafts, even short-term patency may be sufficient to allow healing of an ischemic ulcer or amputation site or to avoid amputation altogether.[137] However, tibial recanalization is much less effective when in-line run-off (continuous flow to the pedal arch) is not reestablished or when heroic procedures are performed on patients with severe, widespread infrapopliteal disease because they are poor surgical candidates.

Endovascular options include conventional balloon angioplasty, bare stent placement, or drug-eluting

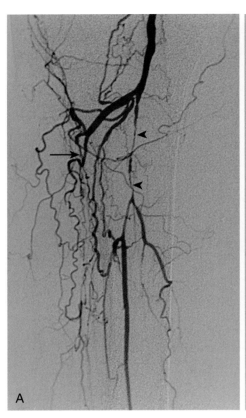
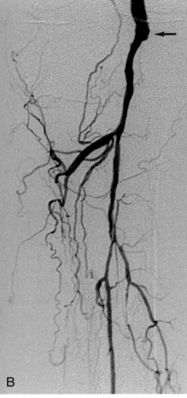

FIGURE 8-31   Severe infrapopliteal disease in a patient with a nonhealing right foot ulcer and patent femoropopliteal graft. **A,** The tibioperoneal trunk has critical stenoses *(arrowheads),* and the posterior and anterior tibial arteries *(arrow)* are occluded proximally. **B,** A 2.5-mm angioplasty balloon was used to reestablish continuous run-off to the foot through the peroneal artery. Notice the below-knee distal graft anastomosis *(arrow).*

stent insertion. The latter measures are clearly appropriate for angioplasty failures.[138,139] Limited evidence to date supports DES over bare stents for this application.[139,140] Technical success can be anticipated for most stenotic lesions (see Table 8-3). Outcomes are better for stenoses than occlusions (patency at 1 year, 68% vs. 48%, respectively).[141] Liberal use of heparin is important to maintain vessel patency after angioplasty. Intraprocedural intraarterial vasodilators may prevent or limit vessel spasm.

COMPLICATIONS

Although most angioplasty and stent procedures proceed without incident, several problems can arise (see Chapter 3).

Vasospasm is most frequently encountered during angioplasty below the knee (Fig. 8-32). Spasm may be largely prevented by giving a vasodilator (e.g., nitroglycerin 100 to 200 μg) immediately before dilation. If severe spasm occurs, more heparin is administered immediately (as needed) to prevent occlusion. Spasm usually resolves with additional intraarterial vasodilator and time.

Repeat angioplasty is performed for acute thrombosis immediately after angioplasty. If the occlusion is long, a brief trial of thrombolytic therapy followed by repeat angioplasty and stent placement often is successful.

For arterial rupture, the balloon is advanced across the torn artery and reinflated. Some ruptures close with this maneuver. If not, placement of a covered stent is usually effective. Otherwise, surgical repair may be needed if the vessel continues to bleed.

Surgical Therapy

For aortoiliac occlusions, surgical options include an AFB graft, extraanatomic graft, or (rarely) endarterectomy.[142] When the external iliac artery is patent, the distal anastomosis is made in an end-to-side fashion to the CFA to maintain perfusion to the pelvis and left colon (Fig. 8-33). Extraanatomic conduits include *axillobifemoral, axillofemoral,* and *femorofemoral grafts* (Fig. 8-34). These grafts are preferred in patients with unilateral iliac disease, high surgical risk, severe scarring from multiple prior vascular procedures, abdominal or groin infections, or chronic occlusion of one limb of an AFB. The 5-year patency of an AFB placed for occlusive disease is 85% to 95%.[142] Complications of bypass grafts are discussed in a later section.

Infrainguinal arterial occlusions not suitable for endovascular therapy are treated with a bypass graft. The large BASIL study confirmed the conventional wisdom that late outcomes (>2 years) were better with infrainguinal surgical bypass than angioplasty as first treatment, although results with prosthetic graft

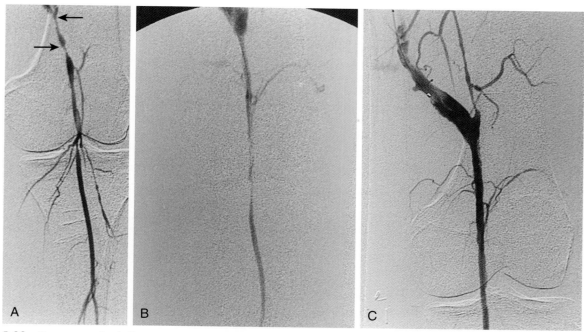

FIGURE 8-32   Vasospasm after balloon angioplasty. **A,** Tight stenoses of the popliteal artery are just beyond a bypass graft anastomosis *(arrows).* **B,** Severe vasospasm occurred after initial angioplasty with a 4-mm balloon. **C,** The vasospasm resolved with additional heparin, intraarterial nitroglycerin (200 μg), and time.

material were poor.[143,144] The indications for an above-knee synthetic (PTFE) bypass graft are vanishing. Two other randomized studies found that patients with SFA occlusive disease had comparable benefit from this form of bypass and ePTFE/nitinol self-expanding stent placement.[145,146] Thus all above-knee femoropopliteal and distal below-knee femoropopliteal, tibial, and pedal grafts should be constructed with vein. If suitable vein is not available, an endovascular approach is generally favored.

Reversed saphenous vein grafts are created by ligating all major tributaries of the vessel, harvesting the graft, and then reversing it so that blood can flow through the valves. *In situ saphenous vein grafts* are constructed by ligating all main tributaries of the dissected vein, anastomosing the proximal and distal ends to the appropriate arteries, and destroying the valves with an endoluminal valvulotome to permit antegrade flow. When the ipsilateral saphenous vein is not suitable, the choices are among short or accessory saphenous veins, the contralateral great saphenous vein, or superficial upper arm vein.[147] A critical step in preoperative planning is to identify a target vessel for distal bypass. Ideally, the selected tibial artery has continuous in-line run-off to the pedal arch.

More than 70% to 80% of in situ lower extremity saphenous vein grafts are patent 5 years after placement.[148] Outcomes are less favorable with prosthetic material and poor with umbilical vein conduit.[149] Good results are expected with distal pedal bypass procedures if patients are properly selected, with 3-year patency and limb salvage rates of about 60% and 90%, respectively.[150-152]

Acute Lower Extremity Ischemia (Online Cases 28, 43, and 99)

Etiology

The most frequent reasons for acute lower extremity ischemia are embolization, thrombosis of diseased native arteries, and occlusion of bypass grafts[14,153] (Box 8-6). Less common causes include trauma and peripheral aneurysm thrombosis or distal embolization. The severity of symptoms is largely determined by the maturity of the collateral circulation. If blood flow is markedly compromised and revascularization is delayed, the result may be muscle/skin necrosis or nerve injury. Acute limb ischemia is a very serious condition. Even in contemporary reports, the mortality rate approaches 20%.[14]

Macroemboli typically arise from the heart in patients with some form of cardiac disease. Less often, clot or large plaque fragments migrate from a proximal artery.[154] Immediately after the embolic event, downstream arteries constrict. Clot then propagates proximally or distally to the next large collateral branch(es). *Microemboli* are minute particles composed of cholesterol crystals, fibrin-platelet deposits, or cellular thrombi that break off from proximal ulcerated plaques or aneurysms[155,156] (see

Chapter 1). The source usually is the aorta or iliac arteries.[157,158] *Cholesterol embolization syndrome* is an acute, life-threatening event usually precipitated by catheterization or aortic manipulation. *Blue toe syndrome* is a more subacute or chronic condition resulting from spontaneous embolization of microemboli. Recurrent embolic showers are the rule, resulting in necrosis and tissue loss in about 60% of cases.

In a native artery or a bypass graft, acute thrombotic occlusion usually is superimposed on underlying disease. If blood flow has been compromised long enough for collateral channels to develop, the patient may present with chronic symptoms rather than sudden onset of ischemia. *In situ thrombosis* without underlying disease virtually always occurs in patients with a thrombophilic state (see Chapter 1 and Boxes 1-4 and 1-5).

Clinical Features

By convention, acute lower extremity ischemia implies symptoms of less than 2 weeks' duration.[14] The physician can usually elicit a history of cardiac disease, atrial dysrhythmias, claudication, or prior bypass graft placement.

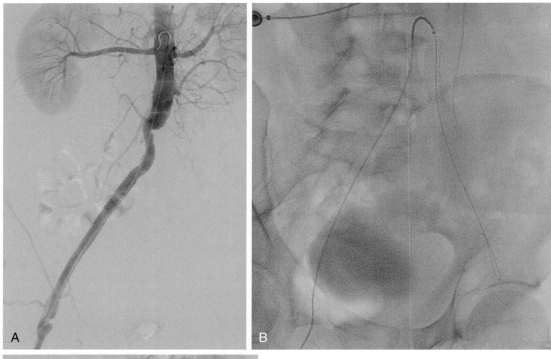

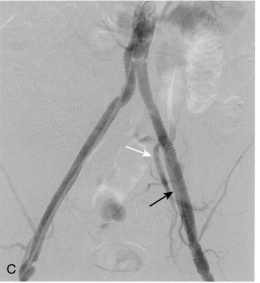

FIGURE 8-33   Thrombosed left limb of aortobifemoral bypass graft placed for aortoiliac occlusive disease. Patient has severe acute left leg ischemic symptoms. **A,** The graft begins near the distal aorta. The right limb is patent. The left limb is occluded. A stent had been placed in the left limb previously for proximal obstructive disease. **B,** Due to the hairpin turn from right to left iliac limb, a 5-French catheter could not be advanced into the left side. Therefore a coaxial Micro Mewi multi-sidehole infusion microcatheter was directed into the left limb of the graft **(B)**, and thrombolysis with tissue plasminogen activator 1 mg/hr begun. After about 14 hours, repeat arteriography shows a widely patent graft **(C).** Patient's symptoms resolved. Note retrograde flow up the left external iliac artery *(black arrow)* and into the internal iliac artery *(white arrow).*

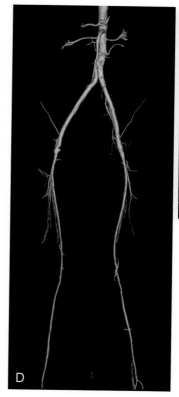

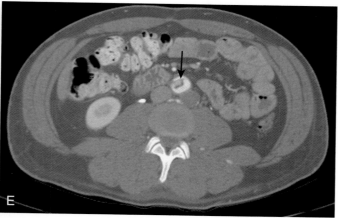

FIGURE 8-33, cont'd **D,** Follow-up reformatted contrast-enhanced shaded surface display computed tomography angiogram shows patent graft and proximal left iliac stent. **E,** However, a liplike defect persists where the two limbs join the native aorta *(arrow).*

The classic "5 *P*s" of a "cold leg" from acute ischemia are pain, pulselessness, pallor, paresthesia, and paralysis. The pulse examination helps determine the level of obstruction. The grade of acute ischemia is determined by physical examination and Doppler signal in the foot (Table 8-6). Classification is critical because it guides the mode of therapy.

The dramatic presentation of cholesterol embolization syndrome is the abrupt onset of a painful, white, marbled extremity ("livido reticularis"), often accompanied by acute renal failure or mesenteric ischemia.

Imaging

COMPUTED TOMOGRAPHY AND MAGNETIC RESONANCE ANGIOGRAPHY

For some patients, immediate surgery without preoperative imaging is appropriate. If the degree of ischemia is relatively mild and intervention is contemplated, CT or MR angiography can be used to confirm the diagnosis and tailor the operative strategy.

CATHETER ANGIOGRAPHY

The majority of patients with acute lower extremity ischemia will benefit from initial endovascular therapy. Therefore, catheter arteriography should be the first study after presentation. Traditionally, the diagnostic arteriogram is done from the contralateral groin (Fig. 8-35). However, if recent imaging studies document normal aortoiliac inflow, direct antegrade CFA puncture on the affected side can simplify thrombolysis and subsequent angioplasty, as long as there is sufficient room to enter the CFA below the inguinal ligament and select the graft or artery (see Chapter 3).

Embolism may be impossible to differentiate from acute thrombosis, although certain angiographic features are characteristic (Fig. 8-36 and see Fig. 1-12; see also Box 1-8). Most macroemboli lodge in the femoral or popliteal artery. Total occlusion can hide an unusual cause for thrombosis, such as a popliteal artery aneurysm (see Fig. 8-14). Rarely, the thoracic aorta is a source of lower extremity emboli (see Fig. 8-36). In situ thrombosis often appears as wormlike filling defects that simulate emboli (see Fig. 1-11).

In patients with microembolization syndromes, proximal atherosclerotic disease (particularly shaggy, ulcerated plaques) or aneurysms usually are detected in the abdominal aorta, iliac arteries, or SFA (Fig. 8-37). It is sometimes impossible to determine which of multiple lesions is responsible for embolic events. Although a continuous channel usually exists between the presumed source and the feet, microemboli can pass through collateral beds around major arterial obstructions.

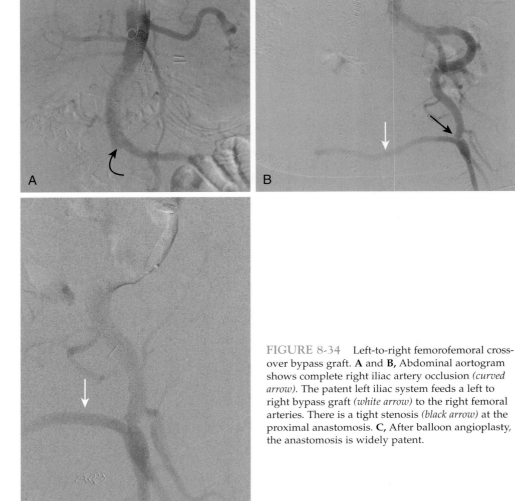

FIGURE 8-34   Left-to-right femorofemoral cross-over bypass graft. **A** and **B,** Abdominal aortogram shows complete right iliac artery occlusion *(curved arrow).* The patent left iliac system feeds a left to right bypass graft *(white arrow)* to the right femoral arteries. There is a tight stenosis *(black arrow)* at the proximal anastomosis. **C,** After balloon angioplasty, the anastomosis is widely patent.

Treatment

Immediate full-dose anticoagulation is indicated in almost every case.[14] The choice between endovascular treatment and immediate operation hinges on the ischemic grade[14,159] (see Table 8-6). The thrombotic or embolic nature of the occlusion may also be an important factor.[160]

- Rutherford category I: a "viable" limb can undergo thrombolysis or urgent operation.
- Rutherford category III: irreversible ischemia ("dead leg") is a contraindication to revascularization—amputation is usually necessary. Only about 10% of patients present in this serious state.[14]

Thrombolysis is futile and potentially dangerous; a life-threatening reperfusion syndrome can result.
- Rutherford category II: the "immediately threatened" limb can be a therapeutic dilemma. Thrombolysis is appropriate if it can be instituted almost immediately. Otherwise, emergent operation is advisable.
- About 50% of patients with a popliteal artery aneurysms initially present with acute limb ischemia.[161-164] The frequency of limb loss in this situation is high (20% to 60%). Except in young individuals, aneurysm should be suspected in all cases of popliteal artery occlusion. An on-table

BOX 8-6

CAUSES OF ACUTE LOWER EXTREMITY ARTERIAL OCCLUSION

- Embolism
  - Macroembolization
    - Heart
    - Proximal atherosclerotic plaque or aneurysm thrombus
    - Catheterization or surgery
    - Paradoxical embolization (through right-to-left shunts)
  - Microembolization
- Thrombosis
  - Secondary to preexisting obstructive disease
  - Arterial bypass grafts
  - Aneurysm thrombosis (e.g., popliteal artery aneurysm)
- In situ thrombosis (thrombophilic states)
- Trauma
- Dissection
- Vasculitis
- Extrinsic compression
  - Popliteal artery entrapment
  - Cystic adventitial disease

ultrasound confirms or excludes the diagnosis. Many experts support catheter-directed thrombolysis before definitive aneurysm treatment[14] (see later section).

Endovascular Therapy

Enzymatic thrombolysis, mechanical thrombectomy, or thromboaspiration are used to manage many acute lower extremity arterial occlusions[165-174] (see Chapter 3). Clot dissolves easily because it is relatively fresh; fibrinolytic agents lyse small vessel thrombus that is inaccessible to surgical removal. In some cases, thrombolysis and angioplasty or stent placement afford definitive treatment without the need for operation. With embolic occlusions, however, fibrinolytic infusion cannot lyse the nidus if it is composed of organized clot or plaque material. There is also the remote possibility that systemic effects of the drug might release more clot from the original embolic source. Even so, most embolic occlusions respond favorably (see Fig. 8-36).

PATIENT SELECTION

Thrombolytic therapy has proven effective in patients with limb-threatening ischemia from an acute occlusion (<14 days old) of native lower extremity arteries and bypass grafts.[175-177] It is sometimes valuable in cases of subacute thrombosis when endovascular therapy is safer than open operation. It has no proven benefit in chronic occlusions (>6 months old).

Selection of patients based on degree of ischemia or nature of the obstruction is discussed earlier. Patients are screened for contraindications to therapy, including risks from thrombolytic agents, anticoagulants, and contrast material (see Boxes 2-2, 2-3, 2-7, and 2-8). Any patient suspected to harbor infected thrombus requires operative clot removal; thrombolysis could precipitate life-threatening sepsis. Finally, success is much more likely if a guidewire can be negotiated through the entire occlusion before beginning lytic therapy ("guidewire traversal test").[178]

TECHNIQUE

The options for endovascular removal of acute lower extremity arterial thrombus include the following:

- Catheter-directed fibrinolytic drug infusion
- Pharmacomechanical thrombolysis (e.g., Trellis device)
- Ultrasound-enhanced catheter-directed thrombolysis[179]
- Mechanical thrombectomy (e.g., AngioJet device)
- Aspiration thrombectomy

The details and relative merits of these various methods are considered in Chapter 3. Strict adherence to recent

TABLE 8-6   Rutherford Classification of Acute Limb Ischemia

Category	Definition	Prognosis	PHYSICAL EXAMINATION		DOPPLER SIGNAL	
			Sensory	Muscle	Arterial	Venous
I	Viable	Salvageable	Intact	Full	+	+
IIA	Threatened, marginal	Salvageable with prompt treatment	Mild loss	Full	±	+
IIB	Severe	Salvageable with immediate treatment	Rest pain	Weak	−	+
III	Irreversible	Permanent tissue loss or nerve damage	Anesthetic	Paralysis	−	−

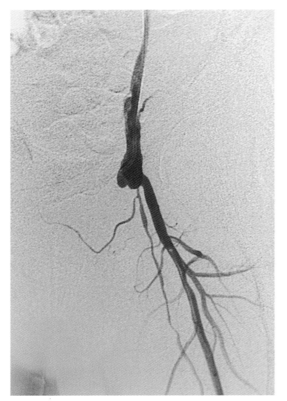

FIGURE 8-35 Acute occlusion of a left in situ saphenous vein femoropopliteal bypass graft that was placed to remedy superficial femoral artery occlusion. Notice the residual graft "nipple" at the bottom of the common femoral artery. Antegrade puncture on this side for recanalization would be difficult because of the short distance between the external iliac artery and graft origin.

guidelines for fibrinolytic agent dosing is necessary to avoid undue bleeding complications.* No single fibrinolytic agent in current use is superior to the others[183-187] (see Table 3-5). Surprisingly, one randomized trial evaluating the direct plasminogen activator *alfimeprase* failed to show any benefit over placebo.[188]

Antiplatelet and antithrombin agents play an important role during this procedure. Unless contraindicated, all patients should receive aspirin 325 mg orally before thrombolysis. Heparin is given in doses that depend on operator preference. In the setting of heparin allergy or history of heparin-induced thrombocytopenia, a direct thrombin inhibitor (e.g., bivalirudin) is an excellent substitute.

Recently, there has been some enthusiasm for use of potent intravenous $\alpha_{IIb}\beta3$ integrin (GP IIb/IIIa) receptor inhibitors to improve the efficacy and speed of lysis[189-191] (see Chapter 3 and Table 3-3). However, none of three randomized trials (PROMPT, APART, and RELAX) that evaluated these agents in acute peripheral arterial

thrombolysis offered convincing support for their routine use.[192-194] Therefore many interventionalists reserve them for special circumstances (e.g., slow response to fibrinolytic agents, presence of a thrombophilic state, and below-knee treatment). If they are used at all, anticoagulant and fibrinolytic doses should be adjusted downward, and platelet counts should be monitored periodically. Sudden and profound thrombocytopenia can occur with some of these drugs.

Before the long fibrinolytic infusion begins, some operators will inject a bolus dose of agent through the multiside hole catheter to accelerate the lytic process (Fig. 8-38). The infusion is then continued while the patient is carefully monitored for local or remote bleeding (e.g., headache or altered mental status) and the condition of treated extremity. Most interventionalists follow hemoglobin, hematocrit, and coagulation parameters every 4 to 6 hours. If fibrinogen levels are monitored, drug infusion is slowed or stopped if the serum level drops below about 100 to 150 mg/dL. Transient worsening of ischemic symptoms is common as clot lyses and small emboli shower distally. In most cases, thrombolysis should still be continued. The patient is reevaluated every 6 to 12 hours by angiography for progression of lysis. When the clot burden is less than 5% or so, any underlying stenoses are treated with angioplasty and/or stent placement. Drug infusion is continued when significant thrombus remains; if substantial lysis has not occurred with 24 hours, further therapy usually is fruitless. Angiography of the distal arteries is always performed to identify subclinical emboli that may need treatment.

Mechanical thrombectomy catheters (see Chapter 3) are popular as primary or adjunctive tools for acute arterial occlusions* (Fig. 8-39). These devices have the potential to shorten procedure times and reduce bleeding complications. They may also be employed in patients with a contraindication to fibrinolytic agents. Potential disadvantages include direct vessel injury, distal embolization, and the cost of the devices. There is very limited published experience with any of these catheters in this setting. Aspiration thrombectomy is especially popular among some interventionalists as first-line treatment for acute arterial thrombosis.[198]

RESULTS

Technical success is achieved in about 75% to 85% of attempts. Although some refined techniques (e.g., pulse-spray injection, high dose infusion, addition of GP IIb/IIIa inhibitors) may accelerate lysis, there is no evidence that their routine use alters limb salvage rates or need for additional interventions. Common reasons for technical failure include inability to traverse the obstruction, the

---

*See references 166-169, 174, 180-182.

*See references 153, 170, 171, 195-197.

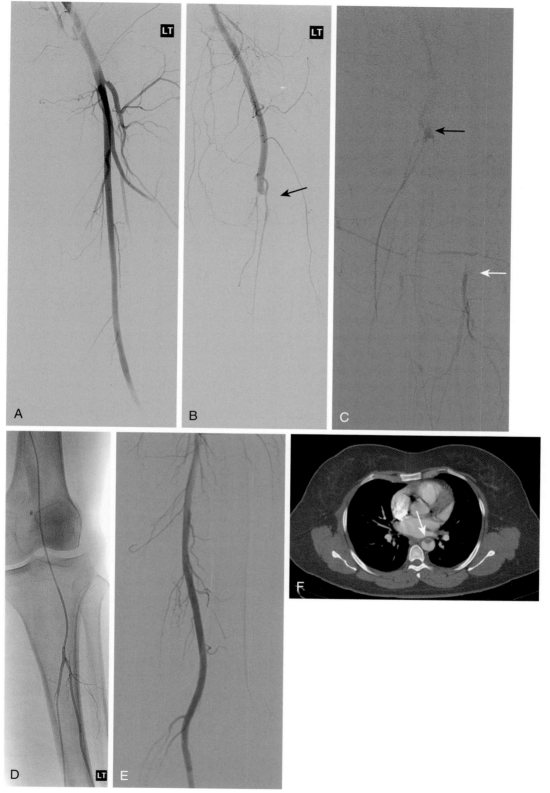

FIGURE 8-36   Thrombolysis of a left popliteal artery embolus. **A** through **C,** Left leg arteriography shows a filling defect in the above-knee popliteal artery *(black arrow).* The collateral circulation is very immature. The proximal femoral arteries are entirely normal. There is distal reconstitution of the tibioperoneal trunk *(white arrow).* **D,** A multiside hole infusion catheter now spans the occlusion. **E,** After overnight thrombolysis with tissue plasminogen activator at 1 mg/hr, the thrombus is completely lysed with no underlying disease. **F,** Later, contrast-enhanced computed tomography scan shows the probable culprit thrombus in the descending thoracic aorta *(white arrow).*

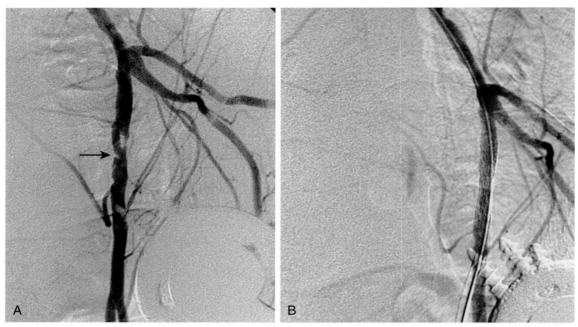

FIGURE 8-37   Iliac artery stent placement for left-sided blue toe syndrome. **A,** A complex, ulcerated plaque is detected in the distal left external iliac artery *(arrow).* **B,** Primary stent placement was done to remodel and cover the plaque to prevent recurrent microembolization.

presence of organized clot, inadequate anticoagulation, a thrombophilic state, and poor run-off.

Three randomized clinical trials (STILES, TOPAS, University of Rochester) have substantiated the equivalence of catheter-directed thrombolysis and surgery in patients with acute lower extremity arterial ischemia with respect to limb salvage and mortality.[165,175-177,199] In patients suffering from microembolization syndromes, PTA and stents are sometimes effective in remodelling, removing, or covering the embolic surface and preventing recurrent showering of particles[200] (see Fig. 8-37).

COMPLICATIONS

The most important adverse events from lower extremity thrombolytic therapy are outlined in Table 3-6. Major complications are relatively frequent in some series. Causes of bleeding are multifactorial and include a systemic "lytic state" from fibrinogen depletion, lysis of hemostatic plugs (e.g., in the brain) by fibrin-specific agents, effects of anticoagulants or antiplatelet agents, and patient-related factors. Other problems include pericatheter thrombosis, reperfusion or compartment syndrome, drug reaction, and vessel or graft extravasation.

About 15% of patients require fasciotomy for *compartment syndrome* following revascularization of an ischemic limb.[14] This disorder reflects increased capillary permeability and fluid accumulation within the anterior (and less often posterior) fascial space following

restoration of blood flow. The diagnosis is suggested by pain, sensory deficits, and swelling. Fasciotomy is usually necessary when the intracompartment pressure exceeds 20 mm Hg.

Reperfusion syndrome is a consequence of massive *rhabdomyolysis,* which is manifested by a spike in serum creatine kinase (>5000 units/L), myoglobinuria (with tea-colored urine), and acute renal failure.[14] Standard treatment is vigorous IV hydration and alkalinization of the urine.

Surgical Therapy

Operative revascularization entails bypass procedures almost identical to those used for chronic limb ischemia (see previous discussion). For acute embolic occlusions, Fogarty balloon thromboembolectomy or intraoperative fibrinolytic infusion are used. Ultimately, the offending source of emboli must be removed, remodeled, or excluded by endovascular or operative means.

Arterial Bypass Graft Failure (Online Cases 43 and 97)

Etiology and Clinical Features

Immediate complications of an AFB graft include occlusion, bleeding, colonic ischemia, and spinal cord ischemia. Late complications include infection, pseudoaneurysm formation, partial or complete thrombosis, and *aortoenteric*

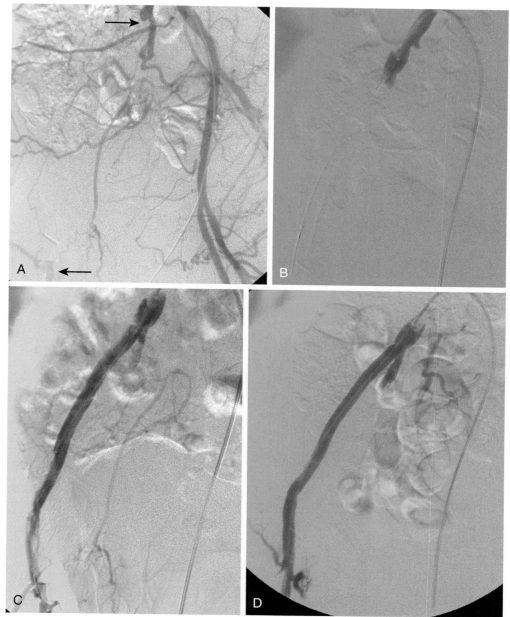

FIGURE 8-38 Iliac artery thrombolysis for acute ischemic symptoms. **A,** Right posterior oblique pelvic angiogram shows complete occlusion of a graft *(between arrows)* from the right external iliac artery to the deep femoral artery. **B,** A guiding sheath was placed over the aortic bifurcation and the occlusion traversed with an angled hydrophilic guidewire. A pulse-spray catheter with multiple side slits spans the lesion. **C,** After 35 minutes of periodic injection of tissue plasminogen activator to a dose of 4 mg, there is substantial lysis. **D,** Following additional overnight infusion of the drug at 0.5 mg/hr, the graft is widely patent.

fistula (see Fig. 7-13). Early graft thrombosis often is the result of an operative error. Late graft thrombosis is caused by neointimal hyperplasia at graft anastomoses, progressive atherosclerosis, pseudoaneurysm formation, or infection.

Early or subacute infrainguinal bypass graft failure has several causes (Box 8-7). The major reasons for delayed infrainguinal graft failure are graft stenosis from neointimal hyperplasia, progression of atherosclerosis, and poor run-off. About half of the obstructions develop within the graft, and the remainder occur at the anastomoses or within native arteries.[201]

Most patients with acute graft thrombosis present with sudden onset of ischemia (see earlier). However, less than 50% of individuals with graft dysfunction and impending failure are symptomatic.

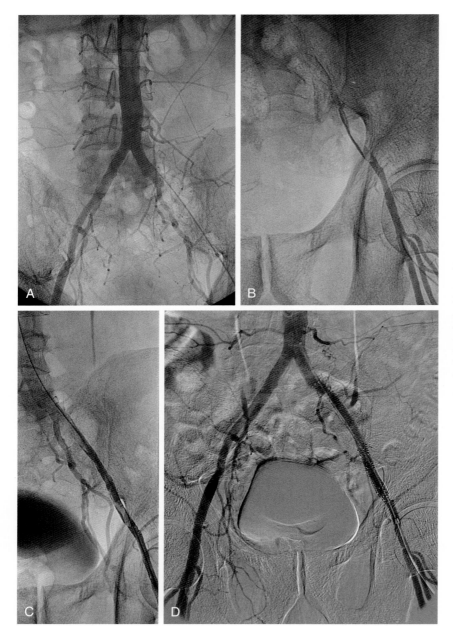

FIGURE 8-39   Iliac artery mechanical thrombectomy and stent placement for acute ischemic symptoms. **A** and **B,** Pelvic arteriograms show near-total left external iliac artery occlusion. A guidewire passed easily from the left common femoral artery puncture site. **C,** After use of the AngioJet thrombectomy device, there is moderate clot removal. **D,** Tandem balloon expandable stents were placed over the entire occlusion to restore essentially normal flow.

Imaging

NONINVASIVE SCREENING

Routine surveillance of infrainguinal venous bypass grafts is necessary to identify conditions that predispose to complete occlusion. Screening entails periodic measurement of the ABI and color Doppler sonography of the graft.[202,203] An angiographic study (noninvasive or catheter-based) is warranted when one or more of the following criteria are met (Figs. 8-40 and 8-41):

- A fall in ABI by 0.15 to 0.20, or 10% of baseline
- Graft body peak systolic velocity (PSV) of less than 40 to 45 cm/second

- Peak systolic velocity greater than 300 cm/sec at a stenosis detected with color imaging
- Systolic velocity ratio greater than 3.5 at the site of a suspected stenosis versus adjacent normal graft

Surveillance programs extend the longevity of infrainguinal venous bypass grafts; in addition, conduits are much more durable after detected stenoses are repaired than after thrombosed grafts are recanalized.[201,204]

CROSS-SECTIONAL TECHNIQUES

CT and MR angiography are at least as accurate as color Doppler sonography for screening.[35,205,206] However, because of the longer procedure time and greater expense, they are only used when there is other evidence for graft dysfunction. Cross-sectional angiography guides operation when endovascular repair is not contemplated.

CATHETER ANGIOGRAPHY

The findings with a failing or occluded bypass graft include complete thrombosis, focal or long segment stenoses, clamp injuries, arteriovenous fistulas (AVFs),

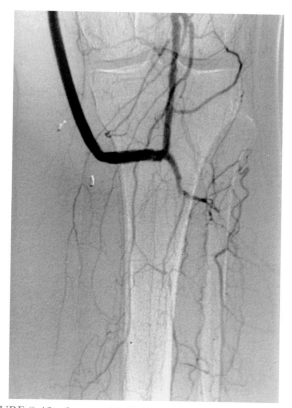

FIGURE 8-40 Sonographic detection of a failing left femoropopliteal bypass graft. Sonography showed diffuse decreased velocities in the range of 20 to 30 cm/sec. The angiogram shows a widely patent graft and anastomoses but almost no distal run-off.

retained valve cusps, anastomotic native arterial stenoses, pseudoaneurysms, and poor distal run-off (Figs. 8-42 through 8-44; see also Figs. 8-33 through 8-35, 8-40, and 8-41).

Endovascular Therapy

Percutaneous treatment is generally inferior to surgical revision or a new bypass.[207,208] However, the secondary patency of most endovascular procedures for stenotic lesions is excellent. Thus angioplasty or stent insertion is a reasonable first (and sometimes definitive) step for bypass graft stenoses[209] (see Fig. 8-34). Factors that predict poor outcome with endovascular methods are long lesion length (>2 cm), multiple stenoses, and early stenoses (within 3 months of construction).[151] If antegrade puncture of the common femoral artery feeding an infrainguinal graft is not feasible, angioplasty is done from the opposite groin with the aid of a guiding catheter advanced over the aortic bifurcation. Many graft-related stenoses are quite fibrotic and require multiple, prolonged balloon inflations or use of a cutting balloon.[210] Some AVFs may be closed with embolotherapy (see Fig. 8-43).

Acute thrombosis of an AFB is often amenable to thrombolytic therapy (see Fig. 8-33). On the other hand, the role of thrombolysis for clotted infrainguinal bypass grafts is questionable.[211,212] Although revascularization is initially successful in more than 90% of cases, long-term results are dismal (20% to 60% patency at 1 year).[151,211-214] Still, these results are not much worse than those for surgical thrombectomy and revision. Most interventionalists have abandoned this procedure unless surgical options are exhausted (see Chapter 3).

Surgical Therapy

Failing grafts are repaired with a patch graft or graft extension. Retained valves are obliterated with an endoluminal valvulotome. Clotted grafts require surgical thrombectomy and revision or complete graft replacement. With infrainguinal conduits, the 2-year patency rate for the former approach is less than 40%.[211]

Aneurysms (Online Cases 28 and 81)

Etiology

Pelvic and lower extremity artery aneurysms may be true (e.g., degenerative [atherosclerosis-associated]) or false (e.g., post-traumatic)[215-217] (Box 8-8). For lower extremity *degenerative aneurysms*, bilaterality is the rule; individuals with popliteal and CFA aneurysms often have such lesions at other sites.

Popliteal artery aneurysms (PAA) (vessel diameter ≥1 cm) account for more than two thirds of lower extremity degenerative aneurysms.[218,219] PAA are bilateral in about one half of cases and are associated with abdominal aortic aneurysms (AAA) in about one third

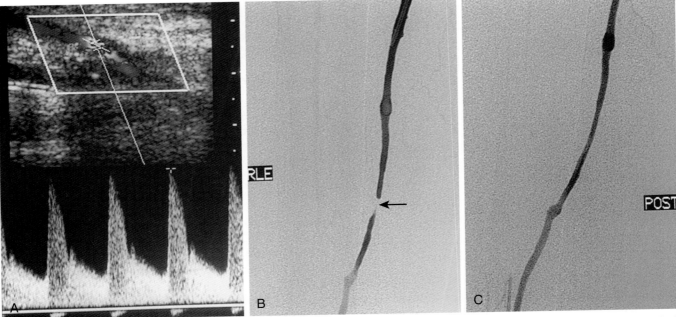

FIGURE 8-41   Stenosis of an in situ saphenous vein bypass graft in an asymptomatic patient. **A,** The sonogram detected overall diminished velocities (13 to 28 cm/sec) but a markedly increased velocity (512 cm/sec) in the middle thigh. **B,** A critical intragraft stenosis was discovered at catheter angiography *(arrow).* **C,** It was treated successfully with a 4-mm balloon.

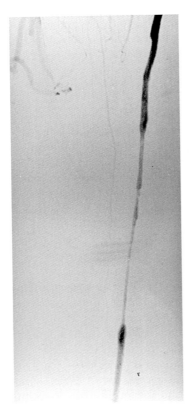

FIGURE 8-42   Long-segment fibrosis of a right saphenous vein infrainguinal bypass graft.

of cases.[220,221] The major clinical sequelae are thrombosis and distal embolization. Symptomatic extrinsic compression of the popliteal vein or tibial nerve is infrequent. Rupture is quite rare.

Common iliac artery (CIA) aneurysm is present when the vessel diameter exceeds 1.5 to 2 cm.[217,222] Some are isolated; others reflect extensions of AAA (see Fig. 7-11). CIA aneurysms are at particular risk for rupture when they are larger than 3.5 cm.[217] Ilioiliac or iliocaval fistula is a much rarer complication. In one series, the relative frequency of *isolated* common, internal, and external iliac aneurysms was 89%, 10%, and 1%, respectively[223] (Fig. 8-45). *Common femoral artery aneurysms* are unusual. True aneurysms of the SFA, DFA, and infrapopliteal artery are rare.[216]

Most false aneurysms of lower extremity arteries are post-traumatic (e.g., postcatheterization femoral artery pseudoaneurysms). Although some of these lesions close spontaneously, expansion and rupture is a significant concern for large or persistent lesions. *Infectious (mycotic) aneurysms* can occur anywhere but have a predilection for the iliac and common femoral vessels.[224] The offending organism usually is *Salmonella* or *Staphylococcus* species. Pseudoaneurysms at graft anastomoses often are a consequence of indolent infection.[225]

Clinical Features

Pelvic and lower extremity degenerative aneurysms are very much a disease of men.[216,217] Many patients with iliac artery aneurysms are asymptomatic. In particular,

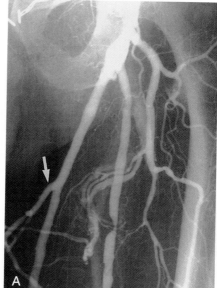

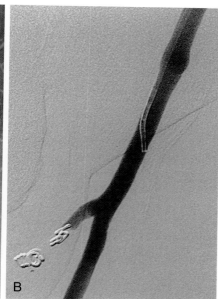

FIGURE 8-43 Arteriovenous graft fistula. **A,** The left in situ saphenous vein bypass graft has a large, nonligated tributary *(arrow)*. **B,** A 5-French catheter was advanced into the tributary from the contralateral groin and used to embolize the branch.

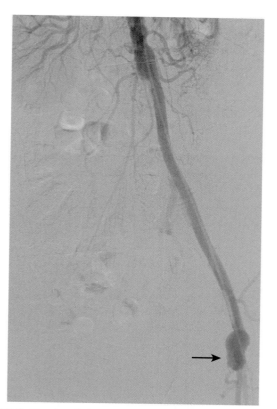

FIGURE 8-44 Aortobifemoral bypass graft with pseudoaneurysm of left distal anastomosis *(arrow)* and complete occlusion of right limb.

internal iliac artery aneurysms often are silent until they rupture.[223,226] Warning symptoms are related to compression of adjacent structures or (rarely) fistulization with a pelvic organ. Up to one third of popliteal artery aneurysms are unsuspected at the time of diagnosis.[220]

Some are detected by physical examination. Degenerative CFA aneurysms may present with local swelling and pain or evidence for distal embolization; a substantial number of patients are also asymptomatic. Catheterization-related pseudoaneurysms can produce a pulsatile, expanding mass. Classically, patients with mycotic aneurysms have fever, local tenderness, and a risk factor for bacteremia or groin infection (e.g., intravenous drug abuse).

Imaging

CROSS-SECTIONAL TECHNIQUES

For aneurysm detection and surveillance, MR or CT imaging is used for the iliac arteries and color Doppler sonography for the infrainguinal arteries.[227] Sonography is essentially 100% accurate in the diagnosis of postcatheterization pseudoaneurysms. These lesions are characterized by swirling color flow in the aneurysm sac and to-and-fro flow at the aneurysm neck (see Figs. 3-10 and 3-12). On MR or CT angiography, a pelvic or peripheral aneurysm may display intimal calcification, fusiform widening of the artery, and mural thrombus[228] (Figs. 8-45 through 8-48). Popliteal artery aneurysms usually spare the distal segment of the artery.

CATHETER ANGIOGRAPHY

Degenerative aneurysms are typically fusiform and may be solitary or multiple. Aneurysms that are saccular, eccentric, or atypical in location should raise the suspicion of an unusual cause, such as infection or trauma (see Fig. 8-48). Aneurysms can be missed at angiography

---

BOX 8-8

CAUSES OF PELVIC AND LOWER EXTREMITY ANEURYSMS

True Aneurysms

- Degenerative
- Infectious (mycotic)
- Noninflammatory vasculopathy
  - Marfan syndrome
  - Ehlers-Danlos syndrome
  - Human immunodeficiency virus arteriopathy
- Vasculitis
  - Behçet disease
  - Polyarteritis nodosa
- Congenital

False Aneurysms

- Traumatic
  - Iatrogenic
  - Accidental
  - Anastomotic
- Infectious
- Erosive (e.g., extrinsic compression by osteophytes)

---

if they are noncalcified and thrombosed or lined with mural thrombus (see Fig. 8-14).

Endovascular Therapy

When anatomically feasible, common iliac artery aneurysms (contained or ruptured) are usually repaired by endovascular means with stent grafts. Preemptive embolization of the ipsilateral internal iliac artery may be necessary to avoid a type II endoleak (see Chapter 7) after device deployment. Published results (including patency rates and subsequent rupture rates) have been excellent.[217,229-232]

The rationale for repair of popliteal artery aneurysms is prevention of ischemia and limb loss from aneurysm thrombosis or distal embolization. Elective treatment of asymptomatic lesions is usually recommended when the aneurysm is greater than 2 cm or mural thrombus is detected.[233-235] However, the presence of symptomatic nerve or vein compression mandates operation. Stent grafts have become very popular among interventionalists in this setting, especially in individuals at high risk for operation or who lack suitable vein for bypass. The ePTFE-nitinol Viabahn device is favored by many operators. Deployment is usually done with an antegrade femoral artery puncture. The graft is oversized to no more than 10% to 15% of the nominal diameter of the vessel. Stents should be inserted with knowledge of the vascular flexion point

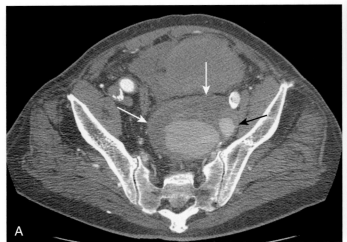
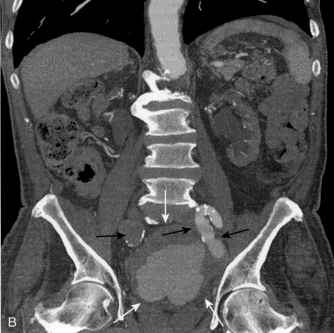

FIGURE 8-45   Ruptured, isolated left internal iliac artery aneurysm. **A** and **B,** Axial and reformatted coronal computed tomography images show aneurysmal enlargement of the calcified left internal iliac artery *(black arrows)*. A pseudoaneurysm has been produced from contained rupture. Surrounding low-density fluid suggests prior leak *(white arrows)*. A right iliac artery aneurysm is also noted *(most rightward black arrow).*

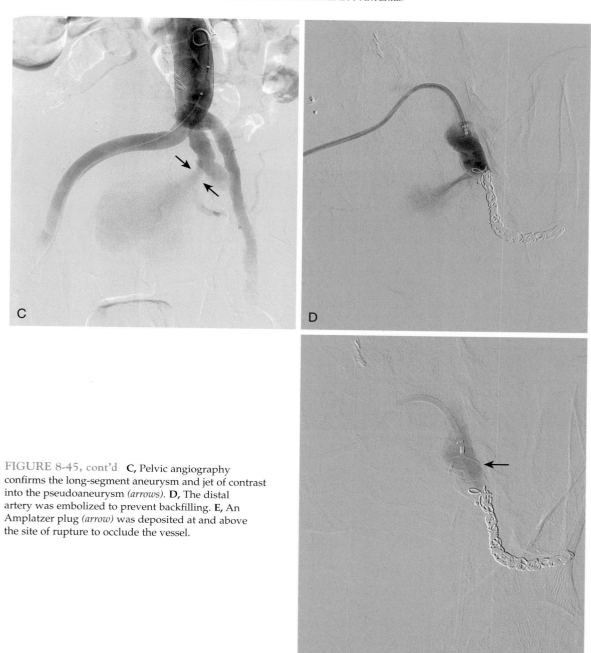

FIGURE 8-45, cont'd **C,** Pelvic angiography confirms the long-segment aneurysm and jet of contrast into the pseudoaneurysm *(arrows).* **D,** The distal artery was embolized to prevent backfilling. **E,** An Amplatzer plug *(arrow)* was deposited at and above the site of rupture to occlude the vessel.

as determined at fluoroscopy. Proximal and distal landing zones of at least 2 cm are necessary.[234] Tandem grafts should have at least 2 cm overlap in case of delayed component separation. Aspirin and clopidogrel are prescribed for at least 3 months afterward to optimize patency. Patients are followed with periodic imaging for late complications including graft thrombosis and endoleak (types II, I or III; see Chapter 7). A recent metaanalysis of the existing literature and one randomized controlled trial showed no significant

difference in primary or secondary patency rates at 3 years for open and endovascular treatment.[219,236] In patients with acute ischemia from popliteal artery aneurysm thrombosis or distal embolization, thrombolysis before definitive repair is now standard of care[161,163,234,237] (see Fig. 8-14).

Internal iliac artery aneurysms are notorious for completely unexpected rupture; elective repair is indicated in most cases. They can be obliterated with complete internal iliac artery embolization (see Fig. 8-45) or

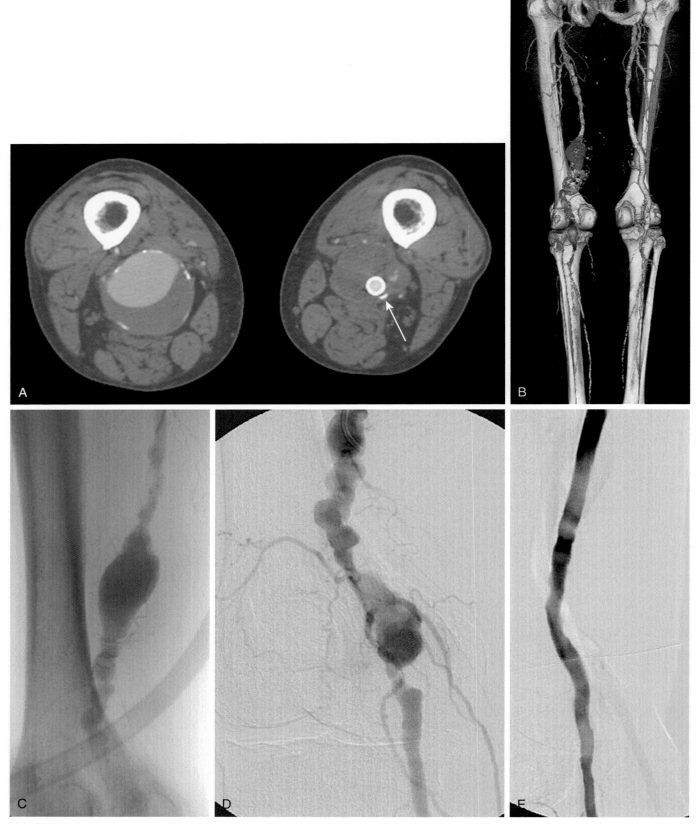

FIGURE 8-46   Popliteal artery (PA) aneurysm. **A** and **B,** Axial and reformatted shaded-surface display computed tomography images show a large, bipartite, above-knee, right PA aneurysm with wall calcification and mural thrombus. A left-sided aneurysm had been previously repaired with a prosthetic bypass graft *(arrow).* **C** and **D,** Right leg angiography shows the tandem degenerative PA aneurysms with diffuse arteriomegaly in the intervening segments. **E,** The aneurysms were treated by endovascular Viabahn stent graft placement, which has restored a normal lumen.

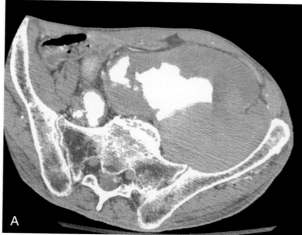

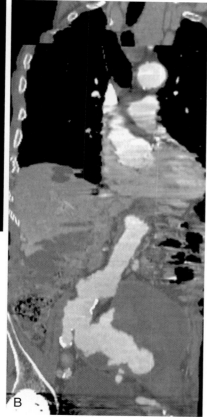

FIGURE 8-47 Ruptured left common iliac artery aneurysm. The patient presented with pelvic pain and hypotension. Transverse **(A)** and reformatted coronal **(B)** computed tomography images show a massive aneurysm with ill-defined hyperattenuation in the thrombus, indicating active extravasation.

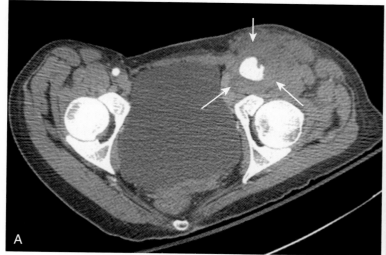

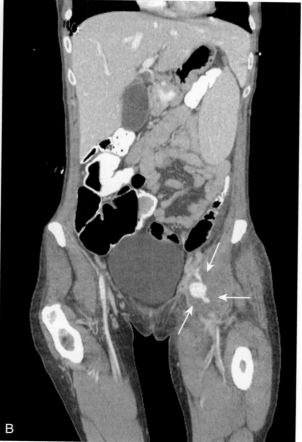

FIGURE 8-48 Mycotic left common femoral artery (CFA) aneurysm in an intravenous drug user. **A** and **B,** Axial and reformatted coronal contrast-enhanced computed tomography images show a large saccular aneurysm of the left CFA with surrounding low-density tissue representing prominent inflammatory reaction *(arrows).*

distal occlusion of the vessel followed by placement of a covered stent over its origin.[238,239] Distal embolization is necessary to prevent aneurysm backfilling through pelvic collaterals. Treatment of postcatheterization pseudoaneurysms[240-242] is described in Chapter 3.

Surgical Therapy

Iliac and CFA aneurysms are excluded with a bypass graft. Postcatheterization femoral artery pseudoaneurysms are operated only if percutaneous thrombin injection or ultrasound-guided neck compression fails and the aneurysm continues to expand. Open PAA repair involves saphenous vein bypass grafting with proximal and distal aneurysm ligation.[161-164,237] The mean 5-year patency rate is about 72%.[219]

Pelvic Trauma (Online Cases 54 and 80)

Etiology and Clinical Features

Because the branches of the internal iliac artery run close to the bony and ligamentous structures of the pelvis, they are frequently injured during severe blunt pelvic trauma from motor vehicle crashes, falls from a height, and crush accidents. The mechanism of injury in the subgroup with persistent arterial bleeding often is severe anteroposterior compression (with diastasis of the symphysis pubis, pubic rami fractures, and sacroiliac joint disruption) or lateral compression (with sacral and pubic rami fractures).[243,244]

Most patients with pelvic arterial hemorrhage are hypotensive, and some have extensive multiorgan injury. The initial decision to opt for conservative management, angiographic evaluation, or operation is often a difficult one.

Imaging

CROSS-SECTIONAL IMAGING

In most trauma centers, focused abdominal sonography in trauma (FAST) has replaced diagnostic peritoneal lavage (DPL) to identify abdominal bleeding that requires immediate operation. CT scanning is also extremely valuable in this setting.[245] It delineates pelvic fractures, associated hematomas, active arterial or venous bleeding, and any associated internal organ injury. However, the place of CT in initial pelvic trauma management is still debated.

CATHETER ANGIOGRAPHY

Evaluation starts with nonselective arteriography of the entire pelvis and femoral regions. This step provides a road map for further catheterization and identifies massive bleeding that must be addressed first. Then the following sources of bleeding should be considered:

- Bilateral internal iliac arteries and branches. Identification of one bleeding vessel does not end the search for other lesions
- Bilateral external iliac arteries and branches[246] (e.g., inferior epigastric artery, anomalous origin of obturator artery; Fig. 8-49 and see Fig. 8-4)
- Lumbar arteries[247] (Fig. 8-50)
- Visceral arteries if there is any suspicion of hemorrhage from a solid organ

Arterial hemorrhage is marked by discrete and focal, or multiple punctate sites of contrast extravasation (see Fig. 1-37). Additional findings include abrupt vessel occlusion and severe tapering from vasospasm. Care must be taken not to mistake bowel activity, hypervascularity, or "road dirt" for a bleeding site. The most commonly injured vessels are the superior gluteal and internal pudendal arteries.

Treatment

Management begins with immediate resuscitation followed by clinical and imaging assessment for associated injuries. Venous and minor arterial bleeding often stop with external compressive fixation of the pelvis done in a variety of ways. In isolated pelvic trauma, surgery is generally avoided, because it is almost impossible to find the bleeding vessels at operation and because exploration releases the tamponading effect of the hematoma below the pelvic peritoneum. Angiography with intent to embolize is indicated for the following[244,248]:

- Hemodynamically unstable patients with negative FAST or presence of pelvic hematoma on CT
- Hemodynamically stable patient with active bleeding on pelvic CT scan and no evidence of hollow viscus injury that would demand operation
- Identification of pelvic hematoma at laparotomy with persistent hypotension
- Elderly patients or long duration of hypotension whether stable or unstable (controversial)[249]

ENDOVASCULAR THERAPY

Embolization is the definitive therapy for traumatic pelvic arterial hemorrhage (see Figs. 8-49 and 8-50). If the patient is exsanguinating and massive extravasation is seen, bleeding must be stopped with alacrity by rapidly depositing stainless steel coils, Gelfoam, or both in the proximal internal iliac artery. In most situations, however, there is time for selective embolization of the damaged arteries. If multiple bleeding sites are found, "scatter (shower) embolization" with small Gelfoam

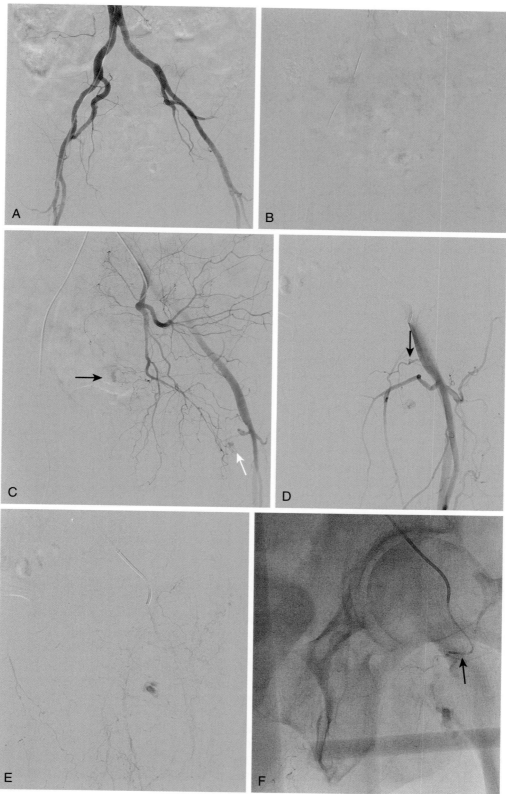

FIGURE 8-49 Arterial bleeding from pelvic injury due to a motor vehicle collision. **A** and **B,** The initial pelvic arteriogram did not show bleeding. **C,** Left internal iliac arteriography shows probable extravasation *(white arrow)* but it did not appear to arise from that vessel. A focal density in the left medial pelvis *(black arrow)* proved to be artifactual. **D** and **E,** Left external iliac arteriography identifies the external pudendal artery as the likely culprit *(arrow),* which was proven with coaxial microcatheterization of that vessel. **F,** The vessel was embolized with microcoils and a single small Gelfoam piece.

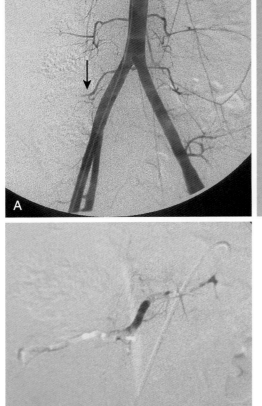

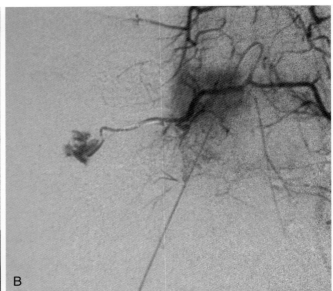

FIGURE 8-50   Lumbar artery embolization for pelvic trauma. **A,** Pelvic arteriogram reveals truncation of the right fourth lumbar artery *(arrow).* Neither selective internal iliac artery study showed extravasation or abnormal vessels. **B,** Shetty catheter was used to engage the common L4 trunk; active bleeding is evident. **C,** The vessel was embolized to stasis with Gelfoam torpedoes via a selective microcatheter.

pieces often is appropriate (see Chapter 3). Some interventionalists embolize truncated or narrowed arteries that are not actively bleeding on the grounds that hemorrhage may have come or may resume from these injured vessels. The vascular beds that should be examined are outlined previously. After embolotherapy is complete, it is wise to reinject both internal iliac arteries to confirm that hemorrhage has stopped and that collateral branches are not reconstituting the bleeding vessel. In the unlikely event that the common or external iliac artery itself is lacerated, placement of a stent graft can be curative (Fig. 8-51).

A significant fraction of patients with initially negative angiography but clinical or imaging evidence for persistent bleeding will show extravasation at repeat angiography.[250] Even bilateral internal iliac artery embolization is well tolerated in most individuals; the collateral circulation usually is sufficient to prevent ischemia of the pelvic organs. However, buttock and thigh paresthesia can occur.[251] Skin sloughing is rare but can be serious. Sexual dysfunction (which is frequent

after pelvic fractures) is probably related to the injury itself rather than embolization.[252]

Lower Extremity Trauma (Online Case 5)

Etiology and Clinical Features

Lower extremity arteries are subject to injury from penetrating objects, blunt trauma, medical procedures (e.g., catheterization), and bone fractures or joint dislocations.[253] Postcatheterization abnormalities include pseudoaneurysm or AVF formation, dissection, and thrombosis. Any long bone fracture can damage a major artery; posterior knee dislocations are a classic cause of popliteal artery injury[254] (Fig. 8-52).

Some patients have symptoms that strongly predict a clinically significant arterial injury ("hard signs"), including active bleeding, diminished distal pulses, expanding or pulsatile hematoma, neurologic deficit, or evidence of distal ischemia.[255] Others have less convincing findings, namely proximity of the injury to a major artery, small hematoma, or unexplained hypotension.

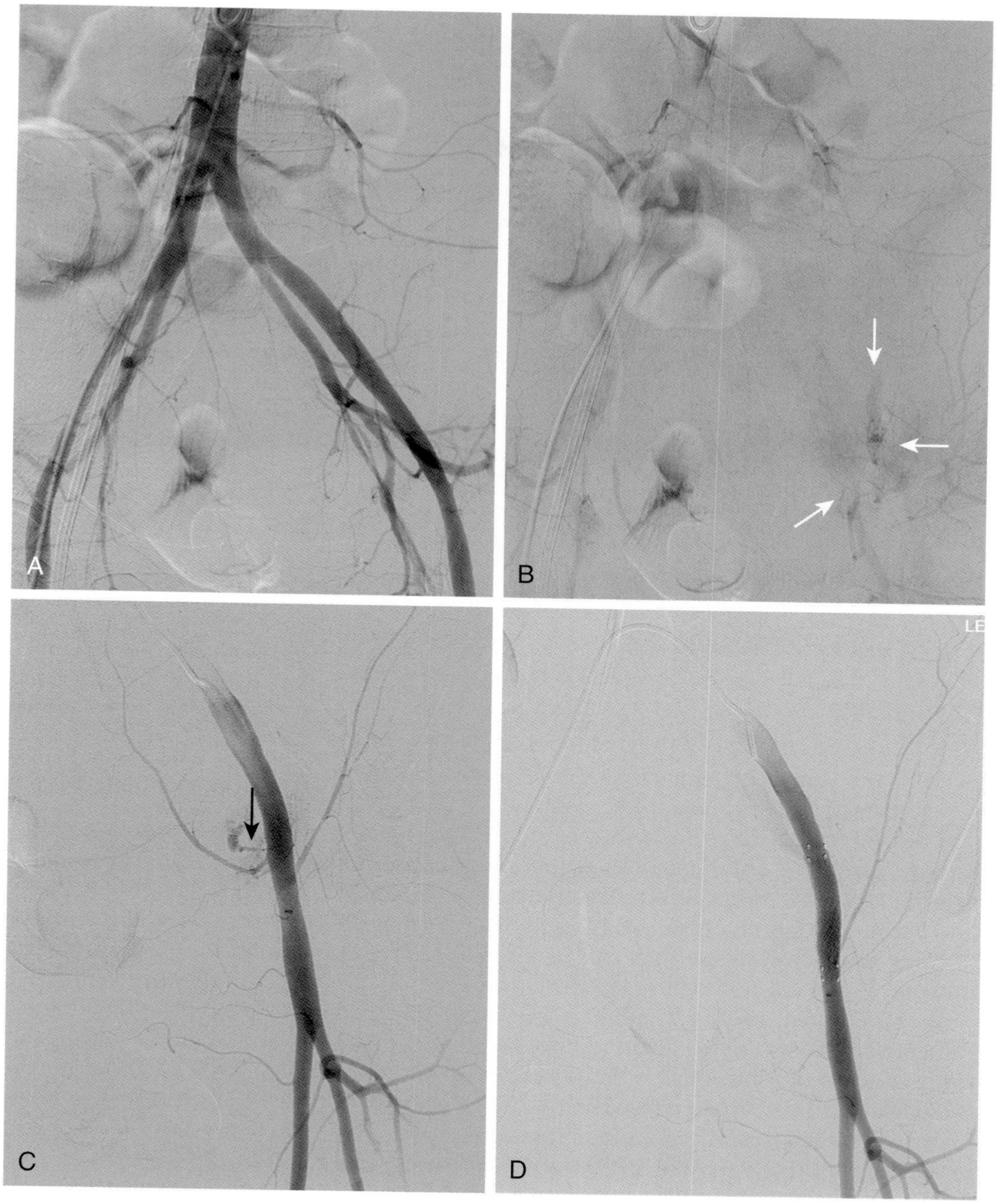

FIGURE 8-51 External iliac artery tear with massive hemorrhage from attempted dialysis catheter placement. **A** and **B,** Pelvic arteriography shows diffuse extravasation in the left lower pelvis *(arrows)* but does not identify the precise bleeding point. **C,** Selective left external iliac arteriography show the point of leak just above the inferior epigastric artery *(black arrow).* **D,** The leak was sealed with a covered stent.

AVFs may become apparent long after the traumatic event.

Imaging

Several large clinical studies have shown that the frequency of arterial injuries that require endovascular or surgical intervention in the absence of hard signs is only 0% to 3%.[255,256] Therefore this population should be screened before CT or catheter angiography or surgical exploration based on the physical examination findings and quick noninvasive tests. In one widely used algorithm, patients with intact distal pulses, an ABI greater than 1.00, and no hard signs are managed conservatively. Well-accepted indications for imaging include the following[255,257,258]:

- Abnormal ABI (<1.0)
- Blunt or penetrating trauma with hard signs
- Penetrating trauma in the setting of a shotgun injury, projectile path that follows a major artery for a long distance, history of PAD, or extensive limb injury
- Postoperative evaluation
- Delayed diagnosis

There is a short therapeutic window (about 6 to 8 hours) between acute injury and the possibility of permanent

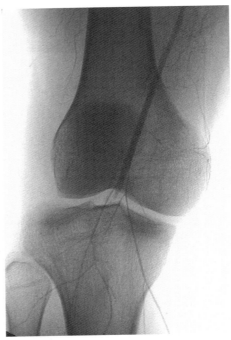

FIGURE 8-52   Complete popliteal artery occlusion after posterior knee dislocation.

nerve injury due to ischemia; therefore definitive imaging (or operation) must proceed without delay.

Color Doppler sonography is a standard tool for detecting iatrogenic and some accidental lower extremity arterial injuries[259] (Figs. 8-53 and 8-54 and see Figs. 3-10 and 3-12). Sonography also is extremely useful for identifying venous injuries, which can be a major source of morbidity and are not visible at arteriography.[260]

For the most part, CT angiography has replaced catheter arteriography in evaluation of blunt and penetrating extremity trauma.[261-263] The latter is reserved for endovascular repair procedures. The spectrum of findings at angiography includes intimal tears, intraluminal thrombus, vasospasm, intramural hematoma, dissection, transection with or without thrombosis, vessel deviation, AVF, pseudoaneurysm, and slow flow (which can be seen with a compartment syndrome) (Fig. 8-55; see Figs. 8-52 through 8-54; see also Figs. 1-3, 1-21, 1-34, 3-10 and 3-11).

Treatment

ENDOVASCULAR THERAPY

Embolotherapy is used to treat pseudoaneurysms, AVFs, or extravasation arising from minor arterial branches.[264] The neck of a pseudoaneurysm or AVF must be completely excluded from the circulation (distally and proximally) to prevent delayed backfilling through collateral vessels (see Fig. 8-54). Gelfoam pieces and coils are the most commonly used agents. Bleeding tibial ar-

teries can be embolized if at least one (and preferably two) calf arteries are intact.[265]

Stent-grafts are effective in closing major artery pseudoaneurysms, AVFs, and rupture that would not be amenable to embolotherapy[266] (see Fig. 8-51).

SURGICAL THERAPY

Significant injury to a named artery is sometimes managed by direct repair or bypass graft placement, ideally with autologous vein. Isolated tibial artery injuries are sometimes left alone. Many trauma surgeons simply observe minor vascular injuries such as nonocclusive intimal flaps, intramural hematomas, small (<1 cm) pseudoaneurysms, and small asymptomatic AVFs.[267] These lesions usually have a benign course.

OTHER DISORDERS

Dissection

Lower extremity arterial dissection most often results from extension of an abdominal aortic dissection or a medical procedure such as catheterization (see Chapters 3 and 7).

Retroperitoneal Bleeding

Retroperitoneal hemorrhage (RPH) may be either spontaneous or post-traumatic. Most patients with "spontaneous" bleeding have a coagulopathic condition due to an underlying illness or anticoagulant medication. Blood may accumulate in the retroperitoneal space or rectus sheath (*rectus sheath hematoma*).[268] The diagnosis is based on clinical suspicion (localized pain or mass, hypotension, falling hemoglobin) and CT imaging (Fig. 8-56). Many of the afflicted patients are older. If the individual is hemodynamically stable, fluid resuscitation, blood products, and correction of the coagulopathy is often sufficient.[269] If these measures fail, the patient should undergo catheter angiography with intention to embolize any bleeding arteries.[270] Contrary to popular teaching, an actively bleeding vessel (most often a lumbar artery) can be detected and embolized in most cases.

Vasculitis and Mimics (Online Case 74)

Buerger disease (thromboangiitis obliterans) is a rare systemic inflammatory disorder affecting small and medium-sized arteries and veins[271,272] (see Chapter 1). Large arteries (proximal to the tibial vessels) are relatively spared. The disease involves the lower extremity in 90% of cases; the upper extremity is affected in about 50%. It is a common cause of PAD in smokers (usually male) younger than 40 years of age. Patients complain of symptoms of chronic

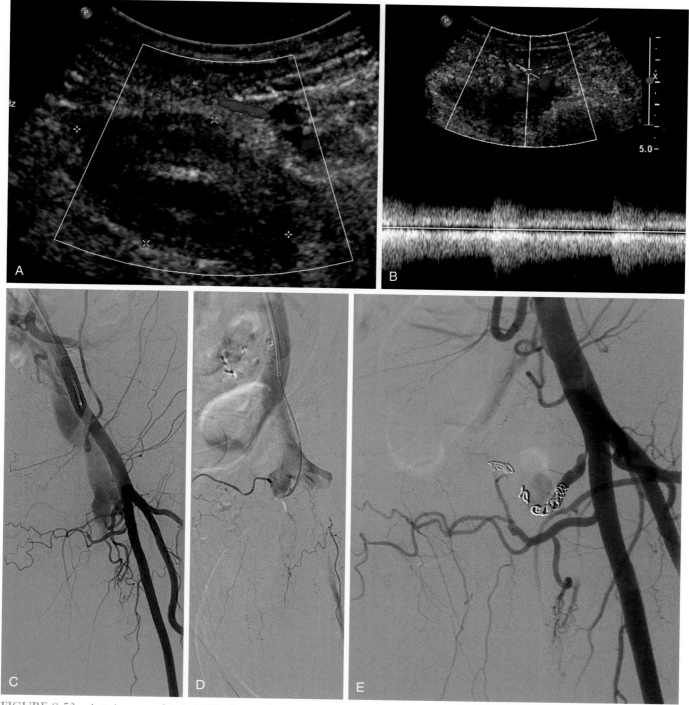

FIGURE 8-53 Arteriovenous fistula (AVF) after cardiac catheterization. Color Doppler ultrasound shows a large left groin hematoma **(A)** and vessel with turbulent arterial flow **(B)** suggesting a fistula. **C,** Selective left iliac arteriography confirms the iatrogenic AVF. In this unusual instance, the communication is through a small branch **(D),** which could be catheterized and embolized **(E)** to abolish the fistula.

limb ischemia and Raynaud phenomenon. The classic angiographic features are abrupt occlusions of tibial and pedal arteries with normal intervening segments, tortuous "corkscrew" collaterals, and relative sparing of proximal arteries (see Fig. 8-19).

If the patient continues to smoke, gangrene and amputation may result. If the patient stops smoking, stabilization and some improvement in symptoms can be expected. Pharmacologic treatment with the prostacyclin analogue iloprost is effective in some cases.

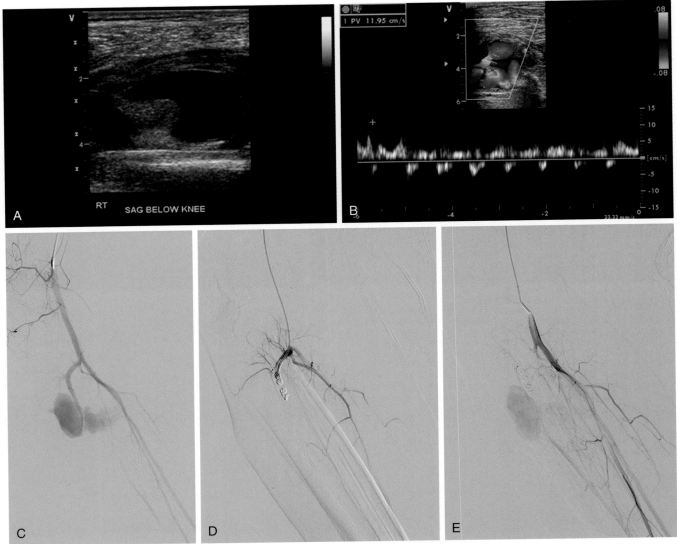

FIGURE 8-54   Traumatic anterior tibial artery pseudoaneurysm from criminal stab wound. **A** and **B,** Color Doppler ultrasound shows a large vascular structure in the right calf with to-and-fro flow characteristic of a pseudoaneurysm. **C,** Selective angiography confirms the diagnosis, with origin from the proximal right anterior tibial artery. **D,** Embolization with coils was done proximally, but later phase of the arteriogram showed continued pressurization of the pseudoaneurysm through the distal artery via collateral channels **(E).** At this point, ultrasound-guided percutaneous thrombin injection was recommended.

Thrombolytic therapy has had mixed results.[273] Surgical options include sympathectomy, bypass grafting (when feasible), and, ultimately, amputation.

Vasospasm of the lower extremity arteries is seen with a variety of disorders (see Figs. 1-3 and 8-55). Functional arterial narrowing occurs when proximal arteries are obstructed. Chronic use or abuse of certain vasospastic agents can cause ischemic symptoms, diminished pulses, and occasionally gangrene.[274] The characteristic finding of drug-induced vasospasm is bilateral, symmetric, abrupt narrowing of the iliac, femoral, or popliteal arteries that resolves after discontinuation of the drug. Vasospasm

from any source is partially or completely relieved with vasodilators, removal of the causative factor, and time.

Standing waves are periodic oscillations in an arterial segment that are occasionally seen during lower extremity CT, MR, or catheter arteriography (see Fig. 1-5). The regular, corrugated appearance should not be confused with other entities. A leading hypothesis invokes secondary retrograde flow (typical in high resistance arteries) as the explanation for this temporary oscillating pattern.[275,276]

Fibromuscular dysplasia is a set of related disorders in which noninflammatory fibrotic tissue proliferates in

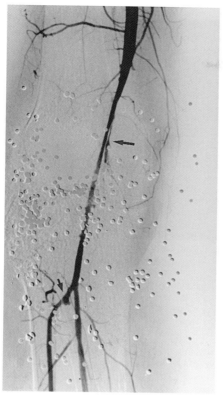

FIGURE 8-55   A shotgun blast to the right knee caused diffuse spasm or intramural hematoma in the popliteal artery, a focal dissection *(long arrow)*, and an anterior tibial artery pseudoaneurysm *(short arrow)*.

mass associated with pain, varices, or a thrill or bruit over the lesion. Color Doppler sonography and MRI are the primary tools for diagnosis and staging of suspected extremity AVMs[283,284] (Figs. 8-57 and 8-58). Catheter angiography (arteriography or direct lesion puncture) is reserved for embolotherapy or operative planning.

VMs are the most common type of vascular malformation.[285] They are distinguished by slightly dilated or nondilated inflow arteries, variable flow patterns, and large spongy venous spaces. *AVMs* are distinguished by marked dilation of the feeding vessels, hypervascularity, numerous arteriovenous connections around the nidus, early venous filling, and rapid venous washout (see Fig. 8-58). AVMs typically pass through several stages, from dormancy, to expansion with associated pulsation and thrill, to destruction with pain, bleeding or ulceration, to decompensation and possibly heart failure. Trauma, hormonal changes, and ischemia seem to encourage growth; the latter response is one of several reasons to avoid proximal occlusion of feeding arteries. *Hemangiomas* are marked by normal-caliber feeding vessels, large vascular channels, and early filling of amorphous vascular spaces that persists through the venous phase of a contrast imaging study (see Figs. 8-57 and 1-32).

It is almost impossible to completely eradicate lower extremity malformations without surgical extirpation. Invasive measures should only be undertaken to relieve pain, bleeding, ulceration, severe deformity, or high-output cardiac failure. When feasible, the treatment of choice is embolotherapy by an intraarterial or direct percutaneous route[286-289] (see Chapter 3). Embolization is performed in stages to limit nontarget tissue loss. The often unattainable goal is permanent obliteration of the AVM nidus.

Proximal embolization must be strictly avoided. Depending on the subtype of AVM (e.g., arterial, venous), the agents of choice are absolute alcohol, sodium tetradecyl sulfate (SDS) 3% foam, cyanoacrylates (glue), or ethylene vinyl alcohol copolymer (Onyx).[289-294] For hemangiomas and venous malformations, direct injection with a sclerosing agent (e.g., SDS or absolute alcohol) can be extremely effective[288] (see Fig. 8-57). Amputation is ultimately required for some lower extremity high-flow AVMs, even after multiple aggressive percutaneous treatment sessions.[287]

Pelvic AVMs include true congenital AVMs (often arising from the uterus) and acquired lesions (from gestational trophoblastic disease, prior surgery, tumor, or other causes)[291,295] (see Chapter 13). These malformations, which are typically seen in young to middle-aged women, cause pelvic pain, vaginal bleeding, spontaneous abortion, and occasionally congestive heart failure. Congenital lesions are supplied by numerous vessels, including branches of the internal iliac, ovarian, and inferior mesenteric arteries. Acquired

one or more layers of the arterial wall (see Chapter 1). It is an uncommon cause of renal artery stenosis; it is a rare cause of carotid or iliac artery disease.[277,278] The medial fibroplasia type of fibromuscular dysplasia produces a "string of beads" appearance, with alternating constriction and dilation of the vessel (see Fig. 8-17).

Radiation arteritis can develop years after high-dose radiotherapy for pelvic malignancy[279,280] (see Chapter 1 and Fig. 8-20). Patients with preexisting PAD are more susceptible to radiation arteritis. The typical angiographic findings are focal or diffuse stenoses and occlusions within the radiation field.

Arteriovenous Communications

Vascular anomalies are relatively rare, but the pelvis and legs are among the most commonly affected sites. These lesions encompass both classic vascular malformation (e.g., *congenital venous [VM]* and *arteriovenous [AVM] malformations*) and *hemangiomas,* which are actually vascular tumors.[281,282] These often confusing and always challenging entities are considered in greater detail in Chapter 1. Patients usually present as children or young adults with a cutaneous vascular lesion or enlarging leg

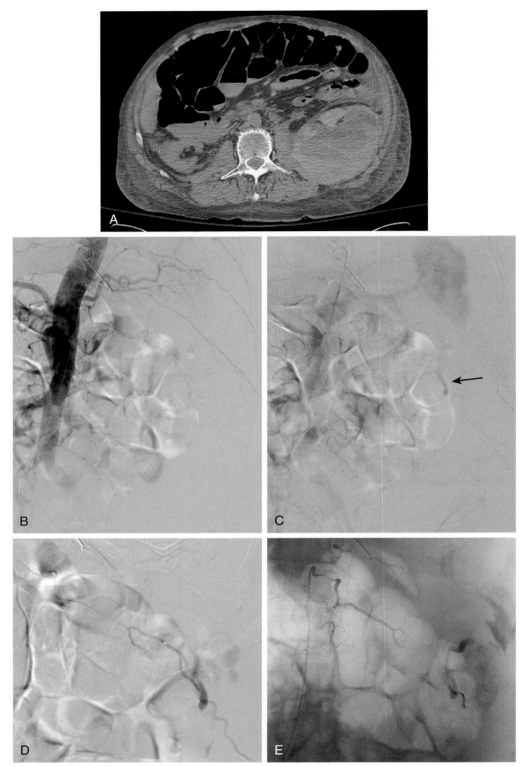

FIGURE 8-56 Spontaneous retroperitoneal hemorrhage in a patient with sudden onset of back pain and drop in hematocrit. **A,** Computed tomography scan shows large heterogenous bleed in left retroperitoneal space. **B** and **C,** Abdominal aortography shows a bleeding site *(arrow)* but not the source vessel. Sequential arteriography of all left-sided lumbar arteries identified the culprit vessel **(D),** which was embolized distally with coils and Gelfoam **(E).** Bleeding stopped.

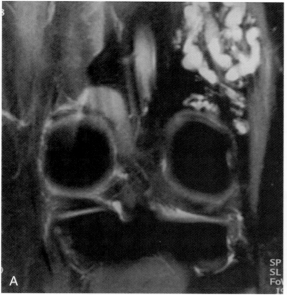
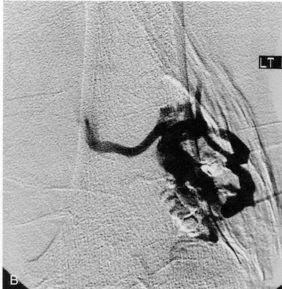
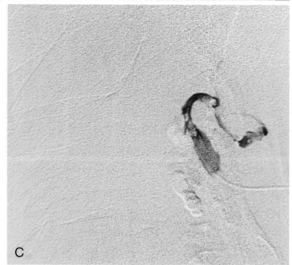

FIGURE 8-57   Hemangioma of the lower left thigh in a 35-year-old woman with pain. **A,** The magnetic resonance angiogram shows dilated vascular spaces above the lateral femoral condyle. **B,** Direct percutaneous contrast injection through an Angiocath opacifies the vascular channels. **C,** The lesion was obliterated after injection of 3 mL of sodium tetradecyl sulfate (Sotradecol) while a blood pressure cuff was inflated around the upper thigh to retain sclerosant in the lesion for 10 minutes.

lesions may be supplied entirely by the uterine arteries. Surgical resection is only possible in a minority of cases and often requires hysterectomy. Embolotherapy is more effective for palliation and may allow preservation of the uterus. A variety of embolic agents has been tried, including polyvinyl alcohol particles or microspheres, absolute alcohol, and Gelfoam.

AVFs in the lower extremity are almost always caused by accidental or iatrogenic trauma (see Fig. 8-53). Physiologic arteriovenous shunts are present throughout most vascular beds.[296] They are occasionally seen during lower extremity angiography in patients with PAD and after angioplasty of arterial stenoses (see Fig. 1-35).

Popliteal Artery Disorders (Online Case 70)

The popliteal artery is affected by a fairly unique set of diseases. In older patients, occlusion of this vessel should always raise the suspicion of underlying aneurysm (see previous discussion). In younger patients with popliteal artery lesions, several distinctive entities should be considered (Box 8-9).

Cystic adventitial disease is a rare condition in which mucin collects in the adventitial layer of the popliteal artery, and rarely in other vessels (femoral, axillary, iliac, and forearm arteries).[228,297-299] It is largely a disease of young to middle-aged men who complain of sudden onset of popliteal fossa pain and claudication.

about 50% of the general population.[305] A small percentage of individuals with *functional* narrowing suffer chronic injury to the artery and frank entrapment syndrome. However, most patients with this disorder have a congenital, *anatomic* basis for disease, described by one of four distinct abnormal relationships between the artery and adjacent muscular bundles.[302,306] The most common form (type I) involves abnormal fetal migration of the medial head of the gastrocnemius muscle, which displaces the artery medially. Type V describes patients with popliteal vein entrapment. Entrapment is bilateral in about one third of cases. Men are affected more often than women, and many of them are athletes or exercise regularly.

Popliteal artery entrapment is usually confirmed and staged with MR or CT angiography. Typical findings include narrowing and medial (or occasionally lateral) deviation of the midportion of the popliteal artery.[306,307] Sometimes, the artery appears normal in a neutral position. The imaging study is then repeated with *active, prolonged plantar flexion* or passive dorsiflexion of the foot, which should provoke the compression (Fig. 8-60). Left untreated, the condition can lead to aneurysm formation, thrombosis, or distal embolization. The standard therapy is popliteal fossa exploration with myotomy or muscular/tendinous release along with vein bypass grafting if the artery is diseased.

Iliac Artery Endofibrosis

External iliac artery endofibrosis is an obscure disorder in which the vascular intima is thickened by collagen, smooth muscle cells, and fibroblasts without any histologic evidence for atherosclerosis or inflammation. Endofibrosis is almost exclusively confined to the first few centimeters of the external iliac artery, and it is virtually

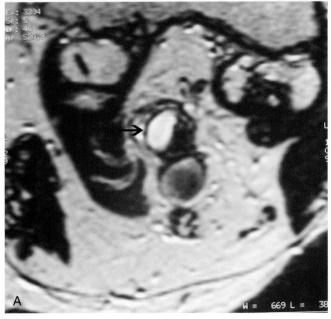
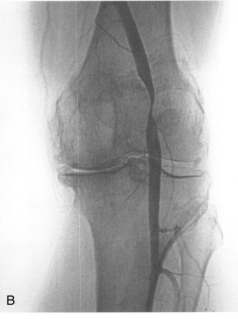

FIGURE 8-59   Cystic adventitial disease of the popliteal artery. **A,** T2-weighted transverse magnetic resonance image shows a cystic lesion *(arrow)* compressing the normal popliteal artery. **B,** Catheter angiogram reveals the classic hourglass appearance of the lesion. *(Courtesy of Thomas Velling, MD, Newport Beach, Calif.)*

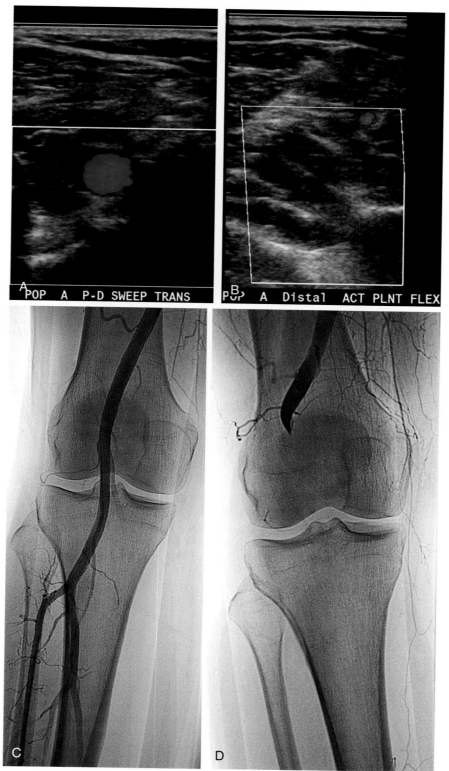

FIGURE 8-60 Popliteal artery entrapment syndrome. **A,** Color Doppler ultrasound of right popliteal fossa shows widely patent artery. **B,** With active plantar flexion of the ankle, the artery is occluded. Selective left leg arteriography shows a normal popliteal artery at rest **(C),** but complete compression with active plantar flexion **(D).**

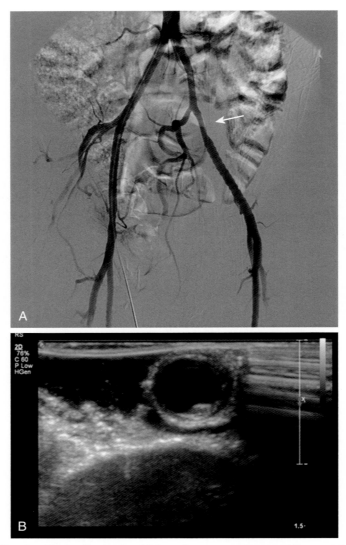

FIGURE 8-61 Iliac artery endofibrosis with claudication in a high-performance cyclist. **A,** Oblique pelvic arteriography shows short segment proximal narrowing of the left external iliac artery *(arrow)*. Note "standing waves" below this level; this is a functional phenomenon. **B,** Ultrasound at the level of the affected artery shows typical heaped-up arterial wall causing only minimal narrowing at rest.

only seen in high-performance athletes (particularly racing cyclists)[308-311] (Fig. 8-61). The cause is unknown. Patients are only symptomatic with vigorous activity. Screening is done with segmental blood pressure measurements during and after extreme exercise. Sonography or CT angiography confirms the diagnosis. The standard treatment is saphenous vein patch angioplasty or bypass graft placement.[310]

Neoplasms

Catheter angiography has almost no role in the evaluation of neoplasms of the lower extremity. Occasionally, patients with highly vascular tumors undergo arteriography as part of an embolization procedure to minimize bleeding during surgery. Women with gynecologic tumors complicated by pelvic or vaginal bleeding may also be treated with embolotherapy (see Chapter 13).

References

1. Caridi JG, Hawkins Jr IF, Klioze SD, et al. Carbon dioxide digital subtraction angiography: the practical approach. *Tech Vasc Interv Radiol* 2001;**4**:57.

2. Dowling K, Kan H, Siskin G, et al. Safety of limited supplemental iodinated contrast administration in azotemic patients undergoing CO2 angiography. *J Endovasc Ther* 2003;**10**:312.

3. Shaw DR, Kessel DO. The current status of the use of carbon dioxide in diagnostic interventional angiographic procedures. *Cardiovasc Intervent Radiol* 2006;**29**:32.3

4. Huber PR, Leimbach ME, Lewis WL, et al. CO2 angiography. *Catheter Cardiovasc Interv* 2002;**55**:398.

5. Collins P, editor. Embryology and development. In: Williams PL, Bannister LH, Berry MM, et al, editors. *Gray's anatomy* . 38th ed. New York: Churchill Livingstone; 1995, p. 320.

6. Gabella G, editor. Cardiovascular system. In: Williams PL, Bannister LH, Berry MM, et al, editors. *Gray's anatomy.* 38th ed. New York: Churchill Livingstone; 1995, p. 1558.

7. Mauro MA, Jaques PF, Moore M. The popliteal artery and its branches: embryologic basis of normal and variant anatomy. *AJR Am J Roentgenol* 1988;**150**:435.

8. Santaollala V, Bernabe MH, Hipola Ulecia JM, et al. Persistent sciatic artery. *Ann Vasc Surg* 2010;**24**:e7.

9. Mousa A, Rapp Parker A, Emmett MK, et al. Endovascular treatment of symptomatic persistent sciatic artery aneurysm: report and review of literature. *Vasc Endovasc Surg* 2010;**44**:312.

10. Javerliat I, Rouanet A, Bourguigon T, et al. Duplication of superficial femoral artery: an uncommon variation of the lower limb arterial system. *Ann Vasc Surg* 2010;**24**:e1.

11. Piral T, Germain M, Princ G. Absence of the posterior tibial artery: implications for free transplants of the fibula. *Surg Radiol Anat* 1996;**18**:155.

12. Lutz BS, Wei FC, Ng SH, et al. Routine donor leg angiography before vascularized free fibula transplantation is not necessary: a prospective study in 120 clinical cases. *Plast Reconstr Surg* 1999;**103**:121.

13. Tindall AJ, Shetty AA, James KD, et al. Prevalence and surgical significance of a high-origin anterior tibial artery. *J Orthop Surg (Hong Kong)* 2006;**14**:13.

14. Norgren L, Hiatt WR, Dormandy JA, et al. Inter-Society Consensus for the Management of Peripheral Arterial Disease (TASC II). *Eur J Vasc Endovasc Surg* 2007;**33**:S1.

15. Olin JW, Sealove BA. Peripheral arterial disease: current insight into the disease and its diagnosis and management. *Mayo Clin Proc* 2010;**85**:678.

16. Selvin E, Erlinger TP. Prevalence of and risk factors for peripheral arterial disease in the United States: results from the National Health and Nutrition Examination Survey, 1999-2000. *Circulation* 2004;**110**:738.

17. Blair JM, Glagov S, Zarins CK. Mechanism of superficial femoral artery adductor canal stenosis. *Surg Forum* 1990;**41**:359.

18. Wood NB, Zhao SZ, Zambanini A, et al. Curvature and tortuosity of the superficial femoral artery: a possible risk factor for peripheral arterial disease. *J Appl Physiol* 2006;**101**:1412.

19. Rutherford RB, Becker GJ. Standards for evaluating and reporting the results of surgical and percutaneous therapy for peripheral arterial disease. *J Vasc Interv Radiol* 1991;**2**:169.

20. Turnipseed WD. Clinical review of patients treated for atypical claudication: a 28-year experience. *J Vasc Surg* 2004;**40**:79.

21. Renshaw A, McCowen T, Waltke EA, et al. Angioplasty with stenting is effective in treating blue toe syndrome. *Vasc Endovascular Surg* 2002;**36**:155.

22. Matchett WJ, McFarland DR, Eidt JF, et al. Blue toe syndrome: treatment with intra-arterial stents and review of therapies. *J Vasc Interv Radiol* 2000;**11**:585.

23. Chan D, Anderson ME, Dolmatch BL. Imaging evaluation of lower extremity infrainguinal disease: role of the noninvasive vascular laboratory, computed tomographic angiography, and magnetic resonance angiography. *Tech Vasc Interv Radiol* 2010;**13**:11.

24. Eiberg JP, Gronvall Rasmussen JB, Hansen MA, et al. Duplex ultrasound scanning of peripheral arterial disease of the lower limb. *Eur J Vasc Endovasc Surg* 2010;**40**:507.

25. Cambria RP, Kaufman JA, L'Italien GJ, et al. Magnetic resonance angiography in the management of lower extremity arterial occlusive disease: a prospective study. *J Vasc Surg* 1997;**25**:380.

26. Nelemans PJ, Leiner T, de Vet HC, et al. Peripheral arterial disease: meta-analysis of the diagnostic performance of MR angiography. *Radiology* 2000;**217**:105.

27. Collins R, Cranny G, Burch J, et al. A systematic review of duplex ultrasound, magnetic resonance angiography and computed tomography angiography for the diagnosis and assessment of symptomatic, lower limb peripheral arterial disease. *Health Technol Assess* 2007;**11**:1.

28. Menke J, Larsen J. Meta-analysis: accuracy of contrast enhanced magnetic resonance angiography for assessing steno-occlusions in peripheral arterial disease. *Ann Intern Med* 2010;**153**:325.

29. Bertschinger K, Cassina PC, Debatin JF, et al. Surveillance of peripheral arterial bypass grafts with three-dimensional MR angiography: comparison with digital subtraction angiography. *AJR Am J Roentgenol* 2001;**176**:215.

30. Khilnani NM, Winchester PA, Prince MR, et al. Peripheral vascular disease: combined 3D bolus chase and dynamic 2D MR angiography compared with x-ray angiography for treatment planning. *Radiology* 2002;**224**:63.

31. Foley WD, Stonely T. CT angiography of the lower extremities. *Radiol Clin North Am* 2010;**48**:367.

32. Duddalwar VA. Multislice CT angiography: a practical guide to CT angiography in vascular imaging and intervention. *Br J Radiol* 2004;**77**:S27.

33. Jakobs TF, Wintersperger BJ, Becker CR. MDCT-imaging of peripheral arterial disease. *Semin Ultrasound CT MR* 2004;**25**:145.

34. Met R, Bipat S, Legemate DA, et al. Diagnostic performance of computed tomography angiography in peripheral arterial disease: a systematic review and meta-analysis. *JAMA* 2009;**301**:415.

35. Heijenbrok-Kal MH, Kock MC, Hunink MG. Lower extremity arterial disease: multidetector CT angiography meta-analysis. *Radiology* 2007;**245**:433.

36. Mohler III ER. Combination antiplatelet therapy in patients with peripheral arterial disease: is the best therapy aspirin, clopidogrel, or both? *Catheter Cardiovasc Intervent* 2009;**74**:S1.

37. Greenhalgh RM, Belch JJ, Brown LC, et al. The adjuvant benefit of angioplasty in patients with mild to moderate intermittent claudication (MIMIC) managed by supervised exercise, smoking cessation advice and best medical therapy: results from two randomized trials for stenotic femoropopliteal and aortoiliac arterial disease. *Eur J Vasc Endovasc Surg* 2008;**36**:680.

38. Mazari FA, Gulati S, Rahman MN, et al. Early outcomes from a randomized, controlled trial of supervised exercise, angioplasty, and combined therapy in intermittent claudication. *Ann Vasc Surg* 2010;**24**:69.

39. Robless P, Mikhalidis DP, Stansby GP. Cilostazol for peripheral arterial disease. *Cochrane Database Syst Rev* 2008;**23**:CD003748.

40. Regensteiner JG, Ware Jr JE, McCarthy WJ, et al. Effect of cilostazol on treadmill walking, community based walking ability, and health-related quality of life in patients with intermittent claudication due to peripheral arterial disease: meta-analysis of six randomized controlled trials. *J Am Geriatr Soc* 2002;**50**:1939.

41. De Backer T, Vander Stichele R, Lehert P, et al. Naftidrofuryl for intermittent claudication: meta-analysis based on individual patient data. *BMJ* 2009;**338**:b603.

42. Spengel F, Clement D, Boccalon H, et al. Findings of the Naftidrofuryl in Quality of Life (NIQOL) European study program. *Int Angiol* 2002;**21**:20.

43. Kieffer E, Bahnini A, Mouren X, et al. A new study demonstrates the efficacy of naftidrofuryl in the treatment of intermittent claudication. Findings of the Naftidrofuryl Clinical Ischemia Study (NCIS). *Int Angiol* 2001;**20**:58.

44. de Vries SO, Visser K, de Vries JA, et al. Intermittent claudication: cost-effectiveness of revascularization versus exercise therapy. *Radiology* 2002;**222**:25.

45. Schillinger M, Exner M, Mlekusch W, et al. Vascular inflammation and percutaneous transluminal angioplasty of the femoropopliteal artery: association with restenosis. *Radiology* 2002;**225**:21.

46. Schillinger M, Exner M, Mlekusch W, et al. Endovascular revascularization below the knee: 6-month results and predictive value of C-reactive protein level. *Radiology* 2003;**227**:419.

47. Dibra A, Mehilli J, Braun S, et al. Association between C-reactive protein levels and subsequent cardiac events among patients with stable angina treated with coronary artery stenting. *Am J Med* 2003;**114**:715.

48. Walton BL, Dougherty K, Mortazavi A, et al. Percutaneous intervention for the treatment of hypoplastic aortoiliac syndrome. *Catheter Cardiovasc Interv* 2003;**60**:329.

49. Audet P, Therasse E, Oliva VL, et al. Infrarenal aortic stenosis: long-term clinical and hemodynamic results of percutaneous transluminal angioplasty. *Radiology* 1998;**209**:357.

50. Therasse E, Cote G, Oliva VL, et al. Infrarenal aortic stenosis: value of stent placement after percutaneous transluminal angioplasty failure. *Radiology* 2001;**219**:655.

51. Schedel H, Wissgott C, Rademaker J, et al. Primary stent placement for infrarenal aortic stenosis: immediate and midterm results. *J Vasc Interv Radiol* 2004;**15**:353.

52. Klonaris C, Katsargyris A, Tsekouras N, et al. Primary stenting for aortic lesion: from single stenoses to total aortoiliac occlusions. *J Vasc Surg* 2008;**47**:310.

53. Simons PC, Nawjin AA, Bruijninckx CM, et al. Long-term results of primary stent placement to treat infrarenal aortic stenosis. *Eur J Vasc Endovasc Surg* 2006;**32**:627.

54. Stoeckelhuber BM, Stoeckelhuber M, Gellissen J, et al. Primary endovascular stent placement for focal infrarenal aortic stenosis: long-term results. *J Vasc Interv Radiol* 2006;**17**:1105.

55. Sheeran SR, Hallisey MJ, Ferguson D. Percutaneous transluminal stent placement in the abdominal aorta. *J Vasc Interv Radiol* 1997;**8**:55.

56. Ligush J, Criado E, Burnham SJ, et al. Management and outcome of chronic atherosclerotic infrarenal aortic occlusion. *J Vasc Surg* 1996;**24**:394.

57. Jongkind V, Akkersdijk GJ, Yeung KK, et al. A systematic review of endovascular treatment of extensive aortoiliac occlusive disease. *J Vasc Surg* 2010;**52**:1376.

58. Burke CR, Henke PK, Hernandez R, et al. A contemporary comparison of aortofemoral bypass and aortoiliac stenting in the treatment of aortoiliac occlusive disease. *Ann Vasc Surg* 2010;**24**:4.

59. Hans SS, DeSantis D, Siddiqui R, et al. Results of endovascular therapy and aortobifemoral grafting for Transatlantic Inter-Society type C and D aortoiliac occlusive disease. *Surgery* 2008;**144**:583.

60. Houston JG, Bhat R, Ross R, et al. Long-term results after placement of aortic bifurcation self-expanding stents: 10 year mortality, stent restenosis, and distal disease progression. *Cardiovasc Intervent Radiol* 2007;**30**:42.

61. Moise MA, Alvarez-Tostado JA, Clair DG, et al. Endovascular management of chronic infrarenal aortic occlusion. *J Endovasc Ther* 2009;**6**:84.

62. Kashyap VS, Pavkov ML, Bena JF, et al. The management of severe aortoiliac occlusive disease: endovascular therapy rivals open reconstruction. *J Vasc Surg* 2008;**48**:1451.

63. Chang RW, Goodney PP, Baek JH, et al. Long-term results of combined common femoral endarterectomy and iliac stenting/stent grafting for occlusive disease. *J Vasc Surg* 2008;**48**:362.

64. AbuRahma AF, Hayes JD, Flaherty SK, et al. Primary iliac stenting versus transluminal angioplasty with selective stenting. *J Vasc Surg* 2007;**46**:965.

65. Klein WM, van der Graaf Y, Seegers J, et al. Dutch iliac stent trial: long-term results in patients randomized for primary or selective stent placement. *Radiology* 2006;**238**:734.

66. Bosch JL, Haaring C, Meyerovitz MF, et al. Cost-effectiveness of percutaneous treatment of iliac artery occlusive disease in the United States. *AJR Am J Roentgenol* 2000;**175**:517.

67. Ponec D, Jaff MR, Swischuk J, et al. The Nitinol SMART stent vs Wallstent for suboptimal iliac artery angioplasty: CRISP-US trial results. *J Vasc Interv Radiol* 2004;**15**:911.

68. Sharafuddin MJ, Hoballah JJ, Kresowik TF, et al. Long-term outcome following stent reconstruction of the aortic bifurcation and the role of geometric determinants. *Ann Vasc Surg* 2008;**22**:346.

69. Smith JC, Watkins GE, Taylor FC, et al. Angioplasty or stent placement in the proximal common iliac artery: is protection of the contralateral side necessary? *J Vasc Interv Radiol* 2001;**12**:1395.

70. Murphy TP, Ariaratnam NS, Carney Jr WI, et al. Aortoiliac insufficiency: long-term experience with stent placement for treatment. *Radiology* 2004;**231**:243.

71. Schurmann K, Mahnken A, Meyer J, et al. Long-term results 10 years after iliac arterial stent placement. *Radiology* 2002;**224**:731.

72. Leung DA, Spinosa DJ, Hagspiel KD, et al. Selection of stents for treating iliac arterial occlusive disease. *J Vasc Interv Radiol* 2003;**14**:137.

73. Hamer OW, Borisch I, Finkenzeller T, et al. Iliac artery stent placement: clinical experience and short-term follow-up regarding a self-expanding nitinol stent. *J Vasc Interv Radiol* 2004;**15**:1231.

74. Timaran CH, Stevens SL, Freeman MB, et al. External iliac and common iliac artery angioplasty and stenting in men and women. *J Vasc Surg* 2001;**34**:440.

75. Park SI, Won JH, Kim BM, et al. The arterial folding point during flexion of the hip joint. *Cardiovasc Intervent Radiol* 2005;**28**:173.

76. Reyes R, Maynar M, Lopera J, et al. Treatment of chronic iliac artery occlusions with guide wire recanalization and primary stent placement. *J Vasc Interv Radiol* 1997;**8**:1049.

77. Vorwerk D, Guenther RW, Schuermann K, et al. Primary stent placement for chronic iliac artery occlusions: follow-up results in 103 patients. *Radiology* 1995;**194**:745.

78. Dyet JF, Gaines PA, Nicholson AA, et al. Treatment of chronic iliac artery occlusions by means of percutaneous endovascular stent placement. *J Vasc Interv Radiol* 1997;**8**:349.

79. Yedlicka Jr JW, Ferral H, Bjarnason H, et al. Chronic iliac artery occlusions: primary recanalization with endovascular stents. *J Vasc Interv Radiol* 1994;**5**:843.

80. Kofoed SC, Bismuth J, Just S, et al. Angioplasty for the treatment of buttock claudication caused by internal iliac artery stenoses. *Ann Vasc Surg* 2001;**15**:396.

81. Thompson K, Cook P, Dilley R, et al. Internal iliac artery angioplasty and stenting: an underutilized therapy. *Ann Vasc Surg* 2010;**24**:23.

82. Paumier A, Abraham P, Mahe G, et al. Functional outcome of hypogastric revascularisation for prevention of buttock claudication in patients with peripheral artery occlusive disease. *Eur J Vasc Endovasc Surg* 2010;**39**:323.

83. Kang JL, Patel VI, Conrad MF, et al. Common femoral artery occlusive disease: contemporary results following surgical endarterectomy. *J Vasc Surg* 2008;**48**:872.

84. Ballotta E, Gruppo M, Mazzalai F, et al. Common femoral artery endarterectomy for occlusive disease: 8 year single center prospective study. *Surgery* 2010;**147**:268.

85. Stricker H, Jacomella V. Stent-assisted angioplasty at the level of the common femoral artery bifurcation: midterm outcomes. *J Endovasc Ther* 2004;**11**:281.

86. Silva JA, White CJ, Ramee SR, et al. Percutaneous profundaplasty in the treatment of lower extremity ischemia: results of long-term surveillance. *J Endovasc Ther* 2001;**8**:75.

87. Dick P, Mlekusch W, Sabeti S, et al. Outcome after endovascular treatment of deep femoral artery stenosis: results in a consecutive patient series and systematic review of the literature. *J Endovasc Ther* 2006;**13**:221.

88. Donas KP, Pitloulas GA, Schwindt A, et al. Endovascular treatment of profunda femoris artery obstructive disease: nonsense or useful tool in selected cases? *Eur J Vasc Endovasc Surg* 2010;**39**:308.

89. Clark TW, Groffsky JL, Soulen MC. Predictors of long-term patency after femoropopliteal angioplasty: results from the STAR registry. *J Vasc Interv Radiol* 2001;**12**:923.

90. Jamsen TS, Manninen HI, Jaakkola PA, et al. Long-term outcome of patients with claudication after balloon angioplasty of the femoropopliteal arteries. *Radiology* 2002;**225**:345.

91. Dick P, Sabeti S, Miekusch W, et al. Conventional balloon angioplasty versus peripheral cutting balloon angioplasty for treatment of femoropopliteal artery in-stent restenosis: initial experience. *Radiology* 2008;**248**:297.

92. Amighi J, Schillinger M, Dick P, et al. De novo superficial femoropopliteal artery lesions: peripheral cutting balloon angioplasty and restenosis rates- randomized controlled trial. *Radiology* 2008;**247**:267

93. Canaud L, Alric P, Berthet JP, et al. Infrainguinal cutting balloon angioplasty in de novo arterial lesions. *J Vasc Surg* 2008;**48**:1182.

94. Rabbi JF, Kiran RP, Gersten G, et al. Early results with infrainguinal cutting balloon angioplasty limits distal dissection. *Ann Vasc Surg* 2004;**18**:640.

95. Laird J, Jaff MR, Biamino G, et al. Cryoplasty for the treatment of femoropopliteal arterial disease: results of a prospective, multi-center registry. *J Vasc Interv Radiol* 2005;**16**:1067.

96. Kortweg MA, van Gils M, Hoedt MT, et al. Cryoplasty for occlusive disease of the femoropopliteal arteries: 1-year follow-up. *Cardiovasc Intervent Radiol* 2009;**32**:221.

97. Spiliopoulos S, Katsanos K, Karnabatidis D, et al. Cryoplasty versus conventional balloon angioplasty of the femoropopliteal artery in diabetic patients: long-term results from a prospective randomized single-center controlled trial. *J Vasc Interv Radiol* 2010;**33**:929.

98. Werk M, Lagner S, Reinkensmeier B, et al. Inhibition of restenosis in femoropopliteal arteries: paclitaxel-coated versus uncoated balloon: femoral paclitaxel randomized pilot trial. *Circulation* 2008;**118**:1358.

99. Tepe G, Zeller T, Albrecht T, et al. Local delivery of paclitaxel to inhibit restenosis during angioplasty of the leg. *N Engl J Med* 2008;**358**:689.

100. Henry TD, Schwartz RS, Hirsch AT. "POBA Plus": will the balloon regain its luster? *Circulation* 2008;**118**:1309.

101. Manzi M, Cester G, Palena LM. Paclitaxel-coated balloon angioplasty for lower extremity revascularization: a new way to fight in-stent restenosis. *J Cardiovasc Surg* (Torino) 2010;**51**:567.

102. Waksman R, Laird JR, Jurkovitz CT, et al. Intravascular radiation therapy after balloon angioplasty of narrowed femoropopliteal arteries to prevent restenosis: results of the PARIS feasibility clinical trial. *J Vasc Interv Radiol* 2001;**12**:915.

103. Krueger K, Zaehringer M, Bendel M, et al. De novo femoropopliteal stenoses: endovascular gamma irradiation following angioplasty—angiographic and clinical follow-up in a prospective randomized controlled trial. *Radiology* 2004;**231**:546.

104. Schillinger M, Minar E. Advances in vascular brachytherapy over the last 10 years: focus on femoropopliteal applications. *J Endovasc Ther* 2004;**11**(Suppl 2):II180.

105. Chung SW, Sharafuddin MJ, Chigurupati R, et al. Midterm patency following atherectomy for infrainguinal occlusive disease: a word of caution. *Ann Vasc Surg* 2008;**22**:358.

106. Keeling WB, Shames ML, Stone PA, et al. Plaque excision with the Silverhawk catheter: early results in patients with claudication or critical limb ischemia. *J Vasc Surg* 2007;**45**:25.

107. Zeller T, Krankenberg H, Steinkamp H, et al. One-year outcome of percutaneous rotational atherectomy with aspiration in infrainguinal peripheral arterial occlusive disease: the multicenter pathway PVD trial. *J Endovasc Ther* 2009;**16**:653.

108. Garcia LA, Lyden SP. Atherectomy for infrainguinal peripheral artery disease. *J Endovasc Ther* 2009;**16**:II105.

109. Sixt S, Rastan A, Beschorner U, et al. Acute and long-term outcome of Silverhawk assisted atherectomy for femoro-popliteal lesions according the TASC classification: a single-center experience. *Vasa* 2010;**39**:229.

110. Ramaiah V, Gammon R, Kiesz S, et al. Midterm outcomes from the TALON Registry: treating peripherals with SilverHawk: outcomes collection. *J Endovasc Ther* 2006;**13**:592.

111. Dearing DD, Patel KR, Compoginis JM, et al. Primary stenting of the superficial femoral and popliteal artery. *J Vasc Surg* 2009;**50**:542.

112. Mewissen MW. Primary nitinol stenting for femoropopliteal disease. *J Endovasc Ther* 2009;**16**:II63.

113. Mwipatayi BP, Hockings A, Hofmann M, et al. Balloon angioplasty compared with stenting for treatment of femoropopliteal occlusive disease: a meta-analysis. *J Vasc Surg* 2008;**47**:461.

114. Twine CP, Coulston J, Shandall A, et al. Angioplasty versus stenting for superficial femoral artery lesions. *Cochrane Database Syst Rev* 2009:CD006767.

115. Becquemin JP, Favre JP, Marzelle J, et al. Systematic versus selective stent placement after superficial femoral artery balloon angioplasty: a multicenter prospective randomized study. *J Vasc Surg* 2003;**37**:487.

116. Laird JR, Katzen BT, Scheinert D, et al. Nitinol stent implantation versus balloon angioplasty for lesions in the superficial femoral artery and proximal popliteal artery: twelve-months results from the RESILIENT randomized trial. *Circ Cardiovasc Interv* 2010;**3**:267.

117. Krankenberg H, Schlueter M, Steinkamp HJ, et al. Nitinol stent implantation versus percutaneous transluminal angioplasty in superficial femoral artery lesions up to 10 cm in length: the femoral artery stenting trial (FAST). *Circulation* 2007;**116**:285.

118. Schillinger M, Sabeti S, Dick P, et al. Sustained benefit at 2 years of primary femoropopliteal stenting compared with balloon angioplasty with optional stenting. *Circulation* 2007;**115**:2745.

119. Iida O, Nanto S, Uematsu M, et al. Influence of stent fracture on the long-term patency in the femoro-popliteal artery: experience of 4 years. *JACC Cardiovasc Interv* 2009;**2**:665.

120. Duda SH, Poerner TC, Wiesinger B, et al. Drug-eluting stents: potential applications for peripheral arterial occlusive disease. *J Vasc Interv Radiol* 2003;**14**:291.

121. Duda SH, Bosiers M, Lammer J, et al. Sirolimus-eluting versus bare nitinol stent for obstructive superficial femoral artery disease: The SIROCCO II trial. *J Vasc Interv Radiol* 2005;**16**:331.

122. Oliva VL, Soulez G. Sirolimus-eluting stents versus the superficial femoral artery: Second round. *J Vasc Interv Radiol* 2005;**16**:313.

123. Zeller T, Macharzina R, Tepe G. The potential role of DES in peripheral in-stent restenosis. *J Cardiovasc Surg* (Torino) 2010;**51**:561.

124. Saxon RR, Dake MD, Vogelzang RL, et al. Randomized, multicenter study comparing expanded polytetrafluoroethylene covered endoprosthesis with percutaneous transluminal angioplasty in the treatment of superficial femoral artery occlusive disease. *J Vasc Interv Radiol* 2008;**19**:823.

125. Jahnke T, Andresen R, Mueller-Huelsbeck S, et al. Hemobahn stent-grafts for treatment of femoropopliteal arterial obstructions: midterm results of a prospective trial. *J Vasc Interv Radiol* 2003;**14**:41.

126. Iida O, Nanto S, Uematsu M, et al. Cilostazol reduces restenosis after endovascular therapy in patients with femoropopliteal lesions. *J Vasc Surg* 2008;**48**:144.

127. Doeffler-Melly J, Koopman MM, Prins MH, et al. Antiplatelet and anticoagulant drugs for prevention of restenosis/reocclusion following peripheral endovascular treatment. *Cochrane Database Syst Rev* 2005:CD002071.

128. Spinosa DJ, Leung DA, Matsumoto AH, et al. Percutaneous intentional extraluminal recanalization in patients with chronic critical limb ischemia. *Radiology* 2004;**232**:499.

129. Met R, van Lienden KP, Koelemay MJ, et al. Subintimal angioplasty for peripheral arterial occlusive disease: a systematic review. *Cardiovasc Intervent Radiol* 2008;**31**:687

130. Spinosa DJ, Harthun NL, Bissonette EA, et al. Subintimal arterial flossing with antegrade-retrograde intervention (SAFARI) for subintimal recanalization to treat chronic critical limb ischemia. *J Vasc Interv Radiol* 2005;**16**:37.

131. Yilmaz S, Sindel T, Yegin A, et al. Subintimal angioplasty of long superficial femoral artery occlusions. *J Vasc Interv Radiol* 2003;**14**:997.

132. Lipsitz EC, Ohki T, Veith FJ, et al. Does subintimal angioplasty have a role in the treatment of severe lower extremity ischemia? *J Vasc Surg* 2003;**37**:386.

133. Beschorner U, Sixt S, Schwarzwaelder U, et al. Recanalization of chronic occlusions of the superficial femoral artery using the Outback re-entry catheter: a single centre experience. *Catheter Cardiovasc Interv* 2009;**74**:934.

134. Etezadi V, Benenati JF, Patel PJ, et al. The reentry catheter: a second chance for endoluminal reentry therapy for difficult lower extremity subintimal arterial recanalizations. *J Vasc Interv Radiol* 2010;**21**:730.

135. Shin SU, Baril D, Chaer R, et al. Limitations of the Outback LTD re-entry device in femoropopliteal chronic total occlusions. *J Vasc Surg* 2011;**53**:1260.

136. Scott EC, Biuckians A, Light RE, et al. Subintimal angioplasty: our experience in the treatment of 506 infrainguinal arterial occlusions. *J Vasc Surg* 2008;**48**:878.

137. Romiti M, Albers M, Brochado-Neto FC, et al. Meta-analysis of infrapopliteal angioplasty for chronic critical limb ischemia. *J Vasc Surg* 2008;**47**:975.

138. Randon C, Jacobs B, deRyck F, et al. Angioplasty or primary stenting for infrapopliteal lesions: results of a prospective randomized trial. *Cardiovasc Intervent Radiol* 2010;**33**:260.

139. Biondi-Zocai GG, Sangiori G, Lotrionte M, et al. Infragenicular stent implantation for below-the-knee atherosclerotic disease: clinical evidence from an international collaborative meta-analysis of 640 patients. *J Endovasc Ther* 2009;**16**:251.

140. Siablis D, Karnabatidis D, Katsanos K, et al. Infrapopliteal application of sirolimus-eluting versus bare metal stents for critical limb ischemia: analysis of long-term angiographic and clinical outcome. *J Vasc Interv Radiol* 2009;**20**:1141.

141. Soder HK, Manninen HI, Jaakkola P, et al. Prospective trial of infrapopliteal artery balloon angioplasty for critical limb ischemia: angiographic and clinical results. *J Vasc Interv Radiol* 2000;**11**:1021.

142. Rutherford RB. Options in the surgical management of aorto-iliac occlusive disease: a changing perspective. *Cardiovasc Surg* 1999;**7**:5.

143. Bradbury AW, Adam DJ, Bell J, et al. Bypass versus Angioplasty in Severe Ischaemia of the Leg (BASIL) trial: an intention-to-treat analysis of amputation-free and overall survival in patients randomized to a bypass surgery first or a balloon angioplasty first strategy. *J Vasc Surg* 2010;**51**:5S.

144. Conte MS. Bypass versus Angioplasty in Severe Ischaemia of the Leg (BASIL) and the (hoped for) dawn of evidence-based treatment for advanced limb ischemia. *J Vasc Surg* 2010;**51**:69S.

145. McQuade K, Gable D, Pearl G, et al. Four year randomized prospective comparison of percutaneous ePTFE/nitinol self-expanding stent graft versus prosthetic femoro-popliteal bypass graft in the treatment of superficial femoral artery occlusive disease. *J Vasc Surg* 2010;**52**:584.

146. Kedora J, Hohmann S, Garrett W, et al. Randomized comparison of percutaneous Viabahn stent grafts vs. prosthetic femoral-popliteal bypass in the treatment of superficial femoral arterial occlusive disease. *J Vasc Surg* 2007;**45**:10.

147. Conte MS. Technical factors in lower-extremity vein bypass surgery: how can we improve outcomes? *Semin Vasc Surg* 2009;**22**:227.

148. Shah DM, Darling RC III, Chang BB, et al. Long-term results of in situ saphenous vein bypass: analysis of 2058 cases. *Ann Surg* 1995;**222**:438.

149. Johnson WC, Lee KK. A comparative evaluation of polytetrafluoroethylene, umbilical vein, and saphenous vein bypass grafts for femoral-popliteal above-knee revascularization: a prospective randomized Department of Veterans Affairs cooperative study. *J Vasc Surg* 2000;**32**:268.

150. Schneider JR, Walsh DB, McDaniel MD, et al. Pedal bypass versus tibial bypass with autogenous vein: a comparison of outcome and hemodynamic results. *J Vasc Surg* 1993;**17**:1029.

151. Berceli SA. Revision of vein bypass grafts: factors affecting durability of interventions. *Semin Vasc Surg* 2009;**22**:261.

152. Conte MS. Challenges of distal bypass surgery in patients with diabetes: patient selection, techniques, and outcomes. *J Vasc Surg* 2010;**52**:96S.

153. Walker TG. Acute limb ischemia. *Tech Vasc Interventional Rad* 2009;**12**:117.

154. Karalis DG, Quinn V, Victor MF, et al. Risk of catheter-related emboli in patients with atherosclerotic debris in the thoracic aorta. *Am Heart J* 1996;**131**:1149.

155. Applebaum RM, Kronzon I. Evaluation and management of cholesterol embolization and blue toe syndrome. *Curr Opin Cardiol* 1996;**11**:533.

156. Bashore TM, Gehrig T. Cholesterol emboli after invasive cardiac procedures. *J Am Coll Cardiol* 2003;**42**:217.

157. Paraskevas KI, Koutsias S, Mikhailidis DP, et al. Cholesterol crystal embolization: a possible complication of peripheral endovascular interventions. *J Endovasc Ther* 2008;**15**:614.

158. Keen RR, McCarthy WJ, Shireman PK, et al. Surgical management of atheroembolization. *J Vasc Surg* 1995;**21**:773.

159. Rutherford RB. Clinical staging of acute limb ischemia as the basis for choice of revascularization method: when and how to intervene. *Semin Vasc Surg* 2009;**22**:5.

160. O'Connell JB, Quinones-Baldrich WJ. Proper evaluation and management of acute embolic versus thrombotic limb ischemia. *Semin Vasc Surg* 2009;**22**:10.

161. Kropman RH, Schrijver AM, Kelder JC, et al. Clinical outcome of acute leg ischaemia due to thrombosed popliteal artery aneurysm: systematic review of 895 cases. *Eur J Vasc Endovasc Surg* 2010;**39**:452.

162. Pulli R, Dorigo W, Troisi N, et al. Surgical management of popliteal artery aneurysms: which factors affect outcomes? *J Vasc Surg* 2006;**43**:481.

163. Huang Y, Gloviczki P, Noel AA. Early complications and long-term outcome after open surgical treatment of popliteal artery aneurysm: is exclusion with saphenous vein bypass still the gold standard? *J Vasc Surg* 2007;**45**:706.

164. Robinson WP 3rd, Belkin M. Acute limb ischemia due to popliteal artery aneurysm: a continuing surgical challenge. *Semin Vasc Surg* 2009;**22**:17.

165. van den Berg JC. Thrombolysis for acute arterial occlusion. *J Vasc Surg* 2010;**52**:512.

166. Valji K. Evolving strategies for thrombolytic therapy of peripheral vascular occlusion. *J Vasc Interv Radiol* 2000;**11**:411.

167. Semba CP, Murphy TP, Bakal CW, et al; The Advisory Panel. Thrombolytic therapy with use of alteplase (rt-PA) in peripheral arterial occlusive disease: review of the clinical literature. *J Vasc Interv Radiol* 2000;**11**:149.

168. Benenati J, Shlansky-Goldberg R, Meglin A, et al. Thrombolytic and antiplatelet therapy in peripheral vascular disease with use of reteplase and/or abciximab. The SCVIR Consultants' Conference. *J Vasc Interv Radiol* 2001;**12**:795.

169. Razavi MK, Lee DS, Hofmann LV. Catheter-directed thrombolytic therapy for limb ischemia: current status and controversies. *J Vasc Interv Radiol* 2004;**15**:13.

170. Wagner H-J, Mueller-Huelsbeck S, Pitton MB, et al. Rapid thrombectomy with a hydrodynamic catheter: results from a prospective, multicenter trial. *Radiology* 1997;**205**:675.

171. Rilinger N, Goerich J, Scharrer-Pamler R, et al. Short-term results with use of the Amplatz thrombectomy device in the treatment of acute lower limb occlusions. *J Vasc Interv Radiol* 1997;**8**:343.

172. Huettl EA, Soulen MC. Thrombolysis of lower extremity embolic occlusions: a study of the results of the STAR registry. *Radiology* 1995;**197**:141.

173. Spence LD, Hartnell GG, Reinking G, et al. Thrombolysis of infrapopliteal bypass grafts: efficacy and underlying angiographic pathology. *AJR Am J Roentgenol* 1997;**169**:717.

174. Rajan DK, Patel NH, Valji K, et al. Quality improvement guidelines for percutaneous management of acute limb ischemia. *J Vasc Interv Radiol* 2005;**16**:585.

175. Weaver FA, Comerota AJ, Youngblood M, et al. Surgical revascularization versus thrombolysis for nonembolic lower extremity native artery occlusions: results of a prospective randomized trial. The STILE Investigators. Surgery versus Thrombolysis for Ischemia of the Lower Extremity. *J Vasc Surg* 1996;**24**:513.

176. Ouriel K, Veith FJ, Sasahara AA. A comparison of recombinant urokinase with vascular surgery as initial treatment for acute arterial occlusion of the legs: Thrombolysis or Peripheral Arterial Surgery (TOPAS) Investigators. *N Engl J Med* 1998;**338**:1105.

177. Ouriel K, Shortell CK, DeWeese JA, et al. A comparison of thrombolytic therapy with operative revascularization in the initial treatment of acute peripheral arterial ischemia. *J Vasc Surg* 1994;**19**:1021.

178. Ouriel K, Shortell CK, Azodo MV, et al. Acute peripheral arterial occlusion: predictors of success in catheter-directed thrombolytic therapy. *Radiology* 1994;**193**:561.

179. Wissgott C, Richter A, Kamusella P, et al. Treatment of critical limb ischemia using ultrasound-enhanced thrombolysis (PARES Trial): final results. *J Endovasc Ther* 2007;**14**:438.

180. Arepally A, Hofmann LV, Kim HS, et al. Weight-based rt-PA thrombolysis protocol for acute native arterial and bypass graft occlusions. *J Vasc Interv Radiol* 2002;**13**:45.

181. Swischuk JL, Fox PF, Young K, et al. Transcatheter intraarterial infusion of rt-PA for acute lower limb ischemia: results and complications. *J Vasc Interv Radiol* 2001;**12**:423.

182. Semba CP, Bakal CW, Calis KA, et al; Advisory Panel on Catheter-Directed Thrombolytic Therapy. Alteplase as an alternative to urokinase. *J Vasc Interv Radiol* 2000;**11**:279.

183. Davidian MM, Powell A, Benenati JF, et al. Initial results of reteplase in the treatment of acute lower extremity arterial occlusions. *J Vasc Interv Radiol* 2000;**11**:289.

184. Burkart DJ, Borsa JJ, Anthony JP, et al. Thrombolysis of occluded peripheral arteries and veins with tenecteplase: a pilot study. *J Vasc Interv Radiol* 2002;**13**:1099.

185. Ouriel K, Katzen B, Mewissen M, et al. Reteplase in the treatment of peripheral arterial and venous occlusions: a pilot study. *J Vasc Interv Radiol* 2000;**11**:849.

186. Castaneda F, Swischuk JL, Li R, et al. Declining-dose study of reteplase treatment for lower extremity arterial occlusions. *J Vasc Interv Radiol* 2002;**13**:1093.

187. Mahler F, Schneider E, Hess H, et al. Recombinant tissue plasminogen activator versus urokinase for local thrombolysis of femoropopliteal occlusions: a prospective, randomized multicenter trial. *J Endovasc Ther* 2001;**8**:638.

188. Han SM, Weaver FA, Comerota AJ, et al. Efficacy and safety of alfimeprase in patients with acute peripheral arterial occlusion (PAO). *J Vasc Surg* 2010;**51**:600.

189. Drescher P, McGuckin J, Rilling WS, et al. Catheter-directed thrombolytic therapy in peripheral artery occlusions: combining reteplase and abciximab. *AJR Am J Roentgenol* 2003;**180**:1385.

190. Ouriel K. Use of concomitant glycoprotein IIb/IIIa inhibitors with catheter-directed peripheral arterial thrombolysis. *J Vasc Interv Radiol* 2004;**15**:543.

191. Shlansky-Goldberg R. Platelet aggregation inhibitors for use in peripheral vascular interventions: what can we learn from the experience in the coronary arteries? *J Vasc Interv Radiol* 2002;**13**:229.

192. Ouriel K, Castaneda F, McNamara T, et al. Reteplase monotherapy and reteplase/abciximab combination therapy in peripheral arterial occlusive disease: results from the RELAX trial. *J Vasc Interv Radiol* 2004;**15**:229.

193. Duda SH, Tepe G, Luz O, et al. Peripheral artery occlusion: treatment with abciximab plus urokinase versus with urokinase alone-a randomized pilot trial (the PROMPT Study). Platelet Receptor Antibodies in Order to Manage Peripheral Artery Thrombosis. *Radiology* 2001;**221**:689.

194. Tepe G, Hopfenzitz C, Dietz K, et al. Peripheral arteries: treatment with antibodies of platelet receptors and reteplase for thrombolysis- APART trial. *Radiology* 2006;**239**:892.

195. Kasirajan K, Gray B, Beavers FP, et al. Rheolytic thrombectomy in the management of acute and subacute limb-threatening ischemia. *J Vasc Interv Radiol* 2001;**12**:413.

196. Kasirajan K, Haskal ZJ, Ouriel K. The use of mechanical thrombectomy devices in the management of acute peripheral arterial occlusive disease. *J Vasc Interv Radiol* 2001;**12**:405.

197. Gorich J, Rilinger N, Sokiranski R, et al. Mechanical thrombolysis of acute occlusion of both the superficial and the deep femoral arteries using a thrombectomy device. *AJR Am J Roentgenol* 1998;**170**:1177.

198. Wagner HJ, Starck EE. Acute embolic occlusions of the infrainguinal arteries: percutaneous aspiration embolectomy in 102 patients. *Radiology* 1992;**182**:403.

199. Kessel DO, Berridge DC, Robertson I. Infusion techniques for peripheral arterial thrombolysis. *Cochrane Database Syst Rev* 2004:CD000985.

200. Vorwerk D, Guenther RW, Wendt G, et al. Ulcerated plaques and focal aneurysms of iliac arteries: treatment with noncovered, self-expanding stents. *AJR Am J Roentgenol* 1994;**162**:1421.

201. Mattos MA, van Bemmelen PS, Hodgson KJ, et al. Does correction of stenoses identified with color duplex scanning improve infrainguinal graft patency? *J Vasc Surg* 1993;**17**:54.

202. Davies AH, Hawdon AJ, Sydes MR, et al. Is duplex surveillance of value after leg vein bypass grafting? Principal results of the Vein Graft Surveillance Randomised Trial (VGST). *Circulation* 2005;**112**:1985.

203. Tinder CN, Bandyk DF. Detection of imminent vein graft occlusion: what is the optimal surveillance program? *Semin Vasc Surg* 2009;**22**:252.

204. Idu MM, Blankenstein JD, deGier P, et al. Impact of a color-flow duplex surveillance program on infrainguinal vein graft patency: a five year experience. *J Vasc Surg* 1993;**17**:42.

205. Meissner OA, Verrel F, Tato F, et al. Magnetic resonance angiography in the follow-up of distal lower-extremity bypass surgery: comparison with duplex ultrasound and digital subtraction angiography. *J Vasc Interv Radiol* 2004;**15**:1269.

206. Loewe C, Cejna M, Schoder M, et al. Contrast material-enhanced, moving-table MR angiography versus digital subtraction angiography for surveillance of peripheral arterial bypass grafts. *J Vasc Interv Radiol* 2003;**14**:1129.

207. Whittemore AD, Donaldson MC, Polak JF, et al. Limitations of balloon angioplasty for vein graft stenosis. *J Vasc Surg* 1991;**14**:340.

208. Perler BA, Osterman FA, Mitchell SE, et al. Balloon dilatation versus surgical revision of infra-inguinal autogenous vein graft stenoses: long-term follow-up. *J Cardiovasc Surg* 1990;**31**:656.

209. Goh RH, Sniderman KW, Kalman PG. Long-term follow-up of management of failing in situ saphenous vein bypass grafts using endovascular intervention techniques. *J Vasc Interv Radiol* 2000;**11**:705.

210. Engelke C, Morgan RA, Belli AM. Cutting balloon percutaneous transluminal angioplasty for salvage of lower limb arterial bypass grafts: feasibility. *Radiology* 2002;**223**:106.

211. Hye RJ, Turner C, Valji K, et al. Is thrombolysis of occluded popliteal and tibial bypass grafts worthwhile? *J Vasc Surg* 1994;**20**:588.

212. Durham JD, Geller SC, Abbott WM, et al. Regional infusion of urokinase into occluded lower-extremity bypass grafts: long-term clinical results. *Radiology* 1989;**172**:83.

213. Sullivan KL, Gardiner Jr GA, Kandarpa K, et al. Efficacy of thrombolysis in infrainguinal bypass grafts. *Circulation* 1991;**83**(Suppl. I):I-99.

214. Seabrook GR, Mewissen MW, Schmitt DD, et al. Percutaneous intra-arterial thrombolysis in the treatment of thrombosis of lower extremity arterial reconstructions. *J Vasc Surg* 1991;**13**:646.

215. Richardson JW, Greenfield LJ. Natural history and management of iliac aneurysms. *J Vasc Surg* 1988;**8**:165.

216. Leon Jr LR, Taylor Z, Psalms SB, et al. Degenerative aneurysms of the superficial femoral artery. *Eur J Vasc Endovasc Surg* 2008;**35**:332.

217. Huang Y, Gloviczki P, Duncan AA, et al. Common iliac artery aneurysm: expansion rate and results of open surgical and endovascular repair. *J Vasc Surg* 2008;**47**:1203.

218. Wolf YG, Kobzantsev Z, Zelmanovich L. Size of normal and aneurysmal popliteal arteries: a duplex ultrasound study. *J Vasc Surg* 2006;**43**:488.

219. Cina CS. Endovascular repair of popliteal aneurysms. *J Vasc Surg* 2010;**51**:1056.

220. Varga ZA, Locke-Edmunds JC, Baird RN, et al. A multicenter study of popliteal aneurysms. *J Vasc Surg* 1994;**20**:171.

221. Dawson I, Sie RB, van Bockel JH. Atherosclerotic popliteal aneurysm. *Br J Surg* 1997;**84**:293.

222. Buckley CJ, Buckley SD. Technical tips for endovascular repair of common iliac artery aneurysms. *Semin Vasc Surg* 2008;**21**:31.

223. Philpott JM, Parker FM, Benton CR, et al. Isolated internal iliac artery aneurysm resection and reconstruction: operative planning and technical considerations. *Am Surg* 2003;**69**:569.

224. Hsu RB, Tsay YG, Wang SS, et al. Surgical treatment for primary infected aneurysm of the descending thoracic aorta, abdominal aorta, and iliac arteries. *J Vasc Surg* 2002;**36**:746.

225. Piffaretti G, Tozzi M, Lomazzi C, et al. Endovascular treatment for para-anastomotic abdominal aortic and iliac aneurysms following aortic surgery. *J Cardiovasc Surg (Torino)* 2007;**48**:711.

226. Fahrni M, Lachat MM, Wildermuth S, et al. Endovascular therapeutic options for isolated iliac aneurysms with a working classification. *Cardiovasc Intervent Radiol* 2003;**26**:443.

227. Helvie MA, Rubin JM, Silver TM, et al. The distinction between femoral artery pseudoaneurysms and other causes of groin masses: value of duplex Doppler sonography. *AJR Am J Roentgenol* 1988;**150**:1177.

228. Wright LB, Matchett WJ, Cruz CP, et al. Popliteal artery disease: diagnosis and treatment. *Radiographics* 2004;**24**:467.

229. Patel NV, Long GW, Cheema ZF, et al. Open vs. endovascular repair of isolated iliac artery aneurysms: a 12-year experience. *J Vasc Surg* 2009;**49**:1147.

230. Hechelhammer L, Rancic Z, Pfiffner R, et al. Midterm outcome of endovascular repair of ruptured isolated iliac aneurysms. *J Vasc Surg* 2010;**52**:1159.

231. Marin ML, Veith FJ, Lyon RT, et al. Transfemoral endovascular repair of iliac artery aneurysms. *Am J Surg* 1995;**170**:179.

232. Razavi MK, Dake MD, Semba CP, et al. Percutaneous endoluminal placement of stent-grafts for the treatment of isolated iliac artery aneurysms. *Radiology* 1995;**197**:801.

233. Tielliu IF, Verhoeven EL, Prins TR, et al. Treatment of popliteal artery aneurysms with the Hemobahn stent-graft. *J Endovasc Ther* 2003;**10**:111.

234. Geraghty PJ. Endovascular treatment of lower extremity aneurysms. *Semin Vasc Surg* 2008;**21**:195.

235. Stiegler H, Mendler G, Baumann G. Prospective study of 36 patients with 46 popliteal artery aneurysms with non-surgical treatment. *Vasa* 2002;**31**:43.

236. Antonello M, Frigatti P, Battocchio P, et al. Open versus endovascular treatment for asymptomatic popliteal artery aneurysm: results of a prospective randomized study. *J Vasc Surg* 2005;**42**:185.

237. Ravn H, Bjorck M. Popliteal artery aneurysm with acute ischemia in 229 patients. Outcome after thrombolytic and surgical therapy. *Eur J Vasc Endovasc Surg* 2007;**33**:690.

238. Hollis Jr HW, Luethke JM, Yakes WF, et al. Percutaneous embolization of an internal iliac artery aneurysm: technical considerations and literature review. *J Vasc Interv Radiol* 1994;**5**:449.

239. Cynamon J, Marin ML, Veith FJ, et al. Endovascular repair of an internal iliac artery aneurysm with use of a stented graft and embolization coils. *J Vasc Interv Radiol* 1995;**6**:509.

240. Paulson EK, Hertzberg BS, Paine SS, et al. Femoral artery pseudoaneurysms: value of color Doppler sonography in predicting which ones will thrombose without treatment. *AJR Am J Roentgenol* 1992;**159**:1077.

241. Morgan R, Belli AM. Current treatment methods for postcatheterization pseudoaneurysms. *J Vasc Interv Radiol* 2003;**14**:697.

242. Krueger K, Zaehringer M, Soehngen FD, et al. Femoral pseudoaneurysms: management with percutaneous thrombin injections-success rates and effects on systemic coagulation. *Radiology* 2003;**226**:452.

243. Dyer GSM, Vrahas MS. Review of the pathophysiology and acute management of haemorrhage in pelvic fracture. *Injury* 2006;**37**:602.

244. Stein DM, O'Toole R, Scalea TM. Multidisciplinary approach for patients with pelvic fractures and hemodynamic instability. *Scand J Surg* 2007;**96**:272.

245. Anderson SW, Soto JA, Lucey BC, et al. Blunt trauma: feasibility and clinical utility of pelvic CT angiography performed with 64-detector row CT. *Radiology* 2008;**246**:410.

246. Yalamanchili S, Harvey SM, Friedman A, et al. Transarterial embolization for inferior epigastric artery injury. *Vasc Endovascular Surg* 2008;**42**:489.

247. Sofocleous CT, Hinrichs CR, Hubbi B, et al. Embolization of isolated lumbar artery injuries in trauma patients. *Cardiovasc Intervent Radiol* 2005;**28**:730.

248. Salim A, Teixeira PG, DuBose J, et al. Predictors of positive angiography in pelvic fractures: a prospective study. *J Am Coll Surg* 2008;**207**:656.

249. Kimbrell BJ, Velmahos GC, Chan LS et al. Angiographic embolization for pelvic fractures in older patients. *Arch Surg* 2004;**139**:728.

250. Shapiro M, McDonald AA, Knight D, et al. The role of repeat angiography in the management of pelvic fractures. *J Trauma* 2005;**58**:227.

251. Travis T, Monsky WL, London J, et al. Evaluation of short-term and long-term complications after emergent internal iliac artery embolization in patients with pelvic trauma. *J Vasc Interv Radiol* 2008;**19**:840.

252. Ramirez JI, Velmahos GC, Best CR, et al. Male sexual function after bilateral internal iliac artery embolization for pelvic fracture. *J Trauma* 2004;**56**:734.

253. Hafez HM, Woolgar J, Robbs JV. Lower extremity arterial injury: results of 550 cases and review of risk factors associated with limb loss. *J Vasc Surg* 2001;**33**:1212.

254. Patterson BM, Agel J, Swiontkowski MF, et al. Knee dislocations with vascular injury: outcomes in the Lower Extremity Assessment Project (LEAP) Study. *J Trauma* 2007;**63**:855.

255. Britt LD, Weireter LJ, Cole FJ. Newer diagnostic modalities for vascular injuries. *Surg Clin North Am* 2001;**81**:1263.

256. Dennis JW, Frykberg ER, Crump JM, et al. New perspectives on the management of penetrating trauma in proximity to major limb arteries. *J Vasc Surg* 1990;**11**:85.

257. Schwartz MR, Weaver FA, Bauer M, et al. Redefining the indications for arteriography in penetrating extremity trauma: a prospective analysis. *J Vasc Surg* 1993;**17**:116.

258. Sadjadi J, Cureton EL, Dozier KC, et al. Expedited treatment of lower extremity gunshot wounds. *J Am Coll Surg* 2009;**209**:740.

259. Knudson MM, Lewis FR, Atkinson K, et al. The role of duplex ultrasound arterial imaging in patients with penetrating extremity trauma. *Arch Surg* 1993;**128**:1033.

260. Gagne PJ, Cone JB, McFarland D, et al. Proximity penetrating extremity trauma: the role of duplex ultrasound in the detection of occult venous injuries. *J Trauma* 1995;**39**:1157.

261. Seamon MJ, Smoger D, Torres DM, et al. A prospective validation of a current practice: the detection of extremity vascular injury with CT angiography. *J Trauma* 2009;**67**:238

262. Peng PD, Spain DA, Tataria M, et al. CT angiography effectively evaluates extremity arterial trauma. *Am Surg* 2008;**74**:103.

263. Pieroni S, Foster BR, Anderson SW, et al. Use of 64-row multidetector CT angiography in blunt and penetrating trauma of the upper and lower extremities. *Radiographics* 2009;**29**:863.

264. Starnes BW, Arthurs ZM. Endovascular management of vascular trauma. *Perspect Vasc Surg Endovasc Ther* 2006;**18**:114.

265. Lopera JE, Suri R, Cura M, et al. Crural artery traumatic injuries: treatment with embolization. *Cardiovasc Intervent Radiol* 2008;**31**:550.

266. Marin ML, Veith FJ, Panetta TF, et al. Transluminally placed endovascular stented graft repair for arterial trauma. *J Vasc Surg* 1994;**20**:466.

267. Hoffer EK, Sclafani SJ, Herskowitz MM, et al. Natural history of arterial injuries diagnosed with arteriography. *J Vasc Interv Radiol* 1997;**8**:43.

268. Cherry WB, Mueller PS. Rectus sheath hematoma: review of 126 cases at a single institution. *Medicine* (Baltimore) 2006;**85**:105.

269. Chan YC, Morales JP, Reidy JF, et al. Management of spontaneous and iatrogenic retroperitoneal haemorrhage: conservative management, endovascular intervention, or open surgery? *Int J Clin Pract* 2008;**62**:1604.

270. Isokangas JM, Perala JM. Endovascular embolization of spontaneous retroperitoneal hemorrhage secondary to anticoagulant treatment. *Cardiovasc Intervent Radiol* 2004;**27**:607.

271. Piazza G, Creager MA. Thromboangiitis obliterans. *Circulation* 2010;**121**:1858.

272. Olin JW, Shih A. Thromboangiitis obliterans (Buerger's disease). *Curr Opin Rheumatol* 2006;**18**:18-24.

273. Hussein EA, Dorri A. Intra-arterial streptokinase as adjuvant therapy for complicated Buerger's disease: early trials. *Int Surg* 1993;**78**:54.

274. McKiernan TL, Bock K, Leya F, et al. Ergot induced peripheral vascular insufficiency, non-interventional treatment. *Cathet Cardiovasc Diagn* 1994;**31**:211.

275. Norton PT, Hagspiel K. Stationary arterial waves in magnetic resonance angiography. *J Vasc Interv Radiol* 2005;**16**:423.

276. Peynircioglu B, Cil BE, Karcaaltincaba M. Standing or stationary arterial waves of the superior mesenteric artery at MR angiography and subsequent conventional arteriography. *J Vasc Interv Radiol* 2007;**18**:1329-1330.

277. Wing RJ, Waugh RC, Harris JP. Treatment of fibromuscular dysplasia of the external iliac artery by percutaneous transluminal angioplasty. *Australas Radiol* 1993;**37**:223.

278. Olin JW, Pierce M. Contemporary management of fibromuscular dysplasia. *Curr Opin Cardiol* 2008;**23**:527-536.

279. Jurado JA, Bashir R, Burket MW. Radiation-induced peripheral artery disease. *Catheter Cardiovasc Interv* 2008;**72**:563.

280. Baerlocher MO, Rajan DK, Ing DJ, et al. Primary stenting of bilateral radiation induced external iliac stenoses. *J Vasc Surg* 2004;**40**:1028-1031.

281. Gloviczki P, Duncan A, Kalra M, et al. Vascular malformations: an update. *Perspect Vasc Surg Endovasc Ther* 2009;**21**:133.

282. Chiller KG, Frieden IJ, Arbiser JL. Molecular pathogenesis of vascular anomalies: classification into three categories based upon clinical and biochemical characteristics. *Lymphat Res Biol* 2003;**1**:267.

283. Fayad LM, Hazirolan T, Bluemke D, et al. Vascular malformations in the extremities: emphasis on MR imaging features that guide treatment options. *Skeletal Radiol* 2006;**35**:127.

284. Konez O, Burrows PE. Magnetic resonance of vascular anomalies. *Magn Reson Imaging Clin N Am* 2002;**10**:363.

285. Arneja JS, Gosain AK. Vascular malformations. *Plast Reconstr Surg* 2008;**121**:195e.

286. Marler JJ, Mulliken JB. Current management of hemangiomas and vascular malformations. *Clin Plast Surg* 2005;**32**:99.

287. White Jr RI, Pollak J, Persing J, et al. Long-term outcome of embolotherapy and surgery for high-flow extremity arteriovenous malformations. *J Vasc Interv Radiol* 2000;**11**:1285.

288. Burrows PE, Mason KP. Percutaneous treatment of low flow vascular malformations. *J Vasc Interv Radiol* 2004;**15**:431.

289. Tan KT, Simons ME, Rajan DK, et al. Peripheral high-flow arteriovenous vascular malformations: a single-center experience. *J Vasc Interv Radiol* 2004;**15**:1071.

290. Pollak JS, White Jr RI. The use of cyanoacrylate adhesives in peripheral embolization. *J Vasc Interv Radiol* 2001;**12**:907.

291. Castaneda F, Goodwin SC, Swischuk JL, et al. Treatment of pelvic arteriovenous malformations with ethylene vinyl alcohol copolymer (Onyx). *J Vasc Interv Radiol* 2002;**13**:513.

292. Orsini C, Brotto M. Immediate pathologic effects on the vein wall of foam sclerotherapy. *Dermatol Surg* 2007;**33**:1250.

293. Ayad M, Eskioglu E, Mericle RA. Onyx: a unique neuroembolic agent. *Expert Rev Med Devices* 2006;**3**:705.

294. Do YS, Park KB, Park HS, et al. Extremity arteriovenous malformations involving the bone: therapeutic outcomes of ethanol embolotherapy. *J Vasc Interv Radiol* 2010;**21**:807.

295. Cura M, Martinez N, Cura A, et al. Arteriovenous malformations of the uterus. *Acta Radiol* 2009;**50**:823.

296. Vallance R, Quin RO, Forrest H. Arterio-venous shunting complicating occlusive atherosclerotic peripheral vascular disease. *Clin Radiol* 1986;**37**:389.

297. Rehman S, Hancock L, Wolfe J. Recurrent cystic adventitial disease of the iliofemoral artery. *Ann Vasc Surg* 2010;**24**:550e1.

298. Levien LJ, Benn CA. Adventitial cystic disease: a unifying hypothesis. *J Vasc Surg* 1998;**28**:193.

299. Elster EA, Hewlett S, DeRienzo DP, et al. Adventitial cystic disease of the axillary artery. *Ann Vasc Surg* 2002;**16**:134.

300. Maged IM, Turba UC, Housseini AM, et al. High spatial resolution magnetic resonance imaging of cystic adventitial disease of the popliteal artery. *J Vasc Surg* 2010;**51**:471.

301. Maged IM, Kron IL, Hagspiel KD. Recurrent cystic adventitial disease of the popliteal artery: successful treatment with percutaneous transluminal angioplasty. *Vasc Endovasc Surg* 2009;**43**:399.

302. Pillai J. A current interpretation of popliteal vascular entrapment. *J Vasc Surg* 2008;**48**:61S.

303. Levien JL, Veller MG. Popliteal artery entrapment syndrome: more common than previously recognized. *J Vasc Surg* 1999;**30**:587.

304. Levien LJ. Popliteal artery entrapment syndrome. *Semin Vasc Surg* 2003;**16**:223.

305. Erdoes LS, Devine JJ, Bernhard VM, et al. Popliteal vascular compression in a normal population. *J Vasc Surg* 1994;**20**:978.

306. Hai Z, Guangrui S, Yuan Z, et al. CT angiography and MRI in patients with popliteal artery entrapment syndrome. *AJR Am J Roentgenol* 2008;**191**:1760.

307. Zhong H, Liu C, Shao G. Computed tomographic angiography and digital subtraction angiography findings in popliteal artery entrapment syndrome. *J Comput Assist Tomogr* 2010;**34**:254.

308. Vink A, Bender MH, Schep G, et al. Histopathological comparison between endofibrosis of the high-performance cyclist and atherosclerosis in the external iliac artery. *J Vasc Surg* 2008;**48**:1458.

309. Scavee V, Stainier L, Deltombe T, et al. External iliac artery endofibrosis: a new possible predisposing factor. *J Vasc Surg* 2003; **38**:180.

310. Abraham P, Bouye P, Quere I, et al. Past, present and future of arterial endofibrosis in athletes: a point of view. *Sports Med* 2004;**34**:419.

311. Giannoukas AD, Berczi V, Anoop U, et al. Endofibrosis of iliac arteries in high-performance athletes: diagnostic approach and minimally invasive endovascular treatment. *Cardiovasc Intervent Radiol* 2006;**29**:866.

CHAPTER
9

Upper Extremity Arteries

Karim Valji

ARTERIOGRAPHY (VIDEO 9-1)

The brachiocephalic, left carotid, and left subclavian arteries are catheterized from a common femoral artery approach with a 4- or 5-French (Fr) vertebral or head-hunter catheter. The catheter is advanced over a guidewire into the ascending thoracic aorta and then simultaneously torqued and withdrawn at the groin until the tip engages the artery of interest (Fig. 9-1). In older patients with ectasia of the aorta and arch vessels, a reverse-curve catheter may be useful (Fig. 9-2). When atherosclerotic disease is present, gentle catheter manipulations are essential to avoid dislodging aortic plaque fragments into the brain or periphery. Even minute air bubbles or clots released during catheterization of arch vessels and their branches may cause a stroke (through the carotid or vertebral arteries) or paraplegia (e.g., through spinal branches of the costocervical artery.) Therefore meticulous double

flushing with uncontaminated saline is done every 60 to 90 seconds *if* blood can be aspirated from the catheter.

During arteriography of the upper extremity, a high origin of the radial artery from the brachial or axillary trunk should be sought (see later discussion). In this situation, the catheter tip is positioned proximal to its take-off. Arteriography of the hand is usually performed with a catheter in the midbrachial artery. The arteries of the hand and forearm are especially prone to vasospasm, which may be prevented or relieved by intraarterial injection of a vasodilator (e.g., 100 to 200 μg of nitroglycerin).

In some instances, arteriography of the forearm and hand is accomplished by direct antegrade brachial artery puncture (see Chapter 3). For example, this approach is useful to evaluate the anastomosis of a dialysis fistula that is not easily accessible directly from the access itself.

ANATOMY (ONLINE CASES 3 AND 17)

Development

In early gestation, the upper limbs are nourished by the axial artery. This vessel evolves into the axillary, brachial, interosseous, and median arteries that feed the hand in the fetus.[1] The ulnar artery is an outgrowth of the brachial artery at the elbow. The radial artery arises from a superficial branch of the proximal brachial artery, but its origin migrates toward the elbow as the fetus grows. In most cases, the distal interosseous and median arteries regress before birth.

Normal Anatomy

The *subclavian arteries* originate from the *brachiocephalic (innominate) artery* on the right and directly from the aortic arch on the left[2] (Fig. 9-3). The artery runs posterior to the subclavian vein and the anterior scalene muscle. It arches over the pulmonary apex within the costoclavicular space

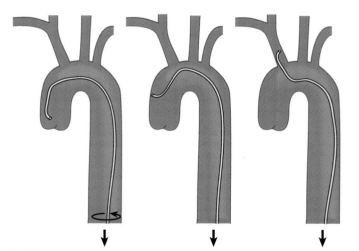

FIGURE 9-1 Steps in catheterization of the arch vessels with a headhunter catheter. The catheter can then be advanced into the right subclavian artery over a guidewire. Further withdrawal of the catheter (third panel) will cause it to jump into the left common carotid and then into the left subclavian artery. (*Adapted from Kadir S. Diagnostic angiography. Philadelphia: WB Saunders, 1986:177.*)

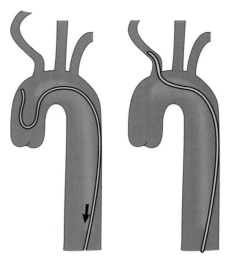

FIGURE 9-2   Steps in catheterization of a tortuous brachiocephalic artery with a Simmons catheter. (*Adapted from Kadir S.* Diagnostic angiography. *Philadelphia: WB Saunders; 1986: p.178.*)

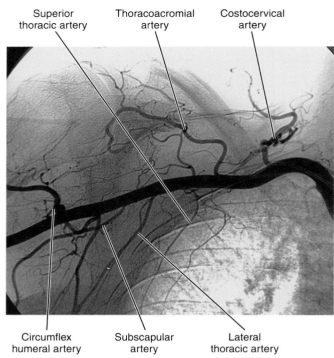

FIGURE 9-4   Arteriogram of the right subclavian and axillary arteries.

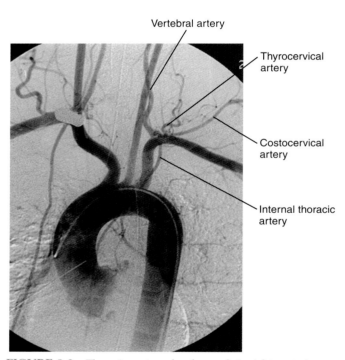

FIGURE 9-3   Thoracic aorta and arch vessels in right posterior oblique projection.

surrounded by nerves of the brachial plexus. The subclavian artery has several major branches (Fig. 9-4):

- The *vertebral artery* exits the superior aspect of the vessel and travels through the bony canal of the cervical transverse processes into the skull.

- The *internal thoracic (mammary) artery* exits the undersurface of the subclavian artery opposite the vertebral artery and runs behind the costosternal junctions (Fig. 9-5). The vessel divides into musculophrenic and superior epigastric branches. The internal thoracic artery and its musculophrenic branch give rise to the anterior intercostal arteries. The musculophrenic and superior epigastric branches have anastomoses with the inferior phrenic and inferior epigastric arteries, respectively, in the abdomen.
- The *thyrocervical trunk* takes off beyond the vertebral artery origin and immediately divides into the inferior thyroid, suprascapular, and superficial cervical arteries.
- The *costocervical trunk* gives rise to the superior intercostal artery (source of the first, second, and, occasionally, third posterior intercostal arteries) and the deep cervical artery. Small branches may supply the anterior spinal artery.
- The *dorsal scapular artery* is the final branch of the subclavian artery.

At the outer edge of the first rib, the subclavian artery becomes the *axillary artery* (see Fig. 9-4). The vessel runs deep to the pectoralis major and minor muscles and lateral to the axillary vein. Its major branches include the superior thoracic, thoracoacromial, lateral thoracic, subscapular, and anterior and posterior humeral circumflex

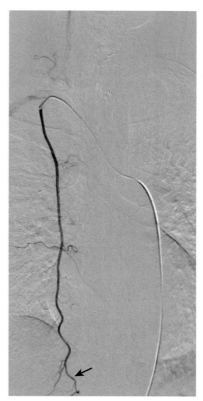

FIGURE 9-5   Right internal thoracic (mammary) arteriography. The vessel continues as the superficial epigastric artery as it enters the abdomen *(arrow)*.

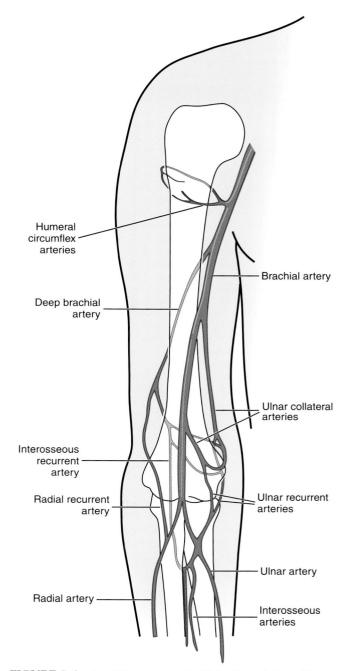

FIGURE 9-6   Arterial anatomy and collateral circulation of the upper arm and elbow.

arteries. These branches supply muscles of the shoulder girdle, humerus, scapula, and chest wall.

At the lateral edge of the teres major muscle (approximately the lateral scapular border), the axillary artery becomes the *brachial artery*. In the mid-upper arm, the artery lies in a fascial sheath along with the basilic vein, paired brachial veins, and the median and ulnar nerves. Its major branches include the deep brachial and the superior and inferior ulnar collateral arteries (Fig. 9-6). At about the level of the radial head, the brachial artery divides into the radial and ulnar arteries (Fig. 9-7). The *radial artery* obviously descends on the radial side of the forearm. The *ulnar artery,* which is usually the larger of the two, gives off the common interosseous artery and then descends on the ulnar side of the forearm. The *interosseous artery* divides into anterior and posterior branches separated by the interosseous membrane. In less than 10% of individuals, the anterior interosseous or *median artery* persists and contributes to the palmar arch.[3]

The arterial anatomy of the hand is extremely variable, and deviations from the classic pattern described here are common.[3,4] The ulnar artery supplies the *superficial palmar arch,* and the radial artery supplies the *deep palmar arch* (Figs. 9-8 and 9-9). The arches often are in continuity with the opposing forearm artery through small branches at the wrist. The superficial arch is dominant and typically forms distal to the deep arch. The princeps pollicis and radialis indicis arteries arise from the radial artery and supply the thumb and index finger, respectively. The superficial palmar arch gives off three or four common palmar digital arteries, and the deep arch gives off the palmar metacarpal arteries. At the bases of the proximal phalanges, adjacent metacarpal vessels from each arch merge and then immediately divide into proper digital

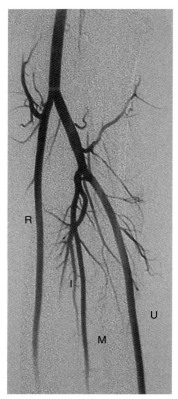

FIGURE 9-7   Right forearm arteriogram. The brachial artery bifurcates into radial *(R)* and ulnar *(U)* arteries. The ulnar artery gives off anterior and posterior interosseous arteries *(I)*. Also note an unusually prominent median artery *(M)*.

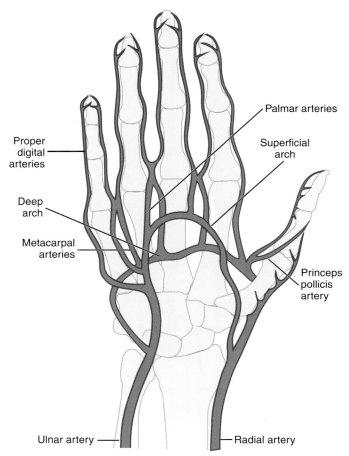

FIGURE 9-8   Arterial anatomy of the hand. *(Adapted from Loring LA, Hallisey MJ. Arteriography and interventional therapy for diseases of the hand.* Radiographics 1995;**15**:1299.)

arteries, which supply apposing surfaces of the fingers. A so-called *incomplete superficial arch,* defined by lack of continuity of the radial artery with the superficial arch and lack of supply of the thumb and medial index finger by the ulnar artery, is found in about 14% to 20% of the population in autopsy studies.[3,4]

Variant Anatomy

Anomalies of the subclavian artery origin are discussed in Chapter 6. In about one third of the population, the superficial cervical and dorsal scapular arteries have a common origin from the thyrocervical artery (i.e., transverse cervical artery). Variations in muscular branches of the axillary or brachial artery are common but do not have much clinical relevance.[5,6]

"High" origin of the radial artery from the axillary or upper brachial artery is an important variant (Fig. 9-10). This anomaly results when the radial artery origin fails to migrate distally toward the elbow during gestation. It was found in 14% of cases in one autopsy series.[6] A high origin of the ulnar artery is far less common. Duplications of the brachial artery and hypoplasia or aplasia of the radial and ulnar arteries are rare variants.

The *persistent median artery* reflects lack of regression of the embryonic median branch of the common interosseous artery (Fig. 9-11). It was identified in 3.4% of cases in one large operative series.[7] This vessel may supply a palmar arch.

Collateral Circulation

With proximal subclavian artery obstruction, blood may flow from the contralateral vertebrobasilar system into the ipsilateral mid-subclavian artery (see later discussion). When the obstruction is more distal, major collateral pathways are present across the thyroidal arterial system, between the internal thoracic and lateral thoracic arteries, and between the thyrocervical trunk and circumflex humeral arteries. With axillary artery obstruction, a rich network of muscular branches around the shoulder girdle provides collateral blood supply into the brachial artery.

In proximal brachial artery obstruction, the subscapular and posterior humeral circumflex arteries provide flow through muscular branches into the distal brachial or

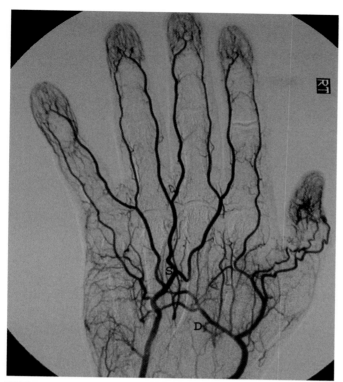

FIGURE 9-9   Normal hand arteriogram. Note superficial *(S)* and deep *(D)* palmar arches.

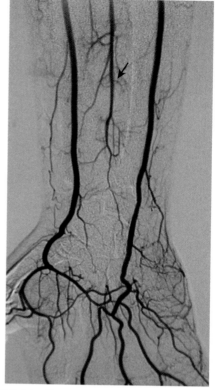

FIGURE 9-11   Prominent persistent median artery *(arrow)*.

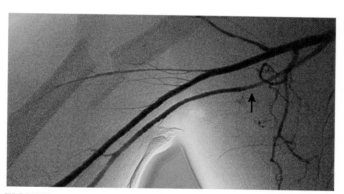

FIGURE 9-10   High origin of the radial artery *(arrow)* from the axillary artery. Note diffuse arterial spasm in the setting of acute fracture of the right humerus.

forearm arteries[2] (see Fig. 9-6). In cases of midbrachial artery occlusion, the deep brachial artery and superior ulnar collateral arteries supply the radial recurrent and ulnar recurrent arteries, respectively, above the elbow. The radial and ulnar recurrent arteries are the chief pathways across the elbow in patients with distal brachial artery occlusions.

When the radial or ulnar artery is obstructed, the opposing forearm artery, along with the anterior interosseous or median artery (if persistent into the wrist), supplies the hand. Collateral circulation with occlusion of the distal

forearm or hand vessels depends on the individual anatomy and continuity of the palmar arches.

MAJOR DISORDERS

Acute Upper Extremity Ischemia (Online Case 64)

Etiology

Acute ischemia is far less common in the arm than in the leg. This disparity is partially explained by the extensive collateral network around the scapula and shoulder and by the smaller muscle mass and metabolic needs of the arm. Emboli account for about 50% of cases of acute arterial occlusion, and most come from the heart[8-10] (Box 9-1). About one fourth of cases result from iatrogenic or accidental trauma leading to arterial thrombosis. In the remainder, acute thrombosis is caused by superimposed atherosclerotic plaque, local extrinsic disease (e.g., thoracic outlet syndrome), aneurysm, or arteritis.

Clinical Features

Most embolic occlusions occur in older patients with a history of cardiac dysrhythmias, myocardial infarction, or valvular heart disease. Sudden and complete upper extremity arterial obstruction causes abrupt onset of arm pain, coolness, cyanosis, pallor, diminished or absent pulses, and, occasionally, sensorimotor deficits. However, some patients are only mildly symptomatic if the underlying disease is chronic (as with thrombosis at a site of preexisting atherosclerotic stenosis) and collateral circulation is robust. The presence of arm swelling should raise the suspicion of severe venous thrombosis (see Chapter 17).

Imaging

Duplex sonography, computed tomography (CT) angiography, and magnetic resonance (MR) angiography are sometimes used in the initial evaluation of patients who do not go directly for operation[11-13] (Fig. 9-12). Catheter angiography is usually reserved for cases in which endovascular treatment is planned. It is customary to investigate the entire circulation from the aortic arch to the digital arteries of the hand to identify potential sources of emboli and to search for occult distal disease. An acute embolus produces a discrete filling defect with reconstitution of the distal vessels. However, it also may appear as a sharp cutoff that mimics a thrombotic occlusion (Fig. 9-13). After the embolic event occurs, clot propagates proximally and distally to the next large collateral branches. Post-traumatic thrombosis results in an abrupt occlusion at or near the site of injury (Fig. 9-14).

Treatment

Blood flow to the arm must be restored promptly (within about 4 to 6 hours after acute occlusion in the absence of preexisting collateral circulation) to avoid ischemic

---

BOX 9-1

SOURCES OF UPPER EXTREMITY ARTERIAL EMBOLI

- Cardiac thrombus (e.g., left atrium in atrial fibrillation)
- Atherosclerotic plaque in aortic arch or proximal arteries
- Aneurysm thrombus (e.g., subclavian artery)
- Proximal in situ thrombosis from thrombophilic state
- Trauma
- Endocarditis
- Paradoxical embolus from venous circulation through right to left shunt

---

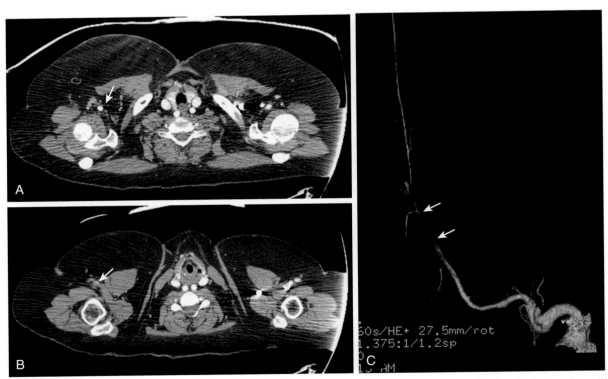

FIGURE 9-12   Brachial artery embolus. **A,** On contrast computed tomography angiography, the patent right brachial artery (*arrow*) becomes filled with thrombus on more distal image (**B,** *arrow*). **C,** On a reformatted image, the short segment brachial artery occlusion (*arrows*) is depicted.

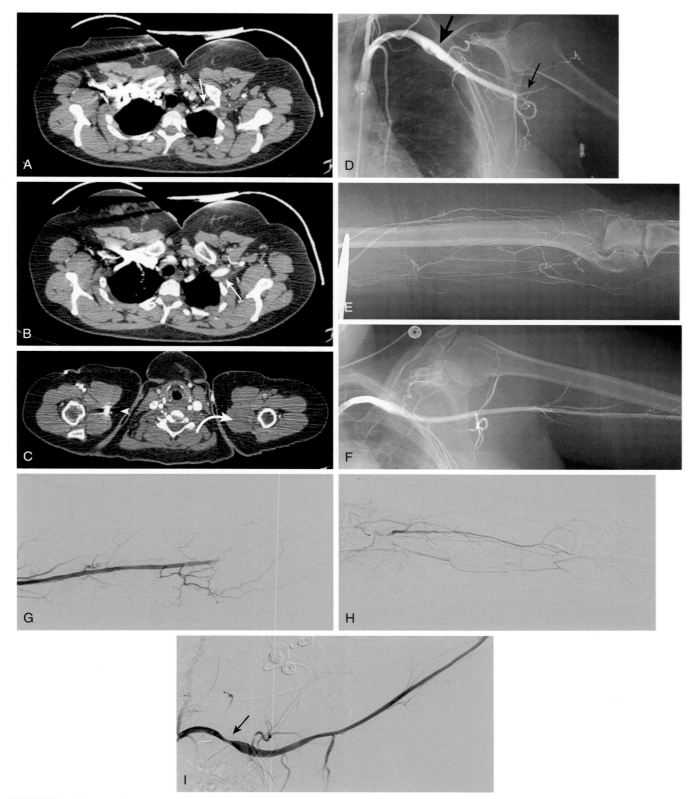

FIGURE 9-13 Embolus to the left brachial artery in a patient with thoracic outlet syndrome. **A** through **C,** Contrast-enhanced computed tomography images show left subclavian artery *(arrow)* abutting callus from an old clavicular fracture with post-stenotic dilation of the artery *(arrow)*. Unlike the right brachial artery *(arrowhead),* the mid left brachial artery is thrombosed *(curved arrow).* **D,** Left subclavian arteriogram shows mural thrombus within the dilated segment of the left subclavian artery *(large arrow)* and complete occlusion of the proximal left brachial artery *(small arrow).* **E,** Weak collateral flow is found in the upper arm. **F,** Following overnight thrombolysis with t-PA at 1 mg/hr, the proximal occlusion is completely gone. Flow is noted to the distal left brachial artery **(G),** with collateral filling of forearm arteries **(H). I,** With the left arm in extreme abduction, narrowing of the subclavian artery is noted *(arrow).*

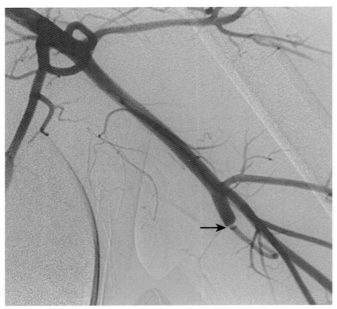

FIGURE 9-14   Thrombosis of the left brachial artery after catheterization.

peripheral neuropathy, irreversible muscle necrosis, and (ultimately) amputation.[14]

SURGICAL THERAPY

Anticoagulation and embolectomy with a Fogarty catheter are standard treatment for embolic occlusions.[8-10,15] If the symptoms are mild and the clot burden is small, the patient can sometimes be managed with anticoagulation alone. Thrombotic occlusions are repaired by direct thrombectomy, patch revision, or bypass grafting.

ENDOVASCULAR THERAPY

Thrombolysis is an attractive alternative to surgery for some acute upper extremity arterial occlusions.[16,17] Acute embolic occlusions are very responsive to enzymatic thrombolysis, which achieves complete or near-complete clot lysis and limb salvage in many cases[18,19] (see Fig. 9-13). Techniques for extremity arterial thrombolysis are considered in Chapter 3. Liberal use of intraarterial vasodilators is recommended to combat vasospasm, which occurs frequently with upper extremity artery manipulations. Because the collateral circulation in the arm and hand is so extensive, even partial lysis of an occlusion may avoid amputation or at least limit its extent. Occlusions less than 48 hours old respond better to thrombolysis than do older ones. An important advantage of lytic infusion over surgery is the ability to lyse clots in small vessels of the forearm and hand. Stroke from embolization of pericatheter clot has been reported with prolonged infusions, but it is a rare complication.

Chronic Upper Extremity Ischemia (Online Case 29)

Etiology

A variety of diseases may cause subacute or chronic upper extremity ischemia[20,21] (Box 9-2). Atherosclerosis usually affects the proximal segments of the subclavian artery and less often the brachiocephalic artery. Oddly, symptomatic disease is far more common in the left than the right subclavian artery. The various sources of thromboemboli were considered in the previous section.

Chronic occlusive disease of the upper extremity arteries is associated with several noteworthy clinical disorders:

- Stenosis or occlusion of the proximal subclavian artery may force blood to flow from the contralateral vertebral artery through the basilar artery, then retrograde in the ipsilateral vertebral artery, and finally into the post-stenotic subclavian artery. These compensatory hemodynamics can lead to cerebral ischemia during arm exercise (subclavian steal syndrome)[22,23] (Fig. 9-15).
- In patients with left internal mammary artery (LIMA) bypass grafts to a coronary artery, a proximal subclavian artery stenosis can result in reversal of flow in the graft during arm exercise (coronary-subclavian steal syndrome)[24,25] (Fig. 9-16).
- Individuals with a hemodialysis access site in the arm are prone to distal ischemia, usually from a combination of graft steal and underlying arterial disease[26,27] (see Chapter 19).
- In patients with extraanatomic bypass conduits (e.g., axillofemoral grafts), subclavian artery stenosis may result in leg ischemia or precipitate graft thrombosis.

BOX 9-2

CAUSES OF OBSTRUCTIVE ARTERIAL DISEASE OF THE ARM

- Atherosclerosis
- Thromboembolism
- Thoracic outlet syndrome
- Trauma
- Dissection
- Vasculitis
- Aneurysm (thrombosis)
- Extrinsic compression by tumor
- Drug-related causes (e.g., illicit drug injections, ergot derivatives)

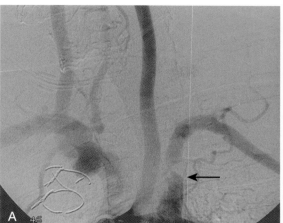

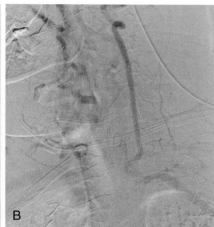

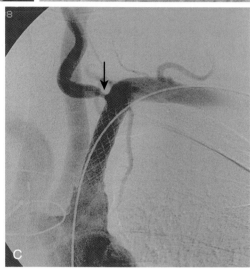

FIGURE 9-15 Subclavian steal syndrome and subclavian artery stent placement. **A,** Arch aortogram shows an irregular stenosis of the proximal left subclavian artery *(arrow)*. **B,** The late-phase arteriogram shows retrograde flow down the left vertebral artery into the subclavian artery beyond the stenosis. **C,** A stent was placed to relieve the obstruction. Note antegrade flow in the diseased vertebral artery *(arrow)*.

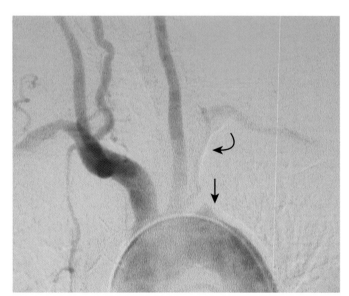

FIGURE 9-16 Coronary-subclavian steal in a patient with a left internal mammary artery (LIMA) coronary bypass graft. Early phase of arch aortogram shows occlusion at the origin of the left subclavian artery *(arrow)* and retrograde flow up the LIMA *(curved arrow)* into the mid left subclavian artery.

Clinical Features

Most patients with atherosclerosis-related thrombosis are older than 50 years of age. Chronic obstructions of the subclavian and axillary arteries may be entirely asymptomatic. Similar percentages of patients suffer arm ischemia and neurologic problems. Arterial obstructions are associated with ischemic symptoms such as exertional arm pain ("claudication"), and less commonly rest pain or tissue loss. Pulse deficits and blood pressure differences between the two arms (usually ≥20 mm Hg systolic) should be sought. Many individuals have neurologic symptoms related to subclavian steal, including dizziness, syncope, visual disturbances, or ataxia. Those with coronary-subclavian steal are at risk for developing angina during arm exercise. Finally, thoracic outlet syndrome is a common cause of arm ischemia, particularly in younger individuals (see later discussion).

Imaging

Duplex sonography, CT angiography, and MR imaging (MRI) play a role in evaluation of patients with suspected proximal arterial obstruction, particularly when they have symptoms of subclavian steal.[11-13,28] Doppler ultrasound signs of obstructive disease include a "parvus et tardus" waveform (downstream lesion) and loss of normal diastolic flow reversal (upstream lesion).[11]

Catheter angiography is performed when noninvasive imaging studies are equivocal (a rare situation) or endovascular therapy is contemplated. Atherosclerotic stenoses are typically found at the origins of the subclavian or brachiocephalic arteries (see Fig. 9-15). With proximal subclavian artery obstruction, flow in the ipsilateral vertebral artery may be reversed. Thrombotic occlusions produce an abrupt vessel cutoff. Arteriographic findings in thoracic outlet syndrome and more unusual causes of chronic obstruction are considered in later sections.

Treatment

ENDOVASCULAR THERAPY

When feasible, catheter-based interventions (usually primary stent placement) are preferred for subclavian and brachiocephalic artery obstructions.[24,29-32] In a minority of cases, direct brachial artery puncture is necessary instead of (or combined with) femoral artery access:

- For proximal left subclavian and brachiocephalic artery stenosis, current practice favors primary stent placement to improve long-term durability. However, data supporting this approach (rather than stent placement for immediate angioplasty failure) are weak. Both technical success (>90%) and long-term results (almost 90% primary patency at 10 years in one large series) are excellent.[32-36] Adverse events are uncommon, and neurologic events are rare.
- Balloon angioplasty alone may be performed in the central segment of the subclavian arteries. If a stent is absolutely necessary, only the self-expanding variety should be considered because of the potential for extrinsic compression by adjacent musculoskeletal structures.
- Treatment is indicated for patients with significant arch vessel obstructions before planned internal thoracic artery bypass to the coronary arteries.
- Thrombolysis has virtually no role in chronic total brachiocephalic and subclavian artery occlusions. Balloon angioplasty alone is not durable.[37] If such lesions can be crossed with a guidewire, primary stent placement (if at a suitable site) is warranted.

SURGICAL THERAPY

The preferred operative method for treating total subclavian artery occlusion is an extrathoracic bypass procedure, such as carotid-subclavian bypass, carotid-subclavian transposition, axilloaxillary bypass, or subclavian-subclavian bypass.[29,38] Brachial artery revascularization is done with autologous vein or synthetic graft material.[39]

Thoracic Outlet Syndrome

Etiology

The various forms of thoracic outlet syndrome are a distinct set of clinical disorders of the upper extremity caused by extrinsic compression of the major nerves and blood vessels exiting or entering the thorax. In more than 90% of affected persons, symptoms are caused by compression of the brachial plexus and related nerves; arterial compression is responsible for less than 5% of cases.[40-42] However, these frequently reported figures are strongly influenced by the composition of referral patterns.

The subclavian and axillary arteries are subject to compression primarily within three well-defined anatomic regions: the interscalene triangle, costoclavicular space, and retropectal (subcoracoid) space (Fig. 9-17). Imaging studies in normal volunteers show that a significant minority of healthy individuals

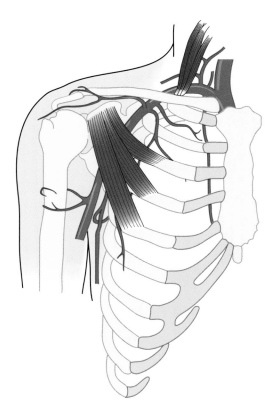

FIGURE 9-17   The major sites of arterial compression in thoracic outlet syndrome are (medial to lateral) the scalene triangle, costoclavicular space, and subcoracoid (retropectal) space.

exhibit arterial constriction within the costoclavicular and retropectal spaces with arm elevation.[43,44] In a small number of patients, however, this physiologic narrowing is exaggerated by one of several musculoskeletal abnormalities. These include cervical ribs, elongated C7 transverse processes, and congenital or acquired pathology of the first rib or clavicle.[45] Sometimes, soft tissue abnormalities alone (e.g., congenital fibromuscular bands, muscular hypertrophy) are responsible.

Chronic and intermittent arterial compression, which is usually exacerbated by particular arm positions, can lead to intimal and ultimately transmural vascular injury. Over time, the result is post-stenotic dilation or frank aneurysm formation, premature atherosclerosis, embolization of platelet-fibrin deposits or thrombus from the diseased wall, or complete occlusion.

Clinical Features

Thoracic outlet syndrome is classically seen in young or middle-aged adults.[46] The arterial form of the disease causes arm pain, weakness, coolness, and pallor. Symptoms often are intermittent and usually provoked by certain arm positions or exercise. There may be evidence for distal embolization, such as digital ulcerations or cyanosis. With associated arm swelling, the venous form of thoracic outlet syndrome should be considered (see Chapter 17).

A host of shoulder movements are reported to reproduce symptoms in some individuals, including the Adson maneuver (i.e., depression of the shoulder with the head turned to the symptomatic side), military position (i.e., shoulders hyperflexed), hyperabduction of the arm, and the so-called surrender position (hands above the head).[45] However, loss of the radial pulse with extreme abduction of the arm is normal in a minority of the population and is not itself diagnostic of the disease. Frankly, it may be difficult to distinguish neurogenic from arterial thoracic outlet syndrome, and sometimes they coexist.

Imaging

PLAIN RADIOGRAPHY

Chest or cervical spine radiographs are inspected for cervical ribs or other bony abnormalities often found with arterial thoracic outlet syndrome.

CROSS-SECTIONAL TECHNIQUES

MR angiography and CT angiography are the primary modalities used to evaluate these patients[43,45-48] (see Fig. 9-13). When thoracic outlet syndrome is suspected, imaging is done first with the arms at the side and then with the arm extended above the head. Sagittal reformations are especially useful in depicting arterial (or

venous) compression along the thoracic outlet. More flagrant findings may also be seen, including post-stenotic arterial dilation, aneurysm formation with or without mural thrombus, distal embolization, or complete thrombosis. MR angiography is particularly helpful in assessing the brachial plexus and fibromuscular abnormalities affecting the blood vessels. Duplex sonography is a complementary tool, but it has distinct limitations compared with MR and CT.[44,45] It is important to realize that compression of the subclavian artery during provocative maneuvers has been identified in a substantial percentage of normal volunteers by Doppler sonography.[44]

CATHETER ANGIOGRAPHY

This procedure is only required for assessment of forearm or hand arteries (if CT or MR angiography is not diagnostic) and when endovascular therapy is contemplated. Arteriographic findings mirror those described above with cross-sectional imaging (see Fig. 9-13). With complete thrombosis of the subclavian or axillary artery, an underlying abnormality rooted in thoracic outlet syndrome may only be revealed after thrombolytic therapy (Fig. 9-18).

Treatment

ENDOVASCULAR THERAPY

Thrombolysis may be used to recanalize an acutely occluded artery from suspected thoracic outlet syndrome (see Figs. 9-13 and 9-18). After flow is restored, anticoagulation is begun. Later, the underlying compressive abnormality is treated operatively. Stents should not be placed at the site of compression.[49]

SURGICAL THERAPY

For patients with mild symptoms and an imaging study showing normal subclavian and axillary arteries or only mild post-stenotic dilation in the neutral position, conservative therapy is often appropriate. For individuals with disabling symptoms, florid imaging findings, or distal embolization, surgery usually is performed.[49] The underlying musculoskeletal abnormality is corrected (e.g., removal of a cervical rib, release of fibrous bands) along with resection of the first rib.[41,42] Subclavian artery aneurysms are treated by resection and bypass.

Digital Ischemia (Online Case 56)

Etiology

Ischemia of the digits may be caused by fixed obstructions of large or small arteries, intermittent vasospasm, or both. Obstruction of large or medium-sized arteries alone occasionally produces digital ischemia (see Box 9-2). More

FIGURE 9-20 Hand ischemia from proximal atheroma embolization. **A,** Right posterior oblique arch aortogram shows a plaque on the inferior surface of the brachiocephalic artery *(arrow).* Also note occlusion of the proximal left subclavian artery. **B,** Hand angiogram shows occlusion of the distal ulnar artery and of multiple proper digital arteries.

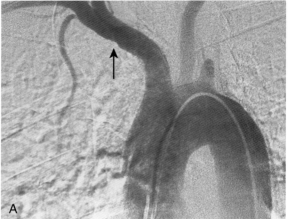
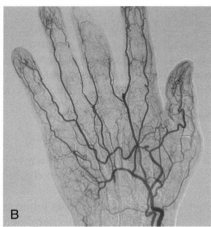

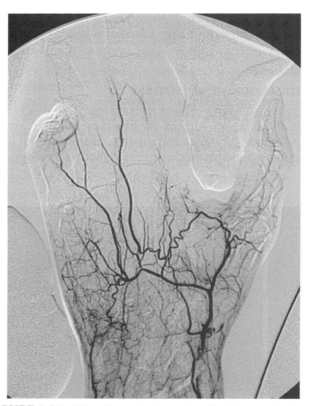

FIGURE 9-21 Scleroderma is characterized by abrupt occlusions of multiple proper digital arteries. The distal radial and ulnar arteries are occluded. Note prior second digit amputation.

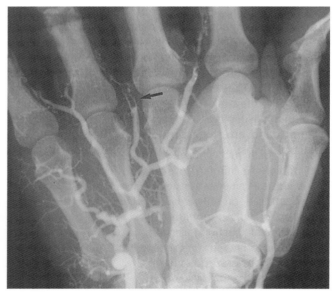

FIGURE 9-22 Hypothenar hammer syndrome. The patient has a pseudoaneurysm of the distal ulnar artery and an embolus in the palmar artery of the third web space *(arrow).*

ENDOVASCULAR THERAPY

Thrombolytic therapy has been used occasionally in some cases of acute or subacute arterial occlusion in the hand.[16,69,70]

Trauma (Online Cases 94 and 109)

Etiology and Clinical Features

The arteries of the upper extremity can be damaged in a variety of ways[71-74] (Box 9-4). In most series, penetrating injury is far more common than blunt injury. Iatrogenic trauma may result from brachial or axillary artery catheterization, attempted vascular access placement in the chest or neck, or radial artery line insertion. The

Vasodilators such as the prostacyclin analogue iloprost have been found to be beneficial in patients with some disorders such as systemic sclerosis and Raynaud phenomenon.[66,67] Operative bypass procedures with autologous vein have been performed successfully for limb-threatening thrombotic or embolic disease involving the forearm arteries.[68]

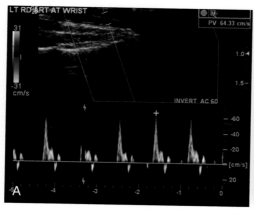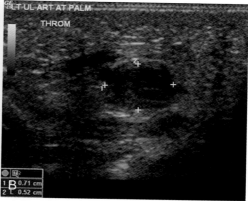

FIGURE 9-23 Hypothenar hammer syndrome. **A,** Ultrasound of distal radial artery is normal, with typical triphasic wave pattern (including reversal of flow at end-diastole). **B,** Ultrasound of distal ulnar artery shows an enlarged artery (5 × 7 mm) filled with clot.

most common complications of axillary or brachial artery catheterization are local hematoma (occasionally with nerve compression) and arterial thrombosis; less commonly, pseudoaneurysms or arteriovenous fistulas may develop[75] (see Chapter 3). Athletic individuals are especially prone to chronic injury to upper extremity arteries.[76] Skeletal disruptions, especially humeral fractures, clavicular fractures, and anterior shoulder dislocations, can cause arterial damage. Chronic use of crutches may expose the axillary artery to injury.

Box 9-5 lists the "hard signs" that strongly suggest clinically important arterial damage.[77-79] Because of the extensive collateral circulation in the arm, some patients with severe proximal arterial injury have normal distal pulses.

Imaging

Over the past several decades, there has been a gradual evolution in the approach to suspected upper extremity arterial damage. Protocols for routine surgical exploration or arteriography for all "proximity" injuries have been abandoned.[80] After clinical evaluation, some patients with hard signs of injury go directly to operation without imaging studies. In most cases, an ankle-brachial index (ABI) or Doppler arterial pressure index (API, ratio of distal pressure in affected versus unaffected arm) is determined. In the absence of hard signs of injury or in the presence of API or ABI greater than 0.90, patients are usually observed.[77]

SONOGRAPHY

In some centers, patients with suspected extremity arterial injuries are routinely evaluated with color Doppler sonography.[78,79] In patients at low risk for significant pathology, the accuracy exceeds 95% in recent reports. Pitfalls of the technique include limited evaluation of the thoracic outlet and confusion in the face of variant anatomy. Sonography is useful also for delayed diagnosis of post-traumatic pseudoaneurysms and arteriovenous fistulas, particularly in the subclavian and axillary arteries (Fig. 9-24).

BOX 9-4

CAUSES OF TRAUMA TO UPPER EXTREMITY ARTERIES

- Penetrating injury
  - Accidental or criminal
  - Iatrogenic (e.g., catheterization procedures)
- Blunt injury
  - Bone fracture or joint dislocation
  - Crush injury
  - Chronic vibrational or pounding injury
  - Use of crutches
- Thermal injury (e.g., frostbite, electrical injury)

BOX 9-5

INDICATIONS FOR VASCULAR IMAGING AFTER UPPER EXTREMITY TRAUMA

- "Hard signs" of vascular injury
  - Obvious arterial bleeding
  - Expanding hematoma
  - Absent or markedly diminished distal pulses
  - Ischemic symptoms
  - Bruit or thrill
  - Neurologic deficit
- Shock in absence of other injuries
- Shotgun blast
- History of peripheral vascular disease
- Thoracic outlet injury
- Extensive bone or soft tissue injury
- Delayed presentation

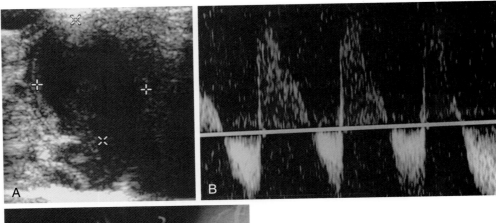

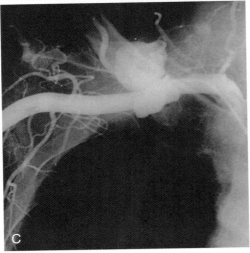

FIGURE 9-24   Subclavian artery pseudoaneurysm resulting from attempted venous access placement. **A,** Sonography shows a rounded, hypoechoic mass adjacent to the mid right subclavian artery. **B,** Spectral tracing shows the typical to-and-fro pattern in the pseudoaneurysm neck. **C,** The arteriogram confirms a large bilobed pseudoaneurysm.

COMPUTED TOMOGRAPHY

CT angiography has become the primary imaging modality in patients with extremity trauma, both upper and lower.[81-85] With state-of-the-art imaging, sensitivity and specificity should approach 95% to 100% and 90% to 100%, respectively, for detecting clinically significant extremity arterial damage. Evaluation includes volume-rendered images (which creates conventional angiographic images useful to the treating surgeon or interventionalist) along with two-dimensional multiplanar reformations. Trauma can produce a wide spectrum of arterial abnormalities, including intimal tears, intraluminal thrombus, vasospasm, intramural hematoma, dissection, transection with or without thrombosis, vessel deviation, arteriovenous fistula formation, pseudoaneurysm formation, and compartment syndrome (which causes slow flow in proximal arteries) (Fig. 9-25). Suspected abnormalities should be confirmed on axial source images.

ANGIOGRAPHY

In many trauma centers with 64-slice CT scanners, diagnostic arteriography has been eliminated in this setting. Catheterization or endovascular repair is reserved for cases in which embolotherapy or endovascular repair is anticipated (see later discussion). Two projections often are needed to exclude subtle findings such as intimal tears (Fig. 9-26).

Treatment

ENDOVASCULAR THERAPY

When feasible, transcatheter therapy is favored over open surgical repair or bypass. Large pseudoaneurysms or arteriovenous fistulas from a branch of a main upper extremity artery are best treated with embolotherapy.[86-89] Embolization usually is performed with Gelfoam pledgets or coils (Fig. 9-27). Pseudoaneurysms from femoral or brachial artery catheterization are usually closed with percutaneous thrombin injection or ultrasound-guided compression repair.[90,91] Traumatic pseudoaneurysms of the central arteries can be covered with stent graft devices.[92,93] However, the operator should consider potential problems from extrinsic compression at these sites before inserting a stent. Balloon catheters may be used to tamponade massive bleeding from a major artery, such as following accidental catheterization of the subclavian or brachiocephalic artery during attempted central venous line placement. In some instances, this

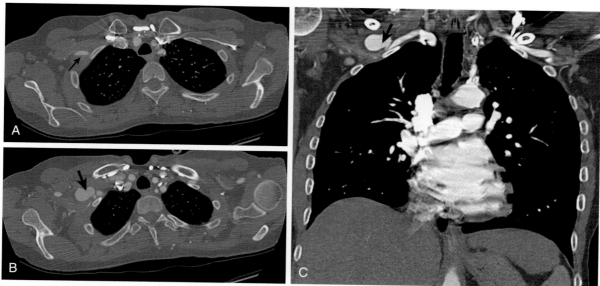

FIGURE 9-25 Subclavian artery pseudoaneurysm resulting from attempted venous access placement without imaging guidance. **A** through **C,** Axial and reformatted coronal contrast-enhanced computed tomography of the upper chest shows a pseudoaneurysm *(large arrow)* arising from the mid right subclavian artery *(small arrow).* There is some surrounding soft tissue density suggesting the presence of blood.

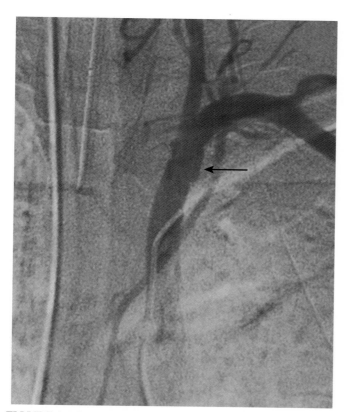

FIGURE 9-26 Small pseudoaneurysm of the proximal left subclavian artery *(arrow)* after motor vehicle accident.

maneuver alone is curative (Fig. 9-28). If not, a stent graft is placed or the balloon is kept inflated until the artery is repaired in the operating room.[94,95]

SURGICAL THERAPY

Significant injuries to major arteries, such as occlusion, laceration, pseudoaneurysm, and flow-limiting dissection, require surgical treatment with resection or bypass grafting if not amenable to endovascular techniques.[96-98] Time is of the essence in repairing occlusive injuries. Permanent ischemic injury can result if revascularization is not accomplished within about 4 to 6 hours of proximal injury (somewhat longer for more distal occlusions).[14] The current trend is toward conservative management of minor vascular injuries such as nonocclusive intimal flaps, intramural hematomas, and small (≤1 cm) pseudoaneurysms.[87] These lesions generally have a benign clinical course.

Aneurysms (Online Case 109)

Etiology and Clinical Features

A variety of diseases can produce true or false aneurysms of the upper extremity arteries (Box 9-6 on p. 278). Compared with the aorta and lower extremity arteries, degenerative aneurysms associated with atherosclerosis are uncommon in the upper extremity (see Chapter 1). They occur most frequently in the brachiocephalic and subclavian arteries.[99] Pseudoaneurysms often are the result of catheterization procedures such as brachial artery

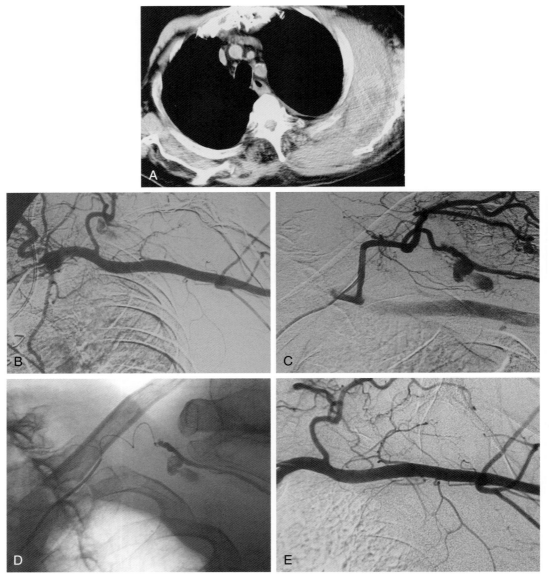

FIGURE 9-27   Older man with hypotension after a fall. **A,** Computed tomography scan shows swelling and high density in left shoulder girdle muscles, suggesting active bleeding. **B,** Left subclavian arteriography shows a pseudoaneurysm arising from a branch of the costocervical trunk, confirmed with selective catheterization **(C). D,** Coaxial microcatheter advanced to the inflow branch. **E,** Following embolotherapy across the aneurysm neck with microcoils and Gelfoam pledgets, bleeding has stopped.

puncture, radial artery line placement, or attempted vascular access placement in the subclavian or jugular vein (see Fig. 9-28). Aneurysms can develop near the site of extrinsic compression in patients with TOS (see Fig. 9-18). In the hand, aneurysms usually are caused by penetrating trauma or chronic blunt trauma (e.g., hypothenar hammer syndrome). Microaneurysms of small vessels of the hand are characteristic of a necrotizing vasculitis such as *polyarteritis nodosa*.

Subclavian artery aneurysms often are asymptomatic. Some patients present with chest pain, shoulder pain, or a pulsatile supraclavicular mass. Others complain of symptoms from distal embolization or aneurysmal thrombosis or have hypotension from rupture. Rarely, patients suffer massive hemoptysis after erosion into the lung.

Imaging and Treatment

Duplex sonography, CT angiography, and MR angiography are used to diagnose central aneurysms[100,101] (see Figs. 9-24 and 9-28). Color Doppler sonography is valuable for detecting aneurysms of the brachial, forearm, and hand arteries.[102] Catheter angiography usually is reserved for cases in which percutaneous

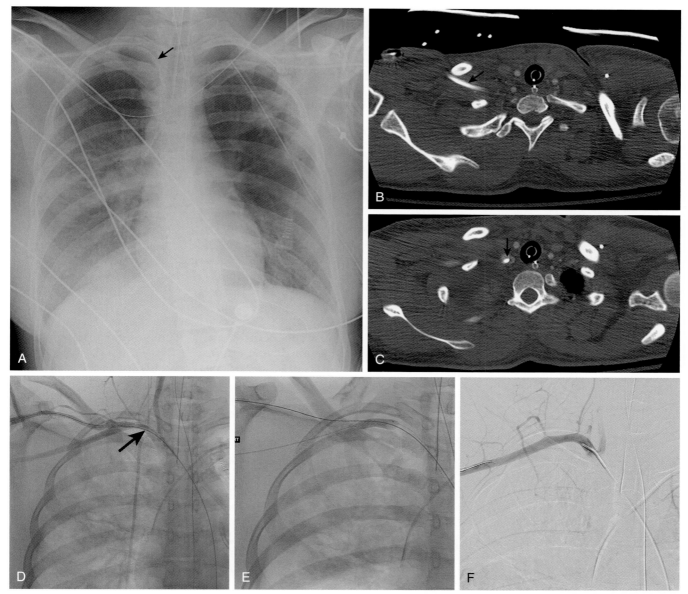

FIGURE 9-28   Balloon tamponade of inadvertent subclavian artery puncture for central venous catheter placement. **A,** Chest radiograph shows the access line in place *(small arrow)*. Pulsatile blood was obtained from the catheter. **B** and **C,** Axial computed tomography images confirm that the catheter is in the right subclavian artery *(small arrows)*. **D,** Transfemoral subclavian arteriography identified the entry site of the errant catheter *(large arrow)*. **E,** Via transbrachial access, a balloon is inflated across the vessel puncture site after the catheter was removed but guidewire left in place. **F,** Final subclavian arteriogram shows that the artery is normal and no leak is evident.

therapy is being considered. Degenerative aneurysms, which are typically located in the brachiocephalic or subclavian arteries, usually are fusiform and calcified. Traumatic or infectious pseudoaneurysms are typically saccular, irregular, or multilobed (see Figs. 9-22, 9-24, 9-25, and 9-27). Aneurysms caused by connective tissue disorders or vasculopathies may be fusiform or saccular (Fig. 9-29).

The standard treatment for upper extremity arterial aneurysms is surgical resection with end-to-end anastomosis or bypass grafting.[103] Percutaneous therapy for post-traumatic aneurysms is described previously. Stent grafts may play a role in rare instances.

OTHER DISORDERS

Vasculitis and Vasculopathies

Several vasculitides and noninflammatory vasculopathic states affect the upper extremity arteries (Fig. 9-30). Their pathogenesis is considered in more depth in Chapter 1.

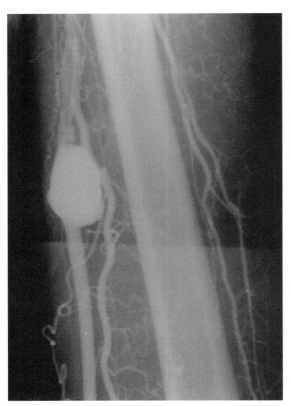

FIGURE 9-29   Brachial artery aneurysm in a patient with Ehlers-Danlos syndrome.

Buerger disease (thromboangiitis obliterans) is an occlusive panarteritis of medium-sized and small arteries and veins of the extremities.[104,105] The disease is classically seen in young to middle-aged men, all of whom are smokers. Buerger disease almost always affects the lower extremities, and arm artery involvement is seen in about 50% of cases. The occlusions usually are bilateral, although symptoms may be confined to one extremity. The proximal vessels (i.e., subclavian, axillary, and upper brachial arteries) are not affected. Abrupt, segmental occlusions begin in the arteries of the forearm. A "corkscrew" appearance of the collateral vessels is said to be characteristic, but this often is not the case. Occlusions of palmar and digital arteries always occur (Fig. 9-31). "Corrugation" of the arteries adjacent to obstructed segments has also been described. Subacute thromboses have been successfully treated with thrombolysis.[70]

Takayasu arteritis is an inflammatory vasculitis affecting large- and medium-sized elastic arteries (see Chapter 1). The disease may cause long segmental stenoses or occlusions of branches of the aorta, especially the subclavian arteries[106-109] (see Fig. 6-25).

Giant cell arteritis has many features that are similar to those of Takayasu arteritis. However, it affects an older population, and the distribution of disease is different.[110,111] The neck and cranial vessels, particularly the carotid and temporal arteries, are most commonly affected. Occasionally, obstruction of the subclavian artery produces ischemic symptoms in the arm. Giant cell arteritis tends to cause long stenoses of the middle to distal segments of the subclavian artery, which may extend into the axillary artery.

Radiation arteritis is a rare complication of high-dose radiation therapy. Pathologic changes include intimal proliferation and fibrotic occlusion. These changes may only become apparent 5 years or more after treatment. Radiotherapy for breast carcinoma and lymphoma has caused obstructions of and, rarely, distal embolization from the subclavian and axillary arteries.[112,113]

Arteriovenous Communications

Vascular anomalies and techniques for percutaneous treatment are discussed in greater detail in Chapters 1 and 3. This set of disorders encompasses vascular malformations, including arteriovenous malformations (AVMs), venous malformations (VM), and lymphatic malformations (LM), hemangiomas, and arteriovenous fistulas (AVFs). AVFs are almost always acquired from accidental or iatrogenic trauma. Congenital AVMs and VMs and hemangiomas are conditions that also may affect the upper extremity.[114-117] Most patients with these lesions present as children or young adults with

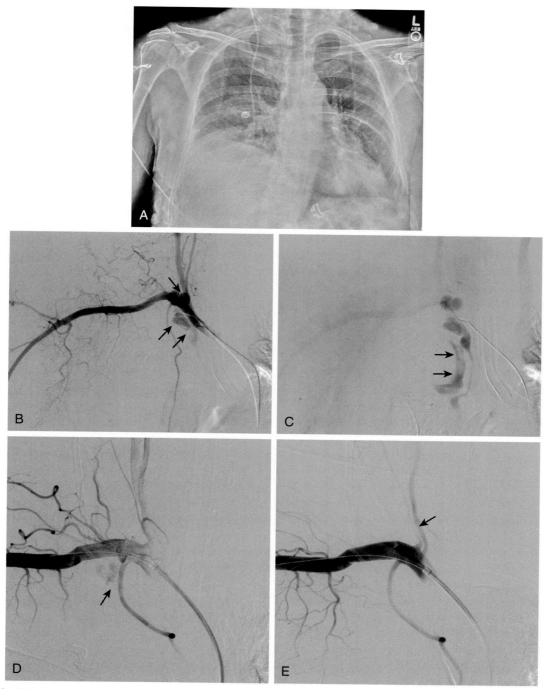

FIGURE 9-30   Subclavian artery aneurysm in a patient with neurofibromatosis. **A,** Chest radiograph shows innumerable cutaneous neurofibromas. **B** and **C,** Right brachiocephalic arteriography shows a bilobed aneurysm *(single arrow)* with massive extravasation into the chest *(double arrows)*. The relationship to the vertebral artery must be determined. **D,** A covered stent was inserted in proper position, but leak persists *(arrow)*. **E,** The stent graft was slightly overdilated, now sealing the pseudoaneurysm and eliminating the leak. Vertebral artery patency was maintained *(arrow)*.

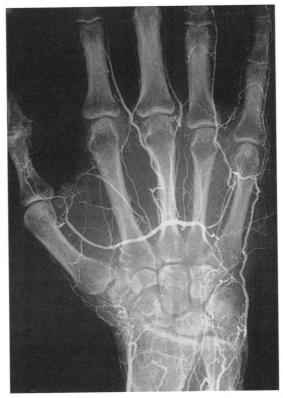

FIGURE 9-31   Buerger disease in this patient is characterized by abrupt occlusions of the distal radial and ulnar arteries and of multiple metacarpal and proper digital arteries. The intervening vessels are normal. Tortuous collaterals, which are most notable around the wrist, are characteristic of the disease.

local hypertrophy, varices, pain, or a thrill or bruit over the site.

Most extremity AVFs are detected by color Doppler sonography. MRI has become the primary tool for diagnosis and staging of extremity vascular malformations and hemangiomas. Angiography (arteriography or direct VM puncture) is reserved for embolotherapy or preoperative management. The angiographic findings vary with the type of AVM. With arterial malformations, markedly dilated inflow arteries, numerous feeding arterioles, pools of contrast within the AVM, and early filling of draining veins may be seen (see Fig. 1-31). VMs have slightly dilated or nondilated inflow arteries, variable flow patterns, and large spongy venous spaces. Occasionally, vascular soft tissue or bony tumors can be confused with these congenital lesions.

Arteriovenous malformations are difficult to cure. None of the available treatments (short of amputation) is likely to give a permanent result, and recurrence is the rule. Therapy should be undertaken only when the patient has significant symptoms, such as bleeding, ulceration, pain, severe deformity, or high-output cardiac failure. When feasible, the treatment of choice is embolotherapy by an intraarterial route (for high flow AVMs) or by direct percutaneous puncture for (low flow VMs).[116-118] Embolization is performed in stages to limit tissue loss. Ideally, the nidus of the AVM is obliterated. A permanent agent that can enter the substance of the AVM should be used, such as cyanoacrylate (glue) or ethylene vinyl alcohol copolymer (Onyx) (see Chapter 3). Proximal embolization must be strictly avoided. For venous malformations, direct injection with a sclerosing agent, such as absolute alcohol, can be extremely effective.

Neoplasms

Arteriography has virtually no role in the evaluation of patients with benign or malignant tumors of the shoulder or arm. Occasionally, patients with highly vascular tumors undergo arteriography for preoperative planning or for embolotherapy to reduce blood loss during surgery.

References

1. Collins P, editor. Embryology and development. In: Williams PL, Bannister LH, Berry MM, et al, editors. *Gray's anatomy*, 38th ed. New York, Churchill Livingstone, 1995: p. 318.
2. Gabella G, editor. Cardiovascular system. In: Williams PL, Bannister LH, Berry MM, et al, editors. *Gray's anatomy*, 38th ed. New York, Churchill Livingstone, 1995: p. 1529.
3. Coleman SS, Anson BJ. Arterial patterns in the hand based on a study of 650 specimens. *Surg Gynecol Obstet* 1961;**113**:409.
4. Bilge O, Pinar Y, Govsa F. A morphometric study on the superficial palmar arch of the hand. *Surg Radiol Anat* 2006;**28**:343.
5. Keen JA. A study of the arterial variations in the limbs with special reference to symmetry of vascular patterns. *Am J Anat* 1961;**108**:245.
6. McCormack LJ, Cauldwell EW, Anson BJ. Brachial and antebrachial arterial patterns: a study of 750 extremities. *Surg Gynecol Obstet* 1965;**96**:43.
7. Lindley SG, Kleinert JM. Prevalence of anatomic variations encountered in elective carpal tunnel release. *J Hand Surg [Am]* 2003;**28**:849.
8. Deguara J, Ali T, Modarai B, et al. Upper limb ischemia: 20 years experience from a single center. *Vascular* 2005;**13**:84.
9. Ueberrueck T, Marusch F, Schmidt H, et al. Risk factors and management of arterial emboli of the upper and lower extremities. *J Cardiovasc Surg* (Torino) 2007;**48**:181.
10. Gossage JA, Ali T, Chambers J. Peripheral arterial embolism: prevalence, outcome, and role of echocardiography in management. *J Endovascular Surg* 2006;**40**:280.
11. Rose SC. Noninvasive vascular laboratory for evaluation of peripheral arterial occlusive disease. Part III—clinical applications: nonatherosclerotic lower extremity arterial conditions and upper extremity arterial disease. *J Vasc Interv Radiol* 2001;**12**:11.
12. Nael K, Villablanca JP, Pope WB, et al. Supraaortic arteries: contrast-enhanced MR angiography at 3.0 T—highly accelerated parallel acquisition for improved spatial resolution over an extended field of view. *Radiology* 2007;**242**:600.
13. Randoux B, Marro B, Koskas F, et al. Proximal great vessels of aortic arch: comparison of three-dimensional gadolinium enhanced MR angiography and digital subtraction angiography. *Radiology* 2003;**229**:697.
14. Newton EJ, Love J. Acute complications of extremity trauma. *Emerg Med Clin N Am* 2007;**25**:751.

15. Licht PB, Balezantis T, Wolff B, et al. Long-term outcome following thromboembolectomy in the upper extremity. *Eur J Vasc Endovasc Surg.* 2004;**28**:508.

16. Johnson SP, Durham JD, Subber SW. Acute arterial occlusions of the small vessels of the hand and forearm: treatment with regional urokinase therapy. *J Vasc Interv Radiol* 1999;**10**:869.

17. Michaels JA, Torrie EP, Galland RB. The treatment of upper limb vascular occlusions using intraarterial thrombolysis. *Eur J Vasc Surg* 1993;**7**:744.

18. Coulon M, Goffette P, Dondelinger RF. Local thrombolytic infusion in arterial ischemia of the upper limb: mid-term results. *Cardiovasc Intervent Radiol* 1994;**17**:81.

19. Cejna M, Salomonowitz E, Wohlschlager. rt-PA thrombolysis in acute thromboembolic upper extremity occlusion. *Cardiovasc Intervent Radiol* 2001;**24**:218.

20. Voyvodic F, Hayward M. Case report. Upper extremity ischaemia secondary to ergotamine poisoning. *Clin Radiol* 1996;**51**:589.

21. Bakken AM, Palchik E, Saad WE, et al. Outcomes of endovascular therapy for ostial disease of the major branches of the aortic arch. *Ann Vasc Surg* 2008;**22**:388.

22. Bauer AM, Amin-Hanjani S, Alaraj A, et al. Quantitative magnetic resonance angiography in the evaluation of the subclavian steal syndrome: report of 5 patients. *J Neuroimaging* 2009;**19**:250.

23. Wu C, Zhang J, Ladner CJ, et al. Subclavian steal syndrome: diagnosis with perfusion metrics from contrast-enhanced MR angiographic bolus-timing examination-initial experience. *Radiology* 2005;**235**:927.

24. Westerband A, Rodriguez JA, Ramaiah VG, et al. Endovascular therapy in prevention and management of coronary-subclavian steal. *J Vasc Surg* 2003;**38**:699.

25. Takach TJ, Reul GJ, Cooley DA, et al. Myocardial thievery: the coronary-subclavian steal syndrome. *Ann Thorac Surg* 2006;**81**:386.

26. Valji K, Hye RJ, Roberts AC, et al. Hand ischemia in patients with hemodialysis access grafts: angiographic diagnosis and treatment. *Radiology* 1995;**196**:697.

27. Salman L, Maya ID, Asif A. Current concepts in the pathophysiology and management of arteriovenous access-induced hand ischemia. *Adv Chronic Kidney Dis* 2009;**16**:371.

28. Peloschek P, Sailer J, Loewe C, et al. The role of multi-slice spiral CT angiography in patient management after endovascular therapy. *Cardiovasc Intervent Radiol* 2006;**29**:756.

29. Palchik E, Bakken AM, Wolford HY, et al. Subclavian artery revascularization: an outcome analysis based on mode of therapy and presenting symptoms. *Ann Vasc Surg* 2008;**22**:70.

30. Patel SN, White CJ, Collins TJ, et al. Catheter-based treatment of the subclavian and innominate arteries. *Catheter Cardiovasc Interv* 2008;**71**:963.

31. Criado FJ. Endovascular techniques for supra-aortic trunk intervention. *Perspect Vasc Surg Endovasc Ther* 2007;**19**:231.

32. Henry M, Henry I, Polydorou A, et al. Percutaneous transluminal angioplasty of the subclavian arteries. *Int Angiol* 2007;**26**:324.

33. Rogers JH, Calhoun II RF. Diagnosis and management of subclavian artery stenosis before coronary artery bypass grafting in the current era. *J Card Surg* 2007;**22**:20.

34. Angle JF, Matsumoto AH, McGraw JK, et al. Percutaneous angioplasty and stenting of left subclavian artery stenosis in patients with left internal mammary-coronary bypass grafts: clinical experience and long-term follow-up. *Vasc Endovascular Surg* 2003;**37**:89.

35. Bates MC, Broce M, Lavigne PS, et al. Subclavian artery stenting: factors influencing long-term outcome. *Catheter Cardiovasc Interv* 2004;**61**:5.

36. Brountzos EN, Malagari K, Kelekis DA. Endovascular treatment of occlusive lesions of the subclavian and innominate arteries. *Cardiovasc Intervent Radiol* 2006;**29**:503.

37. Mathias KD, Lueth I, Haarmann P. Percutaneous transluminal angioplasty of proximal subclavian artery occlusions. *Cardiovasc Intervent Radiol* 1993;**16**:214.

38. Cina CS, Safar HA, Lagana A, et al. Subclavian carotid transposition and bypass grafting: consecutive cohort study and systematic review. *J Vasc Surg* 2002;**35**:422.

39. Roddy SP, Darling RC 3rd, Chang BB, et al. Brachial artery reconstruction for occlusive disease: a 12 year experience. *J Vasc Surg* 2001;**33**:802.

40. Sanders RJ, Hammond SL, Rao NM. Diagnosis of thoracic outlet syndrome. *J Vasc Surg* 2007;**46**:601.

41. Maxey TS, Reece TB, Ellman PI, et al. Safety and efficacy of the supraclavicular approach to thoracic outlet decompression. *Ann Thorac Surg* 2003;**76**:396.

42. Balci AE, Balci TA, Cakir O, et al. Surgical treatment of thoracic outlet syndrome: effects and results of surgery. *Ann Thorac Surg* 2003;**75**:1091.

43. Demondion X, Bacqueville E, Paul C, et al. Thoracic outlet: assessment with MR imaging in asymptomatic and symptomatic populations. *Radiology* 2003;**227**:461.

44. Demondion X, Vidal C, Herbinet P, et al. Ultrasonographic assessment of arterial cross-sectional area in the thoracic outlet on postural maneuvers measured with power Doppler ultrasonography in both asymptomatic and symptomatic populations. *J Ultrasound Med* 2006;**25**:217.

45. Demondion X, Herbinet P, van Sint Jan S, et al. Imaging assessment of thoracic outlet syndrome. *Radiographics* 2006;**26**:1735-50.

46. Atasoy E. Thoracic outlet compression syndrome. *Orthop Clin North Am* 1996;**27**:265.

47. Charon JP, Milne W, Sheppard DG, et al. Evaluation of MR angiographic technique in the assessment of thoracic outlet syndrome. *Clin Radiol* 2004;**59**:588.

48. Remy-Jardin M, Remy J, Masson P, et al. Helical CT angiography of thoracic outlet syndrome: functional anatomy. *AJR Am J Roentgenol* 2000;**174**:1667.

49. Fugate MW, Rotellini-Coltvet L, Freischlag JA. Current management of thoracic outlet syndrome. *Curr Treat Options Cardiovasc Med* 2009;**11**:176.

50. McLafferty RB, Edwards JM, Taylor Jr LM, et al. Diagnosis and long-term clinical outcome in patients diagnosed with hand ischemia. *J Vasc Surg* 1995;**22**:361.

51. Pope JE. The diagnosis and treatment of Raynaud's phenomenon: a practical approach. *Drugs* 2007;**67**:517.

52. Wigley FM. Clinical practice. Raynaud's phenomenon. *N Engl J Med* 2002;**347**:1001.

53. Boin F, Wigley FM. Understanding, assessing and treating Raynaud's phenomenon. *Curr Opin Rheumatol* 2005;**17**:752-60.

54. Cooke JP, Marshall JM. Mechanisms of Raynaud's disease. *Vasc Med* 2005;**10**:293.

55. Blum AG, Zabel JP, Kohlmann R, et al. Pathologic conditions of the hypothenar eminence: evaluation with multidetector CT and MR imaging. *Radiographics* 2006;**26**:1021.

56. Marie I, Herve F, Primard E, et al. Long-term follow-up of hypothenar hammer syndrome: a series of 47 patients. *Medicine* (Baltimore) 2007;**86**:334.

57. McCready RA, Bryant MA, Divelbiss JL. Combined thenar and hypothenar hammer syndromes: case report and review of the literature. *J Vasc Surg* 2008;**48**:741.

58. Hummers LK, Wigley FM. Management of Raynaud's phenomenon and digital ischemia in scleroderma. *Rheum Dis Clin North Am* 2003;**29**:293.

59. Herrick A. Diagnosis and management of scleroderma peripheral vascular disease. *Rheum Dis Clin North Am* 2008;**34**:89.

60. Ketteler M, Westenfeld R, Schlieper G, et al. Pathogenesis of vascular calcification in dialysis patients. *Clin Exp Nephrol* 2005;**9**:265.

61. Meharwal ZS, Trehan N. Functional status of the hand after radial artery harvesting: results in 3,977 cases. *Ann Thorac Surg* 2001; **72**:1557.

62. Lim RP, Storey P, Atanasova IP, et al. Three-dimensional electrocardiographically gated variable flip angle FSE imaging for MR angiography of the hands at 3.0 T: initial experience. *Radiology* 2009; **252**:874.

63. Winterer JT, Moske-Eick O, Markl M, et al. Bilateral ce-MR angiography of the hands at 3.0 T and 1.5T: intraindividual comparison of quantitative and qualitative image parameters in healthy volunteers. *Eur Radiol* 2008;**18**:658.

64. Reisinger C, Gluecker T, Jacob AL, et al. Dynamic magnetic resonance angiography of the arteries of the hand. A comparison between an extracellular and an intravascular contrast agent. *Eur Radiol* 2009; **19**:495.

65. Loring LA, Hallisey MJ. Arteriography and interventional therapy for diseases of the hand. *Radiographics* 1995;**15**:1299.

66. Kawald A, Burmester GR, Huscher D, et al. Low versus high dose iloprost therapy over 21 days in patients with secondary Raynaud's phenomenon and systemic sclerosis: a randomized, open, single center study. *J Rheumatol* 2008;**35**:1830.

67. Pope J, Fenlon D, Thompson A, et al. Iloprost and cisaprost for Raynaud's phenomenon in progressive systemic sclerosis. *Cochrane Database Syst Rev* 2000;**2**:CD000953.

68. Chang BB, Roddy SP, Darling III RC, et al. Upper extremity bypass grafting for limb salvage in end-stage renal failure. *J Vasc Surg* 2003;**38**:1313.

69. Capek P, Holcroft J. Traumatic ischemia of the hand in a tennis player: successful treatment with urokinase. *J Vasc Interv Radiol* 1993;**4**:279.

70. Lang EV, Bookstein JJ. Accelerated thrombolysis and angioplasty for hand ischemia in Buerger's disease. *Cardiovasc Intervent Radiol* 1989;**12**:95.

71. Levy BA, Zlowodzki MP, Graves M, et al. Screening for extremity arterial injury with the arterial pressure index. *Am J Emerg Med* 2005;**23**:689.

72. Doody O, Given MF, Lyon SM. Extremities—indications and techniques for treatment of extremity vascular injuries. *Injury* 2008; **39**:1295.

73. Stone WM, Fowl RJ, Money SR. Upper extremity trauma: current trends in management. *J Cardiovasc Surg* (Torino) 2007;**48**:551.

74. Rose SC, Moore EE. Angiography in patients with arterial trauma: correlation between angiographic abnormalities, operative findings, and clinical outcome. *AJR Am J Roentgenol* 1987;**149**:613.

75. Scalea TM, Sclafani S. Interventional techniques in vascular trauma. *Surg Clin North Am* 2001;**81**:1281.

76. Jackson MR. Upper extremity arterial injuries in athletes. *Semin Vasc Surg* 2003;**16**:232.

77. Britt LD, Weireter LJ, Cole FJ. Newer diagnostic modalities for vascular injuries. *Surg Clin North Am* 2001;**81**:1263.

78. Knudson MM, Lewis FR, Atkinson K, et al. The role of duplex ultrasound arterial imaging in patients with penetrating extremity trauma. *Arch Surg* 1993;**128**:1033.

79. Edwards JW, Bergstein JB, Karp DL, et al. Penetrating proximity injuries—the role of duplex scanning: a prospective study. *Journal of Vascular Technology* 1993;**17**:257.

80. Kaufman JA, Parker JE, Gillespie DL, et al. Arteriography for proximity of injury in penetrating extremity trauma. *J Vasc Interv Radiol* 1992; **3**:719.

81. Pieroni S, Foster BR, Anderson SW, et al. Use of 64-row multidetector CT angiography in blunt and penetrating trauma of the upper and lower extremities. *Radiographics* 2009;**29**:863.

82. Fishman EK, Horton KM, Johnson PT. Multidetector CT and three-dimensional CT angiography for suspected vascular trauma of the extremities. *Radiographics* 2008;**28**:653.

83. Rieger M, Mallohi A, Tauscher T, et al. Traumatic arterial injuries of the extremities: initial evaluation with MDCT angiography. *AJR Am J Roentgenol* 2006;**186**:656.

84. Anderson SW, Lucey BC, Varghese JC, et al. Sixty-four multidetector row computed tomography in multitrauma patient imaging: early experience. *Curr Probl Diagn Radiol* 2006;**35**: 188.

85. Miller-Thomas MM, West OC, Cohen AM, et al. Diagnosing traumatic arterial injury in the extremities with CT angiography: pearls and pitfalls. *Radiographics* 2005;**25**(Suppl. 1):S133.

86. Starnes BW, Arthurs ZM. Endovascular management of vascular trauma. *Perspect Vasc Surg Endovasc Ther* 2006;**18**:114.

87. Frykberg ER, Crump JM, Dennis JW, et al. Nonoperative observation of clinically occult arterial injuries: a prospective evaluation. *Surgery* 1991;**109**:85.

88. Levey DS, Teitelbaum GP, Finck EJ, et al. Safety and efficacy of transcatheter embolization of axillary and shoulder arterial injuries. *J Vasc Interv Radiol* 1991;**2**:99.

89. Herbreteau D, Aymard A, Khayata MH, et al. Endovascular treatment of arteriovenous fistulas arising from branches of the subclavian artery. *J Vasc Interv Radiol* 1993;**4**:237.

90. Skibo L, Polak JF. Compression repair of a postcatheterization pseudoaneurysm of the brachial artery under sonographic guidance. *AJR Am J Roentgenol* 1993;**160**:383.

91. Krueger K, Zaehringer M, Strohe D, et al. Postcatheterization pseudoaneurysm: results of US-guided percutaneous thrombin injection in 240 patients. *Radiology* 2005;**236**:1104.

92. Hilfiker PR, Razavi MK, Kee ST, et al. Stent-graft therapy for subclavian artery aneurysms and fistulas: single center mid-term results. *J Vasc Interv Radiol* 2000;**11**:578.

93. du Toit DF, Lambrechts AV, Stark H, et al. Long-term results of stent graft treatment of subclavian artery injuries: management of choice for stable patients? *J Vasc Surg* 2008;**47**:739.

94. Guilbert MC, Elkouri S, Bracco D, et al. Arterial trauma during central venous catheter insertion: case series, review and proposed algorithm. *J Vasc Surg* 2008;**48**:918.

95. Schoenholz CJ, Uflacker R, de Gregorio MA, et al. Stent-graft treatment of trauma to the supra-aortic arteries. A review. *J Cardiovasc Surg (Torino)* 2007;**48**:537.

96. Franz RW, Goodwin RB, Hartman JF, et al. Management of upper extremity arterial injuries at an urban level I trauma center. *Ann Vasc Surg* 2009;**23**:8.

97. Demetriades D, Asensio JA. Subclavian and axillary vascular injuries. *Surg Clin North Am* 2001;**81**:1357.

98. Rozycki CS, Tremblay LN, Feliciano DV, et al. Blunt vascular trauma in the extremity: diagnosis, management and outcome. *J Trauma* 2003;**55**:814.

99. Dougherty MJ, Calligaro KD, Savarese RP, et al. Atherosclerotic aneurysm of the intrathoracic subclavian artery: a case report and review of the literature. *J Vasc Surg* 1995;**21**:521.

100. Cosottini M, Zampa V, Petruzzi P, et al. Contrast-enhanced three-dimensional MR angiography in the assessment of subclavian artery disease. *Eur Radiol* 2000;**10**:1737.

101. Halldorsson A, Ramsey J, Gallagher C, et al. Proximal left subclavian artery aneurysms: a case report and review of the literature. *Angiology* 2007;**58**:367.

102. Anderson SE, DeMonaco D, Buechler U, et al. Imaging features of pseudoaneurysms of the hand in children and adults. *AJR Am J Roentgenol* 2003;**180**:659.

103. Davidovic LB, Markovic DM, Pejkic SD, et al. Subclavian artery aneurysms. *Asian J Surg* 2003;**26**:7.

104. Olin JW, Shih A. Thromboangiitis obliterans (Buerger's disease). *Curr Opin Rheumatol* 2006;**18**:18.

105. Mills Sr JL. Buerger's disease in the 21st century: diagnosis, clinical features, and therapy. *Semin Vasc Surg* 2003;**16**:179.

106. Seko Y. Giant cell and Takayasu arteritis. *Curr Opin Rheumatol* 2007;**19**:39.

107. Maksimowicz-McKinnon K, Hoffman GS. Takayasu arteritis: what is the long term prognosis? *Rheum Dis Clin North Am* 2007; **33**:777.

108. Ogino H, Matsuda H, Minatoya K, et al. Overview of late outcome of medical and surgical treatment for Takayasu arteritis. *Circulation* 2008;**118**:2738.

109. Tyagi S, Verma PK, Gambhir DS, et al. Early and long-term results of subclavian angioplasty in aortoarteritis (Takayasu disease): comparison with atherosclerosis. *Cardiovasc Intervent Radiol* 1998;**21**:219.

110. Cid MC, Garcia-Martinez A, Lozano E, et al. Five clinical conundrums in the management of giant cell arteritis. *Rheum Dis Clin North Am* 2007;**33**:819.

111. Wang X, Hu Z-P, Lu W, et al. Giant cell arteritis. *Rheumatol Int* 2008;**29**:1.

112. Rubin DI, Schomberg PJ, Shepherd RF, et al. Arteritis and brachial plexus neuropathy as delayed complications of radiation therapy. *Mayo Clin Proc* 2001;**76**:849.

113. Rhodes JM, Cherry Jr KJ, Clark RC, et al. Aortic-origin reconstruction of the great vessels: risk factors of early and late complications. *J Vasc Surg* 2000;**31**:260.

114. Chiller KG, Frieden IJ, Arbiser JL. Molecular pathogenesis of vascular anomalies: classification into three categories based upon clinical and biochemical characteristics. *Lymphat Res Biol* 2003;**1**:267.

115. Konez O, Burrows PE. Magnetic resonance of vascular anomalies. *Magn Reson Imaging Clin N Am* 2002;**10**:363.

116. Arneja JS, Gosain AK. Vascular malformations. *Plast Reconstr Surg* 2008;**121**:195e.

117. Marler JJ, Mulliken JB. Current management of hemangiomas and vascular malformations. *Clin Plast Surg* 2005;**32**:99.

118. White Jr RI, Pollak J, Persing J, et al. Long-term outcome of embolotherapy and surgery for high-flow extremity arteriovenous malformations. *J Vasc Interv Radiol* 2000;**11**:1285.

VISCERAL ARTERIES AND VEINS

Renal Arteries and Veins

Karim Valji

ARTERIOGRAPHY AND VENOGRAPHY (ONLINE VIDEOS 10-1 AND 10-2)

Evaluation of the renal arteries begins with abdominal aortography to detect renal artery ostial disease and accessory arteries before selective catheterization is done. A 4- or 5-French (Fr) pigtail catheter (or similar configuration) is positioned with the side holes at the level of the main renal arteries (approximately the L1 or L2 vertebral body). Images are routinely obtained in an anteroposterior or slight right posterior oblique views.[1] If computed tomography (CT) or magnetic resonance (MR) angiograms are available, they will guide selection of an optimal projection to place the renal artery origins in profile or may replace the catheter aortogram.

Selective renal arteriography is performed with a 4- or 5-Fr cobra or reverse curve (e.g., Sos or Simmons) catheter. The average flow rate in a normal renal artery is 5 to 6 mL/sec. More distal catheterization is done with coaxial microcatheters and microwires. Because the renal artery and its branches are prone to vasospasm and dissection, guidewires and catheters should be manipulated with extreme care.

Renal venography is accomplished with a straight catheter (e.g., cobra shape) or reverse curve catheter (e.g., Simmons 2). Valves at the origin of the veins may cause resistance to catheter passage. The valves can always be crossed with gentle guidewire probing. A wire may be required to seat the catheter well within the vein.

In patients with renal dysfunction (serum creatinine level greater than 1.2 to 1.5 mg/dL), various measures are taken to minimize the risk of contrast-induced nephropathy[2-6] (see Chapter 2).

ANATOMY

Development

In the fetus, the kidneys lie in the pelvis and receive blood from neighboring vessels, including the median sacral and common iliac arteries.[7] With time, lateral splanchnic branches of the aorta begin to perfuse structures arising from the mesonephric ridge: adrenal glands, gonads, and kidneys. With the ascent of the kidneys to the midabdomen, they are ultimately supplied by the more caudal of these lateral splanchnic arteries. Anomalies in the location and number of renal arteries can be explained by incomplete regression of some of these primitive vessels.

Normal Anatomy

The renal arteries arise from the lateral surface of the aorta at about the L1-L2 vertebral level.[8,9] The *right renal artery* runs posterior to the inferior vena cava (IVC) and right renal vein to enter the renal hilum. The *left renal artery* passes behind the left renal vein. The proximal renal arteries have small *inferior adrenal, ureteric,* and *capsular branches,* which often are not seen on imaging studies. At the renal hilum, the artery bifurcates into dorsal and ventral rami (Fig. 10-1). These trunks separate into segmental branches, which then further divide into lobar branches supplying the renal pyramids. The vessels successively branch into the interlobar, arcuate, and interlobular arteries. In the renal cortex, the interlobular arteries divide into afferent arterioles that supply the glomeruli.

The renal venous system follows a branching pattern similar to that of the renal arteries. However, wide anastomoses exist among the intrarenal veins (Fig. 10-2). Both main renal veins run in front of their corresponding arteries. The *right renal vein* passes behind the duodenum and enters the right lateral surface of the IVC.[10] The *left renal vein,* which is about three times as long, runs between the aorta and superior mesenteric artery and then drains into the left lateral wall of the IVC. The *left gonadal vein* enters the left renal vein along its undersurface just to the left of the spine (Fig. 10-3). The *left adrenal vein* enters the left renal vein on its superior surface usually in a combined trunk with the left inferior phrenic vein. The *right adrenal* and *gonadal veins* typically have separate entrances into the IVC at or near the origin of the right renal vein

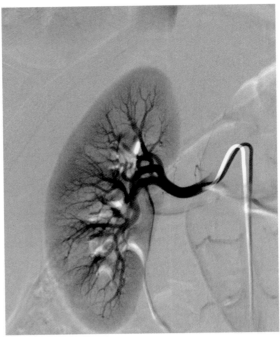

FIGURE 10-1   Arteriogram of a normal right kidney.

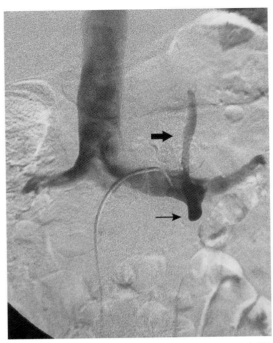

FIGURE 10-3   Normal left renal venogram with partial filling of the left phrenicoadrenal trunk *(thick arrow)* and gonadal vein to the level of the first valve *(thin arrow).*

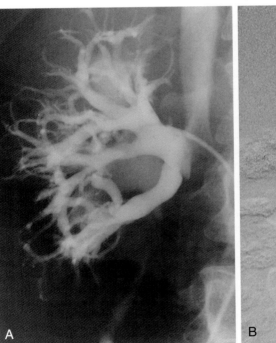

FIGURE 10-2   Normal right renal venograms.

(see Figs. 13-8, 13-9, and 13-13). In most patients, branches of the ascending lumbar and hemiazygous venous systems enter the left renal and left gonadal veins (see Fig. 16-4). Some patients have valves in the renal veins between the hilum and the IVC.

Variant Anatomy (Online Cases 4 and 31)

Accessory renal arteries supply one or both kidneys in about 25% to 35% of the general population.[11-15] Most accessory renal arteries supply the lower pole of the kidney but may originate anywhere from the suprarenal

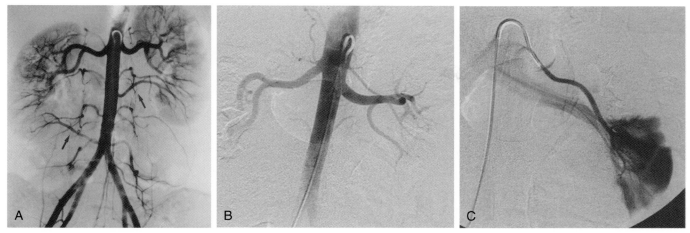

FIGURE 10-4 **A,** Accessory right and left renal arteries *(arrows).* **B,** In another patient, a small artery above the left renal artery is noted. **C,** Selective injection indicates an accessory renal artery feeding the lower pole.

aorta to the iliac artery (Figs. 10-4 through 10-6). Anomalies of position (i.e., ectopia), fusion, or rotation of the kidney are associated with variations in the origin and number of renal arteries. The *horseshoe kidney* usually is fed by three or more arteries arising from the aorta, iliac arteries, or both.

Several renal vein anomalies may be encountered[16-19] (Table 10-1 and Figs. 10-7 through 10-9). That close to one third of the population has multiple (especially right) renal veins is not well appreciated by many interventionalists. The *circumaortic left renal vein* consists of a "preaortic" segment that enters the IVC in the usual location and a "retroaortic" segment between the kidney and the low IVC. The two veins may or may not communicate in the renal hilum. The solitary *retroaortic left renal vein* is a less common variant.[15]

Collateral Circulation

With renal artery stenosis or occlusion, an extensive collateral circulation maintains blood flow to the kidney. Although renal arteries have been described as end arteries, communications between extrarenal arteries and segmental, interlobar, and arcuate vessels do exist. The classic description of collateral arterial flow in the kidney was made by Abrams and Cornell.[20] The intrarenal vessels are primarily supplied by three collateral networks: the capsular, peripelvic, and periureteric arteries. These three systems are ultimately fed by the lumbar arteries, aorta, internal iliac artery, inferior adrenal artery, and other vessels (Fig. 10-10).

In main renal vein obstruction, venous outflow occurs through ureteral, gonadal, adrenal, ascending lumbar, and capsular venous pathways (Fig. 10-11).

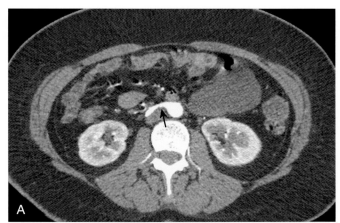

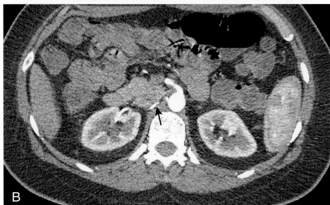

FIGURE 10-5 Accessory right renal artery. **A,** Contrast-enhanced computed tomography shows main right renal artery *(arrow).* **B,** An accessory right renal artery exits the aorta above the main vessel *(arrow).*

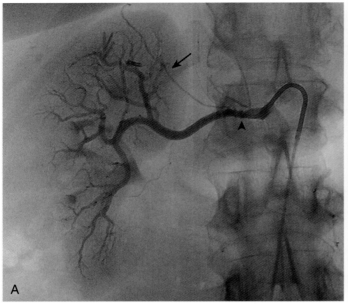
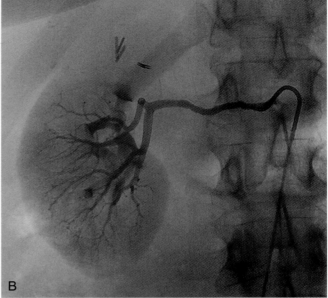

FIGURE 10-6   Accessory right renal artery. **A,** Injection of the main artery demonstrates the beaded appearance of fibromuscular dysplasia *(arrowhead)*. In addition, it shows no crossing of vessels in the hilum and indistinct nephrogram in mid and lower pole, suggesting the presence of an additional artery feeding the dorsal aspect of the kidney **(B).** Also note prominent capsular arteries *(arrow)*.

TABLE 10-1   Renal Venous Anomalies

Type	Reported Frequency (%)
Multiple right renal veins	8 to 24
Circumaortic left renal vein	2 to 10
Retroaortic left renal vein	2 to 7
Right gonadal vein enters right renal vein	<10

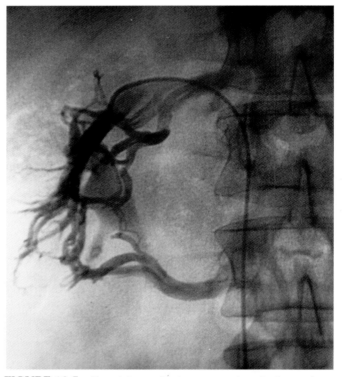

FIGURE 10-7   Two right renal veins communicate in the renal hilum.

MAJOR DISORDERS

Atherosclerotic Renovascular Disease (Online Case 18)

Etiology and Natural History

The renal arterial system plays a critical role in many patients with hypertension and chronic kidney disease. More commonly, long-standing or inadequately treated high blood pressure (from any cause) leads to progressive thickening and luminal narrowing of the small arteries of the kidneys. This *nephrosclerosis* is characterized by global damage of distal intrarenal vessels, which become irregular, tortuous, and pruned (Fig. 10-12). Less commonly, main, accessory, or branch renal artery obstruction (stenosis or occlusion) leads to so-called *renovascular hypertension (RVH)*. The consequent reduction in intrarenal arterial pressure is sensed by the juxtaglomerular apparatus of the afferent arterioles. The renin-angiotensin-aldosterone system is triggered, leading to increased renin production, vasoconstriction of systemic arteries, sodium and water retention, and systemic hypertension. Other factors that sustain hypertension include endothelin release and upregulation of the sympathetic nervous system.[21] Over time, untreated RVH will also cause nephrosclerosis that in and of itself

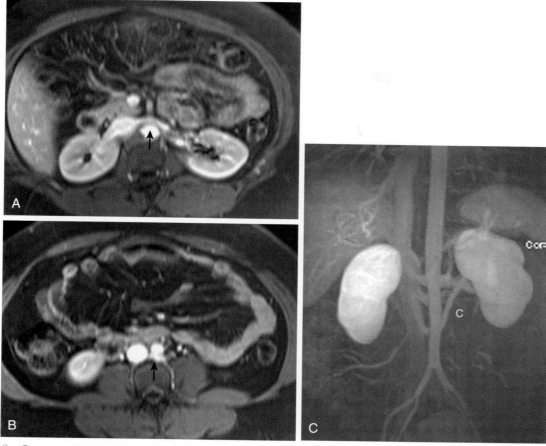

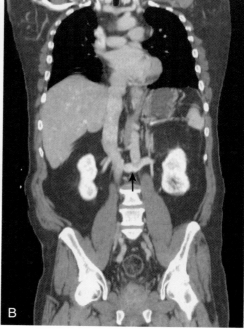

FIGURE 10-8   Circumaortic left renal vein. **A,** Gadolinium-enhanced magnetic resonance angiogram shows main left renal vein *(arrow)* entering the inferior vena cava (IVC). **B,** Circumaortic component passes behind the aorta to join the IVC *(arrow).* **C,** Maximum intensity projection demonstrates the orthotopic and circumaortic *(C)* left renal veins.

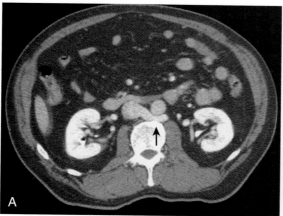

FIGURE 10-9   Retroaortic left renal vein. Axial and reformatted coronal computed tomography scans show the solitary left renal vein *(arrow)* passing behind the aorta well below the expected position of the vessel.

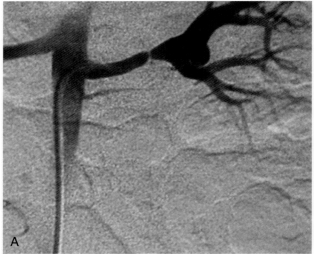

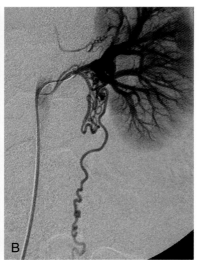

FIGURE 10-10 Significant left renal artery stenosis from intimal or perimedial fibroplasia type fibromuscular dysplasia. **A,** Pretreatment arteriogram shows typical weblike appearance of lesion in the distal left renal artery. **B,** Following angioplasty, inreased flow in the main artery causes antegrade flow in ureteric branches beyond the stenosis, which provided retrograde collateral circulation into the kidney before treatment.

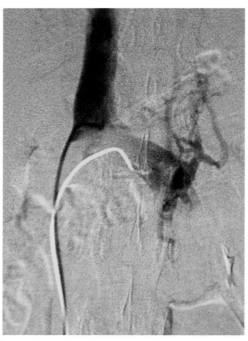

FIGURE 10-11 Venous collaterals with chronic left renal vein stenosis caused by impingement between the superior mesenteric artery and aorta ("nutcracker phenomenon").

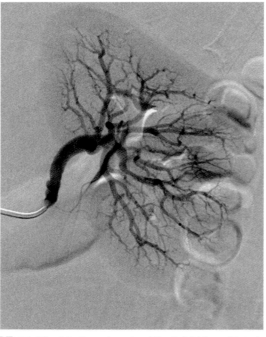

FIGURE 10-12 Nephrosclerosis of the left kidney. Note irregularity and pruning of distal intrarenal branches (compare with Fig. 10-1).

contributes to elevated blood pressure. RVH is reported in about 3% to 5% of cases of hypertension in the general population, although this figure is hotly debated.[22]

Ischemic nephropathy is generally defined as loss of renal function related to hypoperfusion from renal artery disease.[23] Atherosclerotic renal artery disease affecting both renal arteries or the artery to a solitary kidney is a common cause of ischemic nephropathy. Bilateral occlusions may eventually cause end-stage kidney disease. However, diminished central blood flow may be a minor factor in development of chronic kidney disease compared with microvascular changes caused by diabetes, hyperlipidemia, or hypertension itself.[24] Finally, the magnitude of renal artery stenosis has no direct correlation with the severity of kidney disease, unless the artery is completely occluded.[25,26]

Atherosclerosis is responsible for at least two thirds of cases of clinically significant renal artery stenosis.[21] Obstruction usually results from aortic plaque engulfing the renal artery *ostium* (i.e., within 5 to 10 mm of the aortic lumen). Less frequently, plaque develops independently in the *truncal* portion of the renal artery. In several studies, atherosclerotic renal artery stenosis was found to be progressive in more than one third of cases.[27,28] However, conversion to frank thrombosis is uncommon. Atherosclerotic renal artery disease must be distinguished from other causes of renal artery obstruction, particularly *fibromuscular dysplasia (FMD;* see later) (Box 10-1). Other kidney-related conditions that occasionally lead to chronic hypertension include trauma (e.g., Page kidney), cystic disease, renal cell carcinoma (RCC) or pheochromocytoma, renal artery aneurysm, reninoma, and renal infarction.

Clinical Features

Most patients with atherosclerotic RVH or ischemic nephropathy are middle aged or older adults and have one or more risk factors for atherosclerosis. Younger patients are more likely to suffer from one of the less common causes of RVH (see later discussion). Although African Americans suffer from essential hypertension more frequently than do whites, RVH is relatively more common in whites.[29] Patients with thrombosis superimposed on underlying disease often are asymptomatic. However, worsening of hypertension or loss of renal function may occur when there is occlusion of the artery to a solitary functioning kidney.

In the United States, the prevalence of significant renovascular disease (detected by duplex sonography) among individuals older than 65 years is about 7%.[30] Significant atherosclerotic renal artery stenosis is associated with particularly high rates of chronic kidney disease (about 25%), coronary artery disease, peripheral arterial disease, and stroke.[31]

Imaging

Because hypertension is common but RVH is not, screening should be reserved for patients at moderate to high risk for RVH. Box 10-2 lists the criteria proposed by the Joint National Committee on Prevention, Detection, Evaluation, and Treatment of High Blood Pressure.[32] Revised guidelines are currently in preparation.

Several metabolic screening tests may be first performed to exclude other uncommon causes of hypertension (e.g., pheochromocytoma, aldosteronoma). Noninvasive imaging procedures are then used to further screen patients. Catheter arteriography is employed only when results are equivocal or endovascular therapy is being considered. No single screening procedure has emerged as the ideal technique.

COLOR DOPPLER SONOGRAPHY

Ultrasound is one of the principal tools for detecting RVH because it is quick, relatively inexpensive, and completely safe (Fig. 10-13). If the aorta and main renal artery can be imaged, criteria for significant renal artery stenosis include intrastenotic peak systolic velocity (PSV) of greater than 180 cm/sec and PSV renal/aortic ratio of greater than 3.0 to 3.5[33,34] (Fig. 10-14). If these vessels cannot be seen because of technical factors, the intrarenal arteries are interrogated. With significant renal artery stenosis, damping and slowing of the time to peak systole ("parvus et tardus" waveform) is typical.[35] In addition, flow acceleration is diminished and the acceleration time prolonged (<300 to 390 cm/sec^2 and >0.06 to 0.07 sec, respectively).[33,36] The *resistive index*

BOX 10-1

CAUSES OF RENAL ARTERY STENOSIS

- Atherosclerosis
- Fibromuscular dysplasia
- Dissection
- Vasculitis
  - Takayasu arteritis
  - Radiation arteritis
- Coarctation syndromes
  - Neurofibromatosis
  - Congenital rubella
  - Williams syndrome
  - Tuberous sclerosis
  - Midaortic syndrome
- Trauma
- Extrinsic compression

BOX 10-2

SIGNS OF RENOVASCULAR HYPERTENSION

Onset of hypertension in patients <30 or >55 years of age
Resistant hypertension (blood pressure >140/90 mm Hg on appropriate triple drug therapy)
Accelerated hypertension
Recurrent (flash) pulmonary edema
Renal failure of uncertain etiology
Abdominal bruit
Renal insufficiency after ACE or ARB therapy
Significant extrarenal occlusive arterial disease

ACE, angiotensin-converting enzyme inhibitor; *ARB,* angiotensin II receptor blocker

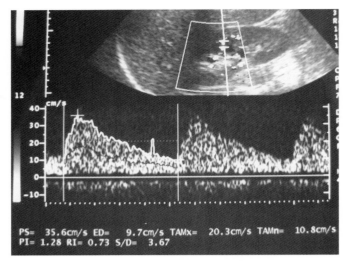

FIGURE 10-13   Normal renal artery duplex ultrasound with sampling of intrarenal branches.

([PSV − diastolic velocity]/PSV) usually is less than 0.45.[34] However, duplex sonography is highly operator dependent, and some studies have failed to confirm the touted accuracy of this technique.[37,38]

COMPUTED TOMOGRAPHY AND MAGNETIC RESONANCE ANGIOGRAPHY

Many centers rely on gadolinium-enhanced MR angiography for screening patients with suspected RVH if renal function is close to normal. Patients with preexisting renal insufficiency are at risk for nephrogenic systemic fibrosis after receiving some gadolinium-based contrast agents. With current techniques, MR angiography can detect main renal artery stenoses with up to 90% to 100% sensitivity and 75% to 100% specificity[38-45] (Figs. 10-15 and 10-16). Weaknesses of the method include identification of disease in accessory and segmental renal arteries and artifacts related to metallic clips, intravascular stents, or patient motion. However, isolated significant

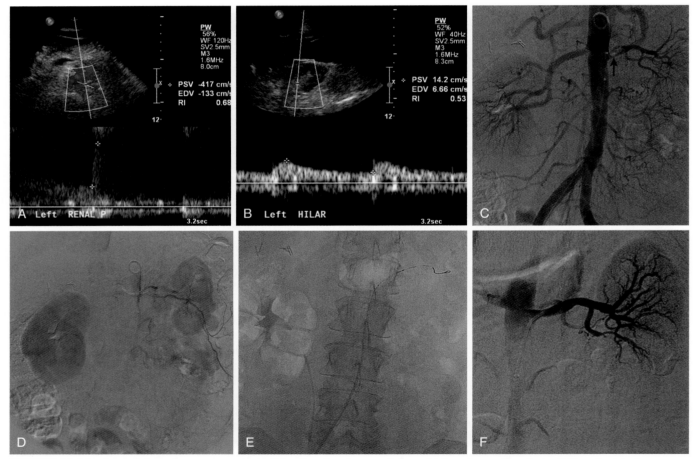

FIGURE 10-14   Severe left renal artery stenosis. **A,** Color Doppler ultrasound shows high peak systolic velocity (417 cm/sec) in the proximal renal artery. **B,** Spectral waveforms of intrarenal arteries depict the "tardus et parvus" waveform expected with a significant upstream stenosis. **C** and **D,** Aortography defines the tight truncal renal artery stenosis *(arrow).* The left kidney is small. **E,** The lesion is crossed with a guidewire, and a balloon expandable stent placed. **F,** Post-stent arteriography shows a widely patent lumen, but embolization of atheroma or thrombus into lower pole vessels is evident.

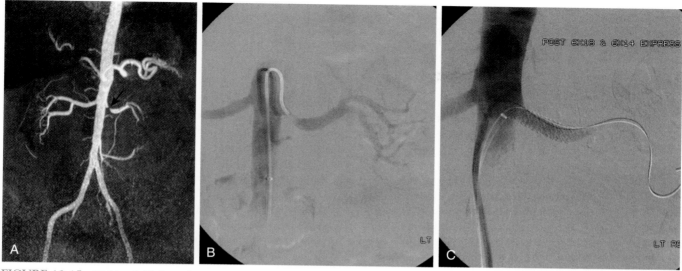

FIGURE 10-15 Tight ostial left renal artery stenosis. **A,** Magnetic resonance angiography depicts the lesion well *(arrow)*. **B,** Catheter arteriography confirms the stenosis, which was treated successfully with a balloon-expandable stent **(C).** Note slight extension of stent into the aorta.

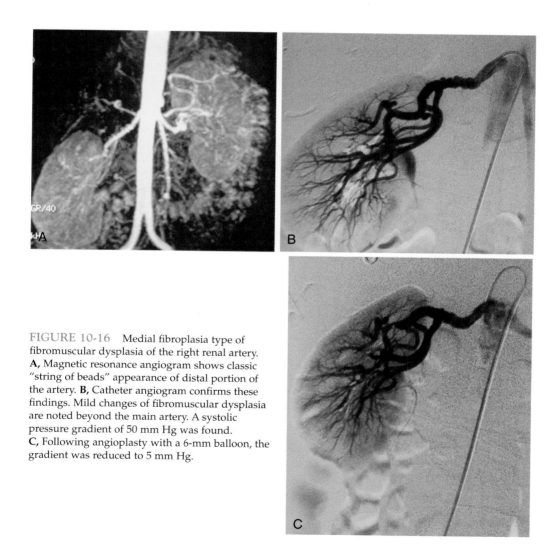

FIGURE 10-16 Medial fibroplasia type of fibromuscular dysplasia of the right renal artery. **A,** Magnetic resonance angiogram shows classic "string of beads" appearance of distal portion of the artery. **B,** Catheter angiogram confirms these findings. Mild changes of fibromuscular dysplasia are noted beyond the main artery. A systolic pressure gradient of 50 mm Hg was found. **C,** Following angioplasty with a 6-mm balloon, the gradient was reduced to 5 mm Hg.

stenoses of accessory arteries in this population are uncommon (<2%).[46]

Multidetector row CT angiography achieves comparable sensitivity and specificity to MR angiography in depicting renal artery stenosis[39,40,44,47] (Fig. 10-17). Sixty-four–detector row CT is almost equivalent to catheter angiography in uncovering in-stent restenosis (which is obscured in MR angiography).[48] Its major disadvantage is the need for iodinated contrast in a population at increased risk for contrast nephropathy.

CAPTOPRIL RENAL SCINTIGRAPHY

To a great extent, this functional rather than anatomic imaging modality has fallen out of favor in routine evaluation of patients with suspected RVH.[40,49]

RENAL VEIN RENIN SAMPLING

Normally, the ratio of renin activity in the renal vein versus the IVC is about 1.24.[50] In a patient with RVH and two functioning kidneys, the affected kidney overproduces renin, and renin secretion from the contralateral kidney is suppressed. Several criteria have been used to diagnose RVH based on renal vein renin values, including a renal vein renin ratio between the involved and uninvolved kidney of greater than 1.5 and a ratio of (renal renin–IVC renin)/IVC renin of greater than 0.48 (Vaughan formula).[51] While renal vein renin sampling was once a mainstay of RVH diagnosis, it is seldom used by interventionalists (Fig. 10-18).

CATHETER ANGIOGRAPHY

Catheter angiography is still the gold standard for the diagnosis of RVH. Initial abdominal aortography may not be necessary if high-quality CT or MR angiography

studies clearly depict the renal artery ostia and identify all renal arteries. Narrowing of accessory renal arteries or intrarenal branches can cause RVH and should be carefully sought; intrarenal stenoses are particularly common in children with RVH (Figs. 10-19 and 10-20). Stenoses may go undetected for several reasons, including oblique origin of the renal artery from the aorta and superimposition of intrarenal branches. Multiple angiographic views may be necessary to identify such hidden lesions.

Atherosclerosis produces irregular narrowing of the renal ostium or proximal renal artery (see Figs. 10-14 and 10-15). Bilateral disease is common, and infrarenal aortic atherosclerosis usually is present. After a stenosis has been identified, its hemodynamic significance must be proved by one of the following criteria[21,52]:

- Reduction in luminal diameter of greater than 75%
- Systolic pressure gradient across stenosis in the main renal artery greater than 10 to 20 mm Hg or greater than 20% of aortic systolic pressure

A stenosis with a 50% to 75% reduction in the luminal diameter may be hemodynamically significant, but in such cases, pressures should be measured.

Treatment

Selection of patients with RVH or ischemic nephropathy for endovascular or operative therapy is highly controversial[21,53] (Box 10-3). Recent improvements in antihypertensive medications and routine lifelong treatment of this population with lipid-lowering "statins" and oral antiplatelet agents may allow many people with RVH and normal or mild renal insufficiency to be treated medically. The mere presence of a significant renal artery stenosis does not by itself warrant treatment, because not all such patients will have a positive clinical outcome from arterial recanalization. In addition, the procedure itself may worsen renal function by contrast nephropathy, atheroembolization, or, rarely, complete vessel occlusion.

RENAL ARTERY STENT PLACEMENT

Over the past two decades, endovascular treatment of renal artery disease has been embraced by interventionalists of all kinds.[54] Advocates point to numerous large historical series that support the value of renal artery stents in treating hypertension or stabilizing (or even reversing) renal insufficiency.[55-58] However, this enthusiasm has been tempered by several recent randomized trials that have failed to show significant benefit, particularly in light of nontrivial adverse events (see later discussion). Although some of these studies are fraught with important drawbacks, many physicians outside

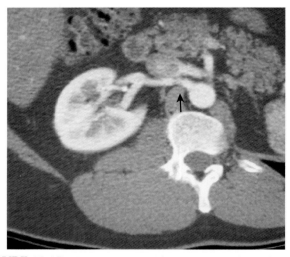

FIGURE 10-17 Transverse image from contrast-enhanced computed tomography scan shows a mild to moderate stenosis of the proximal right renal artery.

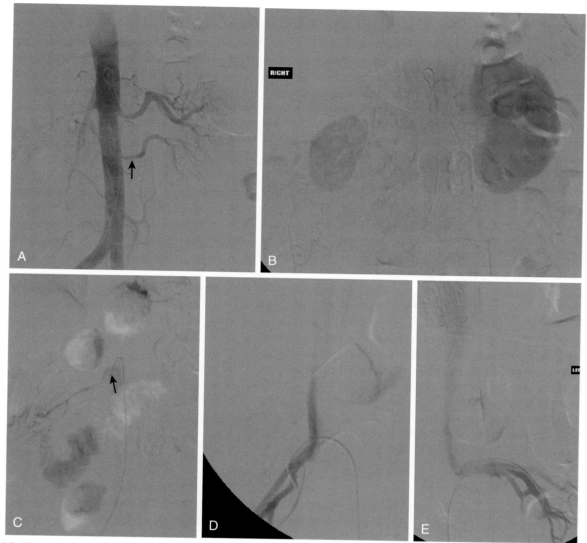

FIGURE 10-18   Renal vein renin analysis in patient with severe uncontrolled hypertension. **A** and **B,** Abdominal aortography shows two left renal arteries, the more inferior of which has an origin stenosis *(arrow)*. The right kidney is very small, and there is only minimal flow through a highly diseased artery *(arrow,* **C)**. Right **(D),** lower pole left **(E),** and upper pole left (not shown) renal vein renins were obtained. Markedly elevated levels from the right kidney prompted right nephrectomy. Blood pressure was then easily controlled.

the interventional community are skeptical of routine application of this aggressive approach.

PATIENT SELECTION   In patients with hypertension, renal artery revascularization is of no proven value for the following:

- Nonsignificant renal artery stenosis
- Incidental finding of significant disease in the absence of hypertension or renal insufficiency
- Significant renal artery stenosis with severe bilateral nephrosclerosis that may be responsible for hypertension

Box 10-3 lists the primary indications for intervention in patients with atherosclerotic RVH or ischemic nephropathy.[21,59] Angioplasty alone is rarely employed in this setting, with the possible exception of focal truncal stenoses.[60] Stents significantly improve the technical success of renal artery angioplasty for atherosclerotic disease, particularly for ostial lesions (from 55% to 70% to more than 95%).[56,60-65] This improvement alone may largely explain the better long-term patency rates associated with stent placement. Use of stents in renal arteries with nominal diameter of less than 5 mm usually is avoided because of the relatively higher rates of clinically significant restenosis in this setting.[66]

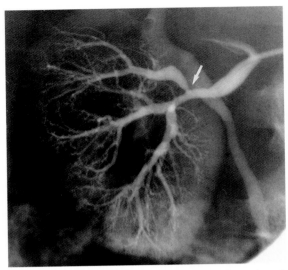

FIGURE 10-19 Intrarenal renal artery stenosis. Stenosis at the origin of a segmental branch *(arrow)* produced renovascular hypertension in this child. The upper pole of the kidney is not filled because of injection into the dorsal ramus of the renal artery.

Revascularization for renal salvage is considered in patients with significant bilateral renal artery disease or disease in a solitary functioning kidney with some functional reserve. Even when the main renal artery is completely occluded, collateral circulation has often developed over time to keep the kidney viable, even up to 6 months or more after occlusion. There is usually no benefit to revascularizing a minimally functioning kidney.

TECHNIQUE (SEE FIG. 10-14) Most interventionalists continue the patient's blood pressure medication until the procedure is completed. The dose of iodinated contrast material should be kept to an absolute minimum. In patients with preexisting renal dysfunction, various measures are taken to protect the kidneys including use of carbon dioxide angiography and administration of *N*-acetyl cysteine and intravenous bicarbonate infusion (see Chapter 2 and Fig. 3-20). All patients should receive aspirin (325 mg orally) or clopidogrel (300 mg oral loading dose) beforehand. If there are no contraindications, the former is continued for the patient's lifetime or the latter for at least 3 to 6 months afterward. Parenteral platelet inhibition may be helpful in minimizing deleterious effects to the kidney from atheroemboli or contrast.[67,68] Full anticoagulation with heparin (or a direct thrombin inhibitor if heparin allergy history exists) is instituted before crossing the obstructive lesion. An intraarterial dose of nitroglycerin (150 to 200 mg) may help prevent guidewire or catheter-induced vasospasm.

The diagnostic catheter is replaced with a 5- or 6-Fr guiding sheath or catheter with distal curve appropriate for the renal artery origin. Traditionally, the stenosis

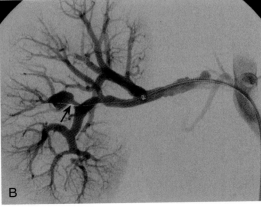

FIGURE 10-20 Neurofibromatosis in an 11-year-old boy with hypertension. **A,** Aneurysms and an intrarenal branch stenosis *(arrow)* are noted. **B,** There is some improvement in the intrarenal obstruction after balloon angioplasty.

was crossed with a floppy 0.035″ guidewire, a 5-Fr catheter advanced beyond the lesion, and the balloon or stent inserted over a stiff 0.035″ Rosen or TAD exchange wire. Most practitioners now favor low-profile platforms.[69] Thus the stenosis is crossed with a steerable 0.014″ to 0.018″ microwire followed by a microcatheter. If difficulty is encountered traversing the lesion, several maneuvers should be tried. Changes in the patient's respiration can dramatically alter the aortorenal artery angle. Stiffer (or sometimes less stiff) guidewires may be helpful.

A heavy-duty microwire with a floppy tip is positioned to give support for the balloon-mounted stent delivery catheter but avoid damage to the distal renal artery branches. Monorail systems that circumvent the need for a long exchange wire are popular. Great care must be taken with wire manipulations because even a small-caliber floppy-tipped nitinol wire can dissect the main vessel or perforate small renal artery branches, leading to occlusion or hemorrhage.

Recent data prove that endovascular renal procedures reliably cause showers of atheroembolic particles into the distal vasculature.[70,71] This embolic burden may negate any positive effect expected from the intervention. Distal embolic protective devices (occlusion balloons or permeable filters) that trap this material may prevent microembolic injury to the treated kidney. These filters are strongly advocated by some experts.

If the lumen is initially so narrow that passage of the guiding sheath or stent device is impossible, predilation of the stenosis with an undersized balloon may be required. Off-label use of a variety of stents is standard practice but is not condoned by the U.S. Food and Drug Administration. The device is usually a nitinol stent that is factory-mounted on a slightly oversized diameter angioplasty balloon. It is chosen by measuring the luminal diameter of the normal portion of the renal artery or contralateral artery on the diagnostic arteriogram. In adults, the usual balloon diameter is 5 to 7 mm. The shortest available stent length is selected to entirely cover the diseased area. The stent may be inserted into the artery within the guiding sheath or directly over the guidewire without sheath protection ("bareback"). The stent is exposed by withdrawing the guiding catheter from the renal artery.

For ostial lesions, the stent is positioned with the proximal end about 1 mm inside the aortic lumen to completely cover the overhanging plaque. Angiograms are obtained through the guiding sheath to ensure precise positioning. The stent is deployed by expansion of the balloon with an inflation device. Additional stents are placed if needed, which is rare. Care should be taken to avoid placing stents into the distal renal artery, which could preclude later surgical revascularization or

damage branch vessels. In the event of vessel rupture, an angioplasty balloon of appropriate size is quickly reinflated within the stent. Placement of a covered stent is usually required. The procedure ends with a completion angiogram and pressure measurements to document satisfactory result.

RESULTS Success in renal artery revascularization for RVH is judged by blood pressure response, with clinical benefit defined as *cure* (i.e., blood pressure lower than 140/90 mm Hg without medication) or *improvement* (i.e., reduced number of medications required to maintain blood pressure below 140/90 mm Hg or a 15-mm Hg reduction in blood pressure on the same or reduced number of medications).[22] In ischemic nephropathy, clinical benefit is defined as reduction or stabilization in serum creatinine or flattening of the renal dysfunction curve (1/creatinine versus time).

A widely patent artery can be created with a metallic stent in greater than 95% of cases.[24,61,63,72,73] In atherosclerotic RVH, actual cure of hypertension is achieved in less than 10% to 20% of individuals whether stents are used or not. Blood pressure control is better in about 50% to 80% of patients. Based on historical series, angioplasty and stent placement lead to improvement or stabilization of renal insufficiency in about 70% of cases; however, in some (but not all) series, that benefit diminished over time.[64,66,72,74] The value of embolic protection is unproven despite some encouraging nonrandomized series.[67,68,75]

The reported angiographic restenosis rate for atherosclerotic lesions is about 20%.[63,66,76,77] However, the reported Doppler sonographic restenosis rate at 9 to 12 months has ranged from 21% to 50%.[78,79] Luminal compromise seems to increase slowly over time. One important predictor of clinically significant restenosis is small initial vessel diameter (<5 mm). Preliminary trials suggest that drug-eluting stents may be of added value in such small caliber arteries.[80,81] Restenosis is treated by repeated balloon angioplasty without or with additional stent placement[82,83] (see Fig. 1-10).

Despite encouraging results from retrospective studies and registries, controlled randomized trials of stent placement versus best medical therapy for patients with atherosclerotic renal artery stenosis have not supported routine endovascular therapy for management of RVH or ischemic nephropathy.[24,53,73,84,85] Critics are quick to note the frequency of major adverse events associated with stent insertion, including loss of renal function after revascularization in 10% to 20% of individuals.[21] These studies had numerous deficiencies, including inclusion of a substantial number of patients with nonsignificant renal artery stenosis and lack of standardization of stent insertion techniques. Nonetheless, the cumulative burden of these recent trials is sobering. There is hope that the ongoing multicenter CORAL and RADAR trials will satisfy both proponents and skeptics of renal artery stent placement.[87,88]

COMPLICATIONS Major complications occur in about 8% to 15% of procedures[22,89] (see Fig. 10-14). Permanent decline in renal function is noted in about 6% of cases and usually is caused by contrast nephropathy and/or microembolization. Periodic surveillance CT angiography or duplex ultrasound is advisable to detect restenosis and the need for further treatment.[48,79]

SURGICAL THERAPY

In patients with RVH or ischemic nephropathy, surgery is reserved for failures of endovascular treatment, cases with associated aortic disease that require open operation, and most renal artery occlusions.[90] If minimal aortic disease is present, the standard procedure is aortorenal bypass grafting with autologous vein. In patients with severe aortic atherosclerosis or an aortic aneurysm, the hepatic or splenic artery may be used as a bypass conduit for the right or left renal artery, respectively.[91,92] If the main renal artery is occluded but the distal artery reconstitutes through collaterals, bypass is sometimes done to improve function or treat RVH. Otherwise, hypertension may be treated by excision of the renin-producing kidney (see Fig. 10-18).

Renal Artery Fibromuscular Dysplasia (Online Case 76)

Etiology and Clinical Features

Fibromuscular dysplasia (FMD) is a group of related noninflammatory disorders of unknown etiology in which affected arteries become narrowed, aneurysmal, or dissected.[93] FMD is not rare; it is found in about 3% to 5% of preoperative imaging studies of potential kidney donors.[94,95] Six types of FMD are described in one traditional classification scheme; the most common type is *medial fibroplasia*[93,96] (Table 10-2). In this form of the disease, the normal media is replaced by fibrous tissue and extracellular matrix. The thickened segments alternate with sites of medial thinning, which produces the classic "string-of-beads" appearance of the lumen on imaging studies. The less common types of FMD cause luminal beading, smooth and tapered stenosis, focal bandlike narrowing, dissection, or aneurysm without stenosis.

FMD is largely a disease of young or middle-aged women. However, it may be seen in men and young children. The disorder is often asymptomatic and only detected on imaging studies obtained for other reasons. Difficult to control hypertension and onset at a younger age should suggest the diagnosis. Renal FMD rarely results in ischemic nephropathy.

TABLE 10-2 Classification of Subtypes of Renal Artery Fibromuscular Dysplasia

Type	Frequency (%)	Morphology
Medial fibroplasia	60 to 70	Alternating narrowing and aneurysms ("string of beads")
Perimedial fibroplasia	15 to 25	Irregular, beaded narrowing
Medial hyperplasia	5 to 15	Tubular, smooth narrowing
Medial dissection	5	False channel in media
Intimal fibroplasia	1 to 2	Focal, smooth narrowing
Periarterial fibroplasia	<1	Tubular, smooth narrowing

Imaging

The approach to imaging of patients with suspected FMD-related renovascular hypertension is similar to that for cases of atherosclerotic-associated disease (see earlier discussion). Most patients are screened with duplex sonography and then referred for CT or MR angiography if ultrasound is positive. The latter modalities approach but do not achieve the accuracy of catheter arteriography in the diagnosis of main renal artery FMD.[97,98] Catheter angiography is still necessary to detect or exclude branch vessel involvement, so the threshold for performing an angiogram should be low when the index of suspicion is high.

FMD typically attacks the middle to distal renal artery and less commonly intrarenal branches. However, proximal (but rarely ostial) lesions do occur. The aorta usually is disease-free. Bilateral FMD is seen in about two thirds of cases; the right kidney is affected more commonly than the left.[99] The classic appearance of the common medial fibroplasia type of FMD is a "string of beads" (see Figs. 1-25 and 10-16). The other forms of FMD have different morphologies (Figs. 10-21 and 10-22; see also Table 10-2). However, the pathologic subtype cannot always be predicted by the angiogram.[100]

Treatment

RENAL ARTERY ANGIOPLASTY

By common consent, balloon angioplasty is the first-line treatment for symptomatic renal FMD (see Figs. 1-25, 10-16, and 10-21).

TECHNIQUE The steps in renal artery angioplasty are almost identical to those for renal artery stent placement (see earlier). It is crucial to obtain pressure measurements before treatment. The apparent luminal narrowing of an FMD lesion may overestimate or underestimate the actual resistance to flow.

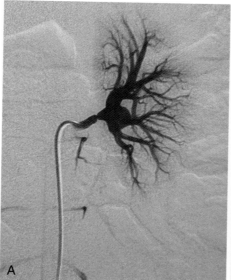
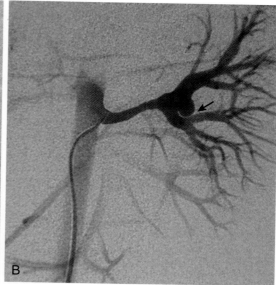

FIGURE 10-21 Intimal or perimedial fibroplasia type of fibromuscular dysplasia before (A) and after (B) angioplasty. Note the intrarenal aneurysm (arrow).

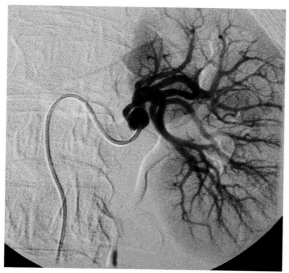

FIGURE 10-22 Probable medial dissection type of fibromuscular dysplasia.

The distal portion of the balloon must be kept away from smaller branch vessels when it is expanded. FMD lesions may require multiple prolonged balloon inflations or pressures in excess of the 4 to 12 mm Hg needed to crack most atherosclerotic plaques. Cutting balloons (see Chapter 3) can be helpful in this situation.[101] If the patient complains of severe pain, the vessel may be overstretched, and the balloon should be immediately deflated. Renal artery perforation is fortunately rare but may be remedied by prolonged balloon inflation or placement of a covered stent.

Angioplasty is considered successful when the residual stenosis is less than 30% and the systolic pressure gradient is less than 10 mm Hg. An irregular "ratty" luminal surface alone is not an indication for stent placement because these vessels often remodel over time. If results are inadequate, stent placement should be considered[102] (see earlier discussion).

RESULTS Technical success occurs in greater than 90% of cases; this figure approaches 100% when stents are used as needed.[102,103] Clinical benefit is noted in about 75% to 90% of cases, and results usually are long lasting. In fact, complete cure of hypertension from medial fibroplasia-type FMD is noted about half the time. However, these figures primarily apply to that common subtype, because large series that focused on the less common subtypes are unavailable. FMD-related renal artery aneurysms have been excluded with covered stents.[104]

COMPLICATIONS Adverse events are reported in 5% to 10% of procedures and include renal artery dissection, thrombosis, rupture, distal thrombus embolization, and access site complications (e.g., groin hematoma). Many complications are related to injury of the renal artery or its branches by guidewires.

Acute Renal Artery Occlusion (Online Case 82)

Etiology and Clinical Features

Box 10-4 lists the primary reasons for complete renal artery occlusion.[105,106] The most common etiology is an embolus, which originates from the heart in about 90% of cases.[107] Thrombosis superimposed on existing atherosclerotic disease is another important cause. Blunt or penetrating abdominal trauma can produce an intimal tear, dissection, or complete avulsion of the renal artery, any of which can result in acute thrombosis. Renal artery dissection is usually an extension of the process arising in the abdominal aorta.

Most patients are older and have an underlying history of a heart condition, particularly atrial fibrillation or coronary artery disease. Individuals with acute occlusion of a previously patent renal artery may complain of sudden flank pain and hematuria. However, embolic obstructions often are silent and may be missed for some time.

Imaging

CROSS-SECTIONAL IMAGING

Color Doppler sonography is the simplest method for detecting renal artery occlusion. If results are equivocal, CT or MR angiography should be performed.[108]

CATHETER ANGIOGRAPHY

Catheter arteriography is performed in the setting of trauma or when endovascular therapy is being considered. An embolus appears as a filling defect or complete occlusion with concave margin (Fig. 10-23). Emboli tend to lodge in the proximal renal artery or at a branch point.[109] When embolization occurs into a normal vessel, the collateral circulation may be inadequate to perfuse the kidney. Embolization of intrarenal vessels leads to segmental infarction. Traumatic occlusions usually produce an abrupt cutoff of the vessel at the site of injury (Fig. 10-24).

Treatment

Although the native human kidney may only be viable for several hours after sudden deprivation of blood flow, renal revascularization following acute occlusion has allowed salvage after much longer intervals.[106,110,111] Collateral flow can preserve some kidney function for weeks or even months after complete obstruction of a previously normal vessel. Therefore treatment should not be withheld based solely on estimated time from occlusion. Scintigraphy and sonography are sometimes used to determine viability and residual mass.

SURGICAL THERAPY

Renal artery thrombus is easily removed by surgical embolectomy. However, there is substantial morbidity and mortality associated with this procedure, mostly related to patients' existing cardiac diseases. Return of renal function can be anticipated in some cases after conservative treatment with anticoagulation and temporary dialysis, as needed.[112] Embolectomy is therefore usually reserved for cases of bilateral embolism or obstruction of a solitary kidney.

ENDOVASCULAR THERAPY

Although catheter-directed thrombolytic therapy can completely dissolve most acute renal artery emboli, long-term kidney salvage is uncommon unless flow

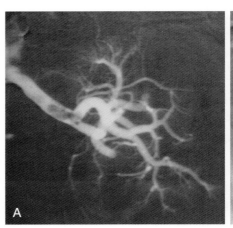
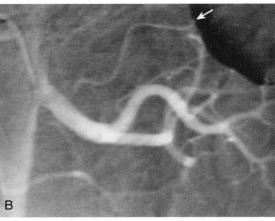

FIGURE 10-23   An embolic renal artery occlusion about 5 days old was treated with thrombolysis. **A,** Left renal angiogram shows a filling defect in the distal artery. **B,** After intraarterial infusion of a fibrinolytic agent, complete lysis has occurred. The renal function of the patient returned.

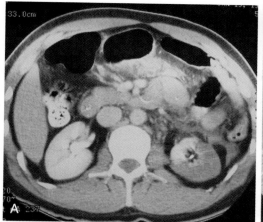

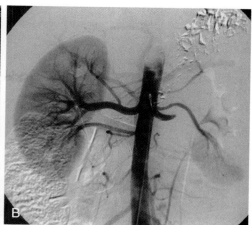

FIGURE 10-24 Traumatic renal artery occlusion after a motor vehicle accident. **A,** Computed tomography shows almost complete lack of enhancement of the left kidney. **B,** Arteriogram shows traumatic occlusion of the main left renal artery and preservation of the accessory artery to the lower pole.

is restored within about 3 hours of occlusion[113] (see Fig. 10-23). Angioplasty and stent placement have been effective in preserving function in some cases when renal viability is proven.[114]

Vascular Complications after Kidney Transplantation (Online Case 92)

Etiology

The harvested kidney is placed into either iliac fossa of the recipient. The donor renal vein is sutured to the native external iliac vein in an end-to-side fashion or the internal iliac vein in an end-to-end fashion. The donor artery is connected in one of two ways. The surgeon may construct an end-to-side anastomosis to the recipient external (or common) iliac artery (Fig. 10-25). In cadaveric transplants, an oval segment of aorta surrounding the donor artery (Carrel patch) may be incorporated. Otherwise, an end-to-end anastomosis to the recipient's

ligated internal iliac artery is made. If the donor kidney has multiple arteries, the accessory branches may be tied individually into the main vessel. Sometimes, more elaborate reconstruction is necessary.

Vascular complications develop in up to 25% of patients after kidney transplantation.[115] *Arterial stenosis* is the most common problem, encountered in about 4% to 10% of transplant recipients.[115-117] Most lesions develop between 3 months and 2 years after placement. The stenosis is usually located at the anastomosis and less often in the recipient or graft artery. Inflow iliac artery obstructions unsuspected before surgery also may contribute to declining allograft function. Stenoses are more common in cadaveric grafts than in organs from living-related donors. Immune-related proliferative narrowing has been postulated as the cause of some cases of graft arterial stenosis.[118]

Arterial thrombosis usually is the result of operative injury to the donor or recipient artery, kinking of the

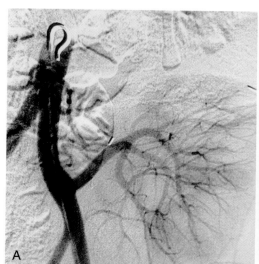

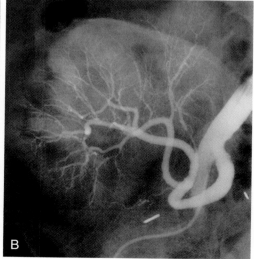

FIGURE 10-25 Kidney transplant arterial connections. **A,** End-to-side anastomosis to the left common iliac artery. **B,** End-to-end anastomosis to the right internal iliac artery. Irregular stenoses and occlusions of distal renal arterial branches are consistent with the clinical diagnosis of chronic rejection.

arterial connection, underlying atherosclerosis, acute rejection, thrombophilic state, or hypotension. Fortunately, the incidence of complete main renal artery thrombosis is less than 1%; thrombosis of accessory branches or segmental infarcts is more common.[119] Transplant *renal vein thrombosis (RVT)* may be caused by intraoperative damage to the vein, hypotension, venous compression by an extrinsic mass (e.g., lymphocele), extension of lower extremity thrombus into the iliac veins, or graft infection.

After operation, many patients require percutaneous biopsy of kidney transplants to assess graft function, and large cores of cortical and medullary tissue are required for analysis. There is a nontrivial risk of vascular injury; the consequence may be significant immediate arterial bleeding or delayed hemorrhage from *pseudoaneurysm* or *arteriovenous fistula (AVF)* formation. Aneurysms or pseudoaneurysms may also follow graft infection or loss of integrity of the arterial anastomosis.

Clinical Features

The most common signs of transplant renal artery obstruction are hypertension, worsening renal function, and a bruit heard over the allograft. Because elevated blood pressure is common after transplantation, only patients with severe or refractory hypertension are evaluated for treatable causes. In addition to arterial stenosis or occlusion, a decline in renal function after transplantation may be caused by acute or chronic rejection, acute tubular necrosis, drug reaction from immunosuppressive agents, or the development of intrinsic disease in the transplant.

The classic signs of transplant RVT are swelling and tenderness of the graft and impaired renal function. Patients with renal artery aneurysms may develop a pulsatile mass over the graft. Self-limited hematuria or small perigraft hematoma is common after percutaneous biopsy. If bleeding is exuberant or persistent, or the patient shows evidence for substantial blood loss (based on vital signs, drop in hemoglobin, or postbiopsy imaging), an angiogram should be performed without delay.

Imaging

Imaging is used to distinguish vascular, medical, and urinary tract complications as the cause of allograft dysfunction.

SONOGRAPHY

Color or power Doppler sonography is the standard tool for screening patients with suspected vascular complications after renal transplantation.[119-121] The criteria for significant arterial stenosis include a PSV ratio of 2:1 or more (stenosis versus adjacent normal segment), color aliasing, and a PSV of greater than 2 m/sec. Spectral analysis of intrarenal vessels may show a marked slowing of acceleration time as an indirect indicator of a proximal stenosis (Fig. 10-26). Segmental infarcts appear as sharply defined regions of absent flow in small parenchymal vessels. Sonography is useful also in detecting renal artery thrombosis, RVT, renal vein kinks, AVFs, and pseudoaneurysms (Fig. 10-27). On color Doppler analysis, the pseudoaneurysm sac is often identified. AVFs show venous turbulence throughout the cardiac cycle.

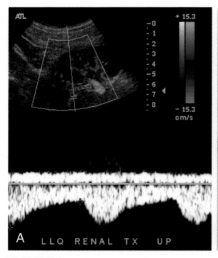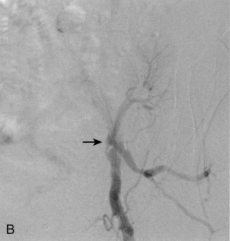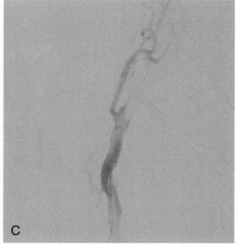

FIGURE 10-26 Transplant renal artery stenosis. **A,** Color Doppler ultrasound of distal arterial system shows typical "parvus et tardus" waveform because of upstream stenosis. **B,** Steep oblique left external iliac arteriogram barely documents the anastomotic stenosis *(arrow).* **C,** After balloon angioplasty, vessel patency is markedly improved.

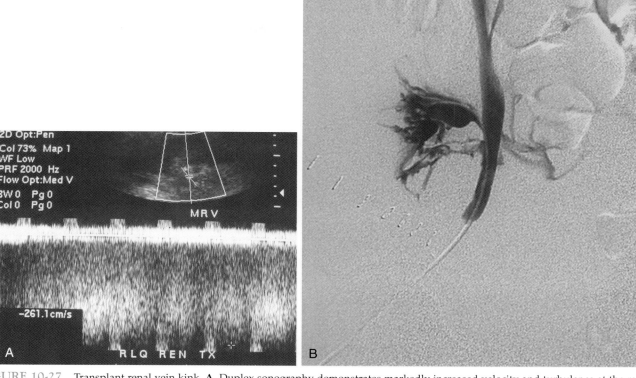

FIGURE 10-27   Transplant renal vein kink. **A,** Duplex sonography demonstrates markedly increased velocity and turbulence at the renal vein anastomosis. **B,** Selective catheter venogram confirms tight narrowing because of a kink in the vessel.

COMPUTED TOMOGRAPHY AND MAGNETIC RESONANCE ANGIOGRAPHY

In the typical setting of underlying renal graft insufficiency, the great concern with contrast-based CT or MR angiography is the associated risks of contrast nephropathy or nephrogenic systemic fibrosis, respectively. Nonetheless, these modalities are often employed before catheter angiography or surgical repair.[121-124] Recently, promising work in this arena has been reported with steady-state free precision (SSFP) MR angiography that totally avoids the risks of contrast materials.[125]

CATHETER ANGIOGRAPHY

Catheter arteriography and venography remain the gold standards for diagnosis. Given reported false-negative rates up to 14% and 18% for MR angiography and color Doppler sonography, respectively, in detection of transplant renal artery stenosis, arteriography should be pursued when clinical suspicion for vascular disease remains high.[126] Grafts with end-to-side anastomoses to the external iliac artery are best approached with a cobra or hockey stick–shaped catheter from the ipsilateral femoral artery. Grafts with end-to-end anastomoses to the internal iliac artery usually are studied with a cobra

or long reverse-curve catheter from the contralateral groin. The renal vein may be approached from the ipsilateral groin. Care must be taken to strictly limit the volume of iodinated contrast material. The risk of contrast nephropathy is completely eliminated when carbon dioxide is used as the contrast agent.[127] Steep oblique projections often are required to lay out the arterial anastomosis (see Fig. 10-26). However, a single pressure gradient across the anastomosis is far more accurate than multiple images for excluding a hemodynamically significant obstruction.

Arterial stenoses usually occur directly at the anastomosis and produce little change in renal blood flow (see Fig. 10-26). Other possible findings include iliac artery stenosis, segmental artery occlusion, main transplant artery stenosis, and vessel kink. Acute or chronic rejection causes markedly diminished flow (<5 to 6 mL/sec), severe pruning of distal intrarenal branches, and a faint or absent nephrogram (Fig. 10-28). Renal artery or vein thrombosis appears as complete or near-complete occlusion of the vessel. Venous kinks also have been described (see Fig. 10-27). AVFs and pseudoaneurysms have a characteristic appearance and are virtually always intrarenal (see later discussion).

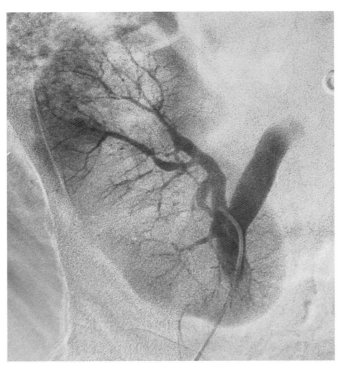

FIGURE 10-28 Acute rejection of a renal transplant is characterized by severe pruning of the intrarenal branches.

Treatment

ENDOVASCULAR THERAPY

Transcatheter techniques are extremely effective in treating most vascular complications of renal transplantation.[128] The techniques for balloon angioplasty and stent deployment are essentially the same as those for atherosclerotic arterial stenoses in a native solitary kidney (see earlier discussion). Primary stent insertion or selective placement for failures of balloon angioplasty afford technical success rates approaching 100%. Long-term graft salvage and improvement in blood pressure is expected 90% or more of the time.[117,126,128-131] Complications, which are uncommon, include arterial dissection, perforation, and rupture; however, loss of the allograft is rare.

On occasion, stents are inserted to open transplant renal vein stenoses.[132] Thrombolytic therapy has been used to treat arterial and venous thromboses of renal transplants. Renal vein clot is lysed with selective intravenous and intraarterial fibrinolytic infusion, alone or in combination.[133,134]

Percutaneous treatment of postbiopsy AVFs and pseudoaneurysms is preferred over surgery[135-137] (see later discussion). Tissue loss is minimized by superselective embolization with microcoils deposited through coaxial microcatheters directly at the site of abnormality.

SURGICAL THERAPY

Operative treatment of arterial stenoses usually is reserved for patients with a poor response to balloon angioplasty or stenting. Surgical thrombectomy and revision may be performed for cases of acute arterial or venous thrombosis, although long-term salvage is uncommon.

Trauma (Online Cases 44, 66, and 82)

Etiology

Injury to the renal artery can occur from blunt trauma (e.g., motor vehicle crashes), penetrating trauma (e.g., criminal assault), or medical procedures (e.g., percutaneous biopsy, percutaneous nephrostomy, nephrolithotomy, open surgery). Blunt trauma is associated with a whole spectrum of renal injuries. The most severe insults disrupt the renal pedicle and include intimal damage, dissection, thrombotic occlusion, or complete avulsion of the artery.[138] A subcapsular hematoma can ultimately produce RVH by a compressive effect *(Page kidney)*.[139] Other traumatic lesions include pseudoaneurysms, AVFs, and frank extravasation.

Penetrating injuries may lead to perirenal hematomas, AVFs, pseudoaneurysms, arteriocaliceal fistulas, or complete arterial occlusion. AVFs can occur after percutaneous renal biopsy, although most of these lesions close spontaneously.[135] Percutaneous nephrostomy is complicated by a significant vascular injury in about 1% of cases.[140] Retroperitoneal hematoma, intrarenal hemorrhage, or urinary tract bleeding may develop from inadvertent laceration of an artery or delayed rupture of a pseudoaneurysm.

Clinical Features

Minor bleeding is common immediately after percutaneous nonvascular renal interventions. Most lesions resolve spontaneously within days to weeks. Patients with persistent or recurrent gross hematuria or evidence of substantial blood loss (based on vital signs, changes in hematocrit, or imaging studies) require direct intervention. In some patients, symptoms occur weeks to months after the injury, particularly in the case of AVFs or pseudoaneurysms that expand and eventually rupture into the kidney parenchyma or collecting system. Left untreated, some of these abnormalities may result in RVH or renal ischemia, leading to acute kidney injury if the kidney is solitary.

Imaging

CROSS-SECTIONAL IMAGING

Patients with blunt abdominal injury are initially evaluated and staged with CT.[141] The American Association for the Surgery of Trauma (AAST) grading scheme is

TABLE 10-3 The American Association for the Surgery of Trauma Organ Injury Scale—Kidney

Grade	Description
I	Subcapsular hematoma without parenchymal laceration
II	Nonexpanding perirenal hematoma
	<1 cm renal cortical laceration, no urinary extravasation
III	>1 cm renal cortical laceration, no collecting system involvement
IV	Laceration from cortex through collecting system
	Main renal artery or vein injury
V	Shattered kidney
	Avulsion of renal hilum, devascularized kidney

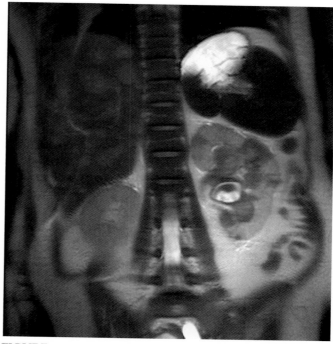

FIGURE 10-29 Postnephrostomy renal artery pseudoaneurysm. Coronal T2-weighted magnetic resonance image shows a round mass in the left renal pelvis with swirling flow, indicating an aneurysm.

outlined in Table 10-3. Findings of vascular trauma include main renal artery occlusion, segmental infarcts, active bleeding, perinephric hematoma, lacerations, AVFs, and pseudoaneurysms (Figs. 10-29 and 10-30). Ultrasound or CT is favored as the initial study after penetrating injuries.

CATHETER ANGIOGRAPHY

Catheter angiography is reserved for the following situations:

- Hematuria with hypotension or falling hematocrit
- Persistent or recurrent hematuria
- Hypotension or hypertension after documented renal injury
- Retroperitoneal hematoma detected by CT or during surgery

An initial abdominal aortogram will identify accessory renal arteries or suggest other sites of injury (e.g., bleeding from a lumbar artery). Angiographic findings vary widely and may include AVF, pseudoaneurysm, frank extravasation, perirenal or retroperitoneal hematoma, intimal injury or dissection, or complete renal artery occlusion (Figs. 10-31 and 10-32; see Fig. 10-30).

Treatment

ENDOVASCULAR THERAPY

Surgery, which almost always leads to unnecessary parenchymal damage, is reserved only for cases that cannot be treated by endovascular means.[136,137,142] As a rule, grade I-III injuries are observed, grade V injuries deserve operative management, and many grade IV injuries are ideal for embolotherapy. Major CT findings that suggest the need for intervention include large perirenal hematoma, frank arterial extravasation of contrast, and medial kidney laceration.[143,144] To minimize tissue loss, the embolic agent should be placed as close to the bleeding vessel as possible (see Figs. 10-30 and 10-31). Gelfoam pieces and microcoils placed through coaxial

microcatheters are favored for embolization of both large and small arterial branches. In patients with AVFs, the coil should be large enough to avoid escape through the fistula into the venous system.[145] Stents are placed to tack down post-traumatic renal artery intimal flaps and avoid thrombosis or distal embolization[146] (see Fig. 10-32).

Postembolization syndrome (fever, flank pain) is seen in a few patients. Nontarget embolization (usually of uninvolved renal vessels) is uncommon. Postembolization hypertension is unusual and usually transient.

Neoplasms (Online Cases 57 and 83)

Etiology

The major benign and malignant neoplasms of the kidney are outlined in Box 10-5. *Renal cell carcinoma (RCC)* is the most common malignant neoplasm of the kidney.[147,148] The most frequent subtype of RCC is clear cell, followed by papillary and chromophobe carcinomas. Clear cell RCC is often encapsulated and extremely vascular. Tumor growth into the renal vein or IVC is characteristic but relatively uncommon (5% to 10% of patients).[149,150] Recent investigations have identified mutations in the von Hippel-Lindau (VHL) gene on chromosome 3 as the underlying defect in many sporadic and familial cases of clear cell RCC.[151,152] Gene dysfunction leads to accumulation of factors that

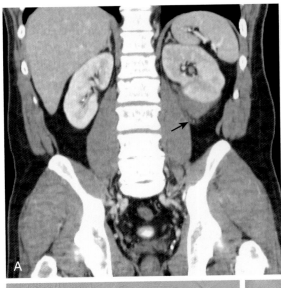
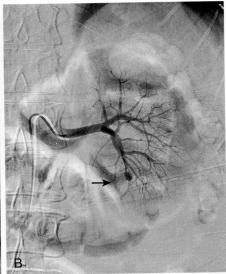
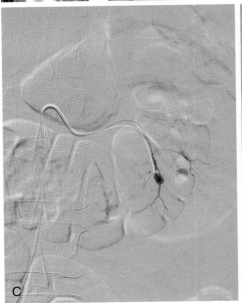
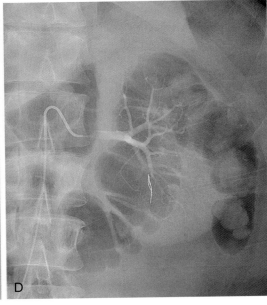

FIGURE 10-30   Pseudoaneurysm of the left kidney after motor vehicle crash. **A,** Reformatted coronal computed tomography shows soft tissue mass displacing left kidney superiorly *(arrow).* **B,** Left renal arteriogram reveals a pseudoaneurysm in the lower pole of the kidney *(arrow).* **C,** After selective microcatheterization, the feeding branch is closed with microcoils, with minimal loss of renal parenchyma **(D).**

promote overproduction of tumorigenic vascular endothelial growth factors and platelet-derived growth factors. This discovery now explains the development of multiple, bilateral tumors in about 40% of patients with *von Hippel-Lindau disease.*[153,154] Worldwide, the true incidence of RCC has been steadily growing over the past several decades; this development is only partly explained by more frequent detection of incidental tumors in asymptomatic patients by cross-sectional imaging.[155]

Wilms tumor is composed of a variety of cellular elements and frequently produces areas of hemorrhage and necrosis.[156] *Angiomyolipoma (AML)* is a renal hamartoma made up of blood vessels, smooth muscle cells, lipid, and connective tissue.[157] Angiomyolipomas may be solitary or multiple and bilateral, as in patients with *tuberous sclerosis. Adenoma* is a benign tumor of epithelial cell origin. *Oncocytoma* is one form of adenoma that features cells with eosinophilic cytoplasm. The lesion usually is solitary, well-defined, and often has a central scar.[158]

Clinical Features

The classic symptom triad of malignant kidney tumors is hematuria, flank pain, and a palpable abdominal mass.[147] Rarely, patients may have hypertension directly related to the tumor. Male patients with neoplastic invasion of the left renal vein may present with a left-sided varicocele.

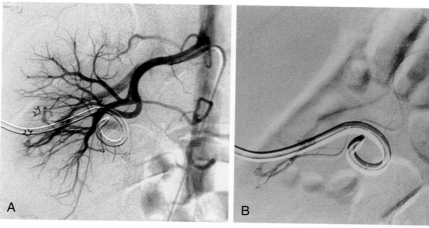

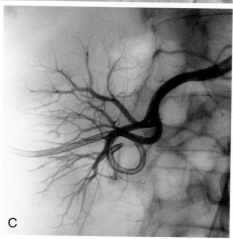

FIGURE 10-31 Arteriovenous fistula in a patient with persistent bleeding after right nephrostomy placement. **A,** The initial arteriogram shows two lower pole fistulas with early venous drainage *(arrows).* **B,** A coaxial microcatheter was advanced to the branch feeding both fistulas. **C,** After placement of two microcoils, the fistulas are closed.

However, many renal neoplasm are now discovered incidentally because of the widespread use of cross-sectional imaging in medicine. Most people with malignant kidney tumors are older than 50 years of age. RCC affects men more frequently than women. On the other hand, angiomyolipomas are commonly seen in middle-aged women. Tumors associated with tuberous sclerosis tend to be more aggressive. Larger tumors are more likely to bleed. Most patients with Wilms tumor are less than 5 years old.

Imaging

COMPUTED TOMOGRAPHY AND MAGNETIC RESONANCE IMAGING

Diagnosis and staging of benign and malignant renal neoplasms is accomplished with CT or MRI[158,159] (Figs. 10-33 and 10-34, and see Fig. 1-29). Clear cell RCC appears as an infiltrating or exophytic hypervascular mass with heterogeneity affected by cystic degeneration, bleeding, or necrosis. The presence of tumor in the renal vein or IVC should be sought (see Fig. 10-33). Papillary RCC is encapsulated and relatively homogenous. Transitional cell carcinoma features an enhancing mass in the renal pelvis or ureter. AML may be difficult to diagnose when small. But when the tumor is large, the hallmark fatty component is distinctive (see Fig. 10-34). Assessing the extent of IVC thrombosis with RCC is crucial to operative planning. The *Nevus classification* stratifies cases with tumor thrombus less than 2 cm above the renal veins (level 1), below the most inferior hepatic vein (level 2), below the diaphragm (level 3), or supradiaphragmatic (level 4).[149,150]

CATHETER ANGIOGRAPHY

In RCC, the typical angiographic features are neovascularity, hypervascularity, dilation of the main renal artery, tumor stain, contrast puddling, displacement of normal renal vessels, and arteriovenous shunts with early venous drainage[160] (see Fig. 10-33). Parasitization of neighboring vessels (e.g., inferior mesenteric or lumbar arteries) is relatively common (Fig. 10-35). Less than 10% of tumors are hypovascular, and most of these are of the papillary type. Invasion of tumor into the renal vein or IVC is characteristic.[161]

In contrast, Wilms tumor usually is moderately vascular. Arteriography shows displacement of normal

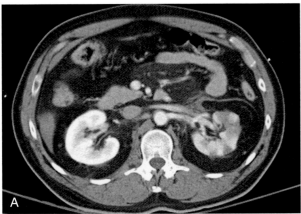

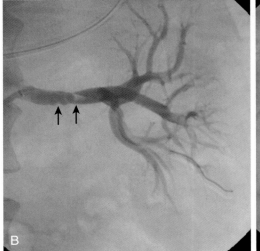

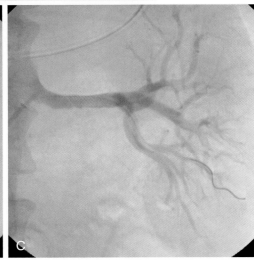

FIGURE 10-32   Dissection of renal artery from blunt trauma. **A,** Computed tomography scan after a fall shows mottled left nephrogram. **B,** Left renal arteriography reveals the spiraling dissection in the main vessel *(arrows).* **C,** A stent was inserted to tack down the flap and prevent arterial thrombosis.

BOX 10-5

MAJOR RENAL NEOPLASMS

Benign Tumors

Adenoma (including oncocytoma)
Angiomyolipoma

Malignant Tumors

Renal cell carcinoma
Transitional cell carcinoma
Wilms tumor
Metastases (including lymphoma)

renal vessels around the tumor mass with encasement or occlusion of vessels. Transitional cell carcinoma is typically hypovascular with encasement of vessels, presence of tumor stain, and fine neovascularity.[162] Lymphoma may be hypovascular or hypervascular.

Angiomyolipomas are solitary or multiple hypervascular masses with bizarre vascularity and multiple small aneurysms[163] (see Fig. 10-34). Renal oncocytoma can have a characteristic angiographic appearance with a dense, homogeneous stain and "spoke-wheel" arrangement of vessels corresponding to the central scar[164] (Fig. 10-36). On rare occasion, intravascular biopsy of difficult-to-categorize tumors may be useful (Fig. 10-37).

Treatment

For many years, a solitary renal mass was removed by radical nephrectomy regardless of the cell type. Percutaneous biopsy was thought to be too inaccurate to preclude operative removal of the tumor. This reasoning held despite reports that found up to 25% of operated renal tumors were benign.[147] Over the past decade, the increasing discovery of small, incidental renal tumors has paralleled improvements in biopsy analysis, push for nephron-sparing surgery, and new percutaneous ablative methods. The consequence is much greater enthusiasm by urologists for pretreatment biopsy (see Chapter 4).

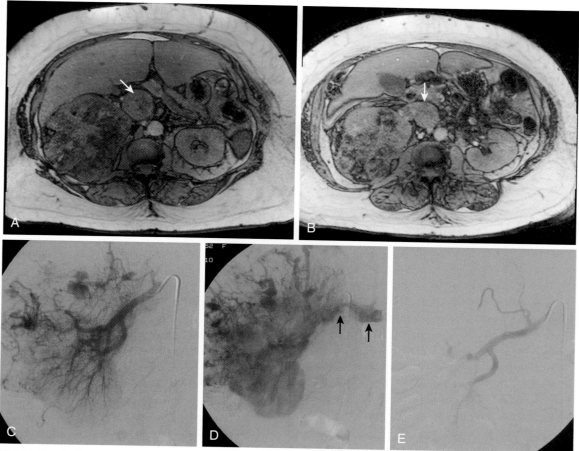

FIGURE 10-33 Renal cell carcinoma invading the renal vein and inferior vena cava (IVC). **A** and **B,** Magnetic resonance images show a huge heterogeneous mass largely replacing the upper right kidney. There is invasion of the right renal vein and IVC, which is massively enlarged *(arrow)*. **C** and **D,** Renal arteriography shows a large mass with bizarre vascularity and numerous amorphous contrast lakes. The deformity in the renal vein *(arrows)* represents tumor thrombus. **E,** After preoperative embolization with small microspheres, there is stasis of flow in the renal artery.

ENDOVASCULAR THERAPY

In patients with renal neoplasms, transcatheter embolization is requested for the following reasons[165-167]:

- Devascularization before open or laparoscopic nephrectomy to ease resection, minimize blood loss, and possibly heighten the immune response against the tumor
- Palliative treatment in patients with unresectable disease
- Treatment or prevention of hemorrhagic complications

For RCC, the preoperative procedure usually is performed within 24 hours of nephrectomy (see Figs. 10-33 and 10-35). However, it is important to realize that the clinical benefits of this maneuver have not been rigorously proven in controlled trials, and urologists are divided on the value of this approach.[165,166,168-170] The most popular embolic agents are absolute ethanol and microspheres. For ethanol ablation, an occlusion balloon is advanced into the distal renal artery beyond adrenal and ureteral branches to avoid reflux of alcohol into the aorta, which may have disastrous consequences. The volume of alcohol can be estimated by measuring the amount of contrast required to fill the renal artery and branches with the occlusion balloon inflated. Alcohol is slowly injected in small aliquots (1 to 5 mL) into the main renal artery. The balloon is kept inflated for several minutes after injection and is then slowly deflated. Patients commonly experience a profound postembolization syndrome, characterized by fever, flank pain, and nausea. For microsphere ablation, microcatheters are used and small particles (e.g., 300- to 500-micron microspheres) are preferred. Accessory or parasitized arteries may be treated in a similar fashion if there is virtually no chance of nontarget embolization.

For patients with AMLs, embolization has emerged as a useful alternative to surgery, particularly for symptomatic lesions and silent tumors larger than 4 cm (which have a propensity to growth and hemorrhage).[163,167,171-175] Tumor shrinkage and pain relief occur in many (but not

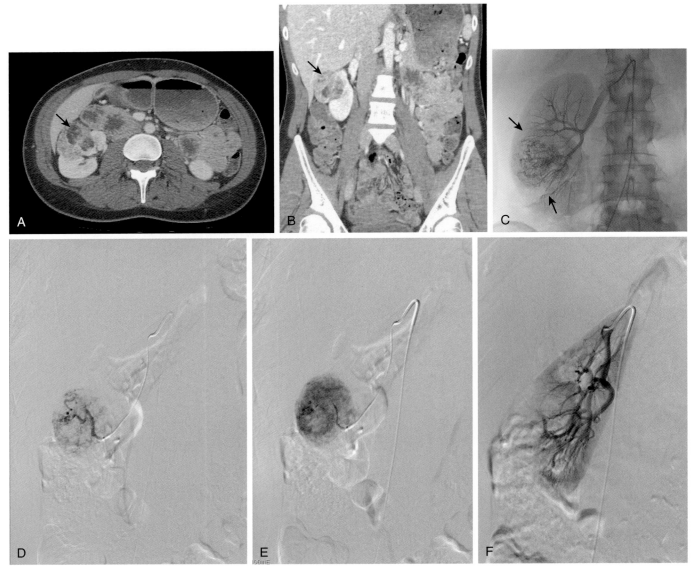

FIGURE 10-34 Angiomyolipoma. **A** and **B,** Axial and coronal reformatted contrast-enhanced computed tomography images show a well-circumscribed largely exophytic mass arising from the upper pole of the right kidney *(arrow).* The mass is heterogeneous, but has some very low density elements similar to fat. No other renal lesions were identified. **C,** Right renal arteriography shows the hypervascular mass. **D** and **E,** Superselective arteriography of the segmental branch feeding the tumor highlights its hypervascular, well-circumscribed nature. **F,** After infusion of 300- to 500-micron Embospheres, the tumor's blood supply is obliterated.

all) cases (see Fig. 10-34). Patients with smaller tumors should be imaged periodically to assess growth.

PERCUTANEOUS ABLATION THERAPY

See Chapter 24 for an in-depth discussion of percutaneous ablation therapy.[176-179]

SURGICAL THERAPY

The standard treatment for RCC is radical nephrectomy with removal of Gerota fascia. The adrenal gland may be spared if there is no involvement of the gland or upper pole of the kidney. Renal vein or IVC invasion does not preclude surgical resection.[161,180,181] Nephron-sparing

procedures are offered to patients with bilateral tumors, malignancy in a solitary kidney, and angiomyolipomas.[147]

Miscellaneous Conditions

Several common renal diseases may been seen as incidental findings at abdominal aortography or renal arteriography. *Renal cysts* produce round, avascular filling defects in the renal parenchyma, with draping of vessels around the cyst. Hypovascular neoplasms rarely mimic benign cysts; sonography or CT is recommended to exclude a hypovascular or cystic tumor. *Hydronephrosis* typically has a "soap bubble" appearance, with displacement of intrarenal

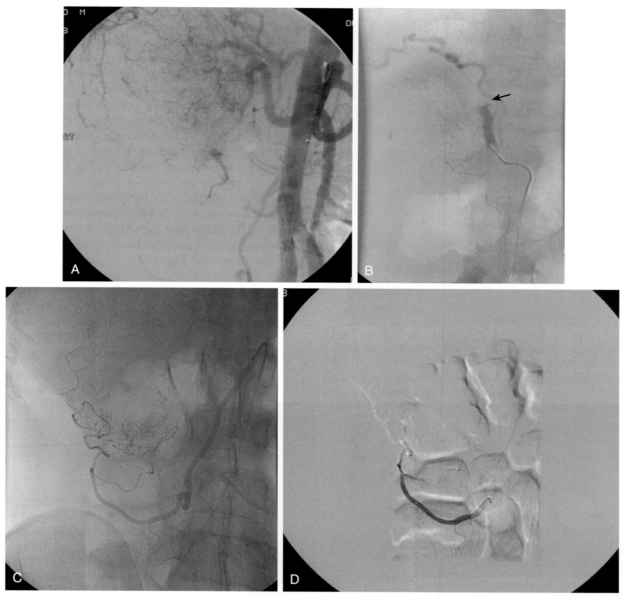

FIGURE 10-35   Renal cell carcinoma parasitizing the right testicular artery. **A,** Abdominal aortography shows the markedly hypervascular tumor. **B,** Following embolization of the distal artery, there is stasis of flow to the kidney, but the proximal superior capsular branch was spared *(arrow)*. **C,** Selective right testicular arteriography shows a markedly dilated vessel with supply to the mass. **D,** The artery was embolized proximal to the mass with coils and Gelfoam.

branches around the dilated collecting system. Late-stage chronic kidney disease causes the kidneys to shrink. Flow into the renal branches is markedly diminished, but the central artery usually remains patent.

OTHER DISORDERS

Aneurysms (Online Case 110)

Extrarenal artery aneurysms are most commonly caused by arterial dysplasia, FMD, arteritis, trauma, infection, or a congenital abnormality (Box 10-6). The "atherosclerotic" changes (e.g., calcification) in some *dysplastic aneurysms* are probably a secondary effect rather than causative. Dysplastic aneurysms typically target the vessel segment near or just beyond the first bifurcation of the main renal artery[182] (Fig. 10-38). These lesions are more frequent on the right side and may be multiple or bilateral. Extrarenal pseudoaneurysms usually are caused by trauma or infection.[183] Intrarenal aneurysms are most commonly caused by a penetrating trauma, necrotizing arteritis (e.g., *poly-arteritis nodosa*), or illicit drug use (e.g., cocaine, methamphetamines), or are associated with tumors such as AML.[184]

BOX 10-6

CAUSES OF RENAL ARTERY ANEURYSMS

True Aneurysms

Dysplastic
Connective tissue disorders
    Ehlers-Danlos syndrome
    Neurofibromatosis
Vasculitis
    Polyarteritis nodosa
    Takayasu arteritis
Fibromuscular dysplasia
Congenital

False Aneurysms

Trauma
Inflammation
    Infection
Post-transplant
Dissection

- Regardless of size in women of child-bearing potential because of the propensity for expansion and fatal rupture.[185] Increased blood flow and effects of estrogen on elastic tissue in arterial media may partially explain this phenomenon.
- To relieve renovascular hypertension caused by compressive effects on adjacent arterial branches. Results of operative repair are clearly beneficial in this regard.[182,189,190]

Virtually all pseudoaneurysms (symptomatic or asymptomatic) are prone to rupture and require treatment.

With main or primary branch arterial aneurysms, repair is first attempted with covered stent placement or embolization of the aneurysm sac.[191-194] With segmental or distal artery aneurysms, embolotherapy is recommended. If these interventions fail or are not feasible, operative aneurysmectomy or bypass is done.

Dissection

Renal artery dissection has a variety of causes (Box 10-7). Patients with acute dissection can present with flank pain, hematuria, or hypertension. Patients with chronic dissection may be hypertensive. Imaging findings include an intimal flap, an irregularly dilated vessel from filling of a false lumen (especially in dissections from FMD), or complete vessel occlusion (Fig. 10-41 and see Fig. 10-32). Branch vessels often are involved. Surgical treatment consists of aortorenal bypass (when feasible) or nephrectomy to treat severe hypertension. Intravascular stents have been used to repair spontaneous renal artery dissections and those extending from an aortic dissection.[195,196]

Arteriovenous Fistulas and Malformations (Online Case 87)

Acquired renal AVFs are most often post-traumatic. Massive renal AVFs can cause high-output heart failure.[197] On the other hand, congenital AVMs of the kidney are exceedingly rare.[198] These lesions consist of numerous dilated, tortuous vessels within the subepithelium of the collecting system. When symptomatic, they cause gross hematuria or less commonly hypertension. Color Doppler sonography, CT, and MRI detect most of these anomalies.[198,199]

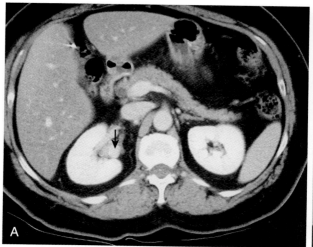
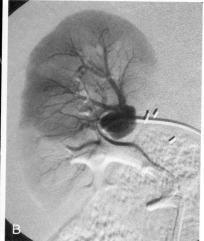

FIGURE 10-38 Dysplastic right renal artery aneurysm. **A,** Computed tomography scan reveals a round vascular mass with rim calcification in the renal pelvis *(arrow).* **B,** Catheter angiogram displays the aneurysm.

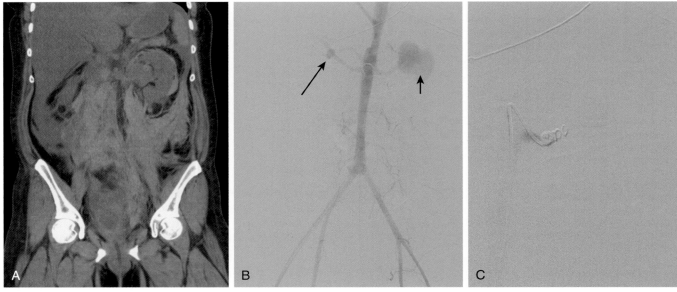

FIGURE 10-39   Bilateral renal artery aneurysms with rupture during pregnancy. **A,** Reformatted coronal computed tomography scan shows massive acute retroperitoneal hemorrhage displacing the left kidney superiorly. **B,** Emergent aortography revealed a large left renal artery aneurysm *(small arrow)* and incidental small right renal artery aneurysm *(large arrow)*. Small caliber of all arteries reflects shock. **C,** The left renal artery was quickly embolized to prevent further bleeding.

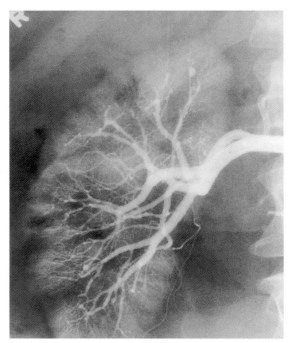

FIGURE 10-40   Polyarteritis nodosa with multiple distal renal artery branch aneurysms.

At catheter angiography, an AVF produces dilation of the feeding branch and early filling of the draining renal vein (Fig. 10-42; see also Fig. 10-31). Numerous segmental or interlobar arteries feed the renal AVM, which is composed of dilated, tortuous channels with rapid shunting into the renal vein and IVC.

BOX 10-7

CAUSES OF RENAL ARTERY DISSECTION

- Extension of aortic dissection
- Trauma
  - Iatrogenic (e.g., catheterization)
  - Blunt or penetrating trauma
- Fibromuscular dysplasia
- Segmental arterial mediolysis
- Spontaneous

Transcatheter embolization is the first-line treatment for renal AVFs.[140,197] Coils are effective for closing fistulas. In AVMs, the nidus must be obliterated using a liquid agent such as cyanoacrylate (glue) or Onyx.[200,201]

Renal Vein Thrombosis

Box 10-8 outlines several etiologies for RVT.[202-204] The most common cause in adults is the nephrotic syndrome, resulting from a variety of renal or systemic disorders, particularly membranous glomerulonephritis. The combination of intravascular volume depletion and a thrombophilic state makes these patients especially prone to RVT.

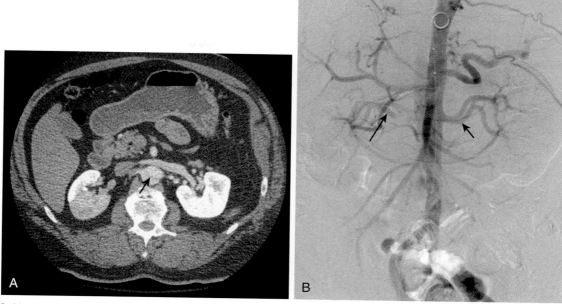

FIGURE 10-41 Renal artery dissection from extension of abdominal aortic dissection. **A,** Contrast-enhanced computed tomography shows a geographic zone of hypoperfusion of the dorsal side of the right kidney as well as a dissection flap in the aorta *(arrow)*. **B,** Aortography through the true lumen shows poor filling of the right renal artery *(large arrow)* but good flow in the left renal artery *(small arrow)*.

FIGURE 10-42 Massive congenital right renal arteriovenous fistula. **A,** Selective arteriogram in early arterial phase shows early filling of large venous structures. **B,** Late arterial phase shows rapid washout through engorged venous channels into the inferior vena cava. **C,** Selective catheterization to the center of the connection. **D,** Following coil embolization, the connection is obliterated. Overall perfusion to the kidney is improved.

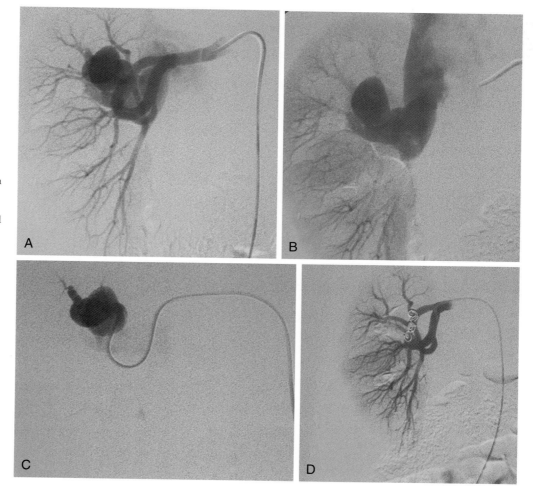

BOX 10-8

CAUSES OF RENAL VEIN THROMBOSIS

- Nephrotic syndrome
- Glomerulonephritis (membranous)
- Renal cell carcinoma
- Extension of clot or tumor from the inferior vena cava
- Dehydration (in children)
- Thrombophilic states
- Lupus nephropathy
- Diabetic nephropathy
- Amyloidosis
- Extrinsic renal vein compression
- Trauma (e.g., postoperative)
- Idiopathic causes

Many afflicted individuals have bilateral venous obstruction. Concurrent IVC or iliofemoral vein thrombosis and pulmonary embolism are relatively common.[205] Acute occlusion leads to kidney swelling, flank pain, and hematuria. Although hemorrhagic infarction is possible, the disease usually follows a more benign course. Collateral channels have time to develop when thrombus progression is limited, and kidney loss is avoided.

The diagnosis of RVT is made by color Doppler sonography, CT, or MR venography.[206,207] A filling defect or flow void is noted in the main renal vein (see Figs. 10-33 and 10-37). Distention of the vein suggests acute thrombus. Vein retraction and abundant collaterals suggest chronic occlusion. The appearance at catheter venography is varied. Clot may extend to the IVC and preclude catheterization. Nonocclusive thrombus may fill part of the main renal vein or intrarenal branches. In patients with chronic RVT, the venous branches are small and irregular, and collateral vessels or varices are opacified.

The standard treatment for acute RVT is anticoagulation. In selected cases, surgical thrombectomy or endovascular therapy may be advisable. Several reports have described successful treatment of acute native RVT with thrombolytic infusion or mechanical thrombectomy directly in the renal vein.[208,209] Intraarterial injection may assist in lysis of thrombi within small intrarenal veins. Retrievable suprarenal IVC filter placement is warranted in patients with a contraindication to anticoagulation or history of recurrent pulmonary embolism.

Renal Vein Varices (Online Case 107)

Renal vein varices may develop for many reasons (Box 10-9). Varices virtually always occur in relation to the left kidney. It has been postulated that compression of the left renal vein between the superior mesenteric artery and the aorta (nutcracker phenomenon) may be responsible for renal vein hypertension and development of varices in some cases[210-212] (see Fig. 10-11).

Renal vein varices may be asymptomatic. When patients develop intermittent or persistent hematuria and flank pain, hemorrhage can be localized to the left kidney by cystoscopy. Varices are among several possible causes of unexplained bleeding from the kidney (Box 10-10). Women also may suffer from *pelvic congestion syndrome* (pelvic pain, dyspareunia, dysmenorrhea) because of impeded outflow from the left ovarian vein[210] (see Chapter 13).

The diagnosis is initially made by noninvasive vascular imaging.[213] Angiographic features include a pressure gradient across the left renal vein of 4 mm Hg or greater and dilated intrarenal veins and venous collaterals (Fig. 10-43). The treatment is either surgical (bypass or stent placement) or endovascular stent placement.[210,214-216]

BOX 10-9

CAUSES OF RENAL VEIN VARICES

- Chronic renal vein thrombosis
- Renal vein hypertension (nutcracker syndrome)
- Portal hypertension with development of splenorenal or other shunts
- Compressed retroaortic left renal vein
- Congenital anomalies
- Idiopathic causes

BOX 10-10

CAUSES OF OCCULT RENAL BLEEDING

- Neoplasm (e.g., renal cell carcinoma, angiomyolipoma)
- Arteriovenous malformation
- Arteriovenous fistula
- Renal artery aneurysm
- Renal vein varices
- Arteritis (e.g., polyarteritis nodosa)

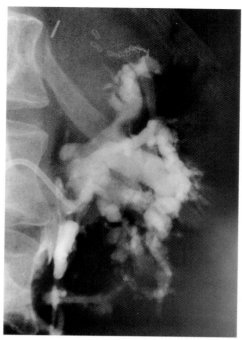

FIGURE 10-43   Renal vein varices with a 5-mm Hg gradient across the left renal vein. The patient had intermittent hematuria localized to the left kidney.

Vasculitis and Coarctation Syndromes

Several types of vasculitis can attack the renal arteries, including *Takayasu arteritis, radiation-induced arteritis,* and *polyarteritis nodosa.*[217-220] The congenital abdominal coarctation syndromes are an extremely rare cause for narrowing of the renal arteries in children and young adults[221-223] (see Fig. 10-20 and 7-27). Renal artery stenosis may provoke renovascular hypertension. Endovascular treatment with angioplasty alone or combined with stent placement (if necessary) is appropriate and effective in selected cases.[217,224-226] These disorders are considered further in Chapters 1 and 7.

Polyarteritis nodosa produces multiple microaneurysms in the kidney and many other vascular beds (see Figs. 1-23 and 10-40). Large- and medium-vessel aneurysms are seen less frequently.[227] Patients may present with spontaneous perinephric bleeding.[228,229] Catheter angiography usually is required for definitive diagnosis and has been used to treat aneurysm hemorrhage.[230]

Segmental Arterial Mediolysis

Segmental arterial mediolysis is an extremely rare disorder (which may be related to FMD) that primarily attacks the coronary, splanchnic, and renal arteries.[231,232] SAM begins with destruction of medial smooth muscle and replacement by fibrin and granulation tissue. Extension to other layers of the arterial wall can lead to spontaneous dissection or aneurysm formation. The cause is unknown.

References

1. Verschuyl E-J, Kaatee R, Beek FJA, et al. Renal artery origins: best angiographic projection angles. *Radiology* 1997;**205**:115.
2. Navaneethan SD, Singh S, Appasamy S, et al. Sodium bicarbonate therapy for prevention of contrast-induced nephropathy: a systematic review and meta-analysis. *Am J Kid Dis* 2009;**53**:617.
3. Briguori C, Airoldi F, D'Andrea D, et al. Renal insufficiency following contrast media administration trial (REMEDIAL): a randomized comparison of 3 preventative strategies. *Circulation* 2007;**115**:1211.
4. Stenstrom DA, Muldoon LL, Armijo-Medina H, et al. N-acetylcysteine use to prevent contrast medium-induced nephropathy: premature phase III trials. *J Vasc Interv Radiol* 2008;**19**:309.
5. Jo S-H, Koo B-K, Park J-S, et al. N-acetylcysteine versus Ascorbic acid for preventing contrast-induced nephropathy in patients with renal insufficiency undergoing coronary angiography: NASPI study- a prospective controlled trial. *Am Heart J* 2009;**157**:576.
6. Caridi JG, Stavropoulos SW, Hawkins Jr IF. CO_2 digital subtraction angiography for renal artery angioplasty in high-risk patients. *AJR Am J Roentgenol* 1999;**173**:1551.
7. Collins P, editor. Embryology and development. In: Williams PL, Bannister LH, Berry MM, et al, editors. *Gray's anatomy*, 38th ed. New York, Churchill Livingstone, 1995;**204**:318.
8. Gabella G, editor. Cardiovascular system. In: Williams PL, Bannister LH, Berry MM, et al, editors. *Gray's anatomy*, 38th ed. New York, Churchill Livingstone; 1995: p. 1557.
9. Dyson M, editor. Urinary system. In: Williams PL, Bannister LH, Berry MM, et al, editors. *Gray's anatomy*, 38th ed. New York, Churchill Livingstone; 1995: p. 1826.
10. Gabella G, editor. Cardiovascular system. In: Williams PL, Bannister LH, Berry MM, et al, editors. *Gray's anatomy*, 38th ed. New York, Churchill Livingstone; 1995: p. 1601.
11. Shokeir AA, el-Diasty TA, Nabeeh A, et al. Digital subtraction angiography in potential live-kidney donors: a study of 1000 cases. *Abdom Imaging* 1994;**19**:461.
12. Gupta A, Tello R. Accessory renal arteries are not related to hypertension risk: a review of MR angiography data. *AJR Am J Roentgenol* 2004;**182**:1521.
13. Platt JF, Ellis JH, Korobkin M, et al. Helical CT evaluation of potential kidney donors: findings in 154 subjects. *AJR Am J Roentgenol* 1997;**169**:1325.
14. Rankin SC, Jan W, Koffman CG. Noninvasive imaging of living related kidney donors: evaluation of CT angiography and gadolinium enhanced MR angiography. *AJR Am J Roentgenol* 2001;**177**:349.
15. Raman SS, Pojchamarnwiputh S, Muangsomboon K, et al. Surgically relevant normal and variant renal parenchymal and vascular anatomy in preoperative 16-MDCT evaluation of potential laparoscopic renal donors. *AJR Am J Roentgenol* 2007;**188**:105.
16. Kaufman JA, Waltman AC, Rivitz SM, et al. Anatomical observations on the renal veins and inferior vena cava at magnetic resonance angiography. *Cardiovasc Intervent Radiol* 1995;**18**:153.
17. Hicks ME, Malden ES, Vesely TM, et al. Prospective anatomic study of the inferior vena cava and renal veins: comparison of selective renal venography with cavography and relevance in filter placement. *J Vasc Interv Radiol* 1995;**6**:721.
18. Trigaux JP, Vandroogenbroek S, deWispelaere JF, et al. Congenital anomalies of the inferior vena cava and left renal vein: evaluation with spiral CT. *J Vasc Interv Radiol* 1998;**9**:339.
19. Aljabri B, MacDonald PS, Satin R, et al. Incidence of major venous and renal anomalies relevant to aortoiliac surgery as demonstrated by computed tomography. *Ann Vasc Surg* 2001;**15**:615.
20. Abrams HL, Cornell SH. Patterns of collateral flow in renal ischemia. *Radiology* 1965;**84**:1001.

21. Textor SC. Current approaches to renovascular hypertension. *Med Clin North Am* 2009;**93**:717.
22. Martin LG, Rundback JH, Sacks D, et al. Quality improvement guidelines for angiography, angioplasty, and stent placement in the diagnosis and treatment of renal artery stenosis in adults. *J Vasc Interv Radiol* 2003;**4**:S297.
23. Rundback JH, Murphy TP, Cooper C, et al. Chronic renal ischemia: pathophysiologic mechanisms of cardiovascular and renal disease. *J Vasc Interv Radiol* 2002:**13**:1085.
24. Bax L, Woittierz AJ, Kouwenberg HJ, et al. Stent placement in patients with atherosclerotic renal artery stenosis and impaired renal function: a randomized trial. *Ann Intern Med* 2009;**150**:840.
25. Suresh M, Laboi P, Mamtora H, et al. Relationship of renal dysfunction to proximal renal arterial disease severity in atherosclerotic renovascular disease. *Nephrol Dial Transplant* 2000;**12**:631.
26. Wright Jr JT, Bakris G, Greene T, et al. Effect of blood pressure lowering and antihypertensive drug class on progression of hypertensive kidney disease: results from the AASK trial. *JAMA* 2002;**288**:2421.
27. Schreiber MJU, Pohl MA, Novick AC. The natural history of atherosclerotic and fibrous renal artery disease. *Urol Clin North Am* 1984;**11**:383.
28. Caps MT, Zierler RE, Polissar NL, et al. Risk of atrophy in kidneys with atherosclerotic renal artery stenosis. *Kidney Int* 1998;**53**:735.
29. Ram CV, Clagett GP, Radford LR. Renovascular hypertension. *Semin Nephrol* 1995;**15**:152.
30. Hansen KJ, Edwards MS, Craven TE, et al. Prevalence of renovascular disease in the elderly: a population-based study. *J Vasc Surg* 2002;**36**:443.
31. Kalra PA, Guo H, Kausz AT, et al. Atherosclerotic renovascular disease in United States patients aged 67 years or older: risk factors, revascularization, and prognosis. *Kidney Int* 2005;**68**:293.
32. Chobanian AV, Bakris GL, Black HR, et al. Seventh report of the Joint National Committee on Prevention, Detection, Evaluation, and Treatment of High Blood Pressure. *Hypertension* 2003;**42**:1206.
33. House MK, Dowling RJ, King P, et al. Using Doppler sonography to reveal renal artery stenosis: an evaluation of optimal imaging parameters. *AJR Am J Roentgenol* 1999;**173**:761.
34. Zucchelli PC. Hypertension and atherosclerotic renal artery stenosis: diagnostic approach. *J Am Soc Nephrol* 2002;**13**:S184.
35. Patriquin HB, Lafortune M, Jequier J-C, et al. Stenosis of the renal artery: assessment of slowed systole in the downstream circulation with Doppler sonography. *Radiology* 1992;**184**:479.
36. Qanadli SD, Soulez G, Therasse E, et al. Detection of renal artery stenosis: prospective comparison of captopril-enhanced Doppler sonography, captopril-enhanced scintigraphy, and MR angiography. *AJR Am J Roentgenol* 2001;**177**:1123.
37. Stavros AT, Parker SH, Yakes WF, et al. Segmental stenosis of the renal artery: pattern recognition of tardus and parvus abnormalities with duplex sonography. *Radiology* 1992;**184**:487.
38. Vasbinder GB, Nelemans PJ, Kessels AG, et al. Diagnostic tests for renal artery stenosis in patients suspected of having renovascular hypertension: meta-analysis. *Ann Intern Med* 2001;**135**:401.
39. Vasbinder GB, Nelemans PJ, Kessels AG, et al. Accuracy of computed tomographic angiography and magnetic resonance angiography for diagnosing renal artery stenosis. *Ann Intern Med* 2004;**141**:674.
40. Eklof H, Ahlstrom H, Magnusson A, et al. A prospective comparison of duplex sonography, captopril renography, MRA and CTA in assessing renal artery stenosis. *Acta Radiol* 2006;**47**:764.
41. Leiner T, Michaely H. Advances in contrast-enhanced MR angiography of the renal arteries. *Magn Reson Imaging Clin N Am* 2008;**16**:561.
42. Fain SB, King BF, Breen JF, et al. High-spatial resolution contrast-enhanced MR angiography of the renal arteries: a prospective comparison with digital subtraction angiography. *Radiology* 2001;**218**:481.
43. DeCobelli F, Venturini M, Vanzulli A, et al. Renal arterial stenosis: prospective comparison of color Doppler US and breath-hold, three dimensional dynamic, gadolinium-enhanced MR angiography. *Radiology* 2000;**214**:373.
44. Willmann JK, Wildermuth S, Pfammatter T, et al. Aortoiliac and renal arteries: prospective intraindividual comparison of contrast-enhanced three-dimensional MR angiography and multi-detector row CT angiography. *Radiology* 2003;**226**:798.
45. Soulez G, Paswicz M, Benea G, et al. Renal artery stenosis evaluation: diagnostic performance of gadobenate dimeglumine-enhanced MR angiography- comparison with DSA. *Radiology* 2008;**247**:273.
46. Bude RO, Forauer AR, Caoili EM, et al. Is it necessary to study accessory arteries when screening the renal arteries for renovascular hypertension? *Radiology* 2003;**226**:411.
47. Pannu HK, Fishman EK. Multidetector computed tomographic evaluation of the renal artery. *Abdom Imaging* 2002;**27**:611.
48. Steinwender C, Schuetzenberg W, Fellner F, et al. 64-detector CT angiography in renal artery stent evaluation: prospective comparison with selective catheter angiography. *Radiology* 2009;**252**:299.
49. Huot SJ, Hansson JH, Dey H, et al. Utility of captopril renal scans for detecting renal artery stenosis. *Arch Intern Med* 2002;**162**:1981.
50. Vaughan Jr ED, Buehler FR, Laragh JH, et al. Renovascular hypertension: renin measurements to indicate hypersecretion and contralateral suppression, estimate renal plasma flow, and score for surgical curability. *Am J Med* 1973;**55**:402.
51. Vaughan Jr ED. Renin sampling: collection and interpretation *N Engl J Med* 1974;**290**:1195.
52. de Bruyne B, Manoharan G, Pijls NHG, et al. Assessment of renal artery stenosis severity by pressure gradient measurements. *J Am Coll Cardiol* 2006;**48**:1851.
53. Dworkin LD, Cooper CJ. Clinical practice. Renal artery stenosis. *N Engl J Med* 2009;**361**:1972.
54. Kiernan TJ, Yan BP, Jaff MR. Renal artery revascularization: collaborative approaches for specialists. *Adv Chronic Kidney Dis* 2008;**15**:363.
55. Rees CR. Stents for atherosclerotic renovascular disease. *J Vasc Interv Radiol* 1999;**10**:689.
56. Burket MW, Cooper CJ, Kennedy DJ, et al. Renal artery angioplasty and stent placement: predictors of favorable outcome. *Am Heart J* 2000;**139**:64.
57. Beutler JJ, van Ampting JM, vandeVen PJ, et al. Long-term effects of arterial stenting on kidney function for patients with ostial atherosclerotic renal artery stenosis and renal insufficiency. *J Am Soc Nephrol* 2001;**12**:1475.
58. Harden PN, MacLeod MJ, Rodger RS, et al. Effect of renal artery stenting on progression of renovascular renal failure. *Lancet* 1997;**349**:1133.
59. American Heart Association Atherosclerotic Peripheral Vascular Disease Symposium recommendations. *Circulation* 2008;**118**:2873.
60. Baumgartner I, von Aesch K, Do DD, et al. Stent placement in ostial and nonostial atherosclerotic renal arterial stenoses: a prospective follow-up study. *Radiology* 2000;**216**:498.
61. van de Ven PJ, Kaatee R, Beutler JJ, et al. Arterial stenting and balloon angioplasty in ostial atherosclerotic renovascular disease: a randomized trial. *Lancet* 1999;**353**:282.
62. Kashyap VS, Sepulveda RN, Bena JF, et al. The management of renal artery atherosclerosis for renal salvage: does stenting help? *J Vasc Surg* 2007;**45**:101.

63. Blum U, Krumme B, Fluegel P, et al. Treatment of ostial renal-artery stenoses with vascular endoprostheses after unsuccessful balloon angioplasty. *N Engl J Med* 1997;**336**:459.

64. Leertouwer TC, Gussenhoven EJ, Bosch JL, et al. Stent placement for renal arterial stenosis: where do we stand? A meta-analysis. *Radiology* 2000;**216**:78.

65. van Jaarsveld BC, Krijnen P, Pieterman H, et al. The effect of balloon angioplasty on hypertension in atherosclerotic renal artery stenosis. Dutch Renal Artery Stenosis Intervention Cooperative Study Group. *N Engl J Med* 2000;**342**:1007.

66. Lederman RJ, Mendelsohn FO, Santos R, et al. Primary renal artery stenting: characteristics and outcomes after 363 procedures. *Am Heart J* 2001;**142**:314.

67. Cooper CJ, Haller ST, Colyer W, et al. Embolic protection and platelet inhibition during renal artery stenting. *Circulation* 2008;**27**:2752.

68. Kanjwal K, Haller S, Steffes M, et al. Complete versus partial distal embolic protection during renal artery stenting. *Catheter Cardiovasc Interv* 2009;**73**:725.

69. Sapoval M, Zaehringer M, Pattynama P, et al. Low profile stent system for treatment of atherosclerotic renal artery stenosis: the GREAT trial. *J Vasc Interv Radiol* 2005;**16**:1195.

70. Holden A, Hill A, Jaff MR, et al. Renal artery stent revascularization with embolic protection in patients with ischemic nephropathy. *Kidney Int* 2006;**70**:948.

71. Henry M, Henry I, Polydorou A, et al. Embolic protection for renal artery stenting. *J Cardiovasc Surg (Torino)* 2008;**49**:571.

72. Gill KS, Fowler RC. Atherosclerotic renal arterial stenosis: clinical outcomes of stent placement for hypertension and renal failure. *Radiology* 2003;**226**:821.

73. Rocha-Singh K, Jaff MR, Rosenfield K. Evaluation of the safety and effectiveness of renal artery stenting after unsuccessful balloon angioplasty: the ASPIRE-2 study. *J Am Coll Cardiol* 2005;**46**:776.

74. Rundback JH, Gray RJ, Rozenblit G, et al. Renal artery stent placement for the management of ischemic nephropathy. *J Vasc Interv Radiol* 1998;**9**:413.

75. Thatipelli MR, Misra S, Sanikommu SR, et al. Embolic protection device use in renal artery stent placement. *J Vasc Interv Radiol* 2009;**20**:58.

76. Bakker J, Goffette PP, Henry M, et al. The Erasme study: a multicenter study on the safety and technical results of the Palmaz stent used for the treatment of atherosclerotic ostial renal artery stenosis. *Cardiovasc Intervent Radiol* 1999;**22**:468.

77. Henry M, Amor M, Henry I, et al. Stent placement in the renal artery: three-year experience with the Palmaz stent. *J Vasc Interv Radiol* 1996;**7**:343.

78. Corriere MA, Edwards MS, Pearce JD, et al. Restenosis after renal artery angioplasty and stenting: incidence and risk factors. *J Vasc Surg* 2009;**50**:813.

79. Rocha-Singh K, Jaff MR, Lynne Kelley E, et al. Renal artery stenting with noninvasive duplex ultrasound follow-up: 3 year results from the RENNAISANCE renal stent trial. *Catheter Cardiovasc Interv* 2008;**72**:853.

80. Misra S, Thatipelli MR, Howe PW, et al. Preliminary study of the use of drug-eluting stents in atherosclerotic renal artery stenoses 4 mm in diameter or less. *J Vasc Interv Radiol* 2008;**19**:833.

81. Zaehringer M, Sapoval M, Pattynama PM, et al. Sirolimus-eluting versus bare-metal low profile stent for renal artery treatment (GREAT trial): angiographic followup after 6 months and clinical outcome up to 2 years. *J Endovasc Ther* 2007;**14**:460.

82. Bax L, Mali WP, Van De Ven PJ, et al. Repeated intervention for in-stent restenosis of the renal arteries. *J Vasc Interv Radiol* 2002;**13**:1219.

83. Davies MG, Saad WA, Bismuth JX, et al. Outcomes of endoluminal reintervention for restenosis after percutaneous renal angioplasty and stenting. *J Vasc Surg* 2009;**49**:946.

84. The ASTRAL investigators. Revascularization versus medical therapy for renal artery stenosis. *N Engl J Med* 2009;**361**: 1953.

85. Balk E, Raman G, Chung M, et al. Effectiveness of management strategies for renal artery stenosis: a systematic review. *Ann Intern Med* 2006;**145**:901.

86. Balzer KM, Pfeiffer T, Rossbach S, et al. Prospective randomized trial of operative vs. interventional treatment for renal artery ostial occlusive disease. *J Vasc Surg* 2009;**49**:667.

87. Schwartzwaelder U, Hauk M, Zeller T. RADAR—a randomised multi-centre prospective study comparing best medical treatment versus best medical treatment plus renal artery stenting in patients with haemodynamically relevant atherosclerotic renal artery stenosis. *Trials* 2009;**10**:60.

88. Dubel GJ, Murphy TP. The role of percutaneous revascularization for renal artery stenosis. *Vasc Med* 2008;**12**:141.

89. Ivanovic V, McKusick MA, Johnson III CM, et al. Renal artery stent placement: complications at a single tertiary care center. *J Vasc Interv Radiol* 2003;**14**:217.

90. Hassen-Khodja R, Sala F, Declemy S, et al. Renal artery revascularization in combination with infrarenal aortic reconstruction. *Ann Vasc Surg* 2000;**14**:577.

91. Rigdon EE, Durham JR, Massop DW, et al. Hepatorenal and splenorenal artery bypass for salvage of renal function. *Ann Vasc Surg* 1991;**5**:133.

92. Geroulakos G, Wright JG, Tober JC, et al. Use of the splenic and hepatic artery for renal revascularization in patients with atherosclerotic renal artery disease. *Ann Vasc Surg* 1997;**11**:85.

93. Olin JW, Pierce M. Contemporary management of fibromuscular dysplasia. *Curr Opin Cardiol* 2008;**23**:527.

94. Neymark E, LaBerge J, Hirose R, et al. Arteriographic detection of renovascular disease in potential renal donors: incidence and effect on donor surgery. *Radiology* 2000;**214**:755.

95. Cragg AH, Smith TP, Thompson BH, et al. Incidental fibromuscular dysplasia in potential renal donors: long-term clinical follow-up. *Radiology* 1989;**172**:145.

96. Luescher TF, Lie JT, Stanson AW, et al. Arterial fibromuscular dysplasia. *Mayo Clin Proc* 1987;**62**:931.

97. Sabharwal R, Vladica P, Coleman P. Multidetector spiral CT angiography in the diagnosis of renal artery fibromuscular dysplasia. *Eur J Radiol* 2007;**61**:520.

98. Willoteaux S, Faivre-Pierret M, Moranne O, et al. Fibromuscular dysplasia of the main renal arteries: comparison of contrast-enhanced MR angiography with digital subtraction angiography. *Radiology* 2006;**241**:922.

99. Stanley JC, Fry WJ. Renovascular hypertension secondary to arterial fibrodysplasia in adults. Criteria for operation and results of surgical therapy. *Arch Surg* 1975;**110**:922.

100. Scott JA, Rabe FE, Becker GJ, et al. Angiographic assessment of renal artery pathology: how reliable? *AJR Am J Roentgenol* 1983;**141**:1299.

101. Tanaka R, Higashi M, Naito H. Angioplasty for non-arteriosclerotic renal artery stenosis: the efficacy of cutting balloon angioplasty versus conventional angioplasty. *Cardiovasc Intervent Radiol* 2007;**30**:601.

102. Davies MG, Saad WE, Peden EK, et al. The long-term outcomes of percutaneous therapy for renal artery fibromuscular dysplasia. *J Vasc Surg* 2008;**48**:865.

103. Alhadad A, Mattiasson I, Ivancev K, et al. Revascularization of renal artery stenosis caused by fibromuscular dysplasia: effects on blood pressure during 7-year follow-up are influenced by duration of hypertension and branch artery stenosis. *J Hum Hypertens* 2005;**19**:761.

104. Sciacca L, Ciocca RG, Eslami MH, et al. Endovascular treatment of renal artery aneurysm secondary to fibromuscular dysplasia: a case report. *Ann Vasc Surg* 2009;**23**:e9.

105. van der Wal MA, Wisselink W, Rauwerda JA, et al. Traumatic bilateral renal artery thrombosis: case report and review of the literature. *Cardiovasc Surg* 2003;**11**:527.

106. Wright MPJ, Persad RA, Cranston DW. Renal artery occlusion. *BJU Int* 2001;**87**:9.

107. Kansal S, Feldman M, Cooksey S, et al. Renal artery embolism: a case report and review. *J Gen Intern Med* 2008;**23**:644.

108. Glockner JF, Vrtiska TJ. Renal MR and CT angiography: current concepts. *Abdom Imaging* 2007;**32**:407.

109. Ouriel K, Andrus CH, Ricotta JJ, et al. Acute renal artery occlusion: when is revascularization justified? *J Vasc Surg* 1987;**5**:348.

110. Towne JB, Bernhard VM. Revascularization of the ischemic kidney. *Arch Surg* 1978;**113**:216.

111. Morris D, Kisly A, Stoyka CG, et al. Spontaneous bilateral renal artery occlusion associated with chronic atrial fibrillation. *Clin Nephrol* 1993;**39**:257.

112. Nicholas GG, DeMuth Jr WE. Treatment of renal artery embolism. *Arch Surg* 1984;**119**:278.

113. Blum U, Billmann P, Krause T, et al. Effect of local low-dose thrombolysis on clinical outcome in acute embolic renal artery occlusion. *Radiology* 1993;**189**:549.

114. Dwyer KM, Vrazas JI, Lodge RS, et al. Treatment of acute renal failure caused by renal artery occlusion with renal artery angioplasty. *Am J Kidney Dis* 2002;**40**:189.

115. Singh AK, Sahani DV. Imaging of the renal donor and transplant recipient. *Radiol Clin North Am* 2008;**46**:79.

116. Bruno S, Remuzzi G, Ruggenenti P. Transplant renal artery stenosis. *J Am Soc Nephrol* 2004;**15**:134.

117. Henning BF, Kuchlbauer S, Boeger CA, et al. Percutaneous transluminal angioplasty as first-line treatment of transplant renal artery stenosis. *Clin Nephrol* 2009;**71**:543.

118. Wong F, Fynn SP, Higgins RM, et al. Transplant renal artery stenosis in 77 patients—does it have an immunological cause? *Transplantation* 1996;**61**:215.

119. Claudon M, Lefevre F, Hestin D, et al. Power Doppler imaging: evaluation of vascular complications after renal transplantation. *AJR Am J Roentgenol* 1999;**173**:41.

120. Irshad A, Ackerman SJ, Campbell AS, et al. An overview of renal transplantation: current practice and use of ultrasound. *Semin Ultrasound CT MR* 2009;**30**:298.

121. Baxter GM. Imaging in renal transplantation. *Ultrasound Q* 2003;**19**:123.

122. Huber A, Heuck A, Scheidler J, et al. Contrast-enhanced MR angiography in patients after kidney transplantation. *Eur Radiol* 2001;**11**:2488.

123. Rajiah P, Lim YY, Taylor P. Renal transplant imaging and complications. *Abdom Imaging* 2006;**31**:735.

124. Fany YC, Siegelman ES. Complications of renal transplantation: MR findings. *J Comput Assist Tomogr* 2001;**25**:836.

125. Lanzman RS, Voiculescu A, Walther C, et al. ECG-gated nonenhanced steady-state free precision MR angiography in assessment of transplant renal arteries: comparison with DSA. *Radiology* 2009;**252**:914.

126. Pappas P, Zavos G, Kaza S, et al. Angioplasty and stenting of arterial stenosis affecting renal transplant function. *Transplant Proc* 2008;**40**:1391.

127. Kuo PC, Petersen J, Semba C, et al. CO_2 angiography—a technique for vascular imaging in renal allograft dysfunction. *Transplantation* 1996;**61**:652.

128. Libicher M, Radeleff B, Grenacher L, et al. Interventional therapy of vascular complications following renal transplantation. *Clin Transplant* 2006;**20**:55.

129. Beecroft JR, Rajan DK, Clark TW, et al. Transplant renal artery stenosis: outcome after percutaneous intervention. *J Vasc Interv Radiol* 2004;**15**:1407.

130. Hagen G, Wadstrom J, Magnusson M, et al. Outcome after percutaneous transluminal angioplasty of arterial stenoses in renal transplant patients. *Acta Radiol* 2009;**50**:270.

131. Valpreda S, Messina M, Rabbia C. Stenting of transplant renal artery stenosis: outcome in a single center study. *J Cardiovasc Surg* (Torino) 2008;**49**:565.

132. Obed A, Uihlein DC, Zorger N, et al. Severe renal vein stenosis of a kidney transplant with beneficial clinical course after successful percutaneous stenting. *Am J Transplant* 2008;**8**:2173.

133. Modrall JG, Teitelbaum GP, Diaz-Luna H, et al. Local thrombolysis in a renal allograft threatened by renal vein thrombosis. *Transplantation* 1993;**56**:1011.

134. Melamed ML, Kim HS, Jaar BG, et al. Combined percutaneous mechanical and chemical thrombectomy for renal vein thrombosis in kidney transplant recipients. *Am J Transplant* 2005;**5**:621.

135. deSouza NM, Reidy JF, Koffman CG. Arteriovenous fistulas complicating biopsy of renal allografts: treatment of bleeding with superselective embolization. *AJR Am J Roentgenol* 1991;**156**:507.

136. Perini S, Gordon RL, LaBerge JM, et al. Transcatheter embolization of biopsy-related vascular injury in the transplant kidney: immediate and long-term outcome. *J Vasc Interv Radiol* 1998;**9**:1011.

137. Maleux G, Messiaen T, Stockx L, et al. Transcatheter embolization of biopsy-related vascular injuries in renal allografts. Long-term technical, clinical, and biochemical results. *Acta Radiol* 2003;**44**:13.

138. Smith JK, Kenney PJ. Imaging of renal trauma. *Radiol Clin North Am* 2003;**41**:1019.

139. Dopson SJ, Jayakumar S, Velez JC. Page kidney as a rare cause of hypertension: case report and review of the literature. *Am J Kidney Dis* 2009;**54**:334.

140. Beaujeux R, Saussine C, Al-Fakir A, et al. Superselective endovascular treatment of renal vascular lesions. *J Urol* 1995;**153**:14.

141. Alonso RC, Nacenta SB, Martinez PD, et al. Kidney in danger: CT findings of blunt and penetrating renal trauma. *Radiographics* 2009;**29**:2033.

142. Eastham JA, Wilson TG, Larsen DW, et al. Angiographic embolization of renal stab wounds. *J Urol* 1992;**148**:268.

143. Dugi III DD, Morey AF, Gupta A, et al. American Association for the Surgery of Trauma grade 4 renal injury substratification into grades 4a (low risk) and 4b (high risk). *J Urol* 2010;**183**:592.

144. Nuss GR, Morey AF, Jenkins AC, et al. Radiographic predictors of need for angiographic embolization after traumatic renal injury. *J Trauma* 2009;**67**:578.

145. Loffroy R, Guiu B, Lambert A, et al. Management of post-biopsy renal allograft arteriovenous fistulas with selective arterial embolization: immediate and long-term outcome. *Clin Radiol* 2008;**63**:657.

146. Whigham Jr CJ, Bodenhamer JR, Miller JK. Use of the Palmaz stent in primary treatment of renal artery intimal injury secondary to blunt trauma. *J Vasc Interv Radiol* 1995;**6**:175.

147. Patard J-J. Incidental renal tumours. *Curr Opin Urol* 2009;**19**:454.

148. Garcia JA, Cowey CL, Godley PA. Renal cell carcinoma. *Curr Opin Oncol* 2009;**21**:266.

149. Oto A, Herts BR, Remer EM, et al. Inferior vena cava tumor thrombus in renal cell carcinoma: staging by MR imaging and impact on surgical treatment. *AJR Am J Roentgenol* 1998;**171**:1619.

150. Lawrentschuk N, Gani J, Riordan R, et al. Multidetector computed tomography vs. magnetic resonance imaging for defining the upper limit of tumour thrombus in renal cell carcinoma: a study and review. *BJU Int* 2005;**96**:291.

151. Saylor PJ, Michaelson MD. New treatments for renal cell carcinoma: targeted therapies. *J Natl Compr Canc Netw* 2009;**7**:645.

152. Clark PE. The role of VHL in clear cell renal cell carcinoma and its relation to targeted therapy. *Kidney Int* 2009;**76**:939.

153. Miller DL, Choyke PL, Walther MM, et al. von Hippel-Lindau disease: inadequacy of angiography for identification of renal cancers. *Radiology* 1991;**179**:833.

154. Meister M, Choyke P, Anderson C, et al. Radiological evaluation, management, and surveillance of renal masses in von Hippel-Lindau disease. *Clin Radiol* 2009;**64**:589.

155. Chow WH, Devesa SS. Contemporary epidemiology of renal cell cancer. *Cancer J* 2008;**14**:288.

156. Davidoff AM. Wilms' tumor. *Curr Opin Pediatr* 2009;**21**:357.

157. Seyam RM, Bissada NK, Kattan SA, et al. Changing trends in presentation, diagnosis, and management of renal angiomyolipoma: comparison of sporadic and tuberous sclerosis complex-associated forms. *Urology* 2008;**72**:1077.

158. Prasad SR, Surabhi VR, Menias CO, et al. Benign renal neoplasms in adults: cross-sectional imaging findings. *AJR Am J Roentgenol* 2008;**190**:158.

159. Pedrosa I, Sun MR, Spencer M, et al. MR imaging of renal masses: correlation with findings at surgery and pathologic analysis. *Radiographics* 2008;**28**:985.

160. Watson RC, Fleming RJ, Evans JA. Arteriography in the diagnosis of renal carcinoma. Review of 100 cases. *Radiology* 1968;**91**:888.

161. Karnes RJ, Blute ML. Surgery insight: management of renal cell carcinoma with associated inferior vena cava thrombus. *Nat Clin Pract Urol* 2008;**5**:329.

162. Rabinowitz JG, Kinkhabwala M, Himmelfarb E, et al. Renal pelvic carcinoma: an angiographic re-evaluation. *Radiology* 1972;**102**:551.

163. Han Y-M, Kim J-K, Roh B-S, et al. Renal angiomyolipoma: selective arterial embolization-effectiveness and changes in angiomyogenic components in long-term follow-up. *Radiology* 1997;**204**:70.

164. Quinn MJ, Hartman DS, Friedman AC, et al. Renal oncocytoma: new observations. *Radiology* 1984;**153**:49.

165. Bakal CW, Cynamon J, Lakritz PS, et al. Value of preoperative renal artery embolization in reducing blood transfusion requirements during nephrectomy for renal cell carcinoma. *J Vasc Interv Radiol* 1993;**4**:727.

166. Park JH, Kim SH, Han JK, et al. Transcatheter arterial embolization of unresectable renal cell carcinoma with a mixture of ethanol and iodized oil. *Cardiovasc Intervent Radiol* 1994;**17**:323.

167. Harabayashi T, Shinohara N, Katano H, et al. Management of renal angiomyolipomas associated with tuberous sclerosis complex. *J Urol* 2004;**171**:102.

168. May M, Brookman-Amissah S, Pflanz S, et al. Pre-operative renal arterial embolisation does not provide survival benefit in patients with radical nephrectomy for renal cell carcinoma. *Br J Radiol* 2009;**82**:724.

169. Schwartz MJ, Smith EB, Trost DW, et al. Renal artery embolization: clinical indications and experience from over 100 cases. *BJU Int* 2007;**99**:881.

170. Subramanian Vs, Stephenson AJ, Goldfarb DA, et al. Utility of preoperative renal artery embolization for management of renal tumors with inferior vena caval thrombi. *Urology* 2009;**74**:154.

171. Soulen MC, Faykus Jr MH, Shlansky-Goldberg RD, et al. Elective embolization for prevention of hemorrhage from renal angiomyolipomas. *J Vasc Interv Radiol* 1994;**5**:587.

172. Lee SY, Hsu HH, Chen YC, et al. Evaluation of renal function of angiomyolipoma patients after selective transcatheter arterial embolization. *Am J Med Sci* 2009;**337**:103.

173. Lenton J, Kessel D, Watkinson AF. Embolization of renal angiomyolipoma: immediate complications and long-term outcomes. *Clin Radiol* 2008;**63**:864.

174. Ramon J, Rimon U, Garniek A, et al. Renal angiomyolipoma: long-term results following selective arterial embolization. *Eur Urol* 2009;**55**:1155.

175. Williams JM, Racadio JM, Johnson ND, et al. Embolization of renal angiomyolipoma in patients with tuberous sclerosis complex. *Am J Kidney Dis* 2006;**47**:95.

176. Gervais DA, McGovern FJ, Arellano RS, et al. Renal cell carcinoma: clinical experience and technical success with radio-frequency ablation of 42 tumors. *Radiology* 2003;**226**:417.

177. Matlaga BR, Zagoria RJ, Clark PE, et al. Radiofrequency ablation of renal tumors. *Curr Urol Rep* 2004;**5**:39.

178. Farrell MA, Charboneau WJ, DiMarco DS, et al. Imaging-guided radiofrequency ablation of solid renal tumors. *AJR Am J Roentgenol* 2003;**180**:1509.

179. Mayo-Smith WW, Dupuy DE, Parikh PM, et al. Imaging-guided percutaneous radiofrequency ablation of solid renal masses: technique and outcomes of 38 treatment sessions in 32 consecutive patients. *AJR Am J Roentgenol* 2003;**180**:1503.

180. Wotkowicz C, Wszolek MF, Libertino JA. Resection of renal tumors invading the vena cava. *Urol Clin North Am* 2008;**35**:657.

181. Wang GJ, Carpenter JP, Fairman RM, et al. Single center experience of caval thrombectomy in patients with renal cell carcinoma with tumor thrombus extension into the inferior vena cava. *Vasc Endovascular Surg* 2008;**42**:335.

182. Henke PK, Cardneau JD, Welling TH III, et al. Renal artery aneurysms. A 35-year clinical experience with 252 aneurysms in 168 patients. *Ann Surg* 2001;**234**:454.

183. Lee RS, Porter JR. Traumatic renal artery pseudoaneurysm: diagnosis and management techniques. *J Trauma* 2003;**55**:972.

184. Henke PK, Stanley JC. Renal artery aneurysms: diagnosis, management, and outcomes. *Minerva Chir* 2003;**58**:305.

185. Cohen JR, Shamash FS. Ruptured renal artery aneurysms during pregnancy. *J Vasc Surg* 1987;**6**:51.

186. Tham G, Ekelund L, Herrlin K, et al. Renal artery aneurysms. Natural history and prognosis. *Ann Surg* 1983;**197**:348.

187. Henriksson C, Lukes P, Nilson AE, et al. Angiographically discovered, non-operated renal artery aneurysms. *Scand J Urol Nephrol* 1984;**18**:59.

188. Hubert Jr JP, Pairolero PC, Kazmier FJ. Solitary renal artery aneurysms. *Surgery* 1980;**88**:557.

189. Dzsinich C, Gloviczki P, McKusick MA, et al. Surgical management of renal artery aneurysms. *Cardiovasc Surg* 1993;**1**:243.

190. Lumsden AB, Salam TA, Walton KG. Renal artery aneurysm: a report of 28 cases. *Cardiovasc Surg* 1996;**4**:185.

191. Bui BT, Oliva VL, Leclerc G, et al. Renal artery aneurysm: treatment with percutaneous placement of a stent-graft. *Radiology* 1995;**195**:181.

192. Routh WD, Keller FS, Gross GM. Transcatheter thrombosis of a leaking saccular aneurysm of the main renal artery with preservation of renal blood flow. *AJR Am J Roentgenol* 1990;**154**:1097.

193. Rundback JH, Rizvi A, Rozenblit GN, et al. Percutaneous stent-graft management of renal artery aneurysms. *J Vasc Interv Radiol* 2000;**11**:1189.

194. Bisschops RHC, Popma JJ, Meyerovitz MF. Treatment of fibromuscular dysplasia and renal artery aneurysm with use of a stent-graft. *J Vasc Interv Radiol* 2001;**12**:757.

195. Starnes BW, O'Donnell SD, Gillespie DL, et al. Endovascular management of renal ischemia in a patient with acute aortic dissection and renovascular hypertension. *Ann Vasc Surg* 2002;**16**:368.

196. Lee SH, Lee HC, Oh SJ, et al. Percutaneous intervention of spontaneous renal artery dissection complicated with renal infarction: a case report and literature review. *Catheter Cardiovasc Interv* 2003;**60**:335.

197. Khawaja AT, McLean GK, Srinivasa V. Successful intervention for high-output cardiac failure caused by massive renal arteriovenous fistula—a case report. *Angiology* 2004;**55**:205.

198. Crotty KL, Orihuela E, Warren MM. Recent advances in the diagnosis and treatment of renal arteriovenous malformations and fistulas. *J Urol* 1993;**150**:1355.

199. Takebayashi S, Aida N, Matsui K. Arteriovenous malformations of the kidneys: diagnosis and follow-up with color Doppler sonography in six patients. *AJR Am J Roentgenol* 1991;**157**:991.

200. Allione A, Pomero F, Valpreda S, et al. Worsening of hypertension in a pregnant women with renal arteriovenous malformation: a successful superselective embolization after delivery. *Clin Nephrol* 2003;**60**:211.

201. Takebayashi S, Hosaka M, Ishizuka E, et al. Arteriovenous malformations of the kidneys: ablation with alcohol. *AJR Am J Roentgenol* 1988;**150**:587.

202. Asghar M, Ahmed K, Shah SS, et al. Renal vein thrombosis. *Eur J Vasc Endovasc Surg* 2007;**34**:217.

203. Singhal R, Brimble KS. Thromboembolic complications in the nephrotic syndrome: pathophysiology and clinical management. *Thromb Res* 2006;**118**:397.

204. Lau KK, Stoffman JM, Williams S, et al. Neonatal renal vein thrombosis: a review of the English language literature between 1992 and 2006. *Pediatrics* 2007;**120**:e1278.

205. Llach F, Arieff AI, Massry SG. Renal vein thrombosis and nephrotic syndrome: a prospective study of 36 adult patients. *Ann Intern Med* 1975;**83**:8.

206. Kawashima A, Sandler CM, Ernst RD, et al. CT evaluation of renovascular disease. *Radiographics* 2000;**20**:1321.

207. Butty S, Hagspiel KD, Leung DA, et al. Body MR venography. *Radiol Clin North Am* 2002;**40**:899.

208. Huang AB, Glanz S, Hon M, et al. Renal vein thrombolysis with selective simultaneous renal artery and renal vein infusions. *J Vasc Interv Radiol* 1995;**6**:581.

209. Kim HS, Fine DM, Atta MG. Catheter-directed thrombectomy and thrombolysis for acute renal vein thrombosis. *J Vasc Interv Radiol* 2006;**17**:815.

210. Scultetus AH, Villavicencio JL, Gillespie DL. The nutcracker syndrome: its role in the pelvic venous disorders. *J Vasc Surg* 2001;**34**:812.

211. Menard MT. Nutcracker syndrome: when should it be treated and how? *Perspect Vasc Surg Endovasc Ther* 2009;**21**:117.

212. Rudloff U, Holmes RJ, Prem JT, et al. Mesoaortic compression of the left renal vein (nutcracker syndrome): case reports and review of the literature. *Ann Vasc Surg* 2006;**20**:120.

213. Takebayashi S, Ueki T, Ikeda N, et al. Diagnosis of the nutcracker syndrome with color Doppler sonography: correlation with flow patterns on retrograde left renal venography. *AJR Am J Roentgenol* 1999;**172**:39.

214. Chiesa R, Anzuini A, Marone EM, et al. Endovascular stenting for the nutcracker phenomenon. *J Endovasc Ther* 2001;**8**:652.

215. Wei SM, Chen ZD, Zhou M. Intravenous stent placement for treatment of the nutcracker syndrome. *J Urol* 2003;**170**:1934.

216. Hartung O, Grisoli D, Boufi M, et al. Endovascular stenting in the treatment of pelvic vein congestion caused by nutcracker syndrome: lessons learned from the first five cases. *J Vasc Surg* 2005;**42**:275.

217. Sharma S, Thatai D, Saxena A, et al. Renovascular hypertension resulting from nonspecific aortoarteritis in children: midterm results of percutaneous transluminal renal angioplasty and predictors of restenosis. *AJR Am J Roentgenol* 1996;**166**:157.

218. Chuang VP. Radiation-induced arteritis. *Semin Roentgenol* 1994;**29**:64.

219. Samarkos M, Loizou S, Vaiopoulos G, et al. The clinical spectrum of primary renal vasculitis. *Semin Arthritis Rheum* 2005;**35**:95.

220. Kissin EY, Merkel PA. Diagnostic imaging in Takayasu arteritis. *Curr Opin Rheumatol* 2004;**16**:31.

221. Itzchak Y, Katznelson D, Boichis H, et al. Angiographic features of arterial lesions in neurofibromatosis. *AJR Am J Roentgenol* 1974;**122**:643.

222. Sumboonnananda A, Robinson BL, Gedroyc WMW, et al. Middle aortic syndrome: clinical and radiological findings. *Arch Dis Child* 1992;**67**:501.

223. Lin YJ, Hwang B, Lee PC, et al. Mid-aortic syndrome: a case report and review of the literature. *Int J Cardiol* 2008;**123**:348.

224. Both M, Jahnke T, Reinhold-Keller E, et al. Percutaneous management of occlusive arterial disease associated with vasculitis: a single center experience. *Cardiovasc Intervent Radiol* 2003;**26**:19.

225. Lee BB, Laredo J, Neville R, et al. Endovascular management of Takayasu arteritis: is it a durable option? *Vascular* 2009;**17**:138.

226. Bayrak AH, Numan F, Cantasdemir M, et al. Percutaneous balloon angioplasty of renovascular hypertension in pediatric cases. *Acta Chir Belg* 2008;**108**:708.

227. Brogan PA, Davies R, Gordon I, et al. Renal angiography in children with polyarteritis nodosa. *Pediatr Nephrol* 2002;**17**:277.

228. Nguan C, Leone E. A case of spontaneous perirenal hemorrhage secondary to polyarteritis nodosa. *Can J Urol* 2002;**9**:1704.

229. Allen AW, Waybill PN, Singh H, et al. Polyarteritis nodosa presenting as spontaneous perirenal hemorrhage: angiographic diagnosis and treatment with microcoil embolization. *J Vasc Interv Radiol* 1999;**10**:1361.

230. Hidalgo J, Crego M, Montlleo M, et al.: Embolization of a bleeding aneurysm in a patient with spontaneous perirenal hematoma due to Polyarteritis nodosa. *Arch Esp Urol* 2005;**58**:694.

231. Slavin RE. Segmental arterial mediolysis: course, sequelae, prognosis, and pathologic-radiologic correlation. *Cardiovasc Pathol* 2009;**18**:352.

232. Soulen MC, Cohen DL, Itkin M, et al. Segmental arterial mediolysis: angioplasty of bilateral renal artery stenoses with 2-year imaging follow-up. *J Vasc Interv Radiol* 2004;**15**:763.

Mesenteric Arteries

Karim Valji

ARTERIOGRAPHY
(ONLINE VIDEOS 11-1 TO 11-3)

A wide variety of catheters are available for mesenteric arteriography; the Sos and cobra shapes are popular (see Figs. 3-14 and 3-15). The celiac and superior mesenteric arteries are engaged by searching the anterior aortic wall at about the T12 and L1 levels, respectively. The inferior mesenteric artery (IMA) typically originates from the left anterolateral surface of the aorta at about the L3-L4 level. If the desired vessel is not easily found, aortography will often show an obstructed origin or atypical location. Inadvertent dissection of a mesenteric arterial trunk or branch can have serious consequences. Therefore great care should be taken with catheter and guidewire manipulations. Large contrast injections are only made after secure intravascular location is documented and good backflow of blood is observed.

Most practitioners use coaxial microcatheters and microwires for selective catheterization of mesenteric artery branches. Occasionally, a larger catheter or sheath must be negotiated into a second- or third-order vessel to allow an intervention. In this situation, the catheter may be advanced using steerable, hydrophilic guidewires or an exchange done with a more suitably shaped catheter and wire. There are several methods for engaging the left gastric artery (LGA); one traditional technique is outlined in Figure 11-1.

ANATOMY
(ONLINE CASES 6 AND 19)

Development

In the fetus, a series of vitelline arteries arising from the fused dorsal aortae supply the abdominal viscera.[1] These branches are initially connected by a ventral anastomotic channel (Fig. 11-2). The celiac, superior mesenteric, and inferior mesenteric arteries originate

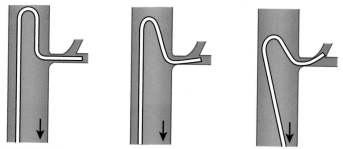

FIGURE 11-1 Selective catheterization of the left gastric artery. As the sidewinder-shaped catheter with its tip well into the celiac artery is withdrawn at the groin, the tip begins to point upward and eventually engages the left gastric artery.

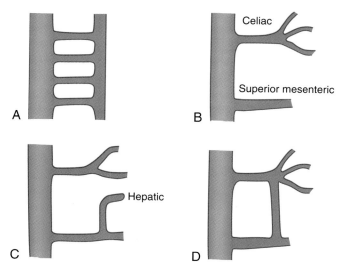

FIGURE 11-2 Embryologic development of the mesenteric arteries (right lateral view). **A,** In the fetus, the dorsal aorta on the left and the ventral anastomotic channel on the right are connected by a series of vitelline arteries. **B,** Normal anatomy at birth. **C,** Failure of a portion of the ventral anastomosis to regress causes the hepatic artery to be "replaced" to the superior mesenteric artery. **D,** Failed regression of a segment of the ventral anastomosis between the celiac and superior mesenteric arteries leaves a direct collateral pathway (i.e., arc of Buehler). *(Adapted from Reuter SR, Redman HC, Cho KJ: Gastrointestinal angiography. 3rd ed. Philadelphia: WB Saunders; 1986: p. 34.)*

from three of these vitelline segments; the remaining segments regress before birth. Common variants in mesenteric artery anatomy can be explained by abnormal persistence of vitelline remnants or portions of the ventral anastomosis.

Normal Anatomy

The *celiac artery* exits the anterior surface of the aorta at about the T12 level[2-4] (Fig. 11-3). The main trunk can take an upward, downward, or forward course. Just beyond its origin, the celiac artery gives off the LGA and then divides into the common hepatic and splenic arteries. Sometimes, the inferior phrenic or dorsal pancreatic artery arises directly from the celiac trunk.

The *common hepatic artery* runs toward the liver. After giving off the *gastroduodenal artery (GDA)*, it becomes the *proper hepatic artery*, which itself divides into *right* and *left* (and occasionally *middle*) *hepatic arteries*. Hepatic arterial anatomy is detailed in Chapter 12. The *right gastric artery* usually takes off from the proper or left hepatic artery but sometimes is not visualized on nonselective angiograms. It supplies the pylorus and the lesser curvature of the stomach and communicates with distal branches of the LGA. The *cystic artery* usually originates from the right hepatic artery, although it may arise more proximally.

The *GDA* runs between the neck of the pancreas and the duodenum. Its first major branch is the *posterior superior pancreaticoduodenal artery*. This vessel gives off branches to the pancreas on the left and to the duodenum on the right. The GDA then divides into its terminal branches, the *anterior superior pancreaticoduodenal artery* and the *right gastroepiploic artery*.

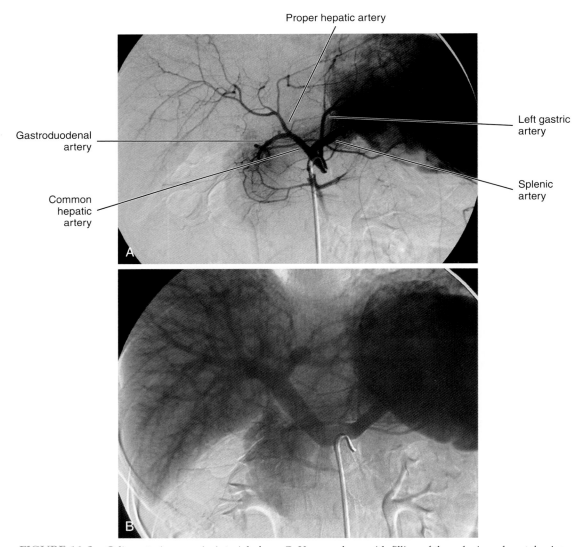

FIGURE 11-3   Celiac arteriogram. **A,** Arterial phase. **B,** Venous phase with filling of the splenic and portal veins.

The superior pancreaticoduodenal arteries lead into an arterial network that supplies the head of the pancreas. These vessels have rich anastomoses with the corresponding branches of the inferior pancreaticoduodenal artery, which originates from the superior mesenteric artery (SMA). The right gastroepiploic artery runs along the greater curvature of the stomach and communicates with the *left gastroepiploic branch* of the splenic artery.

The *splenic artery* supplies the spleen, pancreas, and stomach (see Chapter 12). It runs dorsal to the upper border of the pancreas along with the splenic vein. Its branches usually include the *dorsal pancreatic, pancreatica magna, short gastric,* and *polar arteries.* The splenic artery divides into superior and inferior branches near the splenic hilum. The inferior polar artery gives rise to the left gastroepiploic artery, which courses along the greater curvature of the stomach.

The *LGA* exits the upper surface of the celiac artery and runs toward the cardia of the stomach (Fig. 11-4). At this point, it divides into several branches that supply the distal esophagus and fundus of the stomach. These vessels communicate with short gastric branches of the splenic artery, the right gastric artery, and the left inferior phrenic artery.

The *SMA* supplies the bowel from the distal duodenum to the mid-transverse colon (Fig. 11-5). It courses behind the body of the pancreas and then enters the root of the mesentery. The *superior mesenteric vein* runs along the right side of the artery. The *inferior pancreaticoduodenal artery* is the first branch of the SMA,

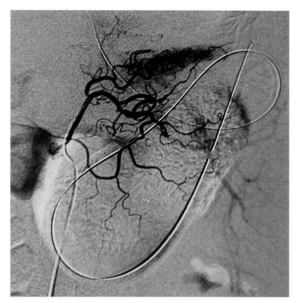

FIGURE 11-4   Left gastric arteriogram.

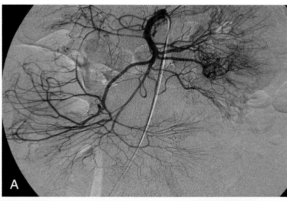

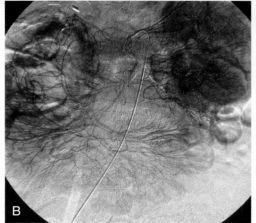

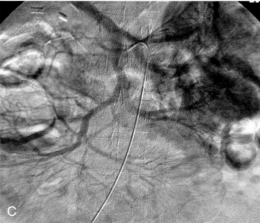

FIGURE 11-5   Superior mesenteric arteriogram. **A,** Arterial phase. There is variable enhancement of bowel wall. **B,** Capillary phase. **C,** Venous phase.

although it may arise in a common trunk with the first jejunal artery. It passes to the right and superiorly into the head of the pancreas, where it communicates with the superior pancreaticoduodenal branches of the GDA. A series of jejunal and ileal branches occupy most of the main trunk of the SMA. Usually, these vessels fan out from the left upper quadrant to the right lower quadrant. A system of elaborate arcades between these branches feed the vasa recta that directly supply the wall of the bowel. The *ileocolic artery* is the terminal continuation of the SMA. It gives off branches to the ileum, appendix, cecum, and right colon. The *right* and *middle colic arteries* arise separately or as a common trunk on the right side of the SMA. These vessels supply the ascending and transverse colon, respectively. Small bowel branches of the SMA can be differentiated from colonic branches by their more extensive arcade system and longer vasa recta (see Fig. 11-5).

The *IMA* supplies the colon from its mid-transverse segment to the rectum (Fig. 11-6). The vessel runs inferiorly for several centimeters and then gives off the *left colic artery*. An ascending branch of this artery joins the middle colic branch of the SMA. *Descending colic (sigmoid) branches* originate from the left colic artery and distal IMA to supply the lower descending and sigmoid colon. The terminal branch of the IMA is the *superior rectal (hemorrhoidal) artery*, which divides into right and left branches that supply blood to the rectum.

Variant Anatomy

Anomalies in the origins of the central mesenteric arteries are rare, but anomalies in the branching patterns of the mesenteric arteries are common. It is vital to be alert to potential variants when performing angiographic procedures. Table 11-1 outlines the important variants formulated by the classic anatomic studies of Michel and coworkers[5,6] (Figs. 11-7 through 11-9; see also Fig. 7-4). The reported frequencies vary somewhat in postmortem and angiographic studies.

A *replaced* hepatic artery exists when an entire hepatic lobe is supplied by a vessel with an aberrant origin. An *accessory* hepatic artery exists when a portion of the affected lobe is supplied by a vessel with an aberrant origin. Accessory hepatic arteries supply isolated hepatic segments and are not redundant arteries. As a rule of thumb, a replaced or accessory hepatic artery arises from the LGA in 20% of patients and from the SMA in 20%.

Other rare variants include common origin of the celiac artery and SMA (*celiomesenteric trunk*, Fig. 11-10), separate origin of one or more major celiac branches from the aorta, and splenic artery arising from the SMA (Figs. 11-11 and 11-12).

Collateral Circulation

The intestinal tract has an extensive collateral network that prevents or limits bowel ischemia when central arteries become obstructed. The more important pathways[6] are outlined in Table 11-2 and shown in Figures 11-13 through 11-16. The different collateral routes between the SMA and IMA are often confused.

Text continued on p.332

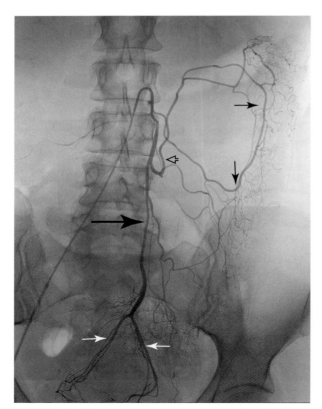

FIGURE 11-6 Inferior mesenteric arteriogram. Note left colic artery *(open arrow)*, descending colic artery *(large arrow)*, superior rectal artery *(white arrows)*, and marginal artery *(black arrows)*.

TABLE 11-1   Important Anomalies of the Mesenteric Arteries

Artery	Anomalous Origin	Frequency (%)
Replaced common hepatic	Superior mesenteric	2.5
Replaced right hepatic	Superior mesenteric	10
Accessory right hepatic	Superior mesenteric	6
Replaced left hepatic	Left gastric	10 to 12
Accessory left hepatic	Left gastric	8 to 13
Inferior phrenic	Celiac	35
Right gastric	CHA, RHA, GDA	15
Dorsal pancreatic	Celiac	22
Gastroduodenal	Right or left hepatic	18
Left gastric, splenic, hepatic	Aorta	<1
Celiomesenteric trunk	Aorta	<1
Middle colic	Dorsal pancreatic, splenic, hepatic	<1

CHA, *common hepatic artery*; GDA, *gastroduodenal artery*; RHA, *right hepatic artery*.

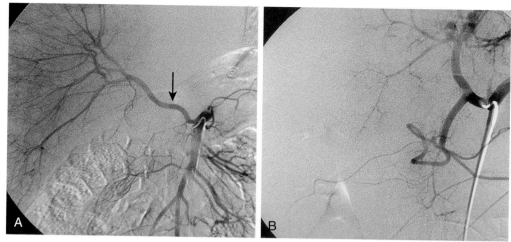

FIGURE 11-7 **A,** Replaced right hepatic artery *(arrow)* to the superior mesenteric artery. **B,** No filling of the right hepatic branches is seen on the celiac arteriogram.

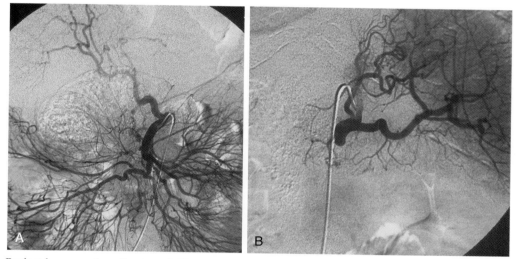

FIGURE 11-8 Replaced common hepatic artery. **A,** The common hepatic artery originates from the superior mesenteric artery. **B,** At celiac angiography, only the left gastric and splenic arteries are seen.

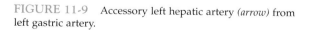

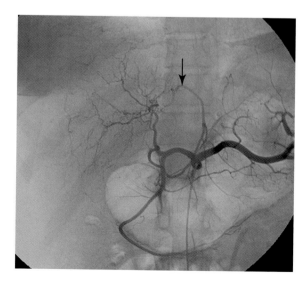

FIGURE 11-9 Accessory left hepatic artery *(arrow)* from left gastric artery.

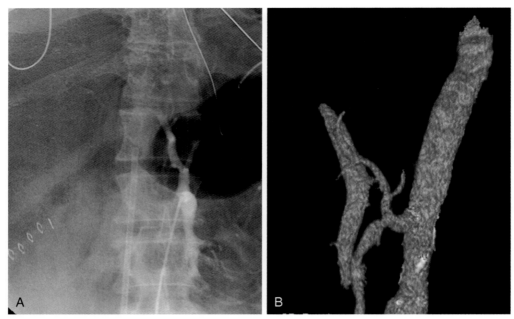

FIGURE 11-10   Common celiomesenteric trunk on mesenteric arteriography **(A)** and sagittal shaded surface display CT angiography **(B).**

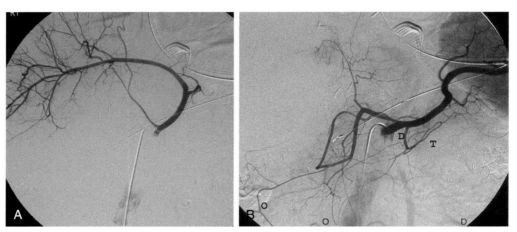

FIGURE 11-11   Right hepatic artery takes off directly from the aorta **(A),** separate from the celiac trunk **(B).** The dorsal pancreatic artery *(D)*, transverse pancreatic artery *(T)*, and omental branches *(O)* are seen.

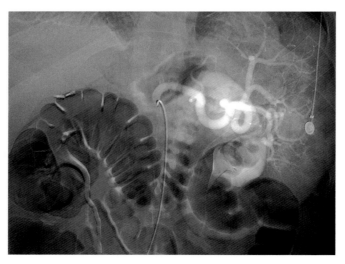

FIGURE 11-12   Separate origin of splenic artery from the aorta.

TABLE 11-2   Major Mesenteric Arterial Collateral Pathways

Pathway	Communication	Pathway	Communication
CELIAC AND SUPERIOR MESENTERIC ARTERIES (SEE FIG. 11-13)		**SUPERIOR AND INFERIOR MESENTERIC ARTERIES (SEE FIG. 11-15)**	
Pancreatic arcade	Gastroduodenal and inferior pancreaticoduodenal arteries	Marginal artery	Branches of middle and left colic arteries (of Drummond)
Arc of Buehler	Direct embryologic pathway	Arc of Riolan	Central vessel from middle to left colic artery
INTRACELIAC BRANCHES (SEE FIG. 11-14)		**INFERIOR MESENTERIC AND ILIAC ARTERIES**	
Gastric arcade	Left and right gastric arteries	Rectal (hemorrhoidal)	Superior and middle/inferior rectal arteries arcade
Gastroepiploic arcade	Left and right gastroepiploic arteries		
Arc of Barkow	Left and right epiploic arteries (within omentum)		

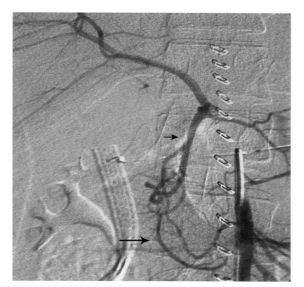

FIGURE 11-13   Pancreatic arcade collateral network with celiac artery occlusion. Superior mesenteric arterial injection fills dilated inferior pancreaticoduodenal arteries *(long arrow)* and pancreatic arcades. Retrograde flow in the gastroduodenal artery *(short arrow)* then backfills the hepatic artery.

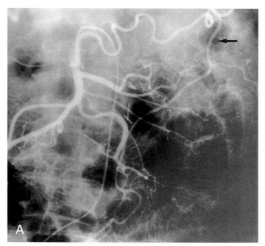

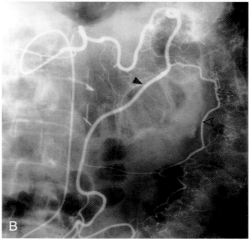

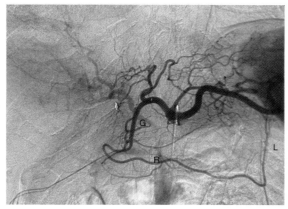

FIGURE 11-14   Gastroepiploic arcade. The right gastroepiploic artery *(R)*, the terminal branch of the gastroduodenal artery *(G)*, continues to the left gastroepiploic artery *(L)* in the splenic hilum. This pathway provides collateral circulation with splenic artery obstruction. Also note the replaced right hepatic artery.

FIGURE 11-15   Marginal artery of Drummond and arc of Riolan with inferior mesenteric artery (IMA) occlusion. **A,** Superior mesenteric arteriogram shows dilation of the middle colic artery with flow into the IMA distribution *(arrow).* **B,** Selective middle colic artery injection shows filling of the arc of Riolan *(arrowhead)* and the marginal artery *(open arrowhead).*

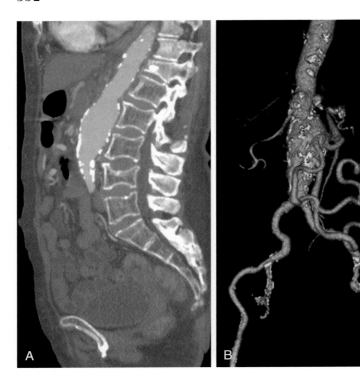

FIGURE 11-16   Meandering mesenteric artery in superior mesenteric artery (SMA) and celiac artery occlusion. **A,** Reformatted sagittal computed tomography angiogram shows highly calcified aorta and no evidence for celiac artery or SMA origin. **B,** Shaded surface display image depicts large tortuous branch of the inferior mesenteric artery which ultimately supplies SMA distribution.

BOX 11-1

CAUSES OF ACUTE MESENTERIC ISCHEMIA (GLOBAL OR SEGMENTAL)

- Embolism
- Superior mesenteric artery thrombosis
- Superior mesenteric vein thrombosis
- Nonocclusive mesenteric ischemia
- Dissection
- Trauma
- Surgery
- Celiac artery compression (median arcuate ligament) syndrome
- Radiation therapy
- Vasculitis (Buerger disease, Takayasu arteritis, polyarteritis nodosa)
- Tumor
- Cholesterol embolization
- Crohn disease
- Diabetes mellitus
- Retroperitoneal fibrosis
- Bowel strangulation or intussusception
- Drugs (e.g., cocaine)
- Fibromuscular dysplasia
- Aneurysm rupture

The *marginal artery (of Drummond)* is a longitudinal vessel formed by trunks or distal branches of the right, middle, and left colic arteries. When fully formed, it runs along the entire mesenteric border of the colon. The *arc of Riolan* is a central vessel embedded in the root of the mesentery that directly connects the middle colic artery with the left colic artery.

MAJOR DISORDERS

Acute Mesenteric Ischemia

Etiology

It is noteworthy that sudden obstruction of the celiac artery or IMA rarely causes symptomatic mesenteric ischemia, as long as adequate collaterals exist. Several vascular diseases that reduce blood flow to or from the intestinal arteries or veins can lead to acute mesenteric ischemia[7-11] (Box 11-1). *SMA embolism* is one of the most common causes of acute mesenteric vascular obstruction. Most emboli come from the heart. The embolus typically lodges in the SMA just below the origin of the middle colic artery, although single or multiple emboli may pass into the distal SMA trunk or its branches. The arteries beyond the obstruction undergo reflex vasoconstriction, which further worsens bowel ischemia. *SMA thrombosis* is another frequent cause for acute intestinal ischemia. Thrombosis is usually superimposed on severe atherosclerotic disease near the origin of the SMA.

Nonocclusive mesenteric ischemia is responsible for some cases of bowel ischemia.[11-12] The disorder is caused by hypotension or hypovolemia in the setting of acute cardiac disease, sepsis, liver or kidney disease, and after recent surgery. Certain drugs (including digitalis, dopamine, and vasopressin) have also been implicated. Regardless of the cause, the result is persistent vasoconstriction of the SMA and its branches leading to intestinal hypoxia. This entity is particularly lethal; the 30-day mortality rate despite surgery in one large contemporary series was 80%.[13]

Superior mesenteric vein thrombosis may be spontaneous... secondary to portal hypertension, thrombophilic... trauma, abdominal surgery, inflammatory bowel... epsis, neoplasm, or pancreatitis.[14] If the venous... circulation is inadequate, the bowel wall... ematous, and arterial inflow is diminished... sion of an *aortic dissection* into main mes... is an important reason for inadequate... el.

...acute mesenteric ischemia are... associated conditions such... oronary artery disease, val-... thmias, or hypotension... cute onset of moderate... imes accompanied by... tinal bleeding. Clas-... ortion to the rela-... ination. Often, a... resent. If bowel... nal condition... nt to avoid... d sepsis,... cclusion... devel-... rate

...n shows... as in the wall... wing overnight

...of the mesenteric ves-... ntestinal ischemia. The... ction is atherosclerotic... ses are often caused by... tic wall that engulf the... s. Subacute or chronic su-... bosis can mimic chronic... older woman with one or... clerosis. The classic symptom... f abdominal pain after eating... f food, and weight loss. Some

central mesenteric vessels. Findings on CT or MRI include bowel distention and wall thickening, edema of the mesentery, intramural gas, and, sometimes, diminished bowel wall enhancement. Filling defects in the major mesenteric arteries and veins should be carefully sought (Figs. 11-17 and 11-18).

CATHETER ANGIOGRAPHY

Arteriography is indicated when noninvasive imaging is equivocal, nonocclusive mesenteric ischemia is suspected, or endovascular treatment is contemplated. Arteriographic findings depend on the cause of occlusive disease. A fresh embolus produces a discrete filling defect (see Fig. 11-17). In some cases, residual flow is seen around the clot. Reconstitution of the distal SMA is usually poor or nonexistent. Occasionally, small clots are seen in distal SMA branches or other abdominal and pelvic arteries. Thrombotic occlusion causes complete obstruction in the most proximal portion of the SMA trunk (see Fig. 11-16). Because thrombosis usually occurs at a site of previous narrowing, the collateral circulation is often well developed. Despite certain distinguishing features, it may be impossible to differentiate thrombotic and embolic occlusions by angiography.

Nonocclusive mesenteric ischemia is characterized by slow flow in the SMA, diffuse narrowing of SMA branches and arcades, segments of alternating spasm and dilation of these branches, and poor filling of the vasa recta[11,22] (Fig. 11-19). Contrast persists in intestinal branches for greater than 2 seconds after the injection has ended. Profound systemic hypotension ("shock bowel") and certain vasoconstricting drugs can produce similar findings (see later discussion).

Superior mesenteric vein thrombosis is diagnosed by the presence of numerous collateral channels in place of the superior mesenteric vein during the late-phase SMA arteriogram. Sometimes a filling defect in the main trunk of the vein is seen. Venous obstruction is usually associated with slow flow in the SMA and slow washout of mesenteric branches. However, chronic mesenteric artery or vein occlusion may be an incidental finding in patients with acute abdominal pain from other causes.

Treatment

SURGICAL THERAPY

te SMA occlusion is treated by embolectomy, thromarterectomy, patch angioplasty, or bypass grafting with resection of infarcted bowel.[7,8] Many still require a "second look" operation to iden... onal ischemic bowel that must be removed. e early and aggressive treatment, 30-day mortality still close to 30%.[23,24]

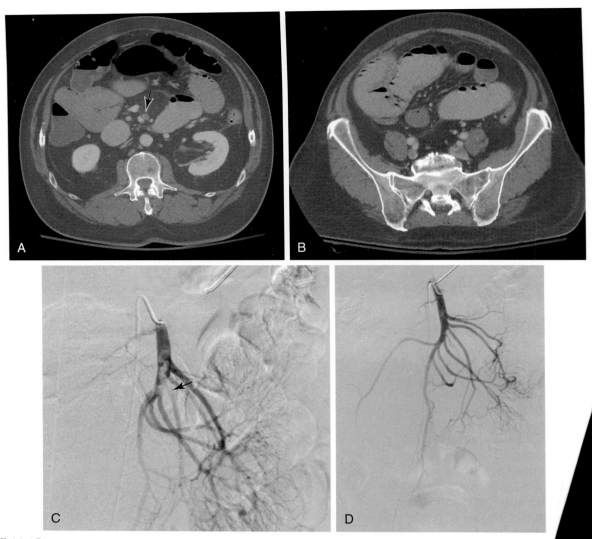

FIGURE 11-17   Embolus to the superior mesenteric artery (SMA). **A** and **B,** Contrast-enhanced computed tomography sc[ ] filling defect in proximal SMA trunk *(arrow).* Also note multiple loops of very dilated, fluid-filled small bowel with possible [ ] **C,** SMA angiography reveals the nonocclusive SMA embolus with extension into at least one jejunal branch *(arrow).* **D,** Foll[ ] thrombolysis with t-PA at 1 mg/hr, there is near complete resolution of clot. Patient's symptoms resolved.

ENDOVASCULAR THERAPY

Infusion of the vasodilator *papaverine* directly into the SMA (60-mg bolus followed by an infusion at 30 to 60 mg/hr) is sometimes effective as primary treatment for nonocclusive mesenteric ischemia or as a preoperative maneuver for other forms of acute mesenteric ischemia.[22] Thrombolysis has also been used effectively for acute SMA embolism and acute superior mesenteric venous thrombosis[25,26] (see Fig. 11-17). It may be particularly appropriate in patients without evidence of frank bowel necrosis. Balloon angioplasty with stent placement is also an attractive alternative to surgery in very high-risk patients with critical stenoses or extensions of dissection.[27,28] Immediate clinical benefit is the rule, but long-term durability has not been established.

Chronic Mesenteric Ischemia (Online Case 67)

Etiology and Clinical Features

Symptomatic chronic obstruction[ ] sels is less common than acute i[ ] primary cause of chronic obstr[ ] disease[8,10,14,15] (Box 11-2). Steno[ ] plaques on the abdominal a[ ] ostia of the mesenteric arterie[ ] perior mesenteric vein thro[ ] arterial obstruction.

The typical patient is a[ ] more risk factors for atheros[ ] complex is a long history [ ] ("intestinal angina"), fear [ ]

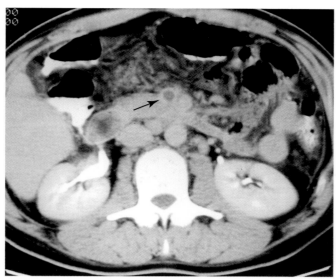

FIGURE 11-18   Superior mesenteric vein thrombosis. The computed tomography scan shows a clot in the superior mesenteric vein *(arrow)* and dilated, thickened small bowel loops.

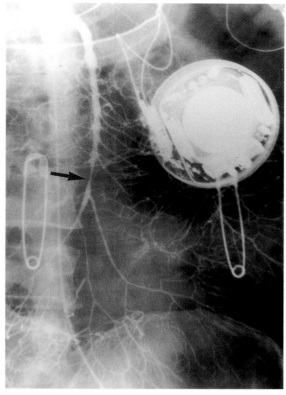

FIGURE 11-19   Nonocclusive mesenteric ischemia. There is slow flow in the superior mesenteric artery (SMA), constriction of intestinal branches, and alternating segments of dilation and narrowing in the distal SMA *(arrow)*.

BOX 11-2

CAUSES OF CHRONIC MESENTERIC ISCHEMIA

- Atherosclerosis
- Thrombotic occlusion
- Celiac artery compression (median arcuate ligament) syndrome
- Dissection
- Extrinsic compression
- Vasculitis
- Tumor
- Inflammatory mass
- Coarctation syndromes
- Vasoconstricting drugs
- Fibromuscular dysplasia

---

patients have diarrhea, nausea, or intermittent vomiting. The abdominal examination is usually unimpressive, although an epigastric bruit may be heard.

Imaging

CROSS-SECTIONAL TECHNIQUES

Because the symptoms of chronic mesenteric ischemia are often vague and intermittent, the diagnosis is often delayed. Duplex sonography is the primary imaging tool for screening in suspected cases. Criteria for diagnosis include major vessel occlusion, high-grade stenosis, or peak systolic velocities in the celiac and superior mesenteric arteries of greater than 200 cm/sec and greater than 275 cm/sec in

the fasting state, respectively[29-31] (Fig. 11-20). CT or MR angiography more thoroughly depicts mesenteric vascular stenoses and occlusions[17,18] (Fig. 11-21). It is commonly accepted that at least two of the three mesenteric arteries must have significant stenoses or occlusions to make the diagnosis of chronic mesenteric ischemia. On the other hand, the mere presence of severe multivessel mesenteric artery disease can be an incidental finding in a patient with other causes for abdominal pain.

CATHETER ANGIOGRAPHY

Arteriography is usually a prelude to percutaneous or open repair. Several entities should be considered in the differential diagnosis of mesenteric artery narrowing (see Box 11-2). Because of the chronic nature of the disease, the collateral circulation is usually extensive. Obstruction of the IMA is suggested by enlargement of the marginal artery (or arc of Riolan) with retrograde flow into the IMA trunk (see Fig. 11-15).

Treatment

Revascularization is performed to relieve chronic ischemic symptoms, prevent the development of life-threatening acute mesenteric ischemia, or avoid postoperative ischemia if the IMA is to be sacrificed during an aortic operation or intervention.

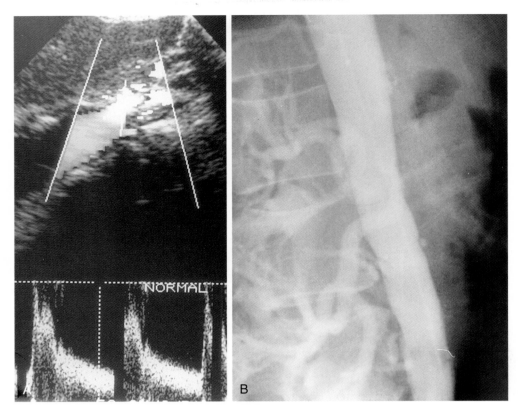

FIGURE 11-20   Chronic mesenteric ischemia. **A,** Duplex sonography shows a stenosis at the origin of the superior mesenteric artery (SMA) with a peak systolic velocity of 302 cm/sec. **B,** The lateral aortogram 3 weeks later showed complete occlusion of the celiac artery and SMA. The inferior mesenteric artery supplied the entire bowel.

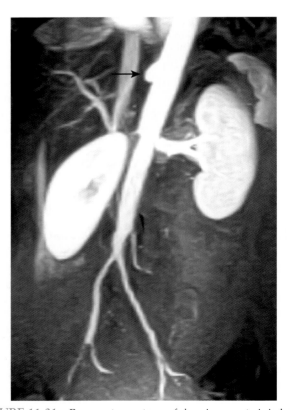

FIGURE 11-21   Recurrent symptoms of chronic mesenteric ischemia after celiac/superior mesenteric artery bypass. Gadolinium-enhanced magnetic resonance angiogram in oblique sagittal projection shows stump of bypass *(arrow)* with no filling of central mesenteric arteries.

SURGICAL THERAPY

The most common procedures for mesenteric revascularization are transaortic thromboendarterectomy, aortovisceral bypass, and arterial reimplantation.[23,32]

ENDOVASCULAR THERAPY

Balloon angioplasty with stenting of the celiac artery and SMA is an acceptable alternative to surgery in some cases, particularly when the patient is at high risk for operative complications[8,32-36] (Fig. 11-22). Technical success is reported in 30% to 90% of cases. However, major complications occur frequently (16% to 33%) in some series.[34] Surgery is more effective than endovascular repair; it affords more durable results and requires fewer reinterventions to maintain patency. Angioplasty and stent insertion is not useful in patients with celiac artery compression syndrome.

Acute Gastrointestinal Bleeding (Online Cases 32 and 103)

The diagnosis and treatment of acute gastrointestinal bleeding have undergone a revolution over the past several decades.[37,38] The widespread use of histamine (H_2) blockers and "proton pump" inhibitors has markedly reduced the incidence of peptic ulcer disease and associated bleeding. Fiberoptic endoscopy

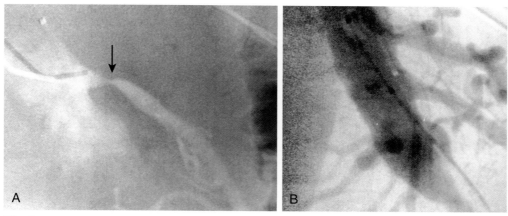

FIGURE 11-22   Superior mesenteric artery (SMA) angioplasty and stent placement in a patient with an abdominal aortic aneurysm and occlusion of the inferior mesenteric artery. **A,** The lateral aortogram shows a tight proximal SMA stenosis *(arrow)*. **B,** After placement of a stent mounted on a 6-mm angioplasty balloon using a brachial approach, the stenosis is relieved. The residual systolic pressure gradient was 7 to 8 mm Hg.

has largely supplanted angiography in the management of upper gastrointestinal hemorrhage.[39] Upper endoscopy, colonoscopy, and push or double balloon enteroscopy have taken the dominant role in the evaluation and treatment of lower intestinal tract bleeding.[40,41] Nonetheless, angiography is still required in a small subset of patients with this difficult clinical problem.

Etiology

For several reasons, acute gastrointestinal bleeding is typically categorized as being from an upper gastrointestinal source (from the esophagus to the ligament of Treitz) or a lower gastrointestinal source (from the small bowel, colon, or rectum).

Box 11-3 outlines the major causes of acute upper gastrointestinal bleeding.[42] The most common are duodenal or gastric ulcer disease, gastritis, endoscopic biopsy, Mallory-Weiss tear, and gastroesophageal varices.

- *Gastroesophageal varices* are a common source of upper gastrointestinal bleeding in patients with portal hypertension (see Chapter 12). However, patients with varices may bleed for other reasons. Variceal bleeding is usually detected by endoscopy. Angiography may show the varices but rarely shows active bleeding.
- *Mallory-Weiss tear* is a laceration at the gastroesophageal junction, often seen in patients with alcoholism after repeated episodes of vomiting.[43]
- *Pseudoaneurysms* of the gastroduodenal, pancreaticoduodenal, and splenic arteries may develop in patients with pancreatitis or trauma and lead to bleeding into the gut.[44]

BOX 11-3

CAUSES OF ACUTE UPPER GASTROINTESTINAL BLEEDING

- Peptic ulcer disease
- Varices
- Gastritis or esophagitis
- Tumor
- Mallory-Weiss tear
- Postoperative anastomotic (marginal) ulcer
- Endoscopic sphincterotomy
- Hemobilia
- Hemosuccus pancreaticus
- Arteriovenous malformation or telangiectasia
- Aneurysm or pseudoaneurysm
- Duodenal diverticulum
- Aortoenteric fistula
- Dieulafoy lesion
- AIDS-related conditions

AIDS, acquired immunodeficiency syndrome.

- *Hemobilia* often becomes apparent from acute gastrointestinal hemorrhage as a consequence of trauma, percutaneous liver biopsy, biliary drainage procedures, or hepatic surgery.[45] Bleeding can be immediate or delayed. *Hemosuccus pancreaticus* can result from a pancreatitis-related pseudoaneurysm which bleeds into the pancreatic duct and then into the duodenum.[46]

- *Aortoenteric fistula* occurs in less than 1% of patients after aortic graft placement. The fistula develops between the bowel (usually the transverse duodenum) and the graft as a consequence of infection.[47]
- *Marginal ulcers* occasionally complicate surgical gastrojejunostomy.[48] Ulcers are located on the jejunal side of the anastomosis; however, bleeding may occur from branches of the celiac artery or SMA.
- *Dieulafoy disease* is a noninflammatory disorder in which a small superficial gastric mucosal erosion covers a submucosal artery and may result in bleeding.[49,50] The lesion is usually found in the cardia or fundus of the stomach, but is rarely seen in the colon or small bowel.

Box 11-4 outlines the major causes of lower gastrointestinal bleeding.[51] Based on two large epidemiologic studies, the most common causes of lower gastrointestinal bleeding among inpatients are diverticular disease, colitis, neoplasms and anorectal disorders.[38,52,53] However, in angiographic series the most common sources are diverticulosis, angiodysplasia, and polyps or cancer (spontaneous lesional hemorrhage or postendoscopic biopsy). At least two thirds of cases are localized to the large bowel. About 10% of the time, apparent lower gastrointestinal bleeding is attributable to rapid hemorrhage from an upper source.[54,55]

- *Diverticular disease* is sometimes complicated by hemorrhage. Bleeding is minor and stops spontaneously in most cases. Massive or recurrent bleeding is an indication for angiography. Hemorrhage occurs from a branch of the vasa recta in continuity with the body of the diverticulum.[56] Diverticula are most common in the sigmoid and left colon. For several reasons, colonoscopy identifies more left-sided bleeding diverticula and angiography more right-sided diverticula.[52,53,56]
- *Angiodysplasia (vascular ectasia)* is a developmental vascular anomaly consisting of clusters of dilated submucosal veins and capillaries in the bowel wall, most frequently in the ascending colon.[55] The cause is unknown. There is speculation that intermittent elevation in intraluminal pressure causes venous obstruction, which over time leads to venous engorgement and bleeding. Lesions are often multiple. Angiodysplasia is relatively common in the elderly and may be an incidental finding in patients with other sources for gastrointestinal bleeding. Although bleeding usually stops spontaneously, rebleeding occurs in the majority of untreated lesions.[54]
- Acquired immunodeficiency syndrome can cause lower or upper gastrointestinal hemorrhage. A wide variety of lesions may bleed, including Kaposi sarcoma, lymphoma, and a host of opportunistic infections.[58]
- *Meckel diverticulum* is a congenital remnant of the fetal omphalomesenteric (vitelline) duct that is seen in about 2% of the general population. The outpouching occurs about 2 feet proximal to the ileocecal valve. Gastric or pancreatic mucosa in the lesion may be detected by ^{99m}Tc scanning. It is a common cause for lower gastrointestinal bleeding in children.

Clinical Features

Upper gastrointestinal bleeding is much more common than lower tract hemorrhage, but interventionalists encounter the latter more often. Patients with significant upper gastrointestinal bleeding have bright red or coffee-ground hematemesis or melena. Patients with lower gastrointestinal bleeding present with hematochezia or melena. However, about 10% of individuals with major upper gastrointestinal hemorrhage have hematochezia suggesting a lower tract source.[55] At least 75% of patients with acute gastrointestinal bleeding respond to supportive measures and minor blood transfusions alone. The remainder require direct intervention.

BOX 11-4

CAUSES OF ACUTE LOWER GASTROINTESTINAL BLEEDING

- Diverticular disease
- Angiodysplasia (vascular ectasia)
- Neoplasms (benign polyps or malignant tumor)
  - Spontaneous
  - Bleeding after endoscopic biopsy or polypectomy
- Anorectal disorders (hemorrhoids, fissures, radiation proctitis, trauma)
- Inflammatory bowel disease
- Ischemic bowel
- Arteriovenous malformations or telangiectasia
- Radiation enteritis
- Vasculitis
- Colonic or small bowel varices
- AIDS-related conditions
- Ulcer
- Aortoenteric fistula
- Meckel diverticulum

AIDS, acquired immunodeficiency syndrome

Imaging

After the patient is resuscitated, endoscopy or anoscopy is usually performed to identify and possibly treat a culprit lesion. In most individuals, minor or moderate bleeding stops spontaneously. In a minority, a source is actually found (and often treated) with endoscopy/colonoscopy. Contrary to popular teaching, colonoscopy after rapid cleansing is often useful in patients with active lower gastrointestinal bleeding.[38,40,41] Radionuclide scans or CT angiography are appropriate for assessing hemodynamically stable patients with moderate to severe but intermittent bleeding. The scan may localize the hemorrhage and determine whether it is brisk enough to be seen at catheter angiography. Patients with *continuous* rapid bleeding, transfusion of more than four to six units of packed red blood cells over 24 hours, or hemodynamic instability should undergo angiography without delay.

RADIONUCLIDE SCANNING

Scintigraphy is most often done with ^{99m}Tc-labeled red blood cells.[60,61] The threshold for detection of gastrointestinal bleeding is quoted as ranging from 0.05 to 0.4 mL/min, compared with a rate of about 0.5 to 1.0 mL/min with angiography.[62-64] However, these figures are based on animal models, phantom studies, and estimated transfusion requirements and are only approximations. Criteria for a positive study include progressive accumulation of activity corresponding to a segment of bowel and movement over time because of tracer transit[60,61,65] (Fig. 11-23). One important advantage of red cell scintigraphy is the ability to detect intermittent bleeding over a 24-hour period. Patients with a negative scan are observed. Patients with a positive scan should go to an interventional suite immediately. Localization by scintigraphy may guide arteriography but is sometimes misleading.[66]

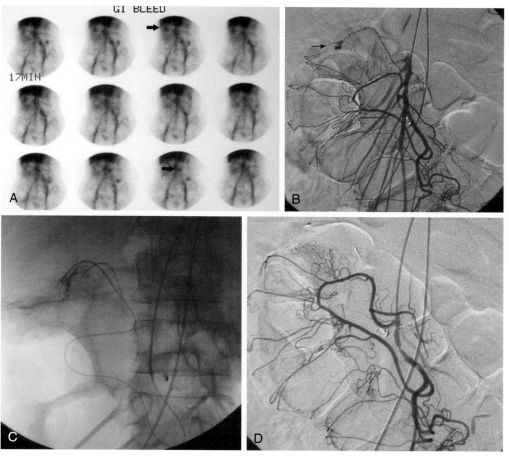

FIGURE 11-23   Right colonic bleed. **A,** Scintigraphy with ^{99m}Tc-labeled red blood cells shows early uptake in the right upper quadrant, which is consistent with hepatic flexure bleed *(arrow)*. **B,** The superior mesenteric arteriogram shows extravasation from a branch of the right colic artery *(arrow)*. **C,** Coaxial microcatheter is advanced to the site of bleeding. **D,** After placement of several microcoils and small Gelfoam pieces, bleeding has stopped.

COMPUTED TOMOGRAPHY ANGIOGRAPHY

Recently, contrast enhanced CT has become a popular method for noninvasive localization of gastrointestinal bleeding[67-71] (Fig. 11-24). The diagnosis requires the presence of hyperattenuated contrast material (compared with the noncontrast scans) within the bowel lumen. A recent metaanalysis of published work calculated a pooled mean sensitivity and specificity of 89% and 85%, respectively, for CT angiography. In the future, this more robust modality may entirely replace red cell scintigraphy in the imaging workup for this clinical situation.

CATHETER ANGIOGRAPHY

Nusbaum and Baum[72] pioneered the angiographic technique for evaluating gastrointestinal hemorrhage. The vessel most likely to supply the bleeding site (based on clinical scenario and results of endoscopy, scintigraphy, or CT angiography) is studied first. Upper gastrointestinal bleeding is evaluated by celiac arteriography, followed by superior mesenteric arteriography. If no bleeding site is found, selective left gastric or gastroduodenal arteriography may detect a subtle bleed. If results

of all these studies are negative, inferior mesenteric arteriography should be considered. Presumed lower gastrointestinal bleeding requires both superior mesenteric and inferior mesenteric arteriography. Some practitioners prefer to study the latter vessel first to minimize obscuration by the contrast-filled bladder. If results of both studies are negative, celiac arteriography is warranted. Aortography is needed only when ostial disease or variant anatomy makes catheterization difficult or when the examiner is trying to find other aortic branches that may be the source of bleeding (e.g., inferior phrenic artery). The entire length of bowel supplied by the injected artery must be visualized by using careful patient positioning and multiple angiographic runs. Selective injections are used to confirm suspicious findings on nonselective angiograms. Patients with suspected aortoenteric fistulas are studied by CT rather than angiography.

The hallmark of gastrointestinal hemorrhage is extravasation of contrast material into the bowel (see Fig. 11-23). Occasionally, extravasated contrast has a curvilinear shape that mimics a vascular structure ("pseudovein" sign) (Fig. 11-25). Several entities can be confused with

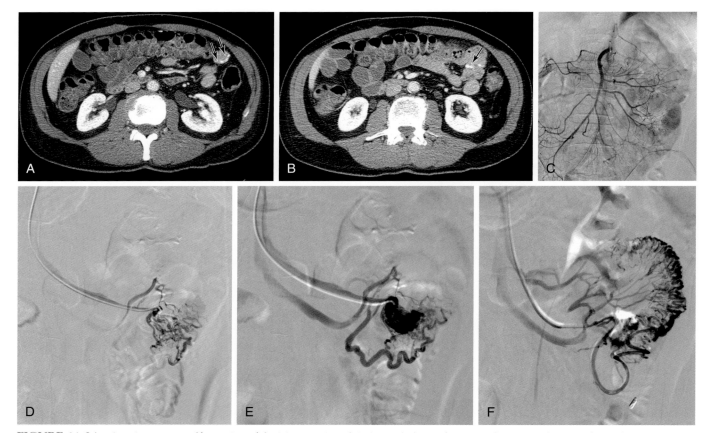

FIGURE 11-24   Arteriovenous malformation of the jejunum. **A** and **B,** Arterial phase of computed tomography scan shows dense round bumps on the wall of the jejunum *(arrows).* **C,** Superior mesenteric arteriography fails to show lesion prospectively. **D** and **E,** After sequential interrogation of jejunal branches, the vascular malformation is identified. **F,** More selective injection reveals the extent of the lesion.

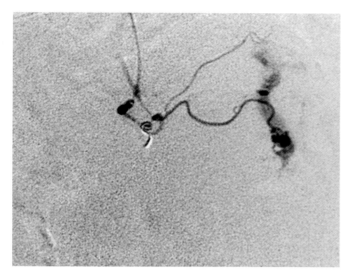

FIGURE 11-25 "Pseudovein" sign of gastrointestinal hemorrhage. The curvilinear, wormlike density in the middle descending colon persisted through the venous phase.

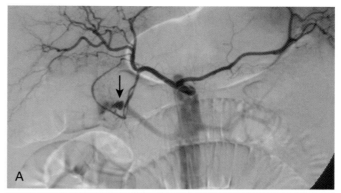

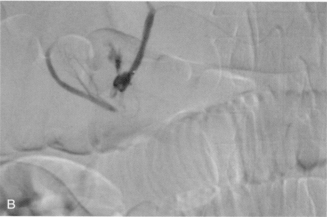

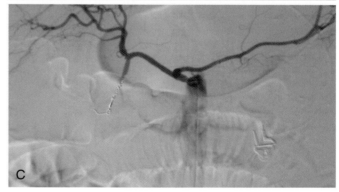

FIGURE 11-26 Duodenal ulcer hemorrhage. **A,** Extravasation *(arrow)* has occurred from duodenal branches of the gastroduodenal artery. **B,** Coils are placed across the gastroduodenal artery to isolate the bleeding vessels and prevent backflow from the superior mesenteric artery. **C,** Bleeding has ceased.

extravasation, including bowel subtraction artifact, hypervascular mucosa, parts of the renal collecting system, and adrenal gland opacification. The angiogram often can identify the bleeding site but usually provides no clue to the underlying condition (Fig. 11-26).

In some situations, frank extravasation of contrast is not seen but a pathologic finding points to the source of bleeding. For example, filling of varices at unsuspected sites (e.g., duodenum, cecum) may suggest a possible source for hemorrhage (see Fig. 12-14). Likewise, angiodysplasia is diagnosed by early and then persistent filling of a draining vein and by an abnormal cluster of vessels in the bowel wall (Fig. 11-27). Contrast extravasation usually is not seen. Lesions can be multiple. This anomaly is identified by early venous return out of a segment bowel or a "tram track" sign from simultaneous opacification of the feeding artery and draining vein. Because angiodysplasia is relatively common in elderly patients and may be an incidental finding, other sources of bleeding should also be considered. Congenital arteriovenous malformations can look identical.

Angiography identifies a bleeding source in upward of 50% of cases.[73-78] Higher rates in older reports probably reflect the inclusion of patients with more obvious bleeding sites now picked up by endoscopy. Not surprisingly, one lower gastrointestinal bleeding clinical series found positive studies in more than 80% of unstable patients with significant transfusion requirements (more than five units packed red cells) but in less than 20% of stable individuals.[74] The angiogram may be normal if bleeding has stopped, is intermittent, or is below the threshold for detection.[79] In some of these cases, provocative angiography may be warranted (see later discussion). Other reasons for a negative angiographic procedure include venous bleeding, failure to inject the correct artery, or bleeding outside the field of imaging.

Treatment

VASOPRESSIN INFUSION THERAPY

Once the mainstay of endovascular therapy for GI bleeding, vasopressin infusion is now relegated to a very minor (and mostly historic) role. Among other effects, the

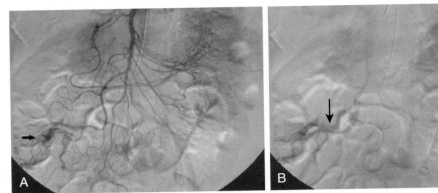

FIGURE 11-27   Angiodysplasia of the cecum. **A,** Early phase of superior mesenteric arteriogram shows a tangle of vessels in the cecum *(arrow).* **B,** Capillary phase exhibits early opacification of draining vein *(arrow).* Note that no venous drainage is seen from other portions of the bowel.

natural hormone *vasopressin (Pitressin)* causes constriction of smooth muscle of the bowel wall and splanchnic blood vessels. Infusion of the drug proximal to a bleeding mesenteric artery reduces blood flow, lowers the pulse pressure, and allows a clot to form.[80] Vasopressin is not useful for bleeding directly from a large artery (e.g., gastroduodenal bleed, splenic artery pseudoaneurysm) or at sites with dual blood supply (e.g., pyloroduodenal bleeding). It is contraindicated in patients with severe coronary artery disease, dysrhythmias, or malignant hypertension.

The catheter is placed in the central vessel feeding the bleeding site (celiac artery, LGA, SMA, or IMA). Vasopressin is infused at 0.2 units per minute. After 20 to 30 minutes, arteriography is repeated to look for residual bleeding and the presence of some direct or collateral blood flow to the viscera (see Fig. 1-4). If bleeding has stopped, the infusion is continued while the patient is monitored in an intensive care unit. If bleeding persists, the infusion rate is increased to 0.3 or 0.4 units per minute, and arteriography is repeated 20 to 30 minutes later. If the lesion is still bleeding, alternate forms of therapy should be pursued. Vasopressin therapy is continued for 6 to 24 hours and then gradually tapered over 12 to 48 hours.

Vasopressin therapy is initially very effective for certain types of gastrointestinal hemorrhage, particularly colonic diverticular and gastric mucosal hemorrhage. Initial success rates range from 60% to 90%.[81-83] However, rebleeding is the rule, and major adverse events are reported in up to 20% of cases.[84,85]

EMBOLIZATION

The goal of embolotherapy is to stop blood flow to the bleeding artery while maintaining viability of the bowel. For many years, embolization, particularly in the small intestine and colon, was avoided by angiographers because of the fear of bowel infarction.

However, with the development of coaxial microcatheters (which can be navigated directly to the site of bleeding) and newer embolic agents (e.g., microcoils), the risk of significant bowel ischemia is now very low.[86] Embolotherapy has the advantage of immediate and theoretically permanent control of bleeding without the risks of vasopressin infusion or prolonged catheterization. For these reasons, the procedure has become widely popular as first-line therapy for acute gastrointestinal hemorrhage.[86,87] Even in the absence of extravasation, empiric embolization of the LGA or GDA often is done to prevent recurrent bleeding in patients with massive upper gastrointestinal bleeding but negative angiograms[88-91] (Fig. 11-28).

Embolotherapy is feasible because of the extensive intestinal collateral circulation (particularly in the upper tract) through arterial arcades, communications between vasa recta, and submucosal interconnections. However, embolization is risky in the setting of previous gastric or bowel surgery or radiation therapy or when the collateral circulation is otherwise inadequate.[92]

Acute hemorrhage from angiodysplasia or arteriovenous malformations may initially respond to embolotherapy.[93,94] Contrary to popular wisdom, several recent series found that distal microembolization provided relatively durable obstruction for angiodysplasia in over 50% of cases.[93-95] Still, bleeding can recur, and those lesions should be removed operatively. In the case of right-sided angiodysplasia, a right hemicolectomy is performed to eliminate the bleeding lesion and any other occult lesions. Small bowel arteriovenous malformations are notoriously difficult to find at surgery. The involved segment of bowel is much easier to locate if a coil is deposited in a distal feeding branch or a coaxial microcatheter is left in place for methylene blue injection during the operation.[96,97]

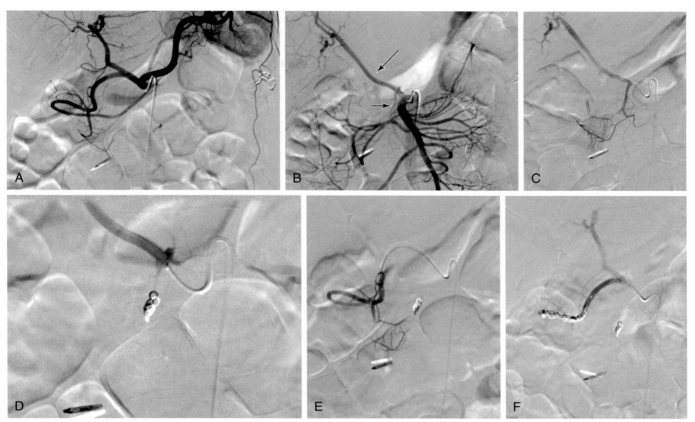

FIGURE 11-28 Prophylactic embolization for a young woman with graft vs. host disease and failed endoscopic clipping of an upper intestinal hemorrhage after duodenal biopsy. **A,** No active bleeding is seen on the celiac arteriogram. **B,** Superior mesenteric arteriography reveals a replaced right hepatic artery *(long arrow)*. A proximal branch *(short arrow)* was determined to be an anomalous pancreaticoduodenal vessel **(C). D,** Microcoils were deposited to occlude this potential bleeding source. Then, the gastroduodenal artery was selectively engaged with a microcatheter **(E)** and completely blocked with multiple microcoils **(F).** The patient did not bleed again.

TECHNIQUE A microcatheter is placed coaxially into the diagnostic catheter residing in the main trunk of the primary mesenteric artery. A steerable microwire is negotiated to the culprit arterial branch. It may be challenging to pick out the particular branch that is bleeding, so sequential injection into multiple vessels often is necessary. The optimal site for depositing embolic material is now established. Early teaching favored proximal occlusion.[98] Experts now recommend more peripheral embolization just proximal to the vasa recta feeding the bleeding site to minimize the length of bowel at risk for ischemia.[86,87,99]

The most commonly used embolic agents are microcoils, Gelfoam pieces, microparticles and cyanoacrylate (glue)[100,101] (Figs. 11-29 through 11-31). Coils can be delivered with precision and are permanent. Recanalization seems to be more frequent when microcoils are used alone.[91] Both large and small PVA particles (threshold 300 μm) have been used safely by some groups. Material is deposited until the bleeding has stopped.

If a lesion is situated within an arcade fed by two mesenteric arteries, angiography is performed at both levels. For example, after embolizing the GDA for a duodenal ulcer hemorrhage, a superior mesenteric arteriogram is done to evaluate the inferior pancreaticoduodenal supply to the duodenum. Embolization of the "back door" to the arcade may be necessary, although this increases the risk of ischemia[102,103] (Fig. 11-32). Before finishing the case, the proximal mesenteric artery is restudied to be certain there is no extravasation through collateral vessels.

RESULTS In contemporary series, embolotherapy successfully stops gastrointestinal bleeding in about 80% of patients.[54,94,95,104-112] The primary reason for technical failure is inability to obtain proper microcatheter position.[54] Recurrent hemorrhage (within 30 days of treatment) occurs in about 20% of cases (Box 11-5). Rebleeding may be more frequent with inflammatory lesions and arteriovenous malformations. If it occurs, repeat angiography (and embolization) may improve success rates by identification of recanalized sites and new sources of bleeding (see Fig. 11-32).

COMPLICATIONS Major adverse events occur in less than 5% of patients.[95] Patients should be monitored closely for clinical signs of ischemia (e.g., abdominal pain, elevated serum lactate), which occurs in well under 20% of cases.[95,100,113,114] In most instances, small areas of infarction are well tolerated and do not require surgery. With current interventional techniques, clinically significant bowel ischemia or infarction is reported in about 1% to 2% of cases.[54,87]

SURGICAL THERAPY

Emergency operation for acute gastrointestinal bleeding has a mortality of greater than 10%.[115,116] Surgery may be necessary when the disease cannot be treated definitively by transcatheter means (e.g., arteriovenous malformations) or when the lesion is malignant. Even in these cases, embolotherapy may be employed to stop or slow hemorrhage and allow the operation to be postponed until the patient is stabilized and the bowel is cleansed.

Chronic and Occult Gastrointestinal Bleeding (Online Case 77)

About 5% of patients with GI hemorrhage suffer from persistent, intermittent bleeding that may be difficult to localize (so-called obscure bleeding).[117-119] Arteriovenous malformations and neoplasms account for most of these cases (Box 11-6). These people typically have recurrent episodes of (usually lower) gastrointestinal bleeding that persist for months or years. Iron deficiency anemia is characteristic. The majority of responsible lesions are ultimately found in the small bowel or ascending colon, which are the most difficult sites to inspect with standard fiberoptic endoscopy. However, relatively new methods

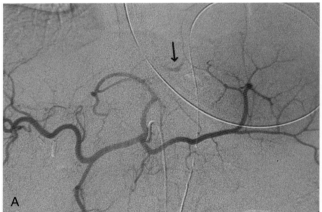

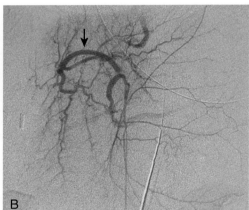

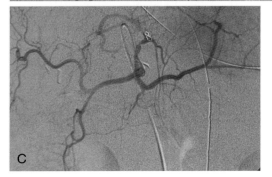

FIGURE 11-29   Gastric fundus bleeding. **A,** Celiac arteriogram shows extravasation from a branch of the left gastric artery *(arrow).* **B,** Left gastric arteriogram confirms bleeding. Also note replaced left hepatic artery *(arrow).* **C,** After Gelfoam and microcoil embolization, bleeding has stopped.

of push and double balloon enteroscopy and especially video capsule endoscopy are quite effective for localizing disease at these remote sites.[120]

Most patients have been through an exhaustive workup before an angiogram is requested. The approach to this vexing clinical problem is similar to the study of acute gastrointestinal hemorrhage. A bleeding source (i.e., pathologic finding or extravasation) is found in about half of examinations.[118,119] It is sometimes fruitful to repeat the angiogram at a later date if first study is unrewarding. *Provocative angiography* is advocated by some aggressive interventionalists to induce hemorrhage through full anticoagulation, intraarterial injection of vasodilators, and/or intraarterial fibrinolytic infusion.[121-126] This somewhat risky maneuver will undercover a bleeding site in one third to half of patients studied. Before attempting to

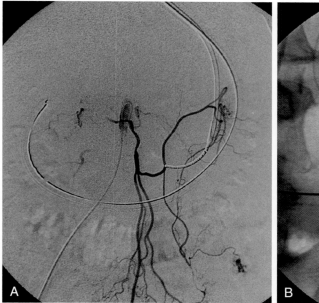

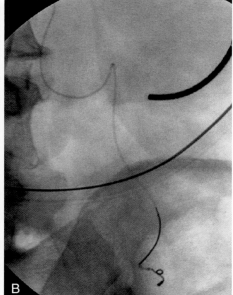

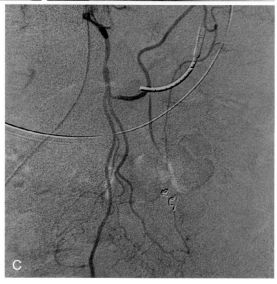

FIGURE 11-30 Massive lower gastrointestinal hemorrhage was treated with microcoil embolization. **A,** The inferior mesenteric arteriogram shows extravasation in the distal left colon. **B,** A coaxial microcatheter has been advanced to a site proximal to the vasa recta supplying the bleed. A second microcoil is being deployed. **C,** Extravasation has stopped on repeat injection of the inferior mesenteric artery, with preservation of flow to the remainder of the bowel.

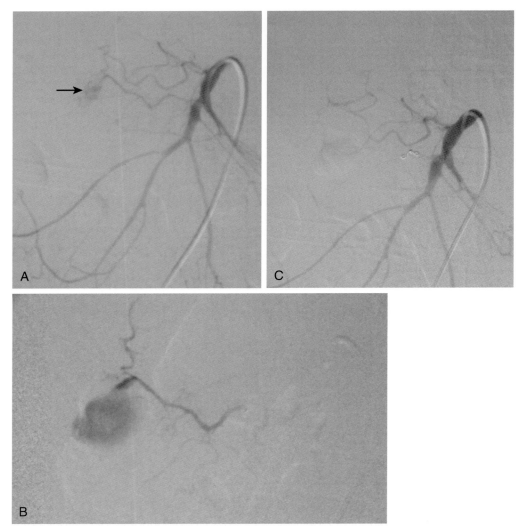

FIGURE 11-31   Duodenal hemorrhage after endoscopic sphincterotomy during endoscopic retrograde cholangiopancreatography. **A,** Superior mesenteric arteriogram shows extravasation *(arrow)* from a duodenal branch of the first jejunal artery. **B,** A microcatheter is advanced into the feeding vessel. **C,** After embolization, hemorrhage has stopped.

provoke bleeding, blood products and surgical backup should be available.

Neoplasms

Angiography plays no role in the evaluation of patients with suspected mesenteric neoplasms unless gastrointestinal bleeding occurs. Hypervascular intestinal tumors include leiomyomas, leiomyosarcomas, adenomas, adenocarcinomas with inflammatory reaction, and hypervascular metastases (e.g., choriocarcinoma, melanoma). Adenocarcinomas and most metastatic lesions are hypovascular. *Carcinoid* of the small intestine has a characteristic appearance. Because the tumor liberates hormones that incite an infiltrating, desmoplastic reaction in the mesentery, the arteries are retracted, narrowed, irregular, or obstructed.[127] Tumors outside the intestinal tract can invade mesenteric vessels.

OTHER DISORDERS

Celiac Artery Compression (Median Arcuate Ligament) Syndrome (Online Case 46)

The root of the celiac artery is draped by the *median arcuate ligament*, which connects the crura of the diaphragm. Mild to moderate compression of the superior aspect of the artery by this ligament is seen frequently on CT or MR angiograms in patients without intestinal symptoms[128,129] (Fig. 11-33). A few patients with severe compression or occlusion of the artery also complain of abdominal pain, weight loss, and nausea. The resulting clinical syndrome is classically seen in young, asthenic women. Compression is exaggerated during *expiration.*

The relationship between celiac artery compression and the associated clinical syndrome is controversial.[130,131]

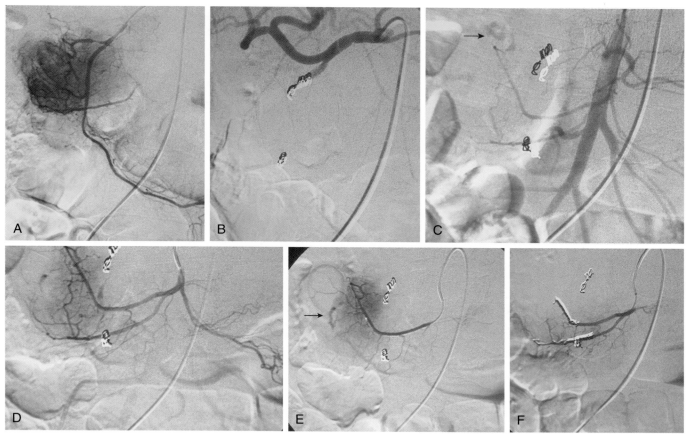

FIGURE 11-32   Recurrent upper gastrointestinal bleeding due to collateral arcade circulation. **A,** Initial gastroduodenal arteriogram shows marked hypervascularity without frank extravasation. The feeding branches could not be selectively catheterized. **B,** Embolization was performed across the gastroduodenal artery. **C,** Patient developed recurrent bleeding. Repeat gastroduodenal arteriography confirmed persistent occlusion (not shown). Superior mesenteric arteriography is suspicious for bleeding from the inferior pancreaticoduodenal artery *(arrow).* **D,** Selective catheterization confirms the bleeding. **E,** The first of two feeding vessels is selected up to the site of bleeding *(arrow).* **F,** After embolization of both distal vessels, bleeding has stopped.

The SMA and IMA are usually patent in these patients, and the existing collateral circulation should be adequate to prevent intestinal ischemia. Nonetheless, symptoms have been attributed to visceral ischemia or to compression of the celiac neural plexus. Surgical treatment, which may include division of the crus, release of sympathetic nerve fibers, and revascularization, is often curative, although the results may not be durable.[130,132]

Aneurysms

Aneurysms of the mesenteric arteries are uncommon. Splenic and hepatic artery aneurysms, which are the most common splanchnic aneurysms, are considered in Chapter 12. The very rare SMA and celiac artery aneurysms (both true and false) are caused by atherosclerosis, a degenerative vasculopathy, infection, or trauma[133-137] (Fig. 11-34). A few patients present with abdominal discomfort, but most are diagnosed incidentally on imaging studies. The natural history of these aneurysms is that of progressive expansion, rupture, or thrombosis. Stent graft placement is often employed when feasible.

Gastric, duodenal, or pancreaticoduodenal artery pseudoaneurysm is a rare complication of an adjacent inflammatory process (e.g., pancreatitis, peptic ulcer disease), trauma, or hyperdynamic state[138] (Fig. 11-35). Many of these patients present with gastrointestinal tract or intraabdominal bleeding and abdominal pain (see Fig. 13-6). The growth rate is unpredictable, and such aneurysms are often lethal without treatment. The preferred therapy is transcatheter embolization.[139,140]

Vasculitis

Mesenteric arteritis is rare. A wide variety of small vessel vasculitides may cause nonspecific findings on CT and MR (segments of bowel wall thickening and enhancement, bowel distention, venous thrombosis) related to inflammation, ulcerations, ischemia, and perforation.[141,142] These include Wegener granulomatosis, microscopic

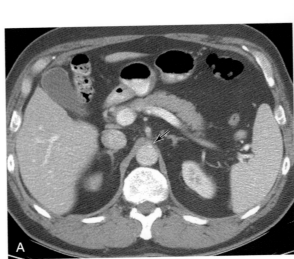
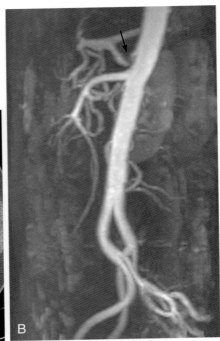

FIGURE 11-33   Celiac artery compression in an asymptomatic patient. **A,** Transverse computed tomography image reveals impingement of diaphragmatic crus on the superior aspect of the celiac artery origin *(arrow)*. **B,** Gadolinium-enhanced magnetic resonance angiogram in sagittal projection depicts proximal celiac artery stenosis *(arrow)*.

polyangiitis, Henoch-Schönlein purpura, collagen vascular diseases, and Behçet syndrome.

Takayasu arteritis is an inflammatory vasculitis of large- and medium-sized arteries[143,144] (see Chapter 1). Stenosis or, rarely, complete occlusion of the mesenteric arteries associated with abdominal aortic narrowing occurs in about 20% of cases.

Polyarteritis nodosa (PAN) is a necrotizing vasculitis that can affect distal branches of the mesenteric arteries, producing multiple small saccular aneurysms.[145] Some of these patients present with abdominal pain, gastrointestinal hemorrhage, or ischemia. Branches of the renal, hepatic, splenic, and pancreatic arteries often are involved.

Radiation arteritis can develop after high-dose radiation therapy for abdominal or pelvic malignancies. The condition may lead to irregular narrowing and occlusion of mesenteric arteries and veins.[146]

Buerger disease is an occlusive vasculitis that primarily affects small vessels of the extremities (see Chapter 1). However, mesenteric artery involvement has been described.[147]

Arteriovenous Malformations

Arteriovenous malformations are congenital lesions that can occur at any site in the intestinal tract. They may cause chronic, intermittent gastrointestinal hemorrhage

(see Fig. 11-24). *Angiodysplasia* (i.e., *vascular ectasia*) is an acquired anomaly of submucosal veins found primarily in the ascending colon (see Fig. 11-27). *Telangiectasias* and *angiomas* are usually associated with congenital or hereditary syndromes, including hereditary hemorrhagic telangiectasia, Klippel-Trenaunay syndrome, and blue rubber nevus syndrome.[148,149] In these disorders, multiple, punctate hypervascular lesions are typically scattered throughout the bowel (Fig. 11-36). In advanced cases, vascular tangles and arteriovenous shunting may be seen. *Arteriovenous fistulas* are acquired lesions that usually result from penetrating trauma.[150]

Trauma

Most injuries are caused by penetrating trauma, although SMA or superior mesenteric vein disruption can occur with blunt or decelerating trauma or catheterization procedures.[151,152] Patients with penetrating trauma to the central mesenteric arteries usually die before reaching medical care. Those who survive present with massive hemoperitoneum or mesenteric hematoma and usually undergo emergency laparotomy without imaging evaluation. Trauma may also lead to vascular occlusion, arteriovenous fistula, or pseudoaneurysm (Fig. 11-37). Isolated mesenteric artery injuries have been successfully treated with embolotherapy.[150,153]

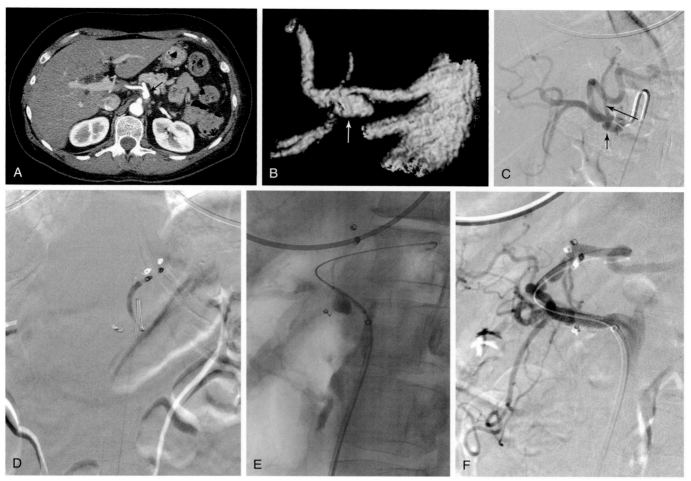

FIGURE 11-34   Dysplastic celiac artery aneurysm. **A** and **B,** Contrast-enhanced axial and shaded surface display sagittal reformatted computed tomography images show a saccular aneurysm arising from the undersurface of the celiac artery *(arrow)*. **C,** Lateral celiac arteriogram displays the aneurysm *(short arrow)*. Note origin of left gastric artery (LGA, *long arrow*) across from aneurysm. The LGA is embolized first to prevent retrograde flow from pressurizing the aneurysm after a stent graft covers the aneurysm neck **(D).** The balloon expandable covered stent is positioned across the aneurysm neck **(E),** and final arteriogram shows aneurysm exclusion **(F).**

Segmental Arterial Mediolysis and Fibromuscular Dysplasia

These rare noninflammatory conditions may be related.[154,155] Unlike classic fibromuscular dysplasia (which is rarely seen in the mesenteric arteries [Fig. 11-38]), segmental arterial mediolysis primarily affects the visceral and coronary arteries. Pathologically, it is characterized by patchy destruction of medial smooth muscles cells that are replaced by fibrin, collagen, and granulation tissue. The weakened arterial wall is predisposed to aneurysm formation and spontaneous dissection (Fig. 11-39). In the abdomen, patients present with vessel rupture and massive bleeding. Celiac artery branches are most commonly affected.[156-158] Multiple lesions may be present. Embolotherapy of affected vessels has been reported.[159]

Coarctation Syndromes

The abdominal coarctation syndromes are rare congenital disorders that can narrow the abdominal aorta and its major branches (see Chapters 1 and 7). Abdominal coarctation is seen in patients with neurofibromatosis, congenital rubella, Williams syndrome, and tuberous sclerosis. Although renovascular hypertension from renal artery stenoses is common, mesenteric ischemia is rare.

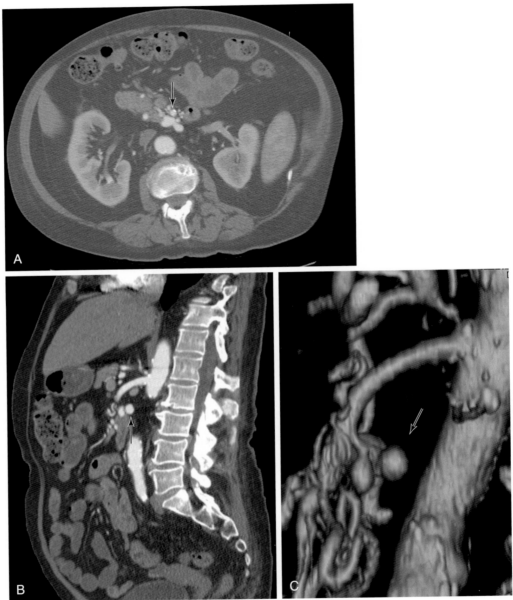

FIGURE 11-35 Pancreaticoduodenal artery aneurysms because of hyperdynamic flow from celiac artery occlusion. Axial **(A)**, reformatted sagittal **(B)**, and shaded surface display **(C)** computed tomography angiograms show dilated aneurysms in the pancreaticoduodenal arcade bed *(arrows)*. The celiac artery is occluded, so flow in the arcade has markedly increased and caused aneurysm formation.

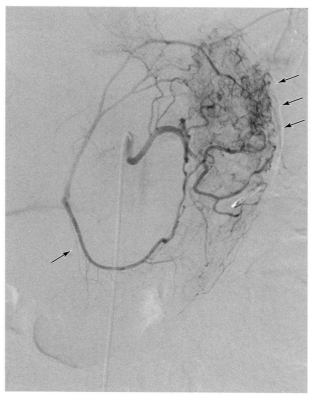

FIGURE 11-36 Multiple telangiectasias of the stomach *(arrows)* in a patient with hereditary hemorrhagic telangiectasia. Note the communication of the injected left gastric artery with the right gastric artery *(single arrow)*.

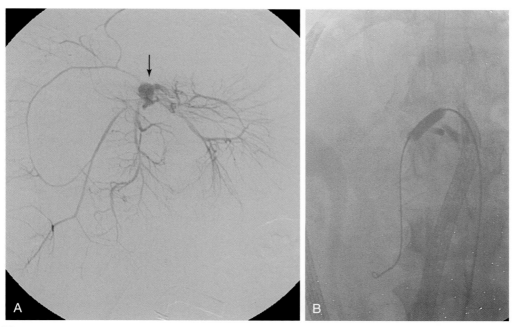

FIGURE 11-37 Superior mesenteric artery (SMA) root pseudoaneurysm from blunt trauma. Patient sent to interventional radiology directly from emergent laparotomy because of uncontrollable hemorrhage. **A,** SMA angiography shows large pseudoaneurysm of SMA root *(arrow)*. **B,** A balloon was inflated to stop bleeding while the patient returned to the operating room.

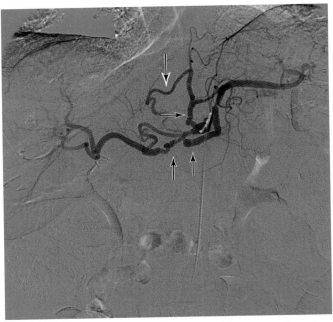

FIGURE 11-38   Fibromuscular dysplasia of the common hepatic, left gastric, and proximal splenic arteries *(short arrows.)* Note accessory left hepatic artery from the left gastric artery *(long arrow)*.

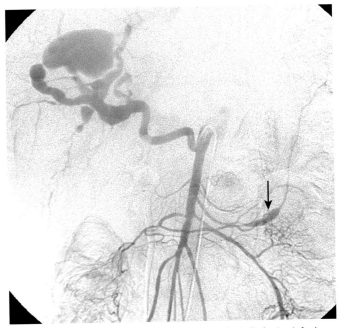

FIGURE 11-39   Probable segmental arterial mediolysis. A fusiform aneurysm of the middle colic artery is identified *(arrow)*. Also seen are multiple saccular aneurysms of branches of the replaced right hepatic artery.

References

1. Collins P, editor. Embryology and development. In: Williams PL, Bannister LH, Berry MM, et al, editors. *Gray's anatomy*. 38th ed. New York: Churchill Livingstone; 1995: p.318.

2. Gabella G, editor. Cardiovascular system. In: Williams PL, Bannister LH, Berry MM, et al, editors. *Gray's anatomy*, 38th ed. New York, Churchill Livingstone; 1995: p. 1548.

3. Kornblith PL, Boley SJ, Whitehouse BS. Anatomy of the splanchnic circulation. *Surg Clin North Am* 1992;**72**:1.

4. Liu DM, Salem R, Bui JT, et al. Angiographic considerations in patients undergoing liver-directed therapy. *J Vasc Interv Radiol* 2005;**16**:911.

5. Hazirolan T, Metin Y, Karaosmanoglu AD, et al. Mesenteric arterial variations detected at MDCT angiography of abdominal aorta. *AJR Am J Roentgenol* 2009;**192**:1097.

6. Michels NA, Siddharth P, Kornblith PL, et al. Routes of collateral circulation of the gastrointestinal tract as ascertained in a dissection of 500 bodies. *Int Surg* 1968;**49**:8.

7. Berland T, Oldenburg WA. Acute mesenteric ischemia. *Curr Gastroenterol Rep* 2008;**10**:341.

8. Herbert GS, Steele SR. Acute and chronic mesenteric ischemia. *Surg Clin North Am* 2007;**87**:1115.

9. Hassoun Z, Lacrosse M, DeRonde T. Intestinal involvement in Buerger's disease. *J Clin Gastroenterol* 2001;**32**:85.

10. Osorio J, Farreras N, Ortiz De Zarate L, et al. Cocaine-induced mesenteric ischemia. *Dig Surg* 2000;**17**:648.

11. Bassiouny HS. Non-occlusive mesenteric ischemia. *Surg Clin North Am* 1997;**77**:319.

12. Kolkman JJ, Mensink PB. Non-occlusive mesenteric ischemia: a common disorder in gastroenterology and intensive care. *Best Pract Res Clin Gastroenterol* 2003;**17**:457.

13. Park WM, Gloviczki P, Cherry Jr KJ, et al. Contemporary management of acute mesenteric ischemia: factors associated with survival. *J Vasc Surg* 2002;**35**:445.

14. Paterno F, Longo WE. The etiology and pathogenesis of vascular disorders of the intestine. *Radiol Clin North Am* 2008;**46**:877.

15. Chang JB, Stein TA. Mesenteric ischemia: acute and chronic. *Ann Vasc Surg* 2003;**17**:323.

16. Schoots IG, Koffeman GI, Legemate DA, et al. Systematic review of survival after acute mesenteric ischaemia according to disease aetiology. *Br J Surg* 2004;**91**:17.

17. Kim JK, Ha HK, Byun JY, et al. CT differentiation of mesenteric ischemia due to vasculitis and thromboembolic disease. *J Comput Assist Tomogr* 2001;**25**:604.

18. Horton KM, Fishman EK. Multidetector CT angiography in the diagnosis of mesenteric ischemia. *Radiol Clin North Am* 2007; **45**:275.

19. Shih MC, Angle JF, Leung DA, et al. CTA and MRA in mesenteric ischemia: part 2, normal findings and complications after surgical and endovascular treatment. *AJR Am J Roentgenol* 2007;**188**:462.

20. Furukawa A, Kanasaki S, Kono N, et al. CT diagnosis of acute mesenteric ischemia from various causes. *AJR Am J Roentgenol* 2009;**192**:408.

21. Bradbury MS, Kavanagh PV, Bechtold RE, et al. Mesenteric venous thrombosis: diagnosis and non-invasive imaging. *Radiographics* 2002;**22**:527.

22. Trompeter M, Brazda T, Remy CT, et al. Non-occlusive mesenteric ischemia: etiology, diagnosis, and interventional therapy. *Eur Radiol* 2002;**12**:1179.

23. Schermerhorn ML, Giles KA, Hamdan AD, et al. Mesenteric revascularization: management and outcomes in the United States, 1988-2006. *J Vasc Surg* 2009;**50**:341.

24. Kouglas P, Lau D, El Sayed HF, et al. Determinants of mortality and treatment outcome following surgical interventions for acute mesenteric ischemia. *J Vasc Surg* 2007;**46**:467.

25. Schoots IG, Levi MM, Reekers JA, et al. Thrombolytic therapy for acute superior mesenteric artery occlusion. *J Vasc Interv Radiol* 2005;**16**:317.

26. Train JS, Ross H, Weiss JD, et al. Mesenteric venous thrombosis: successful treatment by intraarterial lytic therapy. *J Vasc Interv Radiol* 1998;**9**:461.

27. Vedantham S, Picus D, Sanchez LA, et al. Percutaneous management of ischemic complications in patients with type B aortic dissection. *J Vasc Interv Radiol* 2002;**14**:181.

28. Patel HJ, Williams DM, Meerkov M, et al. Long term results of percutaneous management of malperfusion in acute type B aortic dissection: implications for thoracic aortic endovascular repair. *J Thorac Cardiovasc Surg* 2009;**138**:300.

29. Moneta GL, Lee RW, Yeager RA, et al. Mesenteric duplex scanning: a blinded, prospective study. *J Vasc Surg* 1993;**17**:79.

30. Lim HK, Lee WJ, Kim SH, et al. Splanchnic arterial stenosis or occlusion: diagnosis at Doppler US. *Radiology* 1999;**211**:405.

31. Moneta GL. Screening for mesenteric vascular insufficiency and follow-up of mesenteric artery bypass procedures. *Semin Vasc Surg* 2001;**14**:186.

32. Rose SC, Quigley TM, Raker EJ. Revascularization for chronic mesenteric ischemia: comparison of operative arterial bypass grafting and percutaneous transluminal angioplasty. *J Vasc Interv Radiol* 1995;**6**:339.

33. Brown DJ, Schermerhorn ML, Powell RJ, et al. Mesenteric stenting for chronic mesenteric ischemia. *J Vasc Surg* 2005;**42**:268.

34. Atkins MD, Kwolek CJ, LaMuraglia GM, et al. Surgical revascularization versus endovascular therapy for chronic mesenteric ischemia: a comparative experience. *J Vasc Surg* 2007;**45**:1162.

35. Sharafuddin MJ, Olson CH, Sun S, et al. Endovascular treatment of celiac and mesenteric arteries stenoses: applications and results. *J Vasc Surg* 2003;**38**:692.

36. Sarac TP, Altinel O, Kashyap V, et al. Endovascular treatment of stenotic and occluded visceral arteries for chronic mesenteric ischemia. *J Vasc Surg* 2008;**47**:485.

37. Barnert J, Messmann H. Diagnosis and management of lower gastrointestinal bleeding. *Nat Rev Gastroenterol Hepatol* 2009;**6**:637.

38. Farrell JJ, Friedman LS. The management of lower gastrointestinal bleeding. *Aliment Pharmacol Ther* 2005;**21**:1281.

39. Cappell MS, Friedel D. Acute nonvariceal upper gastrointestinal bleeding: endoscopic diagnosis and therapy. *Med Clin North Am* 2008;**92**:511.

40. Chaudry V, Hyser MJ, Gracias VH, et al. Colonoscopy: the initial test for acute lower gastrointestinal bleeding. *Am Surg* 1998;**64**:723.

41. Ohyama T, Sakurai Y, Ito M, et al. Analysis of urgent colonoscopy for lower gastrointestinal tract bleeding. *Digestion* 2000;**61**:189.

42. van Leerdam ME. Epidemiology of acute upper gastrointestinal bleeding. *Best Pract Res Clin Gastroenterol* 2008;**22**:209.

43. Higuchi N, Akahoshi K, Sumida Y, et al. Endoscopic band ligation therapy for upper gastrointestinal bleeding related to Mallory-Weiss syndrome. *Surg Endosc* 2006;**20**:1431.

44. Hyare H, Desigan s, Brookes JA, et al. Endovascular management of major arterial hemorrhage as a complication of inflammatory pancreatic disease. *J Vasc Interv Radiol* 2007;**18**:591.

45. Srivastava DN, Sharma S, Pal S, et al. Transcatheter arterial embolization in the management of hemobilia. *Abdom Imaging* 2006;**31**:439.

46. Dasgupta R, Davies NJ, Williamson RC, et al. Haemosuccus pancreaticus: treatment by arterial embolization. *Clin Radiol* 2002;**57**:1021.

47. Busuttil SJ, Goldstone J. Diagnosis and management of aortoenteric fistula. *Semin Vasc Surg* 2001;**14**:302.

48. Oglevie SB, Smith DC, Mera SS. Bleeding marginal ulcers: angiographic evaluation. *Radiology* 1990;**174**:943.

49. Durham JD, Kumpe DA, Rothbarth LJ, et al. Dieulafoy disease: arteriographic findings and treatment. *Radiology* 1990;**174**:937.

50. Baxter M, Aly EH. Dieulafoy's lesion: current trends in diagnosis and management. *Ann R Coll Surg Engl* 2010;**92**:548.

51. Zuccaro G. Epidemiology of lower gastrointestinal bleeding. *Best Pract Res Clin Gastroenterol* 2008;**22**:225.

52. Longstreth GF. Epidemiology and outcome of patients hospitalized with acute lower gastrointestinal hemorrhage: a population-based study. *Am J Gastroenterol* 1997;**92**:419.

53. Vernava AM, Longo WE, Virgo KS. A nationwide study of the incidence and etiology of lower gastrointestinal bleeding. *Surg Res Commun* 1996;**18**:113.

54. Weldon DT, Burke SJ, Sun S, et al. Interventional management of lower gastrointestinal bleeding. *Eur Radiol* 2008;**18**:857.

55. Jensen DM, Machicado GA. Diagnosis and treatment of severe hematochezia. The role of emergent colonoscopy after purge. *Gastroenterology* 1988;**95**:1569.

56. Lewis M. Bleeding colonic diverticula. *J Clin Gastroenterol* 2008;**42**:1156.

57. Boley SJ, Brandt LJ. Vascular ectasias of the colon—1986. *Dig Dis Sci* 1986;**31**(Suppl. 9):26S.

58. Sharma VS, Valji K, Bookstein JJ. Gastrointestinal hemorrhage in AIDS: arteriographic diagnosis and transcatheter treatment. *Radiology* 1992;**185**:447.

59. Olson DE,Kim YW, Donnelly LF. CT findings in children with Meckel diverticulum. *Pediatr Radiol* 2009;**39**:659.

60. Howarth DM. The role of nuclear medicine in the detection of acute gastrointestinal bleeding. *Semin Nucl Med* 2006;**36**:133.

61. Zink SI, Ohki SK, Stein B, et al. Noninvasive evaluation of active lower gastrointestinal bleeding: comparison between contrast-enhanced MDCT and 99m Tc-labeled RBC scintigraphy. *AJR Am J Roentgenol* 2008;**191**:1107.

62. Smith R, Copely DJ, Bolen FH. 99mTc RBC scintigraphy: correlation of gastrointestinal bleeding rates with scintigraphic findings. *AJR Am J Roentgenol* 1987;**148**:869.

63. Chandeysson PL, Hanson RJ, Watson CE, et al. Minimum gastrointestinal bleeding rate detectable by abdominal scintigraphy (abstract). *J Nucl Med* 1983;**24**:P97.

64. Nusbaum M, Baum S. Radiographic demonstration of unknown sites of gastrointestinal bleeding. *Surg Forum* 1963;**14**:374.

65. Holder LE. Radionuclide imaging in the evaluation of acute gastrointestinal bleeding. *Radiographics* 2000;**20**:1153.

66. Hunter JM, Pezim ME. Limited value of technetium 99m-labeled red cell scintigraphy in localization of lower gastrointestinal bleeding. *Am J Surg* 1990;**159**:504.

67. Sabharwal R, Vladica P, Chou R, et al. Helical CT in the diagnosis of acute lower gastrointestinal haemorrhage. *Eur J Radiol* 2006;**58**:273.

68. Wu LM, Xu JR, Yin Y, et al. Usefulness of CT angiography in diagnosing acute gastrointestinal bleeding: a meta-analysis. *World J Gastroenter* 2010;**16**:3957.

69. Yoon W, Jeong YY, Shin SS, et al. Acute massive gastrointestinal bleeding: detection and localization with arterial phase multidetector row helical CT. *Radiology* 2006;**239**:160.

70. Laing CJ, Tobias T, Rosenblum DI, et al. Acute gastrointestinal bleeding: emerging role of multidetector CT angiography and review of current imaging techniques. *Radiographics* 2007;**27**:1055.

71. Jaeckle T, Stuber G, Hoffmann MH, et al. Detection and localization of acute upper and lower gastrointestinal bleeding with arterial phase multi-detector row helical CT. *Eur Radiol* 2008;**18**:1406.

72. Nusbaum M, Baum S, Blakemore W, et al. Demonstration of intraabdominal bleeding by selective arteriography. *JAMA* 1965;**191**:117.

73. Whitaker SC, Gregson RHS. The role of angiography in the investigation of acute or chronic gastrointestinal haemorrhage. *Clin Radiol* 1993;**47**:382.

74. Abbas SM, Bissett IP, Holden A, et al. Clinical variables associated with positive angiographic localization of lower gastrointestinal bleeding. *ANZ J Surg* 2005;**75**:953.

75. Browder W, Cerise EJ, Litwin MS. Impact of emergency angiography in massive lower gastrointestinal bleeding. *Ann Surg* 1986; **204**:530.

76. Millward SF. ACR Appropriateness Criteria on treatment of acute nonvariceal gastrointestinal tract bleeding. *J Am Coll Radiol* 2008;**5**:550.

77. Allison DJ, Hemingway AP, Cunningham DA. Angiography in gastrointestinal bleeding. *Lancet* 1982;**2**:30.

78. Wagner HE, Stain SC, Gilg M, et al. Systematic assessment of massive bleeding of the lower part of the gastrointestinal tract. *Surg Gynecol Obstet* 1992;**175**:445.

79. Sos TA, Lee JG, Wixson D, et al. Intermittent bleeding from minute to minute in acute massive gastrointestinal hemorrhage: arteriographic demonstration. *AJR Am J Roentgenol* 1978;**131**:1015.

80. Baum S, Athanasoulis CA, Waltman AC. Angiographic diagnosis and control of large-bowel bleeding. *Dis Colon Rectum* 1974;**17**:447.

81. Athanasoulis CA, Baum S, Roesch J, et al. Mesenteric arterial infusions of vasopressin for hemorrhage from colonic diverticulosis. *Am J Surg* 1975;**129**:212.

82. Gomes AS, Lois JF, McCoy RD. Angiographic treatment of gastrointestinal hemorrhage: comparison of vasopressin infusion and embolization. *AJR Am J Roentgenol* 1986;**146**:1031.

83. Eckstein MR, Kelemouridis V, Athanasoulis CA, et al. Gastric bleeding: therapy with intraarterial vasopressin and transcatheter embolization. *Radiology* 1984;**152**:643.

84. Conn HO, Ramsby GR, Storer EH. Selective intra-arterial vasopressin in the treatment of upper gastrointestinal hemorrhage. *Gastroenterology* 1972;**63**:634.

85. Roberts C, Maddison FE. Partial mesenteric arterial occlusion with subsequent ischemic bowel damage due to pitressin infusion. *AJR Am J Roentgenol* 1976;**126**:829.

86. Funaki B. Superselective embolization of lower gastrointestinal hemorrhage: a new paradigm. *Abdom Imaging* 2004;**29**:434.

87. Darcy M. Treatment of lower gastrointestinal bleeding: vasopressin infusion versus embolization. *J Vasc Interv Radiol* 2003;**14**:535.

88. Lang EV, Picus D, Marx MV, et al. Massive upper gastrointestinal hemorrhage with normal findings at arteriography: value of prophylactic embolization of the left gastric artery. *AJR Am J Roentgenol* 1992;**158**:547.

89. Morris DC, Nichols DM, Connell DG, et al. Embolization of the left gastric artery in the absence of angiographic extravasation. *Cardiovasc Intervent Radiol* 1986;**9**:195.

90. Padia SA, Geisinger MA, Newman JS, et al. Effectiveness of coil embolization in angiographically detectable versus non-detectable sources of upper gastrointestinal hemorrhage. *J Vasc Interv Radiol* 2009;**20**:461.

91. Aina R, Oliva VL, Therasse E, et al. Arterial embolotherapy for upper gastrointestinal hemorrhage: outcome assessment. *J Vasc Interv Radiol* 2001;**12**:195.

92. Roesch J, Keller FS, Kozak B, et al. Gelfoam powder embolization of the left gastric artery in treatment of massive small-vessel gastric bleeding. *Radiology* 1984;**151**:365.

93. Defreyne L, Vanlangenhove P, DeVos M, et al. Embolization as a first approach with endoscopically unmanageable acute nonvariceal gastrointestinal hemorrhage. *Radiology* 2001;**218**:739.

94. Funaki B, Kostelic JK, Lorenz J, et al. Superselective microcoil embolization of colonic hemorrhage. *AJR Am J Roentgenol* 2001;**177**:829.

95. Bandi R, Shetty PC, Sharma RP, et al. Superselective arterial embolization for the treatment of lower gastrointestinal hemorrhage. *J Vasc Interv Radiol* 2001;**12**:1399.

96. Athanasoulis CA, Moncure AC, Greenfield AJ, et al. Intraoperative localization of small bowel bleeding sites with combined use of angiographic methods and methylene blue injection. *Surgery* 1980;**87**:77.

97. Schmidt SP, Boskind JF, Smith DC, et al. Angiographic localization of small bowel angiodysplasia with use of platinum coils. *J Vasc Interv Radiol* 1993;**4**:737.

98. Palmaz JC, Walter JF, Cho KJ. Therapeutic embolization of the small-bowel arteries. *Radiology* 1984;**152**:377.

99. Okazaki M, Furui S, Higashihara H, et al. Emergent embolotherapy of small intestinal hemorrhage. *Gastrointest Radiol* 1992;**17**:223.

100. Guy GE, Shetty PC, Sharma R, et al. Acute lower gastrointestinal hemorrhage: treatment by superselective embolization with polyvinyl alcohol particles. *AJR Am J Roentgenol* 1992;**159**:521.

101. Frodsham A, Berkmen T, Ananian C, et al. Initial experience using N-butyl cyanoacrylate for embolization of lower gastrointestinal hemorrhage. *J Vasc Interv Radiol* 2009;**20**:1312.

102. Bell SD, Lau KY, Sniderman KW. Synchronous embolization of the gastroduodenal artery and the inferior pancreaticoduodenal artery in patients with massive duodenal hemorrhage. *J Vasc Interv Radiol* 1995;**6**:531.

103. Okazaki M, Higashihara H, Ono H, et al. Embolotherapy of massive duodenal hemorrhage. *Gastrointest Radiol* 1992;**17**:319.

104. Defreyne L, Vanlangenhove P, deVos M, et al. Embolization as a first approach with endoscopically unmanageable acute nonvariceal gastrointestinal hemorrhage. *Radiology* 2001;**218**:739.

105. Eriksson LG, Ljungdahl M, Sundbom M, et al. Transcatheter arterial embolization versus surgery in the treatment of upper gastrointestinal bleeding after therapeutic endoscopic failure. *J Vasc Interv Radiol* 2008;**19**:1413.

106. Schenker MP, Duszak R, Soulen MC, et al. Upper gastrointestinal hemorrhage and transcatheter embolotherapy: clinical and technical factors impacting success and survival. *J Vasc Interv Radiol* 2001;**12**:1263.

107. Kuo WT, Lee DE, Saad WE, et al. Superselective microcoil embolization for the treatment of lower gastrointestinal hemorrhage. *J Vasc Interv Radiol* 2003;**14**:1503.

108. Maleux G, Roeflaer F, Heye S, et al. Long-term outcome of transcatheter embolotherapy for acute lower gastrointestinal hemorrhage. *Am J Gastroenterol* 2009;**104**:2042.

109. Khanna A, Ognibene SJ, Koniaris LG. Embolization as first-line therapy for diverticulosis-related massive lower gastrointestinal bleeding: evidence from a meta-analysis. *J Gastrointest Surg* 2005;**9**:343.

110. d'Othee BJ, Surapaneni P, Rabkin D, et al. Microcoil embolization for acute lower gastrointestinal bleeding. *Cardiovasc Intervent Radiol* 2006;**29**:49.

111. Neuman HB, Zarzaur BL, Meyer AA, et al. Superselective catheterization and embolization as first-line therapy for lower gastrointestinal bleeding. *Am Surg* 2005;**71**:539.

112. Kickuth R, Rattunde H, Gschossmann J, et al. Acute lower gastrointestinal hemorrhage: minimally invasive management with microcatheter embolization. *J Vasc Interv Radiol* 2008;**19**:1289.

113. Gillespie CJ, Sutherland AD, Mossop PJ, et al. Mesenteric embolization for lower gastrointestinal bleeding. *Dis Colon Rectum* 2010;**53**:1258.

114. Rosenkrantz H, Bookstein JJ, Rosen RJ, et al. Postembolic colonic infarction. *Radiology* 1982;**142**:47.

115. Bohhari M, Vernava AM, Ure T, et al. Diverticular hemorrhage in the elderly—is it well tolerated? *Dis Colon Rectum* 1996;**39**:191.

116. Wagner HE, Stain SC, Gilg M, et al. Systematic assessment of massive bleeding of the lower part of the gastrointestinal tract. *Surg Gynecol Obstet* 1992;**175**:445.

117. Singh V, Alexander JA. The evaluation and management of obscure and occult gastrointestinal bleeding. *Abdom Imaging* 2009;**34**:311.

118. Concha R, Amaro R, Barkin JS. Obscure gastrointestinal bleeding: diagnostic and therapeutic approach. *J Clin Gastroenterol* 2007;**41**:242.

119. Lin S, Rockey DC. Obscure gastrointestinal bleeding. *Gastroenterol Clin North Am* 2005;**34**:679.

120. Triester SL, Leighton JA, Leontiadis GI, et al. A meta-analysis of the yield of capsule endoscopy compared to other diagnostic

modalities in patients with obscure gastrointestinal bleeding. *Am J Gastroenterol* 2005;**100**:2407.

121. Malden ES, Hicks ME, Royal HD, et al. Recurrent gastrointestinal bleeding: use of thrombolytics with anticoagulation in diagnosis. *Radiology* 1998;**207**:147.

122. Kim CY, Suhocki PV, Miller Jr MJ, et al. Provocative mesenteric angiography for lower gastrointestinal hemorrhage: results from a single-institution study. *J Vasc Interv Radiol* 2010;**21**:477.

123. Roesch J, Keller FS, Wawrukiewicz AS, et al. Pharmacoangiography in the diagnosis of recurrent massive lower gastrointestinal bleeding. *Radiology* 1982;**145**:615.

124. Widlus DM, Salis AL. Reteplase provocative visceral arteriography. *J Clin Gastroenterol* 2007;**41**:83.

125. Johnston C, Tuite D, Pritchard R, et al. Use of provocative angiography to localize site in recurrent gastrointestinal bleeding. *Cardiovasc Intervent Radiol* 2007;**30**:1042.

126. Ryan JM, Key SM, Dumbleton SA, et al. Nonlocalized lower gastrointestinal bleeding: provocative bleeding studies with intraarterial tPA, heparin, and tolazoline. *J Vasc Interv Radiol* 2001;**12**:1273.

127. Boijsen E, Kaude J, Tylen U. Radiologic diagnosis of ileal carcinoid tumors. *Acta Radiol* 1974;**15**:65.

128. Lee VS, Morgan JN, Tan AG, et al. Celiac artery compression by the median arcuate ligament: a pitfall of end-expiratory MR imaging. *Radiology* 2003;**228**:437.

129. Horton KM, Talamani MA, Fishman EK. Median arcuate ligament syndrome: evaluation with CT angiography. *Radiographics* 2005;**25**:1177.

130. Gloviczki P, Duncan AA. Treatment of celiac artery compression syndrome: does it really exist? *Perspect Vasc Surg Endovasc Ther* 2007;**19**:259.

131. Kalapatapu VR, Murray BW, Palm-Cruz K, et al. Definitive test to diagnose median arcuate ligament syndrome: injection of vasodilator during angiography. *Vasc Endovascular Surg* 2009;**43**:46.

132. Geelkerken RH, vanBockel JH, deRoos WK, et al. Coeliac artery compression syndrome: the effect of decompression. *Br J Surg* 1990;**77**:807.

133. Saltzberg SS, Maldonado TS, Lamparello PJ, et al. Is endovascular therapy the preferred treatment for all visceral artery aneurysms? *Ann Vasc Surg* 2005;**19**:507.

134. Sachdev U, Baril DT, Ellozy SH, et al. Management of aneurysms involving branches of the celiac and superior mesenteric arteries: a comparison of surgical and endovascular therapy. *J Vasc Surg* 2006;**44**:718.

135. Tulsyan N, Kashyap VS, Greenberg RK, et al. The endovascular management of visceral artery aneurysms and pseudoaneurysms. *J Vasc Surg* 2007;**45**:276.

136. Appel N, Duncan JR, Schuerer DJ. Percutaneous stent-graft treatment of superior mesenteric and internal iliac artery pseudoaneurysms. *J Vasc Interv Radiol* 2003;**14**:917.

137. Miller MT, Comerota AJ, Disalle R, et al. Endoluminal embolization and revascularization for complicated mesenteric pseudoaneurysms: a report of two cases and a literature review. *J Vasc Surg* 2007;**45**:381.

138. Eckhauser FE, Stanley JC, Zelenock GB, et al. Gastroduodenal and pancreaticoduodenal artery aneurysms: a complication of pancreatitis causing spontaneous gastrointestinal hemorrhage. *Surgery* 1980;**88**:335.

139. Guijt M, Delden OM, Koedam NA, et al. Rupture of true aneurysms of the pancreaticoduodenal arcade: treatment with transcatheter arterial embolization. *Cardiovasc Intervent Radiol* 2003; **26**:166.

140. Boudghene F, L'Hermine C, Bigot JM. Arterial complications of pancreatitis: diagnostic and therapeutic aspects in 104 cases. *J Vasc Interv Radiol* 1993;**4**:551.

141. Ha HK, Lee SH, Rha SE, et al. Radiologic features of vasculitis involving the gastrointestinal tract. *Radiographics* 2000;**20**:779.

142. Ahn E, Luk A, Chetty R, et al. Vasculitides of the gastrointestinal tract. *Semin Diagn Pathol* 2009;**26**:77.

143. Ogino H, Matsuda H, Minatoya K, et al. Overview of late outcome of medical and surgical treatment for Takayasu arteritis. *Circulation* 2008;**118**:2738.

144. Hata A, Noda M, Moriwaki R, et al. Angiographic findings of Takayasu arteritis: new classification. *Int J Cardiol* 1996;**54** (Suppl):S155.

145. Ebert EC, Hagspiel KD, Nagar M, et al. Gastrointestinal involvement in polyarteritis nodosa. *Clin Gastroenterol Hepatol* 2008; **6**:960.

146. Dencker H, Holmdahl KH, Lunderquist A, et al. Mesenteric angiography in patients with radiation injury of the bowel after pelvic irradiation. *AJR Am J Roentgenol* 1972;**114**:476.

147. Cho YP, Kwon YM, Kwon TW, et al. Mesenteric Buerger's disease. *Ann Vasc Surg* 2003;**17**:221.

148. Wilson CL, Song LM, Chua H, et al. Bleeding from cavernous angiomatosis of the rectum in Klippel-Trenaunay syndrome: report of three cases and literature review. *Am J Gastroenterol* 2001;**96**:2783.

149. Jennings M, Ward P, Maddocks JL. Blue rubber bleb naevus disease: an uncommon cause of gastrointestinal tract bleeding. *Gut* 1988;**29**:1408.

150. Repasky RG, Tisnado J, Freedman AM. Transcatheter embolization of a superior mesenteric artery pseudoaneurysm and arteriovenous fistula. *J Vasc Interv Radiol* 1993;**4**:241.

151. Asensio JA, Forno W, Roldan G, et al. Visceral vascular injuries. *Surg Clin North Am* 2002;**82**:1.

152. Asensio JA, Chahwan S, Hanpeter D, et al. Operative management and outcome of 302 abdominal vascular injuries. *Am J Surg* 2000;**180**:528.

153. Gabata T, Matsui O, Nakamura Y, et al. Transcatheter embolization of traumatic mesenteric hemorrhage. *J Vasc Interv Radiol* 1994;**5**:891.

154. Slavin RE, Inada K. Segmental arterial mediolysis with accompanying venous angiopathy: a clinical pathologic review, report of 3 new cases, and comments on the role of endothelin-1 in its pathogenesis. *Int J Surg Pathol* 2007;**15**:121.

155. Sandmann W, Schulte KM. Multivisceral fibromuscular dysplasia in childhood: case report and review of the literature. *Ann Vasc Surg* 2000;**14**:496.

156. LaBerge JM, Kerlan Jr RK. Segmental arterial mediolysis (SAM) resulting in spontaneous dissections of the middle colic and left renal arteries and occlusion of the SMA. *J Vasc Interv Radiol* 1999;**10**:509.

157. Lee SI, Chew FS. Splanchnic segmental arterial mediolysis. *AJR Am J Roentgenol* 1998;**170**:122.

158. Michael M, Widmer U, Wildermuth S, et al. Segmental arterial mediolysis: CTA findings at presentation and follow-up. *AJR Am J Roentgenol* 2006;**187**:1463.

159. Shimohira M, Ogino H, Sasaki S, et al. Transcatheter arterial embolization for segmental arterial mediolysis. *J Endovasc Ther* 2008; **15**:493.

12

Hepatic, Splenic, and Portal Vascular Systems

Karim Valji

ARTERIOGRAPHY AND VENOGRAPHY

Techniques for celiac and superior mesenteric arteriography are described in Chapter 11. Splenic or common hepatic arteriography is performed with a variety of catheters, including cobra and sidewinder shapes. Steerable, hydrophilic guidewires simplify catheter placement. Alternatively, high-flow coaxial microcatheters are used to select the main splenic or hepatic arteries and their branches.

The hepatic veins are studied from an internal jugular (IJ) vein approach using a multipurpose angiographic or cobra-shaped catheter. In a small percentage of patients, a femoral route is necessary because of the downgoing orientation of the main hepatic vein entering the inferior vena cava (IVC). This situation may occur after some liver transplantations or with hepatic vein anomalies (see later discussion). Wedged hepatic vein manometry and venography are done with a balloon occlusion catheter inflated within a peripheral hepatic vein branch or a 5-French (Fr) endhole catheter advanced into a peripheral vein until resistance is met. A flat pressure waveform indicates a wedged position. Measurements should be obtained before contrast injection, which may spuriously elevate the sinusoidal pressure. Overinjection can produce subcapsular extravasation and liver perforation. Retrograde filling of the portal vein is enhanced when CO_2 is used as the contrast agent (30 to 60 cc of gas injected rapidly).

The splenic, superior mesenteric, and portal veins are visualized on the late phases of celiac or superior mesenteric arteriography ("indirect portography"). Direct splenoportography is rarely required in the evaluation of patients with portal hypertension.[1] Iodinated contrast or CO_2 (15 to 20 cc) is injected through a micropuncture catheter inserted into the substance of the spleen with ultrasound guidance. The tract is embolized with Gelfoam as the catheter is withdrawn.[2,3]

ANATOMY

Development

The liver bud develops between the pericardial cavity and the stalk of the primitive yolk sac.[4] Liver cords insinuate between tributaries of the vitelline and umbilical veins to form the hepatic sinusoids. Branches of the right vitelline veins around the duodenum develop into the central portal veins.[5] The right umbilical vein involutes, and the left umbilical vein becomes the primary inflow vessel to the liver. The hepatic venous outflow is directed toward the upper portion of the right vitelline vein, which ultimately forms the hepatic veins and the intrahepatic portion of the IVC. The ductus venosus connects the left umbilical vein (portal venous inflow) to the right vitelline vein (hepatic outflow). Shortly after birth, the ductus venosus and left umbilical vein close and form the ligamentum venosum and ligamentum teres, respectively.

Normal Anatomy

Liver

With the advent of living-related split-liver donor transplants, more ambitious surgical techniques for segmental hepatic resection, and transcatheter methods for treatment of liver tumors, a detailed understanding of the normal, variant, and collateral hepatic circulations is critical for the vascular interventionalist. For preoperative planning, high-quality computed tomography (CT) or magnetic resonance (MR) arteriography and venography are both extremely accurate.[6-9] For transarterial therapy, selective digital angiography is required, including celiac and superior mesenteric arteriography, right and left hepatic arteriography, and often more subselective catheterization.[10,11]

The liver is divided into right and left lobes separated by the major fissure. The *right lobe* has anterior and posterior segments; the *left lobe* has medial and lateral segments. The *caudate lobe* is anatomically distinct from the right and left lobes. By convention, segmental anatomy is based on the original system of Couinaud demarcated by the three main hepatic veins and a transverse plane at the level of the portal vein bifurcation[12,13] (Fig. 12-1). However, the relationship between these landmarks identified on cross-sectional imaging and the true anatomic segmental anatomy is only approximate.

The liver is supplied by the common hepatic artery and portal vein. Normally, about three fourths of the blood supply to the liver comes from the portal vein. Any reduction in hepatic arterial or portal venous blood flow leads to a compensatory increase in flow through the companion system. The biliary tree is nourished by branches of the hepatic arteries.

The *common hepatic artery* arises from the celiac artery (Fig. 12-2). After giving off the gastroduodenal artery, it

becomes the *proper hepatic artery*. This vessel enters the porta hepatis and divides into the *right hepatic artery (RHA)* and *left hepatic artery (LHA)*, which feed their respective lobes. The RHA supplies segments V to VIII (and sometimes segment I, caudate lobe). The LHA supplies segments II, III, IVa, and IVb. The inconsistent *middle hepatic artery*, which, if present, supplies segments IVa and IVb, usually originates from the right hepatic artery or forms a true trifurcation. Variations in hepatic arterial anatomy are common (see later discussion). Although the hepatic arteries are considered end arteries, intrahepatic and extrahepatic anastomoses do exist. The origins of important branches are outlined in Table 12-1.

The *portal vein (PV)* is formed by the confluence of the *superior mesenteric vein (SMV)* and *splenic vein*[14] (Fig. 12-3). It is valveless. Normal main portal vein pressure is about

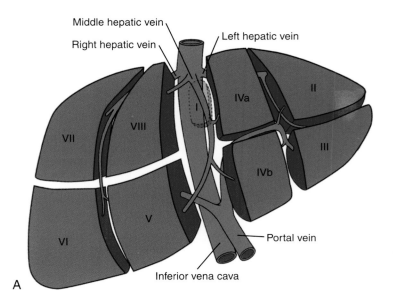

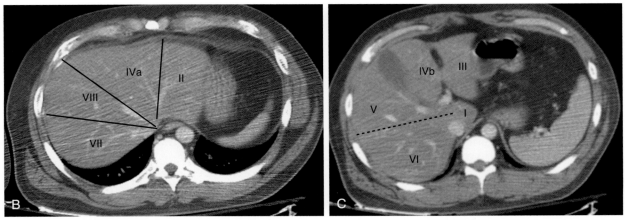

FIGURE 12-1 Segmental anatomy of the liver. **A,** Schematic drawing shows segmental divisions along with portal vein inflow and hepatic vein outflow. Segment I (caudate lobe) lies posterior to segments III and IV and in front of the inferior vena cava. Computed tomography scans through the upper **(B)** and lower **(C)** aspects of the liver, with segments noted. (**A,** *Adapted with permission from the website of the American Hepato-Pancreato-Biliary Association, www.ahpba.org.*)

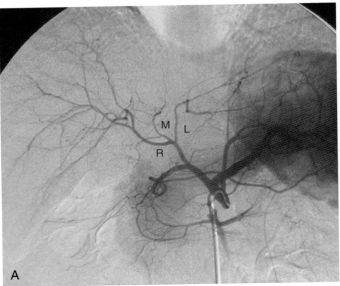

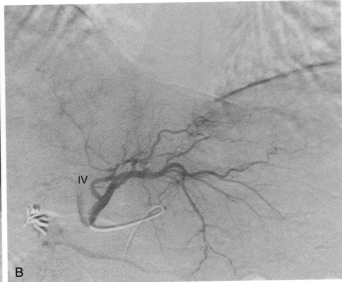

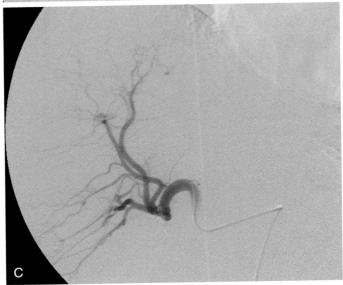

FIGURE 12-2   Normal hepatic arterial anatomy. **A,** Celiac arteriography shows right *(R),* middle *(M),* and left *(L)* hepatic arteries. Normal left **(B)** and right **(C)** hepatic arteriograms in another patient. IV indicates the branch to segment IV.

TABLE 12-1   Important Branches of the Hepatic Arteries

Vessel	Typical and Atypical Origins
Right gastric artery	PHA or LHA
	CHA, RHA, GDA, MHA
Cystic artery	RHA
	Replaced/accessory RHA
	LHA or CHA
	GDA
Supraduodenal artery	GDA, CHA, LHA, RHA, cystic
Dorsal pancreatic artery	SA
	Celiac artery, RHA, SMA
Falciform artery	MHA, LHA

CHA, common hepatic artery; GDA, gastroduodenal artery; LGA, left gastric artery; LHA, left hepatic artery; MHA, middle hepatic artery; PHA, proper hepatic artery; RHA, right hepatic artery; SA, splenic artery; SMA, superior mesenteric artery.

3 to 5 mm Hg. The SMV has numerous jejunal, ileal, and colonic tributaries. The *inferior mesenteric vein (IMV)* joins the splenic vein or the SMV.[15] The right gastroepiploic, pancreaticoduodenal, and right colonic veins often merge into a common gastrocolic trunk that drains into the right side of the SMV near its junction with the PV. The *right and left gastric (coronary) veins* join the superior surface of the main portal or central splenic vein. Multiple coronary veins often exist.

The portal vein runs anterior to the IVC and posterior to the head of the pancreas before entering the liver. The PV bifurcation is outside the liver capsule in about half of the population.[16] The right and left PVs and their branches follow the hepatic artery into the liver. The left PV supplies segments I to IV.[17] The right anterior PV supplies segments V and VIII; the right posterior PV supplies

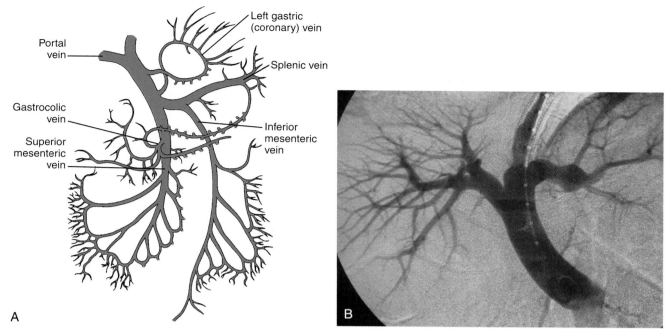

FIGURE 12-3   Portal venous anatomy. **A,** Schematic drawing. **B,** Direct transhepatic portogram through an obstructed transjugular intrahepatic portosystemic shunt. (**A,** *From Lundell C, Kadir S. The portal venous system and hepatic vein. In: Kadir S, editor.* Atlas of normal and variant angiographic anatomy. *Philadelphia: WB Saunders; 1991, p. 370.*)

segments VI and VII. The caudate lobe is usually fed by branches of the left PV. The remnant of the umbilical vein (ligamentum teres) is connected to the left PV. A patent *paraumbilical vein* arising from the left PV is sometimes seen in patients with portal hypertension.

The liver is drained by the hepatic veins. The *right* and *left hepatic veins* run between the segments of the right and left lobes of the liver, and the *middle hepatic vein* lies in the main lobar fissure (Fig. 12-4). These vessels converge into the IVC within several centimeters of the diaphragm. The right hepatic vein (draining segments VI and VII) joins the right posterolateral surface of the IVC. The middle hepatic vein (draining segments V and VIII) and left hepatic vein (draining segments II and III) confluence enters the anteromedial surface of the IVC. Segments IVa and IVb are drained by the left or middle hepatic vein. The caudate lobe empties independently into the intrahepatic IVC.

The liver parenchyma is composed of *hepatic lobules,* which contain the hepatocytes and sinusoidal spaces that form the functional units of the liver[18] (Fig. 12-5). Neighboring lobules are organized into *acini.* Hepatic arterial, portal venous, and biliary duct branches follow the borders of the lobules. Hepatic arterioles feed the sinusoids directly and through communications with portal venules that perforate the lobules. Normally, blood flows freely between acini. Central veins at the core of each lobule drain the sinusoids. These venules coalesce into the hepatic veins.

Spleen

The *splenic artery* supplies the spleen and portions of the pancreas and stomach[19] (Fig. 12-6). It follows the superior edge of the pancreas along with the splenic vein. With advancing age, the splenic artery can become extremely tortuous. Near the splenic hilum, the artery usually divides into superior and inferior branches. *Superior* and *inferior polar arteries* often arise from the midsplenic artery and supply their respective splenic segments. The left gastroepiploic artery originates from the distal inferior polar artery and then courses along the greater curvature of the stomach. Numerous short gastric branches feed the fundus of the stomach. The splenic artery also has numerous branches to the body and tail of the pancreas. The largest of these vessels are the *dorsal pancreatic artery* (which may originate on the celiac trunk) and the *pancreatica magna artery* (see Fig. 12-6).

The *splenic vein* lies behind the upper border of the pancreas below the splenic artery (see Fig. 12-6B). Its tributaries include the short gastric, left gastroepiploic, pancreatic, and inferior mesenteric veins (see Fig. 12-3).

Variant Anatomy

Anomalies of hepatic artery origin and number are common[10,20-23] (Table 12-2). The most frequent variants are *accessory* and *replaced hepatic arteries,* such as the right

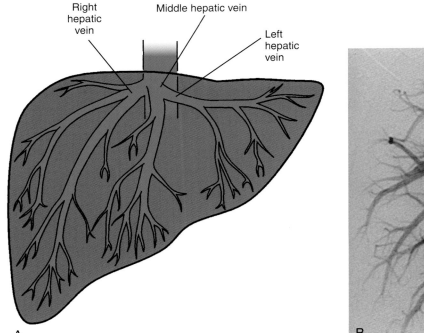

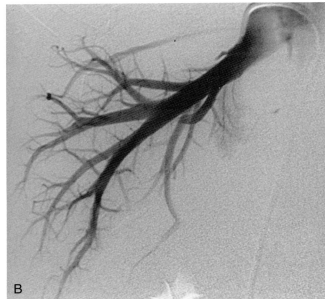

FIGURE 12-4   Hepatic venous anatomy. **A,** Schematic drawing. **B,** Normal right hepatic venogram.

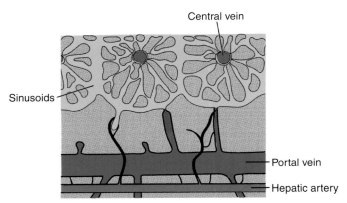

FIGURE 12-5   Microarchitecture of the hepatic sinusoids.
(Adapted from Cho KJ, Lunderquist A. The peribiliary vascular plexus: the microvascular architecture of the bile duct in the rabbit and in clinical cases. Radiology *1983;**147**:357.)*

TABLE 12-2   Variant Hepatic Arterial Anatomy

Type	Michels (%)	Recent Series (%)
I: Classic Anatomy	55	58-79
II: Replaced LHA	10	3-12
III: Replaced RHA	11	6-15
IV: Replaced RHA and LHA	1	1-2
V: Accessory LHA from LGA	8	3-11
VI: Accessory RHA from SMA	7	3-12
VII: Accessory RHA and LHA	1	0-1
VIII: Accessory RHA/LHA replaced LHA or RHA	2	1-3
IX: Replaced CHA to SMA	4.5	1-2
X: Replaced CHA to LGA	0.5	0
Double hepatic artery		1-4
Triple hepatic artery		0-7
Separate CHA origin from aorta		0.4-2
Replaced PHA to SMA, GDA origin from aorta		0.3
Other		1.5-4

CHA, *common hepatic artery;* GDA, *gastroduodenal artery;* LGA, *left gastric artery;* LHA, *left hepatic artery;* PHA, *proper hepatic artery;* RHA, *right hepatic artery;* SMA, *superior mesenteric artery.*

hepatic from the superior mesenteric artery (SMA), the left hepatic from the left gastric, and the common hepatic from the SMA (Fig. 12-7; see also Figs. 11-7 through 11-9). *Accessory* hepatic arteries are those in which a portion of the affected lobe is supplied by a vessel with an aberrant origin. *Replaced* hepatic arteries are those in which the entire lobe is supplied by a vessel with an aberrant origin. Accessory hepatic arteries supply isolated hepatic segments and are believed by most authorities not to be redundant arteries.[24]

Rarely, the hepatic or splenic artery originates directly from the aorta (see Figs. 11-11 and 11-12). An accessory left gastric artery may arise from the proximal splenic artery. Important organ anomalies include an accessory spleen (usually located in the tail of the pancreas), asplenia, polysplenia, and the ectopic or "wandering" spleen.[25]

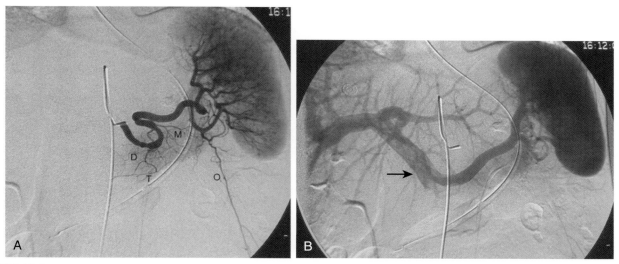

FIGURE 12-6   **A,** Normal splenic arteriogram showing the dorsal pancreatic *(D)*, transverse pancreatic *(T)*, pancreatica magna *(M)*, and omental *(O)* branches. Proxaimal irregularity is guidewire-related spasm. **B,** Late-phase indirect splenoportogram. Diminished density in the main portal vein *(arrow)* is caused by unopacified inflow from the superior mesenteric vein.

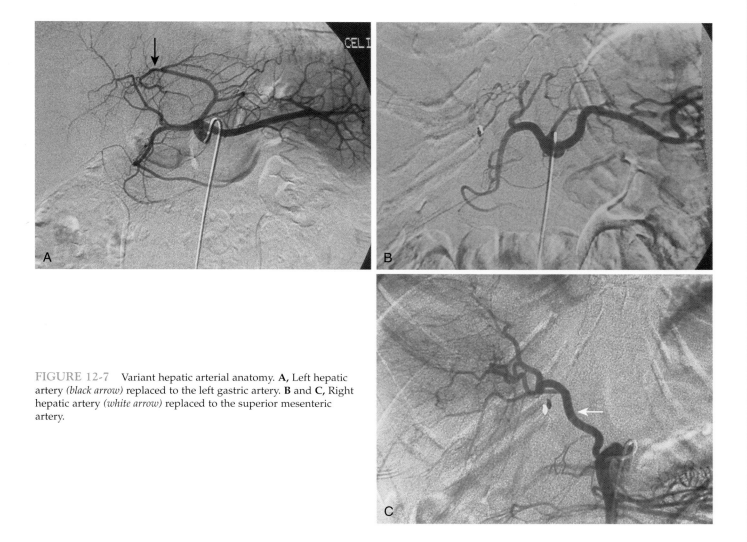

FIGURE 12-7   Variant hepatic arterial anatomy. **A,** Left hepatic artery *(black arrow)* replaced to the left gastric artery. **B** and **C,** Right hepatic artery *(white arrow)* replaced to the superior mesenteric artery.

Classic PV anatomy is found in 65% to 75% of the population. Surgically significant variants involve trifurcation of the main PV (type 2, 9% to 16%), origin of the right posterior branch from the main PV (type 3 or "Z type," 8% to 13%), and separate segment VI or VII branches from the right portal vein (types 4 and 5, 7%).[17,26]

Accessory right hepatic veins are found in 25% or more of the population (Fig. 12-8). In about 3% of individuals, an *inferior right hepatic vein* (entering the IVC well below the diaphragm) is the dominant venous drainage for the right lobe.[16]

Collateral Circulation

With extrahepatic arterial obstruction, the major collateral pathways into the liver are from:

- SMA to pancreaticoduodenal arcades and choledochal arteries (see Fig. 11-13)
- Diaphragmatic inferior phrenic branches to intrahepatic arteries (Fig. 12-9)
- Splenic artery to pancreatic, gastric, and gastroepiploic branches

With intrahepatic arterial obstruction, the liver is primarily supplied by accessory hepatic arteries (if present) and extracapsular branches.

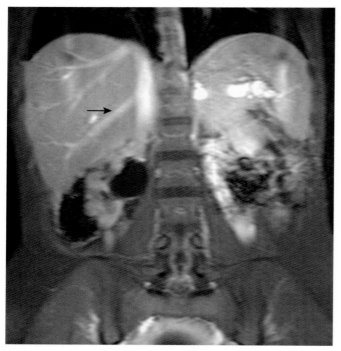

FIGURE 12-8   Accessory inferior right hepatic vein *(arrow)* on coronal maximum intensity projection magnetic resonance venogram.

With splenic artery obstruction, several collateral routes are available:

- Left gastric to short gastric arteries
- Right gastroepiploic to left gastroepiploic artery (see Fig. 11-14)
- Pancreatic arcades or dorsal pancreatic artery to distal pancreatic arteries

Patterns of collateral flow in the portal and hepatic venous systems are discussed subsequently.

MAJOR DISORDERS

Cirrhosis and Portal Hypertension (Online Case 68)

Etiology

Cirrhosis is a progressive liver disease characterized by generalized necrosis, regeneration, and widespread fibrosis.[27] Initially, inflammation or steatosis predominates. Fibrotic tissue then infiltrates the sinusoidal spaces and obstructs central veins while preserving portal venules. Masses (either micronodular or macronodular) begin to form, including regenerative, dysplastic, and malignant lesions. As the vascular resistance in the liver increases, PV pressure rises, but flow is still directed into the liver *(hepatopetal)*. An imbalance in the relative activity of vasodilators (e.g., nitric oxide) and vasoconstrictors (e.g., endothelin-1) is responsible for the disturbances in hepatic, splanchnic, and peripheral hemodynamics that follow.[28,29] With progression of cirrhosis, systemic and splanchnic vasodilation occurs, leading to increased cardiac output (a hyperdynamic circulatory state) and humorally mediated renal and hepatic vasoconstriction, which further impedes liver blood flow.[30,31] Extrahepatic portal flow increases while intrahepatic portal flow decreases; in a compensatory fashion, hepatic arterial flow is augmented.

With end-stage cirrhosis, the liver shrinks, and portal venules and hepatic arterial branches are severely compressed by fibrotic infiltration and regenerating nodules. Hepatic vein outflow drops substantially. Intrahepatic pressure becomes so great that the portal system is decompressed through portosystemic collateral channels (see later discussion). Ultimately, flow in the PV is completely reversed *(hepatofugal)*.

Although cirrhosis is by far the most frequent cause of portal hypertension, many other diseases can produce similar physiologic effects. *Portal hypertension* is traditionally classified by the site of obstruction relative to the hepatic sinusoids[32] (Boxes 12-1 through 12-5). Some diseases affect one level and then extend to others. Disorders that cause elevated portal pressures proximal to or beyond the hepatic sinusoids are considered later in this chapter.

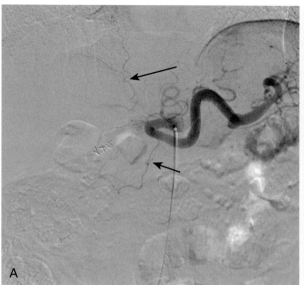
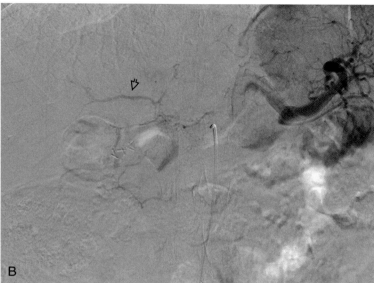

FIGURE 12-9 Acute occlusion of liver transplant hepatic artery (HA). **A** and **B,** Celiac arteriography shows complete HA obstruction along with collateral circulation from the right inferior phrenic artery *(long arrow)* and dorsal pancreatic artery *(short arrow)* into the intrahepatic branches *(open arrow).*

BOX 12-1

FORMS OF PORTAL HYPERTENSION

- Extrahepatic portal vein obstruction (see Box 12-2)
- Presinusoidal intrahepatic obstruction (see Box 12-3)
- Sinusoidal intrahepatic obstruction (see Box 12-4)
- Postsinusoidal obstruction (see Box 12-5)
- Hyperdynamic portal hypertension

BOX 12-2

CAUSES OF PORTAL VEIN OBSTRUCTION

- Thrombosis (bland or neoplastic invasion)
- Extrinsic compression
  - Tumor
  - Inflammatory mass
- Postoperative
- Congenital

BOX 12-3

CAUSES OF PRESINUSOIDAL INTRAHEPATIC OBSTRUCTION

- Hepatitis
- Biliary cirrhosis
  - Primary form
  - Chronic obstruction
- Schistosomiasis
- Toxic agents (e.g., vinyl chloride, cytotoxic drugs)
- Metabolic disorders (e.g., hemochromatosis)
- Malignancies
  - Myeloproliferative disorders
  - Reticuloendothelial tumors
- Sarcoidosis
- Congenital hepatic fibrosis
- Idiopathic portal hypertension

BOX 12-4

CAUSES OF SINUSOIDAL INTRAHEPATIC OBSTRUCTION

- Cirrhosis
  - Alcoholic
  - Cryptogenic
  - Congestive
  - Postnecrotic
- Hepatitis
  - Viral (hepatitis C, B, A)
- Hepatocellular carcinoma
- Sclerosing cholangitis
- Felty syndrome

BOX 12-5

CAUSES OF POSTSINUSOIDAL HEPATIC OBSTRUCTION

- Hepatic vein thrombosis (classic Budd-Chiari disease)
- Hepatic venoocclusive disease
- Inferior vena cava or hepatic vein outflow obstruction
- Hepatic vein or inferior vena cava tumor
- Constrictive pericarditis
- Right atrial tumor

Worldwide, *hepatitis B* and *C infections* are the leading cause of liver cirrhosis.[33] *Alcoholic cirrhosis* is the other common form of the disease in the United States and elsewhere. It evolves from an initial stage of fatty liver to sinusoidal scarring, formation of regenerative nodules (i.e., micronodular cirrhosis), and finally widespread fibrosis with liver shrinkage. Along with diabetes and metabolic syndrome, one consequence of the epidemic of obesity is the rapidly growing incidence of *nonalcoholic fatty liver disease (NAFLD)*, including the particularly aggressive form of *nonalcoholic steatohepatitis (NASH)*. These infiltrative conditions are now responsible for a significant fraction of cases of liver cirrhosis.[34,35]

Primary biliary cirrhosis is a cholestatic liver disease of immunologic origin that results in diffuse bile duct obstruction.[36] It is typically seen in middle-aged women.

In patients with chronic bile duct obstruction, portal fibrosis rather than diffuse cirrhosis is the cause for portal hypertension. *Hepatic schistosomiasis*, which is endemic in Africa and parts of Asia, causes infiltration of portal venules and periportal spaces, leading to presinusoidal obstruction.[37] *Congenital hepatic fibrosis* presents in late childhood with features of portal hypertension but normal liver function. *Idiopathic portal hypertension* and *noncirrhotic portal fibrosis* are rare conditions in which PV pressure is elevated without underlying liver disease.[38] Destruction of intrahepatic portal radicles, portal fibrosis, and liver atrophy are characteristic. *Cryptogenic cirrhosis* encompasses all cases without an identifiable etiology, although many of these patients may have NAFLD or NASH.

Hyperdynamic portal hypertension, defined as increased flow through the portal venous system in the absence of resistive changes, is an unusual reason for elevated portal pressure. Two lesions that produce this physiology are an *arterioportal fistula* (which is often the result of penetrating trauma) or rupture of a hepatic artery aneurysm.[39] In such cases, embolization of the fistula may be curative.

Clinical Features

The most devastating consequence of portal hypertension is bleeding from ruptured gastroesophageal varices that serve as portosystemic collaterals to decompress the fibrotic liver.[31] Varices develop in about half of patients with cirrhosis, but only about one third of those will bleed. Hemorrhagic risk correlates with variceal size, intraluminal pressure, and the patient's *Child-Pugh score* (Table 12-3). Between 40% and 70% of patients die of the first episode of variceal hemorrhage. Bleeding is unlikely when the portosystemic pressure gradient is less than 12 mm Hg.[40]

Fiberoptic endoscopy is performed routinely in all patients with suspected variceal bleeding to document

TABLE 12-3 Modified Child-Pugh Classification for Hepatic Failure

Determinant	Threshold*
Ascites	Controlled medically
Encephalopathy	Controlled medically
INR	1.7-2.2
Bilirubin	2-3 mg/dL
Albumin	2.8-3.5 mg/dL

Classification	Points
Class A	5-6
Class B	7-9
Class C	10-15

*Score 2 points if within threshold, score 1 point if better than threshold, and score 3 points if worse than threshold. INR. International Normalized Ratio.

variceal size and stigmata of recent rupture (e.g., red wheals, cherry spots). Endoscopy may also identify an unrelated reason for acute gastrointestinal bleeding.

Ascites is another important complication of portal hypertension. The causes of ascites are manifold. Increased splanchnic blood flow elevates microcirculatory pressures and increases production of lymph, which leaks from the liver and intestines.[41] In addition, peripheral arterial dilation (a response to vasoactive factors liberated from the gastrointestinal tract) leads to a reduction in effective plasma volume and retention of salt and water by the kidneys. The hepatic lymphatic system becomes overwhelmed, causing peritoneal leakage and a vicious cycle of further reduction in the plasma volume and worsening ascites.

Cirrhotic patients also are at risk for *hepatic encephalopathy, spontaneous bacterial peritonitis,* splenomegaly and pancytopenia, hepatocellular carcinoma, and ultimately complete hepatic failure. Less frequent complications include hepatorenal syndrome, hepatopulmonary syndrome, portopulmonary hypertension, and hepatic hydrothorax. Some of these conditions are related to the misregulation of vasodilating and vasoconstricting factors.[42] *Hepatorenal syndrome* is characterized by diffuse splanchnic and peripheral vasodilation and decreased effective plasma volume, prompting reflex renal vasoconstriction.[43] Whereas the chronic form is treatable, the acute type is almost universally fatal (see later discussion).

Imaging and Tissue Diagnosis

Virtually all patients with suspected cirrhosis or portal hypertension undergo radiologic tests to prove the existence and assess the extent of liver disease and to detect occult hepatic malignancies. The primary indications for diagnostic invasive procedures are confirmation or quantitation of portal hypertension and transvenous liver biopsy.

HEPATIC VEIN MANOMETRY

Direct measurement of PV pressure is hardly ever needed for diagnosing portal hypertension; clinical studies have shown that the hepatic vein wedged (HVW) pressure is equal to PV pressure in most patients.[44] The difference between HVW and IVC (or right atrial) pressure is the *corrected sinusoidal pressure,* which reflects the portosystemic gradient. However, the measurements are valid only when the PVs and hepatic sinusoids are in continuity. In patients with extrahepatic PV obstruction, splenic vein obstruction ("segmental" portal hypertension), or presinusoidal portal hypertension, this disconnection leads to a spuriously low HVW pressure. Normally, the portosystemic gradient is less than 5 mm Hg. Portal hypertension is defined as a gradient more than 6 mm Hg. The risk of bleeding from gastroesophageal varices becomes significant when the gradient is greater than 12 mm Hg.[40]

HEPATIC VENOGRAPHY

Free hepatic venography is done to assess the hepatic veins if obstruction is suspected, during the transjugular intrahepatic portosystemic shunt (TIPS) procedure, and sometimes during transvenous liver biopsy. Balloon-occluded or catheter-wedged hepatic venography with CO_2 is routinely performed before creating TIPS to provide a target for the PV puncture. Hepatic veins have a pinnate (feather-like) branching pattern; portal veins branch dichotomously (Fig. 12-10).

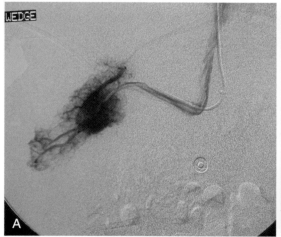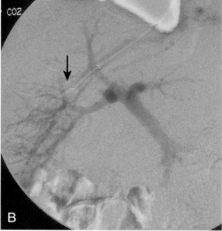

FIGURE 12-10   **A,** Wedged hepatic venography shows homogeneous parenchymal stain and filling of adjacent hepatic venules and veins. **B,** Carbon dioxide wedged hepatic venography using an occlusion balloon *(arrow)* with backfilling of gas that outlines the portal vein.

ARTERIOGRAPHY AND INDIRECT PORTOGRAPHY

With advanced cirrhosis, the hepatic arteries take on a "corkscrew" appearance because of increased arterial flow and liver shrinkage, and the spleen and splenic artery are enlarged (Fig. 12-11). The demand for hepatic artery flow can become so great that flow in the gastroduodenal artery is reversed. Occasionally, arterioportal shunting is seen (Fig. 12-12).

In the early stages of cirrhosis, PV flow is relatively normal. As the disease advances and portal hypertension becomes significant, several changes occur. The most important is the appearance of portosystemic collateral pathways, which include the following principal channels (Fig. 12-13):

- Left gastric (coronary) and short gastric veins through gastroesophageal veins to the azygous venous system
- Left PV through a paraumbilical vein to systemic abdominal wall veins around the umbilicus ("caput medusae") or internal iliac veins
- Splenic or short gastric veins through retroperitoneal branches to the left adrenal/inferior phrenic

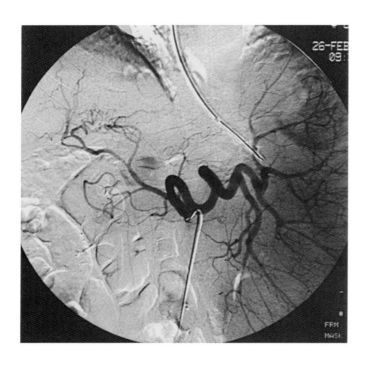

FIGURE 12-11   Advanced cirrhosis. The celiac arteriogram shows "corkscrew" intrahepatic arteries, liver shrinkage, splenic artery enlargement, and massive splenomegaly.

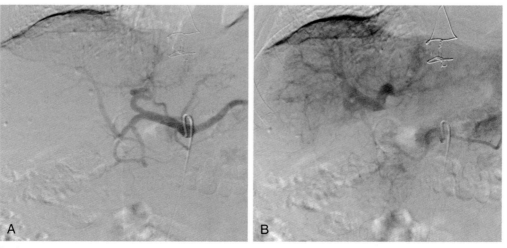

FIGURE 12-12   Advanced cirrhosis with global shunting from hepatic artery **(A)** to portal vein **(B)** seen on celiac arteriography.

veins and then to the left renal vein (*spontaneous splenorenal shunt*)

• IMV through rectal (hemorrhoidal) veins to the internal iliac vein

Less common routes of decompression are gastric veins to pulmonary or intercostal veins, duodenal varices ultimately draining into the right gonadal vein (Fig. 12-14), left colic vein to left renal vein through the left gonadal vein, ileocolic vein to the IVC through hemorrhoidal veins, and intrahepatic portal venous branches to diaphragmatic veins. Gastroesophageal varices may be present but not seen on indirect portography.

The direction of flow in the PV switches as portal hypertension worsens. With mild cirrhosis, PV flow is hepatopetal (see Fig. 12-3). As resistance increases, bidirectional flow in the PV may develop and the PV may not fill at all. With severe portal hypertension, the PV becomes an outflow conduit for the liver, and flow is hepatofugal (Fig. 12-15).

SPLENOPORTOGRAPHY

This imaging study is rarely (if ever) necessary. Before CT and MR angiography became so accurate, direct contrast injection of the splenic parenchyma was occasionally required to document patency of the splenic vein in patients with massive splenomegaly.

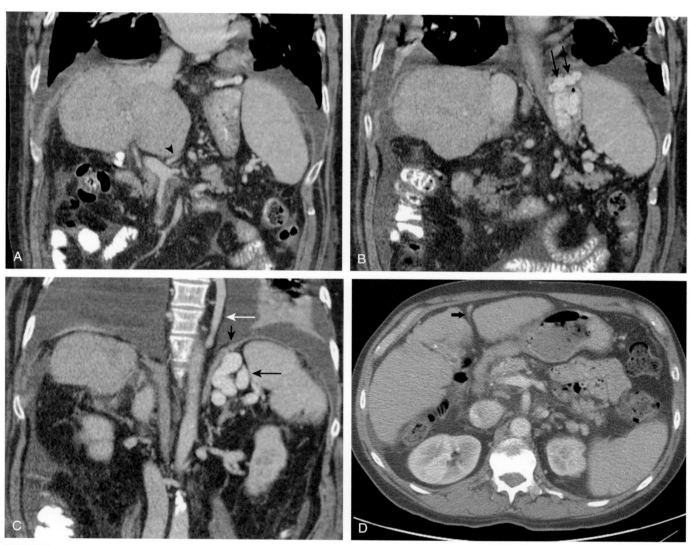

FIGURE 12-13   Portosystemic collateral pathways. **A** through **C,** On reformatted coronal computed tomography (CT) scans, blood is diverted up the coronary vein *(arrowhead),* through large gastroesophageal varices *(black arrows),* and then to the azygous venous system *(white arrow).* Note shrunken nodular liver, enlarged spleen, ascites, and large bilateral pleural effusions. Paraumbilical vein drains the left portal vein through internal iliac venous channels into the inferior vena cava seen on CT scan (**D,** *arrow*).

Continued

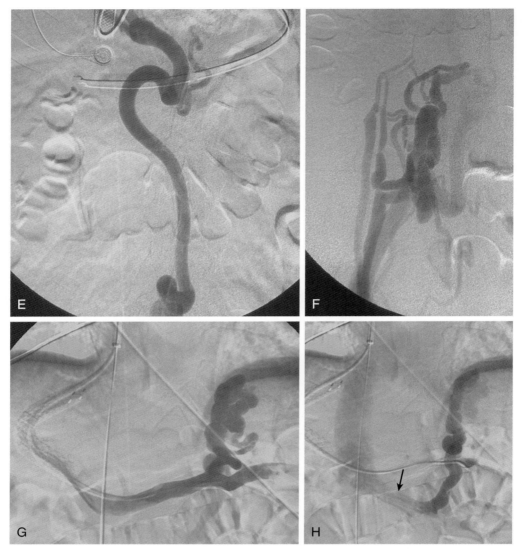

FIGURE 12-13, cont'd **E,** Early and **(F)** late phases of a direct portogram. Splenorenal shunt drains short gastric varices from the splenic hilum into the left renal vein *(arrow),* and then the inferior vena cava on early **(G)** and late **(H)** phases of a direct splenic venogram through a transjugular intrahepatic portosystemic shunt.

TRANSJUGULAR LIVER BIOPSY

PATIENT SELECTION Tissue samples for histologic diagnosis of diffuse liver disease are usually obtained by percutaneous biopsy. For patients with certain conditions, transhepatic biopsy may be relatively unsafe and transvenous biopsy preferred (Box 12-6). This approach is used also in patients already undergoing hepatic vein catheterization for other reasons (e.g., diagnosis of portal hypertension, during the TIPS procedure).

TECHNIQUE From the right (or left) IJ vein, a 40-cm 10-Fr vascular sheath is advanced into the right or middle hepatic vein to the mid-portion of the

---

BOX 12-6

PRIMARY INDICATIONS FOR TRANSJUGULAR LIVER BIOPSY

- Uncorrectable coagulopathy
- Massive ascites
- Morbid obesity
- Grossly shrunken liver

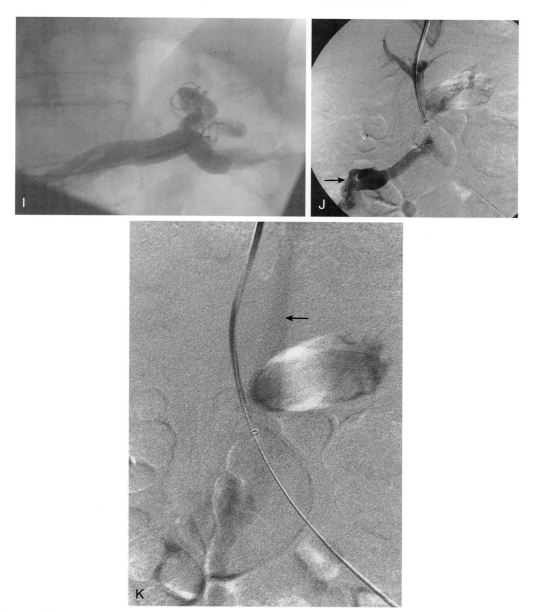

FIGURE 12-13, cont'd   Such shunts are occasionally embolized to prevent bleeding, relieve hepatic encephalopathy, or improve overall liver perfusion **(I).** Cecal varices *(arrow)* fill by direct portal vein injection **(J)** and then drain through systemic pelvic collaterals into the inferior vena cava **(K,** *arrow).*

vessel (Fig. 12-16). A stainless steel stiffening cannula is placed through the sheath. A flexible biopsy needle (e.g., Quick-Core or TLAB Patel set) is then inserted through the cannula and torqued within the hepatic vein until resistance is met. The device is buried in the parenchyma and triggered, and a piece of tissue is removed. Three or four specimens are needed to ensure that sufficient material is obtained for diagnosis.[45,46]

RESULTS AND COMPLICATIONS Liver tissue can be extracted in more than 97% of attempts. It may be slightly more difficult to obtain tissue in liver transplant patients with a "piggyback" type hepatic vein anastomosis[47] (see later discussion). Biopsy samples are adequate for pathologic diagnosis 96% to 97% of the time.[48-52] The major risk of the procedure is liver capsule perforation. Minor complications (including access site bleeding and cardiac dysrhythmias) are reported in up

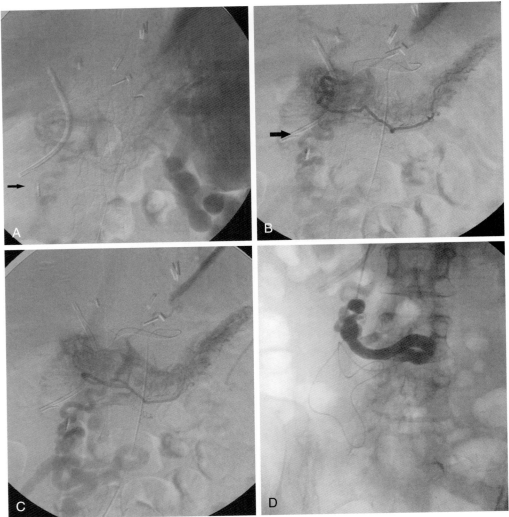

FIGURE 12-14   Duodenal varices treated with embolotherapy. **A,** Late phase of celiac arteriogram shows splenic hilar varices and duodenal varices *(arrow).* **B,** The duodenal varices are better seen with selective gastroduodenal arteriography through a coaxial microcatheter. **C,** Pelvic collaterals were found to drain into the right ovarian vein and then into the inferior vena cava. **D,** The ovarian vein is catheterized, a micro-catheter is negotiated to the site of the varices, and ethanolamine oleate was injected to induce sclerosis.

to 12% of cases. Less than 1% of patients experience seri-ous life-threatening hemorrhage (usually from liver cap-sule perforation with intraperitoneal bleeding).[46,48,49,52]

Treatment
PHARMACOLOGIC THERAPY
Prophylactic treatment with beta-adrenergic blocking agents (often combined with isosorbide nitrate) is routinely prescribed in patients with documented gastroesophageal varices to lower portal venous pressure and thereby pre-vent initial or recurrent bleeding.[53,54] If bleeding occurs, emergent management starts with resuscitation, prophy-lactic antibiotics, and pharmacologic therapy: somatostatin (or its analogue octreotide), vasopressin, or synthetic *terlip-ressin* (which constrict mesenteric arteries and reduces portal venous pressure and flow).[55-57]

ENDOSCOPIC TREATMENT
Variceal band ligation or *sclerotherapy* is highly effective for the initial management and primary or secondary preven-tion of variceal hemorrhage.[53,54,56-59] A sclerosing agent such as ethanolamine oleate or polidocanol injected into or around varices causes variceal thrombosis. Variceal banding is probably safer and more durable.[54,57] About 70% to 90% of patients stop bleeding after one or two treat-ment sessions. However, sclerotherapy does not remedy the underlying hemodynamics of portal hypertension. Rebleeding is observed in about 10% to 15% of cases.[31] Serious complications occur about 10% of the time.

LARGE-VOLUME PARACENTESIS
The standard treatment for cirrhosis-related ascites is so-dium and fluid restriction and diuretic therapy. Some cirrhotics with massive (tense) ascites are largely resistant

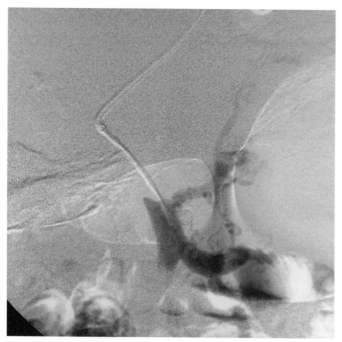

FIGURE 12-15   Hepatofugal flow in the portal vein on direct injection through a TIPS.

to these measures. Intractable ascites can have a marked impact on overall quality of life. In such cases, frequent large volume paracentesis (>4 to 5 L) is necessary to diminish pain, nausea, and respiratory compromise. The application of volume expanders (e.g., intravenous [IV] albumin infusion) in this setting is controversial. However, large volume paracentesis is inconvenient for patients and does have risk.

TRANSCATHETER VARICEAL EMBOLIZATION

Embolization of the coronary vein was quite popular before the widespread use of endoscopic sclerotherapy.[60] Coils, with or without a sclerosing agent, are placed to obstruct the inflow vein. Although immediate results are excellent, rebleeding occurs in more than 50% of cases as new collateral channels develop.[61] This procedure has limited use as an adjunct to TIPS placement (see later discussion) and for obliteration of ectopic varices.[62]

BALLOON-OCCLUDED RETROGRADE TRANSVENOUS OBLITERATION OF GASTRIC AND DUODENAL VARICES

In Japan and other parts of Asia, balloon-occluded retrograde transvenous obliteration (BRTO) has become a popular modality for prevention or control of bleeding from isolated variceal clusters.[63-65] Gastric and duodenal varices are notoriously difficult to treat with endoscopy because of their location and size. In some individuals, these massive shunts can also cause intractable hepatic encephalopathy.

Before BRTO, indirect portography via celiac and SMA arteriography is done to establish the portal venous anatomy and hemodynamics. The outflow vein for the varices (typically the left inferior phrenic/adrenal to left renal vein for gastric varices, right gonadal vein for duodenal varices) is selectively engaged with a diagnostic catheter (see Fig. 12-14). A 6-Fr balloon occlusion catheter (e.g., 11- or 20-mm diameter) is advanced into the main trunk and inflated, and venography is performed to classify the varices and collateral veins.

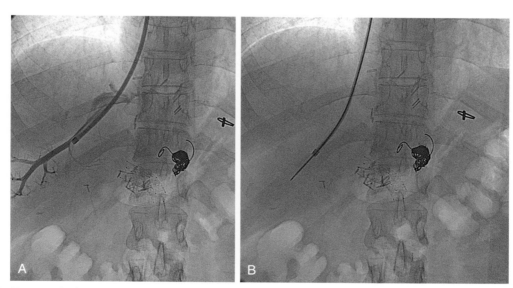

FIGURE 12-16   Transjugular liver biopsy in a posttranplant patient. Note prior coil embolization of gastroesophageal varices and placement of stents for portal vein stenosis. **A,** An angled catheter and sheath have been advanced well into the middle hepatic vein and venography done. **B,** With the metal cannula in place within the sheath, the entire mechanism is rotated anteriorly. The inner biopsy needle is advanced into the liver parenchyma and triggered to obtain liver tissue.

To induce thrombosis of simple varices, 10 mL of ethanolamine oleate 10% mixed with 10 mL of contrast material is slowly injected with the balloon inflated until the dilated veins are completely filled. The agent is left in place from 1 to 24 hours and then aspirated; the balloon is removed. More complex types of variceal communications may require use of a microcatheter or initial partial splenic embolization to reduce flow through the shunts.[63,64] Obliteration of varices is documented with contrast CT.

In experienced hands, BRTO is successful in preventing further bleeding and improving encephalopathy in more than 80% of attempts.[66] A major drawback to this approach is that purposefully closing down these natural shunts causes elevation of portal pressure and greater risk for esophageal variceal bleeding.[67,68] There are some risks to using ethanolamine oleate, including renal failure, pulmonary edema, and anaphylaxis. In Asia it is routine to administer IV haptoglobin, which binds free hemoglobin, to prevent hemolysis-induced kidney damage.

TRANSJUGULAR INTRAHEPATIC PORTOSYSTEMIC SHUNTS

The therapeutic applications of TIPS are discussed later.

SURGICAL THERAPY

Varices can be eliminated by operative ligation or transsection. However, such procedures fail to treat the underlying cause of variceal formation.

In the past, surgical portocaval shunts were commonly recommended for management of these difficult patients.[69,70] Side-to-side portacaval and mesocaval shunts are nonselective conduits that direct all portal blood flow away from the liver and return PV pressure to normal levels. The *distal splenorenal (Warren) shunt* is a selective communication that diverts flow from gastroesophageal varices but maintains intestinal portal flow to the liver. In this procedure, the splenic vein is divided, and the left gastric, right gastric, and gastroepiploic veins are ligated. Surgical mortality rates for all operative shunts are similar (10% to 20%). Rebleeding from varices occurs in about 5% to 15% of cases and is more frequent with selective shunts. Encephalopathy can be problematic.[71] In most centers, operative shunts are rarely performed anymore.

LIVER TRANSPLANTATION

Liver transplantation is the definitive treatment for relieving portal hypertension from chronic liver disease and provides the best long-term outcome compared with all other methods. The current overall 5-year survival rate for primary liver transplantation in the United States is 79%.[72] Not all patients are candidates for transplantation, and donor organs are in short supply.

Transjugular Intrahepatic Portosystemic Shunts (Online Cases 33 and 78)

The TIPS procedure has been in widespread practice for almost two decades and has revolutionized the management of patients with complications related to portal hypertension.

Patient Selection

Current indications for TIPS have been formulated by several expert groups, including the American Association for the Study of Liver Diseases (AASLD)[73-75] (Box 12-7). TIPS is most commonly performed for prevention of recurrent gastroesophageal variceal hemorrhage and management of refractory ascites. Given the inherent risks of the intervention, the fact that many patients with varices will never bleed and that only about half of those who do will rebleed, TIPS is reserved for patients who suffer one or more bleeding episodes that have failed endoscopic methods. However, this stipulation is being questioned. A recent randomized trial in high-risk cirrhotic patients with first variceal hemorrhage compared best medical therapy and endoscopic treatment against initial endoscopic treatment followed by urgent TIPS.[76] Rebleeding was significantly less likely and survival significantly longer in the TIPS arm.

Refractory ascites implies that sodium restriction and maximum diuretic therapy are inadequate therapy. TIPS may afford better quality of life than repeated large-volume paracentesis, but encephalopathy often gets worse and survival is not clearly improved.[77,78]

Several of the secondary indications for TIPS are worthy of comment.

- There is controversy about the value of TIPS as a *bridge to liver transplantation*.[79] Unlike surgical shunts, a TIPS does not interfere with a subsequent transplant (as long as stents are kept out of the retropancreatic portion of the portal vein). In some series, pretransplantation TIPS creation improved the general condition and nutritional status of the patient, reduced operative blood loss and procedure time, and decreased hospital stay.[80]
- TIPS is effective in patients with so-called *ectopic varices* (e.g., colonic, stomal, anorectal) and for portal hypertensive gastropathy.[81-83]
- Isolated gastric varices may not decompress with standard TIPS if the splenic vein is occluded.[84]
- The *hepatorenal syndrome (HRS)* applies to individuals with end-stage liver disease and acute kidney injury without an attributable etiology.[85,86] Ascites must be present, and serum creatinine must exceed 1.5 mg/dL. Type I HRS is the particularly lethal form of the disease, with rapid and severe

BOX 12-7

PATIENT SELECTION FOR THE TRANSJUGULAR INTRAHEPATIC PORTOSYSTEMIC SHUNT PROCEDURE

Accepted Indications

- Acute variceal bleeding unresponsive to medical therapy (including banding/sclerotherapy)
- Prevention of recurrent gastroesophageal variceal bleeding unresponsive to medical therapy (including repeated sclerotherapy/banding)
- Refractory ascites
- Refractory hepatic hydrothorax
- Prevention of rebleeding with gastric and ectopic varices (colonic, stomal, anorectal)
- Budd-Chiari syndrome
- Prevention of recurrent bleeding with portal hypertensive gastropathy on beta-blocker medication

Debated Indications

- Early treatment after first variceal hemorrhage
- Bridge to liver transplantation
- Acute portal vein thrombosis
- Hepatorenal syndrome
- Hepatopulmonary syndrome

Generally Not Acceptable

- Primary prevention of variceal bleeding
- Bleeding from gastric antral vascular ectasia

"Absolute" Contraindications

- Polycystic liver disease
- Severe hepatic failure
- Severe right-sided heart failure
- Severe pulmonary hypertension (mean ≥45 mm Hg)
- Uncontrolled systemic infection or sepsis
- Unrelieved biliary obstruction

Relative Contraindications

- Severe or uncontrollable hepatic encephalopathy
- Chronic portal vein thrombosis
- Severe active infection
- Uncorrectable severe coagulopathy (international normalized ratio >5, platelet count <20,000/L)
- Moderate pulmonary hypertension
- Hepatocellular carcinoma

renal failure brought on by some precipitating event (e.g., spontaneous bacterial peritonitis). Type II HRS is a milder version of the illness. It is difficult to predict which patients with HRS will benefit from a TIPS.

- *Hepatohydrothorax* refers to significant pleural effusion in patients with advanced cirrhosis without underlying unrelated heart or lung disease.[87] Ascites usually accompanies the effusions, which predominate on the right side of the chest in about 85% of cases. The most likely mechanism is seepage of fluid from the abdomen into the chest through diaphragmatic defects. In many cases, the TIPS procedure provides relief.
- Pregnancy does not exclude a woman from the TIPS procedure if it may be life-saving. The perceived radiation risk to the fetus is often overstated.[88]
- Even though *polycystic liver disease* and *hepatic tumors* are relative contraindications to shunt insertion, TIPS creation has been done successfully and safely in these situations[89,90] (Fig. 12-17).
- While AASLD guidelines stipulate *portal vein thrombosis* as a relative contraindication to TIPS insertion, the document recognizes that the procedure is feasible and effective in certain cases[73,91,92] (Fig. 12-18).
- The application of TIPS in Budd-Chiari syndrome is considered in a later section.

The decision to construct a TIPS demands thoughtful consideration by the patient, family, referring physician, and interventionalist. The procedure has a small but significant morbidity, and the immediate mortality rate approaches 1% to 2%. In addition, a substantial number of patients die soon afterward, largely from underlying liver disease but partly as a consequence of diversion of portal venous flow, which can precipitate fulminant hepatic failure.

When counseling patients and referring physicians, it is important to provide a frank assessment of the likelihood of survival following shunt creation. Patients can be stratified in several ways. The severity of liver failure is graded by the Child-Pugh classification (see Table 12-3). The *MELD score* (Mayo Endstage Liver Disease) has been adopted by many centers to predict outcomes in patients being considered for liver transplantation or TIPS. This score incorporates the serum bilirubin, creatinine, international normalized ratio, and recent need for dialysis (for calculation, go to www.mayoclinic.org/gi-rst/mayomodel6.html). Early mortality after TIPS insertion is especially high in patients with a MELD score greater than 18, Child-Pugh score greater than 12 (class C), APACHE severity of illness score greater than 18 to 20, or bilirubin greater than 3 mg/dL.[93-96]

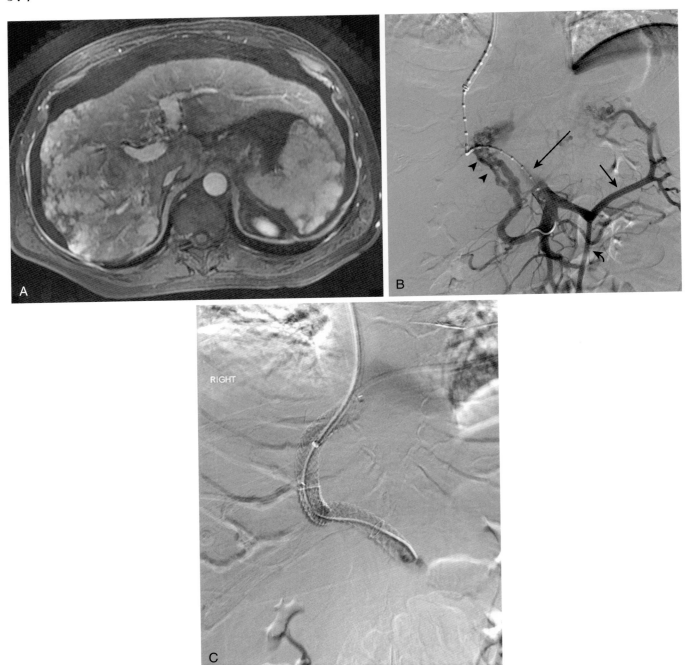

FIGURE 12-17   Transjugular intrahepatic portosystemic shunt (TIPS) procedure with hepatocellular carcinoma and portal vein (PV) throm-bosis. **A,** Contrast-enhanced magnetic resonance image shows a large hypervascular heterogeneous mass invading most of the right lobe of the liver. Right and left main portal veins are patent. Patient suffered several variceal bleeds, and a shunt was requested as a palliative measure. **B,** By the time the TIPS was performed, the tumor had invaded the portal vein *(long arrow)*, and "cavernous transformation" has begun to bypass the obstructed PV *(arrowheads)*. Note retrograde flow into the splenic vein *(short arrow)* and inferior mesenteric vein *(curved black arrow)*. **C,** A portosystemic shunt was created with two Viatorr stent grafts from the patent central portal vein to the inferior vena cava.

Technique

Acute bleeding is controlled with variceal banding or sclerotherapy, systemic terlipressin or octreotide infusion, placement of an esophageal tamponade balloon, or some combination of these measures. Coagulation defects should be corrected and broad-spectrum antibiotics given before the procedure. Some cross-sectional imaging must be obtained beforehand to assess portal vein patency and exclude a large tumor. Color Doppler sonography is adequate. However, three-phase contrast-enhanced CT

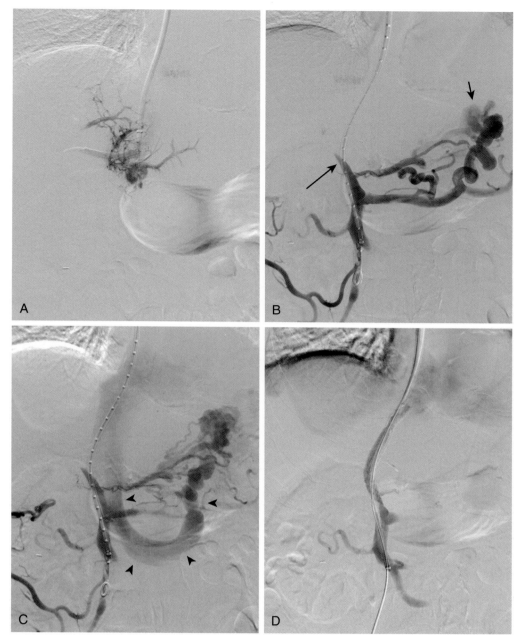

FIGURE 12-18   Transjugular intrahepatic portosystemic shunt procedure with portal vein thrombosis. **A,** Entry is made into a distorted portal venous system. A stiff angled glidewire was ultimately advanced into the main portal vein. **B,** Portography shows tapered occlusion of the main portal vein *(long arrow).* Prominent gastric varices are seen *(short arrow)* along with a splenorenal shunt (**C,** *arrowheads*). **D,** Viatorr stent graft has been inserted; shunt is widely patent.

angiography is certainly better for assessing these parameters (PV patency, status of the hepatic veins, degree of ascites, liver size, presence of liver tumors or polycystic liver disease). Just as important, the operator can determine beforehand the suitability of the individual hepatic veins along with the best trajectory and distance to the portal vein.

The TIPS procedure can be performed with moderate sedation under the direction of the interventionalist.

However, deep sedation or general anesthesia administered by a dedicated anesthesiologist is mandatory in unstable or uncooperative patients and helpful in all cases.

The standard access site is the right IJ vein (Fig. 12-19). The left IJ vein is preferred by some operators and should be considered if a second try is made after a failed first attempt. A 40-cm 10-Fr vascular sheath is advanced into the right atrium. Right atrial and IVC pressures are

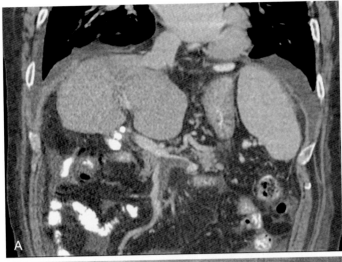

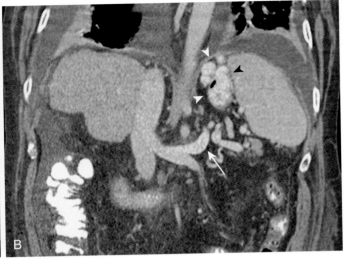

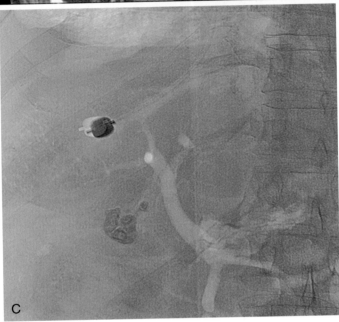

FIGURE 12-19   Transjugular intrahepatic portosystemic shunt procedure. **A** and **B,** Reformatted coronal computed tomography scans show small liver and enlarged spleen along with gastroesophageal varices *(arrowheads)* and a prominent splenorenal portosystemic shunt *(long arrow)*. Also note bilateral pleural effusions. **C,** From the right internal jugular vein, the right hepatic vein has been catheterized. An 8.5-mm occlusion balloon was advanced deep into the vein and inflated. Carbon dioxide wedged hepatic vein injection opacifies the portal venous system to provide a target for portal vein puncture. The Roesch Uchida metal cannula was inserted. The cannula was rotated anteromedially, and the 5-Fr catheter stylet advanced. The crotch of the portal vein was entered.

measured. If right atrial pressure is markedly elevated (>20 to 25 mm Hg), the interventionalist should proceed with caution. Fulminant right heart failure can occur after the shunt is created.

The right or middle hepatic vein is entered with a multipurpose angiographic catheter and steerable guidewire. If the right hepatic vein is small, has a very acute angle with the IVC, or is difficult to catheterize, TIPS can be created from the middle (or even left) hepatic vein. It is important to establish which vein is being used so that the intrahepatic puncture toward the PV is made in the appropriate direction. This step can be accomplished with steep oblique/lateral fluoroscopy or ultrasound interrogation. About 3% of the population has a dominant inferior right hepatic vein. In this situation, TIPS must be formed from the right common femoral vein (Fig. 12-20; see also Fig. 12-8).

Several methods are used to guide the puncture from the hepatic vein toward the PV (Fig. 12-21). The most popular techniques are as follows:

1. Reliance on bony landmarks. The right PV trunk typically runs at the level of the 11th rib, about 0.5 to 1.5 vertebral widths from the lateral border of the spine.[97]
2. Injection of CO_2 through a balloon occlusion catheter to fill the central portal venous system[98] (see Fig. 12-19).
3. Using CT guidance to place a metallic coil adjacent to the intended entry site on the portal vein as a fiduciary marker.
4. Ultrasound-guided catheterization of an enlarged paraumbilical vein. A catheter advanced into the central portal venous system serves as a target for needle passes.[99]

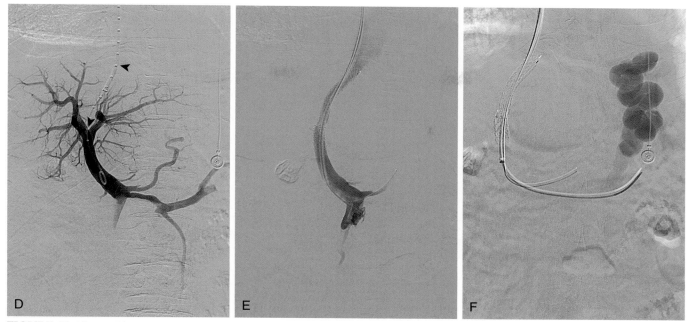

FIGURE 20-19, cont'd   A marking pigtail was advanced for direct portography **(D)**. The distance from portal vein entry to inferior vena cava entry was measured at 6 cm *(arrowheads)*. **E,** A 10 mm × 2 cm × 6 cm Viatorr stent graft was inserted. Repeat portography shows a widely patent shunt with no filling of intrahepatic portal venous branches. Portosystemic gradient was 6 mm Hg. **F,** The coronary vein was catheterized. Gastroesophageal varices still opacify with forced injection, but portal decompression has been achieved and embolization is not necessary.

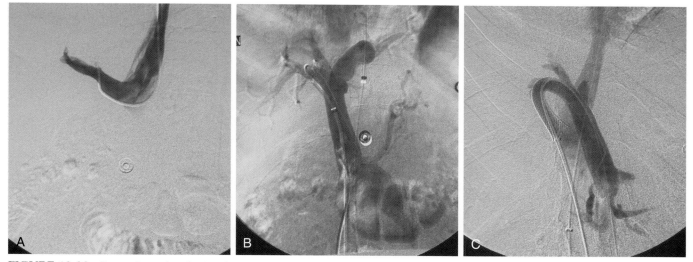

FIGURE 12-20   Femoral transjugular intrahepatic portosystemic shunt (TIPS) procedure. **A,** From right internal jugular vein access, the major draining vein is an inferior right hepatic vein. TIPS cannot be created from above. **B,** Through a right common femoral vein approach, the standard TIPS set is used to enter the right portal vein. **C,** An uncovered Wallstent is placed to create the shunt (procedure done before advent of covered stents).

The site of PV puncture is critical. Because the portal vein bifurcation is extrahepatic in about one half of individuals, entry should be at or peripheral to this point to avoid extrahepatic puncture and the possibility of exsanguinating hemorrhage.[16,100]

After the outer sheath is advanced well into the hepatic vein, the stiffening cannula and catheter-needle system are inserted (e.g., 16-gauge Roesch-Uchida catheter-trocar

set). The catheter-trocar is guided down the protective outer sheath until they are tip to tip. When the right hepatic vein is used, the needle is turned anteromedially toward the right PV, and a brisk needle pass is made. From the middle hepatic vein, either an anterior or posterior throw (toward the left or right portal vein, respectively) may be appropriate. After the sharp stylet is removed, the catheter is slowly withdrawn, and contrast is injected after

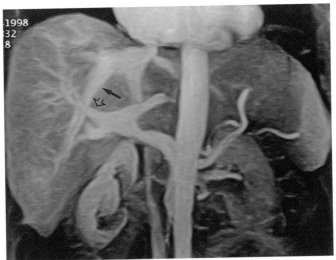

FIGURE 12-21   Relationship between the middle hepatic vein *(arrow)* and the right portal vein *(open arrow)* on coronal gadolinium-enhanced magnetic resonance angiogram.

blood is aspirated. It is common to obtain ascitic fluid or to opacify biliary ducts, hepatic arterial branches, or even lymphatic channels. It is important not to mistake any of them for the portal venous system and inadvertently create a shunt into these structures. When a PV branch fills and the vessel appears suitable, a guidewire (e.g., angled hydrophilic steerable wire) is manipulated into the PV and then into the splenic vein or SMV.

When the TIPS procedure becomes difficult, several steps should be considered (Box 12-8 and Fig. 12-22).

A marking pigtail or straight catheter is placed in the main portal vein for venography and pressure measurements to calculate the initial portosystemic gradient. The suitability of the portal puncture site is confirmed. The parenchymal track is then dilated with an 8- or 10-mm angioplasty balloon or by advancing the covered metal cannula set over a super stiff wire into the portal vein. Ultimately, the 10-Fr outer vascular sheath tip must reside well within the main portal vein.

The Viatorr polytetrafluoroethylene (PTFE) covered stent graft is the best available device based on its superior long-term results (Fig. 12-23). The Wallstent is an inferior choice.

- Graft diameter. The 8-mm–diameter devices are generally too small for adequate portal decompression.[101] The choice between a 10- or 12-mm graft rests on the magnitude of the portosystemic gradient, indication for portal decompression, level of concern for postinsertion encephalopathy, and operator preference.

BOX 12-8

TECHNICAL PEARLS FOR DIFFICULT TRANSJUGULAR INTRAHEPATIC PORTOSYSTEMIC SHUNT

- Exaggerate curve on Roesch-Uchida metal trochar (see Fig. 12-22). Liver scarring and shrinkage markedly distort the anatomic relationship between portal and hepatic veins. For example, the central right portal vein may be almost at the same craniocaudal plane as the right hepatic vein.
- Consider presence of dominant inferior right hepatic vein. If present, femoral vein access may be necessary.
- Switch to Ring set or Angiodynamics set.
- Make needle pass in opposite direction. The cannula may have migrated back centrally and into a different hepatic vein.
- Switch to left internal jugular vein access. Purchase on right/middle hepatic veins and entry angle into portal vein may be more favorable.

- Graft length. The uncovered segment of the stent (always 2 cm) should reside entirely within the portal vein. The remaining PTFE-covered segment (usually 6 or 8 cm) should cover the entire parenchymal track and outflow hepatic vein just into the IVC.

The stent graft is loaded into the outer sheath, which has been advanced into the portal vein. The sheath is withdrawn to expose the uncovered segment (see Fig. 12-23A). The entire unit is pulled back to snug the transition zone (between covered and uncovered stent) against the parenchymal track. The sheath is withdrawn into the right atrium and the release cord is pulled, deploying the remainder of the device. The entire stent is then dilated with a 10- or 12-mm balloon (see Fig. 12-19).

In patients treated for variceal hemorrhage, the conventional endpoint is a portosystemic gradient less than 12 mm Hg. However, there is some evidence that relative reduction of the gradient (e.g., by 50% of baseline) may be sufficient to prevent recurrent variceal rebleeding. The threshold for patients with refractory ascites is controversial. Some experts believe gradients less than 8 mm Hg are necessary; others argue that it is prudent to accept a larger gradient (and thus reduce the risk of encephalopathy and hepatic insufficiency). If balloon diameter is smaller than nominal graft diameter, the shunt can be further dilated at a later time if the clinical response is inadequate.

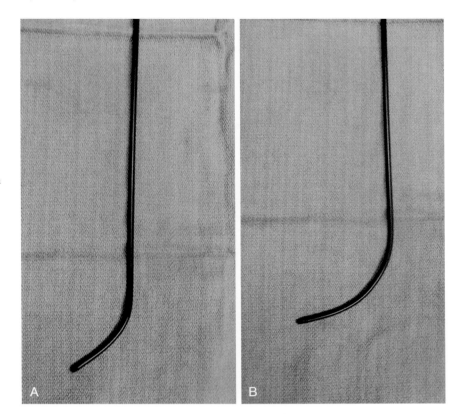

FIGURE 12-22   Adjustment of Roesch-Uchida transjugular intrahepatic portosystemic shunt (TIPS) cannula. **A,** Metal cannula from TIPS set directly out of the package. **B,** The cannula is reshaped to better suit the distorted vascular anatomy of a cirrhotic liver.

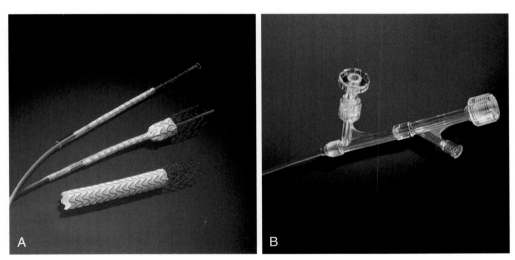

FIGURE 12-23   Viatorr nitinol-ePTFE covered stent graft. **A,** Photograph of fully constrained device *(top)*, partially uncovered device *(middle)*, and fully deployed device *(bottom)*. **B,** Operative end of insertion catheter, with hemostatic valve at end and knob for pulling the "rip cord" to release covered portion of device as a sidearm. *(Courtesy of W.L. Gore and Associates.)*

At the end of the procedure, a portal venogram is done to document shunt patency, lack of filling of intrahepatic PV branches, and nonvisualization of gastroesophageal varices. If the portosystemic gradient remains elevated despite use of a 12-mm balloon, varices continue to fill with portal injection, or the patient recently had massive variceal bleeding, embolization of varices should be considered (Fig. 12-24). On occasion, thrombi will form within the shunt while the procedure is ongoing. The reason is often obscure, but incomplete track coverage, portal vein dissection, or unsuspected thrombophilia are possible. If the patient has not recently bled, full anticoagulation and treatment with fibrinolytic agents may be helpful. If bleeding is

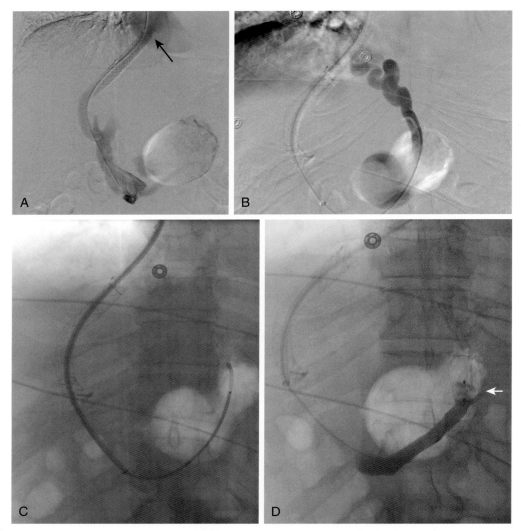

FIGURE 12-24 Variceal embolization after a transjugular intrahepatic portosystemic shunt (TIPS) procedure. **A,** Post-TIPS portography shows a widely patent shunt, which extends up too far into the right atrium *(arrow)*. No varices fill, but patient has suffered very recent massive variceal hemorrhage. **B,** Coronary vein catheterization with an angled catheter outlines the varices. **C,** Through a guiding sheath, an Amplatzer plug is being advanced. **D,** The occluder has been deployed *(arrow),* completely obstructing the coronary vein.

a concern, maceration or mobilization of clot with a dilation or occlusion balloon is appropriate. Overnight anticoagulation is advisable when these steps are necessary.

Postprocedure care includes observation for signs of abdominal bleeding, evaluation of hepatic and renal function, treatment of encephalopathy, and follow-up duplex sonography of the shunt. Because of air trapped in the graft fabric, Viatorr stent visualization by ultrasound is only possible days after deployment.

Early Results

A shunt can be created successfully in more than 90% to 95% of attempts, leaving a portosystemic gradient less than 12 mm Hg or reduced by greater than 50% in most cases.[31,71,73,102,103] In patients treated for variceal hemorrhage, early rebleeding (before 6 months) occurs less than 15% of the time. TIPS is more effective than sclerotherapy or banding in preventing rebleeding, although survival may not be prolonged in all populations.[71,76] About 50% to 75% of individuals treated for refractory ascites have partial or complete resolution within about 1 month of placement.[77,78,104] Early (30-day) mortality after TIPS can be substantial (3% to 45%), but this is largely because of underlying liver disease rather than direct complications of the procedure.[105]

The *direct intrahepatic portosystemic shunt (DIPS)* is an endovascular alternative to TIPS. The portosystemic communication is made between the IVC and the portal vein using intravascular ultrasound (IVUS) guidance.[106] Reported results are promising.

Complications

Major procedure-related complications develop in about 3% to 5% of patients. Table 12-4 lists adverse events.* Other problems include acute renal failure, access site bleeding, cardiac dysrhythmias, and reactions to contrast material.

The riskiest step in the TIPS procedure is the transhepatic needle puncture. Liver capsule perforation and injury to small hepatic artery or bile duct branches are common and usually inconsequential. Rarely, needle passes cause gallbladder perforation, hepatic artery pseudoaneurysms, or arteriovenous fistula formation. Fatal hemorrhage from extracapsular, caval, right atrial, or portal venous perforation is rare. *Acute shunt thrombosis* is reported in about 3% to 4% of cases and has several causes[108,109] (Box 12-9 and Fig. 12-25).

Hepatic encephalopathy is a major concern after any side-to-side portosystemic shunt. With diversion of mesenteric venous blood, nitrogen-containing compounds (among several other substances) produced by bacterial action in the gut are not metabolized by the liver before entering the circulation. Blood ammonia levels can rise sharply and result in encephalopathy. In this population, encephalopathy also may be related to increased protein intake, gastrointestinal bleeding, sepsis, dehydration, or acute hepatitis. This complication is more likely when the residual portosystemic gradient is less than 10 mm Hg.[110] Although about 25% to 30% of patients develop new or worsened encephalopathy, less than 5% to 10% are unresponsive to medical therapy; those individuals may be candidates for shunt reduction (see later discussion).

A transient (and sometimes profound) elevation in liver enzymes is common after TIPS. However, isolated

*See references 73, 102, 103, 105, 107.

persistent hyperbilirubinemia may be related to hemolysis. Fulminant hepatic failure is rare unless the patient already had end-stage liver disease.

The immediate mortality rate is up to 2%, although this figure may be higher for less experienced operators. Early procedure-related death is usually the result of massive bleeding from extracapsular or central vessel perforation, hepatic artery thrombosis with fulminant hepatic failure, or acute right heart failure.

Late Results

In the past, after a TIPS was created with a bare stent (e.g., Wallstent), a layer of pseudointima would slowly cover the track, which protected it from late thrombosis.[111] Cellular and fibrous proliferative tissue lined the walls of the conduit and outflow veins. An inflammatory reaction to injured bile ducts was an important cause of this process.[112] Significant stenoses developed within the body of the stent and the outflow vein; however, PV stenoses were exceedingly uncommon.

Despite excellent short-term results using the uncovered Wallstent, most of these shunts did not remain patent without repeated intervention. The reported primary patency rate for TIPS with these devices is 25% to 66% (average, 50%) at 1 year and 26% to 32% at 2 years.[113-115]

There is incontrovertible evidence that PTFE-covered stent-grafts dramatically improve long-term durability, with 1-year primary patency rates of about 81% to 86%, and 2-year rates of about 80%.[103,107,116] Survival at 5 years after TIPS is about 61% with a 10% rebleeding rate; these outcomes are comparable to those achieved with surgical shunts and are certainly better than best medical therapy and endoscopy.[71,76,117]

TABLE 12-4 Major Complications of the Transjugular Intrahepatic Portosystemic Shunt Procedure

Complication	Frequency (%)
Transcapsular puncture	33
Bleeding	
Intraperitoneal	1-13
Hemobilia	1-4
Liver dysfunction	
Transient worsening	10-20
Fulminant hepatic failure or infarction	3-7
Hepatic encephalopathy	
New onset or worsened	10-44
Uncontrollable	5-10
Sepsis	2-10
Stent malposition or migration	1-3
Other	
Fistula	<1
Infection of TIPS	<1

BOX 12-9

CAUSES OF ACUTE TRANSJUGULAR INTRAHEPATIC PORTOSYSTEMIC SHUNT THROMBOSIS

- Thrombophilia (see Boxes 1-4 and 1-5)
- Uncovered portion of shunt track
- Portal vein dissection
- Low flow (e.g., competing flow through splenorenal shunt)
- Preexisting portal or mesenteric vein thrombus
- Residual shunt stenosis

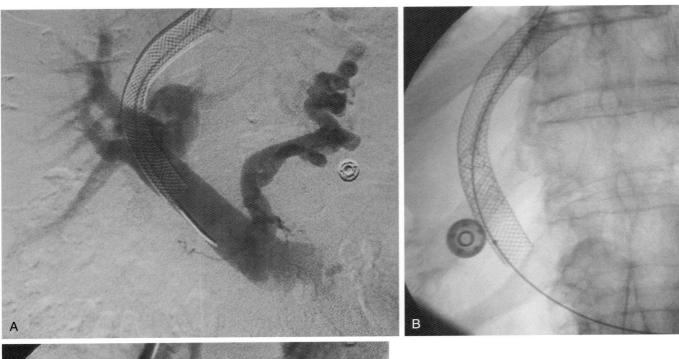

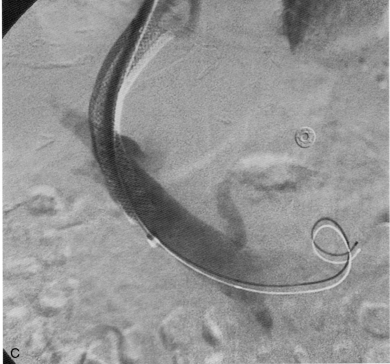

FIGURE 12-25   Acute transjugular intrahepatic portosystemic shunt (TIPS) thrombosis. **A,** Complete shunt occlusion was suspected on the basis of post-TIPS ultrasound findings and confirmed by direct cannulation of the shunt. **B,** A covered Viatorr stent was deployed within the track. **C,** The shunt was recanalized, and portal flow now is hepatofugal.

Surveillance and Shunt Management

Recurrent variceal hemorrhage or return of intractable ascites after TIPS procedure is usually a sign of shunt stenosis or occlusion (see Box 12-9). Because shunt obstruction may be silent, vigorous imaging surveillance programs are routine. CT angiography is helpful in detecting impending TIPS failure, but color Doppler sonography is the best tool for long-term screening because of its simplicity and low cost. Sonography was routinely performed immediately following and 1 month after the TIPS procedure, at 3-month intervals for the first year and at 6- to 12-month intervals thereafter. However, the necessity of this approach has been questioned following widespread adoption of covered stents. In the era of stent grafts, the timing of imaging protocols is hotly debated.[118]

Several findings may signal shunt dysfunction[119-123] (Box 12-10). However, it has recently become apparent that color Doppler sonography is not as accurate in detecting shunt dysfunction as was once thought. Although quite specific in identifying abnormalities (about 90%), sonography is not particularly sensitive in this regard (about 50%).[73] Therefore shunt angiography is advisable if varices reappear at endoscopy or the clinical scenario suggests shunt malfunction.

A direct portal venogram is performed from a right IJ vein approach. A patent shunt almost always can be cannulated with an angiographic catheter (e.g., multipurpose angiographic or cobra shape) and an angled hydrophilic guidewire. Care must taken to avoid unknowingly passing through the interstices (rather than the mouth) of the uncovered portion of the stent. The presence of shunt occlusion, stenosis of greater than 50%, portosystemic gradient of greater than 12 mm Hg, or filling of gastroesophageal varices are indications for intervention. If a bare stent was placed originally, insertion of a Viatorr device that extends from the portal vein up to the IVC is appropriate (Fig. 12-26). With covered stents, in-stent stenosis is much less common. In most cases, lesions develop in unstented portions of the outflow hepatic veins, which then require placement of additional covered stents. Stents should not extend deep into the IVC, because caval thrombosis can result.[124]

Occasionally, patients suffer uncontrollable hepatic encephalopathy or progressive liver failure after the TIPS is placed. In these cases, portal venous flow can be augmented in several ways[125-128] (Fig. 12-27):

- *Shunt occlusion* is accomplished by embolization with coils or an Amplatzer plug. Obviously, the patient will then be at risk for the symptoms of portal hypertension for which he or she was first treated. More importantly, cases of life-threatening or fatal cardiovascular collapse because of abrupt hemodynamic changes have been reported.[129]
- *Shunt reduction* is achieved in several ways, most of which involve placement of a covered, partially constrained stent within the existing shunt. Some of these devices, fashioned sterilely on the interventional table, can later be adjusted using balloons to achieve controlled reduction in shunt flow.
- *Splenorenal shunt embolization* using the BRTO method (see earlier discussion) can be effective in appropriate patients with intractable encephalopathy.

Portal and Splenic Vein Thrombosis

Etiology

Portal vein thrombosis has many causes[130,131] (Box 12-11). It was once thought that most cases were idiopathic. In fact, a precipitating condition can be identified in up to 80% of affected individuals. The etiology is often multifactorial. In children, sepsis is frequently responsible.

PV thrombosis can be confined to the PV itself or include the SMV but spare mesenteric vessels, or it can entail widespread involvement (with or without an adequate collateral circulation).

Splenic vein thrombosis is usually a consequence of pancreatitis, pancreatic neoplasms, splenectomy, thrombophilic states, or trauma.[132,133] With obstruction of the splenic vein, "segmental" or "left-sided" portal hypertension may develop. The spleen then drains through several portoportal collateral routes (see later discussion).

Clinical Features

Classically, patients with acute PV thrombosis complain of fever, abdominal pain, nausea, and (sometimes) new-onset ascites. A few of these cases resolve spontaneously. Patients with chronic PV thrombosis usually present with symptoms related to portal hypertension. Sometimes, the liver size is normal, signs of liver failure are absent, and the liver biopsy is unremarkable. At the other end of the clinical spectrum, bowel infarction is the most devastating outcome. Biliary complications related to mass effect by collateral veins on the extrahepatic bile ducts are also described.

BOX 12-10

SONOGRAPHIC SIGNS OF TRANSJUGULAR INTRAHEPATIC PORTOSYSTEMIC SHUNT DYSFUNCTION

- Absent flow
- Significant rise or fall in shunt velocity (>50 cm/sec) compared with the first post-TIPS study
- Low-peak shunt velocity (<50 to 90 cm/sec)
- High-peak shunt velocity (>190 cm/sec)
- Low main PV velocity (<30 cm/sec or >50% drop from baseline)
- Return of antegrade flow in intrahepatic PVs

PV, portal vein; *TIPS*, transjugular intrahepatic portosystemic shunt.

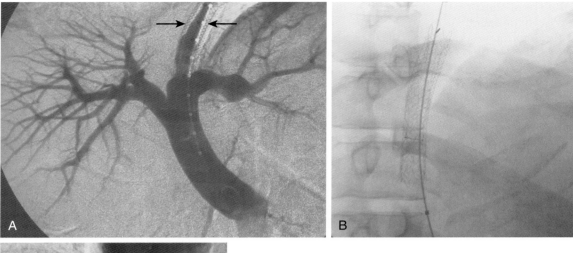

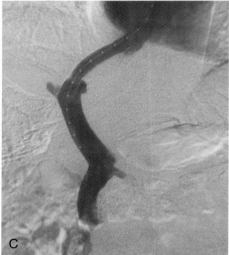

FIGURE 12-26   Covered stent placement for transjugular intrahepatic portosystemic shunt stenosis. **A,** Initial direct portogram revealed in-stent neointimal hyperplasia *(arrows)* and hepatopetal flow. **B,** A Viatorr stent graft is placed across the shunt, taking care to keep the covered portion (above the lower stent markers) within the liver track and hepatic outflow vein. **C,** Widely patent shunt after deployment with no intrahepatic portal venous flow.

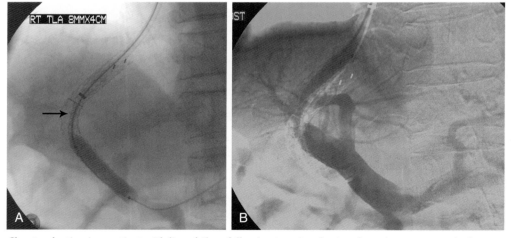

FIGURE 12-27   Shunt reduction in a patient with liver failure following transjugular intrahepatic portosystemic shunt procedure. Initial portogram showed a widely patent shunt. A suture was used to make a waist around the middle of a covered Viatorr stent, which was then inserted into the existing shunt **(A). B,** Follow-up portogram demonstrates flow both in the shunt and the intrahepatic portal vein.

BOX 12-11

CAUSES OF PORTAL VEIN THROMBOSIS

- Neoplasms (hepatic or pancreatic)
- Inflammatory
  - Infection/sepsis
  - Pancreatitis
  - Appendicitis or diverticulitis
  - Schistosomiasis
- Thrombophilic state (see Boxes 1-4 and 1-5)
- Cirrhosis
- Posttraumatic
  - After transplantation
  - After shunt placement
  - After neonatal umbilical vein catheter placement
- Dehydration
- Idiopathic

Patients with isolated splenic vein thrombosis may be asymptomatic or can suffer variceal bleeding or abdominal pain. At endoscopy, bleeding gastric varices without associated esophageal varices are characteristic. However, some patients indeed have coexisting esophageal varices if the left gastric vein drains into the occluded portion of the splenic vein.[132]

Imaging

CROSS-SECTIONAL TECHNIQUES

Portal and splenic vein thrombosis are detected with color Doppler sonography, or CT or MR angiography.[134,135] In the acute phase of the illness, signs of the underlying causes (e.g., neoplasm, cirrhosis, pancreatitis, recent splenectomy) may be evident along with thrombus in the portal, splenic, superior mesenteric, and/or branch mesenteric veins. Ancillary findings are bowel wall edema, varices, and ascites.

In the chronic phase, numerous collateral vascular channels in the porta hepatis and gallbladder fossa will bypass the obstruction and fill intrahepatic PVs. "Cavernous transformation" is a misnomer for this condition—the PV itself remains occluded. Other portoportal and portosystemic collaterals may circumvent the occlusion. Long after the acute event, calcification of the PV, liver atrophy, and splenomegaly are possible.

CATHETER ANGIOGRAPHY

Because the obstruction in portal and splenic vein thrombosis is proximal to the hepatic sinusoids, the normal pressures obtained at HVW manometry do not

reflect true portal hemodynamics. In acute or partial PV thrombosis, a filling defect may be seen on the late-phase celiac or SMA arteriogram. However, a patent PV may not opacify at all if flow is hepatofugal. In cases of subacute or chronic PV thrombosis, changes of "cavernous transformation" are found (Fig. 12-28).

With splenic vein occlusion, the spleen drains through portoportal collateral pathways such as short gastric veins to the left gastric vein, left gastroepiploic vein to the SMV, the venous arc of Barkow running in the greater omentum, IMV to rectal veins (with central splenic vein occlusion), and splenorenal and splenoretroperitoneal shunts. Even with a large-volume contrast injection directly into the splenic artery, a patent splenic vein may not fill in some patients with massive splenomegaly, hepatofugal flow in the splenic vein, or gastroesophageal varices. In such cases, direct splenoportography is helpful.

Treatment

MEDICAL THERAPY

For acute mesenteric vein thrombosis, standard treatment is anticoagulation. Many patients with isolated portal vein thrombus exhibit endogenous lysis.[136]

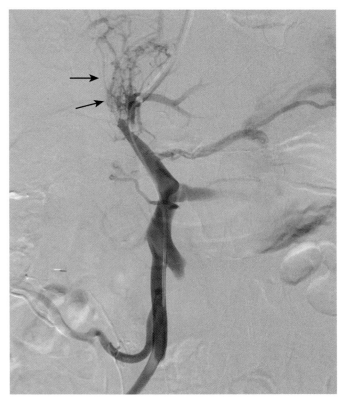

FIGURE 12-28 Cavernous transformation of the portal vein with numerous collateral channels in the gallbladder fossa (*arrow*) is seen on direct portography during transjugular intrahepatic portosystemic shunt procedure.

ENDOVASCULAR THERAPY

Thrombolysis should strongly be considered when acute PV thrombosis is symptomatic or does not quickly improve with anticoagulant therapy. If thrombus is truly acute (≤2 to 4 weeks old), lysis and improvement in symptoms are the rule[136-140] (Fig. 12-29). Adequate thrombolysis often requires several days of tissue plasminogen activator infusion and adjunctive use of a mechanical thrombectomy device. A transhepatic route to the portal veins is sometimes chosen. However, many patients benefit from placement of a TIPS to maintain flow through the newly recanalized PV. With this approach, a transjugular access to the portal veins is made.[141-143] Chronic PV thrombosis rarely responds to thrombolytic therapy; in this setting, TIPS insertion is formidable if not impossible.

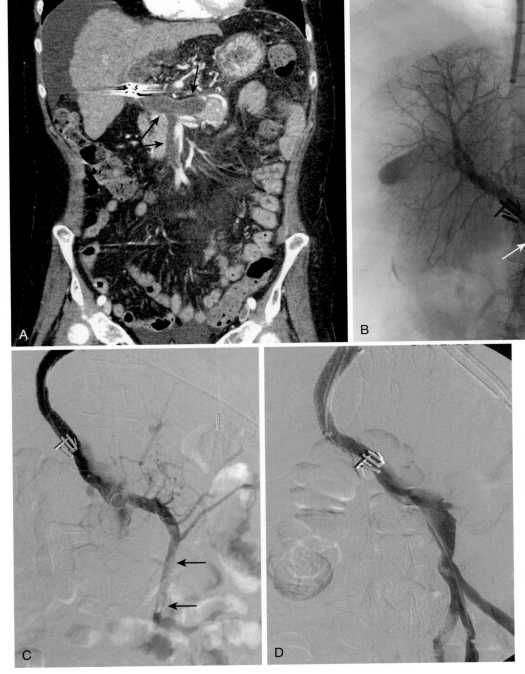

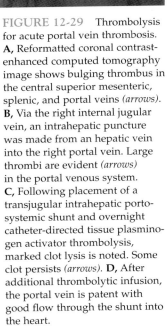

FIGURE 12-29 Thrombolysis for acute portal vein thrombosis. **A,** Reformatted coronal contrast-enhanced computed tomography image shows bulging thrombus in the central superior mesenteric, splenic, and portal veins *(arrows)*. **B,** Via the right internal jugular vein, an intrahepatic puncture was made from an hepatic vein into the right portal vein. Large thrombi are evident *(arrows)* in the portal venous system. **C,** Following placement of a transjugular intrahepatic portosystemic shunt and overnight catheter-directed tissue plasminogen activator thrombolysis, marked clot lysis is noted. Some clot persists *(arrows)*. **D,** After additional thrombolytic infusion, the portal vein is patent with good flow through the shunt into the heart.

Endoscopic banding of isolated gastric varices from splenic vein thrombosis is difficult because of large variceal size and the sharp angles required to access the dilated veins. Some practitioners favor BRTO for this problem (see earlier discussion). Another treatment option is proximal splenic artery embolization with coils to reduce splenic blood flow and thereby variceal flow.[144,145]

SURGICAL THERAPY

Operative treatment of PV thrombosis involves thrombectomy or bowel resection (for acute disease), portomesenteric shunt placement, or liver transplantation.[146] In patients with splenic vein thrombosis, splenectomy may be performed to eliminate variceal flow.

Hepatic Vein Outflow Obstruction (Budd-Chiari Syndrome)

Etiology and Clinical Features

Obstruction to venous drainage of the liver *(Budd-Chiari syndrome)* can occur at several levels[147]:

1. Hepatic venules *(hepatic venoocclusive disease).* This form of venous obstruction usually follows chemotherapy and irradiation for stem cell/bone marrow transplantation.[148-150]
2. Main hepatic veins. Classic *Budd-Chiari disease* reflects widespread clotting of the hepatic veins and is often associated with a thrombophilic state such as polycythemia vera, oral contraceptive use, or malignancy (see Boxes 1-4 and 1-5). Another important cause for hepatic vein (HV) obstruction is neoplastic invasion from hepatocellular carcinoma.
3. Hepatic vein confluence, IVC, or right atrium. Narrowing of the suprahepatic IVC at the hepatic

vein junction is caused by congenital *membranous obstruction of the IVC,* bland thrombus, tumor, or extrinsic compression.[151] Constrictive pericarditis, right heart failure, and right atrial tumors also may cause Budd-Chiari syndrome.

The unifying features of these disparate conditions are hepatic venous hypertension, hypoxic and oxidative hepatocyte injury, and, ultimately, centrilobular necrosis and fibrosis. Early on, symptoms reflect hepatic congestion, but liver function is maintained. With time, cirrhosis, postsinusoidal portal hypertension, and irreversible hepatic failure may ensue.

Fulminant, acute, subacute, and chronic forms of Budd-Chiari syndrome exist. The classic triad of symptoms is hepatomegaly, abdominal pain, and ascites. Some patients are jaundiced and may suffer from variceal bleeding. Others are entirely asymptomatic. In Western countries, central hepatic vein thrombosis is the most common form of the disease and typically is seen in young women. In South Africa and parts of Asia, membranous IVC obstruction is the most frequent cause of Budd-Chiari syndrome.

Imaging
CROSS-SECTIONAL TECHNIQUES

Usually the diagnosis is made by color Doppler sonography, CT, or MRI; each type of study has particular advantages.[152-154] Hepatic vein wall thickening, stenoses or occlusions, and intrahepatic collateral channels are primary characteristic. Secondary findings of ascites, hepatomegaly, areas of necrosis, right lobe atrophy and caudate lobe enlargement (a consequence of its separate and intact venous drainage into the IVC), cirrhosis, and malignancy are well depicted by all modalities[155] (Fig. 12-30).

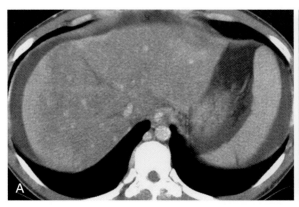
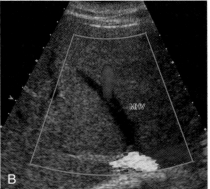

FIGURE 12-30   Budd-Chiari syndrome. **A,** Contrast computed tomography scan shows a mottled parenchymal pattern and lack of filling of central hepatic veins. Ascites is present. **B,** Color Doppler ultrasound fails to identify flow in the middle hepatic vein.

CATHETER ANGIOGRAPHY

Venography and hepatic vein manometry are required when cross-sectional studies are equivocal, when transcatheter therapy is contemplated, and in some patients before shunt procedures. Bone marrow transplantation patients with suspected venoocclusive disease can go directly to percutaneous or transvenous liver biopsy (with hepatic venography and manometry).[156] With contrast injection in the hepatic vein orifice, the "spider-web" pattern of bizarre intrahepatic venous collaterals is pathognomonic of central Budd-Chiari disease (Fig. 12-31). The intrahepatic IVC often is narrowed by ascites or an enlarged caudate lobe. Membranes, webs, and thrombus (bland or neoplastic) also

may be identified. In the advanced stages of the illness, patients will have features of portal hypertension.

Treatment

The goals of treatment are prevention of fulminant hepatic failure and management of complications related to portal hypertension, including variceal bleeding and ascites.

ENDOVASCULAR THERAPY

For central hepatic vein or IVC obstruction, catheter-directed thrombolysis (in the acute setting), angioplasty, and stent placement have been used effectively in selected patients with acute or chronic disease.[157-160]

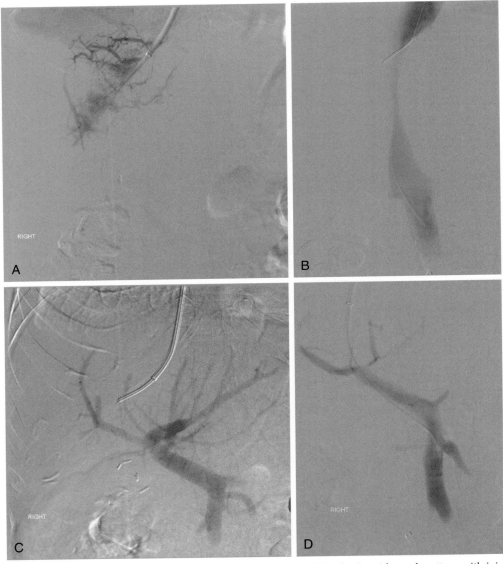

FIGURE 12-31 Budd-Chiari syndrome from central hepatic vein thrombosis. **A,** The classic spider-web pattern with injection of the right hepatic vein is caused by innumerable intrahepatic venous collaterals. **B,** Inferior venacavogram shows severe compression of its intrahepatic segment because of a markedly enlarged caudate lobe. **C,** During TIPS procedure, carbon dioxide wedged hepatic injection outlines the portal vein, providing a target for puncture. **D,** The portal vein has been entered. A Viatorr stent graft was subsequently placed.

The TIPS procedure is valuable in many patients with Budd-Chiari syndrome, sometimes as a bridge to transplantation[148,161-163] (see Fig. 12-31). A shunt improves venous drainage from the liver.

SURGICAL THERAPY

Operative treatment options include mesenteric-systemic shunts (e.g., mesoatrial shunt) and liver transplantation.

Malignant Liver Neoplasms (Online Cases 58, 79, 89, and 113)

The liver is affected by a wide variety of benign and malignant tumors (Box 12-12). Benign liver tumors are considered below. The role of the interventionalist in the management of malignant lesions in adults[164-167] is discussed in Chapter 24.

BOX 12-12

LIVER NEOPLASMS

- Benign
  - Hemangioma
  - Adenoma
  - Focal nodular hyperplasia
  - Regenerating nodule
  - Biliary cystadenoma
- Malignant
  - Hepatocellular carcinoma
  - Cholangiocarcinoma
  - Angiosarcoma
  - Biliary carcinoma
  - Lymphoma
- Metastatic
  - Gastrointestinal tract
  - Breast
  - Pancreas
  - Lung
  - Kidney
  - Islet cell (i.e., pancreas)
  - Carcinoid
- Pediatric
  - Metastases (e.g., neuroblastoma, Wilms tumor)
  - Hepatoblastoma
  - Hemangioendothelioma
  - Hemangioma
  - Hepatocellular carcinoma

Hepatic and Splenic Trauma (Online Case 108)

Etiology and Clinical Features

The liver and spleen are particularly susceptible to injury from blunt or penetrating abdominal trauma. Open or laparoscopic surgical procedures are responsible for a significant number of cases. Arterial laceration can result in parenchymal or peritoneal bleeding, subcapsular hematoma, pseudoaneurysms, or arteriovenous fistulas.[168,169] Although most patients with significant vascular injuries are symptomatic, some show little evidence of massive bleeding.

Imaging

CROSS-SECTIONAL IMAGING

In most centers, focused abdominal sonography in trauma (FAST) has replaced diagnostic peritoneal lavage as the screening tool for detecting posttraumatic intraabdominal hemorrhage.[170] CT is the primary imaging study for stable patients with blunt trauma. CT can accurately stage the extent of injury to the liver or spleen (Tables 12-5 and 12-6) and detect other abdominal or pelvic injuries.[171-174] Management decisions (observation, angiography, operation) are based on the clinical picture and CT grade (Fig. 12-32).

CATHETER ANGIOGRAPHY

With blunt trauma, arteriography shows extravasation, subcapsular or parenchymal hematomas, arterial occlusion, or diffuse punctuate injury (Fig. 12-33 and see Fig. 12-32). With penetrating trauma, typical findings include extravasation, pseudoaneurysms, and arteriovenous fistulas (Fig. 12-34).

TABLE 12-5   AAST Computed Tomography Classification for Liver Trauma

Grade	Injury Type
I	Subcapsular hematoma, <10% surface area
	Capsular tear, <1 cm deep
II	Subcapsular hematoma, 10% to 50% surface area, <10 cm diameter
	Capsular tear, 1-3 cm deep, <10 cm length
III	Subcapsular hematoma, >50% surface area
	Intraparenchymal hematoma, >10 cm or expanding
	Laceration >3 cm deep
IV	Parenchymal laceration 25% to 75% of lobe or 1-3 Couinaud segments
V	Parenchymal laceration >75% of lobe or >4 Couinaud segments
	Juxtahepatic vein injury
VI	Avulsion of liver

AAST, *American Association for the Surgery of Trauma.*

TABLE 12-6   AAST Computed Tomography Classification for Splenic Trauma

Grade	Injury Type
I	Subcapsular hematoma, <10% surface area
	Capsular tear, <1 cm deep
II	Subcapsular hematoma, 10% to 50% surface area, <5 cm diameter
	Capsular tear, 1-3 cm deep, no trabecular vessels
III	Subcapsular hematoma, >50% surface area or expanding
	Ruptured subcapsular or parenchymal hematoma
	Intraparenchymal hematoma, >5 cm or expanding
	Laceration >3 cm deep or trabecular vessel
IV	Laceration of segmental or hilar vessels with major devascularization (>25%)
V	Shattered spleen
	Hilar vascular injury devascularizes spleen

AAST, *American Association for the Surgery of Trauma.*

Treatment

Hemodynamically unstable patients go directly to the operating room. Stable patients with blunt hepatic injuries usually are not explored. Most of them do well with close observation. In fact, this more conservative approach has been associated with decreased transfusion requirements, fewer infectious and biliary complications, and increased survival.[175,176] Management of splenic trauma is somewhat more controversial. Although laparotomy and total splenectomy is an option, the significant risk of late sepsis after splenectomy has encouraged less aggressive strategies.[177]

ENDOVASCULAR THERAPY

Indications for catheter angiography in patients with suspected hepatic or splenic trauma are listed in Box 12-13. Angiography is also appropriate in patients with delayed *hemobilia*, which is often because of hepatic artery pseudoaneurysm, arterioportal fistula, or arteriovenous fistula. Embolization is the first-line treatment for most significant arterial injuries.[168,169,174-182] Embolotherapy is safe in the liver because of its dual blood supply and in the spleen because of the rich collateral circulation. Pseudoaneurysms and fistulas are closed with coils or Gelfoam pledgets (see Figs. 12-32 through 12-34). In the liver, embolic material is placed directly across the site of injury to minimize organ ischemia and prevent backflow into the damaged artery through collateral vessels. In the spleen, more proximal embolization with coils often is sufficient to stop hemorrhage; embolic material such as microcoils or Gelfoam pieces also can be deposited in intrasplenic branches that feed a bleeding site.

Embolotherapy stops hemorrhage in 80% to 100% of cases. Complications include abscess formation, tissue infarction, bleeding, and nontarget embolization.[183] After embolization, many patients with liver trauma develop

---

BOX 12-13

INDICATIONS FOR ANGIOGRAPHIC EVALUATION OF HEPATIC AND SPLENIC TRAUMA

Blunt Injury

- Nonoperative stable patients with evidence for active bleeding or large hemoperitoneum on CT
- Unstable patients with isolated liver injury or co-existent trauma requiring angiography (e.g., pelvic fractures)
- Failure of nonoperative management
- Persistent bleeding after operation
- Falling hemoglobin, ongoing transfusion requirements

Penetrating Injury

- Hemodynamic instability
- CT evidence for active bleeding or bleeding source (e.g., pseudoaneurysm)

---

biliary leaks, bilomas, abscesses, or hepatic necrosis.[184] However, these sequelae are likely related to the injury rather than the therapy.

SURGICAL THERAPY

Operative repair for liver injuries involves gauze packing, oversewing, or partial hepatic resection. In most patients, splenectomy after abdominal trauma is unnecessary. Operation is reserved for patients who are hemodynamically unstable or who fail embolotherapy.

Vascular Complications After Liver Transplantation (Online Cases 55 and 106)

Liver transplantation is the definitive treatment for patients with nonreversible hepatic failure, complications of cirrhosis and portal hypertension, certain metabolic liver diseases, and hepatocellular carcinoma. The interventionalist has two primary roles in this setting: (1) to provide a bridge to transplantation by portal decompression (e.g., TIPS creation) or tumor ablation, and (2) to help manage vascular complications afterward.[185,186] In the former situation, the goal of intervention is to maintain the patient as a transplant candidate. Extensive preoperative imaging (usually with MR angiography and cholangiography) is necessary to determine the suitability for transplantation with regard

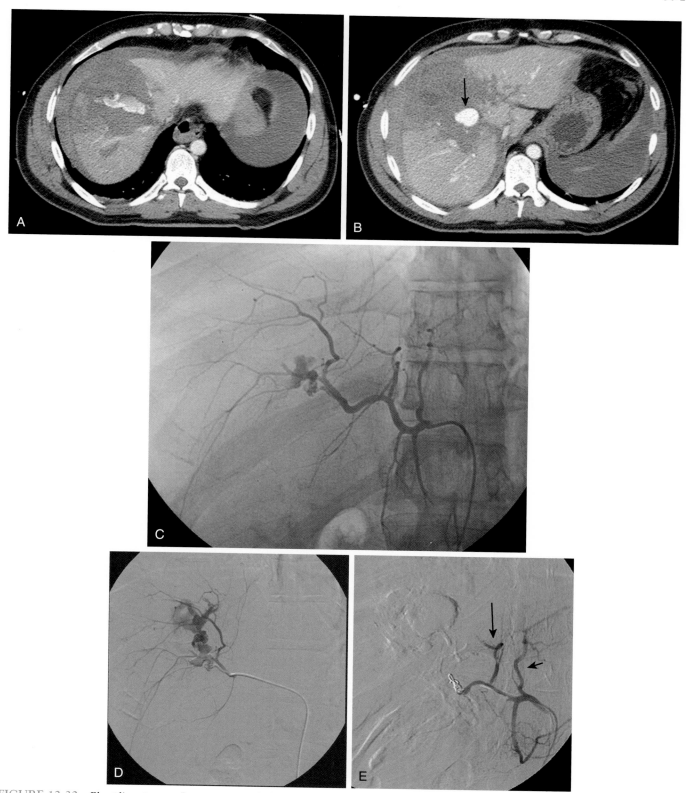

FIGURE 12-32　Blunt liver trauma from a motor vehicle crash. **A** and **B**, Contrast-enhanced computed tomography images show grade IV liver injury with active bleeding and probable pseudoaneurysm *(arrow)*. Also note perihepatic blood and left upper quadrant bleeding. **C** and **D**, Common and selective right hepatic (RHA) arteriography show massive bleeding from the proximal RHA. **E**, The entire vessel was embolized, and bleeding has ceased. No extravasation is noted from branches of the middle *(long arrow)* or left *(short arrow)* hepatic arteries.

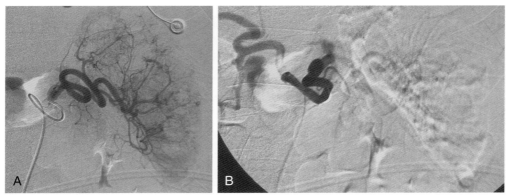

FIGURE 12-33   Splenic artery embolization for abdominal trauma following a motor vehicle collision. **A,** Splenic arteriogram reveals diffuse injury with irregular branch vessels and areas of gross and punctate extravasation. **B,** Following shower embolization with Gelfoam pieces, the artery is occluded and bleeding is no longer seen.

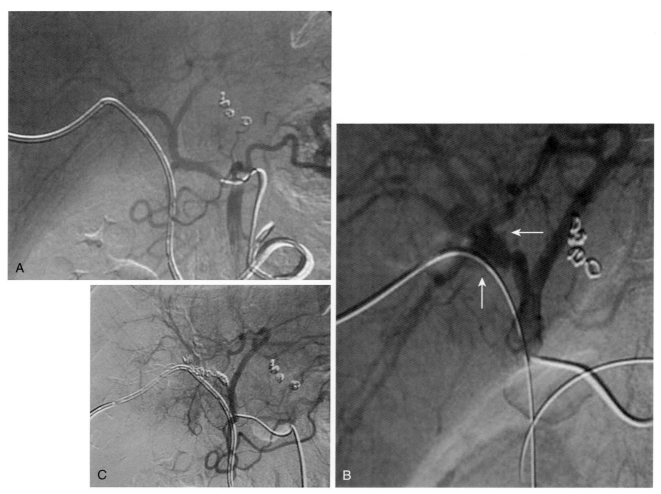

FIGURE 12-34   Bleeding hepatic artery pseudoaneurysm from percutaneous biliary drainage. Patient developed exuberant hemobilia through the drainage catheter about one week after insertion. **A,** Hepatic arteriogram (done via SMA for replaced common hepatic artery) shows no evidence of bleeding or culprit lesion. **B,** Tube was removed over a guidewire. Repeat angiography now reveals a pseudoaneurysm *(arrows)*. **C,** The involved branch was embolized distal and proximal to the lesion. Posttreatment angiography shows exclusion of the aneurysm.

to liver size, underlying liver disease, and vascular/biliary anatomic variants.[187,188] Rarely, catheter angiography is required before reduced-size transplants to identify arterial variants, segmental blood supply, and the size of the donor artery.

Operative Procedures

In the classic orthotopic liver transplant procedure, the hepatic arterial anastomosis is made between the donor celiac axis or common hepatic artery and the recipient common hepatic artery. When the recipient has two arteries supplying the liver (e.g., replaced right hepatic artery), a common trunk is created. Occasionally, an infrarenal iliac artery homograft is used (Fig. 12-35). The PV anastomosis is created in an end-to-end fashion. An iliac vein interposition graft to the SMV may be required if the recipient PV is diseased. The IVC connection can be fashioned with both suprahepatic and infrahepatic anastomoses. However, many transplant surgeons now use the "piggyback technique" in which an end-to-side anastomosis is formed using the suprahepatic donor segment and the hepatic vein confluence of the recipient.

Segmental (reduced or split) liver transplantation allows for pediatric or adult transplants from either cadaveric or living donors and increases the overall number of available grafts.[189] Surgical options include removal of the left lateral liver (segments II and III), right trisegmentectomy (segments IV to VIII), left lobe (segments II, III, IVa, and IVb), or right lobe (segments V to VIII).[190] The interventionalist must understand the precise operative anatomy in a particular case before proceeding with diagnostic or interventional procedures.

Complications

Up to 15% of patients suffer vascular complications after liver transplantation. Because often they are initially silent and the clinical course may be hard to differentiate from graft rejection or primary nonfunction, routine imaging of transplants with noninvasive imaging (ultrasound, CT, or MR) is crucial.[191-194]

HEPATIC ARTERY THROMBOSIS

The most frequent vascular complication after liver transplant is hepatic artery thrombosis, which occurs in 3% to 5% of cases, and more frequently in children.[192,195-198] The common causes are operative errors, progressive hepatic artery stenosis, rejection, and arterial kinking. With the exception of some children, no extrahepatic arterial collaterals initially support the graft. Coupled with some loss of the normal reciprocal relationship between portal and arterial liver flow, the graft will be in jeopardy. Since the biliary tree is

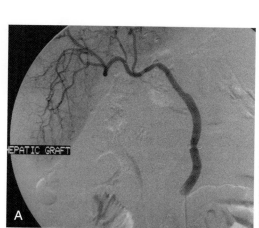
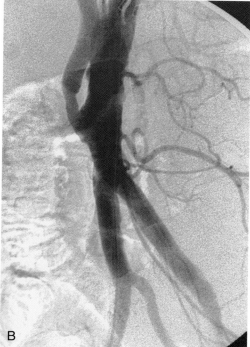

FIGURE 12-35 Orthotopic liver transplant with the donor hepatic artery (**A**) fed by an iliac artery homograft anastomosed to the recipient's distal abdominal aorta (**B**).

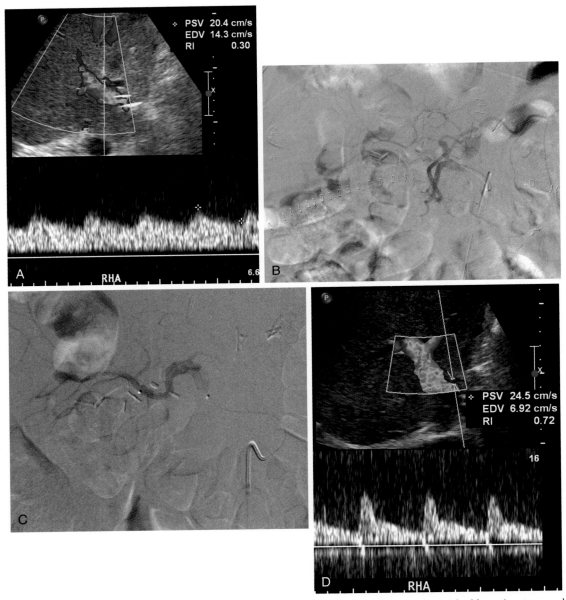

FIGURE 12-36   Liver transplant hepatic artery thrombosis. **A,** Color Doppler ultrasound shows diminished hepatic artery peak velocity, low resistive index, and "parvus et tardus" waveform. **B,** Catheter angiography confirms complete hepatic artery occlusion with minimal collateral flow into the liver. The occlusion could not be crossed with a guidewire, but thrombolysis was done through a proximal microcatheter. After about 12 mg of tissue plasminogen activator was infused, flow is restored in the hepatic artery **(C). D,** Ultrasound the following day shows more normal appearance of waveform and improved resistive index.

exclusively supplied by the hepatic artery, bile duct ischemia occurs frequently without treatment, resulting in strictures, bilomas, or mucosal sloughing (ischemic cholangiopathy).

Hepatic artery thrombosis usually happens within 2 to 3 months of transplantation. Patients often show signs of fulminant liver failure, biliary leak, or sepsis. The diagnosis is made with Doppler ultrasound or contrast-enhanced CT imaging. Catheterization is sometimes required for confirmation. Endovascular thrombolysis, angioplasty, and stent placement may allow graft salvage, but many patients require immediate revascularization to avoid the need for retransplantation[195,199,201] (Fig. 12-36).

HEPATIC ARTERY STENOSIS

Hepatic artery stenosis is less common than frank occlusion.[192,196,198] Most obstructions occur at the anastomosis and are because of technical errors, intimal hyperplasia, or graft rejection. Even when stenoses do not threaten graft viability, biliary duct ischemia complicated by stricture formation is common (see earlier discussion). Sonographic signs of hepatic artery stenosis include a "parvus et tardus" waveform, focal peak hepatic artery velocity of greater than 200 to 300 cm/sec, a resistive index less than 0.5, and a systolic acceleration time greater than 0.08 second in the intrahepatic arteries[202-204] (Fig. 12-37).

Angioplasty of hepatic artery stenoses is technically successful in about 80% of cases.[205,206] However, stenoses in fresh grafts (≤2 weeks old) may rupture if opened with a balloon. Reported rates of restenosis have been highly variable; stents may improve on these results[207,208] (see Fig. 12-37). Transplant hepatic arteries are very prone to vasospasm and thrombosis. Only floppy microwires (e.g., Synchro wire) should be used. If occlusion occurs, liberal use of intraarterial nitroglycerin (100 to 200 μg), additional heparin, small doses of tissue plasminogen activator, and "tincture of time" usually resolve the problem.

PORTAL VEIN THROMBOSIS OR STENOSIS

Significant portal vein (PV) stenosis or thrombosis is uncommon (up to 7% of pediatric recipients; 1% to 3% of adults).[185,198,209] At sonography, PV obstruction is signaled by absence of flow, focal areas of stenosis with increased peak velocity, or alterations in normal flow patterns and phasicity.[210] Contrast CT usually depicts the lesion convincingly (Fig. 12-38). When repair is indicated, direct catheter-based pressure measurements confirm the significance of the narrowing (≥5 mm Hg). Stenoses respond extremely well to angioplasty and selective stent placement.[211,213] However, the majority of thrombotic obstructions require operative repair.[192]

INFERIOR VENA CAVA/HEPATIC VEIN OBSTRUCTION

IVC and hepatic venous obstructions are virtually unheard of after traditional orthotopic liver transplantation, in that no hepatic vein anastomosis is created. However, stenoses are a serious problem in 1% to 17% of split liver or "piggyback" transplants.[209,213-216] Early postoperative lesions are usually technical problems such as a tight suture line or venous kinking; late stenoses are a consequence of fibrosis or neointimal hyperplasia around the anastomosis. Suggestive symptoms and signs are worsening ascites, abdominal pain, leg edema, and signs of graft dysfunction.

These obstructions are readily detected on Doppler sonography or CT angiography. Direct catheter-based pressure gradients are needed to confirm cross-sectional imaging findings (gradient >5 to 6 mm Hg). Because reoperation in this situation is technically difficult, most surgeons favor endovascular treatment. Stent placement usually is necessary for durable results in adults[217-220] (Fig. 12-39). Operators should be aware that stent placement in this location is treacherous (see Chapter 16 and Fig. 16-31).

HEPATIC ARTERY PSEUDOANEURYSMS

These lesions may present some time after transplantation with fever, hemobilia, unexplained bleeding, graft dysfunction, or arterial occlusion.[185] Extrahepatic arterial pseudoaneurysms are rare and potentially catastrophic. They develop at the hepatic arterial anastomosis and may have an infectious origin (Fig. 12-40). Intrahepatic pseudoaneurysms and arteriovenous fistulas usually are caused by a postoperative percutaneous procedure.[221,222]

OTHER DISORDERS

Hemangiomas and Other Benign Liver Tumors (Online Case 89)

Hemangioma is the most common benign mass found in the liver. These lesions are vascular tumors characterized by collections of blood spaces lined with an endothelium[223] (see Chapter 1). They are usually small (≤ 3 cm in diameter), may be multiple, and are more common in women than men. Hemangiomas often are silent, although the mass can cause abdominal pain or hemorrhage. On CT imaging, hemangiomas show peripheral enhancement in the arterial phase of contrast injection, with gradual fill-in through the portal and equilibrium phases (Fig. 12-41). On MRI, they have a similar pattern and are intensely bright on T2-weighted and gadolinium-enhanced images.[224-226] The angiographic appearance is almost pathognomonic, with a normal-caliber feeding artery, absence of neovascularity, and pooling of contrast in amorphous

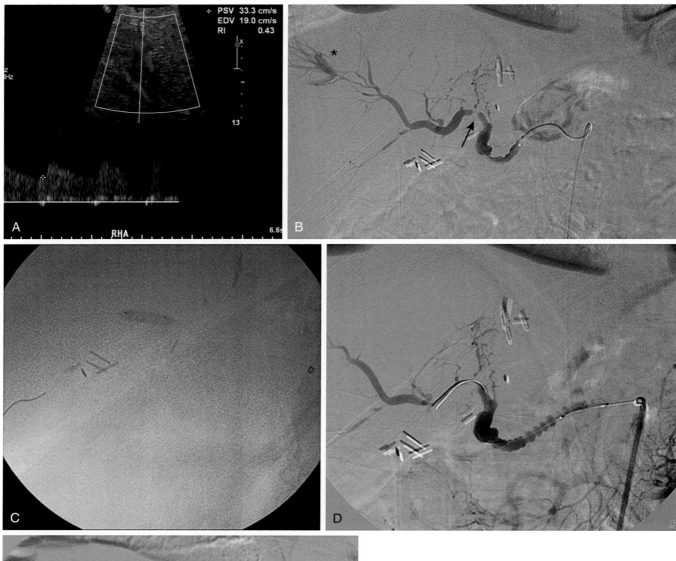

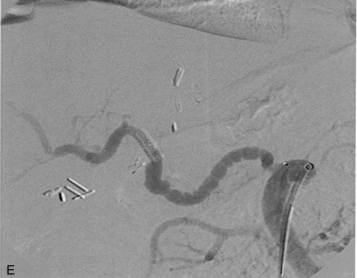

FIGURE 12-37 Liver transplant hepatic artery stenosis. **A,** Color Doppler ultrasound of right hepatic artery shows typical "parvus et tardus" spectral waveform suggesting upstream obstruction. **B,** Common hepatic angiography (arising aberrantly from the superior mesenteric artery) confirms a critical anastomotic stenosis *(arrow)*. Note guidewire-induced spasm in the proximal hepatic artery. A posttraumatic arterioportal fistula is also evident *(asterisk)*. The intrahepatic arterial branches are markedly irregular. Following balloon angioplasty **(C),** the vessel is still narrowed **(D).** Diffuse spasm is noted despite prophylactic vasodilators. Therefore a balloon expandable stent was inserted **(E),** markedly improving patency.

spaces (see Fig. 12-41). Contrast puddles linger well into the venous phase of the arteriogram because of slow flow in the lesion. These features differentiate hemangioma from hepatocellular carcinoma. Although surgery is rarely indicated, transcatheter embolization is done preoperatively for large, symptomatic masses and emergently for actively bleeding ones.[227-229]

Hepatic adenoma is a rare benign liver tumor that is largely a disease of young to middle-aged women who take oral contraceptives. Other associations included androgen hormonal therapy in men and glycogen storage diseases.[230] Most patients are asymptomatic. Certain imaging findings are characteristic, but distinction from other liver lesions may be problematic. Resection is often recommended for two reasons: (1) the risk for rupture (particularly when the tumor is greater than 4 to 5 cm), and (2) the rare possibility for malignant degeneration.[231] Prophylactic or urgent endovascular embolotherapy has also been employed in small series of patients, with tumor regression observed in most cases.[230,232]

Focal nodular hyperplasia is another uncommon benign hepatic mass with demographic pattern and imaging features similar to hepatic adenoma. Symptoms usually arise from mass effect causing abdominal pain. On imaging studies, a central scar or septations are fairly specific. While operative resection is the treatment of choice in most patients, embolization has been effective in selected individuals.[233,234]

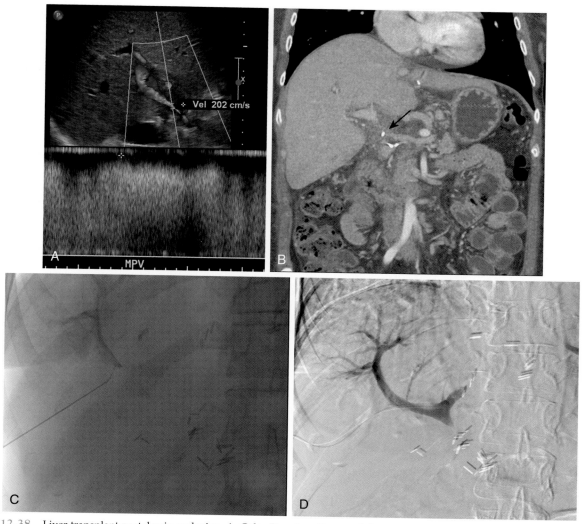

FIGURE 12-38 Liver transplant portal vein occlusion. **A,** Color Doppler ultrasound demonstrates high-velocity jet with turbulent flow at the portal vein anastomosis. **B,** Reformatted coronal contrast-enhanced CT shows the likely obstruction *(arrow).* **C,** A right portal vein radicle was punctured from the midaxillary line. **D,** Transhepatic portography reveals progression to total occlusion. *Continued*

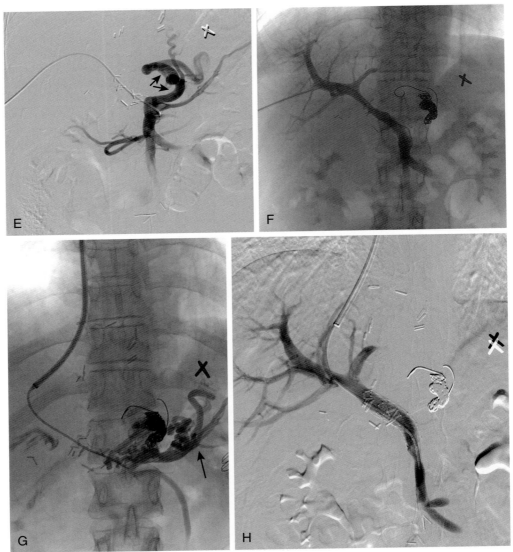

FIGURE 20-38, cont'd   Total occlusion traversed with an angled glidewire **(E).** Central portography shows a large coronary vein *(arrows).* The varices were embolized with coils, and the portal vein dilated with a 10-mm balloon. Although the technical results look good **(F),** repeat CT scanning about 4 months later showed reocclusion. This time, with a transjugular intrahepatic approach, the diseased portal vein was reentered **(G).** Embolized varices remain obstructed, but new ones are developing *(arrow).* Balloon-expandable stents were placed across the portal vein anastomosis **(H).**

Arteriovenous Communications

A wide variety of disorders can form or accentuate arteriovenous shunts in the liver[235,236] (Box 12-14; see Figs. 12-12, 12-37, and 1-36). Massive *arterioportal shunting* is one cause of hyperdynamic portal hypertension. Portohepatic vein fistulas are rare and usually congenital. Intrahepatic fistulas may be closed by transcatheter embolotherapy.[237-239]

Splenic arteriovenous fistulas are rare lesions caused by rupture of a splenic artery aneurysm, a congenital malformation, or previous splenectomy.[240,241] Hyperdynamic portal hypertension may result.

In a minority of patients with *hereditary hemorrhagic telangiectasia,* liver AVMs predominate and become responsible for abdominal ischemia, heart or liver failure, or portal hypertension (Fig. 12-42). Staged embolization has been used with success, but fatalities from this procedure have also been reported.[242-244]

Obstructive Arterial Diseases

Atherosclerosis may affect the hepatic and splenic arteries, but clinically significant disease is rare. Several other entities can mimic atherosclerotic plaque (Box 12-15).

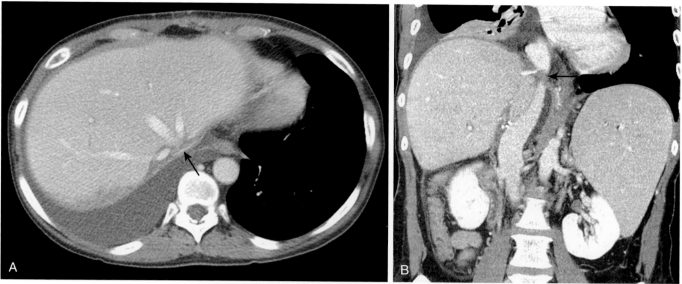

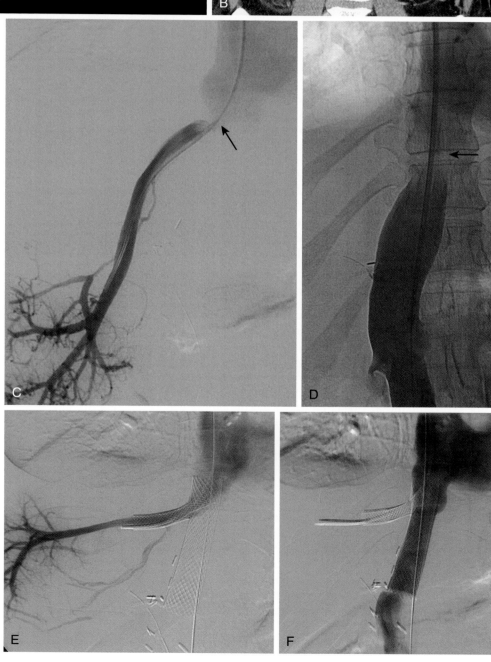

FIGURE 12-39   Liver transplant hepatic vein and inferior vena cava (IVC) stenoses. **A** and **B,** Axial and reformatted coronal computed tomography images suggest narrowing at the piggyback hepatic vein anastomosis *(arrow).* Middle hepatic venography (**C,** *arrow*) and inferior venacavography (**D,** *arrow*) show the focal narrowing. Through femoral access, a Wallstent was placed into the IVC. Through jugular access, the hepatic veins were entered through the IVC stent interstices, and two Wallstents placed in a Y-configuration. At the end of the procedure, both hepatic vein outflow (**E**) and IVC (**F**) are widely patent.

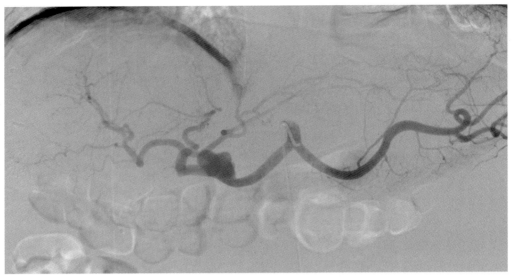

FIGURE 12-40   Posttransplant hepatic artery aneurysm. Celiac arteriogram shows a large bilobed aneurysm at the transplant arterial anastomosis. The etiology is not clear.

Marked elongation, tortuosity, and calcification of the splenic artery is a frequent finding in older patients. Atherosclerosis may progress to complete thrombotic occlusion (Box 12-16). However, the extensive collateral pathways to the spleen and the dual blood supply of the liver usually prevent organ infarction. Splenic infarction is generally the result of hematologic disorders or acute embolization (usually from the heart)[245] (Fig. 12-43). Dissection of the hepatic or splenic artery may be posttraumatic (iatrogenic) or spontaneous (e.g., extension of a celiac artery dissection)[246,247] (see Fig. 3-25).

Aneurysms (Online Cases 7 and 47)

The splenic and hepatic circulations are the most common sites for visceral artery aneurysms.[248,249] True visceral artery aneurysms are rare. They are usually small and asymptomatic when detected, and slow-growing but lethal when they do rupture.[248,250,251] Visceral artery pseudoaneurysms are slightly more common and typically symptomatic at presentation.[249,252] The causes are myriad (Box 12-17). The pathogenesis of dysplastic visceral aneurysm is not well understood. Women are afflicted more often than men. Patients with splenic artery aneurysms may have abdominal pain or hypotension from bleeding. Hepatic artery aneurysms can cause abdominal pain, hemobilia, or jaundice.

On noninvasive studies, a focally enlarged, enhancing vessel is seen (Fig. 12-44). Fluid or soft tissue adjacent to the lesion suggests an inflammatory pseudoaneurysm. At catheter angiography, dysplastic visceral artery aneurysms are often saccular, sometimes multiple, and may be calcified. Hepatic artery aneurysms usually are solitary and extrahepatic. In patients with *polyarteritis*

nodosa, numerous intrahepatic or intrasplenic microaneurysms are characteristic (Fig. 12-45).

Although the natural history of some visceral aneurysms is one of slow growth and eventual rupture, it is difficult to predict which ones will ultimately leak. Hemorrhage may occur into the peritoneal space, lesser sac (splenic aneurysms), or biliary system (hepatic aneurysms). The following indications for treatment are fairly well established:

- Based on several large natural history studies, asymptomatic dysplastic splenic artery aneurysms larger than 2 cm in diameter warrant repair.[251,253,254]
- No clear size cutoff has been established for treating dysplastic hepatic artery aneurysms.[255-257] Aneurysm leak with exsanguinating hemorrhage is more common with extrahepatic aneurysms; therefore most authorities favor early repair in almost all cases.
- All symptomatic or rapidly expanding true aneurysms are repaired.
- Visceral aneurysms in pregnant women are especially prone to rupture.[253,258] Fetal and maternal mortality exceed 75%, so all visceral artery aneurysms in women of childbearing potential deserve treatment.[259]
- Most experts endorse repair of all visceral artery pseudoaneurysms based on their unpredictable growth pattern and high mortality rates when they leak.[249]
- Because of the excessive risk of rupture of visceral aneurysms in patients with portal hypertension, these lesions are treated in candidates for or recipients of liver transplant.[260]

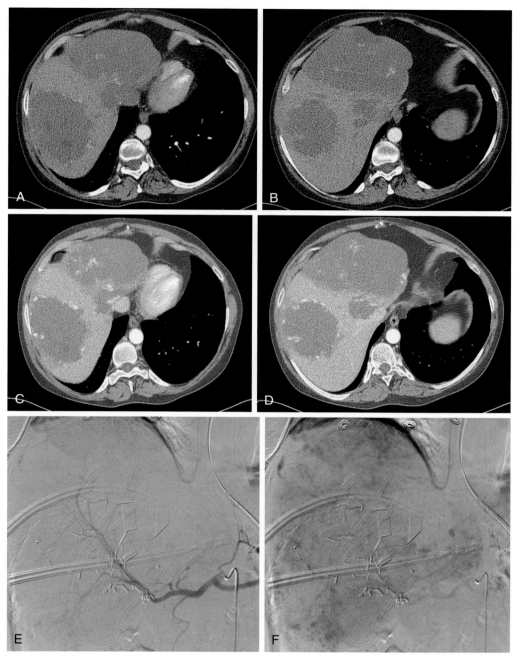

FIGURE 12-41 Cavernous hemangioma of the liver. Arterial phase (**A** and **B**) and slightly delayed (**C** and **D**) CT scans show two huge hypodense masses in the right and left liver lobes with nodular peripheral enhancement that migrates centrally and persists into the later phase. **E** and **F,** Early and later phase of celiac arteriogram demonstrate huge masses occupying large parts of the liver with innumerable contrast puddles that remain in the venous phase of the study. Note the normal-caliber hepatic artery and lack of any hypervascularity or neovascularity.

Transcatheter embolization is the treatment of choice for most intrahepatic and splenic artery aneurysms and pseudoaneurysms.[248,249,261] The preferred embolic agent is a coil; Gelfoam pledgets can be used to accelerate thrombosis. When feasible, embolization across the aneurysm neck is important to prevent delayed retrograde flow into the sac through collateral vessels feeding the distal artery ("closing the back door"). Even with properly performed large vessel embolotherapy, about 40% of patients treated for splenic artery aneurysms will suffer partial or complete splenic infarction (which may be quite symptomatic) or pancreatitis.[252,262,263] If the parent artery allows delivery of an appropriately sized sheath, covered stent

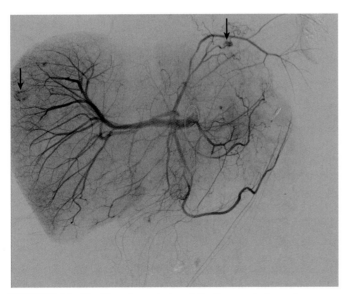

FIGURE 12-42   Vascular ectasias of the liver and stomach on celiac arteriography *(arrows)* in a patient with hereditary hemorrhagic telangiectasia.

placement is a better alternative to exclude the aneurysm but maintain vessel patency.[264]

Surgery (by exclusion, excision, or bypass grafting) is required for some extrahepatic artery aneurysms and for failures of embolotherapy. Rarely, splenic artery aneurysms require splenectomy and aneurysm removal or proximal and distal vessel ligation.

Vasculitis

Several forms of arteritis are seen in the liver and spleen. *Polyarteritis nodosa* and illicit drug use can produce a necrotizing vasculitis that may involve the liver, kidneys, intestinal tract, and extremities (see Fig. 12-45). Liver involvement with giant cell arteritis also has been described.[265]

Hypersplenism

In *hypersplenism*, the physiologic destruction of cellular blood elements by the spleen is exaggerated because of reticuloendothelial hyperplasia in the organ. The syndrome is associated with cirrhosis and portal

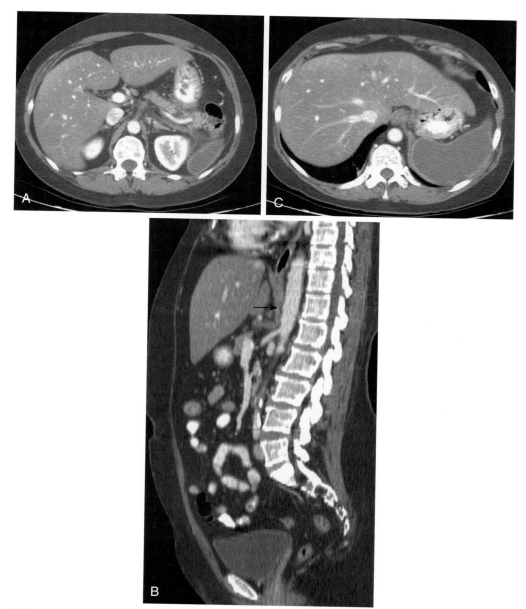

FIGURE 12-43   Celiac artery embolism. **A,** Transverse contrast-enhanced computed tomography (CT) scan shows lack of opacification of the celiac axis, which is confirmed on a sagittal reformatted image (**B,** *arrow*). **C,** CT scan shows splenic infarction because of the acute ischemic insult.

hypertension, thalassemia, idiopathic thrombocytopenic purpura, and several other disorders.[145,266,267] Signs of hypersplenism include splenomegaly and pancytopenia.

Splenic artery embolization often is requested before open or laparoscopic splenectomy to minimize intraoperative blood loss. Although splenectomy will eradicate hypersplenism, the risk of postoperative sepsis makes it a less than ideal plan of attack. Partial splenic embolization is an accepted alternative for reducing organ size and the inhibitory effects on platelets and red blood cells while maintaining some splenic activity

to prevent postprocedure sepsis.[266-269] Embolization is performed from the distal splenic artery beyond the pancreatic and gastric branches. Gelfoam pledgets, polyvinyl alcohol particles, or microspheres may be used. The goal is splenic volume reduction by 60% to 80%. Some interventionalists prefer to stage the procedure over several weeks.

Patients are given broad-spectrum antibiotics beforehand and are treated for postembolization syndrome for days afterward. The spleen shrinks markedly over 3 to 4 months. The procedure increases total blood cell

---

BOX 12-17

CAUSES OF SPLENIC AND HEPATIC ARTERY ANEURYSMS AND PSEUDOANEURYSMS

True Aneurysms

- Arterial dysplasia
- Degenerative (atherosclerosis-associated)
- High flow states (e.g., portal hypertension, hypersplenism)
- Connective tissue disorders
  - Ehlers Danlos syndrome
  - Marfan syndrome
  - Behçet syndrome
  - Neurofibromatosis
- Vasculitis
  - Polyarteritis nodosa
  - Takayasu arteritis
- Congenital

False Aneurysms

- Inflammation
  - Pancreatitis
- Infection (mycotic)
- Trauma
- Posttransplant
- Dissection

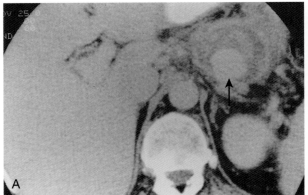
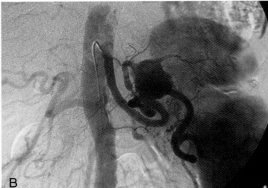
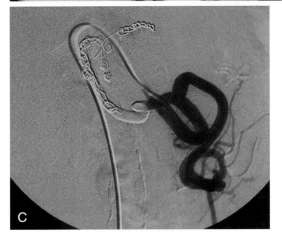

FIGURE 12-44 Splenic artery pseudoaneurysm caused by pancreatitis. **A,** Contrast-enhanced computed tomography scan shows a round, enhancing mass in the tail of the pancreas *(arrow)* surrounded by a larger, inhomogeneous soft tissue collection. **B,** Celiac arteriography in another patient shows a large midsplenic artery pseudoaneurysm. **C,** The branch feeding the aneurysm has been embolized with coils, and flow to the spleen was preserved.

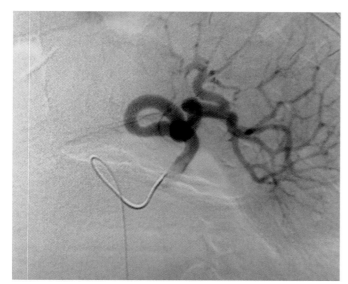

FIGURE 12-45 Polyarteritis nodosa with multiple microaneurysms of intrasplenic arteries.

counts and improves qualitative platelet activity.[270] The results are long lasting in many patients, although repeat embolization is often necessary if less than 50% of splenic volume is eliminated initially. Complications, including splenic abscess formation and splenic vein thrombosis, are unlikely if complete organ infarction is avoided.[271]

Peliosis

Peliosis hepatis is a rare disorder in which multiple blood-filled cavities develop within the liver or the spleen. Although the cause is unknown in many cases, peliosis is associated with androgen hormone-replacement therapy and *Bartonella* infections.[272,273] The diagnosis can be made with cross-sectional imaging.[274] The innumerable lucent spaces scattered throughout the liver are distinctive.

Segmental Arterial Mediolysis

Segmental arterial mediolysis is an exceedingly rare disease of unknown etiology characterized by destruction of arterial medial smooth muscle cells and eventual replacement by fibrin and granulation tissue.[275] Over time, extension to the entire arterial wall can lead to multiple spontaneous dissections and/or aneurysms. It has been postulated that segmental arterial mediolysis is related to fibromuscular dysplasia. Segmental arterial mediolysis primarily affects mesenteric, renal, and coronary arteries (see Fig. 11-39).

References

1. Brazzini A, Hunter DW, Darcy MD, et al. Safe splenoportography. *Radiology* 1987;**162**:607.
2. Burke CT, Weeks SM, Mauro MA, et al. CO_2 splenoportography for evaluating the splenic and portal veins before or after liver transplantation. *J Vasc Interv Radiol* 2004;**15**:1161.
3. Caridi JG, Hawkins Jr IF, Cho K, et al. CO_2 splenoportography: preliminary results. *AJR Am J Roentgenol* 2003;**180**:1375.
4. Sadler TW, editor. *Langman's medical embryology*. Baltimore: Williams & Wilkins; 1995, p. 254.
5. Sadler TW, editor. *Langman's medical embryology*. Baltimore: Williams & Wilkins; 1995, p. 219.
6. Takahashi S, Murakami T, Takamura M, et al. Multi-detector row helical CT angiography of hepatic vessels: depiction with dual-arterial phase acquisition during single breath hold. *Radiology* 2002;**222**:81.
7. Lee VS, Morgan GR, Teperman LW, et al. MR imaging as the sole preoperative imaging modality for right hepatectomy: a prospective study of living adult-to-adult liver donor candidates. *AJR Am J Roentgenol* 2001;**176**:1475.
8. Lavelle MT, Lee VS, Rofsky NM, et al. Dynamic contrast-enhanced three-dimensional MR imaging of liver parenchyma: source images and angiographic reconstructions to define hepatic arterial anatomy. *Radiology* 2001;**218**:389.
9. Guiney MJ, Kruskal JB, Sosna J, et al. Multi-detector row CT of relevant vascular anatomy of the surgical plane in split-liver transplantation. *Radiology* 2003;**229**:401.
10. Liu DM, Salem R, Bui JT, et al. Angiographic considerations in patients undergoing liver-directed therapy: a comprehensive review. *J Vasc Interv Radiol* 2005;**16**:911.
11. Lewandowski RJ, Sato KT, Atassi B, et al. Radioembolization with 90Y microspheres: angiographic and technical considerations. *Cardiovasc Intervent Radiol* 2007;**30**:571.
12. The Terminology Committee of the IHPBA. The Brisbane 2000 terminology of hepatic anatomy and resections. *HPB*. 2000; **2**:333.
13. Abdel-Misih SR, Bloomston M. Liver anatomy. *Surg Clin North Am* 2010;**90**:643.
14. Pieters PC, Miller WJ, DeMeo JH. Evaluation of the portal venous system: complementary roles of invasive and non-invasive imaging strategies. *Radiographics* 1997;**17**:879.
15. Graf O, Boland GW, Kaufman JA, et al. Anatomic variants of mesenteric veins: depiction with helical CT venography. *AJR Am J Roentgenol* 1997;**168**:1209.
16. LaBerge JM. Anatomy relevant to the transjugular intrahepatic portosystemic shunt procedure. *Semin Intervent Radiol* 1995;**12**:337.
17. Covey AM, Brody LA, Getrajdman GI, et al. Incidence, patterns, and clinical relevance of variant portal vein anatomy. *AJR Am J Roentgenol* 2004;**183**:1055.
18. McCuskey RS. The hepatic microvascular system in health and its response to toxicants. *Anat Rec* (Hoboken) 2008;**291**:661.
19. Gabella G, editor. Cardiovascular system. In: Williams PL, Bannister LH, Berry MM, et al, editors. *Gray's anatomy*, 38th ed. New York: Churchill Livingstone; 1995, p. 1551.
20. Ishigami K, Zhang Y, Rayhill S, et al. Does variant hepatic artery anatomy in a liver transplant recipient increase the risk of hepatic artery complications after transplantation? *AJR Am J Roentgenol* 2004;**183**:1577.
21. Koops A, Wojciechowski B, Broering DC, et al. Anatomic variations of the hepatic arteries in 604 selective celiac and superior mesenteric angiographies. *Surg Radiol Anat* 2004;**26**:239.
22. Kopka L, Rodenwaldt J, Vosshenrich R, et al. Hepatic blood supply: comparison of optimized dual phase contrast-enhanced three-dimensional MR angiography and digital subtraction angiography. *Radiology* 1999;**211**:51.

23. Michels NA. *Blood supply and anatomy of the upper abdominal organs with descriptive atlas.* Philadelphia: Lippincott; 1955.

24. Covey AM, Brody LA, Maluccio MA, et al. Variant hepatic arterial anatomy revisited: digital subtraction angiography performed in 600 patients. *Radiology* 2002;**224**:542.

25. Gayer G, Hertz M, Strauss S, et al. Congenital anomalies of the spleen. *Semin Ultrasound CT MR* 2006;**27**:358.

26. Carr JC, Nemcek Jr AA, Abecassis M, et al. Preoperative evaluation of the entire hepatic vasculature in living liver donors with use of contrast-enhanced MR angiography and true FAST imaging with steady-state precession. *J Vasc Interv Radiol* 2003;**14**:441.

27. Ramachandran P, Iredale JP. Reversibility of liver fibrosis. *Ann Hepatol* 2009;**8**:283.

28. Shah V. Molecular mechanisms of increased intrahepatic resistance in portal hypertension. *J Clin Gastroenterol* 2007;**41**:S259.

29. Zipprich A. Hemodynamics in the isolated cirrhotic liver. *J Clin Gastroenterol* 2007;**41**:S254.

30. Vaughan RB, Chin-Dusting JP. Current pharmacotherapy in the management of cirrhosis: focus on the hyperdynamic circulation. *Expert Opin Pharmacother* 2003;**4**:625.

31. Garcia-Tsao G, Bosch J. Management of varices and variceal hemorrhage in cirrhosis. *N Engl J Med* 2010;**362**:823.

32. de Franchis R, Primignani M. Natural history of portal hypertension in patients with cirrhosis. *Clin Liver Dis* 2001;**5**:645.

33. Perz JF, Armstrong GL, Farrington LA, et al. The contributions of hepatitis B virus and hepatitis C virus infections to cirrhosis and primary liver cancer worldwide. *J Hepatol* 2006;**45**:529.

34. Lim YS, Kim WR. The global impact of hepatic fibrosis and end-stage liver disease. *Clin Liver Dis* 2008;**12**:733.

35. Starley BQ, Calcagno CJ, Harrison SA. Nonalcoholic fatty liver disease and hepatocellular carcinoma: a weighty connection. *Hepatology* 2010;**51**:1820.

36. Invernizzi P, Selmi C, Gershwin ME. Update on primary biliary cirrhosis. *Dig Liver Dis* 2010;**42**:401.

37. Manzella A, Ohtomo K, Monzawa S, et al. Schistosomiasis of the liver. *Abdom Imaging* 2008;**33**:144.

38. Chawla Y, Dhiman RK. Intrahepatic portal venopathy and related disorders of the liver. *Semin Liver Dis* 2008;**28**:270.

39. Defreyne L, De Schrijver I, Vanlangenhove P, et al. Detachable balloon embolization of an aneurysmal gastroduodenal arterioportal fistula. *Eur Radiol* 2002;**12**:231.

40. Reynolds TB. Interrelationships of portal pressure, variceal size, and upper gastrointestinal bleeding. *Gastroenterology* 1980;**79**:1332.

41. Salerno F, Guevara M, Bernardi M, et al. Refractory ascites: pathogenesis, definition and therapy of a severe complication in patient with cirrhosis. *Liver Int* 2010;**30**:937.

42. Menon KV, Kamath PS. Regional and systemic hemodynamic disturbances in cirrhosis. *Clin Liver Dis* 2001;**5**:617.

43. Mackelaite L, Alsauskas ZC, Ranganna K. Renal failure in patients with ascites. *Med Clin North Am* 2009;**93**:855.

44. Reynolds TB, Ito S, Iwatsuki S. Measurement of portal pressure and its clinical application. *Am J Med* 1970;**49**:649.

45. Cholongitas E, Qualgia A, Samonakis D, et al. Transjugular liver biopsy: how good is it for accurate histological interpretation? *Gut* 2006;**55**:1789.

46. Vibhakorn S, Clolongitas E, Kalambokis G, et al. A comparison of four- versus three-pass transjugular biopsy using a 19G Tru-Cut needle and a randomized study using a cassette to prevent biopsy fragmentation. *Cardiovasc Intervent Radiol* 2009;**32**:508.

47. Miller MJ, Smith TP, Kuo PC, et al. Transjugular liver biopsy results in the transplanted liver: comparison of two surgical hepatic venous anastomotic configurations in 269 consecutive biopsies over a 14-year period. *J Vasc Interv Radiol* 2010;**21**:508.

48. Soyer P, Fargeaudou Y, Boudiaf M, et al. Transjugular liver biopsy using ultrasonographic guidance for jugular vein puncture and an automated device for hepatic tissue sampling: a retrospective analysis of 200 consecutive cases. *Abdom Imaging* 2008;**33**:627.

49. Mammen T, Keshava SN, Eapen CE, et al. Transjugular liver biopsy: a retrospective analysis of 601 cases. *J Vasc Interv Radiol* 2008;**19**:351.

50. Kim KR, Ko GY, Sung KB, et al. Transjugular liver biopsy in patient with living donor liver transplantation: comparison with percutaneous biopsy. *Liver Transpl* 2008;**14**:971.

51. Kalambokis G, Manousou P, Vibhakorn S, et al. Transjugular liver biopsy- indications, adequacy, quality of specimens, and complications- a systematic review. *J Hepatol* 2007;**47**:284.

52. Ahmad A, Hasan F, Abdeen S, et al. Transjugular liver biopsy in patients with end-stage renal disease. *J Vasc Interv Radiol* 2004;**15**:257.

53. Gonzalez R, Zamora J, Gomez-Caramero J, et al. Meta-analysis: combination endoscopic and drug therapy to prevent variceal rebleeding in cirrhosis. *Ann Intern Med* 2008;**149**:109.

54. Kravetz D. Prevention of recurrent esophageal variceal hemorrhage: review and current recommendations. *J Clin Gastroenterol* 2007;**41**:S318.

55. D'Amico G, Pagliaro L, Pietrosi G, et al. Emergency sclerotherapy versus vasoactive drugs for bleeding oesophageal varices in cirrhotic patients. *Cochrane Database Syst Rev* 2010:CD002233.

56. Sass DA, Chopra KB. Portal hypertension and variceal hemorrhage. *Med Clin North Am* 2009;**93**:837.

57. Bendtsen F, Krag A, Moeller S. Treatment of acute variceal bleeding. *Dig Liver Dis* 2008;**40**:328.

58. Villanueva C, Minana J, Ortiz J, et al. Endoscopic ligation compared with combined treatment with nadolol and isosorbide mononitrate to prevent recurrent variceal bleeding. *N Engl J Med* 2001;**345**:647.

59. Lui HF, Stanley AJ, Forrest EH, et al. Primary prophylaxis of variceal hemorrhage: a randomized controlled trial comparing band ligation, propranolol, and isosorbide mononitrate. *Gastroenterology* 2002;**123**:735.

60. Lunderquist A, Vang J. Transhepatic catheterization and obliteration of the coronary vein in patients with portal hypertension and esophageal varices. *N Engl J Med* 1974;**291**:646.

61. L'Hermine CL, Chastanet P, Delemazure O, et al. Percutaneous transhepatic embolization of gastroesophageal varices: results in 400 patients. *AJR Am J Roentgenol* 1989;**152**:755.

62. Thouveny F, Aube C, Konate A, et al. Direct percutaneous approach for endoluminal glue embolization of stomal varices. *J Vasc Interv Radiol* 2008;**19**:774.

63. Kiyosue H, Mori H, Matsumoto S, et al. Transcatheter obliteration of gastric varices. Part 1. Anatomic classification. *Radiographics* 2003;**23**:911.

64. Hirota S, Matsumoto S, Tomita M, et al. Retrograde transvenous obliteration of gastric varices. *Radiology* 1999;**211**:349.

65. Sonomura T, Horihata K, Yamahara K, et al. Ruptured duodenal varices successfully treated with balloon-occluded retrograde transvenous obliteration: usefulness of microcatheters. *AJR Am J Roentgenol* 2003;**181**:725.

66. Fukuda T, Hirota S, Sugimura K. Long-term results of balloon-occluded retrograde transvenous obliteration for the treatment of gastric varices and hepatic encephalopathy. *J Vasc Interv Radiol* 2001;**12**:327.

67. Tanihata H, Minamiguchi H, Sato M, et al. Changes in portal systemic pressure gradient after balloon-occluded retrograde transvenous obliteration of gastric varices and aggravation of esophageal varices. *Cardiovasc Intervent Radiol* 2009;**32**:1209.

68. Choi YS, Lee JH, Sinn DH, et al. Effect of balloon-occluded retrograde transvenous obliteration on the natural history of coexisting esophageal varices. *J Clin Gastroenterol* 2008;**42**:974.

69. Warren WD, Millikan Jr WJ, Henderson JM, et al. Ten years portal hypertensive surgery at Emory. *Ann Surg* 1982;**195**:530.

70. Orloff MJ, Orloff MS, Orloff SL, et al. Three decades of experience with emergency portacaval shunt for acutely bleeding esophageal varices in 400 unselected patients with cirrhosis of the liver. *J Am Coll Surg* 1995;**180**:257.

71. Khan S, Tudur Smith C, Williamson P, et al. Portosystemic shunts versus endoscopic therapy for variceal rebleeding in patients with cirrhosis. *Cochrane Database Syst Rev* 2006:CD000553.

72. http://www.ustransplant.org/annual_reports/current/914b_state_li.htm

73. Boyer TD, Haskal ZJ. The role of transjugular intrahepatic portosystemic shunt (TIPS) in the management of portal hypertension: update 2009. *Hepatology* 2010;**51**:306.

74. Shiffman ML, Jeffers L, Hoofnagle JH, et al. The role of transjugular intrahepatic portosystemic shunt for treatment of portal hypertension and its complications: a conference sponsored by the National Digestive Diseases Advisory Board. *Hepatology* 1995;**22**:1591.

75. Haskal ZJ, Martin L, Cardella JF, et al. Quality improvement guidelines for transjugular intrahepatic portosystemic shunts. *J Vasc Interv Radiol* 2003;**14**:S265.

76. Garcia-Pagan JC, Caca K, Bureau C, et al. Early use of TIPS in patients with cirrhosis and variceal bleeding. *N Engl J Med* 2010;**362**:2370.

77. Salerno F, Camma C, Enea M, et al. Transjugular intrahepatic portosystemic shunt for refractory ascites: a meta-analysis of individual patient data. *Gastroenterology* 2007;**133**:825.

78. Saab S, Nieto JM, Lewis SK, et al. TIPS versus paracentesis for cirrhotic patients with refractory ascites. *Cochrane Database Syst Rev* 2006;CD004889.

79. Cosenza CA, Hoffman AL, Friedman ML, et al. Transjugular intrahepatic portosystemic shunt: efficacy for the treatment of portal hypertension and impact on liver transplantation. *Am Surgeon* 1996;**62**:835.

80. Menegaux F, Keeffe EB, Baker E, et al. Comparison of transjugular and surgical portosystemic shunts on the outcome of liver transplantation. *Arch Surg* 1994;**129**:1018.

81. Haskal ZJ, Scott M, Rubin RA, et al. Intestinal varices: treatment with transjugular intrahepatic portosystemic shunt. *Radiology* 1994;**191**:183.

82. Trevino HH, Brady CE 3rd, Schencker S. Portal hypertensive gastropathy. *Dig Dis* 1996;**14**:258.

83. Vidal V, Joly L, Perreault P, et al. Usefulness of transjugular intrahepatic portosystemic shunt in the management of bleeding ectopic varices in cirrhotic patients. *Cardiovasc Intervent Radiol* 2006;**29**:216.

84. Lo GH, Liang HL, Chen WC, et al. A prospective, randomized controlled trial of transjugular intrahepatic portosystemic shunt versus cyanoacrylate injection in the prevention of gastric variceal rebleeding. *Endoscopy* 2007;**39**:679.

85. Wong F. Hepatorenal syndrome: current management. *Curr Gastroenterol Rep* 2008;**10**:22.

86. Wadel HM, Mai ML, Ahsan N. Hepatorenal syndrome: pathophysiology and management. *Clin J Am Soc Nephrol* 2006;**1**:1066.

87. Dhanasekaran R, West JK, Gonzales PC, et al. Transjugular intrahepatic portosystemic shunt for symptomatic refractory hepatic hydrothorax in patients with cirrhosis. *Am J Gastroenterol* 2010;**105**:635.

88. Savage C, Patel J, Lepe MR, et al. Transjugular intrahepatic portosystemic shunt creation for recurrent gastrointestinal bleeding during pregnancy. *J Vasc Interv Radiol* 2007;**18**:902.

89. Wallace M, Swaim M. Transjugular intrahepatic portosystemic shunts through hepatic neoplasms. *J Vasc Interv Radiol* 2003;**14**:501.

90. Shin ES, Darcy MD. Transjugular intrahepatic portosystemic shunt placement in the setting of polycystic liver disease: questioning the contraindication. *J Vasc Interv Radiol* 2001;**12**:1099.

91. Senzolo M, Tibbals J, Cholongitas E, et al. Transjugular intrahepatic portosystemic shunt for portal vein thrombosis with and without cavernous transformation. *Aliment Pharmacol Ther* 2006;**23**:767.

92. Jiang ZB, Shan H, Shen XY, et al. Transjugular intrahepatic portosystemic shunt for palliative treatment of portal hypertension secondary to portal vein tumor thrombosis. *World J Gastroenterol* 2004;**10**:1881.

93. Ferral H, Patel NH. Selection criteria for patients undergoing transjugular intrahepatic portosystemic shunt procedures: current status. *J Vasc Interv Radiol* 2005;**16**:449.

94. Ferral H, Vasan R, Speeg KV, et al. Evaluation of a model to predict poor survival in patients undergoing elective TIPS procedures. *J Vasc Interv Radiol* 2002;**13**:1103.

95. Rajan DK, Haskal ZJ, Clark TW. Serum bilirubin and early mortality after transjugular intrahepatic portosystemic shunts: results of a multivariate analysis. *J Vasc Interv Radiol* 2002;**13**:155.

96. Schepke M, Roth F, Fimmers R, et al. Comparison of MELD, Child-Pugh, and Emory model for the prediction of survival in patients undergoing transjugular intrahepatic portosystemic shunting. *Am J Gastroenterol* 2003;**98**:1167.

97. Darcy MD, Sterling KM. Comparison of portal vein anatomy and bony anatomic landmarks. *Radiology* 1996;**200**:707.

98. Maleux G, Nevens F, Heye S, et al. The use of carbon dioxide wedged hepatic venography to identify the portal vein: comparison with direct catheter portography with iodinated contrast medium and analysis of predictive factors influencing level of opacification. *J Vasc Interv Radiol* 2006;**17**:1771.

99. Chin MS, Stavas JM, Burke CT, et al. Direct puncture of the recanalized paraumbilical vein for portal vein targeting during transjugular intrahepatic portosystemic shunt procedures: assessment of technical success and safety. *J Vasc Interv Radiol* 2010;**21**:671.

100. Schultz SR, LaBerge JM, Gordon RL, et al. Anatomy of the portal vein bifurcation: intra- versus extrahepatic location-implications for transjugular intrahepatic portosystemic shunts. *J Vasc Interv Radiol* 1994;**5**:457.

101. Riggio O, Ridola L, Angeloni S, et al. Clinical efficacy of transjugular intrahepatic portosystemic shunt created with covered stents with different diameters: results of a randomized controlled trial. *J Hepatol* 2010;**53**:267.

102. Coldwell DM, Ring EJ, Rees CR, et al. Multicenter investigation of the role of transjugular intrahepatic portosystemic shunt in management of portal hypertension. *Radiology* 1995;**196**:335.

103. Charon J-P, Alaeddin FH, Pimpalwar SA, et al. Results of a retrospective multicenter trial of the Viatorr expanded polytetrafluoroethylene-covered stent-graft for transjugular intrahepatic portosystemic shunt creation. *J Vasc Interv Radiol* 2004;**15**:1219.

104. Ochs A, Roessle M, Haag K, et al. The transjugular intrahepatic portosystemic stent-shunt procedure for refractory ascites. *N Engl J Med* 1995;**332**:1192.

105. Freedman AM, Sanyal AJ, Tisnado J, et al. Complications of the transjugular intrahepatic portosystemic shunt: a comprehensive review. *Radiographics* 1993;**13**:1185.

106. Hoppe H, Wang SL, Petersen BD. Intravascular US-guided direct intrahepatic portocaval shunt with an expanded polytetrafluoroethylene-covered stent-graft. *Radiology* 2008;**246**:306.

107. Angermayr B, Cejna M, Koenig F, et al. Survival in patients undergoing transjugular intrahepatic portosystemic shunt: ePTFE-covered stent grafts versus bare stents. *Hepatology* 2003;**38**:1043.

108. Darcy MD, Vesely TM, Picus D, et al. Percutaneous revision of an acutely thrombosed transjugular intrahepatic portosystemic shunt. *J Vasc Interv Radiol* 1992;**3**:77.

109. Schmitz-Rode T, Vorwerk D, Marschall H-U, et al. Portal vein thrombosis after occlusion of a transjugular intrahepatic portosystemic shunt: recanalization with the impeller catheter. *J Vasc Interv Radiol* 1994;**5**:467.

110. Riggio O, Merlli M, Pedretti G, et al. Hepatic encephalopathy after transjugular intrahepatic portosystemic shunt: incidence and risk factors. *Dig Dis Sci* 1996;**41**:578.

111. LaBerge JM, Ferrell LD, Ring EJ, et al. Histopathologic study of transjugular intrahepatic portosystemic shunts. *J Vasc Interv Radiol* 1991;**2**:549.

112. Saxon RR, Mendel-Hartvig J, Corless CL, et al. Bile duct injury as a major cause of stenosis and occlusion in transjugular intrahepatic portosystemic shunts: comparative histopathologic analysis in humans and swine. *J Vasc Interv Radiol* 1996;**7**:487.

113. Lind CD, Malisch TW, Chong WK, et al. Incidence of shunt occlusion or stenosis following transjugular intrahepatic portosystemic shunt placement. *Gastroenterology* 1994;**106**:1277.

114. Haskal ZJ, Pentecost MJ, Soulen MC, et al. Transjugular intrahepatic portosystemic shunt stenosis and revision: early and midterm results. *AJR Am J Roentgenol* 1994;**163**:439.

115. Sterling KM, Darcy MD. Stenosis of transjugular intrahepatic portosystemic shunts: presentation and management. *AJR Am J Roentgenol* 1997;**168**:239.

116. Bureau C, Pagan JC, Layrargues GP, et al. Patency of stents covered with polytetrafluoroethylene in patients treated by transjugular intrahepatic portosystemic shunts: long-term results of a randomized multicentre study. *Liver Int* 2007;**27**:742.

117. Henderson JM, Boyer TD, Kutner MH, et al. Distal splenorenal shunt versus transjugular intrahepatic portosystemic shunt for variceal bleeding: a randomized trial. *Gastroenterology* 2006;**130**:1643.

118. Carr CE, Tuite CM, Soulen MC, et al. Role of ultrasound surveillance of transjugular intrahepatic portosystemic shunts in the covered stent era. *J Vasc Interv Radiol* 2006;**17**:1297.

119. Cura M, Cura A, Suri R, et al. Causes of TIPS dysfunction. *AJR Am J Roentgenol* 2008;**191**:1751.

120. Kanterman RY, Darcy MD, Middleton WD, et al. Doppler sonographic findings associated with transjugular intrahepatic portosystemic shunt malfunction. *AJR Am J Roentgenol* 1997;**168**:467.

121. Foshager MC, Ferral H, Nazarian GK, et al. Duplex sonography after transjugular intrahepatic portosystemic shunts (TIPS): normal hemodynamic findings and efficacy in predicting shunt patency and stenosis. *AJR Am J Roentgenol* 1995;**165**:1.

122. Feldstein VA, Patel MD, LaBerge JM. Transjugular intrahepatic portosystemic shunts: accuracy of Doppler US in determination of patency and detection of stenoses. *Radiology* 1996;**201**:141.

123. Abraldes JG, Gilabert R, Turnes J, et al. Utility of color Doppler ultrasonography predicting TIPS dysfunction. *Am J Gastroenterol* 2005;**100**:2696.

124. Hoxworth JM, LaBerge MM, Gordon RL, et al. Inferior vena cava thrombosis after transjugular intrahepatic portosystemic shunt revision with a covered stent. *J Vasc Interv Radiol* 2004;**15**:995.

125. Madoff DC, Wallace MJ, Ahrar K, et al. TIPS-related hepatic encephalopathy: management options with novel endovascular techniques. *Radiographics* 2004;**24**:21.

126. Kaufman L, Itkin M, Furth EE, et al. Detachable balloon-modified reducing stent to treat hepatic insufficiency after transjugular intrahepatic portosystemic shunt creation. *J Vasc Interv Radiol* 2003;**14**:635.

127. Sze DY, Hwang GL, Kao JS, et al. Bidirectionally adjustable TIPS reduction by parallel stent and stent-graft deployment. *J Vasc Interv Radiol* 2008;**19**:1653.

128. Kroma G, Lopera J, Cura M, et al. Transjugular intrahepatic portosystemic shunt flow reduction with adjustable polytetrafluoroethylene-covered balloon-expandable stents. *J Vasc Interv Radiol* 2009;**20**:981.

129. Paz-Fumagalli R, Crain MR, Mewissen MW, et al. Fatal hemodynamic consequences of therapeutic closure of a transjugular intrahepatic portosystemic shunt. *J Vasc Interv Radiol* 1994;**5**:831.

130. Parikh S, Shah R, Kapoor P. Portal vein thrombosis. *Am J Med* 2010;**123**:111.

131. Webster GJ, Burroughs AK, Riordan SM. Portal vein thrombosis—new insights into aetiology and management. *Aliment Pharmacol Ther* 2005;**21**:1.

132. Weber SM, Rikkers LF. Splenic vein thrombosis and gastrointestinal bleeding in chronic pancreatitis. *World J Surg* 2003;**27**:1271.

133. Stamou KM, Toutouzas KG, Kekis PB, et al. Prospective study of the incidence and risk factors of postsplenectomy thrombosis of the portal, mesenteric, and splenic veins. *Arch Surg* 2006;**141**:663.

134. Horton KM, Fishman EK. CT angiography of the mesenteric circulation. *Radiol Clin North Am* 2010;**48**:331.

135. Cakmak O, Elmas N, Tamsel S, et al. Role of contrast-enhanced 3D magnetic resonance portography in evaluating portal venous system compared with color Doppler ultrasonography. *Abdom Imaging* 2008;**33**:65.

136. Plessier A, Darwish-Murad S, Hernandez-Guerra M, et al. Acute portal vein thrombosis unrelated to cirrhosis: a prospective multicenter follow-up study. *Hepatology* 2010;**51**:210.

137. Hollingshead M, Burke CT, Mauro MA, et al. Transcatheter thrombolytic therapy for acute mesenteric and portal vein thrombosis. *J Vasc Interv Radiol* 2005;**16**:651.

138. Henao EA, Bohannon WT, Silva Jr MB. Treatment of portal venous thrombosis with selective superior mesenteric artery infusion of recombinant tissue plasminogen activator. *J Vasc Surg* 2003;**38**:1411.

139. Lopera JE, Correa G, Brazzini A, et al. Percutaneous transhepatic treatment of symptomatic mesenteric venous thrombosis. *J Vasc Surg* 2002;**36**:1058.

140. Hidajat N, Stobbe H, Griesshaber V, et al. Portal vein thrombosis: etiology, diagnostic strategy, therapy and management. *Vasa* 2005;**34**:81.

141. Perarnau JM, Baju A, D'alteroche L, et al. Feasibility and long-term evolution of TIPS in cirrhotic patients with portal thrombosis. *Eur J Gastroenterol Hepatol* 2010;**22**:1093.

142. Bauer J, Johnson S, Durham J, et al. The role of TIPS for portal vein patency in liver transplant patients with portal vein thrombosis. *Liver Transpl* 2006;**12**:1544.

143. van Ha TG, Hodge J, Funaki B, et al. Transjugular intrahepatic portosystemic shunt placement in patients with cirrhosis and concomitant portal vein thrombosis. *Cardiovasc Intervent Radiol* 2006;**29**:785.

144. McDermott VG, England RE, Newman GE. Case report: bleeding gastric varices secondary to splenic vein thrombosis successfully treated by splenic artery embolization. *Br J Radiol* 1995;**68**:928.

145. Koconis KG, Singh H, Soares G. Partial splenic embolization in the treatment of patients with portal hypertension: a review of the English language literature. *J Vasc Interv Radiol* 2007;**18**:463.

146. Klempnauer J, Grothues F, Bektas H, et al. Results of portal thrombectomy and splanchnic thrombolysis for the surgical management of acute mesentericoportal thrombosis. *Br J Surg* 1997;**84**:129.

147. Menon KV, Shah V, Kamath PS. The Budd-Chiari syndrome. *N Engl J Med* 2004;**350**:578.

148. Smith FO, Johnson MS, Scherer LR, et al. Transjugular intrahepatic portosystemic shunting (TIPS) for treatment of severe hepatic veno-occlusive disease. *Bone Marrow Transplant* 1996;**18**:643.

149. Coppell JA, Richardson PG, Soiffer R, et al. Hepatic veno-occlusive disease following stem cell transplantation: incidence, clinical course, and outcome. *Biol Blood Marrow Transplant* 2010;**16**:157.

150. Imran H, Tleyjeh IM, Zirakzadeh A, et al. Use of prophylactic anticoagulation and the risk of hepatic veno-occlusive disease in patients undergoing hematopoietic stem cell transplantation: a systematic review and meta-analysis. *Bone Marrow Transplant* 2006;**37**:677.

151. Ciesek S, Rifai K, Bahr MJ, et al. Membranous Budd-Chiari syndrome in Caucasians. *Scand J Gastroenterol* 2010;**45**:226.

152. Lee BB, Villavicencio L, Kim YW, et al. Primary Budd-Chiari syndrome: outcome of endovascular management for suprahepatic venous obstruction. *J Vasc Surg* 2006;**43**:101.

153. Sheth S, Fishman EK. Imaging of the inferior vena cava with MDCT. *AJR Am J Roentgenol* 2007;**189**:1243.

154. Plessier A, Valla DC. Budd-Chiari syndrome. *Semin Liv Dis* 2008;**28**:259.

155. Gwon 2nd D, Ko GY, Yoon HK, et al. Hepatocellular carcinoma associated with membranous obstruction of the inferior vena cava: incidence, characteristics, risk factors, and clinical efficacy of TACE. *Radiology* 2010;**254**:617.

156. Chahal P, Levy C, Litzow MR, et al. Utility of liver biopsy in bone marrow transplant patients. *J Gastroenterol Hepatol* 2008;**23**:222.

157. Beckett D, Olliff S. Interventional radiology in the management of Budd Chiari syndrome. *Cardiovasc Intervent Radiol* 2008;**31**:839.

158. Li T, Zhai S, Pang Z, et al. Feasibility and midterm outcomes of percutaneous transhepatic balloon angioplasty for symptomatic Budd-Chiari syndrome secondary to hepatic venous obstruction. *J Vasc Surg* 2009;**50**:1079.

159. Cura M, Haskal Z, Lopera J. Diagnosis and interventional radiology for Budd-Chiari syndrome. *Radiographics* 2009;**29**:669.

160. Amarapurkar DN, Punamiya SJ, Patel ND. Changing spectrum of Budd-Chiari syndrome in India with special reference to non-surgical management. *World J Gastroenterol* 2008;**14**:278.

161. Gandini R, Konda D, Simonetti G. Transjugular intrahepatic portosystemic shunt patency and clinical outcome in patients with Budd-Chiari syndrome: covered versus uncovered stents. *Radiology* 2006;**241**:298.

162. Garcia-Pagan JC, Heydtmann M, Raffa S, et al. TIPS for Budd-Chiari syndrome: long-term results and prognostic factors in 124 patients. *Gastroenterology* 2008;**135**:808.

163. Ryu RK, Durham JD, Krysl J, et al. Role of TIPS as a bridge to hepatic transplantation in Budd-Chiari syndrome. *J Vasc Interv Radiol* 1999;**10**:799.

164. Hendlisz A, van den Eynde M, Peeters M, et al. Phase III trial comparing protracted intravenous fluorouracil infusion alone or with yttrium-90 resin microspheres radioembolization for liver-limited metastatic colo-rectal cancer refractory to standard chemotherapy. *J Clin Oncol* 2010;**28**:3687.

165. Brunello F, Veltri A, Carucci P, et al. Radiofrequency ablation versus ethanol injection for early hepatocellular carcinoma: a randomized controlled trial. *Scand J Gastroenterol* 2008;**43**:727.

166. Lo CM, Ngan H, Tso WK, et al. Randomized controlled trial of transarterial lipiodol chemoembolization for unresectable hepatocellular carcinoma. *Hepatology* 2002;**35**:1164.

167. Llovet JM, Real MI, Montana X, et al. Arterial embolisation or chemoembolisation versus symptomatic treatment in patients with unresectable hepatocellular carcinoma: a randomised controlled trial. *Lancet* 2002;**359**:1734.

168. Schwartz RA, Teitelbaum GP, Katz MD, et al. Effectiveness of transcatheter embolization in the control of hepatic vascular injuries. *J Vasc Interv Radiol* 1993;**4**:359.

169. Sclafani SJA, Shaftan GW, Scalea TM, et al. Nonoperative salvage of computed tomography-diagnosed splenic injuries: utilization of angiography for triage and embolization for hemostasis. *J Trauma* 1995;**39**:818.

170. Griffin XL, Pullinger R. Are diagnostic peritoneal lavage or focused abdominal sonography for trauma safe screening investigations for hemodynamically stable patients after blunt abdominal trauma? A review of the literature. *J Trauma* 2007;**62**:779.

171. Shanmuganathan K. Multi-detector row CT imaging of blunt abdominal trauma. *Semin Ultrasound CT MR* 2004;**25**:180.

172. Tinkoff G, Esposito TJ, Reed J, et al. American Association for the Surgery of Trauma Organ Injury Scale I: spleen, liver, and kidney validation based on the National Trauma Data Bank. *J Am Coll Surg* 2008;**207**:646.

173. Demetriades D, Hadjizacharia P, Constantinou C, et al. Selective nonoperative management of penetrating abdominal solid organ injuries. *Ann Surg* 2006;**244**:620.

174. Schroeppel TJ, Croce MA. Diagnosis and management of blunt abdominal solid organ injury. *Curr Opin Crit Care* 2007;**13**:399.

175. Velmahos GC, Toutouzas KG, Radin R, et al. Nonoperative treatment of blunt injury to solid abdominal organs: a prospective study. *Arch Surg* 2003;**138**:844.

176. Christmas AB, Wilson AK, Manning B, et al. Selective management of blunt hepatic injuries including nonoperative management is a safe and effective strategy. *Surgery* 2005;**138**:606.

177. Haan JM, Bochicchio GV, Kramer N, et al. Nonoperative management of blunt splenic injury: a 5-year experience. *J Trauma* 2005;**58**:492.

178. Monnin V, Sengel C, Thony F, et al. Place of arterial embolization in severe blunt hepatic trauma: a multidisciplinary approach. *Cardiovasc Intervent Radiol* 2008;**31**:875.

179. Mohr AM, Lavery RF, Barone A, et al. Angiographic embolization for liver injuries: low mortality, high morbidity. *J Trauma* 2003;**55**:1077.

180. Asensio JA, Roldan G, Petrone P, et al. Operative management and outcomes in 103 AAST-OIS grades IV and V complex hepatic injuries: trauma surgeons still need to operate, but angioembolization helps. *J Trauma* 2003;**54**:647.

181. Haan JM, Biffl W, Knudson MM, et al. Splenic embolization revisited: a multicenter review. *J Trauma* . 2004;**56**:542.

182. Wahl WL, Ahrns KS, Chen S, et al. Blunt splenic injury: operation versus angiographic embolization. *Surgery* 2004;**136**:891.

183. Killeen KL, Shanmuganathan K, Boyd-Kranis R, et al. CT findings after embolization for blunt splenic trauma. *J Vasc Interv Radiol* 2001;**12**:209.

184. Dabbs DN, Stein DM, Scalea TM. Major hepatic necrosis: a common complication after angioembolization for treatment of high grade liver injuries. *J Trauma* 2009;**66**:621.

185. Karani JB, Yu DF, Kane PA. Interventional radiology in liver transplantation. *Cardiovasc Intervent Radiol* 2005;**28**:271.

186. Fontana RJ, Hamidullah H, Nghiem H, et al. Percutaneous radiofrequency thermal ablation of hepatocellular carcinoma: a safe and effective bridge to liver transplantation. *Liver Transpl* 2002;**8**:1165.

187. Lee VS, Morgan GR, Lin JC, et al. Liver transplant donor candidates: associations between vascular and biliary anatomic variants. *Liver Transpl* 2004;**10**:1049.

188. Erbay N, Raptopoulos V, Pomfret EA, et al. Living donor liver transplantation in adults: vascular variants important in surgical planning for donors and recipients. *AJR Am J Roentgenol* 2003;**181**:109.

189. Renz JF, Yersiz H, Reichert PR, et al. Split-liver transplantation: a review. *Am J Transplant* 2003;**3**:1323.

190. Renz JF, Emond JC, Yersiz H, et al. Split-liver transplantation in the United States: outcomes of a national survey. *Ann Surg* 2004;**239**:172.

191. Crossin JD, Muradali D, Wilson SR. US of liver transplants: normal and abnormal. *Radiographics* 2003;**23**:1093.

192. Duffy JP, Hong JC, Farmer DG, et al. Vascular complications of orthotopic liver transplantation: experience in more than 4200 patients. *J Am Coll Surg* 2009;**208**:896.

193. Saad WE, Lin E, Ormanoski M, et al. Noninvasive imaging of liver transplant complications. *Tech Vasc Interv Radiol* 2007;**10**:191.

194. Brancatelli G, Katyal S, Federle MP, et al. Three-dimensional multislice helical computed tomography with the volume rendering technique in the detection of vascular complications after liver transplantation. *Transplantation* 2002;**73**:237.

195. Pareja E, Cortes M, Navarro R, et al. Vascular complications after orthotopic liver transplantation: hepatic artery thrombosis. *Transplant Proc* 2010;**42**:2970.

196. Vivarelli M, Cucchetti A, La Barba G, et al. Ischemic arterial complications after liver transplantation in the adult: multivariate analysis of risk factors. *Arch Surg* 2004;**139**:1069.

197. Martin SR, Atkison P, Anand R, et al. Studies of Pediatric Liver Transplantation 2002: patient and graft survival and rejection in pediatric recipients of a first liver transplant in the United States and Canada. *Pediatr Transplant* 2004;**8**:273.

198. Singh AH, Nachiappan AC, Verma HA, et al. Postoperative imaging in liver transplantation: what radiologists should know. *Radiographics* 2010;**30**:339.

199. Pinna AD, Smith CV, Furukawa H, et al. Urgent revascularization of liver allografts after early hepatic artery thrombosis. *Transplantation* 1996;**62**:1584.

200. Boyvat F, Aytekin C, Harman A, et al. Endovascular stent placement in patients with hepatic artery stenoses or thromboses after liver transplant. *Transplant Proc* 2008;**40**:22.

201. Singhal A, Stokes K, Sebastian A, et al. Endovascular treatment of hepatic artery thrombosis following liver transplantation. *Transpl Int* 2010;**23**:245.

202. Zheng R-Q, Mao R, Ren J, et al. Contrast-enhanced ultrasound for the evaluation of hepatic artery stenosis after liver transplantation: potential role in changing the clinical algorithm. *Liver Transpl* 2010;**16**:729.

203. Dodd GD III, Memel DS, Zajko AB, et al. Hepatic artery stenosis and thrombosis in transplant recipients: Doppler diagnosis with resistive index and systolic acceleration time. *Radiology* 1994;**192**:657.

204. Platt JF, Yutzy GG, Bude RO, et al. Use of Doppler sonography for revealing hepatic artery stenosis in liver transplant recipients. *AJR Am J Roentgenol* 1997;**168**:473.

205. Orons PD, Zajko AB, Bron KM, et al. Hepatic artery angioplasty after liver transplantation: experience in 21 allografts. *J Vasc Interv Radiol* 1995;**6**:523.

206. Saad WE. Management of hepatic artery steno-occlusive complications after liver transplantation. *Tech Vasc Interv Radiol* 2007;**10**:207.

207. Denys AL, Qanadli SD, Durand F, et al. Feasibility and effectiveness of using coronary stents in the treatment of hepatic artery stenoses after orthotopic liver transplantation: preliminary report. *AJR Am J Roentgenol* 2002;**178**:1175.

208. Ueno T, Jones G, Martin A, et al. Clinical outcomes from hepatic artery stenting in liver transplantation. *Liver Transpl* 2006;**12**:422.

209. Buell JF, Funaki B, Cronin DC, et al. Long-term venous complications after full-size and segmental pediatric liver transplantation. *Ann Surg* 2002;**236**:658.

210. Vaidya S, Dinghe M, Kolokythas O, et al. Liver transplantation: vascular complications. *Ultrasound Q* 2007;**23**:239.

211. Funaki B, Rosenblum JD, Leef JA, et al. Percutaneous treatment of portal venous stenosis in children and adolescents with segmental hepatic transplants: long-term results. *Radiology* 2000;**215**:147.

212. Woo DH, Laberge JM, Gordon RL, et al. Management of portal venous complications after liver transplantation. *Tech Vasc Interv Radiol* 2007;**10**:233.

213. Aucejo F, Winans C, Henderson JM, et al. Isolated right hepatic vein obstruction after piggyback liver transplantation. *Liver Transpl* 2006;**12**:808.

214. Darcy MD. Management of venous outflow complications after liver transplantation. *Tech Vasc Interv Radiol* 2007;**10**:240.

215. Navarro F, LeMoine MC, Fabre JM, et al. Specific vascular complications of orthotopic liver transplantation with preservation of the retrohepatic vena cava: review of 1361 cases. *Transplantation* 1999;**68**:646.

216. Parrilla P, Sanchez-Bueno F, Figueras J, et al. Analysis of the complications of the piggy-back technique in 1,112 liver transplants. *Transplantation* 1999;**67**:1214.

217. Ko GY, Sung KB, Yoon HK, et al. Early posttransplant hepatic venous outflow obstruction: long-term efficacy of primary stent placement. *Liver Transpl* 2008;**14**:1505.

218. Wang SL, Sze DY, Busque S, et al. Treatment of hepatic venous outflow obstruction after piggyback liver transplantation. *Radiology* 2005;**236**:352.

219. Carnavale FC, Machado AT, Moreira AM, et al. Midterm and long-term results of percutaneous endovascular treatment of venous outflow obstructions after pediatric liver transplantations. *J Vasc Interv Radiol* 2008;**19**:1439.

220. Lee JM, Ko GY, Sung KB, et al. Long-term efficacy of stent placement for treating inferior vena cava stenosis following liver transplantation. *Liver Transp l* 2010;**16**:513.

221. Elias G, Rastellini C, Nsier H, et al. Successful long-term repair of hepatic artery pseudoaneurysm following liver transplantation with primary stent-grafting. *Liver Transpl* 2007;**13**:1346.

222. Saad WE. Management of nonocclusive hepatic artery complications after liver transplantation. *Tech Vasc Interv Radiol* 2007;**10**:221.

223. Bioulac-Sage P, Laumonier H, Laurent C, et al. Benign and malignant vascular tumors of the liver in adults. *Semin Liver Dis* 2008;**28**:302.

224. Soussan M, Aube C, Bahrami S, et al. Incidental focal solid liver lesions: diagnostic performance of contrast-enhanced ultrasound and MR imaging. *Eur Radiol* 2010;**20**:1715.

225. Silva AC, Evans JM, McCullough AE, et al. MR imaging of hypervascular liver masses: a review of current techniques. *Radiographics* 2009;**29**:385.

226. Winterer JT, Kotter E, Ghanem N, et al. Detection and characterization of benign focal liver lesions with multislice CT. *Eur Radiol* 2006;**16**:2427.

227. Giavroglou C, Economou H, Ioannidis I. Arterial embolization of giant hepatic hemangiomas. *Cardiovasc Intervent Radiol* 2003;**26**:92.

228. Vassiou K, Rountas H, Liakou P, et al. Embolization of giant hepatic hemangioma before urgent liver resection. Case report and review of the literature. *Cardiovasc Intervent Radiol* 2007;**30**:800.

229. Duxbury MS, Garden OJ. Giant hemangioma of the liver: observation or resection? *Dig Surg* 2010;**27**:7.

230. Kim YI, Chung CW, Park JH. Feasibility of transcatheter arterial chemoembolization for hepatic adenoma. *J Vasc Interv Radiol* 2007;**18**:862.

231. Deneve JL, Pawlik TM, Cunningham S, et al. Liver cell adenoma: a multicenter analysis of risk factors for rupture and malignancy. *Ann Surg Oncol* 2009;**16**:640.

232. Stoot JH, van der Linden E, Terpstra OT, et al. Life-saving therapy for haemorrhaging liver adenomas using selective arterial embolization. *Br J Surg* 2007;**94**:1249.

233. Amesur N, Hammond JS, Zajko AB, et al. Management of unresectable symptomatic focal nodular hyperplasia with arterial embolization. *J Vasc Interv Radiol* 2009;**20**:543.

234. Vogl TJ, Own A, Hammerstingl R, et al. Transarterial embolization as a therapeutic option for focal nodular hyperplasia in four patients. *Eur Radiol* 2006;**16**:670.

235. Park CM, Cha SH, Kim DH, et al. Hepatic arterioportal shunts not directly related to hepatocellular carcinoma: findings on CT during hepatic arteriography, CT arterial portography and dual phase spiral CT. *Clin Radiol* 2000;**55**:465.

236. Itai Y, Saida Y, Irie T, et al. Intrahepatic portosystemic venous shunts: spectrum of CT findings in external and internal subtypes. *J Comput Assist Tomogr* 2001;**25**:348.

237. Roux P, Hebert T, Anghelescu D, et al. Endovascular treatment of arterioportal fistula with the Amplatzer occlusion device. *J Vasc Interv Radiol* 2009;**20**:685.

238. Ozyer U, Kirbas I, Aytekin C, et al. Coil embolization of a congenital intrahepatic arterioportal fistula: increasing experience in management. *Pediatr Radiol* 2008;**38**:1253.

239. Huang MS, Lin Q, Jiang ZB, et al. Comparison of long-term effects between intra-arterially delivered ethanol and Gelfoam for the treatment of severe arterioportal shunt in patients with hepatocellular carcinoma. *World J Gastroenterol* 2004;**10**:825.

240. Silberzweig JE, Matissen D, Khorsandi AS. Splenic arteriovenous fistula with pseudoaneurysm as a complication of splenectomy. *AJR Am J Roentgenol* 2006;**187**:W548.

241. Siablis D, Papathanassiou ZG, Karnabatidis D, et al. Splenic arteriovenous fistula and sudden onset of portal hypertension as complications of a ruptured splenic artery aneurysm: successful treatment with transcatheter arterial embolization. A case study and review of the literature. *World J Gastroenterol* 2006;**12**:4264.

242. Larson AM. Liver disease in hereditary hemorrhagic telangiectasia. *J Clin Gastroenterol* 2003;**36**:149.

243. Chavan A, Caselitz M, Gratz KF, et al. Hepatic artery embolization for treatment of patients with hereditary hemorrhagic telangiectasia and symptomatic hepatic vascular malformations. *Eur Radiol* 2004;**14**:2079.

244. Whiting Jr JH, Korzenik JR, Miller Jr FJ, et al. Fatal outcome after embolotherapy for hepatic arteriovenous malformations of the liver in two patients with hereditary hemorrhagic telangiectasia. *J Vasc Interv Radiol* 2000;**11**:855.

245. Frippiat F, Donckier J, Vandenbossche P, et al. Splenic infarction: report of three cases of atherosclerotic embolization originating in the aorta and retrospective study of 64 cases. *Acta Clin Belg* 1996;**51**:395.

246. Matsuo R, Ohta Y, Ohya Y, et al. Isolated dissection of the celiac artery—a case report. *Angiology* 2000;**51**:603.

247. Yoon DY, Park JH, Chung JW, et al. Iatrogenic dissection of the celiac artery and its branches during transcatheter arterial embolization for hepatocellular carcinoma: outcome in 40 patients. *Cardiovasc Intervent Radiol* 1995;**18**:16.

248. Chiesa R, Astore D, Guzzo G, et al. Visceral artery aneurysms. *Ann Vasc Surg* 2005;**19**:42.

249. Tessier DJ, Stone WM, Fowl RJ, et al. Clinical features and management of splenic artery pseudoaneurysm: case series and cumulative review of literature. *J Vasc Surg* 2003;**38**:969.

250. Carr SC, Mahvi DM, Hoch JR, et al. Visceral artery aneurysm rupture. *J Vasc Surg* 2001;**33**:806.

251. Abbas MA, Stone WM, Fowl RJ, et al. Splenic artery aneurysms: two decades experience at Mayo clinic. *Ann Vasc Surg* 2002;**16**:442.

252. Tulsyan N, Kashyap VS, Greenberg RK, et al. The endovascular management of visceral artery aneurysms and pseudoaneurysms. *J Vasc Surg* 2007;**45**:276.

253. Mattar SG, Lumsden AB. The management of splenic artery aneurysms: experience with 23 cases. *Am J Surg* 1995;**169**:580.

254. Trastek VF, Pairolero PC, Joyce JW, et al. Splenic artery aneurysms. *Surgery* 1982;**91**:694.

255. Lumsden AB, Mattar SG, Allen RC, et al. Hepatic artery aneurysms: the management of 22 patients. *J Surg Res* 1996;**60**:345.

256. Pasha SF, Gloviczki P, Stanson AW, et al. Splanchnic artery aneurysms. *Mayo Clin Proc* 2007;**82**:472.

257. Abbas MA, Fowl RJ, Stone WM, et al. Hepatic artery aneurysm: factors that predict complications. *J Vasc Surg* 2003;**38**:41.

258. Asokan S, Chew EK, Ng KY, et al. Post partum splenic artery aneurysm rupture. *J Obstet Gynaecol Res* 2000;**26**:199.

259. Holdsworth RJ, Gunn A. Ruptured splenic artery aneurysm in pregnancy: a review. *Br J Obstet Gynaecol* 1992;**99**:595.

260. Lee PC, Rhee RY, Gordon RY, et al. Management of splenic artery aneurysms: the significance of portal and essential hypertension. *J Am Coll Surg* 1999;**189**:483.

261. McDermott VG, Shlansky-Goldberg R, Cope C. Endovascular management of splenic artery aneurysms and pseudoaneurysms. *Cardiovasc Intervent Radiol* 1994;**17**:179.

262. Saltzberg SS, Maldonado TS, Lamparello PJ, et al. Is endovascular therapy the preferred treatment for all visceral artery aneurysms? *Ann Vasc Surg* 2005;**19**:507.

263. Sachdev U, Baril DT, Ellozy SH, et al. Management of aneurysms involving branches of the celiac and superior mesenteric arteries: a comparison of surgical and endovascular therapy. *J Vasc Surg* 2006;**44**:718.

264. Rami P, Williams D, Forauer A, et al. Stent-graft treatment of patients with acute bleeding from hepatic artery branches. *Cardiovasc Intervent Radiol* 2005;**28**:153.

265. Ilan Y, Ben-Chetrit E. Liver involvement in giant cell arteritis. *Clin Rheumatol* 1993;**12**:219.

266. Zhu K, Meng X, Quian J, et al. Partial splenic embolization for hypersplenism in cirrhosis: a long-term outcome in 62 patients. *Dig Liver Dis* 2009;**41**:411.

267. Kimura F, Itoh H, Ambiru S, et al. Long-term results of initial and repeated partial splenic embolization for the treatment of chronic idiopathic thrombocytopenic purpura. *AJR Am J Roentgenol* 2002;**179**:1323.

268. Palsson B, Hallen M, Forsberg AM, et al. Partial splenic embolization: long-term outcome. *Langenbecks Arch Surg* 2003;**387**:421.

269. Amin MA, el-Gendy MM, Dawoud IE, et al. Partial splenic embolization versus splenectomy for the management of hypersplenism in cirrhotic patients. *World J Surg* 2009;**33**:1702.

270. Noguchi H, Hirai K, Aoki Y, et al. Changes in platelet kinetics after a partial splenic arterial embolization in cirrhotic patients with hypersplenism. *Hepatology* 1995;**22**:1682.

271. Sakai T, Shiraki K, Inoue H, et al. Complications of partial splenic embolization in cirrhotic patients. *Dig Dis Sci* 2002;**47**:388.

272. Tsirigotis P, Sella T, Shapira MY, et al. Peliosis hepatis following treatment with androgen-steroids in patients with bone marrow failure syndromes. *Haematologica* 2007;**92**:e106.

273. Koehler JE, Sanchez MA, Garrido CS, et al. Molecular epidemiology of Bartonella infections in patients with bacillary angiomatosis-peliosis. *N Engl J Med* 1997;**337**:1876.

274. Torabi M, Hosseinzadeh K, Federle MP. CT of nonneoplastic hepatic vascular and perfusion disorders. *Radiographics* 2008;**28**:1967.

275. Ryan JM, Suhocki PV, Smith TP. Coil embolization of segmental arterial mediolysis of the hepatic artery. *J Vasc Interv Radiol* 2000;**11**:865.

Endocrine, Exocrine, and Reproductive Systems

Karim Valji

PANCREAS

ARTERIOGRAPHY

Angiography of the vasculature encompassing pancreatic disease begins with celiac or superior mesenteric arteriography using a 5-French (Fr) cobra or sidewinder-shaped (e.g., Sos) catheter. Selective catheterization of the gastroduodenal, splenic, dorsal pancreatic, inferior pancreaticoduodenal, or other branches is usually accomplished with coaxial microcatheters (see Chapters 11 and 12). The major veins surrounding the pancreas are visualized on late-phase superior mesenteric artery (SMA) and celiac artery injections.

ANATOMY AND PHYSIOLOGY

The pancreas is supplied by branches of the celiac and superior mesenteric arteries.[1,2] The head and uncinate process are fed by the *anterior* and *posterior superior pancreaticoduodenal arteries* (arising from the gastroduodenal artery) and the *anterior* and *posterior inferior pancreaticoduodenal (IPDA) arteries* (arising from the SMA) (Fig. 13-1). Rather than originating as the first branch of the SMA, the IPDA sometimes accompanies the first or second jejunal artery. All of these vessels form a rich network within the pancreatic head; they also serve important collateral pathways between the celiac artery and SMA (see Fig. 11-13).

The body and tail of the pancreas are supplied by the *dorsal pancreatic artery* and by numerous smaller branches of the splenic artery, including the *pancreatica magna* and *caudal pancreatic arteries* (see Fig. 13-1). A right branch of the dorsal pancreatic communicates with the anterior superior pancreaticoduodenal artery. The left branch becomes the *transverse pancreatic artery* and runs through the inferior portion of the distal end of the gland. The dorsal pancreatic artery may exit the celiac artery or other vessels (e.g., splenic artery).

The venous outflow from the pancreas largely follows the corresponding arteries. The anterior superior pancreaticoduodenal vein enters the *gastrocolic vein,* which is a major venous tributary of the superior mesenteric vein (see Fig. 12-3). The other pancreaticoduodenal veins have separate entrances into the portal venous system. The body and tail of the pancreas drain into the splenic and inferior pancreatic veins. The latter may empty into the inferior mesenteric, superior mesenteric, or splenic vein.

The junction of the portal and superior mesenteric veins lies behind the head and neck of the pancreas. The splenic artery and vein run behind the body and tail. The celiac axis and common hepatic artery are just superior to the gland. A replaced right or common hepatic artery may course behind the head and neck of the pancreas. Inflammatory or neoplastic diseases of the pancreas often encroach on one or more of these vessels.

The pancreas has both endocrine and exocrine functions.[3] Digestive proteins are generated by epithelial cells that form the pancreatic *acini,* which ultimately drain into the pancreatic ducts. Hormones are liberated from five cell types that form *islets of Langerhans:* α cells (glucagon), β cells (insulin), γ cells (pancreatic polypeptide, PP), δ cells (somatostatin), and ϵ cells (ghrelin, which controls appetite and release of growth hormone).

MAJOR DISORDERS

Nonendocrine Pancreatic Tumors

Etiology and Clinical Features

The pancreas is affected by a variety of benign and malignant tumors (Box 13-1). *Adenocarcinoma* arising from the ductal epithelium is the most common.[4,5] This usually lethal tumor grows primarily by local infiltration and invasion, and more than 50% occur in the

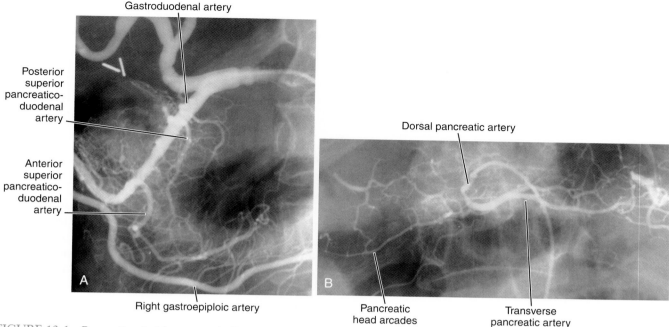

FIGURE 13-1   Pancreatic arterial anatomy. **A,** Gastroduodenal arteriogram. **B,** Dorsal pancreatic arteriogram from the undersurface of the celiac artery.

BOX 13-1

MAJOR NEOPLASMS
OF THE PANCREAS

- Ductal adenocarcinoma
- Neuroendocrine (islet cell) tumors
- Cystic epithelial tumors
- Solid and papillary epithelial tumors
- Metastases
- Lymphoma

pancreatic head. Even a small mass at this site can cause symptomatic biliary duct obstruction. Tumors in the body and tail often reach a large size before they become clinically evident. The most common risk factors for pancreatic adenocarcinoma are smoking, diabetes, and chronic pancreatitis.[5]

The much less common cystic neoplasms of the pancreas include a variety of cell types.[6,7] *Mucinous cystic neoplasms* and *intraductal papillary mucinous neoplasms* are the largest categories. The former type is seen almost exclusively in women and has a propensity for the tail of the gland. Most are benign and slow growing, but a small number have the potential for malignant transformation.

When a nonendocrine pancreatic malignancy is detected at an early stage, it usually has caused biliary obstruction and jaundice. Otherwise, the tumor must become large before the patient notices vague symptoms of fatigue, abdominal pain, and weight loss.

Imaging

Radiologic detection and staging of pancreatic tumors is critical for diagnosis and to avoid extensive surgery in patients with local spread or distant metastatic disease. Classic signs of unresectability include tumor extension to the boundary of the gland or to adjacent structures, extracapsular spread, major extrapancreatic vascular involvement, and distant metastases.[8] However, absolute criteria for unresectability differ among institutions. Unfortunately, most patients have nonoperable disease at the time of presentation. Computed tomography (CT), magnetic resonance imaging (MRI), and endoscopic sonography are most widely used for staging nonendocrine pancreatic tumors.[8-11]

Treatment

Pancreatic adenocarcinoma has a dismal prognosis. Despite long-running efforts at various forms of targeted therapy, mean survival remains about 1 year and fewer than 5% to 10% of patients are alive at 5 years.[12,13] An operation is undertaken to palliate symptoms or for potential (albeit rare) cure in patients without evidence for unresectability. Surgical options include the *Whipple procedure* (i.e., radical pancreaticoduodenectomy, cholecystectomy, choledochojejunostomy, and gastrojejunostomy), pylorus-preserving Whipple, total pancreatectomy, and palliative diversion for biliary obstruction (i.e., choledochojejunostomy) or duodenal obstruction (i.e., gastrojejunostomy). Preoperative or postoperative adjuvant radiation therapy and chemotherapy are used in some centers.[14,15]

Pancreatic Neuroendocrine (Islet Cell) Tumors

Etiology and Clinical Features

Islet cells in and around the pancreas are subject to neoplastic transformation into a variety of rare tumors. These lesions release excess amounts of one or more hormones that are either normal products of the pancreas (e.g., insulin) or normal secretions of the fetal pancreas or other glands (e.g., gastrin).[16-19] Neuroendocrine tumors generally are slow growing and small when found; symptoms arise from hormone imbalance rather than mass effect. About 15% are "nonfunctioning," although these lesions may liberate certain hormones that are not responsible for the particular clinical picture.

Insulinoma is the most common islet cell tumor of the pancreas. The mass is usually quite small (≤1 cm) when first discovered.[20] With a fairly even distribution throughout the pancreas, about 10% are multiple, and 10% are malignant.[19] Most patients are women with symptoms reflecting episodic hypoglycemia, namely weakness, shaking, tachycardia, lightheadedness, and fatigue. Serum levels of insulin and C-peptide are elevated. Rarely, insulinoma is part of the *multiple endocrine neoplasia type 1 (MEN 1)* syndrome. This rare autosomal dominant disease is attributed to mutations of the *MEN 1* tumor suppressor gene and features adenomas of the pancreas, parathyroid, and pituitary.[21,22]

Gastrinomas cause Zollinger-Ellison syndrome, which is characterized by hypersecretion of gastric acid, upper gastrointestinal tract ulcers, and diarrhea. These rare tumors are frequently malignant and usually small at presentation (≤1 cm).[23] About one third of cases are associated with the MEN 1 syndrome and have multiple foci. Most lesions are located within the "gastrinoma triangle," which is bordered by the cystic and common bile ducts, the junction between the pancreatic head and neck, and the second and third portions of the duodenum.[24] Often, the mass is buried in the duodenal wall.

Whereas *carcinoids* are the most common neuroendocrine tumors of the gastrointestinal system, they arise far more often from the gut than the pancreas.

Other exceedingly rare islet cell tumors include[18]:

- *VIPomas* cause *w*atery *d*iarrhea, *h*ypokalemia, *h*ypotension, and skin flushing (WDHA syndrome).
- *Glucagonomas* produce a migratory rash, glucose intolerance, anemia, and weight loss.

- *Somatostatinomas* are associated with gallstones, diabetes, and weight loss.
- Nonfunctioning tumors (some of which release pancreatic polypeptide or other obscure hormones) cause symptoms by mass effect (jaundice, abdominal pain) and are, therefore, quite large at presentation. They usually are solitary and malignant but slow growing.

Imaging

The diagnosis of a specific neuroendocrine disorder is based on the clinical scenario and hormonal testing. Finding the culprit tumor may require a whole gamut of cross-sectional imaging and invasive procedures (including endoscopic sonography).[18,22,25-28] Despite skepticism by some surgeons about the value of an exhaustive search before resection, preoperative localization can be accomplished in more than 90% of patients with the most common subtypes.[19,29,30]

NONINVASIVE IMAGING

Options for tumor localization include CT, MR, ultrasound, positron emission tomography (PET)/CT, and somatostatin receptor scintigraphy (SRS). The latter entails injection of ^{111}In-labeled *octreotide*, a synthetic somatostatin analogue, which is taken up by somatostatin receptors expressed on most of these tumors (with the exception of some insulinomas). Primary and metastatic tumors are then detected by single photon emission tomographic imaging. Most islet cell tumors are high signal on T2-weighted MR images and hyperdense on contrast-enhanced CT images, although hypodense lesions have been described (Figs. 13-2 and 13-3). For neuroendocrine tumors, the reported sensitivity and specificity of the available imaging modalities vary widely and depend largely on the particular population under study and the experience of the imagers.[22,25-27,29-31]

CATHETER ANGIOGRAPHY

Because noninvasive studies are less sensitive for islet cell tumor detection than for most other solid neoplasms, angiography continues to have a role (albeit small) in tumor detection.[17,18] The angiographic appearance of most islet cell tumors is that of a round, well-circumscribed, hypervascular mass within the substance of the pancreas or an adjacent organ (Fig. 13-4; see also Fig. 13-2). Neuroendocrine tumors should not be confused with an accessory spleen, hypervascular region of normal pancreatic tissue, or nodal metastases.

Presently, the most widely used angiographic protocol entails catheter-directed injection of a specific secretagogue into various arteries supplying the pancreas. For example, *calcium* or *secretin* infusion will cause an

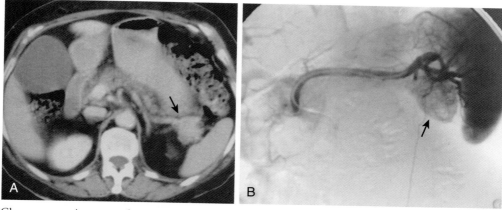

FIGURE 13-2 Glucagonoma. A computed tomography scan (**A**) and late phase splenic arteriogram (**B**) show a hyperdense mass in the tail of the pancreas *(arrow)*.

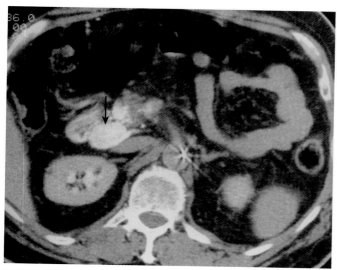

FIGURE 13-3 Gastrinoma. Computed tomography arteriogram with contrast injection into the celiac artery shows a densely enhancing mass adjacent to the duodenum and pancreatic head *(arrow)*.

insulinoma or gastrinoma (respectively) to liberate large quantities of hormone. Blood samples are obtained soon thereafter for hormonal analysis from the hepatic veins, which ultimately drain most islet cell neoplasms. A significant step-up compared with peripheral venous levels will localize the lesion to the vascular territory of the injected artery. In experienced hands, arterial stimulation with venous sampling is close to 100% accurate in preoperative detection of gastrinomas and insulinomas.[31-38]

Treatment

Standard management of solitary, localized pancreatic neuroendocrine tumors is surgical resection.[17,18,20] Nonoperable individuals are relegated to medical therapy, which aims to block the disabling hormonal effects with somatostatin analogues such as long-acting release *octreotide*.[39,40] Interferon has also been tried in this setting. Radiofrequency ablation (RFA) and chemoembolization have important roles in management of symptomatic liver metastases from a variety of neuroendocrine tumors, particularly carcinoid[41-46] (see Chapters 12 and 24).

Inflammatory Diseases

Etiology and Clinical Features

Acute pancreatitis is the consequence of autodigestion of the gland after release of proteolytic enzymes into itself.[47] An intense inflammatory reaction ensues, leading to hemorrhage and fat necrosis. If the patient survives the acute episode, the disease can progress to phlegmon, abscess, or pseudocyst formation, any of which may spread widely throughout the abdomen or pelvis. *Chronic pancreatitis* follows repeated bouts of acute pancreatitis or chronic pancreatic duct obstruction and is characterized by diffuse fibrosis, gland calcification, and pseudocyst formation.

In the United States, the most common risk factors for acute and chronic pancreatitis are alcohol abuse and biliary tract obstruction (e.g., gallstones). Other causes include trauma, surgery, biliary cirrhosis, infection, drugs, hyperparathyroidism, and hyperlipidemia. Acute pancreatitis can become a medical emergency with severe abdominal pain and shock. Both serum amylase and lipase levels are helpful in diagnosis.

Vascular complications follow about 10% of cases of severe pancreatitis.[48-50] They include splenic or portal vein thrombosis, pseudocyst hemorrhage, formation of small intrapancreatic or large vessel pseudoaneurysms from enzymatic destruction or severe inflammation, and pseudoaneurysm rupture. Blood may leak into the peritoneal cavity, retroperitoneum, or gastrointestinal tract (directly into bowel or via the biliary

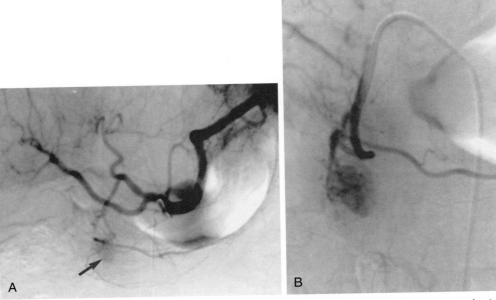

FIGURE 13-4   Insulinoma. **A,** A region of hypervascularity in the pancreatic head is identified by celiac arteriography *(arrow)*. **B,** After intraarterial injection of 1 mEq of calcium gluconate, the islet cell tumor is readily seen during gastroduodenal artery injection.

system [*hemosuccus pancreaticus*]). Thus, hemorrhage is signaled by gastrointestinal blood, falling hemoglobin, or hypotension. In a patient with a history of pancreatitis, erosion of a pseudoaneurysm or pseudocyst into the portal vein can produce hyperdynamic portal hypertension.

Imaging

Vascular sequelae of pancreatitis are first identified by CT, sonography, or (less often) MRI.[51,52] Arteriography is exclusively reserved for patients with a suspected vascular event who may require endovascular intervention. Large pseudoaneurysms, bleeding pseudocysts, and free extravasation are readily seen on CT and angiography (Fig. 13-5). A thorough search for the culprit lesion may require angiography of the splenic, hepatic, gastroduodenal, dorsal pancreatic, and pancreaticoduodenal arteries.

Treatment

Embolization is the optimal treatment for most hemorrhagic complications of pancreatitis, particularly because many of these patients are very poor surgical candidates[53-57] (see Fig. 13-5). The most sensible approach is endovascular deposition of coils and Gelfoam pledgets. Occasionally, other materials and routes are used, including direct percutaneous thrombin injection.[58] Blockade across the neck of a pseudoaneurysm is necessary to prevent backfilling from the distal segment of the

damaged artery through collateral channels (Fig. 13-6). Embolization generally is safe in the upper gastrointestinal tract. Occlusion of small or large bowel branches (e.g., jejunal arteries, middle colic artery arising from the dorsal pancreatic artery) poses some risk of bowel infarction. Permanent control of hemorrhage is achieved in about 75% of attempts.[53-56] However, a significant number of patients require second-look angiography to identify new bleeding sites.[57] Even with aggressive coordinated multispecialty care, mortality is still substantial.

OTHER DISORDERS

Pancreas Transplant Complications

Transplantation of the pancreas (often combined with kidney grafting) is performed for selected patients with type 1 diabetes. In one operative approach, the donor's iliac artery is harvested along with the pancreas and its arterial supply from the splenic artery and SMA. Off the operating field, the transplant splenic artery and SMA are connected to the internal and external iliac artery stumps, respectively.[59] The common iliac artery trunk of the resulting Y-graft is then anastomosed to the recipient's external iliac artery (Fig. 13-7). The donor portal vein is connected to the recipient external iliac vein.

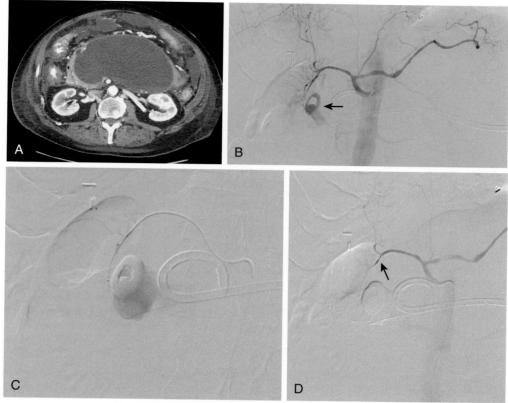

FIGURE 13-5 Pancreatic pseudocyst causing upper gastrointestinal bleeding. **A,** Contrast-enhanced computed tomography scan shows a huge hypodense mass occupying the retroperitoneal space surrounded by pancreatic tissue. A percutaneous drain was subsequently placed. Several days later, massive upper intestinal bleeding occurred. **B,** Celiac arteriogram shows the hemorrhage from the gastroduodenal artery *(arrow)*. Profound constriction of all celiac branches is because of shock. **C,** Microcatheterization of the bleeding vessel was done, followed by microcoil and Gelfoam embolization. **D,** The artery is obstructed *(arrow)*, and bleeding has ceased.

Vascular complications of pancreatic transplantation, although uncommon, can jeopardize the graft.[60,61] The most important of these are venous thrombosis, arterial thrombosis, and pseudoaneurysm formation. Early arterial occlusion usually is caused by improper formation of the anastomosis or graft damage after harvesting. Gadolinium-enhanced MRI and color Doppler sonography are the preferred methods for imaging these patients.[59,62-64] Angiography is rarely needed for diagnostic purposes. Endovascular thrombolysis or embolotherapy has been applied for related complications.[65-67]

Aneurysms

Aneurysms of the pancreatic and pancreaticoduodenal arteries are rare, and most are pseudoaneurysms caused by pancreatitis[53] (Box 13-2). Indications for treatment include rapidly increasing size, persistent symptoms, or rupture into the peritoneal cavity, retroperitoneum, or intestinal tract. An unusual but noteworthy cause of pancreaticoduodenal aneurysms is obstruction of the

---

BOX 13-2

CAUSES OF ANEURYSMS OF PANCREATIC ARTERIES

- Inflammation (i.e., pancreatitis)
- Trauma
- Infection
- Degenerative (atherosclerosis-related) causes
- High-flow state with celiac or superior mesenteric artery obstruction
- Tumor
- Vasculitis

---

celiac artery or SMA (see Fig. 11-35). Massive dilation of the collateral route through the pancreatic bed has been reported to produce frank aneurysm formation.[68] Treatment of certain types of pancreatic artery aneurysms has been discussed previously.[69,70]

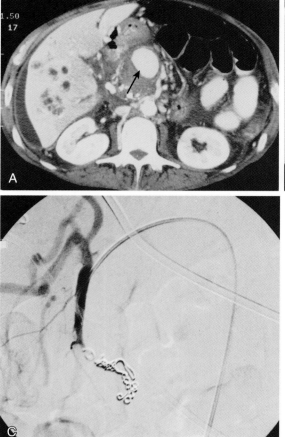

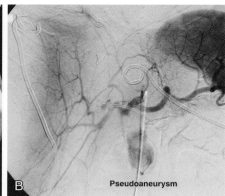

FIGURE 13-6   Gastroduodenal artery pseudoaneurysm. **A,** Computed tomography scan shows a large mass in the head of the pancreas with central dense enhancement *(arrow)*. Subcapsular fluid and numerous cystic hepatic lesions are also seen. **B,** Celiac arteriogram shows the gastroduodenal artery pseudoaneurysm. Subcapsular hepatic fluid has compressed the parenchyma. **C,** Microcoils were placed distal and proximal to the aneurysm neck to exclude it.

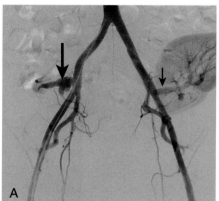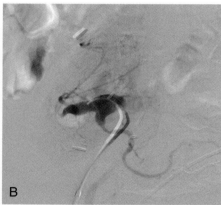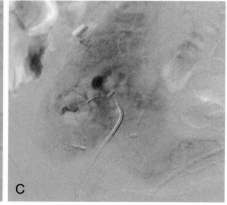

FIGURE 13-7   Pancreas and kidney transplant. **A,** Pelvic angiography shows the right external iliac artery anastomosis to the pancreas *(large arrow)* and left external iliac artery connection to the kidney *(small arrow)*. Early **(B)** and late **(C)** selective pancreatic arteriography shows the vascular anatomy and opacification of the entire gland.

Arteriovenous Malformations

Congenital vascular anomalies of the pancreas are exceedingly rare.[71] However, pancreatic arteriovenous malformations (AVMs) and telangiectasias can be detected in a substantial number of patients with hereditary hemorrhagic telangiectasia if they are sought.[72] Pancreatic AVMs may be found incidentally or after rupture into the gastrointestinal tract. These lesions are diagnosed by CT, MRI, or color Doppler sonography. Angiography is required occasionally to confirm the diagnosis. The usual treatment is operative removal.

ADRENAL GLANDS

ANGIOGRAPHY (VIDEO 13-1)

The only remaining indication for adrenal arteriography is embolotherapy of tumors with collateral supply from adrenal artery branches (e.g., renal cell carcinoma). Venography is required only to document location during adrenal venous sampling. Its major risk is extravasation with infarction from overinjection of contrast, which can lead to complete nonfunction of the gland.[73]

Adrenal venous sampling is a crucial technique for evaluating hormonally active tumors of the gland.[74] Before catheterization of these small caliber vessels, it is wise to partially anticoagulate the patient with heparin 3000 units intravenously. A top hole is punched about 5 mm proximal to the distal tip of the angiographic catheter; this side hole allows aspiration even if the catheter tip is occlusive. The right adrenal gland is catheterized with a renal double curve or sidewinder catheter by searching the posterior or right posterior aspect of the inferior vena cava (IVC) near the upper pole of the kidney (Fig. 13-8). The right adrenal vein must be differentiated from small, upwardly directed hepatic veins. The left adrenal vein, which is much easier to find, is sampled with a Simmons 2 catheter (see Fig. 13-8). First, the catheter is advanced well into the left renal vein. Then, it is withdrawn slowly with the tip pointing up until it engages the left phrenicoadrenal trunk. Blood samples are obtained after a small contrast injection is made to document catheter position. Finally, peripheral and/or IVC blood aliquots are drawn for comparison with selective samples.

ANATOMY

Classically, three arteries feed each adrenal gland[75]:

- *Superior adrenal artery* from the inferior phrenic artery
- *Middle adrenal artery* directly from the aorta above the renal artery (see Fig. 7-1)
- *Inferior adrenal artery* from the proximal renal artery (see Fig. 10-6)

The right adrenal gland has three main venous tributaries that converge into a single vessel entering the posterolateral IVC above the right renal vein (see Fig. 13-8). A central vein runs through the substance of the left adrenal gland. It joins the left inferior phrenic vein to form a common trunk, which then empties into the upper surface of the left renal vein just lateral to the vertebrae (see Fig. 13-8). Anomalous origins of the adrenal arteries are relatively common. On the other hand, venous anomalies are uncommon (e.g., right adrenal vein may join a hepatic vein or enter directly into the right renal vein). Still, knowledge of the typical variants is critical for successful adrenal vein sampling[76] (Fig. 13-9).

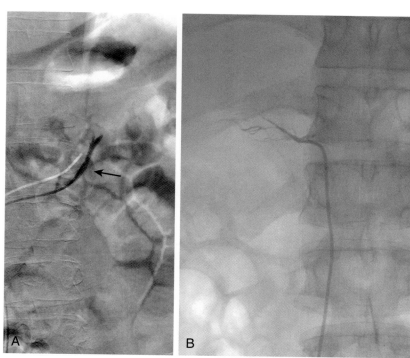

FIGURE 13-8   Bilateral adrenal vein sampling for hyperaldosteronism. Patient had difficult-to-control hypertension and right adrenal adenoma on CT imaging. **A,** Left adrenal venography *(arrow)* at the origin of the phrenicoadrenal trunk. **B,** Right adrenal vein has a "delta" configuration. Hormonal assay showed bilateral adrenal hyperplasia (see Table 13-3).

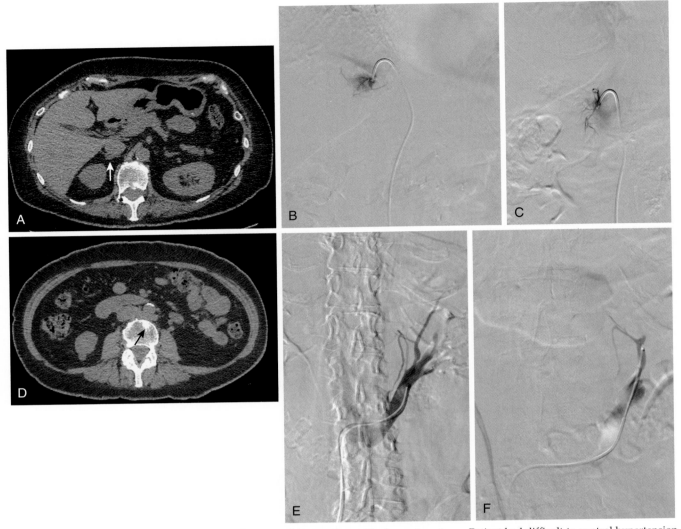

FIGURE 13-9   Bilateral adrenal vein sampling for hyperaldosteronism with aberrant anatomy. Patient had difficult-to-control hypertension. **A,** Computed tomography scan shows large right adrenal mass *(arrow)*. **B,** Catheterization of a small hepatic vein. Note homogenous liver stain. **C,** Right adrenal venography. The left renal vein could not be easily found. **D,** Computed tomography scan shows presence of retroaortic left renal vein *(arrow)*. This vein was catheterized **(E)**, and the adrenal vein sampled **(F)**. Hormonal assay proved active aldosteronoma (see Table 13-4). This was confirmed at operation.

MAJOR DISORDERS

Cushing Syndrome

Hypercortisolism has several causes[77] (Table 13-1). Benign adenomas tend to be small, but functioning adrenal carcinomas often are quite large at the time of presentation. Cushing syndrome occurs in both adults and children.[77] Patients classically suffer from hypertension, hirsutism, abdominal striae, obesity, diabetes, and mental disturbances. By definition, the serum cortisol level is elevated. A high-dose *dexamethasone suppression test* will discriminate between adrenocorticotropin hormone (ACTH)–dependent adrenal hyperplasia from a pituitary tumor and an ACTH-independent adrenal tumor.

TABLE 13-1   Causes of Hypercortisolism

ACTH DEPENDENT (ABOUT 80% OF CASES)

Pituitary adenoma *(Cushing disease)*
Ectopic cortisol-releasing hormone tumor

ACTH INDEPENDENT (ABOUT 20% OF CASES)

Adrenocortical adenoma
Bilateral adrenal hyperplasia
Adrenal carcinoma
Excess cortisol intake

ACTH, *adrenocorticotropin hormone.*

If a pituitary mass is found, *inferior petrosal sinus sampling* confirms the corticotropin gradient and is often requested before operative removal.[78] Otherwise, an adrenal mass is sought with sonography, CT, MRI, or radionuclide-based PET/CT.[79-82] If routine imaging studies are nondiagnostic, adrenal venous sampling should be performed.[34] A unilateral cortisol gradient is diagnostic of adrenal adenoma or adenocarcinoma.[83] The preferred therapy is adrenalectomy.

Aldosteronism (Video 13-1)

Etiology and Clinical Features

Primary aldosteronism has several causes[84] (Table 13-2). In the past, aldosteronism was reported as the cause for hypertension in about 1% to 2% of the general population. However, new evidence supports a higher prevalence (5% to 13%) even among unselected groups.[85-88] A hyperfunctioning adrenal adenoma is the culprit in about 35% of cases.[87-89] These adenomas tend to be smaller ($\leq$2 cm) than those seen with Cushing syndrome. Secondary aldosteronism usually is a consequence of renal artery stenosis, which elevates renin levels and activates the renin-angiotensin-aldosterone system.

Patients with primary or secondary aldosteronism are hypertensive. Hypokalemia, metabolic alkalosis, and elevated urinary aldosterone metabolites are characteristic. A serum aldosterone/renin ratio greater than 20 to 25 is often used as a threshold for further investigation.[90]

Imaging

The distinction between a functioning tumor and bilateral adrenal hyperplasia is essential, because the former is treated with surgery or ablation for cure and the latter is treated medically with aldosterone antagonists. CT, MR, and radionuclide-based PET/CT are the primary imaging options for lesion detection. However, nonfunctioning adrenal adenomas ("incidentalomas") are commonly detected on CT and MR and can be mistaken for a functional aldosteronoma.[91]

Adrenal venous sampling is essential to establish with near certainty that a suspicious adrenal lesion is the culprit.[34] In one recent report, CT or MRI mistook a nonfunctioning adrenal adenoma for a functioning tumor in 38% of cases before classification with venous sampling.[91] Among experienced practitioners, sampling is accurate in more than 90% of attempts.[89,92,93] Novices should not initially expect such reliable outcomes. High-quality CT

TABLE 13-2 Causes of Hyperaldosteronism

Hormonally active adrenal adenoma (*Conn syndrome*)
Bilateral (or rarely unilateral) adrenal hyperplasia
Adrenal carcinoma
Familial hyperaldosteronism
Ectopic tissue

TABLE 13-3 Adrenal Vein Sampling after Cortrosyn Stimulation Results for Figure 13-8

Site	Aldosterone	Cortisol	Aldosterone/Cortisol Ratio
Right adrenal vein	960	428	2.2
Left adrenal vein	1300	648	2.0
Inferior vena cava	21	26	0.8

TABLE 13-4 Adrenal Vein Sampling after Cortrosyn Stimulation Results for Figure 13-9

Site	Aldosterone	Cortisol	Aldosterone/Cortisol Ratio
Right adrenal vein	1800	302	6.0
Left adrenal vein	430	804	0.5
Inferior vena cava	74	37	2.0

scans can be extremely helpful in identifying the precise location of the right adrenal vein connection with the IVC. The technique for adrenal vein sampling is described earlier. Blood aliquots are obtained from the right and left adrenal veins and from the IVC for aldosterone and cortisol analysis. High cortisol levels confirm that the correct vein was catheterized. Many experts believe that sampling should be done after (and possibly before) ACTH stimulation with cosyntropin (Cotrosyn 250 μg IV). In fact, it is the relative suppression of aldosterone from the uninvolved gland that is most predictive of a positive outcome from surgery.[93] An aldosterone/cortisol ratio from the suspected side more than four to five times greater than the ratio in the contralateral vein is diagnostic (Tables 13-3 and 13-4 and see Figs. 13-8 and 13-9). Sequential (rather than simultaneous dual catheter) sampling does not appear to diminish accuracy despite normal temporal fluctuations in hormone release.[92]

Treatment

Bilateral hyperplasia is managed with drug therapy. *Spironolactone (Aldactone)* is a particularly effective competitive inhibitor of aldosterone activity in the renal tubules. Functioning adenomas and adrenal carcinomas are treated by open adrenalectomy or laparoscopic techniques. The evidence to support percutaneous ablation by arterial embolotherapy (e.g., with alcohol sometimes admixed with contrast material) or RFA is only anecdotal.[94-96]

OTHER DISORDERS

Adrenogenital Syndromes

Virilization, or, less frequently, feminization in adults usually is the result of a gonadal tumor or adrenal disease (i.e., adenoma, carcinoma, or bilateral hyperplasia). Polycystic ovary syndrome and certain *ovarian* neoplasms are rarely associated with excess testosterone production. Virilizing *adrenal* tumors typically release dehydroepiandrosterone (DHEA) and dehydroepiandrosterone sulfate.[97] Urinary 17-ketosteroid levels are markedly elevated in either situation. Affected women complain of hirsutism, menstrual dysfunction, acne, and obesity.

CT, transvaginal sonography, or MRI is recommended for evaluation of this vexing clinical problem. If the results are equivocal, bilateral adrenal and ovarian venous sampling should be performed.[98] Various hormonal levels are measured, including testosterone, DHEA, and androstenedione. Virilizing adrenal or ovarian tumors are distinguished by the abnormally high hormone ratio between the ipsilateral vein and a peripheral blood sample.

Pheochromocytoma

Rare tumors of chromaffin cells of the sympathetic nervous system originate in the adrenal medulla *(pheochromocytoma)* or extraadrenal sites *(paraganglionomas* or *chemodectomas).*[99] The disorder is tagged with the "10% rule," whereby 10% of lesions are extraadrenal, metastatic, bilateral, cystic, or associated with MEN-2 syndrome. In fact, the likelihood of ectopic location and malignancy varies with the existence of inherited links to the disease.[100] Almost a third of affected individuals (including sporadic cases) have an identifiable genetic defect. Symptoms are related to excess production of catecholamines (including epinephrine and norepinephrine) in addition to other hormones from the pathologic tissue.

The diagnosis of pheochromocytoma or paraganglionoma usually is made with metaiodobenzylguanidine scintigraphy, MRI, or CT scanning.[101] Iodinated contrast material given by any route may precipitate a potentially lethal hypertensive crisis.[102] Patients with suspected pheochromocytoma should be pretreated with alpha-adrenergic and possibly beta-adrenergic antagonists. A typical regimen includes *phenoxybenzamine* for several days before the procedure (20 mg orally twice daily) and *phentolamine* (5 to 15 mg IV) as needed during the procedure.

CT-guided RFA or percutaneous ethanol injection (PEI) have been employed on occasion for treatment of these lesions.[96,103]

PARATHYROID GLANDS

ANGIOGRAPHY

Parathyroid arteriography is a procedure of the past.[104,105] Parathyroid venous sampling is still done on rare occasions, and it can be a demanding and complex procedure.[34,105] A complete study requires selective catheterization of inferior, superior, and middle thyroid veins along with the thymic and internal jugular veins. Central large vein sampling (i.e., bilateral internal jugular and brachiocephalic veins) is simpler but may be less accurate.[106-108] Small contrast injections are made after obtaining blood aliquots to document catheter position. In postoperative patients, the vertebral veins also are sampled at several sites.

ANATOMY

The primary routes of venous drainage from the normal parathyroid glands are as follows:

- *Inferior thyroid vein* to the upper surface of the left brachiocephalic or right internal jugular vein
- *Superior* and *middle thyroid veins* to the internal jugular vein
- *Thymic vein* to the undersurface of the left brachiocephalic vein

During surgery for parathyroid disease, the thyroidal veins often are ligated.[109] The thyroid bed then empties through collateral channels that join the vertebral veins.

MAJOR DISORDERS

Hyperparathyroidism

Etiology and Clinical Features

Primary hyperparathyroidism is a disorder of excess secretion of parathyroid hormone (PTH) from solitary or multiple parathyroid adenomas, bilateral gland hyperplasia, or parathyroid carcinoma.[110] Adenomas account for about 80% of cases. Patients with either MEN-1 or MEN-2 may suffer from active parathyroid adenomas.[100] The resulting hypercalcemic state is responsible for kidney stones, abdominal pain, renal dysfunction, and dehydration seen in this disease. Conventional management entails surgical resection of the offending adenoma or subtotal parathyroidectomy for glandular hyperplasia. In a few individuals, symptoms persist or recur after surgery because of ectopic or supernumerary glands or incomplete removal of hyperplastic tissue. Residual tumors usually are found in the tracheoesophageal groove of the superior mediastinum, in the thymus, or within the thyroid gland.

Imaging

Patients with hyperparathyroidism are first evaluated with the most sensitive imaging modalities available, namely sonography (with or without fine-needle aspiration of detected masses for PTH levels), ^{99m}Tc-sestamibi scintigraphy, or ^{11}C-methionine PET/CT of the neck and mediastinum.[111-115] When two studies are positive for a solitary adenoma, most surgeons proceed with removal. CT and MRI are second-tier imaging options. If detection remains elusive, selective parathyroid venous sampling may be diagnostic.[108] A 2:1 PTH ratio between a sampled site and a peripheral vein is diagnostic of excess hormone production from the drained site. If symptoms persist after surgery or parathormone levels remain elevated, reoperation is usually preceded by a more aggressive workup, especially selective venous sampling (Fig. 13-10).[116-118] In one large contemporary series, ectopic glandular tissue was found in close to one third of reoperations for disease.[113]

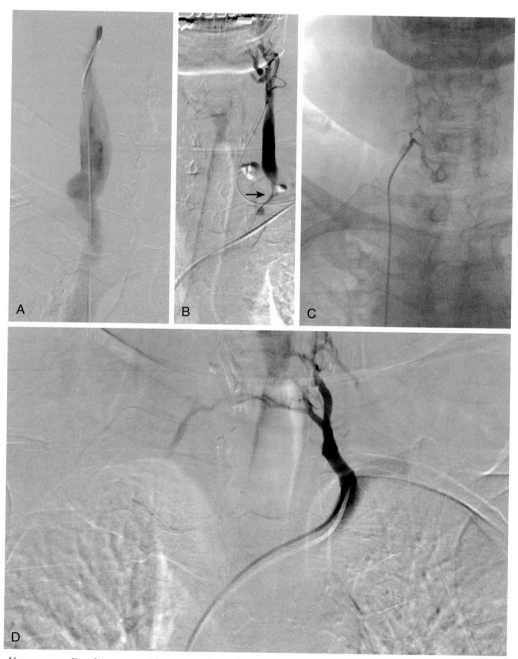

FIGURE 13-10 Venous sampling for recurrent hyperparathyroidism. **A,** Samples for parathormone assay are obtained at various levels of the right internal jugular (IJ) vein **B,** Left internal jugular vein via a collateral (central IJ vein is obstructed, *arrow*). **C,** Right middle thyroid vein. **D,** Inferior thyroid vein.

Treatment

Minimally invasive surgery (sometimes with intraoperative sonography) is preferred by many experienced operators.[119] The recent availability of ultrarapid PTH assay now makes intraoperative hormone analysis practical in guiding open or laparoscopic parathyroid resection.[107] Reoperation is curative in greater than 90% of cases when a robust imaging sequence is followed.[112,113,117,120]

Transcatheter arterial ablation of residual parathyroid adenomas has been described.[117,121] Injection of absolute alcohol is usually sufficient to destroy the lesion. The procedure should be performed only if some parathyroid tissue is preserved to prevent hypoparathyroidism.

MALE REPRODUCTIVE SYSTEM

ARTERIOGRAPHY AND VENOGRAPHY

In the evaluation of men with high-flow priapism or penile trauma, a pelvic arteriogram serves as a roadmap for selective catheterization. The internal pudendal artery is easily catheterized using a 5-Fr ultralong reverse-curve (Bookstein or Roberts) catheter (see Chapter 3). Alternatively, a cobra catheter can be negotiated into the bilateral internal pudendal arteries. Embolization of penile arteries is accomplished with a coaxial microcatheter.

For evaluation of trauma to the corpora cavernosa, cavernosography is performed by injecting dilute, isosmolar contrast material at a rate of 1 to 2 mL/sec through a small butterfly needle inserted into one corpus cavernosum just proximal to the glans penis. Both corpora fill because of normal perforations in the intercavernosal septum.

For varicocele embolization, the operator may choose between right internal jugular and femoral vein access. The left internal spermatic vein is catheterized with a cobra or similarly shaped catheter. The right internal spermatic vein is engaged with a sidewinder or Simmons catheter from the groin or a reshaped headhunter catheter from the neck. The terminal valve is crossed with a hydrophilic guidewire, and selective venography is obtained to map the vein and collateral routes. A left renal venogram may be done with the table tilted slightly head-up or during a Valsalva maneuver to encourage reflux into the left internal spermatic vein. Lead shielding of the testes is important.

ANATOMY

The penis is usually fed by the bilateral *internal pudendal arteries*, which are major branches of the anterior divisions of the internal iliac arteries[122] (Fig. 13-11).

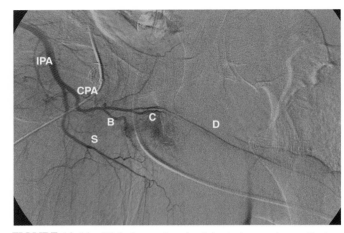

FIGURE 13-11 Right internal pudendal arteriogram in a patient with peroneal trauma and possible arteriocavernosal fistula causing priapism. The cavernosal artery is truncated beyond its origin. Staining of the bulb of the corpus spongiosum is normal. *B*, artery to the bulb; *C*, cavernosal artery; *CPA*, common penile artery; *D*, dorsal penile artery; *IPA*, internal pudendal artery; *S*, scrotal branches.

However, the penile arteries sometimes arise from anomalous vessels such as the obturator, inferior gluteal, external pudendal, or inferior epigastric artery.[123] The internal pudendal artery gives off scrotal vessels, after which it becomes the *common penile artery*. The *artery to the bulb* supplies the corpus spongiosum and the urethra. The penile artery divides into two terminal branches. The *dorsal penile artery* runs in the superficial fascia of the penis; the *cavernosal artery* enters the substance of the corpus cavernosum. Helicine arterioles directly supply the lacunar spaces of the corpora.

The corpora cavernosa drain through a deep system (i.e., deep dorsal vein) and a superficial system (i.e., superficial dorsal vein) into the crural and preprostatic plexuses. These networks empty into the internal pudendal and other deep pelvic veins (Fig. 13-12).

The testes are fed by the *testicular arteries*, which arise from the anterolateral surface of the aorta just at or below the renal artery origins (see Fig. 10-35). Blood drains from the testis and epididymis through the *pampiniform plexus*.[124] At the superficial inguinal ring, this complex forms three or four tributaries that enter the pelvis. These veins eventually converge into two and then into a single internal spermatic vein running in front of the ureter and alongside the gonadal artery. It is common for the main venous channel to have medial and lateral components; the lateral branch often terminates in renal capsular, mesenteric, colonic, or retroperitoneal veins. The *right internal spermatic vein* enters the IVC just below the right renal vein (Fig. 13-13). The *left internal spermatic vein* joins the undersurface of the left renal vein lateral to the vertebral column (see Fig. 10-3). Variant anatomy is seen in about 20% of

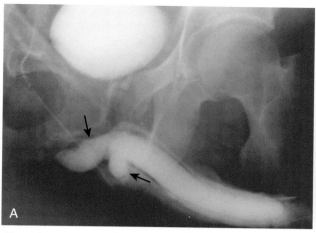
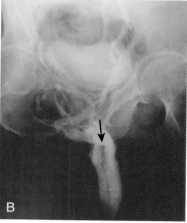

FIGURE 13-12   Normal cavernosography. **A,** Both corpora cavernosa are filled to the crura *(arrows),* and the deep dorsal vein is filled. **B,** The intercavernosal septum *(arrow)* is seen in another patient. The cavernosa drain into the preprostatic plexus and then into internal pudendal and other deep pelvic veins.

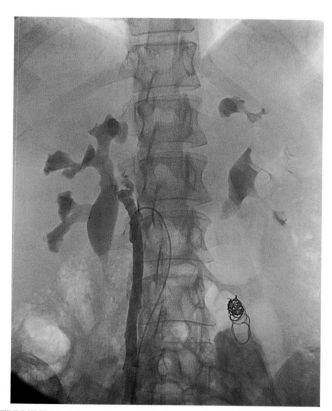

FIGURE 13-13   Right gonadal venogram. The vein is dilated and shows significant reflux.

cases.[125] Important anomalies include drainage of the right internal spermatic vein into the right renal vein (8%) and multiple terminal gonadal veins (15% to 20%). Valves are present in most but not all internal spermatic veins.

MAJOR DISORDERS

Male Varicocele

Etiology

Varicocele is a dilation of the pampiniform plexus in the scrotum with or without central venous dilation.[126] The disorder affects about 15% of the general adult male population.[127] Most cases occur on the left side of the body. The right side is involved in up to 10% of affected men, although some reports note a much higher frequency.[128,129]

The origin of *primary* varicocele is debated.[126,130,131] Various theories have been proposed, including absence or abnormal formation of internal spermatic vein valves and compression of the left renal vein, causing internal spermatic vein hypertension. Regardless of the cause, venous reflux and chronic venous hypertension are the result. *Secondary* varicocele is caused by abdominal or pelvic masses that impede drainage of the pampiniform plexus. The sudden onset of varicocele in an older man or the presence of a right-sided varicocele should raise the suspicion of a neoplasm (e.g., left renal vein invasion from renal cell carcinoma).

Clinical Features

Although more than 80% of patients with varicocele are asymptomatic and do not have a specific problem with fertility, the remainder can suffer from scrotal pain and swelling.[132] Up to 40% of men evaluated in infertility clinics are found to have a varicocele.[133] The explanation for diminished fertility in this population is controversial. The leading hypotheses invoke elevations in scrotal temperature or backflow of renal or adrenal metabolites as a cause for testicular dysfunction and suboptimal sperm production or function. As such, abnormalities of total sperm count, sperm density, and sperm motility are found in many patients with varicocele.

Imaging

Most varicoceles can be detected by physical examination alone. When the diagnosis is equivocal or a subclinical varicocele is suspected (i.e., infertility with abnormal sperm activity but a nonpalpable varicocele), the scrotum is evaluated with duplex sonography.[134] Spermatic venography is reserved for patients undergoing embolotherapy.

Treatment

The commonly (but not universally) accepted indications for invasive varicocele obliteration are scrotal pain, massive size, testicular hypoplasia in adolescent boys, and infertility with laboratory evidence for sperm dysfunction.*

SURGICAL THERAPY

Operation for varicocele entails surgical interruption of the internal spermatic vein and collateral vessels. Classically, ligation is performed at the retroperitoneal, internal

*See references 126, 127, 129, 130, 132, 135.

inguinal ring (Ivanissevitch procedure), or subinguinal level (Marmor procedure). Laparoscopic varicocelectomy is favored by many surgeons.[136,137]

VARICOCELE EMBOLIZATION

Technique A diagnostic venogram on the affected side is obtained to document valvular incompetence, reflux of contrast, venous dilation, and filling of collateral tributaries (see Fig. 13-13 and Fig. 13-14). Catheterization of the gonadal veins may be difficult if variant anatomy is present.[138] The preferred obliterative material is coils with or without adjuvant sclerosing agent such as 3% sodium tetradecyl sulfate foam. Cyanoacrylates (glue) and polidocanol are alternative agents.[139-143]

The internal spermatic vein is first occluded at the level of the superior pubic ramus. Material is then deposited in stages up to the vein origin, taking care not to allow coil springs to extend into the renal vein or IVC. Venography is repeated periodically to identify collateral channels that also may require obliteration. Nitroglycerin (100 to 200 μg) is given to relieve venospasm. In patients with solitary left-sided varicocele, right-sided embolization is performed only when the right internal spermatic vein is incompetent and the goal is improved fertility.

Results Embolotherapy is technically successful in more than 90% of cases.[139-150] No particular embolic agent or combination has proven most effective. The usual reasons for initial failure are inability to cannulate

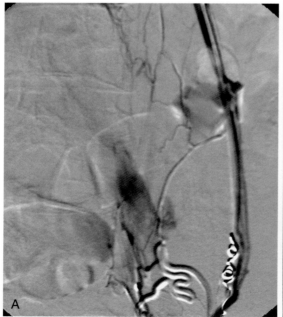
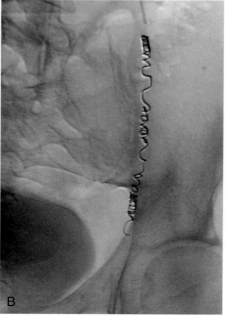

FIGURE 13-14   Varicocele embolization. **A,** Selective catheterization of the lower left internal spermatic vein about the inguinal ligament. Several platinum coils and Gelfoam pieces were placed. Because several collateral channels opacified, sodium morrhuate was injected as a liquid sclerosant. **B,** Additional platinum coils separated by Gelfoam pieces were deposited along the course of the vein up to its orifice at the left renal vein.

the internal spermatic vein or traverse a competent valve, venospasm, and the presence of multiple central collateral veins. Pain relief is almost invariable.[141] The late recurrence rate is 4% to 12%, primarily because of the development of collateral channels.[141,145,148,151] Overall, results of embolotherapy are comparable to surgery and excellent after failed surgical ligation.[152-156] One study found that duplication of the gonadal vein deep in the pelvis was a common finding in men with recurrent or persistent varicocele after operation who were referred for embolotherapy.[139]

At present, the value of embolotherapy or surgery for varicocele in infertile men is being contested. Early reports claimed significant improvement in sperm density and motility in most cases; about one fourth to one third of couples become pregnant in follow-up studies.* Recent studies have failed to show increased likelihood of pregnancy or association of pregnancy with improved sperm quality after varicocele embolization.[158,159] In fact, aggregate analysis of reported randomized trials of treated versus untreated infertile men failed to identify any benefit from varicocele embolization in this regard.[160] Still, many practitioners dispute this wholesale rejection of these methods.[131,135]

Complications Minor flank or scrotal pain, low-grade fever, and transient numbness over the anterior thigh are minor side effects of the procedure. Vein rupture with extravasation usually is self-limited. Adverse events specific to embolotherapy are uncommon (5% to 10%) and include migration of coils to the lung, thrombosis of the pampiniform plexus, and aspermia.[136]

OTHER DISORDERS

Trauma

Direct penile injury can be caused by blunt or penetrating trauma or during sexual activity (e.g., penile fracture). Potential sequelae include penile deformity, urethral damage, or impotence.[161-163] Cavernosography may be requested to delineate the damage to the corpora cavernosa and venous drainage (see earlier discussion).

Priapism refers to sustained penile erection without direct stimulation or sexual desire. *Low-flow priapism* is caused by sludging of blood in the corpora and impeded venous outflow.[164,165] Corporal blood aspirates will be relatively hypoxic. The list of precipitating factors is long, but the consequence is effectively penile ischemia that must be relieved *emergently* or risk necrosis of the corpora cavernosa. Blunt perineal or penile trauma is rarely followed by *high-flow priapism* from a direct arteriocavernous fistula. In this case, corporal blood

*See references 141, 142, 148, 152-154, 157.

remains well oxygenated. The fistula can be confirmed with angiography and obliterated by superselective embolization of the cavernosal arteries with either temporary (e.g., Gelfoam) or permanent agents (e.g., coils or small particles) (Fig. 13-15). Resolution of priapism and maintenance of normal erections is the rule, but recurrence rates are significant.[166-169]

When imaging for potentially treatable vascular causes of erectile dysfunction seems necessary, duplex sonography is the best option. Angiography has no role unless a post-traumatic arteriovenous fistula is suspected or surgical bypass is being considered in a relatively young patient.

FEMALE REPRODUCTIVE SYSTEM

ANATOMY

The ovaries are fed by the *ovarian arteries*, which exit the anterolateral surface of the aorta below the renal arteries (see Fig. 7-1). The vessels descend into the pelvis and then enter the broad ligament of the uterus. The *right ovarian vein* empties directly into the IVC below the right renal vein. The *left ovarian vein* drains into the undersurface of the left renal vein. Variant anatomy is seen in a minority of cases.[170]

The uterus is primarily supplied by the *uterine arteries*, which usually take off as separate branches of the anterior divisions of the internal iliac arteries.[170] They course medially in the broad ligament and then ascend along the lateral border of the uterus. These vessels have anastomoses with branches of the ovarian arteries (see later discussion).

MAJOR DISORDERS

Uterine Leiomyomas (Fibroids) (Online Case 21 and Video 13-2)

Etiology

Uterine leiomyomas (fibroids) are the most common tumor affecting the female reproductive organs and occur in about 20% to 25% of all women.[171] Histologically, they are benign neoplasms composed primarily of whorls of smooth muscle cells and fibrous stroma. These discrete lesions are classified by location as *intramural, subserosal,* or *submucosal.* Uterine fibroids are usually silent and do not require treatment.

As the tumors enlarge, cystic degeneration and calcific deposits can result. Fibroids also may become pedunculated, with long stalks that allow them to migrate

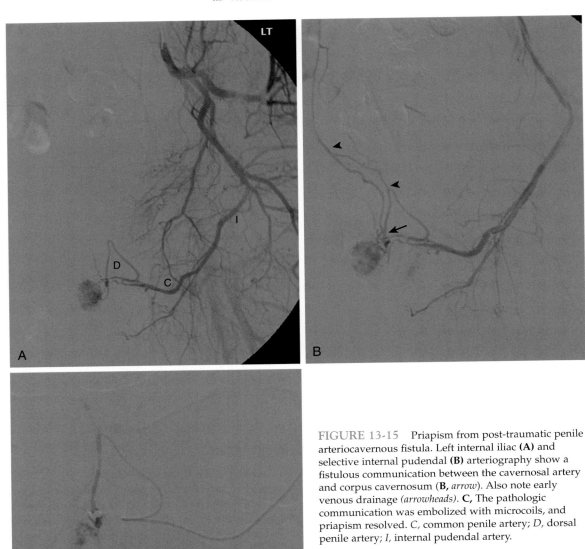

FIGURE 13-15 Priapism from post-traumatic penile arteriocavernous fistula. Left internal iliac **(A)** and selective internal pudendal **(B)** arteriography show a fistulous communication between the cavernosal artery and corpus cavernosum **(B,** *arrow).* Also note early venous drainage *(arrowheads).* **C,** The pathologic communication was embolized with microcoils, and priapism resolved. *C,* common penile artery; *D,* dorsal penile artery; *I,* internal pudendal artery.

into the cervix, vagina, or abdomen. Degeneration into *leiomyosarcoma* is rare but has been described. Leiomyomas must be distinguished from their malignant relative and from *adenomyosis,* which refers to benign invasion of endometrial gland tissue into the myometrium that causes generalized uterine enlargement. Isolated foci of adenomyosis also can mimic leiomyoma.

Clinical Features

Fibroids are up to three times more common in African-American women than in Caucasian women. Most symptomatic patients are between the ages of 35 and 50 years. Development and growth of these lesions is attributed to both genetic and hormonal factors. Because

they are hormonally sensitive, fibroids enlarge rapidly during pregnancy and usually regress after menopause.

Most fibroids do not produce symptoms. When they do, it is primarily by mass effect on the bladder, ureters, and adjacent pelvic structures. Women may suffer from pain, pressure, or heaviness in the pelvis, back, perineum, or legs; heavy menstrual bleeding; abdominal bloating; urinary frequency or incontinence; and ureteral obstruction.[172] Submucosal fibroids can interfere with normal endometrial activity and lead to prolonged menses, infertility, or prolapse into the cervix. Other diseases (including gynecologic malignancies such as ovarian cancer) may cause similar symptoms; they must be excluded by imaging studies or other means.

Imaging

Transabdominal or transvaginal sonography is sensitive in depicting uterine fibroids and in identifying concurrent disease or other causes for symptoms. However, MRI is superior to sonography in assessing the number, size, and location of fibroids; internal architecture and vascularity; effect on adjacent structures; and presence of coexisting adenomyosis or other pathology. For most experienced practitioners, it is the preferred study before and after uterine artery embolization (UAE).

Fibroids appear as discrete round masses with heterogeneous low signal on T2-weighted images and isointense with myometrium on T1-weighted images.[173] Lesions enhance variably on T1-weighted images after gadolinium (Fig. 13-16). In one study, favorable tumor shrinkage after UAE was predicted by lower signal intensity on T1-weighted and higher intensity on T2-weighted scans.[174] Adenomyosis appears as widening of the junctional zone with bright signals in the myometrium on T2-weighted images.

Treatment

The choice between endovascular and operative treatment should be made jointly by the patient, gynecologist, and interventionalist after all available treatment modalities have been considered. Only symptomatic patients in whom other causes for disease have been excluded (including a recent Papanicolaou test) should undergo embolotherapy. The interventionalist or surgeon is obligated to become the primary physician

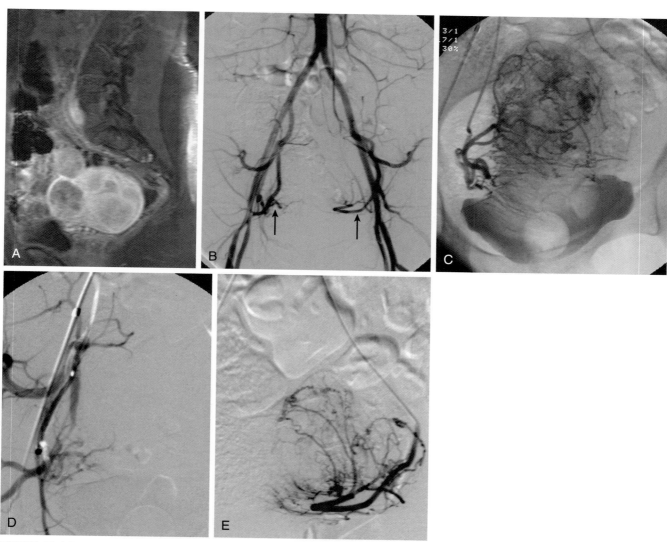

FIGURE 13-16 Uterine artery embolization. **A,** Sagittal gadolinium-enhanced magnetic resonance image shows multiple intramural and submucosal fibroids. **B,** Pelvic arteriogram demonstrates bilaterally enlarged uterine arteries *(arrows)*. **C,** Selective right uterine arteriography through a 4-Fr Roberts catheter shows the hypervascular fibroids. **D,** Following embolization with 300- to 500-μm particles, there is stasis of flow. **E,** Similar findings in the left uterine artery before embolization.

caring for the patient in preprocedure consultation, hospital recovery, and all outpatient management.

UTERINE ARTERY EMBOLIZATION

First reported in 1995, UAE entails small vessel occlusion of feeding arteries, which causes fibroid infarction and eventual shrinkage, ideally providing symptom relief.[175] Because of the organ's naturally rich collateral circulation, normal uterine tissue remains viable in most women.

Patient Selection Absolute or relative contraindications include pregnancy, active or recent pelvic infection, gynecologic malignancy (unless palliation is the goal), uncorrectable coagulopathy, severe allergy to contrast material, and prior pelvic surgery or radiation therapy.[176] No guarantee should be made regarding fertility afterward, although pregnancy can occur following UAE. Some interventionalists are cautious about treating subserosal pedunculated fibroids with relatively narrow stalks despite generally good outcomes for this subgroup.[177]

Technique Gonadotropin-releasing hormones that may have been prescribed as medical therapy for the condition should be stopped at least 3 months beforehand. These drugs cause uterine artery constriction and can make catheterization difficult. A thorough consultation with the interventionalist is crucial well before the procedure. Because pain is expected afterward, moderate sedation and patient-controlled analgesia are used liberally. Although there is no consensus about prophylactic antibiotics in this setting, many practitioners choose to use them (e.g., cephazolin, 1 g IV). Radiation exposure should be kept to a minimum by limiting use of prolonged acquisition, magnification, oblique projections, and wide fields of view. Fluoroscopy time and air kerma dose must be measured and recorded.

A Foley catheter is inserted. The common femoral artery is the usual access route.[178] A pelvic arteriogram with the catheter positioned in the infrarenal abdominal aorta is obtained as a roadmap. Selective catheterization of the anterior divisions of the internal iliac arteries is performed with a cobra or ultralong reverse-curve (e.g., Roberts) catheter (see Figs. 3-15 and 13-16). Once the uterine artery is identified and selected, angiography shows the markedly dilated spiral arteries feeding the uterus along with intense hypervascularity. In some cases, the descending portion of the uterine artery can be engaged with the diagnostic catheter. However, vasospasm may be a problem; coaxial placement of a microcatheter directed well into the uterine artery is then necessary.

The preferred agents for embolization are small-caliber particulate matter, including polyvinyl alcohol (PVA) particles (350 to 500 or 500 to 700 μm) or tris-acryl gelatin microspheres (Embospheres, 500 to 700 or 700 to 900 μm).[179-181] The superiority of one agent over another is contested.[181,182] Proximal embolization (e.g., with coils) is inadvisable, because collateral vessels are sure to develop and continue to feed the tumors.

Infusion of the particulate slurry (made with diluted contrast material, see Video 3-18) is continued until there is static flow in uterine artery branches ("pruned-tree" appearance). Regardless of the location of fibroids, *bilateral* embolization is necessary to prevent recruitment of collateral vessels. Completion internal iliac arteriograms are obtained to identify any additional vessels feeding the tumors.

The interventionalist should be observant of variant arterial anatomy and important collateral vessels.[183] In most cases, the ovarian arteries feed the fibroids through anastomoses with the main uterine artery. In about 10% of patients, the uterine artery is the major blood supply to the ovary, or the ovarian artery has significant direct communication with the fibroid[184] (Fig. 13-17). Of course, embolization of these vessels theoretically increases the risk of ovarian infarction. This is particularly true in women who have undergone prior pelvic surgery, had other tubal pathology, or have fundal fibroids.[185]

A postembolization syndrome consisting of pain, nausea and vomiting, and low-grade fever is expected. Most women are hospitalized overnight, although discharge later in the day is possible for some individuals. Pain must be aggressively managed with IV and then oral narcotics.[186] Antiemetics are given prophylactically or as needed. Discharge medications include antiinflammatory drugs (e.g., ketorolac) and potent oral narcotics. Follow-up is done by the interventionalist, including routine clinic evaluation at 1 to 3 weeks after the procedure.

Results Bilateral uterine artery occlusion is technically successful in about 95% of attempts. Incomplete infarction of fibroids risks continued growth.[187] Clinical success with substantial improvement in symptoms is seen in about 80% to 90% of women.[188-192] Submucosal lesions and smaller tumors seem to respond best.[193]

The primary reasons for failure are outlined in Box 13-3. If symptoms persists and the fibroids fail to shrink on imaging studies, repeat UAE (with a concerted search for collateral vessels including the ovarian arteries) is often warranted (see Fig. 13-17). Clinical failure or recurrence at 5 years is identified in about 25% of treated women.[188]

In two randomized multicenter studies, UAE was comparable to surgical myomectomy or hysterectomy in durable symptom relief from fibroids. The EMMY trial observed similar quality of life outcomes between UAE and hysterectomy in women with symptomatic fibroids.[194] The REST trial compared UAE with hysterectomy or myomectomy in a similar population.[195] Duration of

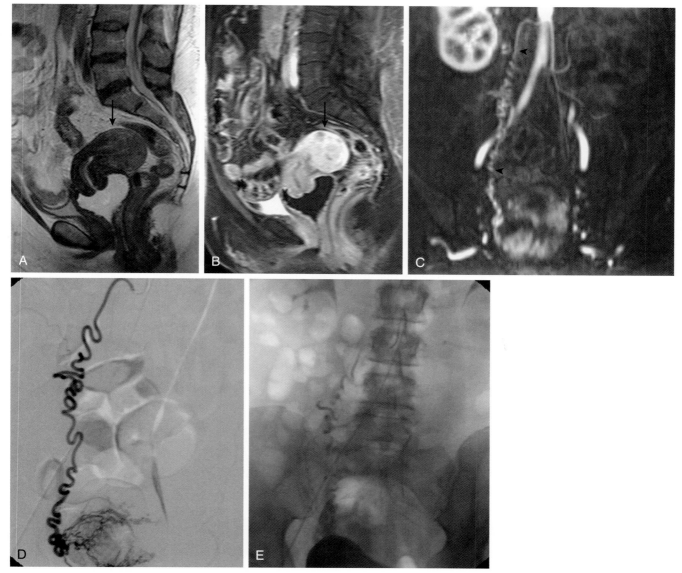

FIGURE 13-17 Ovarian artery embolization for persistent uterine fibroids. T1-weighted **(A)** and gadolinium-enhanced T2-weighted **(B)** parasagittal magnetic resonance (MR) images show persistent enhancing fundal fibroid *(arrow)* several months after bilateral uterine artery embolization. **C,** Coronal MR angiogram identifies a markedly enlarged right ovarian artery feeding the pelvis *(arrowheads)*. **D,** Selective right ovarian arteriogram confirms the presence of this vessel feeding the residual fibroid. **E,** There is stasis of flow after embolization with polyvinyl alcohol particles.

hospital stay was shorter in embolized patients; however, 10% of subjects in that group required a second intervention for initial treatment failure. The most recent report of an American multicenter registry for UAE confirms the value of the procedure.[196] Only 13% of treated individuals ultimately required hysterectomy or myomectomy. These recent papers solidify the evidence from earlier but less robust series in which symptom relief with UAE was comparable to reported rates for surgery but with a smaller risk for complications.[197-200]

Complications Significant intraprocedure and postprocedure pain is the norm with UAE.[201] The most serious complications after embolotherapy are intrauterine infection, uterine ischemia and necrosis, pulmonary embolism, and expulsion of pedunculated submucosal lesions.[202] The overall adverse event rate is about 5%; major complications occur about 1% of the time.[203] Few women have amenorrhea or a significant decrease in follicle-stimulating hormone afterward, although this happens more often in older individuals.[188,190,192,204] Overall, less than 2% of treated women require subsequent hysterectomy for any complications of UAE.[205]

OTHER PERCUTANEOUS METHODS

Studies are currently underway to evaluate the effectiveness of MR- and ultrasound-focused "surgery" to ablate uterine fibroids. In addition, ultrasound-guided cryoablation has been attempted.

Surgical Therapy

For women who still wish to become pregnant, the traditional treatment is open or laparoscopic myomectomy. For women beyond childbearing age, hysterectomy is often recommended.

PELVIC CONGESTION SYNDROME (ONLINE CASE 34)

Ovarian and pelvic vein varices increasingly are being recognized as an important cause of unexplained pelvic pain in women of childbearing age. Hormonal and hemodynamic factors are thought to be responsible for the condition.[206] In a minority of cases, compression of the left renal vein between the aorta and SMA ("nutcracker syndrome") is responsible.[207] Most women with this disorder have borne children. Typical complaints are lower abdominal or perineal pain and fullness, menorrhagia, dyspareunia, bladder urgency, and polymenorrhea.[208] Pain is worse usually with prolonged standing, after intercourse, and just before or during menses. Superficial varicosities often erupt on the vulva and thigh.

Unlike male varicocele, the diagnosis requires imaging studies such as MRI or color Doppler sonography.[207,208] A significant number of asymptomatic women, however, demonstrate ovarian vein enlargement on imaging studies obtained for unrelated reasons.[209] The traditional operation is gonadal vein ligation along with obliteration of collateral pathways.[210] Ovarian and selective internal iliac vein embolization is an attractive alternative to surgery if compression of the renal vein is not responsible.[211-214] At MRI or contrast venography, incompetent ovarian vein valves, main trunk dilation (>1 cm), reflux, and cross-pelvic collateral drainage are characteristic (Fig. 13-18). The majority

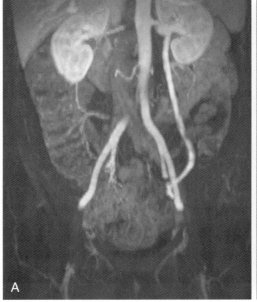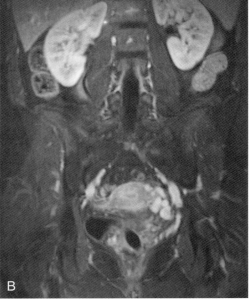

FIGURE 13-18 Pelvic congestion syndrome. **A** and **B,** Gadolinium-enhanced magnetic resonance venography with maximum intensity coronal projection shows reflux down a markedly dilated left ovarian vein with numerous left-sided pelvic varicosities.

of women have reflux down both ovarian and internal iliac veins into a nest of pelvic varicosities. To maximize symptom relief, a thorough search for bilateral ovarian and internal iliac vein reflux and associated variceal complexes must be sought[206,215] (Fig. 13-19). Occlusion of all culprit vessels is accomplished with a variety of agents, including coils, sclerosing agents (e.g., sodium tetradecyl sulfate foam 3%), and glue. Most patients notice improvement or resolution of symptoms soon after the procedure. Procedure-specific complications (which are rare) include embolization of material to the lung and associated thrombophlebitis.[206]

OBSTETRIC AND GYNECOLOGIC BLEEDING (ONLINE CASE 104)

Gynecologic surgery done for any reason can precipitate life-threatening hemorrhage. Massive intrapelvic or vaginal bleeding is also a rare but serious complication of vaginal and cesarean deliveries.[216,217] Significant blood loss may occur also after spontaneous or therapeutic abortion. The major causes of postpartum bleeding are retained products of conception, lacerations, uterine atony, and uterine rupture. Women with

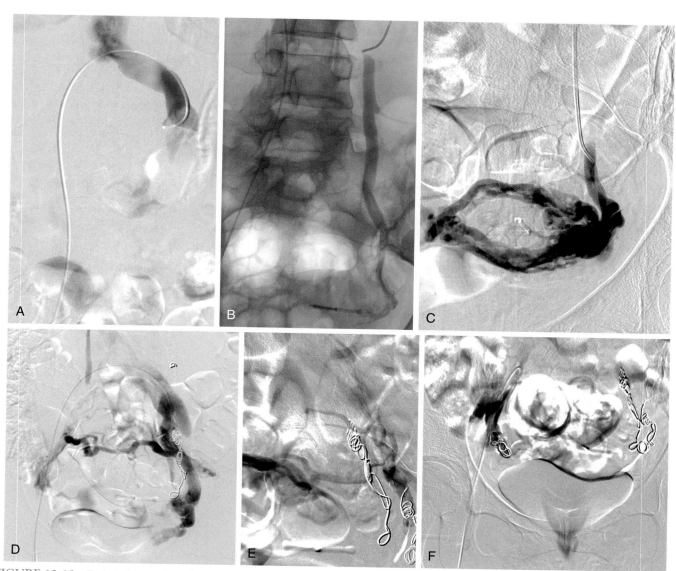

FIGURE 13-19   Embolotherapy for pelvic congestion syndrome. **A** and **B,** Left ovarian venography shows a dilated, patulous vein with reflux into the pelvis. **C,** Varices and transpelvic collaterals are evident. After embolization of the ovarian vein starting in the pelvis, the left internal iliac vein was catheterized. Large veins contributing to the varices **(D)** were then embolized **(E)**. Finally, the right internal iliac vein was embolized **(F)**. The right ovarian vein was relatively normal and therefore not treated.

placental disorders, coexisting leiomyomas, or ectopic pregnancy are at particularly high risk for significant blood loss. Abnormalities of placentation are classified as *placenta accreta* (penetration into the uterine wall), *placenta increta* (penetration through the myometrium), and *placenta percreta* (penetration to the serosa).[218]

Initial management of gynecologic or postpartum bleeding entails uterine massage, drug therapy (e.g., oxytocin), vaginal packing, closure of lacerations, and curettage for retained products. In most cases, bleeding stops with these maneuvers. Hysterectomy is required for life-threatening hemorrhage that cannot be controlled by transcatheter means.

Embolotherapy is extremely effective for most cases of pregnancy-related or post-hysterectomy bleeding.[219-225] The procedure begins with pelvic angiography followed by bilateral internal iliac injections. Occlusion of the branches causing the bleeding is achieved with microcoils or Gelfoam pledgets (Fig. 13-20). The ovarian arteries should be examined if no extravasation is found from pelvic branches. Collateral vessels (i.e., lumbar, femoral circumflex, inferior epigastric, and inferior mesenteric arteries) are other rare potential sources of bleeding, especially in postoperative patients. After embolization, bilateral internal iliac arteriography is repeated to confirm that bleeding does not continue through collateral circulation.

After embolization, hemorrhage stops in almost every case. Complications, including pelvic abscess, organ ischemia, and nerve damage, are reported in less than 10% of procedures. The intervention does not impact fertility and subsequent pregnancy if particulate or liquid agents are avoided.[219,222,225,226]

In pregnant women with abnormal placentation, the standard operation at the time of delivery is cesarean hysterectomy, which is often accompanied by massive hemorrhage and significant mortality. When antenatal diagnosis is made (as is usually the case), some obstetricians elect to have occlusion balloons placed in the proximal internal iliac arteries preoperatively through bilateral femoral artery access. The volume of fluid needed to distend each balloon and completely obstruct flow is recorded by the interventionalist, and balloons are inflated in the operating room, if necessary. However, the evidence is mixed regarding the value of this maneuver in reduced blood loss or lowered mortality.[227-231]

OTHER DISORDERS

Gynecologic Tumors

Women with pelvic malignancies, particularly of the uterus and cervix, occasionally suffer massive hemorrhage from vascular invasion, after radiation therapy, or during surgery. Bleeding may be vaginal or intraabdominal. Embolotherapy is extremely effective in stopping blood loss.[232,233] Because of the progressive nature of the disease, occlusions must be bilateral, and the embolic agent must be *permanent and small* (e.g., PVA particles or microspheres). Rebleeding is a common problem. The major potential complications are pelvic organ ischemia, skin necrosis, and nerve damage (e.g., sciatic neuropathy).

Hormonally active ovarian neoplasms (e.g., the virilizing *Leydig cell tumor*) may be suspected on clinical grounds. Confirmation of the activity of an identified ovarian mass or localization of a difficult-to-find lesion may require bilateral ovarian and adrenal venous sampling (see earlier).[234]

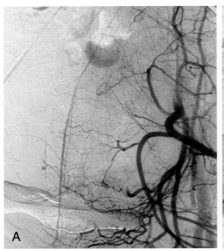
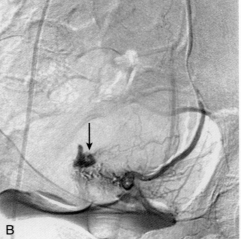
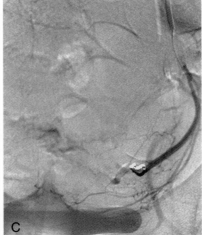

FIGURE 13-20   Massive pelvic bleeding after a vaginal hysterectomy. **A,** The initial left internal iliac arteriogram failed to identify a bleeding site. **B,** Selective injection of a small branch of the anterior division through a coaxial microcatheter shows extravasation *(arrow)*. **C,** Bleeding ceased after placement of several microcoils in the vessel.

FIGURE 13-21 Pelvic arterio-venous malformation in a woman with prior gynecologic instrumentation and massive vaginal bleeding. **A,** Sagittal color Doppler sonography reveals a huge vascular mass within the uterus and extending into the cervix. **B,** Pelvic arteriogram shows the massively dilated inflow arteries and early venous shunting *(arrow)*.

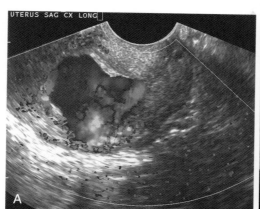

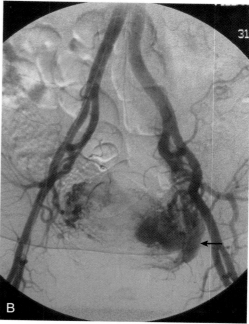

Uterine and Cervical Vascular Malformations

Pelvic AVMs are rare congenital or developmental lesions that can affect the female reproductive organs[235,236] (Fig. 13-21) (see Chapter 8). Many so-called uterine AVMs are actually acquired complex arteriovenous fistulas related to prior pelvic surgery or gestational trophoblastic disease, although the bizarre angiographic appearance is similar to that of an AVM. Vaginal or intraabdominal bleeding may occur. Surgical resection of symptomatic lesions is extremely difficult. Percutaneous embolotherapy is indicated for palliation of symptoms.[237-240] Multiple treatment sessions are often necessary to eradicate these lesions. When embolotherapy fails, an underlying neoplasm should be suspected.

References

1. Gabella G, ed. Cardiovascular system. In: Williams PL, Bannister LH, Berry MM, et al, editors. *Gray's anatomy,* 38th ed. New York: Churchill Livingstone; 1995. p. 1549.
2. Skandalakis LJ, Rowe Jr JS, Gray SW, et al. Surgical embryology and anatomy of the pancreas. *Surg Clin North Am* 1993;**73**:661.
3. Cano DA, Hebrok M, Zenker M. Pancreatic development and disease. *Gastroenterology* 2007;**132**:745.
4. Raimondi S, Maisonneuve P, Lowenfels AB. Epidemiology of pancreatic cancer: an overview. *Nat Rev Gastroenterol Hepatol* 2009;**6**:699.
5. Ghaneh P, Costello E, Neoptolemos JP. Biology and management of pancreatic cancer. *Gut* 2007;**56**:1134.
6. Adsay NV. Cystic neoplasia of the pancreas: pathology and biology. *J Gastrointest Surg* 2008;**12**:401.
7. Scheiman JM. Management of cystic lesions of the pancreas. *J Gastrointest Surg* 2008;**12**:405.
8. Wong JC, Lu DS. Staging of pancreatic adenocarcinoma by imaging studies. *Clin Gastroenterol Hepatol* 2008;**6**:1301.
9. Brennan DD, Zamboni GA, Raptopoulos VD, et al. Comprehensive preoperative assessment of pancreatic adenocarcinoma with 64-section volumetric CT. *Radiographics* 2007;**27**:1653.
10. Ingram M, Arregui ME. Endoscopic ultrasonography. *Surg Clin North Am* 2004;**84**:1035.
11. Vachiranubhap B, Kim YH, Balci NC, et al. Magnetic resonance imaging of adenocarcinoma of the pancreas. *Top Magn Reson Imaging* 2009;**20**:3.
12. Stojadinovic A, Brooks A, Hoos A, et al. An evidence-based approach to the surgical management of resectable pancreatic adenocarcinoma. *J Am Coll Surg* 2003;**196**:954.
13. Diener MK, Heukaufer C, Schwarzer G, et al. Pancreatico-duodenectomy (classic Whipple) versus pylorus-preserving pancreaticoduodenectomy (pp Whipple) for surgical treatment of periampullary and pancreatic carcinoma. *Cochrane Database Syst Rev* 2011;**2**:CD006053.
14. Ghaneh P, Neoptolemos JP. Conclusions from the European Study Group for Pancreatic Cancer adjuvant trial of chemoradiotherapy and chemotherapy for pancreatic cancer. *Surg Oncol Clin N Am* 2004;**13**:567.
15. Miller RC, Iott MJ, Corsini MM. Review of adjuvant radiochemotherapy for resected pancreatic cancer and results from Mayo Clinic for the JUCTS symposium. *Int J Radiat Oncol Biol Phys* 2009;**75**:364.
16. Abood GJ, Go A, Malhotra D, et al. The surgical and systemic management of neuroendocrine tumors of the pancreas. *Surg Clin North Am* 2009;**89**:249.
17. Mansour JC, Chen H. Pancreatic endocrine tumors. *J Surg Res* 2004;**120**:139.
18. Davies K, Conlon KC. Neuroendocrine tumors of the pancreas. *Curr Gastroenterol Rep* 2009;**11**:119.

19. Nakakura EK, Bergsland EK. Islet cell carcinoma: neuroendocrine tumors of the pancreas and periampullary region. *Hematol Oncol Clin North Am* 2007;**21**:457.

20. Mathur A, Gorden P, Libutti SK. Insulinoma. *Surg Clin North Am* 2009;**89**:1105.

21. Marini F, Falchetti A, Del Monte F, et al. Multiple endocrine neoplasia type 1. *Orphanet J Rare Dis* 2006;**1**:38.

22. Horton KM, Hruban RH, Yeo C, et al. Multi-detector row CT of pancreatic islet cell tumors. *Radiographics* 2006;**26**:453.

23. Cisco RM, Norton JA. Surgery for gastrinoma. *Adv Surg* 2007;**41**:165.

24. Norton JA, Jensen RT. Current surgical management of Zollinger-Ellison syndrome (ZES) in patients without multiple endocrine neoplasia-type 1 (MEN1). *Surg Oncol* 2003;**12**:145.

25. Tamm EP, Kim EE, Ng CS. Imaging of neuroendocrine tumors. *Hematol Oncol Clin North Am* 2007;**21**:409.

26. Koopmans KP, Neels OC, Kema IP, et al. Improved staging of patients with carcinoid and islet cell tumors with 18F-dihydroxy-phenyl-alanine and 11C-5-hydroxy-tryptophan positron emission tomography. *J Clin Oncol* 2008;**26**:1489.

27. Zimmer T, Stolzel U, Bader M, et al. Endoscopic ultrasonography and somatostatin receptor scintigraphy in the preoperative localisation of insulinomas and gastrinomas. *Gut* 1996;**39**:562.

28. Imamura M, Komoto I, Ota S. Changing treatment strategy for gastrinoma in patients with Zollinger-Ellison syndrome. *World J Surg* 2006;**30**:1.

29. Guettier JM, Kam A, Chang R, et al. Localization of insulinomas to regions of the pancreas by intraarterial calcium stimulation: the NIH experience. *J Clin Endocrinol Metab* 2009;**94**:1074.

30. Goh BK, Ooi Ll, Cheow PC, et al. Accurate preoperative localization of insulinomas avoids the need for blind resection and reoperation: analysis of a single institution experience with 17 surgically treated tumors over 19 years. *J Gastrointest Surg* 2009;**13**:1071.

31. Morganstein DL, Lewis DH, Jackson J, et al. The role of arterial stimulation and simultaneous venous sampling in addition to cross-sectional imaging for localisation of biochemically proven insulinoma. *Eur Radiol* 2009;**19**:2467.

32. Wiesli P, Brändle M, Schmid C, et al. Selective arterial calcium stimulation and hepatic venous sampling in the evaluation of hyperinsulinemic hypoglycemia: potential and limitations. *J Vasc Interv Radiol* 2004;**15**:1251.

33. Dhillo WS, Jayasena CN, Jackson JE, et al. Localization of gastrinomas by selective intra-arterial calcium injection in patients on proton pump inhibitor or H2 receptor antagonist therapy. *Eur J Gastroenterol Hepatol* 2005;**17**:429.

34. Lau JH, Drake W, Matson M. The current role of venous sampling in the localization of endocrine disease. *Cardiovasc Intervent Radiol* 2007;**30**:555.

35. Doppman JL, Miller DL, Chang R, et al. Gastrinomas: localization by means of selective intraarterial injection of secretin. *Radiology* 1990;**174**:25.

36. Doppman JL, Miller DL, Chang R, et al. Insulinomas: localization with selective intraarterial injection of calcium. *Radiology* 1991;**178**:237.

37. Defreyne L, Koening K, Lerch MM, et al. Modified intra-arterial calcium stimulation with venous sampling test for preoperative localization of insulinomas. *Abdom Imaging* 1998;**23**:322.

38. Jackson JE. Angiography and arterial stimulation venous sampling in the localization of pancreatic neuroendocrine tumours. *Best Pract Res Clin Endocrinol Metab* 2005;**19**:229.

39. Oberg K, Kvols L, Caplin M, et al. Consensus report on the use of somatostatin analogs for the management of neuroendocrine tumors of the gastroenteropancreatic system. *Ann Oncol* 2004;**15**:966.

40. Anthony L, Freda PU. From somatostatin to octreotide LAR: evolution of a somatostatin analogue. *Curr Med Res Opin* 2009;**25**:2989.

41. Kress O, Wagner HJ, Wied M, et al. Transarterial chemoembolization of advanced liver metastases of neuroendocrine tumors—a retrospective single-center analysis. *Digestion* 2003;**68**:94.

42. Yao KA, Talamonti MS, Nemcek A. Indications and results of liver resection and hepatic chemoembolization for metastatic gastrointestinal neuroendocrine tumors. *Surgery* 2001;**130**:677.

43. Amersi FF, McElrath-Garza A, Ahmad A, et al. Long-term survival after radiofrequency ablation of complex unresectable liver tumors. *Arch Surg* 2006;**141**:581.

44. Chamberlain RS, Canes D, Brown KT, et al. Hepatic neuroendocrine metastases: does intervention alter outcomes? *J Am Coll Surg* 2000;**190**:432.

45. Fiorentini G, Rossi S, Bonechi F, et al. Intra-arterial hepatic chemoembolization in liver metastases from neuroendocrine tumors: a phase II study. *J Chemother* 2004;**16**:293.

46. Gee M, Soulen MC. Chemoembolization for hepatic metastases. *Tech Vasc Interv Radiol* 2002;**5**:132.

47. Talukdar R, Vege SS. Recent developments in acute pancreatitis. *Clin Gastroenterol Hepatol* 2009;**7**:S3.

48. Boudghene F, L'Hermine C, Bigot J-M. Arterial complications of pancreatitis: diagnostic and therapeutic aspects in 104 cases. *J Vasc Interv Radiol* 1993;**4**:551.

49. Balachandra S, Siriwardena AK. Systematic appraisal of the management of the major vascular complications of pancreatitis. *Am J Surg* 2005;**190**:489.

50. Mansueto G, Cenzi D, O'Onofrio M, et al. Endovascular treatment of arterial bleeding in patients with pancreatitis. *Pancreatology* 2007;**7**:360.

51. Kim DH, Pickhardt PJ. Radiologic assessment of acute and chronic pancreatitis. *Surg Clin North Am* 2007;**87**:1341.

52. Balci NC, Bienerman BK, Bilgin M, et al. Magnetic resonance imaging in pancreatitis. *Top Magn Reson Imaging* 2009;**20**:25.

53. Nicholson AA, Patel J, McPherson S, et al. Endovascular treatment of visceral aneurysms associated with pancreatitis and a suggested classification with therapeutic implications. *J Vasc Interv Radiol* 2006;**17**:1270.

54. Tessier DJ, Stone WM, Fowl RJ, et al. Clinical features and management of splenic artery pseudoaneurysm: case series and cumulative review of literature. *J Vasc Surg* 2003;**38**:969.

55. Beattie GC, Hardman JG, Redhead D, et al. Evidence for a central role for selective mesenteric angiography in the management of the major vascular complications of pancreatitis. *Am J Surg* 2003;**185**:96.

56. Carr JA, Cho JS, Shepard AD, et al. Visceral pseudoaneurysms due to pancreatic pseudocysts: rare but lethal complications of pancreatitis. *J Vasc Surg* 2000;**32**:722.

57. Hyare H, Desigan S, Brookes JA, et al. Endovascular management of major arterial hemorrhage as a complication of inflammatory pancreatic disease. *J Vasc Interv Radiol* 2007;**18**:591.

58. McErlean A, Looby S, Lee MJ. Percutaneous ultrasound-guided thrombin injection as first-line treatment of pancreatic pseudoaneurysm. *Cardiovasc Intervent Radiol* 2007;**30**:526.

59. Chandra J, Phillips RR, Boardman P, et al. Pancreas transplants. *Clin Radiol* 2009;**64**:714.

60. Spiros D, Christos D, John B, et al. Vascular complications of pancreas transplantation. *Pancreas* 2004;**28**:413.

61. Ciancio G, Cespedes M, Olson L, et al. Partial venous thrombosis of the pancreatic allografts after simultaneous pancreas-kidney transplantation. *Clin Transplant* 2000;**14**:464.

62. Hagspiel KD, Nandalur K, Pruett TL, et al. Evaluation of vascular complications of pancreas transplantation with high spatial resolution contrast-enhanced MR angiography. *Radiology* 2007;**242**:590.

63. Dobos N, Roberts DA, Insko EK, et al. Contrast-enhanced MR angiography for evaluation of vascular complications of the pancreatic transplant. *Radiographics* 2005;**25**:687.

64. Fattahi R, Modanlou KA, Bieneman BK, et al. Magnetic resonance imaging in pancreas transplantation. *Top Magn Reson Imaging* 2009;**20**:49.

65. Stockland AH, Willingham DL, Paz-Fumagalli R, et al. Pancreas transplant venous thrombosis: role of endovascular interventions for salvage. *Cardiovasc Intervent Radiol* 2009;**32**:279.

66. Barth MM, Khwaja K, Faintuch S, et al. Transarterial and transvenous embolotherapy of arteriovenous fistulas in the transplanted pancreas. *J Vasc Interv Radiol* 2008;**19**:1231.

67. Semiz-Oysu A, Gwikiel W. Endovascular management of acute enteric bleeding from pancreas transplant. *Cardiovasc Intervent Radiol* 2007;**30**:313.

68. Uher P, Nyman U, Ivancev K, et al. Aneurysms of the pancreaticoduodenal artery associated with occlusion of the celiac artery. *Abdom Imaging* 1995;**20**:470.

69. Tulsyan N, Kashyap VS, Greenberg RK, et al. The endovascular management of visceral artery aneurysms and pseudoaneurysms. *J Vasc Surg* 2007;**45**:276.

70. Chiang KS, Johnson CM, McKusick MA, et al. Management of inferior pancreaticoduodenal artery aneurysms: a 4-year single center experience. *Cardiovasc Intervent Radiol* 1994;**17**:217.

71. Ogawa H, Itoh S, Mori Y, et al. Arteriovenous malformations of the pancreas: assessment of clinical and multislice CT features. *Abdom Imaging* 2009;**34**:743.

72. Lacout A, Pelage JP, Lesur G, et al. Pancreatic involvement in hereditary hemorrhagic telangiectasia: assessment with multidetector helical CT. *Radiology* 2010;**254**:479.

73. Bookstein JJ, Conn J, Reuter SR. Intra-adrenal hemorrhage as a complication of adrenal venography in primary aldosteronism. *Radiology* 1968;**90**:778.

74. Daunt N. Adrenal vein sampling: how to make it quick, easy, and successful. *Radiographics* 2005;**25**:S143.

75. Gabella G, editor. Cardiovascular system. In: Williams PL, Bannister LH, Berry MM, et al, editors. *Gray's anatomy*. 38th ed. New York: Churchill Livingstone; 1995. p. 1556.

76. Stack SP, Roesch J, Cook DM, et al. Anomalous left adrenal venous drainage directly into the inferior vena cava. *J Vasc Interv Radiol* 2001;**12**:385.

77. Stratakis CA. Cushing syndrome caused by adrenocortical tumors and hyperplasias (corticotropin-independent Cushing syndrome). *Endocr Dev* 2008;**13**:117.

78. Lad SP, Patil CG, Laws Jr ER, et al. The role of inferior petrosal sinus sampling in the diagnostic localization of Cushing's disease. *Neurosurg Focus* 2007;**23**:E2.

79. Hussain HK, Korobkin M. MR imaging of the adrenal glands. *Magn Reson Imaging Clin N Am* 2004;**12**:515.

80. Rockall AG, Babar SA, Sohaib SA, et al. CT and MR imaging of the adrenal glands in ACTH-independent Cushing syndrome. *Radiographics* 2004;**24**:435.

81. Johnson PT, Horton KM, Fishman EK. Adrenal imaging with multidetector CT: evidence-based protocol optimization and interpretation practice. *Radiographics* 2009;**29**:1319.

82. Gross MD, Gauger PG, Djekidel M, et al. The role of PET in the surgical approach to adrenal disease. *Eur J Surg Oncol* 2009;**35**:1137.

83. Young Jr WF, du Plessis H, Thompson GB, et al. The clinical conundrum of corticotropin-independent autonomous cortisol secretion in patients with bilateral adrenal masses. *World J Surg* 2008;**32**:856.

84. Wheeler MH, Harris DA. Diagnosis and management of primary aldosteronism. *World J Surg* 2003;**27**:627.

85. Calhoun DA, Nishizaka MK, Zaman MA, et al. Hyperaldosteronism among black and white subjects with resistant hypertension. *Hypertension* 2002;**40**:892.

86. Strauch B, Zelinka T, Hampf M, et al. Prevalence of primary hyperaldosteronism in the central Europe region. *J Hum Hypertens* 2003;**17**:349.

87. Gordon RD, Stowasser M, Tunny TJ, et al. High incidence of primary aldosteronism in 199 patients referred with hypertension. *Clin Exp Pharmacol Physiol* 1994;**21**:315.

88. Young WF. Primary aldosteronism: renaissance of a syndrome. *Clin Endocrinol* (Oxf) 2007;**66**:607.

89. Thakkar RB, Oparil S. Primary aldosteronism: a practical approach to diagnosis and treatment. *J Clin Hypertens* (Greenwich) 2001; **3**:189.

90. Nishizaka MK, Zaman MA, Calhoun DA. Efficacy of low-dose spironolactone in subjects with resistant hypertension. *Am J Hypertens* 2003;**16**:925.

91. Kempers MJ, Lenders JW, van Outheusden L, et al. Systematic review: diagnostic procedures to differentiate unilateral from bilateral adrenal abnormality in primary aldosteronism. *Ann Intern Med* 2009;**151**:329.

92. Carr CE, Cope C, Cohen DL, et al. Comparison of sequential versus simultaneous methods of adrenal venous sampling. *J Vasc Interv Radiol* 2004;**15**:1245.

93. Doppman JL, Gill Jr JR. Hyperaldosteronism: sampling the adrenal veins. *Radiology* 1996;**198**:309.

94. Inoue H, Nakajo M, Miyazono N, et al. Transcatheter arterial ablation of aldosteronomas with high-concentration ethanol: preliminary and long-term results. *AJR Am J Roentgenol* 1997; **168**:1241.

95. Hokotate H, Inoue H, Baba Y, et al. Aldosteronomas: experience with superselective adrenal arterial embolization in 33 cases. *Radiology* 2003;**227**:401.

96. Mayo-Smith WW, Dupuy DE. Adrenal neoplasms: CT-guided radiofrequency ablation-preliminary results. *Radiology* 2004;**231**:225.

97. Del Gaudio A, Del Gaudio GA. Virilizing adrenocortical tumors in adult women: report of 10 patients, 2 of whom each had a tumor secreting only testosterone. *Cancer* 1993;**72**:1997.

98. Dennedy MC, Smith D, O'Shea D, et al. Investigation of patients with atypical or severe hyperandrogenaemia including androgen-secreting ovarian teratoma. *Eur J Endocrinol* 2010;**162**: 213.

99. Tischler AS. Pheochromocytoma and extra-adrenal paraganglionoma: updates. *Arch Pathol Lab Med* 2008;**132**:1272.

100. Akerstrom G, Stahlberg P. Surgical management of MEN-1 and -2: state of the art. *Surg Clin North Am* 2009;**89**:1047

101. Berglund AS, Hulthen UL, Manhem P, et al. Metaiodobenzylguanidine (MIBG) scintigraphy and computed tomography (CT) in clinical practice. Primary and secondary evaluation for localization of pheochromocytomas. *J Intern Med* 2001;**249**:247.

102. Konen E, Konen O, Katz M, et al. Are referring clinicians aware of patients at risk from intravenous injection of iodinated contrast media? *Clin Radiol* 2002;**57**:132.

103. Wang P, Zuo C, Qian Z, et al. Computerized tomography guided percutaneous ethanol injection for the treatment of hyperfunctioning pheochromocytoma. *J Urol* 2003;**170**:1132.

104. Miller DL, Chang R, Doppman JL, et al. Localization of parathyroid adenomas: superselective arterial DSA versus superselective conventional arteriography. *Radiology* 1989;**170**:1003.

105. Nobori M, Saiki S, Tanaka N, et al. Blood supply of the parathyroid gland from the superior thyroid artery. *Surgery* 1994; **115**:417.

106. Sugg SL, Fraker DL, Alexander R, et al. Prospective evaluation of selective venous sampling for parathyroid hormone concentration in patients undergoing reoperations for primary hyperparathyroidism. *Surgery* 1993;**114**:1004.

107. Broome JT, Schrager JJ, Bilheimer D, et al. Central venous sampling for intraoperative parathyroid hormone monitoring: are peripheral guidelines applicable? *Am Surg* 2007;**73**:712.

108. Elo JA, Mitty H, Genden EM. Preoperative selective venous sampling for nonlocalizing parathyroid adenomas. *Thyroid* 2006; **16**:787.

109. Norton JA. Reoperation for missed parathyroid adenoma. *Adv Surg* 1997;**31**:273.

110. Fraser WD. Hyperparathyroidism. *Lancet* 2009;**374**:145.

111. Mihai R, Simon D, Hellman P. Imaging for primary hyperparathyroidism—an evidence-based analysis. *Langenbecks Arch Surg* 2009;**394**:765.

112. Hessman O, Stalberg P, Sundin A, et al. High success rate of parathyroid reoperation may be achieved with improved localization diagnosis. *World J Surg* 2008;**32**:774.

113. Powell AC, Alexander HR, Chang R, et al. Reoperation for parathyroid adenoma: a contemporary experience. *Surgery* 2009;**146**:1144.

114. Weber AL, Randolph G, Aksoy FG. The thyroid and parathyroid glands. CT and MR imaging and correlation with pathology and clinical findings. *Radiol Clin North Am* 2000;**38**:1105.

115. Sacks BA, Pallotta JA, Cole A, et al. Diagnosis of parathyroid adenomas: efficacy of measuring parathormone levels in needle aspirates of cervical masses. *AJR Am J Roentgenol* 1994;**163**:1223.

116. Seehofer D, Steinmuller T, Rayes N, et al. Parathyroid hormone venous sampling before reoperative surgery in renal hyperparathyroidism: comparison with noninvasive localization procedures and review of the literature. *Arch Surg* 2004;**139**:1331.

117. McIntyre Jr RC, Kumpe DA, Liechty RD. Reexploration and angiographic ablation for hyperparathyroidism. *Arch Surg* 1994;**129**:499.

118. Reidel MA, Schilling T, Graf S, et al. Localization of hyperfunctioning parathyroid gland by selective venous sampling in reoperation for primary or secondary hyperparathyroidism. *Surgery* 2006;**140**:907.

119. Arora S, Balash PR, Yoo J, et al. Benefits of surgeon-performed ultrasound for primary hyperparathyroidism. *Langenbecks Arch Surg* 2009;**394**:861.

120. Jaskowiak N, Norton JA, Alexander HR, et al. A prospective trial evaluating a standard approach to reoperation for missed parathyroid adenoma. *Ann Surg* 1996;**224**:308.

121. Miller DL, Doppman JL, Chang R, et al. Angiographic ablation of parathyroid adenomas: lessons from a ten-year experience. *Radiology* 1987;**165**:601.

122. Bookstein JJ. Penile angiography: the last angiographic frontier. *AJR Am J Roentgenol* 1988;**150**:47.

123. Kawanishi Y, Muguruma H, Sugiyama H, et al. Variations of the internal pudendal artery as a congenital contributing factor to age at onset of erectile dysfunction in Japanese. *BJU Int* 2008;**101**:581.

124. Gabella G, editor. Cardiovascular system. In: Williams PL, Bannister LH, Berry MM, et al, eds. *Gray's anatomy,* 38th ed. New York: Churchill Livingstone; 1995. p. 1600.

125. Lechter A, Lopez G, Martinez C, et al. Anatomy of the gonadal veins: a reappraisal. *Surgery* 1991;**109**:735.

126. Kim HH, Goldstein M. Adult varicocele. *Curr Opin Urol* 2008;**18**:608.

127. Khera M, Lipschultz LI. Evolving approach to the varicocele. *Urol Clin North Am* 2008;**35**:183.

128. Shuman L, White Jr RI, Mitchell SE, et al. Right-sided varicocele: technique and clinical results of balloon embolotherapy from the femoral approach. *Radiology* 1986;**158**:787.

129. Gat Y, Bachar GN, Zukerman Z, et al. Varicocele: a bilateral disease. *Fertil Steril* 2004;**81**:424.

130. Diamond DA. Adolescent varicocele. *Curr Opin Urol* 2007;**17**:263.

131. French DB, Desai NR, Agarwal A. Varicocele repair: does it still have a role in infertility treatment? *Curr Opin Obstet Gynecol* 2008;**20**:269.

132. Bong GW, Koo HP. The adolescent varicocele: to treat or not to treat. *Urol Clin North Am* 2004;**31**:509.

133. Meacham RB, Townsend RR, Rademacher D, et al. The incidence of varicoceles in the general population when evaluated by physical examination, gray scale sonography, and color Doppler sonography. *J Urol* 1994;**151**:1535.

134. Pearl MS, Hill MC. Ultrasound of the scrotum. *Semin Ultrasound CT MR* 2007;**28**:225.

135. Practice Committee of American Society for Reproductive Medicine. Report on varicocele and infertility. *Fertil Steril* 2008;**90**:S247.

136. Bechara CF, Weakley SM, Kougias P, et al. Percutaneous treatment of varicocele with microcoil embolization: comparison of treatment outcome with laparoscopic varicocelectomy. *Vascular* 2009;**17**:S129.

137. Miersch WD, Schoeneich G, Winter P, et al. Laparoscopic varicocelectomy: indications, technique, and surgical results. *Br J Urol* 1995;**76**:636.

138. Tay KH, Martin ML, Mayer AL, et al. Selective spermatic venography and varicocele embolization in men with circumaortic left renal veins. *J Vasc Interv Radiol* 2002;**13**:739.

139. Sze DY, Kao JS, Frisoli JK, et al. Persistent and recurrent postsurgical varicocele: venographic anatomy and treatment with N-butyl cyanoacrylate embolization. *J Vasc Interv Radiol* 2008;**19**:539.

140. Reiner E, Pollak JS, Henderson KJ, et al. Initial experience with 3% sodium tetradecyl sulfate foam and fibered coils for management of adolescent varicocele. *J Vasc Interv Radiol* 2008;**19**:207.

141. Gandini R, Konda D, Reale CA, et al. Male varicocele: transcatheter foam sclerotherapy with sodium tetradecyl sulfate- outcome in 244 patients. *Radiology* 2008;**246**:612.

142. Heye S, Maleux G, Wilms G. Pain experience during internal spermatic vein embolization for varicocele: comparison of two cyanoacrylate glues. *Eur Radiol* 2006;**16**:132.

143. Gazzera C, Rampado O, Savio L, et al. Radiological treatment of male varicocele: technical, clinical, seminal, and dosimetric aspects. *Radiol Med* 2006;**111**:449.

144. Lord DJ, Burrows PE. Pediatric varicocele embolization. *Tech Vasc Interv Radiol* 2003;**6**:169.

145. Shlansky-Goldberg RD, Van Arsdal en KN, Rutter CM, et al. Percutaneous varicocele embolization versus surgical ligation for the treatment of infertility: changes in seminal parameters and pregnancy outcomes. *J Vasc Interv Radiol* 1997;**8**:759.

146. Reyes BL, Trerotola SO, Venbrux AC, et al. Percutaneous embolotherapy of adolescent varicocele: results and long-term follow-up. *J Vasc Interv Radiol* 1994;**5**:131.

147. Di Bisceglie C, Fornengo R, Grosso M, et al. Follow-up of varicocele treated with percutaneous retrograde sclerotherapy: technical, clinical and seminal aspects. *J Endocrinol Invest* 2003;**26**:1059.

148. Zuckerman AM, Mitchell SE, Venbrux AC, et al. Percutaneous varicocele occlusion: long-term follow-up. *J Vasc Interv Radiol* 1994;**5**:315.

149. Mazzoni G, Fiocca G, Minucci S, et al. Varicocele: a multidisciplinary approach in children and adolescents. *J Urol* 1999;**162**:1755.

150. Ferguson JM, Gillespie IN, Chalmers N, et al. Percutaneous varicocele embolization in the treatment of infertility. *Br J Radiol* 1995;**68**:700.

151. Marsman JWP. The aberrantly fed varicocele: frequency, venographic appearance, and results of transcatheter embolization. *AJR Am J Roentgenol* 1995;**164**:649.

152. Sayfan J, Soffer Y, Orda R. Varicocele treatment: prospective randomized trial of 3 methods. *J Urol* 1992;**148**:1447.

153. Yavetz H, Levy R, Papo J, et al. Efficacy of varicocele embolization versus ligation of the left internal spermatic vein for improvement of sperm quality. *Int J Androl* 1992;**15**:338.

154. Schlesinger MH, Wilets IF, Nagler HM. Treatment outcome after varicocelectomy: a critical analysis. *Urol Clin North Am* 1994;**21**:517.

155. Dewire DM, Thomas AJ Jr, Falk RM, et al. Clinical outcome and cost comparison of percutaneous embolization and surgical ligation of varicocele. *J Androl* 1994;**15**(Suppl):38S.

156. Punekar SV, Prem AR, Ridhorkar VR, et al. Post-surgical recurrent varicocele: efficacy of internal spermatic venography and steel-coil embolization. *Br J Urol* 1996;**77**:124.

157. Flacke S, Schuster M, Kovacs A, et al. Embolization of varicoceles: pretreatment sperm motility predicts later pregnancy in partners of infertile men. *Radiology* 2008;**248**:540.

158. Evers JL, Collins JA. Assessment of efficacy of varicocele repair for male subfertility: a systematic review. *Lancet* 2003;**361**:1849.

159. Nabi G, Asterlings S, Greene DR, et al. Percutaneous embolization of varicoceles: outcomes and correlation of semen improvement with pregnancy. *Urology* 2004;**63**:359.

160. Evers JH, Collins J, Clarke J. Surgery or embolisation for varicoceles in subfertile men. *Cochrane Database Syst Rev* 2009;**21**:CD000479.

161. Lurie AL, Bookstein JJ, Kessler WO. Posttraumatic impotence: angiographic evaluation. *Radiology* 1987;**165**:115.

162. Kowalczyk J, Athens A, Grimaldi A. Penile fracture: an unusual presentation with lacerations of bilateral corpora cavernosa and partial disruption of the urethra. *Urology* 1994;**44**:599.

163. Munarriz RM, Yan QR, Nehra A, et al. Blunt trauma: the pathophysiology of hemodynamic injury leading to erectile dysfunction. *J Urol* 1995;**153**:1831.

164. Golijanin D, Singer E, Davis R, et al. Doppler evaluation of erectile dysfunction–part 2. *Int J Imp Res* 2007;**19**:43.

165. Kim SH, Kim SH. Post-traumatic erectile dysfunction: Doppler US findings. *Abdom Imaging* 2005;**31**:598.

166. Savoca G, Pietropaolo F, Scieri F, et al. Sexual function after highly selective embolization of cavernous artery in patients with high flow priapism: long-term followup. *J Urol* 2004;**172**:644.

167. Liu BX, Xin ZC, Zou YH, et al. High-flow priapism: superselective cavernous artery embolization with microcoils. *Urology* 2008;**72**:571.

168. Kim KR, Shin JH, Song HY, et al. Treatment of high flow priapism with superselective transcatheter embolization in 27 patients: a multicenter study. *J Vasc Interv Radiol* 2007;**18**:1222.

169. Alexander Tonseth K, Egge T, Kolbenstvedt A, et al. Evaluation of patients after treatment of arterial priapism with selective micro-embolization. *Scand J Urol Nephrol* 2006;**40**:49.

170. Bannister LH, Dyson M, editors. Reproductive system. In: Williams PL, Bannister LH, Berry MM, et al, eds. *Gray's anatomy*, 38th ed. New York: Churchill Livingstone; 1995. p.1873.

171. Wallach EE, Vlahos NF. Uterine myomas: an overview of development, clinical features, and management. *Obstet Gynecol* 2004;**104**:393.

172. Andrews RT, Spies JB, Sacks D, et al. Patient care and uterine artery embolization for leiomyomata. *J Vasc Interv Radiol* 2004;**15**:115.

173. Szklaruk J, Tamm EP, Choi H, et al. MR imaging of common and uncommon pelvic masses. *Radiographics* 2003;**23**:403.

174. Burn PR, McCall JM, Chinn RJ, et al. Uterine fibroleiomyoma: MR imaging appearances before and after embolization of uterine arteries. *Radiology* 2000;**214**:729.

175. Ravina JH, Herbreteau D, Ciraru-Vigneron N, et al. Arterial embolisation to treat uterine myomata. *Lancet* 1995;**346**:671.

176. Hovsepian DM, Siskin GP, Bonn J, et al. Quality improvement guidelines for uterine artery embolization for symptomatic leiomyomata. *J Vasc Interv Radiol* 2004;**15**:535.

177. Margau R, Simons ME, Rajan DK, et al. Outcomes after uterine artery embolization for pedunculated subserosal leiomyomas. *J Vasc Interv Radiol* 2008;**19**:657.

178. Worthington-Kirsch RL, Andrews RT, et al. Uterine fibroid embolization: technical aspects. *Tech Vasc Interv Radiol* 2002;**5**:17.

179. Banovac F, Ascher SM, Jones DA, et al. Magnetic resonance imaging outcome after uterine artery embolization for leiomyomata with use of tris-acryl gelatin microspheres. *J Vasc Interv Radiol* 2002;**13**:681.

180. Pelage JP, Le Dref O, Beregi JP, et al. Limited uterine artery embolization with tris-acryl gelatin microspheres for uterine fibroids. *J Vasc Interv Radiol* 2003;**14**:15.

181. Spies JB. What evidence should we demand before accepting a new embolic material for uterine artery embolization? *J Vasc Interv Radiol* 2009;**20**:567.

182. Siskin GP, Beck A, Schuster M, et al. Leiomyoma infarction after uterine artery embolization: a prospective randomized study comparing tris-acryl gelatin microspheres versus polyvinyl alcohol microspheres. *J Vasc Interv Radiol* 2008;**19**:58.

183. Pelage JP, Le Dref O, Soyer P, et al. Arterial anatomy of the female genital tract: variations and relevance to transcatheter embolization of the uterus. *AJR Am J Roentgenol* 1999;**172**:989.

184. Razavi MK, Wolanske KA, Hwang GL, et al. Angiographic classification of ovarian artery-to-uterine artery anastomoses: initial observations in uterine fibroid embolization. *Radiology* 2002;**224**:707.

185. Pelage JP, Walker WJ, Le Dref O, et al. Ovarian artery: angiographic appearance, embolization and relevance to uterine fibroid embolization. *Cardiovasc Intervent Radiol* 2003;**26**:227.

186. Siskin GP, Bonn J, Worthington-Kirsch RL, et al. Uterine fibroid embolization: pain management. *Tech Vasc Interv Radiol* 2002;**5**:35.

187. Pelage JP, Guaou NG, Jha RC, et al. Uterine fibroid tumors: long-term MR imaging outcome after embolization. *Radiology* 2004;**230**:803.

188. Spies JB, Bruno J, Czeyda-Pommerscheim F, et al. Long-term outcomes of uterine artery embolization of leiomyomata. *Obstet Gynecol* 2005;**106**:933.

189. Spies JB, Ascher SA, Roth AR, et al. Uterine artery embolization for leiomyomata. *Obstet Gynecol* 2001;**98**:29.

190. Walker WJ, Pelage JP. Uterine artery embolisation for symptomatic fibroids: clinical results in 400 women with imaging follow up. *BJOG* 2002;**109**:1262.

191. Goodwin SC, McLucas B, Lee M, et al. Uterine artery embolization for the treatment of uterine leiomyomata: midterm results. *J Vasc Interv Radiol* 1999;**10**:1159.

192. Pron G, Bennett J, Common A, et al. The Ontario Uterine Fibroid Embolization Trial. Part 2. Uterine fibroid reduction and symptom relief after uterine artery embolization for fibroids. *Fertil Steril* 2003;**79**:120.

193. Spies JB, Roth AR, Jha RC, et al. Leiomyomata treated with uterine artery embolization: factors associated with successful symptom and imaging outcome. *Radiology* 2002;**222**:45.

194. Hehenkamp WJK, Volkers NA, Birnie E, et al. Symptomatic uterine fibroids: treatment with uterine artery embolization or hysterectomy–results from the Randomized Clinical Embolisation versus Hysterectomy (EMMY) trial. *Radiology* 2008;**246**:823.

195. The REST investigators. Uterine artery embolization versus surgery for symptomatic uterine fibroids. *N Engl J Med* 2007;**356**:360.

196. Goodwin SC, Spies JB, Worthington Kirsch R, et al. Uterine artery embolization for treatment of leiomyomata: long-term outcomes from the FIBROID registry. *Obstet Gynecol* 2008;**111**:22.

197. Spies JB, Cooper JM, Worthington-Kirsch R, et al. Outcome of uterine embolization and hysterectomy for leiomyomas: results of a multicenter study. *Am J Obstet Gynecol* 2004;**191**:22.

198. Razavi MK, Hwang G, Jahed A, et al. Abdominal myomectomy versus uterine fibroid embolization in the treatment of symptomatic uterine leiomyomas. *AJR Am J Roentgenol* 2003;**180**:1571.

199. Pinto I, Chimeno P, Romo A, et al. Uterine fibroids: uterine artery embolization versus abdominal hysterectomy for treatment—a prospective, randomized, and controlled clinical trial. *Radiology* 2003;**226**:425.

200. Siskin GP, Shlansky-Goldberg RD, Goodwin SC, et al. A prospective multicenter comparative study between myomectomy and uterine artery embolization with polyvinyl alcohol

microspheres: long-term clinical outcomes in patients with symptomatic uterine fibroids. *J Vasc Interv Radiol* 2006;**17**:1287.

201. Pron G, Mocarski E, Bennett J, et al. Tolerance, hospital stay, and recovery after uterine artery embolization for fibroids: the Ontario Uterine Fibroid Embolization Trial. *J Vasc Interv Radiol* 2003;**14**:1243.

202. Pelage JP, Walker WJ, Dref OL. Uterine necrosis after uterine artery embolization for leiomyoma. *Obstet Gynecol* 2002;**99**:6767.

203. Spies JB, Spector A, Roth AR, et al. Complications after uterine artery embolization for leiomyomas. *Obstet Gynecol* 2002;**100**:873.

204. Spies JB, Roth AR, Gonsalves SM, et al. Ovarian function after uterine artery embolization for leiomyomata: assessment with use of serum follicle stimulating hormone assay. *J Vasc Interv Radiol* 2001;**12**:437.

205. Pron G, Mocarski E, Cohen M, et al. Hysterectomy for complications after uterine artery embolization for leiomyoma: results of a Canadian multicenter clinical trial. *J Am Assoc Gynecol Laparosc* 2003;**10**:99.

206. Ratnam LA, Marsh P, Holdstock JM, et al. Pelvic vein embolisation in the management of varicose veins. *Cardiovasc Intervent Radiol* 2008;**31**:1159.

207. Scultetus AH, Villavicencio JL, Gillespie DL. The nutcracker syndrome: its role in the pelvic venous disorders. *J Vasc Surg* 2001;**34**:812.

208. Park SJ, Lim JW, Ko YT, et al. Diagnosis of pelvic congestion syndrome using transabdominal and transvaginal sonography. *AJR Am J Roentgenol* 2004;**182**:683.

209. Nascimento AB, Mitchell DG, Holland G. Ovarian veins: magnetic resonance imaging findings in an asymptomatic population. *J Magn Reson Imaging* 2002;**15**:551.

210. Grabham JA, Barrie WW. Laparoscopic approach to pelvic congestion syndrome. *Br J Surg* 1997;**84**:1264.

211. Gandini R, Chiocchi M, Konda D, et al. Transcatheter foam sclerotherapy of symptomatic female varicocele with sodium tetradecyl sulfate foam. *Cardiovasc Intervent Radiol* 2008;**31**:778.

212. Ganeshan A, Upponi S, Hon LQ, et al. Chronic pelvic pain due to pelvic congestion syndrome: the role of diagnostic and interventional radiology. *Cardiovasc Intervent Radiol* 2007;**30**:1105.

213. Maleux G, Stockx L, Wilms G, et al. Ovarian vein embolization for the treatment of pelvic congestion syndrome: long-term technical and clinical results. *J Vasc Interv Radiol* 2000;**11**:859.

214. Venbrux AC, Chang AH, Kim HS, et al. Pelvic congestion syndrome (pelvic venous incompetence): impact of ovarian and internal iliac vein embolotherapy on menstrual cycle and chronic pelvic pain. *J Vasc Interv Radiol* 2002;**13**(2 Pt. 1):171.

215. Asciutto G, Asciutto KC, Mumme A, et al. Pelvic venous incompetence: reflux patterns and treatment results. *Eur J Vasc Endovasc Surg* 2009;**38**:381.

216. Banovac F, Lin R, Shah D, et al. Angiographic and interventional options in obstetric and gynecologic emergencies. *Obstet Gynecol Clin North Am* 2007;**34**:599.

217. Salazar GM, Petrozza JC, Walker TG. Transcatheter endovascular techniques for management of obstetrical and gynecologic emergencies. *Tech Vasc Interv Radiol* 2009;**12**:139.

218. Oyelese Y, Smulian JC. Placenta previa, placenta accreta, and vasa previa. *Obstet Gynecol* 2006;**107**:927.

219. Zwart JJ, Dijk PD, van Roosmalen J. Peripartum hysterectomy and arterial embolization for major obstetric hemorrhage: a 2-year nationwide cohort study in the Netherlands. *Am J Obstet Gynecol* 2010;**202**:e1.

220. Pelage JP, Soyer P, Repiquet D, et al. Secondary postpartum hemorrhage: treatment with selective arterial embolization. *Radiology* 1999;**212**:385.

221. Pelage JP, Le Dref O, Mateo J, et al. Life-threatening primary postpartum hemorrhage: treatment with emergency selective arterial embolization. *Radiology* 1998;**208**:359.

222. Eriksson LG, Mulic-Lutvica A, Jangland L, et al. Massive postpartum hemorrhage treated with transcatheter arterial embolization: technical aspects and long-term effects on fertility and menstrual cycle. *Acta Radiol* 2007;**48**:635.

223. Vegas G, Illescas T, Munoz M, et al. Selective pelvic arterial embolization in the management of obstetric hemorrhage. *Eur J Obstet Gynecol Reprod Biol* 2006;**127**:68.

224. Ratman LA, Gibson M, Sandhu C, et al. Transcatheter pelvic arterial embolisation for control of obstetric and gynaecological haemorrhage. *J Obstet Gynaecol* 2008;**28**:573.

225. Ornan D, White R, Pollak J, et al. Pelvic embolization for intractable postpartum hemorrhage: long-term follow-up and implications for fertility. *Obstet Gynecol* 2003;**102**:904.

226. Stancato-Pasik A, Mitty HA, Richard HM, et al. Obstetric embolotherapy: effect on menses and pregnancy. *Radiology* 1997;**204**:791.

227. Kidney DD, Nguyen AM, Ahdoot D, et al. Prophylactic perioperative hypogastric artery balloon occlusion in abnormal placentation. *AJR Am J Roentgenol* 2001;**176**:1521.

228. Levine AB, Kuhlman K, Bonn J. Placenta accreta: comparison of cases managed with and without pelvic artery balloon catheters. *J Matern Fetal Med* 1999;**8**:173.

229. Dubois J, Garel L, Grignon A, et al. Placenta percreta: balloon occlusion and embolization of the internal iliac arteries to reduce intraoperative blood losses. *Am J Obstet Gynecol* 1997;**176**:723.

230. Tan CH, Tay KH, Sheah K, et al. Perioperative endovascular internal iliac artery occlusion balloon placement in management of placenta accreta. *AJR Am J Roentgenol* 2007;**189**:1158.

231. Bodner LJ, Nosher JL, Gribbin C, et al. Balloon-assisted occlusion of the internal iliac arteries in patients with placenta accreta/percreta. *Cardiovasc Intervent Radiol* 2006;**29**:354.

232. Salai M, Garniek A, Rubinstein Z, et al. Preoperative angiography and embolization of large pelvic tumors. *J Surg Oncol* 1999;**70**:41.

233. de Baere T, Ousehal A, Kuoch V, et al. Endovascular management of bleeding iliac artery pseudoaneurysms complicating radiation therapy for pelvic malignancies. *AJR Am J Roentgenol* 1998;**170**:349.

234. Dickerson RD, Putman MJ, Black ME, et al. Selective ovarian vein sampling to localize a Leydig cell tumor. *Fertil Steril* 2005;**84**:218.

235. Cura M, Martinez N, Cura A, et al. Arteriovenous malformations of the uterus. *Acta Radiol* 2009;**50**:823.

236. Calligaro KD, Sedlacek TV, Savarese RP, et al. Congenital pelvic arteriovenous malformations: long term follow-up in two cases and a review of the literature. *J Vasc Surg* 1992;**16**:100.

237. Vogelzang RL, Nemcek Jr AA, Skrtic Z, et al. Uterine arteriovenous malformations: primary treatment with therapeutic embolization. *J Vasc Interv Radiol* 1991;**2**:517.

238. Lim AK, Agarwal R, Seckl MJ, et al. Embolization of bleeding residual uterine vascular malformations in patients with treated gestational trophoblastic tumors. *Radiology* 2002;**222**:640.

239. Ghai S, Rajan DK, Asch MR, et al. Efficacy of embolization in traumatic uterine vascular malformations. *J Vasc Interv Radiol* 2003;**14**:1401.

240. Maleux G, Timmerman D, Heye S, et al. Acquired uterine vascular malformations: radiological and clinical outcome after transcatheter embolotherapy. *Eur Radiol* 2006;**16**:299.

PULMONARY VASCULATURE AND VENOUS SYSTEMS

Pulmonary and Bronchial Arteries

Karim Valji

ARTERIOGRAPHY

Pulmonary Arteriography (Video 14-1)

The remaining indications for catheter angiography of the pulmonary arteries are diagnosis of unusual vascular disorders (e.g., chronic thromboembolic pulmonary hypertension [CTPH], vasculitis) and evaluation as part of endovascular therapy (e.g., embolotherapy of arteriovenous malformations [AVMs]). Before beginning angiography, the interventionalist should inspect a recent electrocardiogram to exclude a left bundle branch block. Right heart catheterization can induce complete heart block in such a case. A temporary transvenous pacemaker may be required before angiography; at a minimum, an external pacing device should be at the ready.

Pulmonary arteriography is performed from a common femoral, internal jugular, or brachial vein in one of several ways:

1. A long 5-French (Fr) *Omniflush catheter* is advanced into the right atrium. When a stiff hydrophilic guidewire is advanced through the catheter, it expands the catheter loop and directs the wire tip toward the right ventricular outflow tract[1] (Fig. 14-1).

2. The preshaped 7-Fr *Grollman catheter* (or the van Aman or Hunter modifications) is designed for easy manipulation into the right ventricle and then into the pulmonary artery[2,3] (Fig. 14-2). When the right atrium is enlarged, a tip-deflecting wire may be needed to advance the catheter fully into the right ventricle. One variant of this approach is to impose a curve on the end of a pigtail catheter with a tip-deflecting wire. As the catheter is fed off the wire, it is directed through the right ventricle and into the ventricular outflow tract, at which point the wire bend is released (Fig. 14-3).

3. A 7-Fr *flow-directed Berman balloon catheter* (with multiple distal side holes) requires insertion through a femoral or internal jugular vein sheath. With the balloon inflated, blood flow guides the advancing catheter from the right atrium into the pulmonary artery.

Extreme care should be taken while traversing the right heart chambers. Short bursts of atrial or ventricular tachycardia almost always stop by quickly repositioning the catheter or guidewire. For sustained or recurrent ventricular tachycardia, amiodarone (150 mg intravenously over 10 minutes) may be required. Cardiac perforation

FIGURE 14-1   Pulmonary arteriography using an Omniflush catheter. **A,** The catheter is positioned in the middle of the right atrium. **B,** When a stiff hydrophilic wire is inserted, the catheter curve opens and points the guidewire toward the right ventricular outflow tract. **C,** The catheter is then advanced into the pulmonary artery. *(Adapted from Velling TE, Brennan FJ, Hall LD. Pulmonary angiography with use of the 5 Fr Omniflush catheter: a safe and efficient procedure with a common catheter. J Vasc Interv Radiol 2000;11:1005.)*

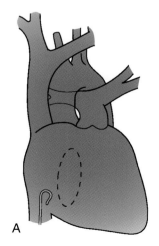
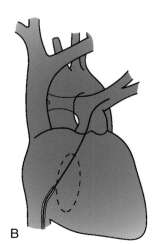
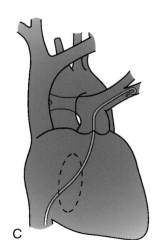

A

B

C

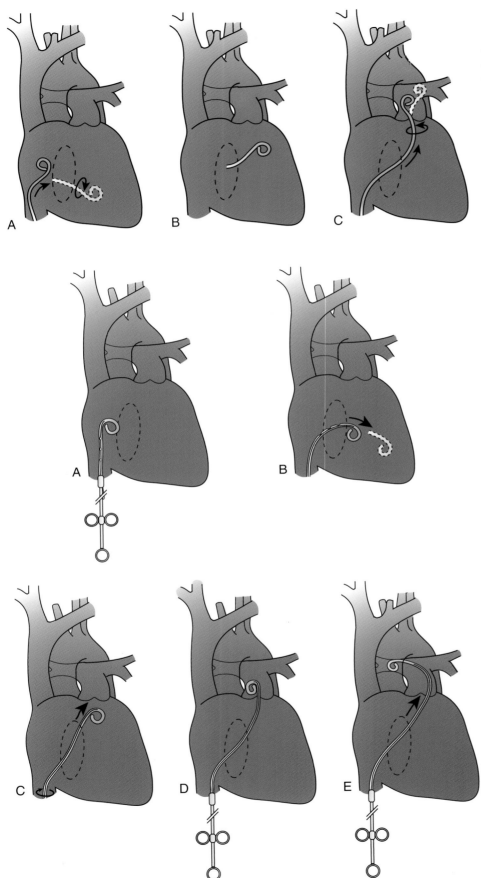

FIGURE 14-2 Pulmonary arteriography using a Grollman catheter. **A,** The catheter is directed through the tricuspid valve into the right ventricle. **B,** The catheter is turned 180 degrees so that the pigtail points up toward the right ventricular outflow tract. **C,** The catheter is advanced into the main pulmonary artery and directed to the right or left. *(Adapted from Kadir S. Diagnostic angiography. Philadelphia: WB Saunders, 1986:591.)*

FIGURE 14-3 Pulmonary arteriography using a pigtail catheter and deflecting wire. **A,** The pigtail is advanced to the right atrium. **B,** While a bend is placed on the tip-deflecting wire, the catheter is fed off into the right ventricle. **C,** The deflection is released, straightening the catheter. **D,** The catheter is rotated and advanced through the right ventricular outflow tract into the main pulmonary artery. **E,** The catheter can be directed into the right or left pulmonary artery by rotating the pigtail toward the desired side and feeding it off the deflected wire. *(Adapted from Kadir S. Diagnostic angiography. Philadelphia: WB Saunders, 1986:590.)*

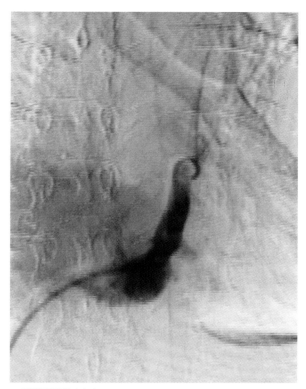

FIGURE 14-4 Pigtail catheter in the coronary sinus.

TABLE 14-1   Normal Right Heart Pressures

	Systolic (mm Hg)	Diastolic (mm Hg)	Mean (mm Hg)
Right atrium			0-8
Right ventricle	15-30	0-8	
Pulmonary artery	15-30	3-12	9-16

BOX 14-1

CAUSES OF PULMONARY ARTERY HYPERTENSION

Group I

- Idiopathic ("primary" pulmonary hypertension)
- Familial
- Secondary
  - Collagen vascular disease
  - Portal hypertension
  - HIV infection
  - Drugs (e.g., fenfluramine-type appetite suppressants, illicit stimulants)
  - Congenital systemic to pulmonary shunt
  - Miscellaneous causes
- Pulmonary venoocclusive disease
- Pulmonary capillary hemangiomatosis

Group II

- Left ventricular or atrial disease
- Left heart valvular disease

Group III

- Chronic interstitial or obstructive lung disease
- Sleep-disordered breathing
- Alveolar hypoventilation syndromes
- Chronic high altitude exposure
- Developmental abnormalities

Group IV

- Chronic thromboembolic disease

Group V

- Pulmonary artery compression
  - Fibrosing mediastinitis
  - Mediastinal tumor
  - Lymphadenopathy
- Miscellaneous causes

From Simonneau G, Galie N, Rubin LJ, et al: Clinical classification of pulmonary hypertension. *J Am Coll Cardiol* 2004; 43 Suppl 1:5S-12S.

---

is avoided by gentle catheter manipulation. Inability to advance the catheter from the right atrium to the right ventricle may result from inadvertent entry into the coronary sinus (Fig. 14-4).

After the catheter has engaged the main pulmonary artery, it is directed to the right or left lung using a standard or stiff hydrophilic guidewire. The side holes of the catheter should rest in the distal main left or right pulmonary artery. Selective catheterization and arteriography of segmental branches usually is performed by exchanging the pigtail catheter for a preshaped headhunter or hockey stick–shaped diagnostic catheter or guiding catheter over a stiff exchange guidewire.

Pulmonary artery pressures are obtained routinely before contrast injection. Table 14-1 lists normal right heart pressures.[4] The pulmonary artery pressure may be elevated for a variety of reasons[5] (Box 14-1). In patients with high right heart pressures, it is prudent to limit each contrast injection to about 20 mL. Interventionalists have personal preferences for tube angulation for pulmonary arteriography. In general, lower lobe vessels are displayed best in the ipsilateral posterior oblique projection.

Adverse events include contrast reaction, transient renal dysfunction, access site hematoma, dysrhythmias, and respiratory distress. In older series, the risks of minor complications, major complications, and death resulting from pulmonary angiography were about 5%, 1%, and 0.2 to 0.5%, respectively.[6] There are conflicting data regarding the increased risk of pulmonary arteriography in patients with pulmonary artery hypertension.[4,5] However, in one recent report, all fatal complications (1.5%) occurred in patients with acute pulmonary artery hypertension.[7] Cardiac perforation is exceedingly rare when appropriate catheters are used.

Bronchial Arteriography

Selective catheterization of the bronchial arteries can be performed with forward-seeking catheters (e.g., spinal or renal double curve catheter) or reverse-curve catheters (e.g., Simmons or Shetty). In any case, the catheter tip must be wall-seeking along the descending thoracic aorta to engage the bronchial arteries. Forward-seeking catheters are easier to maneuver but may be more difficult to seat within the target vessel. Reverse-curve catheters can be more difficult to manipulate, particularly near the aortic arch, but they engage the artery more securely. The bronchial arteries are found by scraping the catheter tip along the aortic wall in the anticipated location of the vessels (level of the fourth to sixth thoracic vertebrae), which corresponds to the position of the left main stem bronchus (Fig. 14-5). A descending thoracic aortogram may be obtained to identify bronchial artery origins if they cannot be catheterized easily. High-quality images are critical to identify small bronchial artery branches that may supply the anterior spinal artery.

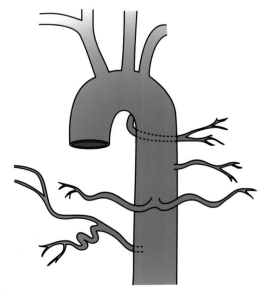

FIGURE 14-5 Common origins of the bronchial arteries from the thoracic aorta.

ANATOMY

Development

Early in fetal development, the lung buds are supplied by a network of vessels arising from the aortic sac, which itself is composed of the paired ventral aortae.[8] The sixth aortic arch becomes the conduit between the pulmonary trunk (which arises from the aortic sac) and the right and left pulmonary arteries (see Fig. 6-1). The ventral segment of the right sixth aortic arch becomes the right pulmonary artery origin. The ventral segment of the left sixth aortic arch develops into part of the pulmonary trunk, and the dorsal segment becomes the ductus arteriosus.

Immediately after birth, the ductus arteriosus constricts. Within several months, this channel is completely obstructed, leaving the ligamentum arteriosum between the origin of the left pulmonary artery and the aortic arch.

Normal Pulmonary Vascular Anatomy and Physiology

The *pulmonary artery* arises from the base of the right ventricle.[9] It courses superiorly to the left of the ascending aorta and then divides below the aortic arch into right and left pulmonary arteries (Fig. 14-6). The bifurcation is located inferior, anterior, and to the left of the tracheal bifurcation.

The *right pulmonary artery* runs horizontally behind the ascending aorta and superior vena cava (SVC) and in front of the tracheal bifurcation and esophagus to reach the hilum of the right lung (Fig. 14-7). It divides behind the SVC into an ascending branch *(truncus anterior)* supplying the right upper lobe and the *descending right pulmonary artery* supplying the middle and lower lobes. The ascending trunk usually has three branches to the segments of the right upper lobe: apical, posterior, and anterior. Occasionally, two segmental branches arise in a common trunk. The descending right pulmonary artery courses behind the intermediate bronchus. This artery commonly gives off an accessory branch to some portion of the right upper lobe. The descending pulmonary artery then provides an anterior branch supplying the right middle lobe and a posterior branch supplying the superior segment of the right lower lobe. The descending pulmonary artery continues inferiorly and then divides. Although the branching pattern is somewhat variable, the relative positions of the segmental branches is fairly predictable on a frontal pulmonary arteriogram going from lateral to medial: anterior, lateral, posterior, medial.

The *left pulmonary artery* courses upward and posteriorly in front of the aorta and the left main stem bronchus (Fig. 14-8). The ascending branch of the left pulmonary artery divides into apical posterior and anterior segmental

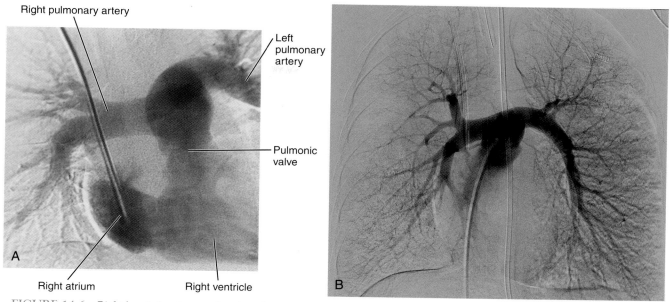

Right pulmonary artery

Left pulmonary artery

Pulmonic valve

Right atrium

Right ventricle

FIGURE 14-6 Right heart chambers and main pulmonary arteries in frontal projection (A) and right posterior oblique projection (B).

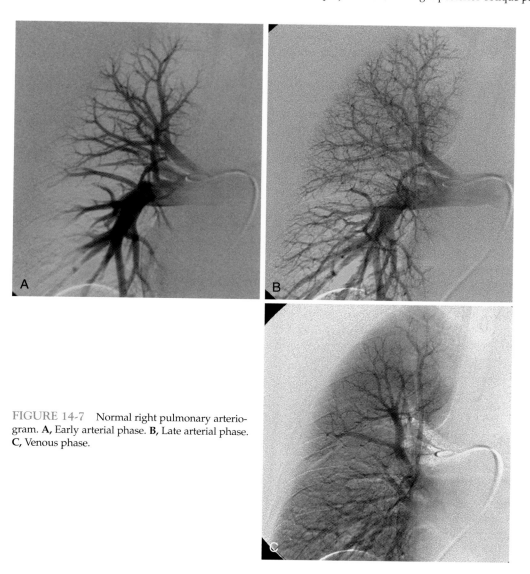

FIGURE 14-7 Normal right pulmonary arteriogram. A, Early arterial phase. B, Late arterial phase. C, Venous phase.

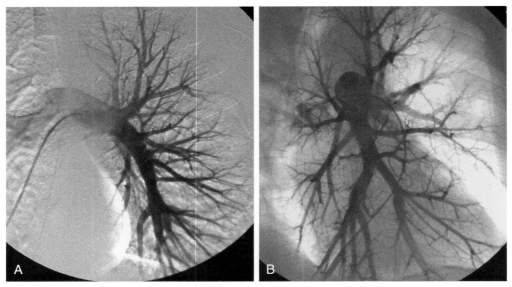

FIGURE 14-8   Normal left pulmonary arteriogram. **A,** Frontal projection. **B,** Left posterior oblique projection lays out lower lobe branches.

arteries. The first one or two branches of the descending left pulmonary artery are the superior and inferior segmental arteries, which supply the lingula. The left pulmonary artery then divides into several vessels supplying the segments of the left lower lobe. The relative location of the terminal portions of the left lower lobe vessels is the mirror image of the pattern just described for the right lung.

Because the venous drainage of the lungs is located within the interlobular septa, the pulmonary veins do not follow the pulmonary arteries and bronchi.[10] The right and left lungs are drained by *superior* and *inferior pulmonary veins* (Fig. 14-9). On each side, the vessels usually enter the left atrium separately, inferior to the pulmonary arteries. In some cases, they form a confluence before draining into the left atrium. The superior pulmonary veins drain the upper and middle (or lingular) lobes of each lung. The inferior pulmonary veins drain the lower lobes.

The pulmonary circulation is a high-flow, low-pressure system with a total resistance about one eighth to one tenth that of the systemic circulation.[11] *Pulmonary vascular resistance (PVR)* is calculated as

$$\frac{([\text{Mean Pulmonary artery pressure} - \text{Pulmonary capillary wedge pressure}] \times 80)}{\text{Cardiac output}}$$

The normal range is 90 to 250 dyne/sec/cm, which in *Wood units* (PVR/80) is 0.7 to 1.1. While standing, blood flows preferentially to the lower lobes. When supine, blood flow is more evenly distributed between the lung bases and apices. Because the system is so distensible and has a large number of reserve vessels, sudden obstruction

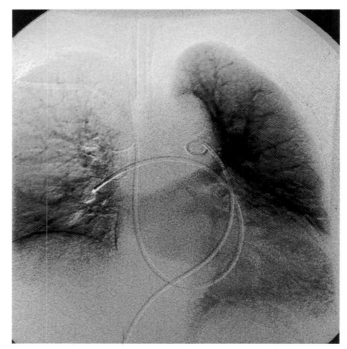

FIGURE 14-9   The late-phase pulmonary arteriogram shows pulmonary veins entering the left atrium.

of one half of the pulmonary circulation in a patient without preexisting cardiopulmonary disease only slightly elevates pulmonary artery pressure. However, in patients with preexisting cardiac or pulmonary disease, which may be associated with elevated right heart pressures and right ventricular dysfunction, acute obstruction of even a small portion of the pulmonary circulation may cause a significant rise in pulmonary artery pressure.

Normal Bronchial Artery Anatomy

The *bronchial arteries* supply the trachea, bronchi, esophagus, and posterior mediastinum, and they also act as the vasa vasorum of the pulmonary arteries. These vessels may not be visible at thoracic aortography in patients without lung disease. However, they become markedly enlarged and serve as an important collateral pathway in patients with certain congenital heart diseases, chronic lung infections, lung tumors, and obstruction of pulmonary arteries or veins.[12] Bronchial artery anatomy is extremely variable.[13-15] Anatomic and angiographic studies differ in the reported pattern and distribution of their origins. As a rule, one or two bronchial arteries supply each lung; however, up to four arteries may supply one side. Several patterns are commonly observed (Fig. 14-10; see also Fig. 14-5):

- Right intercostal-bronchial trunk from the right posterolateral surface of the aorta
- Left bronchial artery from the left anterolateral surface of the aorta
- Common right and left bronchial artery trunk from the anterior surface of the aorta

Rarely, a right intercostal-bronchial artery trunk gives rise to a left bronchial artery. Unusual bronchial artery origins are noted in Box 14-2.

Bronchial arteries may have branches to the *anterior spinal artery*, which supplies the ventral portion of the

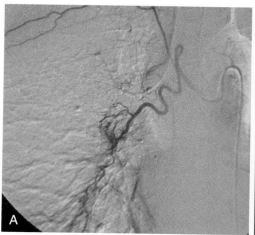
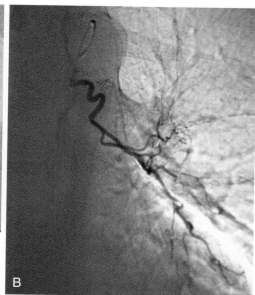
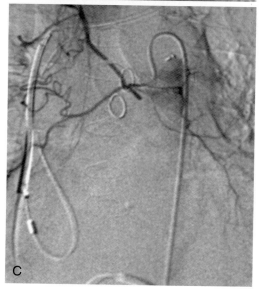

FIGURE 14-10   Bronchial artery patterns. **A,** Right bronchointercostal trunk. **B,** Left bronchial artery. **C,** Common right and left bronchial trunk arising from the anterior surface of the thoracic aorta.

BOX 14-2

ECTOPIC BRONCHIAL ARTERY ORIGINS

- Undersurface or upper surface of aortic arch
- Posterior aortic wall
- Near left subclavian artery origin
- Lower thoracic aorta
- Brachiocephalic artery
- Internal thoracic artery
- Inferior phrenic artery

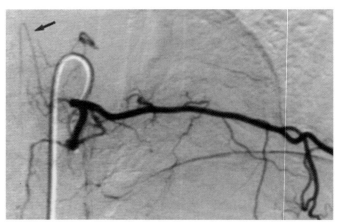

FIGURE 14-11   Spinal artery branch *(arrow)* arising from a left posterior intercostal artery.

BOX 14-3

CONGENITAL ANOMALIES OF THE PULMONARY VESSELS

Main Pulmonary Artery

- Pulmonary valve stenosis
- Pulmonary artery stenosis
- Idiopathic pulmonary artery dilation
- Pulmonary artery aneurysm
- Persistent truncus arteriosus
- Pulmonary atresia
- Aorticopulmonary window
- Absent pulmonic valve

Proximal Pulmonary Arteries

- Patent ductus arteriosus
- Interruption (absence) of right or left pulmonary artery
- Left pulmonary artery sling (with anomalous origin from right pulmonary artery)
- Pulmonary artery stenosis
- Pulmonary artery aneurysm
- Anomalous origin of coronary artery from pulmonary artery
- Crossed pulmonary artery

Distal Pulmonary Arteries

- Peripheral pulmonary artery stenosis

Pulmonary Arteries and Veins

- Arteriovenous malformation
- Pulmonary sequestration
- Hypogenetic lung syndrome
- Anomalous pulmonary venous drainage

spinal cord. In a few individuals, a right bronchointercostal artery (and rarely a right or left bronchial artery) feeds the great anterior radicular artery *(artery of Adamkiewicz)* or a smaller radiculomedullary branch[16] (Fig. 14-11). Although this vessel typically originates at the T9-T12 level, it may have a more superior take-off from the upper thoracic aorta.[17] Very rarely, transverse myelitis with paraplegia may be caused by bronchial artery embolization if this anatomy is present.

Variant Anatomy

A variety of congenital anomalies may affect the pulmonary vasculature[18-20] (Box 14-3).

Pulmonary sequestration is an unusual disorder in which a portion of the lung develops independently and derives its blood supply from a systemic artery.[21] In *intralobar* sequestration, the abnormal tissue lies within the visceral pleura of the adjacent lung. The sequestered segment usually is found in the posterior portion of the lower lobe, more commonly on the left side. The systemic blood

supply to the sequestration comes from the descending thoracic or abdominal aorta (Fig. 14-12). The venous drainage usually is through the pulmonary veins; inferior vena cava (IVC) and azygous drainage also have been described. In *extralobar* sequestration, the abnormal segment is contained within its own pleural membrane. The anomaly occurs when splanchnic branches of the aorta that supply the developing lung buds fail to involute. The sequestered segment develops in the left chest in 90% of cases. The systemic arterial supply is from the descending thoracic or abdominal aorta. The sequestration drains into the IVC, azygous veins, or portal venous system.

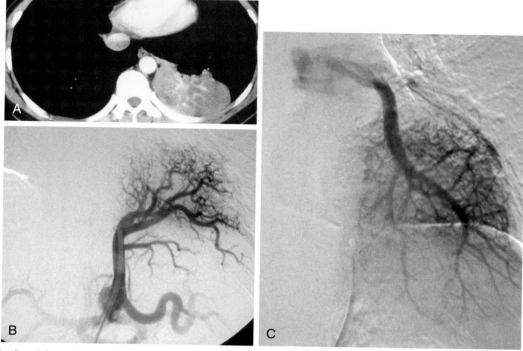

FIGURE 14-12   Intralobar pulmonary sequestration. **A,** A hypervascular multicystic mass in the left lower lobe is identified by computed tomography. **B,** Celiac arteriogram shows a massively enlarged left inferior phrenic artery crossing the hemidiaphragm to supply the sequestration. **C,** The late-phase arteriogram shows venous drainage into the pulmonary veins.

Embolization of the sequestered lung has been performed successfully in neonates.[22]

Hypogenetic lung (scimitar) syndrome features hypoplasia of the right lung and drainage of blood from all or part of the lung into the IVC (or rarely other systemic veins) at the level of the diaphragm.[23] The abnormal lung tissue is fed by branches of the lower thoracic or abdominal aorta. The large draining vein from the mid-right lung to the right cardiophrenic angle produces a C-shaped density on chest radiographs that has been likened to a Turkish sword (scimitar).

Collateral Circulation

The pulmonary artery collateral circulation becomes active with obstruction of a portion of the pulmonary arteries, as a reaction to inflammatory or neoplastic processes in the lung, and in response to regional hypoxia. This situation may occur with acute or chronic emboli, right ventricular outflow or pulmonary artery obstruction (often associated with congenital heart diseases), lung tumors, infections, and vasculitis.

The primary collateral circulations for the pulmonary arteries are the bronchial arteries, small descending thoracic aortic branches (e.g., intercostal arteries), and vessels from major aortic branches.[24] These pathways may fill the pulmonary artery centrally or peripherally.

MAJOR DISORDERS

Acute Pulmonary Embolism (Online Case 8)

Etiology and Natural History

Pulmonary embolism (PE) is a common disorder and one of the leading causes of in-hospital mortality.[25] PE is part of the spectrum of venous thromboembolic disease (see Chapter 1). Most pulmonary emboli arise from the deep veins of the legs. The remainder come from pelvic veins, the IVC and its tributaries, and upper extremity veins. The last is recognized as an increasingly common source of PE, often following venous thrombosis associated with vascular access devices. Lower extremity venous clots usually originate in the soleal sinuses of the deep veins of the calf. In patients with one or more risk factor for thrombosis (Box 14-4), clot may propagate into the calf, popliteal, and femoral veins (see Chapter 15). The risk for PE with untreated "proximal" (femoropopliteal) deep vein thrombosis approaches 50%.[25,26] When embolization occurs, the clot usually shatters while in transit and produces multiple bilateral occlusions of pulmonary artery branches.

Thrombi mechanically impede pulmonary blood flow and lead to the release of a variety of vasospastic activators that intensify the obstruction. The clinical consequences of PE depends on the extent of preexisting cardiopulmonary disease. In patients with previously normal heart and lungs, small emboli produce little effect. However, when the clot burden overwhelms the pulmonary circulation reserve, right ventricular and pulmonary artery pressures rise sharply. This situation may lead to right ventricular dilation, ventricular failure, and ultimately cardiogenic shock. Mortality for patients who present with some hemodynamic compromise is 20% to 30% and approaches 60% in the presence of cardiogenic shock.[27] Although this bleak picture usually accompanies massive PE, even small emboli can start such a chain of events in individuals with underlying heart or lung disease. In some patients, inadequate bronchial artery collateral circulation to the obstructed region results in pulmonary infarction.

In patients who survive the acute insult, the natural history of PE is often endogenous lysis of clot over a period of weeks.[28] About half of patients experience complete resolution of clot; the remainder have partial resolution or chronic obstruction.[29,30] Other nonthrombotic causes of PE include septic foci, fat, air, amniotic fluid, intravascular tumor deposits, and medical devices (e.g., catheter fragments).[31-33]

Clinical Features and Diagnosis

PE is a grossly underdiagnosed problem. Physicians must remain alert to the possibility in any patient with cardiopulmonary symptoms or signs and risk factors for venous thromboembolic disease. The most common complaints are chest pain, shortness of breath, cough, tachypnea, and tachycardia. With massive PE,

patients may present with syncope, dysrhythmias, or cardiogenic shock. The clinical picture often mimics acute myocardial infarction, pneumonia, exacerbation of chronic obstructive lung disease, or congestive heart failure. Because PE is a common disease and symptoms are nonspecific, screening of patients before requesting radiographic studies is useful. Many experts rely on both clinical probability and laboratory tests to guide decisions about imaging in individuals with suspected PE.[25]

D-dimer is a breakdown product of cross-linked fibrin. Serum levels are elevated in the setting of vascular thrombosis among many other conditions (advanced age, trauma, pregnancy, operation, inflammation, neoplasms).[25] The D-dimer test has become a popular screening tool in patients with suspected PE.[34,35] The wide range in reported accuracy speaks to differences in assay methods and thresholds for diagnosis. Using higher cutoff (e.g., >500 ng/mL), the negative predictive value of the test approaches 100%.

Imaging

CHEST RADIOGRAPHY

Chest radiographs are useful for suggesting other diagnoses (e.g., pneumonia or congestive heart failure) and are critical for interpretation of radionuclide lung scans. Many patients have nonspecific abnormalities, such as vague parenchymal densities, areas of atelectasis, or pleural effusions. Findings that are more suggestive of PE are rounded or wedge-shaped pleural-based opacities reflecting pulmonary infarction (Hampton hump), local oligemia (Westermark sign), and central pulmonary artery enlargement (Fig. 14-13).

COMPUTED TOMOGRAPHY ANGIOGRAPHY

In most centers, computed tomography (CT) angiography is the principal imaging study for the diagnosis of acute PE.[36,37] The sensitivity and specificity with helical single or 4-detector row scanners is 83% to 100% and 92% to 100%, respectively[38-44] (Figs. 14-14 and 14-15). Even though the accuracy of commonplace 64-detector row scanners compared with catheter angiography (the gold standard for many decades) has not been rigorously proven, they are considered at least as and probably more accurate for diagnosis than older machines. The negative predictive value of CT angiography approaches 99%.[36,45-48] One prospective study (which used clinical probability and D-dimer testing along with imaging) and a recent metaanalysis of the existing literature evaluated the negative predictive value of CT angiography at 3-month follow-up.[49,50] The results were remarkably consistent: frequency of missed venous thromboembolic events and fatal PE were 1.3% to 1.4% and 0.5%, respectively. Finally, CT provides a thorough evaluation of the lungs, heart, and mediastinum,

FIGURE 14-13   Classic chest radiographic findings for pulmonary embolism. **A,** Diminished vascularity in the right lung (i.e., Westermark sign) and enlargement of the right pulmonary artery suggest pulmonary embolism. **B,** The wedge-shaped, pleural-based density with the apex toward the hilum (i.e., Hampton hump, *arrow*) suggests pulmonary embolism with infarction.

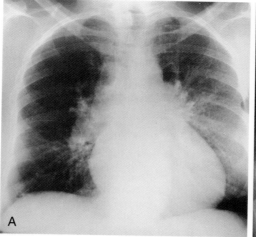
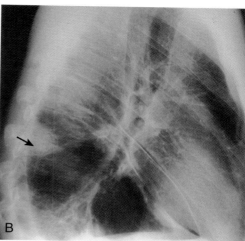

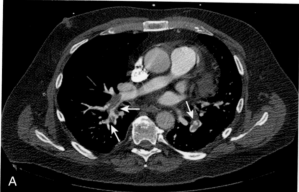
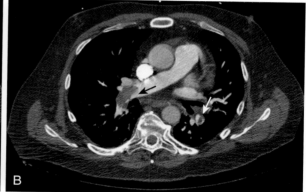

FIGURE 14-14   **A** and **B,** Acute right and left pulmonary artery emboli *(arrows)* are identified by computed tomography angiography.

which allows diagnosis of many other entities that can mimic PE.

In some institutions, chest imaging is followed by CT venography of the lower extremities.[51,52] Specific scanning and contrast injection protocols are required for CT pulmonary angiography. Lung, mediastinal, and embolism-specific displays must be evaluated.[53] Multiplanar reformatted constructions are useful in confirming the diagnosis of clot or the presence of artifacts (see Fig. 14-15). Pulmonary arteries are followed from their origins through the subsegmental branches. Pulmonary artery branches follow their respective bronchi; in the basal segments, medially running pulmonary veins should not be confused with arteries.

Acute emboli appear as complete, partial, or peripheral filling defects sometimes surrounded by contrast (see Figs. 14-14 and 14-15). The affected vessels are often enlarged. These findings must be distinguished from chronic thromboembolic disease (see later discussion). A peripheral wedge-shaped density may represent an infarct (Fig. 14-16). Signs of right ventricular strain (right ventricular dilation or deviation of the intraventricular

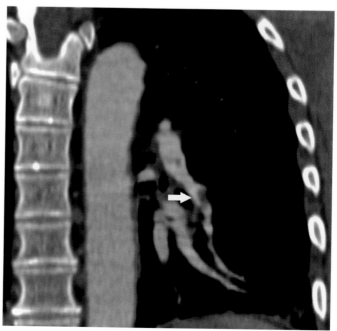

FIGURE 14-15   Multiplanar reformatted computed tomography angiography displays a segmental pulmonary embolus *(arrow).*

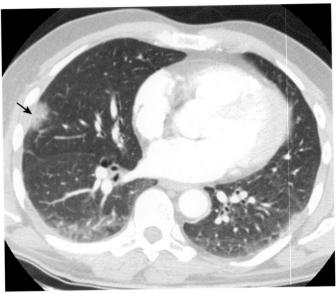

FIGURE 14-16   Peripheral parenchymal density (*arrow*, Hampton hump) distal to segmental pulmonary emboli identified on embolus windows.

TABLE 14-2   Misdiagnosis of Pulmonary Embolism on Computed Tomography Angiography

Cause	Evidence or Response
SIMULATE BLAND ACUTE PULMONARY EMBOLISM	
Respiratory motion artifact	"Seagull sign" from vessel motion
Image noise	Increase detector width in obese patients
Pulmonary artery catheter	Evaluate bone windows
Flow-related artifacts	>78 HU
Lung algorithm artifact	Inspect standard algorithms
Partial volume effect	Evaluate vessels in contiguous images
Partial voluming with lymph nodes	Sagittal and coronal reformatted images
Lucency in peripheral pulmonary veins	Connection with central pulmonary veins
Mucous plug in airway	Note adjacent normal pulmonary artery
Perivascular edema	Other signs of heart failure
Primary pulmonary sarcoma	Lobulated, enhancing, extravascular spread
Tumor emboli (RCC, HCC)	—
Chronic pulmonary embolism	(See text)
MASK PULMONARY EMBOLISM	
Window settings	Window width/level: 700 HU/100 HU
Streak artifact (especially near SVC)	—

HCC, *hepatocellular carcinoma*; HU, *Hounsfield units*; RCC, *renal cell carcinoma*; SVC, *superior vena cava*.

septum) should be sought. Table 14-2 outlines potential pitfalls in diagnosis.[53]

RADIONUCLIDE LUNG SCANNING

For many years, ventilation-perfusion (V/Q) lung scanning was widely used for evaluating patients with suspected pulmonary embolus. Because it is less specific than state-of-the-art CT angiography and a definitive diagnosis cannot be made in a substantial number of cases, it has assumed a minor role in most centers. Nonetheless, V/Q scanning can be useful in some situations:[54]

- History of anaphylactic reaction to contrast material or severe renal dysfunction
- Severe tachypnea or combative patient not suitable for CT angiography
- Pregnancy (first or second trimester)
- Equivocal CT angiography and low clinical probability

Lung perfusion scans are performed by intravenous injection of technetium-99m (^{99m}Tc)–labeled macroaggregated albumin particles. Pulmonary emboli produce localized perfusion defects[55] (Fig. 14-17). Perfusion defects also may be seen in areas of lung consolidation, lung collapse, and vasoconstriction because of hypoxia (e.g., chronic obstructive pulmonary disease), among other reasons. Ventilation scanning is done to exclude such entities by imaging after the patient inhales ^{99m}Tc-diethylenetriamine-pentaacetic acid aerosol.

Several classification schemes have been proposed for interpreting V/Q scans. A widely accepted one is the system established in the Prospective Investigation of Pulmonary Embolism Diagnosis trials (PIOPED-I and -II), which evaluated the diagnostic usefulness of V/Q scanning for acute PE.[56] Two important conclusions can be drawn from the results of the PIOPED-I studies:

1. The likelihood of pulmonary embolus in patients with normal scans (4%) and in patients with low-probability scans plus a low clinical index of suspicion (4%) effectively excludes the diagnosis.
2. The likelihood of pulmonary embolus in patients with high-probability scans (87%) supports definitive treatment if there is no risk factor for anticoagulation.

LOWER EXTREMITY DUPLEX SONOGRAPHY

Because most pulmonary emboli arise from the legs and because treatment of PE is aimed at prevention of recurrent embolism, some practitioners initially perform leg duplex sonography to detect potential sources of recurrent emboli. Deep vein thrombosis of the leg is detected in patients with *suspected* PE less than 25% of the time.[57-59] Likewise, up to 50% of patients with *proven* PE have no sonographic evidence of proximal clot at the time of examination.[27] Sonography may be

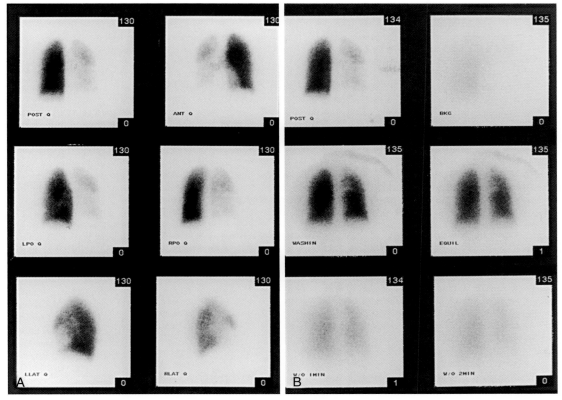

FIGURE 14-17　Ventilation-perfusion lung scan for pulmonary embolism. **A,** The perfusion scan in six projections shows large segmental defects in the right lower lobe. **B,** The ventilation scan in the posterior projection shows that defects are mismatched.

most useful in individuals with equivocal or low probability V/Q scans when clinical signs of deep venous thrombosis or risk factors for venous thromboembolic disease are present.

MAGNETIC RESONANCE IMAGING

Promising results have been obtained with MR angiography for PE diagnosis. The reported sensitivity and specificity of gadolinium-enhanced MR angiography is 77% to 100% and 95% to 98%, respectively.[60-62] However, multidetector row CT is more accurate than MRI because it has better spatial resolution and produces fewer artifacts.[36]

CATHETER ANGIOGRAPHY

For decades, pulmonary arteriography was considered the final arbiter in PE diagnosis, but this is no longer true. Multidetector row CT angiography is probably as accurate; in fact, even expert angiographers misdiagnosed isolated subsegmental emboli in up to one third of cases.[63-65] Because it is invasive, expensive, and requires experienced operators, pulmonary arteriography is now relegated to diagnosis of equivocal cases or planning for endovascular therapy.

The only reliable angiographic sign of acute PE is an intraluminal filling defect at least partially surrounded

by contrast material (Fig. 14-18). Secondary signs of an acute embolus include abrupt vessel cutoff, regional hypoperfusion, slow flow, pruning of vessels, and filling of collateral vessels. Emboli are often multiple and bilateral. They tend to lodge in the lower lobes more often than in the upper lobes.[66] Several other disorders can cause pulmonary artery obstruction, and some may be identified at angiography (e.g., chronic thromboembolic disease, tumor, arteritis)[67] (Fig. 14-19 and Box 14-5).

Treatment

MEDICAL THERAPY

Because many pulmonary emboli undergo spontaneous lysis and most patients survive a single episode of PE, the primary goal of treatment is prevention of recurrent PE and progression of thrombosis in the pulmonary arteries. Anticoagulation with intravenous unfractionated heparin followed by oral warfarin (Coumadin) for 3 to 6 months was the standard therapy for decades. Now, treatment begins with at least 5 days of a low molecular weight heparin (e.g., enoxaparin [Lovenox]) or the pentasaccharide *fondaparinux (Arixtra),* both given by subcutaneous injection without the need for monitoring[68,69] (see Chapter 3). The patient is often switched to Coumadin, which is continued for 3 months or more[70]

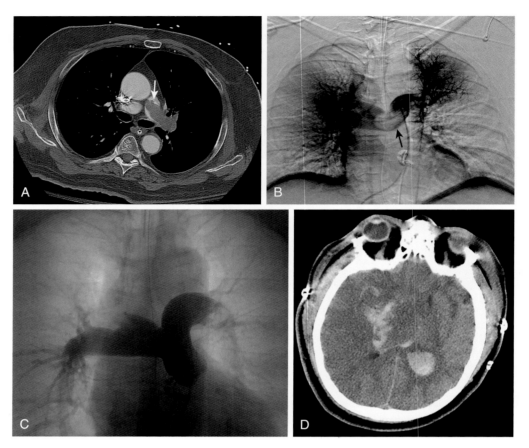

FIGURE 14-18   Massive pulmonary embolism treated with catheter-directed thrombolysis. **A,** Computed tomography (CT) angiography shows a near occlusive saddle embolus extending into both left *(arrow)* and right (not shown) main pulmonary arteries. **B,** These findings are confirmed at catheter angiography *(arrow)*. **C,** On-table thrombolysis was done with intrathrombic injection of tissue plasminogen activator (t-PA) and spinning a pigtail catheter in both pulmonary artery. The result is central clot disruption. The patient's hemodynamics improved markedly. However, within 12 hours, he suddenly became obtunded. **D,** Emergent head CT scan shows massive intracranial bleeding.

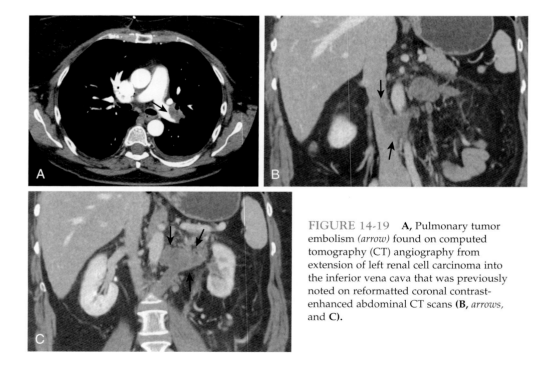

FIGURE 14-19   **A,** Pulmonary tumor embolism *(arrow)* found on computed tomography (CT) angiography from extension of left renal cell carcinoma into the inferior vena cava that was previously noted on reformatted coronal contrast-enhanced abdominal CT scans (**B,** *arrows,* and **C).**

(see Chapter 2). With proper treatment, the mortality rate from PE is reduced from about 30% to less than 5%.[70,71]

The standard management for patients with PE and hemodynamic instability is systemic thrombolysis with intravenous t-PA (100 mg given over 2 hours).[25]

ENDOVASCULAR THERAPY

Patients with a contraindication to anticoagulation, history of bleeding on anticoagulants, or who fail anticoagulation should have an IVC filter placed. As shown in the most rigorous trial to date (PREPIC), filter insertion significantly reduces the risk for further PE[72] (see Chapter 16). The reported recurrent embolism rate is about 3% to 6%.[72-74] The PREPIC investigators also noted an increased likelihood of subsequent lower extremity deep venous thrombosis in the filter group. The switch to retrievable IVC filters may help address this issue.

Aggressive endovascular therapy is usually reserved for patients with massive PE, hemodynamic instability, and (1) a contraindication to full dose systemic fibrinolysis, (2) moribund condition demanding immediate reperfusion, or (3) no response to systemic therapy.[75]

Catheter-directed thrombolysis, mechanical clot fragmentation, or thromboaspiration has been quite effective in selected patients with large clot burden ("massive" PE)[76-83] (see Fig. 14-18). The procedure usually entails pulse spray injection of t-PA (2 to 6 mg or more) into large clots followed or immediately preceded by rotation of a pigtail catheter within the thrombus for fragmentation (see Chapter 3). These maneuvers are continued until there is a significant positive clinical response (improved hemodynamics and oxygen saturation). Residual clot burden on follow-up angiograms may not reflect the actual benefit to the patient. When safe, it is wise to continue local intraarterial thrombolysis and full-dose anticoagulation when the patient returns to the intensive care unit.

Recent metaanalysis of published results of endovascular therapy for massive PE noted 87% overall clinical success (namely, hemodynamic stabilization, improvement in hypoxia, and immediate survival).[75] The overall major adverse event rate was 2.4%. The AngioJet thrombectomy device was associated with significantly more complications (often related to bradyarrhythmias), and therefore its use in this setting is not advisable.

SURGICAL THERAPY

Open pulmonary embolectomy has a substantial mortality rate and is usually a last resort in patients with cardiopulmonary collapse who do not respond rapidly to transcatheter techniques.[70,84]

Hemoptysis (Online Case 22)

Etiology

Mild to moderate hemoptysis is a common clinical problem that usually responds to treatment of the underlying illness. However, several diseases can produce massive hemoptysis that requires more aggressive therapy[15,85,86] (Box 14-6). A minority of individuals will have no identifiable cause for bleeding (so-called cryptogenic hemoptysis).[86] Patients with moderate but recurrent bleeding (e.g., in cystic fibrosis) also may present for angiographic diagnosis and transcatheter therapy. The following bleeding sources should be considered:

- The bronchial arteries are solely or partially responsible for massive hemoptysis in about 90% cases.
- Nonbronchial systemic collateral arteries have an ancillary or solitary role in 30% to 50% of cases.[87-89]
- The pulmonary arterial circulation is rarely the source of bleeding, with the following exceptions: *Rasmussen aneurysm* (classically, erosion of a tuberculosis cavity into a pulmonary artery branch); traumatic pseudoaneurysm (e.g., from a Swan-Ganz catheter); pulmonary AVM; eroding tumor.[90-92]

Clinical Features

To define "massive" hemoptysis, arbitrary 24-hour estimated bleeding rates (e.g., 300 mL) have been proposed. However, the blood loss volume is often difficult to quantitate, and clinical factors are often more important in determining the need for aggressive therapy. Hemoptysis is occasionally mistaken for brisk gastrointestinal or

---

BOX 14-6

CAUSES OF MASSIVE HEMOPTYSIS

- Infection
  - Tuberculosis
  - Fungus (e.g., mycetoma)
  - Chronic pneumonia
  - Abscess
- Cystic fibrosis
- Bronchiectasis or chronic bronchitis
- Neoplasm
- Trauma
  - Iatrogenic (e.g., pulmonary artery balloon catheter)
- Anticoagulant therapy
- Pulmonary arteriovenous malformation
- Vasculitis
- Pulmonary embolus
- Pulmonary hypertension
- Mitral stenosis
- Congestive heart failure
- Congenital
- Idiopathic (cryptogenic)

---

upper airway hemorrhage. Localization of the bleeding site is very helpful before arteriography. Serial changes in chest radiographs or CT scans may suggest the involved lobes. Fiberoptic bronchoscopy often is used to identify the site of bleeding, guide embolotherapy, and, in some cases, coagulate the culprit lesion.[85] Blood transfusion and correction of coagulation deficiencies should be underway at the time of angiography. Airway protection may be necessary if the bleeding is exuberant. Because of the remote possibility of spinal cord injury from bronchial artery embolization, a complete neurologic examination should be documented in the medical record.

Imaging

COMPUTED TOMOGRAPHY

In some centers, CT angiography is replacing flexible bronchoscopy in selected individuals with significant hemoptysis.[93] Properly performed CT angiography is extremely helpful before bronchial arteriography. It identifies ectopic bronchial artery origins, depicts nonbronchial systemic collateral vessels, and detects pulmonary artery origin for bleeding.[94-98] On raw axial images, the bronchial arteries appear as clusters of discrete enhancing dots near the midthoracic aorta that course in a craniocaudal direction (Fig. 14-20).

CATHETER ANGIOGRAPHY

The technique for bronchial arteriography is outlined earlier in this chapter. An empirical search is made for the bronchial arteries on the affected side (see Figs. 14-5 and 14-10). Bronchial arteries arise from the aorta and pass to the hila of the lungs, where they become tortuous and then give off numerous branches. If a bleeding source cannot be found, a descending thoracic aortogram with the catheter placed above the left subclavian artery to identify bronchial or nonbronchial system collateral vessels (especially intercostal or inferior phrenic arteries) may be helpful[99] (Fig. 14-21).

The classic findings with bronchial artery bleeding are enlargement of the main artery (>2 mm), hypervascularity, parenchymal stain, and bronchial to pulmonary artery shunting (Fig. 14-22). *Frank extravasation is uncommon;* it need not be present to warrant embolization. It is critical to look for small branches to the anterior spinal artery, which usually arise from the proximal portion of the vessel and take a characteristic hairpin turn as they pass superiorly and then inferiorly into the anterior spinal cord in the midline (see Fig. 14-11).

After one or more abnormal bronchial arteries is identified and embolized (see later discussion), potential nonbronchial systemic collaterals should be studied (Fig. 14-23 on p. 461). The more common sources are[88,99,100]:

- Internal thoracic (mammary) artery
- Thyrocervical branch of the subclavian artery
- Lateral branches of the subclavian or axillary artery
- Intercostal arteries
- Inferior phrenic artery

As a rule, collaterals come from vessels in proximity to the bleeding site (e.g., lower lobe lesions may be fed by an inferior phrenic artery). Rarely, collateral vessels arising on the opposite side are responsible for bleeding. If neither a bronchial nor nonbronchial systemic arterial source can be found, a pulmonary angiogram is performed to exclude a pulmonary artery lesion (Fig. 14-24).

Treatment

BRONCHIAL ARTERY EMBOLIZATION

PATIENT SELECTION Embolotherapy is the first-line treatment for massive hemoptysis or recurrent intractable hemoptysis.[101,102] Presence of a major spinal artery or radiculomedullary branch from the target artery is considered a contraindication to embolotherapy by some interventionalists, but others perform embolization if a microcatheter can be negotiated well beyond such a vessel.

TECHNIQUE If the diagnostic catheter (without side holes) can be advanced deep into the artery, embolotherapy is performed directly without a significant risk of refluxing material into the aorta. Usually, however,

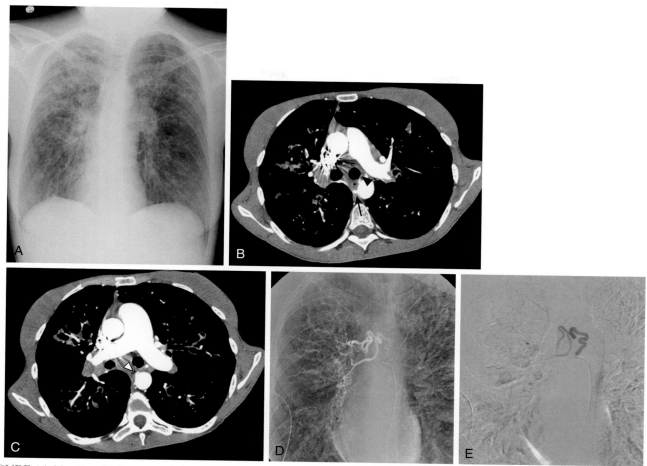

FIGURE 14-20 Bronchial artery embolization for massive hemoptysis from cystic fibrosis. **A,** Chest radiography shows classic pattern of widespread cystic bronchiectasis and large bilateral pulmonary arteries. Bronchoscopy identified active bleeding from the right upper lobe bronchus. **B** and **C,** High-resolution chest computed tomography (CT) shows several possible bronchial artery origins *(arrowheads)* from the descending thoracic aorta. With guidance from the CT images, the responsible vessel was catheterized quickly. Through the 5 Fr catheter, a coaxial microcatheter was advanced well into the bronchial artery **(D).** Note massively enlarged bronchial artery and prominent hypervascularity. **E,** Finally, the vessel was embolized with 300- to 500-μm Embospheres to stasis.

a coaxial microcatheter system is negotiated well into the bronchial artery beyond intercostal or mediastinal branches (Fig. 14-25 on p. 462).

Although a variety of materials has been used for bronchial artery embolization, the most popular agents are polyvinyl alcohol particles (PVA), microspheres (e.g., Embospheres), and Gelfoam pledgets[103-107] (see Chapter 3). PVA and microspheres usually cause long-term occlusion of distal arteries and prevent recruitment of collateral vessels that may lead to rebleeding. Particle sizes between 250 and 700 μm are used. Smaller particles could pass through small spinal artery branches. Patients with large bronchopulmonary artery shunts may require larger sizes to avoid pulmonary infarction or systemic embolization through small arteriovenous shunts.[108] Gelfoam pledgets also have been used successfully by some practitioners, although this material is resorbed over a period of weeks.

A bottle of PVA particles or microspheres is prepared as a slurry made with contrast material (see Video 3-18). A slow and steady injection is made with continuous visualization under fluoroscopy until blood flow is sluggish. Injection is stopped promptly if reflux along the microcatheter is detected. In addition, delayed filling of branches to the anterior spinal artery should be continuously sought. Sometimes, small pledgets of Gelfoam are deployed to complete the embolization. Coils should *not* be used unless they are deposited in side branches before particulate embolization to prevent occlusion of parietal vessels (e.g., intercostal portion of bronchointercostal trunk) (see Fig. 14-23).

In almost 5% of cases, the bleeding source is the pulmonary artery. If CT angiography was not recently done, catheter pulmonary arteriography must be performed if no systemic arterial source is identified. When present, the usual cause is a peripheral aneurysm or pseudoaneurysm.[97]

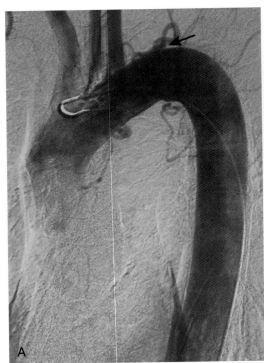
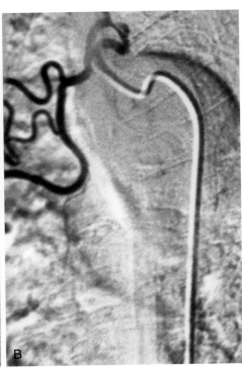

FIGURE 14-21 Unusual origin of a bronchial artery. **A,** Right posterior oblique thoracic aortogram shows an enlarged vessel arising from the upper surface of the descending thoracic aorta *(arrow).* **B,** Selective catheterization proves this vessel is a bronchial artery supplying bleeding in the right lung.

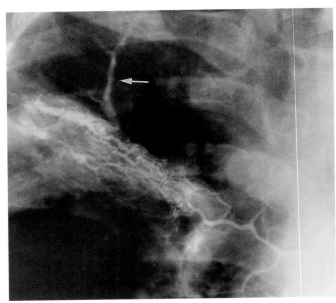

FIGURE 14-22 Right bronchial arteriogram in a patient with massive hemoptysis from actinomycosis. Characteristic findings include bronchial artery enlargement, hypervascularity, and shunting to the pulmonary artery branches *(arrow).* The parenchymal stain is prominent.

RESULTS Bronchial artery embolization is accomplished in more than 90% of cases. Technical failure usually results from an inability to identify bronchial arteries or to successfully catheterize such vessels. Bleeding stops in about 70% to 95% of cases.[15,100-109] Embolotherapy is equally effective when the cause of bleeding is obscure.[86] On the whole, better immediate results have been achieved with PVA and particles than with Gelfoam pledgets. About 20% to 30% of patients suffer recurrent bleeding.[105,111] The usual explanations are incomplete initial embolization, recruitment of collateral vessels, recanalization of embolized vessels, unidentified bleeding arteries, or progression of disease. If rebleeding occurs, a second trial of embolotherapy is worthwhile. The previously treated sites are again studied, and other bronchial and nonbronchial sources of hemorrhage are sought. In some series, early or late rebleeding is particularly common in patients with cystic fibrosis.[107]

COMPLICATIONS Some patients develop a postembolization syndrome consisting of fever, chest wall pain, and, rarely, dysphagia. Symptoms may be severe and can last for up to 1 week. Complications from embolotherapy occur in about 2% to 5% of cases and include nontarget embolization and bronchial or esophageal necrosis. There is a risk of pulmonary infarction if bronchial embolization is performed in the presence of pulmonary artery (or branch) occlusion.[112] The most dreaded but extraordinarily rare complication is transverse myelitis from inadvertent embolization of a branch to the anterior spinal artery.[113]

Embolization of a pulmonary artery aneurysm or pseudoaneurysm is accomplished using coils to cover the neck of the aneurysm[109] (see Fig. 14-24). Some of these cases also require concomitant embolization of bronchial artery branches that may also feed the vascular lesion.

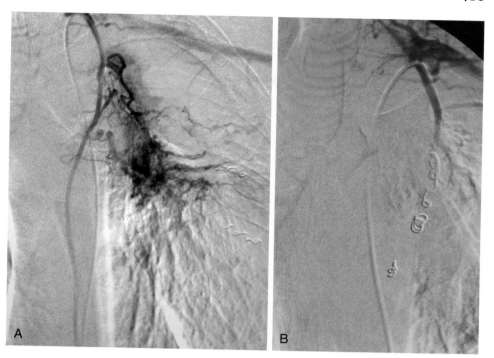

FIGURE 14-23 Nonbronchial systemic collateral arteries. **A,** The left internal thoracic artery supplies numerous hilar vessels. **B,** The distal artery was embolized with coils to prevent nontarget embolization of polyvinyl alcohol particles, which were then delivered to pulmonary branches to complete the occlusion.

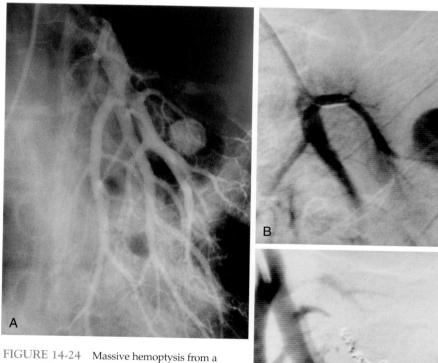

FIGURE 14-24 Massive hemoptysis from a ruptured Rasmussen aneurysm in a patient with disseminated tuberculosis. No bronchial or nonbronchial systemic collateral arteries were identified as a source of the bleeding. **A,** A pseudoaneurysm of a lingular branch of the left pulmonary artery is identified. **B,** Selective catheterization of the feeding branch shows the aneurysm neck. **C,** Embolization with coils across the neck of the pseudoaneurysm led to complete occlusion.

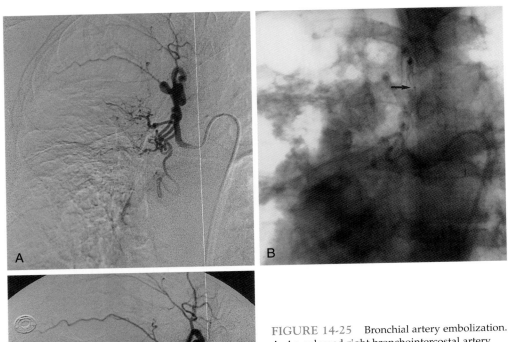

FIGURE 14-25 Bronchial artery embolization. **A,** An enlarged right bronchointercostal artery feeds hypervascular vessels in the right hilum. **B,** Through the 5-Fr Shetty catheter, a 3-Fr microcatheter was placed coaxially into the bronchial artery beyond the intercostal branches (*arrow* indicates the tip). **C,** After embolization with 300- to 500-μm polyvinyl alcohol particles and Gelfoam pledgets, the bronchial branches are occluded but the intercostal arteries are preserved.

SURGICAL THERAPY

An operation to stop bleeding is performed if one or two trials of bronchial artery embolization are unsuccessful. Elective surgery is performed after bleeding is controlled in patients who require definitive treatment of disease.

OTHER DISORDERS

Chronic Thromboembolic Pulmonary Hypertension (CTPH) (Online Case 100)

Almost 50% of patients who survive an episode of acute PE experience total clot lysis, usually within 1 to 3 weeks after the event.[114] About half the time, however, emboli do not completely resolve. Most patients maintain or regain normal gas exchange and pulmonary hemodynamics. However, chronic pulmonary artery hypertension eventually develops in a small fraction (about 0.2%) of individuals as a result of one or more episodes of incompletely resolved PE.[115-119] Symptoms appear many years after the first insult. No specific coagulation abnormalities have been identified in this group. The pathophysiology of the disorder is not related simply to critical luminal obstruction of pulmonary artery branches, but in fact is largely a small vessel vasculopathy that develops in previously unaffected portions of the pulmonary arterial bed.[115] Patients with CTPH usually complain of progressive exertional dyspnea and fatigue. Almost half of them have no documented history of PE or lower extremity deep venous thrombosis.[118,120]

Imaging studies are critical to make the specific diagnosis, determine the extent and sites of disease, and quantify the hemodynamic compromise.[121] Lung V/Q scanning is still mandatory to distinguish CTPH from other causes of global pulmonary artery disease.[115] The

> **BOX 14-7**
>
> ### COMMON COMPUTED TOMOGRAPHY FINDINGS IN PULMONARY HYPERTENSION
>
> - Central pulmonary artery dilation (>29 mm)
> - Globally small peripheral vessels ("mosaic" perfusion pattern)
> - Enlarged bronchial arteries
> - Right ventricular dilation or hypertrophy
> - Right atrial enlargement
> - Contrast reflux into the inferior vena cava or hepatic veins

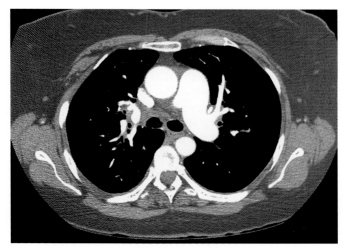

FIGURE 14-26 Chronic pulmonary thromboembolic disease on computed tomography angiography. Bilateral recanalization with narrowed lumens and thickened walls is characteristic.

exam shows multiple bilateral segmental mismatched defects in most patients, although the scan almost always underestimates the extent of disease.[122,123] High-resolution helical CT and (to a lesser extent) gadolinium-enhanced MR angiography are extremely accurate in differentiating this disorder from other causes of chronic pulmonary artery disease and in postoperative follow-up[124-126] (Box 14-7). The spectrum of findings at CT angiography include complete vessel occlusion, vessel narrowing, peripheral crescentic filling defects, diffuse wall thickening, and webs or flaps[53,127-129] (Fig. 14-26). A "mosaic" parenchymal pattern also is typical. The right heart chambers and central pulmonary arteries are markedly enlarged, and prominent mediastinal bronchial artery collateral vessels are seen.

Catheter angiography is still performed before surgery. The findings are characteristic and differ from those of acute PE, idiopathic pulmonary hypertension, or Takayasu arteritis (TA).[130] The disease is virtually always bilateral. The main pulmonary arteries are dilated. Chronic, partially resolved emboli produce webs, luminal irregularities, "pouches," segments of abrupt vessel narrowing, and frank obstructions (Fig. 14-27). The mean pulmonary artery pressure typically is in the range of 35 to 60 mm Hg, and pulmonary vascular resistance is markedly elevated.

CTPH is generally progressive and often fatal. The only successful treatment is pulmonary thromboendarterectomy, which leads to excellent hemodynamic, angiographic, and functional improvement in most patients.[131] Permanent placement of an IVC filter is also recommended. Long-term therapy with certain prostanoids (e.g., epoprostenol [Flolan]), phosphodiesterase-5 inhibitors [sildenafil]) or endothelin receptor antagonists (e.g., bosentan) has shown significant clinical benefit in inoperable patients or as a bridge to surgery.[115]

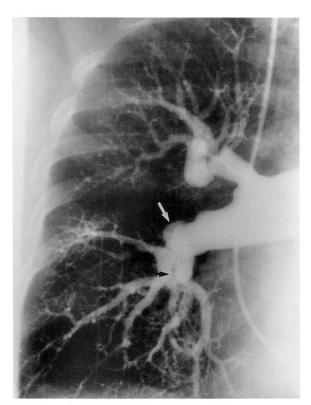

FIGURE 14-27 Chronic pulmonary thromboembolic disease. The classic findings include webs *(black arrow)*, pouches *(white arrow)*, mural irregularity, branch occlusions, areas of diminished perfusion, and central pulmonary artery dilation.

Idiopathic Pulmonary Hypertension

Idiopathic pulmonary artery hypertension (PAH, formerly known as *primary pulmonary hypertension*) is a rare entity in which pulmonary artery pressure is elevated significantly (mean pressure >25 mm Hg, pulmonary capillary wedge pressure <15 mm Hg, and PVR >3 Wood units) without evidence for an underlying cause[132] (see Box 14-1). The cause is unknown; however, a defect in the gene encoding for the bone morphogenetic protein receptor type 2 is the cause of familial PAH and responsible for some sporadic cases[132,133] The common pathologic alteration is widespread thickening or fibrosis of small pulmonary arteries. Idiopathic PAH is more common in women than men, and most present in the fourth decade of life. Typical symptoms are dyspnea, fatigue, chest pain, and syncope. The disease often is progressive and fatal.

Lung V/Q scans usually are interpreted as normal or low probability.[134,135] CT and MR images show a pattern similar to the various of causes of pulmonary hypertension (see Box 14-7) but are helpful in excluding other reasons for the clinical picture.[136,137] When catheter angiography is performed, it shows high pulmonary artery pressures, dilation of the central pulmonary arteries, and widespread tortuosity and severe tapering of distal arterial branches; acute or organized thrombus usually is not seen. Angiograms may be normal in a small percentage of patients.

A variety of drugs are available for palliative treatment. Current standard medical therapy for patients with severe symptoms is continuous IV infusion of epoprostenol (Flolan). Individuals with moderate disability may respond to oral phosphodiesterase-5 inhibitor (e.g., sildenafil) or antagonist to the potent vasoconstrictor and mitogen *endothelin-1* (e.g., bosentan or ambrisentan).[132] Cure is only achieved by lung transplantation.

Vasculitis

A wide variety of vasculitides may attack the pulmonary arteries[138-140] (Box 14-8). *TA* is an inflammatory vasculitis of large- and medium-sized elastic arteries[141,142] (see Chapter 1). The classic disease is seen in young to middle-aged women. Although involvement of the thoracic and abdominal aorta is almost universal, the pulmonary arteries are affected in about 50% of cases.[143] Pulmonary TA is usually bilateral and most commonly targets the segmental branches. Imaging shows wall thickening and enhancement, luminal stenoses and frank occlusions, or aneurysms and patchy areas of parenchymal low attenuation[144] (Fig. 14-28). Both angioplasty and stents have been employed in treating symptomatic patients with chronic pulmonary TA.[145]

The collagen-vascular diseases are associated with a pulmonary vasculitis with fibrotic proliferation in small pulmonary vessels.[146] Pulmonary hypertension may result.

Behçet disease is a multisystem disorder characterized by aphthous ulcers of the mouth and genital area and ocular involvement[147,148] (see Chapter 1). A small percentage of

individuals with Behçet disease (particularly young men) develop solitary or multiple hilar or parahilar pulmonary artery aneurysms that are prone to thrombosis or fatal rupture.[149-151] Endovascular therapy is undertaken to emergently treat or prevent aneurysm rupture.[152-155] Pulmonary artery stenoses have also been reported in this entity (Box 14-9).

Aneurysms

Aneurysms and pseudoaneurysms of the pulmonary arteries have many causes[156,157] (Box 14-10; see also Fig. 14-24). Dilation of the main pulmonary artery usually is seen with left-to-right shunts (*Eisenmenger physiology*) or pulmonary artery hypertension. Post-stenotic dilation from pulmonary valve or root disease can mimic an

---

BOX 14-8

CAUSES OF PULMONARY VASCULITIS

- Takayasu arteritis
- Connective tissue disorders
  - Scleroderma
  - Rheumatoid arthritis
  - Systemic lupus erythematosus
- Behçet disease
- Wegener granulomatosis
- Allergic angiitis and granulomatosis

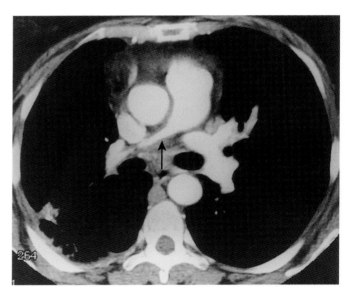

FIGURE 14-28 Takayasu arteritis of the right pulmonary artery. Notice the long, smooth luminal narrowing and wall thickening.

BOX 14-9

CAUSES OF PULMONARY ARTERY STENOSIS

- Chronic thromboembolic disease
- Neoplasm
  - Extravascular (e.g., lung cancer)
- Mediastinal lymphadenopathy
- Inflammatory disease
  - Fibrosing mediastinitis
- Vasculitis
  - Takayasu arteritis
  - Behçet disease
- Radiation therapy
- Congenital disorders

BOX 14-10

CAUSES OF PULMONARY ARTERY ANEURYSMS AND PSEUDOANEURYSMS

- Infection (mycotic)
  - Cavitary tuberculosis (Rasmussen aneurysm)
  - Septic emboli
  - Necrotizing pneumonia
  - Syphilis
- Trauma
  - Pulmonary artery catheterization
- Pulmonary artery hypertension
- Vasculitis
  - Behçet disease
  - Takayasu arteritis
  - Connective tissue disorders
- Noninflammatory vasculopathies
  - Marfan syndrome
- Tumor
- Congenital disorders

aneurysm. Central right or left pulmonary artery aneurysms usually are caused by congenital disorders or vasculitis (e.g., *Behçet disease*). Multiple aneurysms are typical with infection (e.g., septic emboli) and arteritis.[158,159] Large pulmonary artery aneurysms are often incidental findings on chest radiographs or CT scans; on occasion, they are detected when hemoptysis, dyspnea, or chest pain develops. Some aneurysms can be managed successfully with embolization.[90]

Arterial rupture with pseudoaneurysm formation is a rare complication of Swan-Ganz catheter placement.[91,160,161] Several mechanisms of injury have been postulated, including vessel perforation by the catheter tip and over-inflation of the wedge balloon. Those pseudoaneurysms usually are found in the right middle or lower lobe arteries. The first clue to the diagnosis is hemoptysis or a new lung mass identified on imaging studies. When the anatomy is favorable, transcatheter embolization is the treatment of choice and is almost always curative.[152,162,163] The mortality rate without treatment is extremely high.

Bronchial artery aneurysms are rare lesions that may be congenital or caused by inflammation, degeneration, or trauma. Bronchial arteries may also become markedly enlarged when acting as collateral circulation in patients with pulmonary artery hypertension (e.g., CTPH). Rupture into the mediastinum or an airway is the most serious consequence. Endovascular treatment with a variety of agents has been successful.[164-167]

Arteriovenous Malformations (Online Case 48)

Pulmonary AVMs may occur sporadically, but up to 80% to 90% are found in patients with *hereditary hemorrhagic telangiectasia (HHT)*, formerly known as Osler-Weber-Rendu syndrome.[168-170] HHT is an autosomal dominant genetic disorder marked by telangiectasias of the mouth and telangiectasias or AVMs of the gastrointestinal tract, brain, liver, and lung (see Chapter 1). About 30% to 40% of patients with HHT have pulmonary AVMs, and about 60% have multiple lesions.[171,72] Spontaneous epistaxis is the hallmark of the disease. Family members of affected individuals should be evaluated, because about one third of them will also have pulmonary AVMs. Screening is done with contrast (echo-bubble) echocardiography, arterial blood gas measurements, and helical CT scanning.[92]

About 85% of pulmonary AVMs are *simple* (single segmental arterial supply), and 5% to 10% are *complex* (multiple segmental arterial supply).[173-175] They are most commonly found in the lower lobes. *Diffuse* pulmonary AVMs and acquired lesions (e.g., in setting of hepatopulmonary syndrome or trauma) account for the remaining cases.[169,175,176] The AVM causes a right-to-left shunt and provides an open pathway between the venous and arterial circulations. Patients may present in early middle age with dyspnea, fatigue, hemoptysis, hemothorax, stroke, or brain abscess. However, AVMs often are found incidentally on chest radiographs. The primary rationale for obliterating them is prevention of devastating neurologic complications.

CT angiography is exquisitely sensitive for detecting lesions that require treatment (≥3 mm diameter feeding artery)[177] (Fig. 14-29). Pulmonary angiography

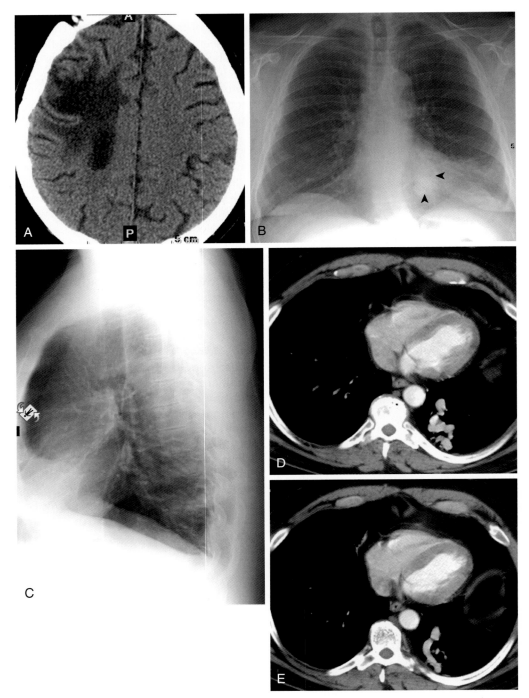

FIGURE 14-29   Symptomatic, complex pulmonary arteriovenous malformation in a patient with hereditary hemorrhagic telangiectasia. **A,** Head computed tomography (CT) documents old bland stroke with no apparent risk factors. Frontal **(B)** and lateral **(C)** chest radiographs show the well-defined lobular mass at the left lung base *(arrowheads).* **D** and **E,** Chest CT scans confirm the arteriovenous malformations, although the vascular anatomy was confusing.

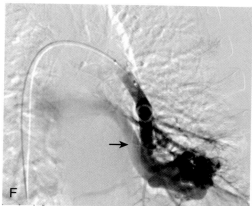

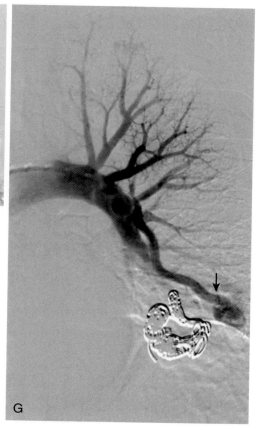

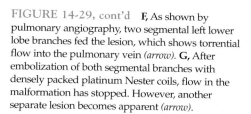

FIGURE 14-29, cont'd   **F,** As shown by pulmonary angiography, two segmental left lower lobe branches fed the lesion, which shows torrential flow into the pulmonary vein *(arrow).* **G,** After embolization of both segmental branches with densely packed platinum Nester coils, flow in the malformation has stopped. However, another separate lesion becomes apparent *(arrow).*

is performed for confirmation and embolotherapy, which is the treatment of choice. Pulmonary artery pressure should be measured; pulmonary hypertension is not uncommon. Selective arteriography in multiple projections is necessary to map out the arterial supply. Great care must be taken to avoid allowing room air into the catheter after it is in a selective position in the segmental artery feeding the malformation. Guidewires are always withdrawn from catheters in a saline bath to prevent even minute air bubbles from escaping into the systemic circulation. Angiography shows one or more dilated segmental arteries (often with several subsegmental branches) feeding an aneurysmally dilated sac with rapid venous outflow (see Fig. 14-29 and Fig. 14-30).

The technique popularized by White utilizes a long guiding catheter (7-Fr Lumax device) along with a 5-Fr diagnostic catheter.[172] Patients are fully heparinized and receive antibiotic prophylaxis with cephazolin. Many devices have been used for occlusion, including coils and detachable balloons. Coils are chosen to be at least 1 to 2 mm larger than the artery being embolized and should be deposited as close as possible to the aneurysmal enlargement near the nidus of the malformation. To ensure a stable coil nest, the first coil is partially deployed in a small sidebranch ("anchor technique"). Alternatively, the first coil is very oversized and composed of stainless steel with high radial force ("scaffold technique"). Nester or tornado platinum coils are good choices for the remainder of the vascular occlusion. These long, highly radiopaque coils can be packed densely into the feeding vessel to prevent recanalization.[179] Recently, the Amplatzer vascular occluder has been used in this setting[180] (see Chapter 3). While initially effective in most cases, late recanalization has been reported.[181] In the minority of individuals with very high flow or dilated arteries, embolization may be done through the endhole of an inflated occlusion balloon. Patients with numerous lesions often require multiple treatment sessions.

The definition of success is controversial. Some experts require near complete fibrosis of the aneurysm sac on follow-up non-enhanced CT; others claim partial success with aneurysm sac size shrinkage to less than 30% and reduction in feeding artery diameter to less than 3 mm.[168,169] Success ranges from 75% to 97%.* Reasons for delayed failure include recanalization of

*See references 168, 169, 174, 178, 182, 183.

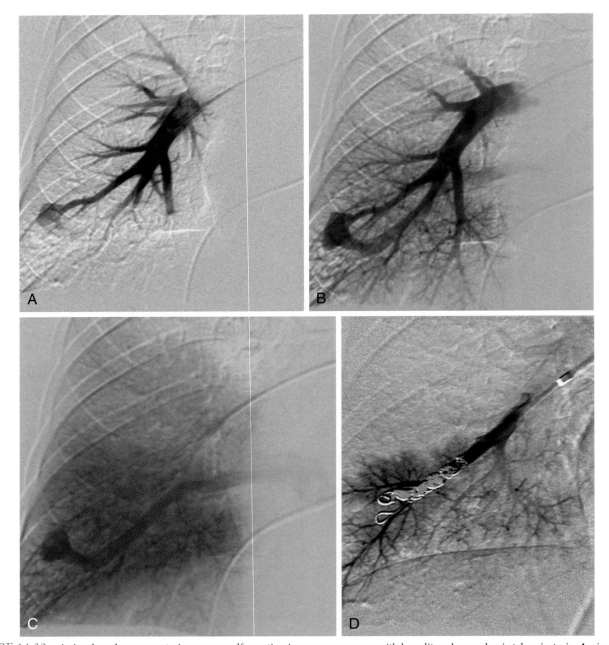

FIGURE 14-30   A simple pulmonary arteriovenous malformation in a young woman with hereditary hemorrhagic telangiectasia. **A,** single enlarged segmental artery feeds the lesion. **B** and **C,** Later phases of angiogram show rapid washout into a huge draining pulmonary vein. **D,** The lesion is occluded with macrocoils.

embolized vessels, visualization of unrecognized feeding vessels in complex AVMs, and development of bronchial artery collaterals that enter the artery beyond the embolization site. A postembolization syndrome with fever or pleuritic chest pain is common (about 15% of cases). Serious complications, including paradoxical embolization of coils or air (which may produce coronary ischemia, transient ischemic attack, or stroke), occur in less than 5% of procedures. The likelihood of major stroke is estimated at 0.5%.[184]

Long-term follow-up CT imaging is important to ensure permanent lesion closure. It is also reported that at least 25% of treated patients will demonstrate subsequent growth of initially undetectable AVMs or enlargement of the feeding artery to previously small lesions that now warrant treatment.[169] A leading expert

in the field recommends noncontrast chest CT 1 year after treatment and every 3 to 5 years thereafter.[169,172] Earlier imaging is mandatory if symptoms develop or pregnancy is planned.

Inflammatory Diseases and Neoplasms

Fibrosing (chronic sclerosing) mediastinitis is a longstanding inflammatory process that can present as a primary (idiopathic) or secondary disorder (usually related to previous *Histoplasma capsulatum* infection).[185] The interventionalist might encounter patients with the focal (rather than diffuse) type of the disease, in which a localized (and sometimes calcified) mass causes obstruction of pulmonary vessels, the superior vena cava, airways, or the esophagus (Fig. 14-31). Endovascular

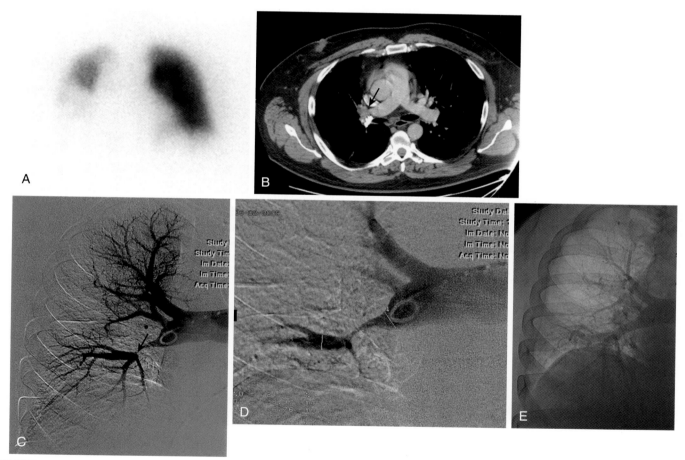

FIGURE 14-31 Pulmonary artery obstruction from fibrosing mediastinitis. **A,** Lung perfusion scan shows markedly diminished blood flow to the right lower lobe. **B,** Chest computed tomography reveals a calcified extrinsic mass impinging on the descending right pulmonary artery, a finding that was confirmed on right pulmonary arteriography *(arrow)* **(C). D,** Measurements of adjacent normal vessel diameter and stenosis length are made, and then a balloon expandable stent was inserted. **E,** Final arteriography shows a widely patent vessel. The patient's exercise tolerance improved markedly soon afterward.

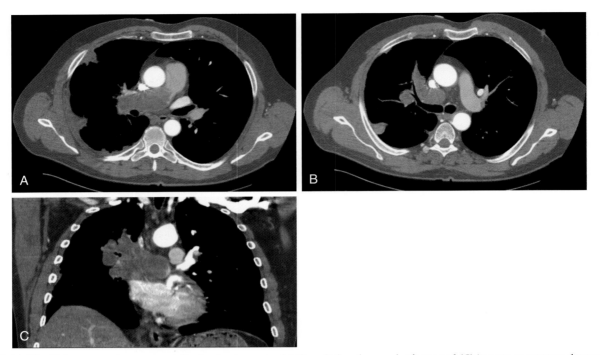

FIGURE 14-32   Pulmonary artery sarcoma. Contrast-enhanced axial **(A** and **B)** and coronal reformatted **(C)** images on computed tomography show tumor extending throughout the main and right pulmonary artery.

stents are sometimes used to relieve symptoms such as dyspnea.

Lung neoplasms are associated with vascular encasement, displacement, or obstruction. Stents and stent-grafts have been used to improve pulmonary artery blood flow in selected symptomatic patients with central obstructions, usually as a palliative measure. Radiofrequency ablation has shown promise in treating patients with unresectable primary and secondary malignancies of the lung (see Chapter 24).

Primary and secondary malignancies of the pulmonary arteries are extremely rare. The most common primary tumor is *pulmonary artery sarcoma*, which usually arises in the main, right, or left pulmonary artery and often is contained within the lumen[186,187] (Fig. 14-32). Differentiation from bland thrombus is occasionally difficult, although prominent expansion of the vessel suggests tumor rather than bland clot. Transvenous biopsy has been used to make the diagnosis.[152,188] Surgical resection with pulmonary artery reconstruction is rarely curative.[189,190]

References

1. Velling TE, Brennan FJ, Hall LD. Pulmonary angiography with use of the 5-F Omni flush catheter: a safe and efficient procedure with a common catheter. *J Vasc Interv Radiol* 2000;**11**:1005.
2. Grollman Jr JH. Pulmonary arteriography. *Cardiovasc Intervent Radiol* 1992;**15**:166.
3. Rosen G, Kowalik KJ, Ganguli S, et al. The Hunter pulmonary angiography catheter for a brachiocephalic vein approach. *Cardiovasc Intervent Radiol* 2005;**29**:997.
4. Grossman W. Cardiac catheterization. In: Braunwald E, editor. *Heart Disease: A Textbook of Cardiovascular Medicine.* 4th ed. Philadelphia: WB Saunders. 1992. p. 180.
5. Simonneau G, Galie N, Rubin LJ, et al. Clinical classification of pulmonary hypertension. *J Am Coll Cardiol* 2004;**43** (Suppl. 1):5S.

6. Stein PD, Athanasoulis C, Alavi A, et al. Complications and validity of pulmonary angiography in acute pulmonary embolism. *Circulation* 1992;**85**:462.
7. Hofmann LV, Lee DS, Gupta A, et al. Safety and hemodynamic effects of pulmonary angiography in patients with pulmonary hypertension: 10-year single-center experience. *AJR Am J Roentgenol* 2004;**183**:779.
8. Collins P, editor. Embryology and development. In: Williams PL, Bannister LH, Berry MM, et al, editors. *Gray's anatomy,* 38th ed. New York: Churchill Livingstone; 1995. p. 312.
9. Gabella G, editor. Cardiovascular system. In: Williams PL, Bannister LH, Berry MM, et al, editors. *Gray's anatomy,* 38th ed. New York: Churchill Livingstone; 1995. p. 1504.
10. Gabella G, editor. Cardiovascular system. In: Williams PL, Bannister LH, Berry MM, et al, editors. *Gray's anatomy,* 38th ed. New York: Churchill Livingstone; 1995. p. 1574.

11. Fishman AP. The pulmonary circulation. In: Fishman AP, editor. *Pulmonary diseases and disorders.* 3rd ed. New York: McGraw-Hill, 1998. p. 1233.

12. Tadavarthy SM, Klugman J, Castaneda-Zuniga WR, et al. Systemic-to-pulmonary collaterals in pathological states. A review. *Radiology* 1982;**144**:55.

13. Cauldwell EW, Siekert RG, Linninger RE, et al. The bronchial arteries: an anatomic study of 150 human cadavers. *Surg Gynecol Obstet* 1948;**86**:395.

14. Liebow AA. Patterns of origin and distribution of the major bronchial arteries in man. *J Anat* 1965;**117**:19.

15. Uflacker R, Kaemmerer A, Picon PD, et al. Bronchial artery embolization in the management of hemoptysis: technical aspects and long-term results. *Radiology* 1985;**157**:637.

16. Kardjiev V, Symeonov A, Chankov I. Etiology, pathogenesis, and prevention of spinal cord lesions in selective angiography of the bronchial and intercostal arteries. *Radiology* 1974;**112**:81.

17. Shamji MR, Maziak DE, Shamji FM, et al. Circulation of the spinal cord: an important consideration for thoracic surgeons. *Ann Thorac Surg* 2003;**76**:315.

18. Rose AG. Diseases of the pulmonary circulation. In: Silver MD, Gotlieb AI, Schoen FJ, editors. *Cardiovascular pathology.* New York: Churchill Livingstone; 2001. p. 166.

19. Castaner E, Gallardo X, Rimola J, et al. Congenital and acquired pulmonary artery anomalies in the adult. Radiologic overview. *Radiographics* 2006;**26**:349.

20. Ellis K. Developmental abnormalities in the systemic blood supply to the lungs. *AJR Am J Roentginol* 1991;**156**:669.

21. Berrocal T, Madrid C, Novo S, et al. Congenital anomalies of the tracheobronchial tree, lung, and mediastinum: embryology, radiology, and pathology. *Radiographics* 2004;**24**:e17.

22. Lee K-H, Sung K-B, Yoon H-K, et al. Transcatheter arterial embolization of pulmonary sequestration in neonates: long-term follow-up results. *J Vasc Interv Radiol* 2003;**14**:363.

23. Zylak CJ, Eyler WR, Spizarny DL, et al. Developmental lung anomalies in the adult: radiologic-pathologic correlation. *Radiographics* 2002;**22**:S25.

24. Lois JF, Gomes AS, Smith DC, et al. Systemic-to-pulmonary collateral vessels and shunts: treatment with embolization. *Radiology* 1988;**169**:671.

25. Tapson VF. Acute pulmonary embolism. *N Engl J Med* 2008;**358**:1037.

26. Huisman MV, Bueller HR, ten Cate JW, et al. Unexpected high prevalence of silent pulmonary embolism in patients with deep venous thrombosis. *Chest* 1989;**95**:498.

27. Goldhaber SZ, Visani L, DeRosa M. Acute pulmonary embolism: clinical outcomes in the International Cooperative Pulmonary Embolism Registry (ICOPER). *Lancet* 1999;**353**:1386.

28. Carlson JL, Kelley MA, Duff A, et al. The clinical course of pulmonary embolism. *New Engl J Med* 1992;**326**:1240.

29. Remy-Jardin M, Louvegny S, Remy J, et al. Acute central thromboembolic disease: posttherapeutic follow-up with spiral CT angiography. *Radiology* 1997;**203**:173.

30. Nijkeuter M, Hovens MMC, Davidson BL, et al. Resolution of thromboemboli in patients with acute pulmonary embolism: a systematic review. *Chest* 2006;**129**:192.

31. Rossi SE, Goodman PC, Franquet T. Nonthrombotic pulmonary emboli. *AJR Am J Roentgenol* 2000;**174**:1499.

32. Brecher CW, Lang EV. Tumor thromboembolism masquerading as bland pulmonary embolism. *J Vasc Interv Radiol* 2004;**15**:293.

33. Vesely T. Air embolism during insertion of central venous catheters. *J Vasc Interv Radiol* 2001;**12**:1291.

34. Stein PD, Hull RD, Patel KC, et al. D-dimer for the exclusion of acute venous thrombosis and pulmonary embolism: a systematic review. *Ann Intern Med* 2004;**140**:589.

35. Di Nisio M, Squizzato A, Rutjes AW, et al. Diagnostic accuracy of D-dimer test for exclusion of venous thromboembolism: a systematic review. *J Thromb Haemost* 2007;**5**:296.

36. Schoepf UJ, Costello P. CT angiography for diagnosis of pulmonary embolism: state of the art. *Radiology* 2004;**230**:329.

37. Kuriakose J, Patel S. Acute pulmonary embolism. *Radiol Clin North Am* 2010;**48**:31.

38. van Rossum AB, Pattynama PMT, Ton ER, et al. Pulmonary embolism: validation of spiral CT angiography in 149 patients. *Radiology* 1996;**201**:467.

39. Teigen CL, Maus TP, Sheedy II PF, et al. Pulmonary embolism: diagnosis with contrast enhanced electron beam CT and comparison with pulmonary angiography. *Radiology* 1995;**194**:313.

40. Goodman LR, Curtin JJ, Mewissen MW, et al. Detection of pulmonary embolism in patients with unresolved clinical and scintigraphic diagnosis: helical CT versus angiography. *AJR Am J Roentgenol* 1995;**164**:1369.

41. Stein PD, Fowler SE, Goodman LR, et al. Multidetector computed tomography for acute pulmonary embolism. *N Engl J Med* 2006;354:2317.

42. Schoepf U, Holzknecht N, Helmberger TK, et al. Subsegmental pulmonary emboli: improved detection with thin-collimation multi-detector row spiral CT. *Radiology* 2002;**222**:483.

43. Raptopoulos V, Boiselle PM. Multi-detector row spiral CT pulmonary angiography: comparison with single-detector row spiral CT. *Radiology* 2001;**221**:606.

44. Patel S, Kazerooni EA, Cascade PN. Pulmonary embolism. optimization of small pulmonary artery visualization at mult-detector row CT. *Radiology* 2003;**227**:455.

45. Goodman LR, Lipchik RJ, Kuzo RS, et al. Subsequent pulmonary embolism: risk after negative helical CT pulmonary angiogram—prospective comparison with scintigraphy. *Radiology* 2000;**215**:535.

46. Garg K, Sieler H, Welsh CH, et al. Clinical validity of helical CT being interpreted as negative for pulmonary embolism: implications for patient treatment. *AJR Am J Roentgenol* 1999;**172**:1627.

47. Tillie-Leblond I, Mastora I, Radenne F, et al. Risk of pulmonary embolism after a negative spiral CT angiogram in patients with pulmonary disease: 1-year clinical follow-up study. *Radiology* 2002;**223**:461.

48. Lomis NN, Moran AG, Miller FJ. Clinical outcomes of patients after negative spiral CT pulmonary arteriogram in the evaluation of acute pulmonary embolism. *J Vasc Interv Radiol* 1999;**10**:707.

49. van Belle A, Bueller HR, Huisman MV, et al. Effectiveness of managing suspected pulmonary embolism using an algorithm combining clinical probability, D-dimer testing, and computed tomography. *JAMA* 2006;**295**:172.

50. Moores LK, Jackson Jr WL, Shorr AF, et al. Meta-analysis: outcomes in patients with suspected pulmonary embolism managed with computed tomographic pulmonary angiography. *Ann Intern Med* 2004;**141**:866.

51. Coche EE, Hamoir XL, Hammer FD, et al. Using dual-detector helical CT angiography to detect deep venous thrombosis in patients with suspicion of pulmonary embolism: diagnostic value and additional findings. *AJR Am J Roentgenol* 2001;**176**:1035.

52. Loud PA, Katz DS, Klippenstein DL, et al. Combined CT venography and pulmonary angiography in suspected thromboembolic disease: diagnostic accuracy for deep venous evaluation. *AJR Am J Roentgenol* 2000;**174**:61.

53. Wittram C, Maher MM, Yoo AJ, et al. CT angiography of pulmonary embolism: diagnostic criteria and causes of misdiagnosis. *Radiographics* 2004;**24**:1219.

54. Stein PD, Woodard PK, Weg JG, et al. Diagnostic pathways in acute pulmonary embolism: recommendations of the PIOPED II investigators. *Am J Med* 2006;**119**:1048.

55. Sostman HD, Stein PD, Gottschalk A, et al. Acute pulmonary embolism: sensitivity and specificity of ventilation-perfusion scintigraphy in PIOPED II study. *Radiology* 2008;**246**:941.

56. Sostman HD, Miniati M, Gottschalk A, et al. Sensitivity and specificity of perfusion scintigraphy combined with chest radiography for acute pulmonary embolism in PIOPED II. *J Nucl Med* 2008;**49**:1741.

57. Rosen MP, Sheiman RG, Weintraub J, et al. Compression sonography in patients with indeterminate or low-probability lung scans: lack of usefulness in the absence of both symptoms of deep-vein thrombosis and thromboembolic risk factors. *AJR Am J Roentgenol* 1996;**166**:285.

58. Beecham RP, Dorfman GS, Cronan JJ, et al. Is bilateral lower extremity compression sonography useful and cost-effective in the evaluation of suspected pulmonary embolism? *AJR Am J Roentgenol* 1993;**161**:1289.

59. Smith LL, Iber C, Sirr S. Pulmonary embolism: confirmation with venous duplex US as adjunct to lung scanning. *Radiology* 1994;**191**:143.

60. Kluge A, Mueller C, Strunk J, et al. Experience in 207 combined MRI examinations for acute pulmonary embolism and deep venous thrombosis. *AJR Am J Roentgenol* 2006;**186**:1686.

61. Stein PD, Woodard PK, Hull RD, et al. Gadolinium-enhanced magnetic resonance angiography for detection of acute pulmonary embolism: an in-depth review. *Chest* 2003;**124**:2324.

62. van Beek EJ, Wild JM, Fink C, et al. MRI for the diagnosis of pulmonary embolism. *J Magn Reson Imaging* 2003;**18**:627.

63. Stein PD, Henry JW, Gottshalk A. Reassessment of pulmonary angiography for the diagnosis of pulmonary embolism: relation of interpreter agreement to the order of the involved pulmonary branch. *Radiology* 1999;**210**:689.

64. Diffin DC, Leyendecker JR, Johnson SP, et al. Effect of anatomic distribution of pulmonary emboli on interobserver agreement in the interpretation of pulmonary angiography. *AJR Am J Roentgenol* 1998;**171**:1085.

65. deMonye W, van Strijen MJL, Hulsman MV, et al. Suspected pulmonary embolism: prevalence and anatomic distribution in 487 consecutive patients. *Radiology* 2000;**215**:184.

66. Oser RF, Zuckerman DA, Gutierrez FR, et al. Anatomic distribution of pulmonary emboli at pulmonary angiography: implications for cross-sectional imaging. *Radiology* 1996;**199**:31.

67. Kayalar N, Leibovich BC, Orszulak TA, et al. Concomitant surgery for renal neoplasm with pulmonary tumor embolism. *J Thorac Cardiovasc Surg* 2010;**139**:320.

68. Garcia DA, Spyropoulos AC. Update in the treatment of venous thromboembolism. *Semin Respir Crit Care Med* 2008;**29**:40.

69. Bueller HR, Davidson BL, Decousus H, et al. Subcutaneous fondaparinux versus intravenous unfractionated heparin in the initial treatment of pulmonary embolism. *N Engl J Med* 2003;**349**:1695.

70. Kearon C, Kahn SR, Agnelli G, et al. Antithrombotic therapy for venous thromboembolic disease: American College of Chest Physicians Evidence-based Clinical Practice Guidelines, 8th ed. *Chest* 2008;**133**:454S.

71. Barritt DW, Jordan SC. Anticoagulant drugs in the treatment of pulmonary embolism: a controlled trial. *Lancet* 1960;**1**:1309.

72. PREPIC Study Group. Eight-year follow-up of patients with permanent vena cava filters in the prevention of pulmonary embolism: the PREPIC randomized study. *Circulation* 2005;**112**:416.

73. Kinney TB. Update on inferior vena cava filters. *J Vasc Interv Radiol* 2003;**14**:425.

74. Ferris EJ, McCowan TC, Carver DK, et al. Percutaneous inferior vena caval filters: follow-up of seven designs in 320 patients. *Radiology* 1993;**188**:851.

75. Kuo WT, Gould MK, Louie JD, et al. Catheter-directed therapy for the treatment of massive pulmonary embolism: systematic review and meta-analysis of modern techniques. *J Vasc Interv Radiol* 2009;**20**:1431.

76. Schmitz-Rode T, Janssens U, Duda SH, et al. Massive pulmonary embolism: percutaneous emergency treatment by pigtail rotation catheter. *J Am Coll Cardiol* 2000;**36**:375.

77. Tajima H, Murata S, Kumazaki T, et al. Hybrid treatment of acute massive pulmonary thromboembolism: mechanical fragmentation with a modified rotating pigtail catheter, local fibrinolytic therapy, and clot aspiration followed by systemic fibrinolytic therapy. *AJR Am J Roentgenol* 2004;**183**:589.

78. Chen L, Gu J, Lou W, et al. Interventional mechanical thrombectomy for acute pulmonary embolism. *J Vasc Interv Radiol* 2008;**17**:468.

79. Uflacker R. Interventional therapy for pulmonary embolism. *J Vasc Interv Radiol* 2001;**12**:147.

80. Zeni PT, Blank BG, Peeler DW. Use of rheolytic thrombectomy in treatment of acute massive pulmonary embolism. *J Vasc Interv Radiol* 2003;**14**:1511.

81. deGregorio MA, Gimeno AJ, Mainar A, et al. Mechanical and enzymatic thrombolysis for massive pulmonary embolism. *J Vasc Interv Radiol* 2002;**13**:163.

82. Eid-Lidt G, Gaspar J, Sandoval J, et al. Combined clot fragmentation and aspiration in patients with acute pulmonary embolism. *Chest* 2008;**134**:54.

83. Kuo WT, van den Bosch MA, Hofmann LV, et al. Catheter-directed embolectomy, fragmentation, and thrombolysis for the treatment of massive pulmonary embolism after failure of systemic thrombolysis. *Chest* 2008;**134**:250.

84. Gray HH, Morgan JM, Paneth M, et al. Pulmonary embolectomy for acute massive pulmonary embolism: an analysis of 71 cases. *Br Heart J* 1988;**60**:196.

85. Fartoukh M, Khalil A, Louis L, et al. An integrated approach to diagnosis and management of severe haemoptysis in patients admitted to the intensive care unit: a case series from a referral centre. *Respir Res* 2007;**15**:11.

86. Savale L, Parrot A, Khalil A, et al. Cryptogenic hemoptysis: from a benign to a life-threatening pathologic vascular condition. *Am J Respir Crit Care Med* 2007;**175**:1181.

87. Jardin M, Remy J. Control of hemoptysis: systemic angiography and anastomoses of the internal mammary artery. *Radiology* 1988;**168**:377.

88. Keller FS, Rosch J, Loflin TG, et al. Nonbronchial systemic collateral arteries: significance in percutaneous embolotherapy for hemoptysis. *Radiology* 1987;**164**:687.

89. Yu-Tang Goh P, Lin M, Teo N, et al. Embolization for hemoptysis: a six-year review. *Cardiovasc Intervent Radiol* 2002;**25**:17.

90. Picard C, Parrot A, Boussaud V, et al. Massive hemoptysis due to Rasmussen aneurysm: detection with helicoidal CT angiography and successful steel coil embolization. *Intensive Care Med* 2003;**29**:1837.

91. Abreu AR, Campos MA, Krieger BP. Pulmonary artery rupture induced by a pulmonary artery catheter: a case report and review of the literature. *J Intensive Care Med* 2004;**19**:291.

92. Cottin V, Plauchu H, Bayle JY, et al. Pulmonary arteriovenous malformations in patients with hereditary hemorrhagic telangiectasia. *Am J Respir Crit Care Med* 2004;**169**:994.

93. Revel MP, Fournier LS, Hennebicque AS, et al. Can CT replace bronchoscopy in detection of the site and cause of bleeding in patients with large or massive hemoptysis? *AJR Am J Roentgenol* 2002;**179**:1217.

94. Remy-Jardin M, Bouaziz N, Dumont P, et al. Bronchial and non-bronchial systemic arteries at multi-detector row CT angiography:

comparison with conventional angiography. *Radiology* 2004; **233**:741.

95. Chung MJ, Lee JH, Lee KS, et al. Bronchial and nonbronchial systemic arteries in patients with hemoptysis: depiction on MDCT angiography. *AJR Am J Roentgenol* 2006;**186**:649.

96. Yoon YC, Lee KS, Yeong YJ, et al. Hemoptysis: bronchial and nonbronchial systemic arteries at 16-detector row CT. *Radiology* 2005;**234**:292.

97. Khalil A, Parrot A, Nedelcu C, et al. Severe hemoptysis of pulmonary arterial origin: signs and role of multidetector row CT angiography. *Chest* 2008;**133**:212.

98. Bruzzi JF, Remy-Jardin M, Delhaye D, et al. Multi-detector row CT of hemoptysis. *Radiographics* 2006;**26**:3.

99. Chun HJ, Byun JY, Yoo SS, et al. Added benefit of thoracic aortography after transarterial embolization in patients with hemoptysis. *AJR Am J Roentgenol* 2003;**180**:1577.

100. Yoon W, Kim YH, Kim JK, et al. Massive hemoptysis: prediction of non-bronchial systemic arterial supply with chest CT. *Radiology* 2003;**227**:232.

101. Yoon W, Kim JK, Kim YH, et al. Bronchial and nonbronchial systemic artery embolization for life-threatening hemoptysis: a comprehensive review. *Radiographics* 2002;**22**:1395.

102. Kalva SP. Bronchial artery embolization. *Tech Vasc Interv Radiol* 2009;**12**:130.

103. Cohen AM, Doershuk CF, Stern RC. Bronchial artery embolization to control hemoptysis in cystic fibrosis. *Radiology* 1990;**175**:401.

104. Hayakawa K, Tanaka F, Torizuka T, et al. Bronchial artery embolization for hemoptysis: immediate and long-term results. *Cardiovasc Intervent Radiol* 1992;**15**:154.

105. Swanson KL, Johnson CM, Prakash UB, et al. Bronchial artery embolization: experience with 54 patients. *Chest* 2002;**121**:789.

106. Poyanli A, Acunas B, Rozanes I, et al. Endovascular therapy in the management of moderate and massive hemoptysis. *Br J Radiol* 2007;**80**:331.

107. Barben JU, Ditchfield M, Carlin JB, et al. Major haemoptysis in children with cystic fibrosis: a 20-year retrospective study. *Cyst Fibros* 2003;**2**:105.

108. Vinaya KN, White RI Jr, Sloan JM. Reassessing bronchial artery embolotherapy with newer spherical embolic materials. *J Vasc Interv Radiol* 2004;**15**:304.

109. Ramakantan R, Bandekar VG, Gandhi MS, et al. Massive hemoptysis due to pulmonary tuberculosis: control with bronchial artery embolization. *Radiology* 1996;**200**:691.

110. Santelli ED, Katz DS, Goldschmidt AM, et al. Embolization of multiple Rasmussen aneurysms as a treatment of hemoptysis. *Radiology* 1994;**193**:396.

111. Katoh O, Kishikawa T, Yamada H, et al. Recurrent bleeding after arterial embolization in patients with hemoptysis. *Chest* 1990;**97**:541.

112. Remy-Jardin M, Wattinne L, Remy J. Transcatheter occlusion of pulmonary arterial circulation and collateral supply: failures, incidents, and complications. *Radiology* 1991;**180**:699.

113. Fraser KL, Grosman H, Hyland RH, et al. Transverse myelitis: a reversible complication of bronchial artery embolisation in cystic fibrosis. *Thorax* 1997;**52**:99.

114. Benotti JR, Dalen JE. The natural history of pulmonary embolism. *Clin Chest Med* 1984;**5**:403.

115. Auger WR, Fedullo PF. Chronic thromboembolic pulmonary hypertension. *Semin Respir Crit Care Med* 2009;**30**:471.

116. Miniati M, Monti S, Bottai M, et al. Survival and restoration of pulmonary perfusion in a long-term follow-up of patients after acute pulmonary embolism. *Medicine* (Baltimore) 2006;**85**:253.

117. Becattini C, Agnelli G, Pesavento R, et al. Incidence of chronic thromboembolic pulmonary hypertension after a first episode of pulmonary embolism. *Chest* 2006;**130**:172.

118. Fedullo PF, Auger WR, Kerr KM, et al. Chronic thromboembolic pulmonary hypertension. *N Engl J Med* 2001;**345**:1465.

119. Pengo V, Lensing AW, Prins MH, et al. Incidence of chronic thromboembolic pulmonary hypertension after pulmonary embolism. *New Engl J Med* 2004;**350**:2257.

120. Simonneau G, Azarian R, Brenot F, et al. Surgical management of unresolved pulmonary embolism: a personal series of 72 patients. *Chest* 1995;**107**:52S.

121. McGoon M, Gutterman D, Steen V, et al. Screening, early detection, and diagnosis of pulmonary arterial hypertension: ACCP evidence-based clinical practice guidelines. *Chest* 2004;**126** (Suppl. 1):14S.

122. Bergin CJ, Hauschildt J, Rios G, et al. Accuracy of MR angiography compared with radionuclide scanning in identifying the cause of pulmonary arterial hypertension. *AJR Am J Roentgenol* 1997;**168**:1549.

123. Ryan KL, Fedullo PF, Davis GB, et al. Perfusion scan findings understate the severity of angiographic and hemodynamic compromise in chronic thromboembolic pulmonary hypertension. *Chest* 1988;**93**:1180.

124. Filipek MS, Gosselin MV. Multidetector pulmonary CT angiography: advances in the evaluation of pulmonary arterial diseases. *Semin Ultrasound CT MR* 2004;**25**:83.

125. Kreitner KF, Ley S, Kauczor HU, et al. Chronic thromboembolic pulmonary hypertension: pre- and postoperative assessment with breath-hold MR imaging techniques. *Radiology* 2004; **232**:535.

126. Ley S, Kauczor HU, Heussel CP, et al. Value of contrast-enhanced MR angiography and helical CT angiography in chronic thromboembolic pulmonary hypertension. *Eur Radiol* 2003;**13**:2365.

127. Cummings KW, Bhalla S. Multidetector computed tomographic pulmonary angiography: beyond acute pulmonary embolism. *Radiol Clin North Am* 2010;**48**:51.

128. Heinrich M, Uder M, Tscholl D, et al. CT scan findings in chronic thromboembolic pulmonary hypertension: predictors of hemodynamic improvement after pulmonary thromboendarterectomy. *Chest* 2005;**127**:1606.

129. Reichelt A, Hoeper MM, Galanski M, et al. Chronic pulmonary thromboembolic pulmonary hypertension: evaluation with 64-detector row CT versus digital subtraction angiography. *Eur J Radiol* 2009;**71**:49.

130. Auger WR, Fedullo PF, Moser KM, et al. Chronic major-vessel thromboembolic pulmonary artery obstruction: appearance at angiography. *Radiology* 1992;**182**:393.

131. Thistlethwaite PA, Madani M, Jamieson SW. Pulmonary thromboendarterectomy surgery. *Cardiol Clin* 2004;**22**:467.

132. Chin KM, Rubin LJ. Pulmonary arterial hypertension. *J Am Coll Cardiol* 2008;**51**:1527.

133. Newman JH, Trembath RC, Morse JA, et al. Genetic basis of pulmonary arterial hypertension: current understanding and future directions. *J Am Coll Cardiol* 2004;**43** Suppl 1:33S.

134. Worsley DF, Palevsky HI, Alavi A. Ventilation-perfusion lung scanning in the evaluation of pulmonary hypertension. *J Nucl Med* 1994;**35**:793.

135. Chapman PJ, Bateman ED, Benatar SR. Primary pulmonary hypertension and thromboembolic pulmonary hypertension-similarities and differences. *Respir Med* 1990;**84**:485.

136. Ley S, Kreitner KF, Fink C, et al. Assessment of pulmonary hypertension by CT and MR imaging. *Eur Radiol* 2004;**14**:359.

137. Hansell DM. Small-vessel diseases of the lung. CT-pathologic correlates. *Radiology* 2002;**225**:639.

138. Brown KK. Pulmonary vasculitis. *Proc Am Thorac Soc* 2006; **3**:48.

139. Seo JB, Im JG, Chung JW, et al. Pulmonary vasculitis: the spectrum of radiological findings. *Br J Radiol* 2000;**73**:1224.

140. Nastri MV, Baptista LP, Baroni RH, et al. Gadolinium-enhanced three-dimensional MR angiography of Takayasu arteritis. *Radiographics* 2004;**24**:773.

141. Liu Y-Q, Jin B-L, Ling J. Pulmonary artery involvement in aortoarteritis: an angiographic study. *Cardiovasc Intervent Radiol* 1994;**17**:2.

142. Yamada I, Shibuya H, Matsubara O, et al. Pulmonary artery disease in Takayasu's arteritis: angiographic findings. *AJR Am J Roentgenol* 1992;**159**:263.

143. Yamada I, Nakagawa T, Himeno Y, et al. Takayasu arteritis: diagnosis with breath-hold contrast-enhanced three-dimensional MR angiography. *J Magn Reson Imaging* 2000;**11**:481.

144. Gotway MB, Araoz PA, Macedo TA, et al. Imaging findings in Takayasu's arteritis. *AJR Am J Roentgenol* 2005;**184**:1945.

145. Tyagi S, Mehta V, Kashyap R, et al. Endovascular stent implantation for severe pulmonary stenosis in aortoarteritis (Takayasu's arteritis). *Catheter Cardiovasc Interv* 2004;**61**:281.

146. Leslie KO, Trahan S, Gruden J. Pulmonary pathology of the rheumatics diseases. *Semin Respir Crit Care Med* 2007;**28**:369.

147. Erkan F, Gul A, Tasali E, et al. Pulmonary manifestations of Behçet's disease. *Thorax* 2001;**56**:572.

148. Yazici H, Fresko I, Yurdakul S. Behçet's syndrome: disease manifestations, management, and advances in treatment. *Nat Clin Pract Rheumatol* 2007;**3**:148.

149. Yazici H, Esen F. Mortality in Behçet's syndrome. *Clin Exp Rheumatol* 2008;**26**:S138.

150. Hamuryudan V, Er T, Seyahi E, et al. Pulmonary artery aneurysms in Behçet syndrome. *Am J Med* 2004;**117**:867.

151. Hiller N, Lieberman S, Chajek-Shaul T, et al. Thoracic manifestations of Behçet disease at CT. *Radiographics* 2004;**24**:801.

152. Pelage J-P, El Hajjam M, Lagrange C, et al. Pulmonary artery interventions: an overview. *Radiographics* 2005;**25**:1653.

153. Cantasdemir M, Kantarci F, Mihmanli I, et al. Emergency endovascular management of pulmonary artery aneurysms in Behçet's disease: report of two cases and review of the literature. *Cardiovasc Intervent Radiol* 2002;**25**:533.

154. Mouas H, Lortholary O, Lacombe P, et al. Embolization of multiple pulmonary arterial aneurysms in Behçet's disease. *Scand J Rheumatol* 1996;**25**:58.

155. Lacombe P, Qanadli SD, Jondeau G, et al. Treatment of hemoptysis in Behçet syndrome with pulmonary and bronchial embolization. *J Vasc Interv Radiol* 1997;**8**:1043.

156. Nguyen ET, Silva CIS, Seely JM, et al. Pulmonary artery aneurysms and pseudoaneurysms in adults: findings at CT and radiography. *AJR Am J Roentgenol* 2007;**188**:W126.

157. Donaldson B, Ngo-Nonga B. Traumatic pseudoaneurysm of the pulmonary artery: case report and review of the literature. *Am Surg* 2002;**68**:414.

158. SanDretto MA, Scanlon GT. Multiple mycotic pulmonary artery aneurysms secondary to intravenous drug abuse. *AJR Am J Roentgenol* 1984;**142**:89.

159. Shin TB, Yoon SK, Lee KN, et al. The role of pulmonary CT angiography and selective pulmonary angiography in endovascular management of pulmonary artery pseudoaneurysms associated with infectious lung disease. *J Vasc Interv Radiol* 2007;**18**:882.

160. Poplausky MR, Rozenblit G, Rundback JH, et al. Swan-Ganz catheter-induced pulmonary artery pseudoaneurysm formation: three case reports and a review of the literature. *Chest* 2001;**120**:2105.

161. Bussieres JS. Iatrogenic pulmonary artery rupture. *Curr Opin Anesthesiol* 2007;**20**:48.

162. Ray Jr CE, Kaufman JA, Geller SC, et al. Embolization of pulmonary catheter-induced pulmonary artery pseudoaneurysms. *Chest* 1996;**110**:1370.

163. Baker CM, McGowan Jr FX, Keane JF, et al. Pulmonary artery trauma due to balloon dilation: recognition, avoidance, and management. *J Am Coll Cardiol* 2000;**36**:1684.

164. Tanaka K, Ihaya A, Horiuci T, et al. Giant mediastinal bronchial artery aneurysm mimicking benign esophageal tumor: a case report and review of 26 cases from literature. *J Vasc Surg* 2003;**38**:1125.

165. Pugnale M, Portier F, Lamarre A, et al. Hemomediastinum caused by rupture of a bronchial artery aneurysm: successful treatment by embolization with N-butyl-2-cyanoacrylate. *J Vasc Interv Radiol* 2001;**12**:1351.

166. Kalva SP, Wicky S. Mediastinal bronchial artery aneurysms: endovascular therapy in two patients. *Catheter Cardiovasc Interv* 2006;**68**:858.

167. Mizuguchi S, Inoue K, Kida A, et al. Ruptured bronchial artery aneurysm associated with bronchiectasis: a case report. *Ann Thorac Cardiovasc Surg* 2009;**15**:115.

168. Remy-Jardin M, Dumont P, Brillet P-Y, et al. Pulmonary arteriovenous malformations treated with embolotherapy: helical CT evaluation of long-term effectiveness after 2-21 year follow-up. *Radiology* 2006:**239**:576.

169. Pollak JS, Saluja S, Thabet A, et al. Clinical and anatomic outcomes after embolotherapy of pulmonary arteriovenous malformations. *J Vasc Interv Radiol* 2006;**17**:35.

170. van den Driesche S, Mummery CL, Westermann CJ. Hereditary hemorrhagic telangiectasia: an update on transforming growth factor beta signaling in vasculogenesis and angiogenesis. *Cardiovasc Res* 2003;**58**:20.

171. Jaskolka J, Wu L, Chan RP, et al. Imaging of hereditary hemorrhagic telangiectasia. *AJR Am J Roentgenol* 2004;**183**:307.

172. White Jr RI. Pulmonary arteriovenous malformations: how do I embolize? *Tech Vasc Interventional Rad* 2007;**10**:283.

173. Remy J, Remy-Jardin M, Giraud F, et al. Angioarchitecture of pulmonary arteriovenous malformations: clinical utility of three-dimensional helical CT. *Radiology* 1994;**191**:657.

174. White RI Jr, Pollak JS, Wirth JA. Pulmonary arteriovenous malformations: diagnosis and transcatheter embolotherapy. *J Vasc Interv Radiol* 1996;**7**:787.

175. Pierucci P, Murphy J, Henderson KJ, et al. New definition and natural history of patients with diffuse pulmonary arteriovenous malformations: twenty-seven-year experience. *Chest* 2008;**133**: 653.

176. Lacombe P, Lagrange C, Beauchet A, et al. Diffuse pulmonary arteriovenous malformations in hereditary hemorrhagic telangiectasia: long-term results of embolization according to the extent of lung involvement. *Chest* 2009;**135**:1031.

177. White RI Jr, Pollak JS. Pulmonary arteriovenous malformations: diagnosis with three-dimensional helical CT: a breakthrough without contrast media. *Radiology* 1994;**191**:613.

178. Mager JJ, Overtoom TT, Blauw H, et al. Embolotherapy of pulmonary arteriovenous malformations: long-term results in 112 patients. *J Vasc Interv Radiol* 2004;**15**:451.

179. Prasad V, Chan RP, Faughnan ME. Embolotherapy of pulmonary arteriovenous malformations: efficacy of platinum versus stainless steel coils. *J Vasc Interv Radiol* 2004;**15**:153.

180. Abdel Asi AK, Hamed MF, Biosca RF, et al. Occlusion time for Amplatzer vascular plug in the management of pulmonary arteriovenous malformations. *AJR Am J Roentgenol* 2009; **192**:793.

181. Fidelman N, Gordon RL, LaBerge JM, et al. Reperfusion of pulmonary arteriovenous malformations after successful embolotherapy with vascular plugs. *J Vasc Interv Radiol* 2008; **19**:1246.

182. Millic A, Chan RP, Cohen JH, et al. Reperfusion of pulmonary arteriovenous malformations after embolotherapy. *J Vasc Interv Radiol* 2005;**16**:1675.

183. Gupta P, Mordin C, Curtis J, et al. Pulmonary arteriovenous malformations: effect of embolization on right-to-left shunt, hypoxemia, and exercise tolerance in 66 patients. *AJR Am J Roentgenol* 2002;**179**:347.

184. Gupta S, Faughnan ME, Bayoumi AM. Embolization for pulmonary arteriovenous malformation in hereditary hemorrhagic telangiectasia. *Chest* 2009;**136**:849.

185. Devaraj A, Griffin N, Nicholson AG, et al. Computed tomography findings in fibrosing mediastinitis. *Clin Radiol* 2007;**62**:781.

186. Yi CA, Lee KS, Choe YH, et al. Computed tomography in pulmonary artery sarcoma: distinguishing features from pulmonary embolic disease. *J Comput Assist Tomogr* 2004;**28**:34.

187. Kaplinsky EJ, Favaloro RR, Pombo G, et al. Primary pulmonary artery sarcoma resembling chronic thromboembolic pulmonary disease. *Eur Respir J* 2000;**16**:1202.

188. Winchester PA, Khilnani NM, Trost DW, et al. Endovascular catheter biopsy of a pulmonary artery sarcoma. *AJR Am J Roentgenol* 1996;**167**:657.

189. Mayer E, Kriegsmann J, Gaumann A, et al. Surgical treatment of pulmonary artery sarcoma. *J Thorac Cardiovasc Surg* 2001;**121**:77.

190. Blackmon SH, Rice DC, Correa AM, et al. Management of primary pulmonary artery sarcoma. *Ann Thorac Surg* 2009;**87**:977.

15

Lower Extremity Veins

Karim Valji

DUPLEX SONOGRAPHY

Color-coded sonography combined with Doppler wave-form analysis ("duplex ultrasound") is the principal imaging tool for evaluation of acute and chronic diseases of the lower extremity veins.[1,2]

For detection of deep venous thrombosis, a high-frequency linear transducer (5 to 10 MHz) with color Doppler capability is used.[3] The patient lies on a table; the leg is externally rotated and the knee slightly flexed. Progressing caudally from the groin, the veins are interrogated for complete color flow saturation of the lumen, which excludes thrombus. The more traditional but time-consuming incremental vein compression test is usually required only to confirm color Doppler flow pattern (Fig. 15-1). The popliteal vein is examined with the patient prone or in the lateral decubitus position. The study then is continued down the calf to assess the three paired tibial veins, preferably with the leg hanging over the examination table. Doppler waveform analysis is used to evaluate flow dynamics which may predict disease within vessels inaccessible to sonography (e.g., deep pelvic veins).

Similar equipment is used for evaluation of patients with suspected venous insufficiency or varicose veins. However, this study is performed with the patient standing and bearing weight on the opposite leg. The leg is slightly flexed at the knee. The great saphenous vein is interrogated from the groin to the level of the lowest varicosity.[1] The vein diameters are measured, and the location of tributaries feeding any varicosities is noted. Following manual calf compression and release, venous reflux is sought from the confluence of the superficial inguinal veins through peripheral perforating veins with color imaging and Doppler waveform analysis (Fig. 15-2). The sine qua non of venous reflux is flow reversal lasting for a predetermined interval. Finally, the short saphenous vein and associated tributaries are examined from a posterior approach.

ANATOMY

Normal Anatomy and Physiology

The leg is drained by superficial and deep venous systems. The deep veins, which are dominant, run alongside their corresponding arteries. The superficial veins are located in the superficial fascia. A network of perforating veins connects these two venous beds. The inconsistent and confusing nomenclature used over the years for lower extremity veins has recently been codified into a new set of standardized terms.[4]

In the foot, the deep plantar arch is formed by the plantar metatarsal veins.[5] The arch forms the medial and lateral plantar veins, which give off branches to the saphenous system and contribute to formation of the tibial veins. The paired posterior tibial, anterior tibial, and peroneal veins constitute the deep system of the calf (Fig. 15-3). These *tibial veins* merge below the knee to establish the *popliteal vein*, which is usually superficial to the popliteal artery. Multiple muscular soleal and gastrocnemius veins also drain into the tibial and popliteal veins. The popliteal vein becomes the *femoral vein (FV,* formerly the superficial femoral vein) at the adductor canal (Fig. 15-4). It runs posterolateral to the artery above the knee and then posteromedial to the artery near the inguinal ligament. The *deep femoral vein* passes alongside the deep femoral artery and joins the FV at a variable distance below the inguinal ligament.

The superficial venous system includes the *great saphenous vein (GSV),* the *small* (formerly short or lesser) *saphenous vein (SSV),* and their numerous tributaries.[4,5] The GSV begins anterior to the medial malleolus. The vessel ascends along the medial aspect of the calf and thigh superficial to the muscular fascia (Fig. 15-5). It then passes through the saphenous opening of the deep fascia and enters the medial side of the femoral vein (also receiving several pelvic venous tributaries) at the *confluence of the superficial inguinal veins* (formerly the *saphenofemoral junction*) (see Fig. 15-4). The SSV originates posterior to the lateral malleolus. It runs behind

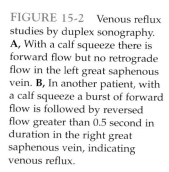

FIGURE 15-1 Normal color Doppler sonography of lower extremity veins. **A,** Normal right common femoral vein, *V.* **B,** Moderate compression with the ultrasound transducer in the transverse plane causes the vein to collapse completely. **C,** Color Doppler imaging of the right femoral vein in a longitudinal plane shows complete saturation of the vessel. **D,** A calf squeeze leads to "augmentation" of flow and aliasing of the signal on spectral waveform analysis.

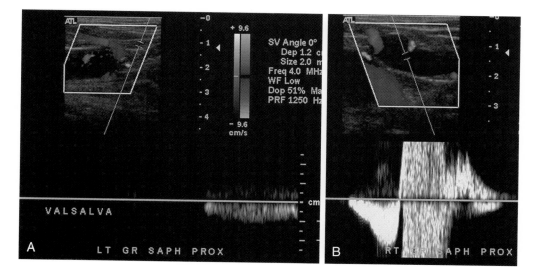

FIGURE 15-2 Venous reflux studies by duplex sonography. **A,** With a calf squeeze there is forward flow but no retrograde flow in the left great saphenous vein. **B,** In another patient, with a calf squeeze a burst of forward flow is followed by reversed flow greater than 0.5 second in duration in the right great saphenous vein, indicating venous reflux.

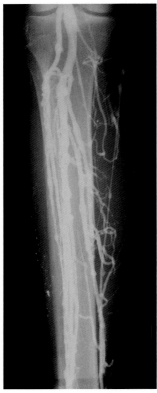

FIGURE 15-3   Normal right lower extremity ascending venography. Three paired tibial veins follow the expected course of the tibial arteries.

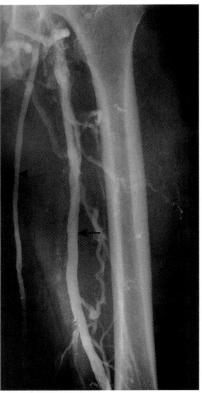

FIGURE 15-4   Ascending venogram of the left leg shows the femoral vein (*arrow*) and great saphenous vein (*arrowhead*). They join at the confluence of the superficial inguinal veins (saphenofemoral junction) in the groin.

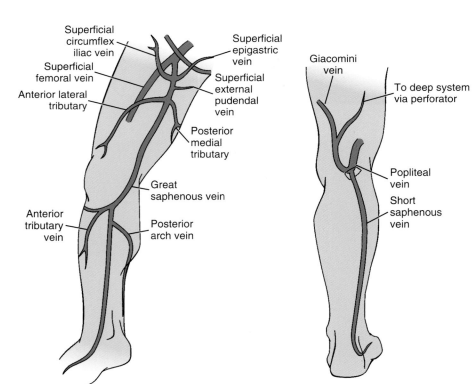

FIGURE 15-5   Superficial venous system of the leg. (*Adapted from Min RJ, Khilnani NM, Golia P. Duplex ultrasound evaluation of lower extremity venous insufficiency. J Vasc Interv Radiol 2003;14:1233.*)

the heads of the gastrocnemius muscle bundles and, in most cases, joins the popliteal vein around the knee at the *saphenopopliteal junction*. In about one third of the population, the SSV communicates with the GSV directly via the *intersaphenous (or Giacomini) vein* or through another tributary.[1]

Numerous *perforating (communicating) veins* connect the superficial and deep veins in the calf and thigh. The most important of these are the *femoral canal perforator* (Hunterian, midthigh, and Dodd, lower thigh), *paratibial perforator* (Boyd, around the knee), and *posterior tibial perforator* (Cockett, in the calf). *Bicuspid valves* are situated throughout the deep, perforating, and superficial veins of the leg up to the groin. They are oriented to direct blood from the superficial to the deep system.

At the inguinal ligament, the *common femoral vein* becomes the *external iliac vein*, which is medial to the iliac artery (Fig. 15-6). Its tributaries include the pubic, deep circumflex iliac, and inferior epigastric veins. The external iliac vein courses over the pelvic brim to the level of the sacroiliac joint, where it joins the *internal iliac vein* to form the common iliac vein. The *right common iliac vein* is first posterior and then lateral to the iliac artery. The *left common iliac vein* has a more horizontal course and lies between the right common iliac artery and the spine. Asymptomatic mild extrinsic compression occurs at this site in up to 60% of the general population[6] (see Fig. 15-6). *Ascending lumbar veins* arise from the upper surface of the common iliac veins. The iliac veins merge at the L4-L5 level to form the inferior vena cava (IVC).

When a person is supine, a pressure gradient (12 to 18 mm Hg on the venous side of capillaries; 4 to 7 mm Hg in right atrium) drives blood toward the heart.[7] In addition, respiratory inspiration accelerates blood flow centrally. In an upright position, however, lower extremity venous drainage against substantial hydrodynamic resistance depends on the following: (1) an intact muscular pump, (2) competent vein valves, and (3) unobstructed outflow. Although the walls of the superficial and muscular leg veins contain smooth muscle and are capable of constriction, blood return to the heart depends largely on extrinsic compression by leg muscles, particularly the "calf pump." At rest, blood flows from the superficial system into the deep veins. Competent valves prevent retrograde flow. With muscular contraction, blood is propelled centrally by forceful emptying of the deep veins.

Variant Anatomy

Duplication of segments of the lower extremity veins is common. *Accessory saphenous veins* (which run in the extrafascial compartment) are described in up to two thirds of the general population.[8] Close to one third of people have duplicated or multiple femoral (or less often, popliteal) veins.[9]

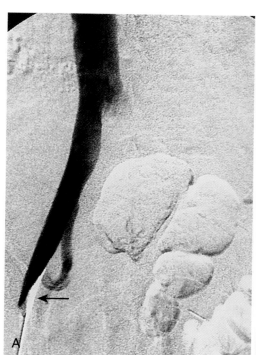
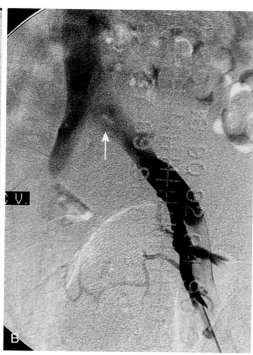

FIGURE 15-6 Normal right **(A)** and left **(B)** pelvic venograms. Retrograde flow is seen in both internal iliac veins, as is apparent narrowing of the right external iliac vein above the catheter tip *(black arrow)* because of coaptation of vein walls from the high-pressure fluid jet (i.e., Venturi effect). Diminished contrast density at the junction of the left common iliac vein and inferior vena cava *(white arrow)* is caused by mild extrinsic compression between the right common iliac artery and spine. Lucency in the left external iliac vein results from unopacified blood entering the vessel.

Klippel-Trénaunay syndrome (KTS) is a rare congenital disorder that features cutaneous capillary malformations, distorted lower extremity veins (multiple varicosities and often an ectopic *marginal vein*), and bone and soft tissue enlargement.[10-12] A similar but distinct condition (*Parkes-Weber syndrome*) includes these elements along with high-flow arteriovenous malformations. Although most cases of KTS are sporadic and not familial, there is some evidence that the disease stems from genetic mutations in the angiogenic protein VG5Q.[13]

A cutaneous "port wine" lesion is characteristic. Symptoms include but are not limited to local pain, swelling, and bleeding. Sonography and computed tomography (CT) or magnetic resonance (MR) venography are useful in mapping the bizarre, disordered venous channels[14] (Fig. 15-7). When present, the marginal vein runs along the lateral aspect of the thigh and drains into the internal iliac or femoral vein. Mild cases of KTS are managed with compressive stocking therapy alone. Sclerotherapy and embolotherapy are used to treat the abnormal venous channels and arteriovenous malformations associated with this syndrome.[10] Surgery is reserved for those patients with functional disabilities or severe bleeding or cutaneous ulcerations.

Persistent sciatic vein is a very rare anomaly in which a remnant of that embryologic vessel remains the primary venous drainage between the adductor canal and the internal iliac vein.[15,16] The vein is markedly dilated and tortuous. The disorder may be an isolated condition but often is associated with KTS.

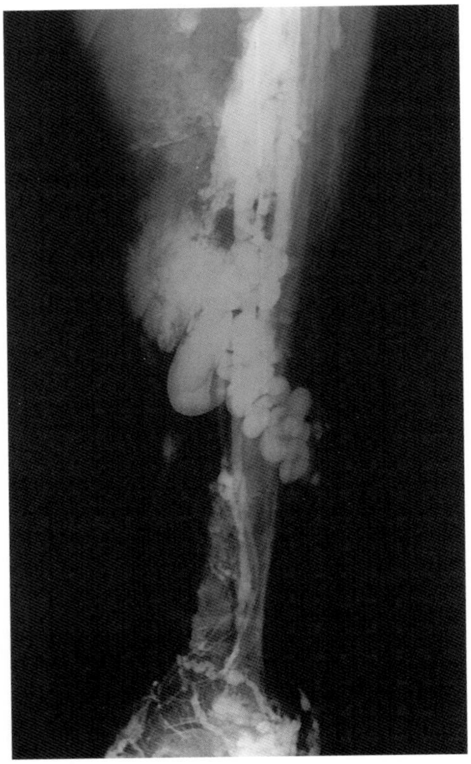

Collateral Circulation

When either the superficial or deep venous system becomes occluded, the complementary network operates as the main collateral pathway. With partial or total iliac vein obstruction, transpelvic and ascending lumbar veins serve as the chief collateral channels (Fig. 15-8).

MAJOR DISORDERS

Acute Deep Venous Thrombosis (Online Case 85)

Etiology and Natural History

Acute lower extremity and pelvic *deep venous thrombosis (DVT)* is part of the spectrum of venous thromboembolic disease (VTE, see also Chapter 1). This disorder also includes *pulmonary embolism* (PE) and *chronic venous insufficiency* (CVI, sometimes called *post-thrombotic* or *postphlebitic syndrome*).[17,18] Acute DVT is a common

FIGURE 15-7   Klippel-Trénaunay syndrome. Bizarre, dilated venous collaterals fill on an ascending venogram in place of a normal deep venous system.

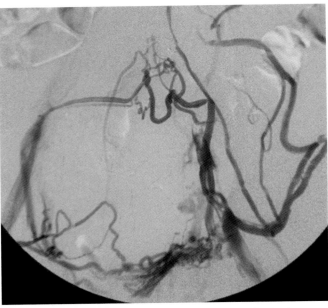

FIGURE 15-8   Chronic left iliac vein occlusion with injection from the left common femoral vein. Transpelvic and circumflex iliac venous collaterals drain the leg.

clinical problem, with an overall lifetime risk of about 2% to 5% of the general population.[19]

In humans, thrombi are constantly forming in the valve sinuses and venous confluences of the muscular calf veins. The endogenous fibrinolytic system usually dissolves these small clots. Thrombus remains confined to the calf veins in about 75% of untreated patients.[20] The risk of symptomatic PE in this situation is low.[21] In the remaining cases, thrombus extends to the "proximal" (femoropopliteal) veins. Most of these individuals have more than one predisposing factor to clot formation, such as sluggish blood flow, vessel injury, or a thrombophilic state (i.e., *Virchow triad*) [7,22] (Box 15-1).

Relative hypercoagulability is the leading culprit in most instances.

Iliac vein thrombosis can occur with propagation of femoropopliteal vein clot. Isolated *iliofemoral venous thrombosis* (encompassing the common femoral and iliac veins) accounts for no more than 20% of cases of lower extremity DVT and usually can be attributed to local factors[23] (Fig. 15-9 and Box 15-2). Left iliac vein compression (*May-Thurner syndrome*) frequently is responsible for left-sided iliofemoral thrombus formation (see later discussion). Iliofemoral DVT is also remarkable for the rarity of complete recanalization, relative resistance to conventional anticoagulative measures, and more profound (and perhaps frequent) symptoms of postthrombotic syndrome (PTS).[24]

In a small subset of patients, extensive peripheral and iliofemoral thrombosis occurs, leading to an edematous, painful white leg (*phlegmasia alba dolens*). If obstruction of collateral channels ensues, venous drainage is almost completely blocked and the patient will suffer from a markedly swollen, painful cyanotic extremity, sometimes with diminished arterial pulses (*phlegmasia cerulea dolens*).[25] This grave condition (which requires immediate intervention) may lead to venous gangrene, massive PE, or death.

Once acute DVT occurs, the fate of the thrombus is variable[7,26] (Box 15-3). The likelihood of a particular outcome depends on many factors, but some important generalizations can be made:

- The risk for PE is quite low with isolated calf DVT. The risk for symptomatic PE is reduced substantially in patients with "proximal" DVT who are given therapeutic anticoagulation (from at least 30% to less than 5%).[22,27,28]
- Recurrent DVT is observed in 25% to 50% of individuals despite adequate treatment.[7,29,30]

BOX 15-1

RISK FACTORS FOR VENOUS THROMBOEMBOLIC DISEASE

- Primary and secondary thrombophilic states (see Boxes 1-4 and 1-5)
- Prior history of venous thromboembolic disease
- Immobilization or bed rest
- Major trauma or surgery
  - Spinal cord injury
- Cancer (and chemotherapy)
- Advanced age
- Central venous catheter
- Obesity
- Use of oral contraceptives or estrogen therapy
- Pregnancy and puerperium
- Congestive heart failure

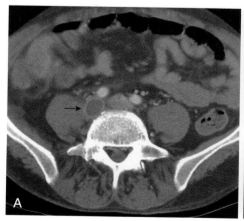
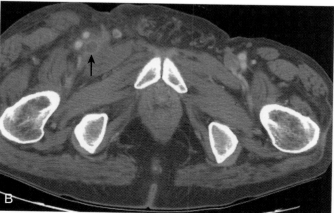

FIGURE 15-9   Right iliofemoral deep venous thrombosis *(arrow)* caused by posttraumatic right thigh and groin hematoma. Contrast-enhanced computed tomography scans through the upper pelvis **(A)** and inguinal region **(B).** The more peripheral veins were normal.

- Complete clot resolution with unscarred veins is much more common in calf and femoropopliteal DVT than often believed. However, recanalization of iliofemoral DVT is uncommon (<30% of cases).[31-33]
- Chronic venous insufficiency and PTS (see later discussion) may result from valve disruption (with associated reflux) or persistent venous occlusion.

Perhaps the most surprising rare sequela of acute DVT is *paradoxical embolism* with thrombus passing through a right-to-left circulatory shunt (e.g., large patent foramen ovale or pulmonary arteriovenous malformation). Arterial embolization is the consequence.

Clinical Features

Patients may complain of acute onset of leg pain, swelling, or tenderness. Less common signs include distention of superficial veins, cyanosis, erythema, palpable calf cords, or Homans' sign (calf pain with forced dorsiflexion of the foot). However, the symptoms and signs of lower extremity deep vein thrombosis are notoriously unreliable. Many patients (particularly in the postoperative setting) with proven DVT are asymptomatic, and many others with classic features do not have the disease. PE can be the first signal of acute DVT. When isolated iliofemoral DVT occurs, symptoms initially may be confined to the pelvis and thigh. Iliofemoral DVT occurs more frequently in the left leg than the right and more frequently in women than men.

Diagnosis

Although individual clinical signs often are misleading, "predictive rules" such as those devised by Wells and colleagues have proven valuable in assessing risk for the disease (Box 15-4). Because the consequences of a missed diagnosis and no treatment can be life-threatening, screening of high-risk asymptomatic patients and accurate diagnosis of symptomatic patients is critical and must depend on risk factor analysis, objective diagnostic tests, and imaging studies, alone or in combination.

BOX 15-2

CAUSES OF ISOLATED ILIOFEMORAL VENOUS THROMBOSIS

- Iliac vein compression (May-Thurner) syndrome
- Prior iliocaval deep venous thrombosis
- Malignancy (benign or malignant)
- Pregnancy
- Surgery
- Inferior vena cava filter
- Indwelling catheter
- Primary thrombophilic state
- Trauma
  - Accidental
  - Iatrogenic (e.g., prior catheterization)
- Benign extrinsic compression (e.g., aneurysm)
- Retroperitoneal fibrosis
- Radiation therapy

BOX 15-3

FATE OF ACUTE LOWER EXTREMITY DEEP VENOUS THROMBOSIS

- Pulmonary embolism
- Complete clot resolution
- Incomplete recanalization with vein scarring, valve injury, and venous reflux
- Thrombus propagation
- Recurrent deep venous thrombosis
- Persistent occlusion

BOX 15-4

CLINICAL PREDICTORS OF ACUTE DEEP VENOUS THROMBOSIS

- Active malignancy
- Paralysis, paresis, or recent lower extremity immobilization
- Bedridden for more than 3 days
- Major surgery within 12 weeks
- Previous deep venous thrombosis
- Localized tenderness
- Complete leg swelling
- Calf swelling 3 cm greater than asymptomatic leg
- Unilateral pitting edema
- Collateral superficial veins (nonvaricose)

Data from Wells PS, Anderson DR, Rodger M, et al. Evaluation of D-dimer in the diagnosis of suspected deep-vein thrombosis. *N Engl J Med* 2003;**349**:1227.

D-dimer is a byproduct of endogenous fibrin degradation, and plasma levels are elevated in patients with venous thrombosis or PE. The D-dimer radioimmunoassay has been useful in excluding acute DVT, particularly when applied along with predictive rules.[19,34,35] For example, a negative result from a high-sensitivity D-dimer test (e.g., serum level <500 ng/mL) and a low Wells score puts the likelihood of acute DVT diagnosis within 3 months at about 0.5%.[36]

Imaging

SONOGRAPHY

Because duplex sonography is extremely accurate, easy to perform, relatively inexpensive, and completely safe, it is the principal imaging study in both symptomatic and asymptomatic groups.[37-40] Several factors are evaluated (Fig. 15-10 and Table 15-1). Sonography also detects other causes for leg symptoms, such as a Baker cyst, lymphadenopathy, hematoma, or popliteal artery aneurysm.

In *symptomatic patients,* compression and color Doppler sonography are about as accurate as traditional contrast venography in the diagnosis of acute proximal DVT, with a sensitivity of 89% to 96% and specificity of 94% to 99%.[37-40] Outcome analyses from two large cohorts of patients with suspected DVT estimated the negative predictive value of a normal compression sonogram at greater than 99.5%.[41,42]

In *asymptomatic patients* with risk factors for DVT, color Doppler sonography is not as accurate (sensitivity 47% to 62%).[38,43] This discrepancy largely is related to the nature of occlusions in this population (i.e., often confined to calf veins, composed of smaller, nonocclusive, segmental thrombi).

Misdiagnosis is usually related to underlying chronic venous disease, isolated clot (iliac vein, calf veins, deep femoral vein, or one limb of a duplicated femoral or popliteal vein) and technical errors. Acute and chronic DVT can be confused at sonography. Certain features are used to differentiate between these entities (Table 15-2). Sometimes, however, it is impossible to distinguish among an acute clot occupying a previously normal vein, a chronic organized clot, and acute clot superimposed on chronic disease (Fig. 15-11). It is for this reason that some experts recommend a follow-up sonogram as a baseline study for all patients with acute DVT in the event that symptoms recur.

The clinical significance of isolated calf vein DVT is controversial.[28,44,45] Compression sonography and color Doppler flow imaging are fairly accurate in detecting calf vein clot.[46,47] In some series, the sensitivity of color Doppler sonography is comparable in the calf veins and

---

TABLE 15-1 Color Doppler Sonography of Acute Deep Vein Thrombosis

Factor	Normal Finding
Color flow	Complete saturation
Compressibility with transducer	Complete coaptation of vein walls (at accessible sites)
Phasicity	Decreased flow with inspiration, increased with expiration (reflects patency of central veins)
Provocative maneuvers	Flow increased with calf compression, decreased with Valsalva (reflects patency of central veins)

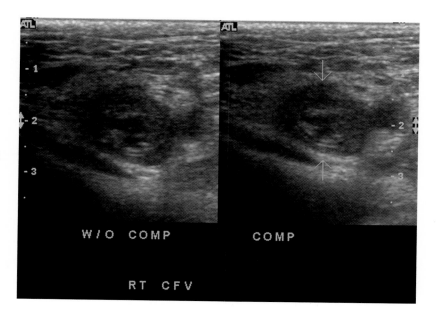

FIGURE 15-10 Acute right common femoral vein thrombosis. The vein is enlarged *(left)*. There is minimal deformity of the vein with transducer compression *(right)*. No color flow was seen at all.

TABLE 15-2   Sonographic Distinction Between Acute and Chronic Deep Venous Thrombosis

Feature	Acute DVT	Chronic DVT
Lumen	Dilated	Narrowed or normal caliber
Luminal flow	Absent or minimal	Residual flow, reflux
Vein wall	Thin	Thickened
Collaterals	Poorly developed	Well developed
Compression	Spongy	Firm resistance

DVT, *deep venous thrombosis.*

proximal veins. But in routine practice, technically inadequate studies of the calf are relatively common.[40,48] Some practitioners opt for serial examinations of the proximal veins to identify propagation into the femoropopliteal system.

COMPUTED TOMOGRAPHY IMAGING

Even though CT venography of the lower extremities is relatively accurate, it is rarely employed as the initial step in routine cases. Some centers favor combined CT venography and CT pulmonary angiography in patients with suspected venous thromboembolic disease.[49] CT venography is more accurate than sonography in the pelvic veins and IVC and may identify the mechanism for isolated iliofemoral DVT.[50-53] Typical findings are luminal filling defects, vein wall enhancement, and filling of collateral veins (see Fig. 15-9). Incomplete opacification of vein segments and beam-hardening artifacts can mimic clot.

MAGNETIC RESONANCE IMAGING

The accuracy of MR venography in the diagnosis of DVT in the leg is similar to contrast venography and duplex sonography.[54-56] However, an MR examination is more costly and time consuming than a sonogram. Still, MR imaging (MRI) is superior to sonography for pelvic vein and IVC disease.

ASCENDING VENOGRAPHY

Although catheter-based contrast venography was once considered the gold standard in the diagnosis of acute and chronic DVT, in fact it was not always reliable.[57] One autopsy study revealed a sensitivity and specificity of 89% and 97%, respectively.[58] Interobserver variability is at least 10% to 15%.[59] The procedure is uncomfortable for the patient, and it has a small risk of significant complications. For these reasons, it rarely is used for diagnosis anymore.

A fresh clot produces an intraluminal, wormlike filling defect (Fig. 15-12). Abrupt occlusion of a vein can reflect acute or chronic thrombosis (see Fig. 15-8).

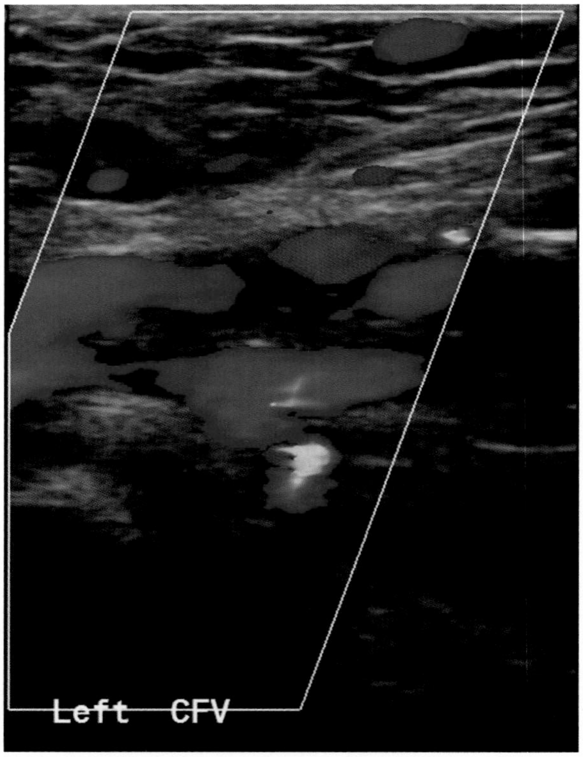

FIGURE 15-11   Chronic left common femoral vein thrombosis. In longitudinal plane, there is partial color saturation with luminal irregularity.

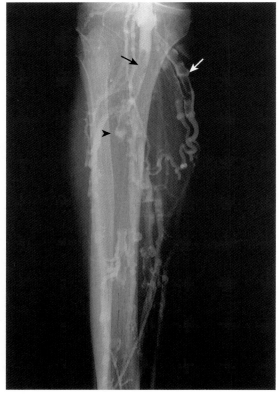

FIGURE 15-12   Acute thrombosis of tibial *(arrowhead),* gastrocnemius *(white arrow),* and popliteal veins *(black arrow).*

Nonfilling of deep veins, preferential filling of superficial veins, and opacification of collateral veins may occur with acute or chronic DVT. Thrombus may be confused with other causes for nonfilling of portions of the deep venous system.

Imaging Strategy

Every physician must develop his or her own algorithm for assessing symptomatic and high-risk patients for acute DVT using a combination of risk-factor analysis, lab testing (D-dimer), color Doppler sonography, and other imaging studies. Periodic surveillance of at-risk populations has uncovered lower extremity DVT in up to 28% of patients, about 80% of whom were asymptomatic.[60-62] Many clinicians order follow-up exams after a normal ultrasound in all cases or at least in those with moderate to high clinical probability of disease. However, only 1% to 2% of patients with initially negative studies subsequently are shown to have developed proximal DVT.[63,64] D-dimer results may be used to withhold ultrasound in patients with low clinical probability.[37] A follow-up study after completion of anticoagulant therapy may be advantageous in higher-risk patients should symptoms recur in order to distinguish chronic disease from recurrent acute DVT.

Treatment

Patients with acute DVT are treated to prevent or limit the major sequelae of venous thrombosis: PE, CVI, and recurrent DVT.[28,65,66]

MEDICAL THERAPY

The cornerstone of treatment is anticoagulation. In addition, class II (30 mm Hg) elastic compression stockings are strongly recommended to lessen the risk for PTS.[67] Anticoagulation does not directly promote fibrinolysis, but it allows endogenous lysis to occur and reduces the likelihood of PE by limiting clot propagation. For many decades, treatment for DVT consisted of unfractionated intravenous heparin (3 to 5 days) and oral warfarin (at least 3 to 6 months).[28,68] In most centers, low molecular weight heparin (e.g., enoxaparin, tinzaparin) or a specific factor Xa inhibitor (e.g., fondaparinux) has replaced initial heparin therapy. Low molecular weight heparins have a more predictable response and a longer duration of action, and they can be given at home once or twice daily as a subcutaneous injection[66,68] (see Chapters 2 and 3). Monitoring of drug effect is unnecessary except in certain situations (e.g., obesity, pregnancy, heart or liver failure). Therapeutic anticoagulation substantially reduces the likelihood of PE. Even with full compliance, however, recurrent DVT still occurs in more than 25% of cases, and at least one fourth will ultimately suffer from chronic PTS.[31,65,69,70]

Treatment of *isolated* calf vein DVT is controversial, because without anticoagulation there is a 20% to 30% risk for clot propagation, a small risk for significant PE, and about a 30% risk for CVI.[31,62,65,69,71] Even without compelling data, many physicians still treat such individuals with a short course of anticoagulation because they are concerned about proximal extension. Those not treated may undergo follow-up Doppler sonography to exclude clot propagation.

IVC FILTER PLACEMENT

If there is a contraindication to or history of complication from anticoagulation, a retrievable IVC filter should be placed instead (see Chapter 16). The detection of free-floating iliofemoral or IVC thrombus deserves special mention. Even with therapeutic anticoagulation, the possibility of PE exceeds 30%; thus insertion of a retrievable IVC filter is prudent.[72]

CATHETER-DIRECTED ILIOFEMORAL VENOUS THROMBOLYSIS

There is ample evidence that following an episode of lower extremity DVT, return of normal valve activity largely is a function of the time to thrombus resolution.[7,73-75] Thus the main reason for aggressive endovascular clot removal in patients with proximal acute DVT is the prevention of CVI and recurrent DVT. A secondary benefit is more rapid symptom relief.

Systemic thrombolytic infusion is moderately successful in this situation, but bleeding complications are frequent.[76-78] Catheter-directed thrombolysis (with or without adjunctive mechanical thrombectomy) offers faster, safer, and more effective treatment for acute venous thrombosis.[79,80]

PATIENT SELECTION Careful case screening is important to avoid subjecting unsuitable patients to this intensive procedure[66,76] (Box 15-5).

- The risk for PTS is relatively low in individuals with isolated calf DVT or asymptomatic DVT; in those patients, thrombolysis is *not* warranted.[81]
- Patients with subacute or chronic venous thrombosis (>2 to 4 weeks), prior ipsilateral proximal DVT, nonambulatory state, or short life expectancy generally do not benefit from thrombolysis.[66,67,79] Individuals with subacute or chronic ilofemoral vein occlusion may benefit from angioplasty and stent placement (Fig. 15-13).
- Individuals with risk factors associated with fibrinolytic agents or full-dose anticoagulants (see Box 3-7) may be suitable for mechanical thrombectomy alone.
- Phlegmasia cerulea dolens is a medical emergency and demands rapid, aggressive treatment.[25,82]

TECHNIQUE Most interventionalists do not place prophylactic IVC filters before thrombolysis unless the consequence of even small pulmonary emboli is great, a large free-floating iliac or IVC clot is found, or mechanical thrombectomy without enzymatic lysis is necessary because of excessive bleeding risks.[31] Many experienced practitioners prefer ultrasound-guided ipsilateral popliteal vein entry. However, solitary or dual access through the internal jugular or femoral veins may sometimes be more appropriate (Fig. 15-14). The entire venous occlusion is traversed with a guidewire and catheter; then, venography is done to document the full extent of thrombus burden.

There are a variety of techniques to treat the clot (see Chapter 3).

- Placement of multiside hole catheter for intrathrombic infusion thrombolysis with

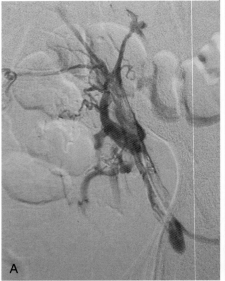
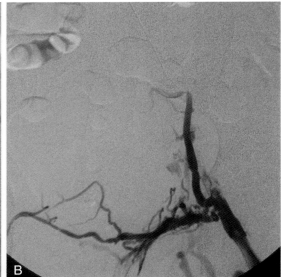
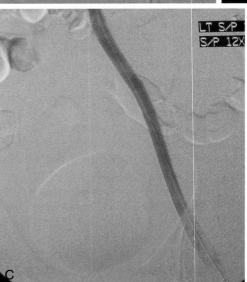

FIGURE 15-13   Chronic iliac vein venous thrombosis unresponsive to thrombolysis (same patient as Figure 15-8). **A,** After overnight infusion with tissue plasminogen activator, some lysis is noted. **B,** After about 48 hours of thrombolytic infusion, persistent occlusion is noted. **C,** Following angioplasty and Wallstent placement, the vein is widely patent.

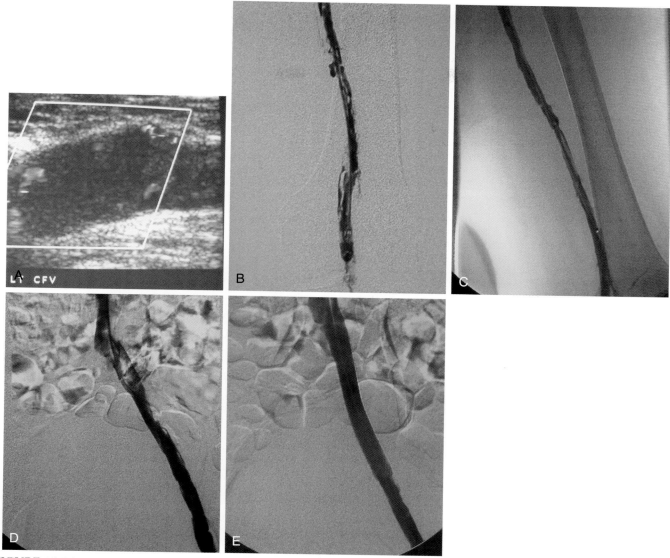

FIGURE 15-14   Iliofemoral deep venous thrombolysis. **A,** Acute thrombus in the left common femoral vein. Disease extends up the iliac vein and down to the popliteal vein. **B,** After 18 hours of tissue plasminogen activator infusion from catheters placed from the popliteal and right internal jugular vein, there is moderate clot dissolution. **C** and **D,** After 36 hours of treatment, there is near complete lysis of the entire diseased segment. **E,** A Wallstent is placed to treat extrinsic disease in the left common iliac vein, with excellent results.

tissue plasminogen activator (or other fibrinolytic agent) at about 1 mg/hr
- Ultrasound-assisted thrombolysis with the EKOS catheter
- "Isolated thrombolysis" with Trellis infusion system
- Enzymatic lysis combined with Arrow-Trerotola or AngioJet mechanical thrombectomy[83-85]

Anticoagulation with heparin is initiated to maintain the partial thromboplastin time (PTT) in the 60- to 80-second range. Thrombolysis alone often requires large doses of a fibrinolytic agent and 2 to 3 days of infusion.[79,86-94] Unfortunately, rapid mechanical thrombectomy alone is not effective in most hands; infusion of a fibrinolytic drug is mandatory, alone or combined with mechanical clot dissolution. Thrombectomy devices may be used initially to reduce the clot burden or employed after lytic infusion to eliminate residual clots.

After the bulk of the clot has been removed, balloon angioplasty and self-expanding stent placement (as needed in the iliac and sometimes femoral veins) are performed to treat residual disease. Because of the availability of large diameter stents and resistance to plastic deformity from extrinsic compression, the Wallstent is still the favored device (Fig. 15-15; see Fig. 15-14). Following the procedure, patients are maintained on

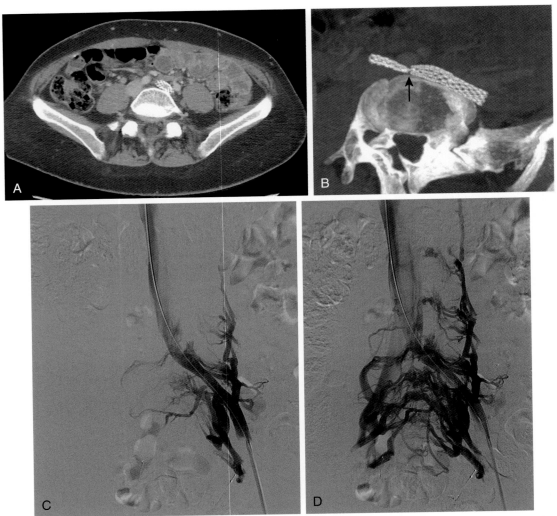

FIGURE 15-15   Collapsed iliac vein stent. Axial **(A)** and magnified **(B)** computed tomography (CT) scans of a previously placed left iliac vein balloon expandable stent shows a crushed device *(arrow)*. **C** and **D,** Left iliac venography demonstrates an the extensive collateral circulation that indicates some degree of obstruction.

aggressive anticoagulation for 6 months to 3 years (or indefinitely if a thrombophilic disorder is identified).[7] Compressive elastic stockings are also strongly recommended for 2 years afterward.

RESULTS   Technical success (using urokinase or tissue plasminogen activator) is achieved in 80% to 95% of cases when the thrombotic disease is acute.* Primary patency at 1 year ranges from 63% to 90% for the iliac segment and 40% to 47% for the femoral segment. There is now very strong evidence for the value of

catheter-directed thrombolysis for reducing PTS after a first episode of acute iliofemoral DVT. The ongoing CaVenT randomized trial is most compelling in this regard.[67] Preliminary findings in the lytic arm included 90% moderate to complete lysis, 2% incidence of major bleeding complications, reduction of venous obstruction at 6 months from 49% to 20%, but no significant difference in incidence of femoral venous insufficiency (60%).

COMPLICATIONS   Major bleeding complications occurred in 11% of cases in the publication from a multiinstitution venous registry.[79] PE attributed to the thrombolytic procedure itself is reported in about 1% of cases.

*See references 80, 84, 88, 89, 95-104.

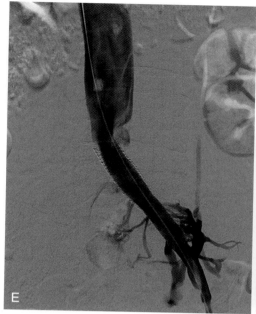

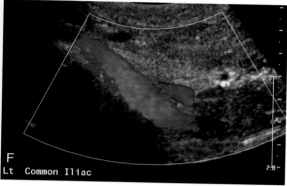

FIGURE 15-15, cont'd **E,** Following additional stent deployment, venography shows excellent flow. **F,** Duplex sonography about 6 months later confirms continued patency.

SURGICAL THERAPY

Endovascular methods largely have supplanted open thrombectomy procedures unless venous gangrene is imminent. Operative techniques for treating iliofemoral DVT include Fogarty embolectomy, thrombectomy, and venovenous bypass. Occasionally, a temporary distal arteriovenous fistula is constructed to improve flow through the newly reconstructed vessels.[7,105]

Post-thrombotic Syndrome (Online Cases 37 and 59)

Etiology and Natural History

If clot does not embolize after an episode of acute leg DVT, it becomes attached to the vein wall within several weeks of formation. When endogenous fibrinolysis occurs at all, it begins in the center of the lumen. Over time, the clot may lyse completely and leave intact vein walls and relatively normal valves. If clot resolution is incomplete, the result is residual vein wall thickening, an irregular intraluminal channel, and incompetence of deep and perforating vein valves.

Even with optimal therapy, more than 25% of individuals who suffer a proximal leg DVT will progress to the potentially disabling post-thrombotic syndrome (PTS). The unifying feature of PTS is *ambulatory venous hypertension*.[106] In most cases, the condition is caused by incompetent valves and abnormal reflux of blood from the deep to the superficial venous system. Less

often, venous outflow obstruction (with or without associated reflux) is the primary cause. Chronically diseased veins remain in half to two thirds of patients who have acute iliofemoral DVT, which is a much higher proportion than observed after femoro-popliteal or isolated calf DVT.[32,107,108] The strongest predictor for development of PTS is recurrent DVT; other factors include obesity, gender, and thrombophilic state.[69,70,109] PTS is more likely when venous recanalization is delayed or slow, rethrombosis occurs, or reflux in the popliteal or saphenous vein ensues.[7,33] Rarely, inadequate function of the calf pump (e.g., in paralyzed patients) contributes to the disorder.

The pathophysiology of CVI is incompletely understood.[33,110] Venous hypertension from reflux and/or obstruction causes capillary damage leading to passage of fluid, proteins, free radicals, and red and white blood cells into the interstitial spaces of the leg. Accumulation of fibrinogen produces a "fibrin cuff" that some think contributes to the classic skin changes associated with the disease. The late effects are local hypoxia, inflammation, and tissue loss.

Clinical Features

Symptoms usually develop months to many years after the acute episode.[110] Some patients give no history of acute DVT. Early signs of CVI include leg "heaviness" or aching or swelling (worsened with standing, improved with leg elevation). Later, skin thickening and erythema *(stasis dermatitis)* are present, characteristically just above the medial malleolus. These changes may progress to skin induration and hyperpigmentation *(lipodermatosclerosis)*. In the late stages, the skin becomes fibrotic and venous ulcers develop. On the other hand, deep ulcers with sharp margins associated with diminished peripheral pulses and abnormal ankle brachial index suggest an ischemic arterial ulcer.[111] So-called venous claudication is deep muscular pain felt in the thigh or calf during exercise and characteristically relieved by rest and leg elevation.

When caused by prior thrombotic disease, symptoms often are unilateral. When caused by primary valve dysfunction, the symptoms usually are bilateral. The clinical exam is in no way a reliable predictor of the site or severity of disease, or the relative contributions of valve dysfunction and venous obstruction.[3] CVI can mimic arterial obstructive disease, neuropathic disorders, congestive heart failure, or kidney disease.

Imaging

Imaging is important in the management of patients with suspected chronic lower extremity venous disease. The most important questions to address are patency of the deep venous system, valvular incompetence in superficial, deep, and perforating veins, the extent of reflux, and the exact sites of incompetent veins.

SONOGRAPHY

Color Doppler sonography is the standard test for studying patients with CVI when invasive therapy is being considered[3,112,113] (see Fig. 15-2). With the aid of provocative measures (e.g., compression of calf veins, Valsalva maneuver), venous reflux, valvular dysfunction, and incompetent perforating veins are detected and mapped. Sonography also identifies persistently occluded or partially recanalized deep veins.

PLETHYSMOGRAPHY

Sonography is an outstanding tool for providing a narrow window on focal venous disease of the leg, but it is relatively useless in assessing the overall dysfunction of the venous circulation. For that, air or strain-gauge plethysmography is needed. Both tests measure changes in limb volume as a reflection of overall venous hemodynamics.[114]

COMPUTED TOMOGRAPHY AND MAGNETIC RESONANCE IMAGING

CT or MR venography can be useful adjuncts to duplex sonography, particularly in the evaluation of chronic pelvic venous disease.

CONTRAST VENOGRAPHY

Ascending venography rarely is needed in this setting. The appearance of chronic DVT can vary from recanalized veins with narrow, irregular, web-filled lumens, distorted valves, and incompetent perforators to nonopacification of deep veins with preferential filling of superficial veins and collateral channels (Figs. 15-16 and 15-17; see also Figs. 15-8 and 15-13).

Treatment

To speak the common language of phlebologists and to choose treatment wisely, the CEAP and VCSS (Venous Clinical Severity Score) classification schemes of the American Venous Forum should be applied to each case[115] (Tables 15-3 and 15-4). The former system categorizes individuals by clinical severity, etiology of disease (primary, secondary, congenital), location (superficial, deep, perforator), and pathophysiology (reflux and obstruction, alone or in combination).

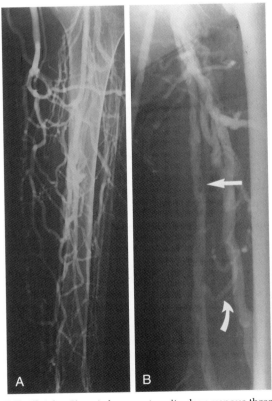

FIGURE 15-16   Chronic lower extremity deep venous thrombosis. **A,** Deep veins of the calf remain completely occluded, and venous drainage is entirely through superficial channels. **B,** Recanalization of a previously occluded left femoral vein. The vein is irregular, contains several webs *(straight arrow)*, is devoid of normal-appearing valves, and communicates with the deep femoral vein *(curved arrow)*.

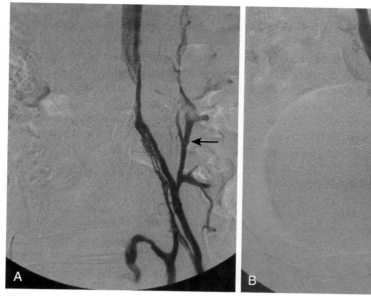

FIGURE 15-17 Patient with symptoms of chronic venous insufficiency. **A,** Pelvic venogram shows recanalized left external and common iliac veins and lower inferior vena cava with luminal irregularity. Ascending lumbar venous collaterals also are present *(arrow).* **B,** After angioplasty with a 10-mm balloon and placement of a 14-mm diameter Wallstent, the vein is widely patent.

TABLE 15-3 Revised CEAP Classification System for Chronic Venous Disease

Class	Stage
0	No signs of venous disease
1	Telangiectasias, reticular veins
2	Varicose veins
3	Lower extremity edema without skin changes
4	Skin pigmentation, lipodermatosclerosis
5	Skin changes with healed ulcer
6	Skin changes with active ulcer

TABLE 15-4 Venous Clinical Severity Score (VCSS) for Chronic Venous Disease

Attribute	Mild	Severe
Pain	Occasional	Limits activities
Varicose veins	Few, scattered	Extensive
Venous edema	Evening, ankle only	All day, most of leg
Pigmentation	Limited area	Wide area
Inflammation	Cellulitis	Severe cellulitis
Induration	Focal (<5 cm)	Entire lower third of lower leg
Number of ulcers	1	3
Ulcer duration	<3 months	>1 year
Ulcer diameter	<2 cm	>6 cm
Compression Rx	Intermittent	Constant

For each attribute, score 0 = none, mild = 1, moderate = 2, severe = 3.

MEDICAL THERAPY

The mainstay of therapy for CVI is leg elevation, exercise, weight reduction, and graded elastic compressive stockings (pressure >20 mm Hg).[33] Simple, semiocclusive, or biologic dressings are applied to the ulcers themselves.

ENDOVASCULAR THERAPY

Patients with CVI primarily because of venous outflow obstruction may benefit from endovascular treatment, particularly when disease is confined to the iliocaval segment.[107,116] Fibrinolysis and mechanical thrombectomy devices generally have no role in this situation. Endovascular recanalization of chronic femoropopliteal disease is frequently not durable.

After gaining vascular access (to the ipsilateral popliteal or femoral vein) with sonographic guidance, the obstruction is crossed with a guidewire and catheter (see Fig. 15-17). If the guidewire will traverse the entire obstruction but a catheter will not follow, the wire may be snared from an access site on the other side of the blocked segment. Tension on the wire from both ends usually permits a catheter to be advanced. Although the wire may be partially in a subintimal location, recanalization is still safe. Full anticoagulation is instituted. Large overlapping stents (e.g., Wallstents) are laid along the entire occlusion. Typical nominal stent diameters are common femoral/external iliac vein 12 mm, common iliac vein 14 to 16 mm, and IVC 16 to 20 mm or more. Ambulation is ordered starting the next day. Compression stockings are mandatory because worsening of venous reflux is the norm. If safe, patients receive clopidogrel for 1 to 3 months, followed by lifelong aspirin, and at least 3 to 6 months of warfarin anticoagulation.

In recent reviews of published experience with this disorder, technical success exceeded 90%, midterm assisted patency exceeded 80%, and complete symptom relief and ulcer healing was observed in about half of cases[117-119] In one large series by a leading investigator in the field, not only did clinical symptoms (particularly venous claudication) abate in the majority of treated individuals, but objective improvement in venous flow and calf pump function also was the rule.[117] Not surprisingly, venous reflux worsened, highlighting the need for compressive stockings. Notably, about one fourth of patients complained of transient back pain afterward.

SURGICAL THERAPY

The nihilistic view of surgery for chronic venous insufficiency was challenged in a recent trial that showed real reduction in venous ulcer recurrence (though not time to healing) after *superficial* vein surgery plus compressive therapy compared with compressive therapy alone.[120] However, the role of surgical repair for *deep* and *perforating* vein incompetence is controversial. Options include vein transfer, internal valvuloplasty, subfascial endoscopic perforator surgery (SEPS), and extrafascial perforator ligations. When endovascular methods fail, iliac vein obstruction can be managed with a femorofemoral vein crossover graft using saphenous vein (Palma procedure).[121] Sometimes, the surgeon will construct a temporary distal arteriovenous fistula to improve patency.

Varicose Veins and Primary Venous Insufficiency

Etiology and Natural History (Video 15-1 and Online Case 98)

Primary venous insufficiency must be distinguished from the secondary form discussed earlier.[122] The precise etiology is obscure, but prevailing research points to underlying structural defects in the vein wall that are ultimately responsible for valve failure and vein enlargement.[123] Regardless of the reason for valve dysfunction, both hydrostatic forces (column of blood acting unopposed on superficial veins) and hydrodynamic ones (calf muscle pump acting on subcutaneous veins in the absence of functional perforating valves) work to

allow superficial venous reflux.[124] In a minority of cases, obstruction and valve incompetence in the deep veins are culpable.[111] Primary superficial venous incompetence can progress to chronic venous insufficiency with associated skin changes, although many of those patients also have chronic deep vein disease (see earlier discussion).

Lower extremity venous insufficiency manifested by telangiectasias and varicose veins afflicts 10% to 20% of men and 25% to 33% of women in Western populations.[1,122] Varicose veins are more common in some families, in obese individuals, in women, and with advancing age.[125]

Clinical Features

The obvious visual signs of the primary venous insufficiency are small telangiectasias and reticular varicosities (CEAP class 1 disease) and later large varicose veins (class 2 disease). Patients also may complain of leg aching, pain, or "heaviness," and eventually postural swelling confined to the foot and ankle (class 3 disease). Symptoms are worse with prolonged standing and at the beginning of the menstrual period. In a minority of cases, pruritic chronic skin changes develop (pigmentation or lipodermatosclerosis, class 4 disease) followed rarely by venous ulcers (class 5 or 6 disease).

Imaging

Ultrasound is the primary modality for assessing patients with superficial venous incompetence and associated symptoms.[1,2,124,126,127] Marked enlargement of the GSV (>4 mm) or SSV (>3 mm) is evident. At the level of major valves, prolonged reversal of flow (>0.5 sec) is observed with Doppler waveform analysis after manual compression of upstream venous beds (see Fig. 15-2). Reflux in the main channels is traced to the level of incompetent tributaries and superficial varicosities. In particular, the anterolateral and posteromedial channels should be assessed. Even following saphenous vein ligation, the sonographer may identify persistent refluxing segments of the GSV or enlarged major tributaries. The most common patterns are insufficiency at the confluence of the superficial inguinal veins, allowing GSV reflux, insufficiency of the femoral canal perforator with lower GSV reflux, external pudendal vein reflux leading to GSV reflux, and incompetence of the intersaphenous vein leading to GSV and SSV reflux. Again, after clinical evaluation and venous imaging, the extent of disease is classified according to the CEAP scheme to optimize communication among providers and guide treatment[115] (see Table 15-3).

Treatment

MEDICAL THERAPY

Patients with mild symptoms will note some relief with compression stockings and elevation of the affected leg.

SURGICAL THERAPY

Saphenous vein ligation and stripping (usually above the knee) combined with stab avulsion phlebectomy or sclerotherapy of varicosities is the standard operation for primary chronic venous insufficiency.[122] However, recurrent symptoms often develop after this procedure, possibly related to neovascularization.[128,129] This open approach is now reserved for failures of endovenous therapy (see later discussion). Lastly, perforator reflux is managed with the SEPS technique.[130]

ENDOVASCULAR THERAPY

Recently, endovascular techniques have become popular in treatment of this common disorder.[124] In fact, they are superior to surgical treatment in almost every way. Two particular methods have emerged, both invoking thermal obliteration of the GSV. A radiofrequency (RF) catheter and generator may be used.[131,132] Alternatively, an endovenous laser ablation probe is applied to the target vessel. Laser energy heats blood; steam bubbles then damage the vein and cause wall thickening with eventual vascular fibrosis. Following either method, residual perforating veins and varicosities are handled with percutaneous sclerotherapy or local phlebectomy.

The absolute requirements for endovenous treatment are clinical evidence of venous insufficiency, imaging proof of reflux lasting longer than 0.5 second, and a patent deep venous system. Contraindications include deep vein thrombosis and presence of arteriovenous malformations.[133] Individuals with restricted ambulation are also not candidates.

Most patients tolerate the procedure with oral anxiolytics alone. Using ultrasound, the entire course of the great saphenous vein and relevant tributaries is marked on the skin. This important first step confirms that the appropriate vessel is being treated and simplifies later imaging. Some practitioners apply anesthetic EMLA cream to the target area about half an hour before the start of the case. Nitropaste (1 to 2 inches) placed on the affected leg may limit vasospasm, which can make the procedure extremely tedious. Ultrasound guided access is gained to the GSV around the knee using a micropuncture set. A guiding sheath of appropriate length is inserted over a standard angiographic guidewire. Using ultrasound guidance and multiple injections, 60 to 120 mL of 0.2% lidocaine with bicarbonate is applied along the entire extravascular course of the GSV ("tumescent anesthesia"). In addition to offering pain relief, this crucial step compresses the vein

wall around the laser tip and creates a "heat-sink" that protects surrounding vital structures. The maximum lidocaine dose is about 5 mg/kg.

An 810 or 940 nm wavelength laser device is inserted through the sheath, which has been advanced to a precise point about 1 to 2 cm below the confluence of the superficial inguinal veins (saphenofemoral junction). The exposed activated tip of the device and guiding sheath then are slowly withdrawn through the length of the vein. For the GSV and other treated vein segments, >70 to 80 Joule/cm is delivered. Peripheral varicose tributaries are then treated by local sclerotherapy. A whole host of sclerosants are available but sodium tetradecyl sulfate (STS) is the most popular. STS foam 3% is appropriate for large varicosities; minute telangiectasias only require 0.125% to 0.25% detergent.

Patients should expect bruising, moderate pain, transient paresthesias, and a palpable cord along the course of the treated vein. Relief is obtained with nonsteroidal antiinflammatory drugs and Neurontin. Compression stockings are prescribed for 3 to 4 weeks afterward, but regular physical activity is also important. Early and long-term outcomes have been uniformly excellent, with more than 90% persistent obliteration at 2-year follow-up.[133-139] A recent metaanalysis of published reports calculated long-term success (mean 32 months) as follows: surgical stripping 78%, endovenous RF ablation 84%, and endovenous laser ablation 94%.[140] Local tenderness or transient paresthesias were observed in 7% to 15% of cases; DVT complicated the procedure less than 3% of the time. True adverse events (including dermal burns, nerve damage, and deep venous thromboembolism) are seen in less than 5% of procedures. These complications are minimized by avoiding probe activation near the common femoral vein or too peripherally in the calf.

OTHER DISORDERS

Iliofemoral Venous Stenoses

Clinically significant stenoses of the lower extremity veins are uncommon. Obstructions usually develop at sites of extrinsic compression or intimal injury (Box 15-6). Most symptomatic stenoses are found in the iliac veins. Some of these patients suffer from pelvic (especially gynecologic) malignancies and have undergone local treatment with surgery or irradiation.

Mild narrowing of the upper left common iliac vein as it passes between the right common iliac artery and the spine is a frequent finding in the normal population (see Fig. 15-6). Severe compression may lead to *iliac vein compression (May-Thurner or Cockett) syndrome*[141-143]

BOX 15-6

CAUSES OF ILIOFEMORAL VEIN NARROWING

- Iliac vein compression (May-Thurner) syndrome
- Pelvic surgery
- Pelvic neoplasm or mass
- Chronic deep venous thrombosis
- Trauma
- Pregnancy
- Retroperitoneal fibrosis
- Venospasm
- Radiation therapy
- Idiopathic causes

(Fig. 15-18). In this disorder, the venous intima has been injured from long-standing compression; webs (bands, "spurs") form in the lumen and obstruct venous flow. Stenosis can progress to complete thrombosis (see earlier). The classic symptoms are left leg swelling and pain in the absence of other risk factors for venous disease.

CT, MRI, or catheter venography is required to make a definitive diagnosis. Stenoses usually are smooth and short but may be long and irregular, particularly when they are caused by chronic DVT. Signs of hemodynamic significance include filling of collateral channels or a focal pressure gradient of 3 to 4 mm Hg or more.[141]

Generally, iliac vein stenoses require stent placement in addition to balloon angioplasty to achieve a durable result. Obstructions may be approached from the right internal jugular vein or either common femoral vein. The

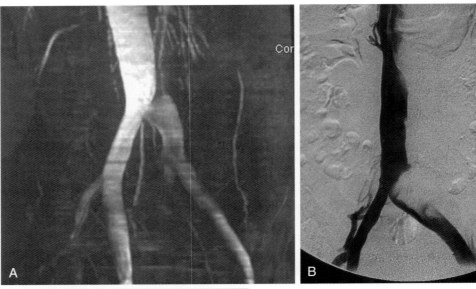

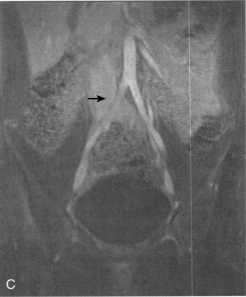

FIGURE 15-18   May-Thurner syndrome. Magnetic resonance (**A**) and catheter (**B**) pelvic venograms (in different patients) show narrowing of the left common iliac vein because of compression between the spine and the right common iliac artery (**C,** *arrow*).

jugular route avoids damage and possible thrombosis of the inflow vein, which could jeopardize the results of the procedure. Patients are heparinized during the intervention. Self-expanding stents (e.g., Wallstents) generally are preferred because many of these lesions have a component of extrinsic compression that could cause permanent plastic deformation and crushing of a balloon-expandable device (see Fig. 15-15). Typically, a 14- to 16-mm diameter stent is necessary in the common and external iliac veins.

Some experts favor anticoagulation with warfarin after stent placement. Recanalization is successful in greater than 90% of cases.[141,144,145] The 1-year primary patency rate ranges from about 50% to 80%. Malignant obstructions are more prone to late occlusion than are benign strictures. Major complications are reported in up to 7% of cases and include access site bleeding, stent malposition, and stent migration. Traditional concerns about placing self-expanding stents across the hip joint may be unfounded.[146]

Trauma

Lower extremity venous trauma requires specific therapy far less often than does arterial trauma, and imaging is rarely needed to evaluate potential injuries[147,148]

(Fig. 15-19). However, occult venous damage is relatively common and ultimately can lead to DVT or PE. Color Doppler sonography is an excellent tool for screening the leg in this population; its accuracy is similar to that of contrast venography.[149] Unsuspected venous trauma may be discovered at the time of surgery for an associated arterial injury. The vein is treated by direct repair, bypass grafting, or ligation.[7,150] As a life-saving measure, an occlusion balloon may be inflated to halt exsanguinating hemorrhage and allow definitive repair.[151]

Aneurysms

Aneurysms of pelvic and extremity veins are exceedingly rare[152,153] (Fig. 15-20). By far, the most common site is the popliteal vein. The diagnosis usually is made by color Doppler sonography. Because of the likelihood for clot formation and subsequent PE, venous reconstruction often is performed.

Venous Malformations

Congenital venous malformations of the legs are considered in Chapter 8.

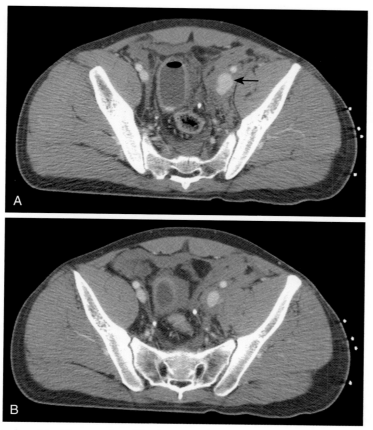

FIGURE 15-19　Iliac vein injury from blunt trauma. **A** and **B,** Contrast-enhanced computed tomography images show abnormal dilation of the left iliac vein *(arrow)* with surrounding density representing blood.

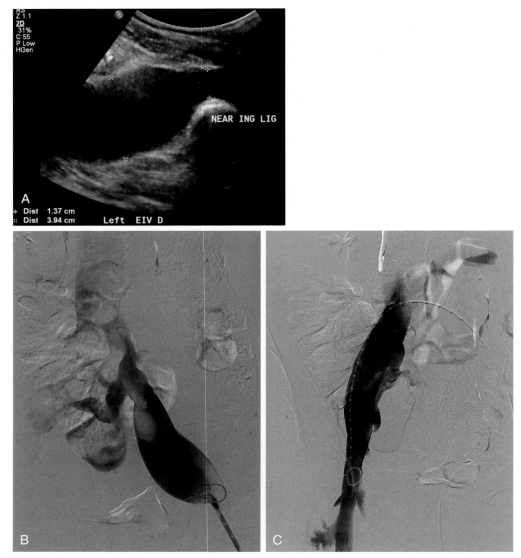

FIGURE 15-20   Iliac vein aneurysm. An incidentally detected massive left external iliac vein aneurysm is noted on a longitudinal ultrasound **(A)** and later on preoperative catheter venography **(B).** The right common and external iliac veins are also dilated **(C).**

References

1. Min RJ, Khilnani NM, Golia P. Duplex ultrasound evaluation of lower extremity venous insufficiency. *J Vasc Interv Radiol* 2003; **14**:1233.

2. Cavezzi A, Labropoulos N, Partsch H, et al. Duplex ultrasound investigation of the veins in chronic venous disease of the lower limbs–UIP consensus document. Part II. Anatomy. *Vasa* 2007; **36**:62.

3. Meissner MH, Moneta G, Burnard K, et al. The hemodynamics and diagnosis of venous disease. *J Vasc Surg* 2007;**46**:4S.

4. Caggiati A, Bergan JJ, Gloviczki P, et al. Nomenclature of the veins of the lower limb: extensions, refinements, and clinical application. *J Vasc Surg* 2005;**41**:719.

5. Gabella G, editor. Cardiovascular system. In: Williams PL, Bannister LH, Berry MM, et al, editors. *Gray's anatomy,* 38th ed. New York: Churchill Livingstone; 1995. p. 1595.

6. Kibbe MR, Ujiki M, Goodwin AL, et al. Iliac vein compression in an asymptomatic population. *J Vasc Surg* 2004;**39**:937.

7. Meissner MH, Wakefield TW, Ascher E, et al. Acute venous disease: venous thrombosis and venous trauma. *J Vasc Surg* 2007; **46**:25S.

8. Cohn JD, Caggiati A, Korver KF. Accessory and great saphenous veins as coronary artery bypass conduits. *Interact Cardiovasc Thorac Surg* 2006;**5**:550.

9. Quinlan DJ, Alikhan R, Gishen P, et al. Variations in lower limb venous anatomy: implications for US diagnosis of deep vein thrombosis. *Radiology* 2003;**228**:443.

10. Gloviczki P, Driscoll DJ. Klippel-Trenaunay syndrome: current management. *Phlebology* 2007;**22**:291.

11. Mavilli E, Ozturk M, Akcali Y, et al. Direct CT venography for evaluation of the lower extremity venous anomalies of Klippel-Trenaunay syndrome. *AJR Am J Roentgenol* 2009;**192**:W311.

12. Bastarrika G, Redondo P, Sierra A, et al. New techniques for the evaluation and therapeutic planning of patients with Klippel-Trenaunay syndrome. *J Am Acad Dermatol* 2007;**56**:242.

13. Tian XL, Kadaba R, You SA, et al. Identification of an angiogenic factor that when mutated causes susceptibility to Klippel-Trenaunay syndrome. *Nature* 2004;**427**:640.

14. Peirce RM, Funaki B. Direct MR venography of persistent sciatic vein in a patient with Klippel-Trenaunay-Weber syndrome. *AJR Am J Roentgenol* 2002;**178**:513.

15. Cherry Jr KJ, Gloviczki P, Stanson AW. Persistent sciatic vein: diagnosis and treatment of a rare condition. *J Vasc Surg* 1996;**23**:490.

16. Caughton JD, Bozlar U, Arslan B, et al. Catheter-directed thrombolysis and mechanical thrombectomy of a thrombosed persistent sciatic vein in a patient with Klippel-Trenaunay syndrome. *J Vasc Interv Radiol* 2007;**18**:1028.

17. American Thoracic Society. The diagnostic approach to acute venous thromboembolism. *Am J Respir Crit Care Med* 1999;**160**:1043.

18. Hyers TM. Management of venous thromboembolism. *Arch Intern Med* 2003;**163**:759.

19. Wells PS, Anderson DR, Rodger M, et al. Evaluation of D-dimer in the diagnosis of suspected deep-vein thrombosis. *N Engl J Med* 2003;**349**:1227.

20. Philbrick JT, Becker DM. Calf deep venous thrombosis. A wolf in sheep's clothing? *Arch Intern Med* 1988;**148**:2131.

21. Moser KM, LeMoine JR. Is embolic risk conditioned by location of deep venous thrombosis? *Ann Intern Med* 1981;**94**:439.

22. Piccioli A, Prandoni P, Goldhaber SZ. Epidemiologic characteristics, management, and outcome of deep venous thrombosis in a tertiary-care hospital: the Brigham and Women's Hospital DVT registry. *Am Heart J* 1996;**132**:1010.

23. Comerota AJ, Gravett MH. Iliofemoral venous thrombosis. *J Vasc Surg* 2007;**46**:1065.

24. Delis KT, Bountouroglou D, Mansfield AO. Venous claudication in iliofemoral thrombosis: long-term effects on venous hemodynamics, clinical status, and quality of life. *Ann Surg* 2004;**239**:118.

25. Tung CS, Soliman PT, Wallace MJ, et al. Successful catheter-directed venous thrombolysis in phlegmasia cerulea dolens. *Gynecol Oncol* 2007;**107**:140.

26. Johnson BF, Manzo RA, Bergelin RO, et al. Relationship between changes in the deep venous system and the development of post thrombotic syndrome after an acute episode of lower limb deep vein thrombosis: one- to six-year followup. *J Vasc Surg* 1995;**21**:307.

27. Barritt DW, Jordan SC. Anticoagulant drugs in the treatment of pulmonary embolism: a controlled trial. *Lancet* 1960;**1**:1309.

28. Bates SM, Ginsberg JS. Treatment of deep-vein thrombosis. *New Engl J Med* 2004;**351**:268.

29. Meissner MH, Caps MT, Bergelin RO, et al. Propagation, rethrombosis, and new thrombus formation after acute deep vein thrombosis. *J Vasc Surg* 1995;**22**:558.

30. Prandoni P, Lensing AW, Prins MH. Residual venous thrombosis as a predictive factor of recurrent venous thromboembolism. *Ann Intern Med* 2002;**137**:955.

31. Vedantham S. Interventional approaches to acute venous thromboembolism. *Semin Respir Crit Care Med* 2008;**29**:56.

32. Akesson H, Brudin L, Dahlstrom JD, et al. Venous function assessed during a 5-year period after acute iliofemoral venous thrombosis treated with anticoagulation. *Eur J Vasc Surg* 1990;**4**:43.

33. Meissner MH, Eklof B, Smith PC, et al. Secondary chronic venous disorders. *J Vasc Surg* 2007;**46**:68S.

34. Stein PD, Hull RD, Patel KC, et al. D-dimer for the exclusion of acute venous thrombosis and pulmonary embolism: a systematic review. *Ann Intern Med* 2004;**140**:589.

35. Caprini JA, Glase CJ, Anderson CB, et al. Laboratory markers in the diagnosis of venous thromboembolism. *Circulation* 2004;**109**(Suppl. 1):I4.

36. Fancher TL, White RH, Kravitz RL. Combined use of D-dimer testing and estimation of clinical probability in the diagnosis of deep vein thrombosis: systematic review. *BMJ* 2004;**329**:821.

37. Tan M, van Rooden CJ, Westerbeek RE, et al. Diagnostic management of clinically suspected acute deep vein thrombosis. *Br J Haematol* 2009;**146**:347.

38. Qaseem A, Snow V, Barry P, et al. Current diagnosis of venous thromboembolism in primary care: a clinical practice guideline from the American Academy of Family Physicians and the American College of Physicians. *Ann Fam Med* 2007;**5**:57.

39. Lewis BD, James EM, Welch TJ, et al. Diagnosis of acute deep venous thrombosis of the lower extremities: prospective evaluation of color duplex flow imaging versus venography. *Radiology* 1994;**192**:651.

40. Hamper UM, DeJong MR, Scoutt LM. Ultrasound evaluation of the lower extremity veins. *Radiol Clin North Am* 2007;**45**:525.

41. Vaccaro JP, Cronan JJ, Dorfman GS. Outcome analysis of patients with normal compression US examinations. *Radiology* 1990;**175**:645.

42. Johnson SA, Stevens SM, Woller SC, et al. Risk of deep vein thrombosis following a single negative whole-leg compression ultrasound: a systematic review and meta-analysis. *JAMA* 2010;**303**:438.

43. Kassai B, Boissel JP, Cucherat M, et al. A systematic review of the accuracy of ultrasound in the diagnosis of deep venous thrombosis in asymptomatic patients. *Thromb Haemost* 2004;**91**:655.

44. Cornuz J, Pearson SD, Polak JF. Deep venous thrombosis: complete lower extremity venous US evaluation in patients without known risk factors—outcome study. *Radiology* 1999;**211**:637.

45. Gottlieb RH, Voci SL, Syed L, et al. Randomized prospective study comparing routine versus selective use of sonography of the complete calf in patients with suspected deep venous thrombosis. *AJR Am J Roentgenol* 2003;**180**:241.

46. Baxter GM, Duffy P, Partridge E. Colour flow imaging of calf vein thrombosis. *Clin Radiol* 1992;**46**:198.

47. Yucel EK, Fisher JS, Egglin TK, et al. Isolated calf venous thrombosis: diagnosis with compression US. *Radiology* 1991;**179**:443.

48. Rose SC, Zwiebel WJ, Murdock LE, et al. Insensitivity of color Doppler flow imaging for detection of acute calf deep venous thrombosis in asymptomatic post-operative patients. *J Vasc Interv Radiol* 1993;**4**:111.

49. Salvolini L, Scaglione M, Guisepetti GM, et al. Suspected pulmonary embolism and deep venous thrombosis: a comprehensive MDCT diagnosis in the acute clinical setting. *Eur J Radiol* 2008;**65**:340.

50. Garg K, Mao J. Deep venous thrombosis: spectrum of findings and pitfalls in interpretation on CT venography. *AJR Am J Roentgenol* 2001;**177**:319.

51. Ghaye B, Szapiro D, Willems V, et al. Pitfalls in CT venography of lower limbs and abdominal veins. *AJR Am J Roentgenol* 2002;**178**:1465.

52. Chung JW, Yoon CJ, Jung SI, et al. Acute iliofemoral deep vein thrombosis: evaluation of underlying anatomic abnormalities by spiral CT venography. *J Vasc Interv Radiol* 2004;**15**:249.

53. Baldt MM, Zontsich T, Stuempflen A, et al. Deep venous thrombosis of the lower extremity: efficacy of spiral CT venography compared with conventional venography in diagnosis. *Radiology* 1996;**200**:423.

54. Fraser DG, Moody AR, Davidson IR, et al. Deep venous thrombosis: diagnosis by using venous enhanced subtracted peak arterial MR venography versus conventional venography. *Radiology* 2003;**226**:812.

55. Spritzer CE, Arata MA, Freed KS. Isolated pelvic deep venous thrombosis: relative frequency as detected with MR imaging. *Radiology* 2001;**219**:521.

56. Kluge A, Mueller C, Strunk J, et al. Experience in 207 combined MRI examinations for acute pulmonary embolism and deep vein thrombosis. *AJR Am J Roentgenol* 2006;**186**:1686.

57. Redman HC. Deep venous thrombosis: is contrast venography still the diagnostic "gold standard"? *Radiology* 1988;**168**:277.

58. Lund F, Diener L, Ericsson JL. Postmortem intraosseous phlebography as an aid in studies of venous thromboembolism. *Angiology* 1969;**20**:155.

59. McLachlan MS, Thomson JG, Taylor DW, et al. Observer variation in the interpretation of lower limb venograms. *AJR Am J Roentgenol* 1979;**132**:227.

60. Headrick JR Jr, Barker DE, Pate LM, et al. The role of ultrasonography and inferior vena cava filter placement in high-risk trauma patients. *Am Surgeon* 1997;**63**:1.

61. Flinn WR, Sandager GP, Silva MB Jr, et al. Prospective surveillance for perioperative venous thrombosis: experience in 2643 patients. *Arch Surg* 1996;**131**:472.

62. Hirsch DR, Ingenito EP, Goldhaber SZ. Prevalence of deep venous thrombosis among patients in medical intensive care. *JAMA* 1995;**274**:335.

63. Cogo A, Lensing AW, Koopman MM, et al. Compression ultrasonography for diagnostic management of patients with clinically suspected deep vein thrombosis: prospective cohort study. *Br Med J* 1998;**316**:17.

64. Heijboer H, Ginsberg JS, Buller HR, et al. The use of the D-dimer test in combination with non-invasive testing versus serial non-invasive testing alone for the diagnosis of deep-vein thrombosis. *Thromb Haemost* 1992;**67**:510.

65. Segal JB, Steiff MB, Hofmann LV, et al. Management of venous thromboembolism: a systematic review for a practice guideline. *Ann Intern Med* 2007;**146**:211.

66. Kearon C, Kahn SR, Agnelli G, et al. Antithrombotic therapy for venous thromboembolic disease: American College of Chest Physicians Evidence-based Clinical Practice Guidelines, 8th ed. *Chest* 2008;**133**:454S.

67. Enden T, Klow NE, Sandvik L, et al. Catheter-directed thrombolysis vs. anticoagulant therapy alone in deep vein thrombosis: results of an open randomized, controlled trial reporting on short term patency. *J Thromb Haemost* 2009;**7**:1268.

68. van Dongen CJ, van den Belt AG, Prins MH, et al. Fixed dose subcutaneous low molecular weight heparin versus adjusted dose unfractionated heparin for venous thromboembolism. *Cochrane Database Syst Rev* 2004;**18**:CD001100.

69. Prandoni P, Lensing AW, Cogo A, et al. The long-term clinical course of acute deep venous thrombosis. *Ann Intern Med* 1996;**125**:1.

70. Prandoni P, Lensing AW, Prins MH, et al. Below-knee elastic compression stockings to prevent the post-thrombotic syndrome: a randomized, controlled trial. *Ann Intern Med* 2004;**141**:249.

71. Protack CD, Bakken AM, Patel N, et al. Long-term outcomes of catheter-directed thrombolysis for lower extremity deep venous thrombosis without prophylactic inferior vena cava filter placement. *J Vasc Surg* 2007;**45**:992.

72. Baldridge E, Martin M, Welling R. Clinical significance of free-floating venous thrombi. *J Vasc Surg* 1990;**11**:62.

73. Koelbel T, Lindh M, Holst J, et al. Extensive acute deep vein thrombosis of the iliocaval segment: mid-term results of thrombolysis and stent placement. *J Vasc Interv Radiol* 2007;**18**:243.

74. O'shaughnessy AM, Fitzgerald DE. The patterns and distribution of residual abnormalities between the individual proximal venous segments after an acute deep vein thrombosis. *J Vasc Surg* 2001;**33**:379.

75. Plate G, Eklof B, Norgren L, et al. Venous thrombectomy for iliofemoral vein thrombosis-10 year results of a prospective randomized study. *Eur J Vasc Endovasc Surg* 1997;**14**:367.

76. Vedantham S. Catheter-directed thrombolysis for deep vein thrombosis. *Curr Opin Hematol* 2010;**17**:464.

77. Lin PH, Zhou W, Dardik A, et al. Catheter-directed thrombolysis versus pharmacomechanical thrombectomy for treatment of symptomatic lower extremity deep venous thrombosis. *Am J Surg* 2006;**192**:782.

78. Turpie AG, Levine MH, Hirsh J, et al. Tissue plasminogen activator (rt-PA) vs. heparin in deep vein thrombosis: results of a randomized trial. *Chest* 1990;**97**(Suppl. 4):172S.

79. Mewissen MW, Seabrook GR, Meissner MH, et al. Catheter-directed thrombolysis for lower extremity deep venous thrombosis: report of a national multicenter registry. *Radiology* 1999;**211**:39.

80. Watson LI, Armon MP. Thrombolysis for acute deep vein thrombosis. *Cochrane Database Syst Rev* 2004:CD002783.

81. Ginsberg JS, Hirsh J, Julian J, et al. Prevention and treatment of postphlebitic syndrome: results of a 3-part study. *Arch Intern Med* 2001;**161**:2105.

82. Robinson DL, Teitelbaum GP. Phlegmasia cerulea dolens: treatment by pulse-spray and infusion thrombolysis. *AJR Am J Roentgenol* 1993;**160**:1288.

83. McLafferty RB. Endovascular management of deep venous thrombosis. *Perspect Vasc Surg Endovasc Ther* 2008;**20**:87.

84. Cynamon J, Stein EG, Dym J, et al. A new method for aggressive management of deep vein thrombosis: retrospective study of the power pulse technique. *J Vasc Interv Radiol* 2006;**17**:1043.

85. O'Sullivan GJ, Lohan DG, Gough N, et al. Pharmacomechanical thrombectomy of acute deep vein thrombosis with the Trellis-8 isolated thrombolysis catheter. *J Vasc Interv Radiol* 2007;**18**:715.

86. Grunwald MR, Hofmann LV. Comparison of urokinase, alteplase, and reteplase for catheter-directed thrombolysis of deep venous thrombosis. *J Vasc Interv Radiol* 2004;**15**:347.

87. Castaneda F, Li R, Young K, et al. Catheter-directed thrombolysis in deep venous thrombosis with use of reteplase: immediate results and complications from a pilot study. *J Vasc Interv Radiol* 2002;**13**:577.

88. O'Sullivan GJ, Semba CP, Bittner CA, et al. Endovascular management of iliac vein compression (May-Thurner) syndrome. *J Vasc Interv Radiol* 2000;**11**:823.

89. Patel NH, Stookey KR, Ketcham DB, et al. Endovascular management of acute extensive iliofemoral deep venous thrombosis caused by May-Thurner syndrome. *J Vasc Interv Radiol* 2000;**11**:1297.

90. Vedantham S, Vesely TM, Parti N, et al. Lower extremity venous thrombolysis with adjunctive mechanical thrombectomy. *J Vasc Interv Radiol* 2002;**13**:1001.

91. Vedantham S, Vesely TM, Sicard GA, et al. Pharmacomechanical thrombolysis and early stent placement for iliofemoral deep vein thrombosis. *J Vasc Interv Radiol* 2004;**15**:565.

92. Kasirajan K, Gray B, Ouriel K. Percutaneous AngioJet thrombectomy in the management of extensive deep venous thrombosis. *J Vasc Interv Radiol* 2001;**12**:179.

93. Wells PS, Forster AJ. Thrombolysis in deep vein thrombosis: is there still an indication. *Thromb Haemost* 2001;**86**:499.

94. Comerota AJ, Throm RC, Mathias SD, et al. Catheter-directed thrombolysis for iliofemoral deep venous thrombosis improves health-related quality of life. *J Vasc Surg* 2000;**32**:130.

95. Elsharawy M, Elzayat E. Early results of thrombolysis vs. anticoagulation in iliofemoral venous thrombosis. A randomised clinical trial. *Eur J Vasc Endovasc Surg* 2002;**24**:209.

96. Vedantham S, Thorpe PE, Cardella JF, et al. Quality improvement guidelines for the treatment of lower extremity deep vein thrombosis with use of endovascular thrombus removal. *J Vasc Interv Radiol* 2006;**17**:435.

97. Comerota AJ, Kagan SA. Catheter directed thrombolysis for the treatment of acute iliofemoral vein thrombosis. *Phlebology* 2001;**15**:149.

98. Bjarnason H, Kruse JR, Asinger DA, et al. Iliofemoral deep venous thrombosis: safety and efficacy outcome during 5 years of catheter directed thrombolytic therapy. *J Vasc Interv Radiol* 1997;**8**:405.

99. Rao AS, Konig G, Leers SA, et al. Pharmacomechanical thrombectomy for iliofemoral deep vein thrombosis: an alternative in patients with contraindications to thrombolysis. *J Vasc Surg* 2009;**50**:1092.

100. Kim BJ, Chung HH, Lee SH, et al. Single session endovascular treatment for symptomatic lower extremity deep vein thrombosis: a feasibility study. *Acta Radiol* 2010;**51**:248.

101. Lee KH, Han H, Lee KJ, et al. Mechanical thrombectomy of acute iliofemoral deep vein thrombosis with use of an Arrow-Trerotola percutaneous thrombectomy device. *J Vasc Interv Radiol* 2006; **17**:487.

102. Baekgaard N, Broholm R, Just S, et al. Long-term results using catheter-directed thrombolysis in 103 lower limbs with acute iliofemoral venous thrombosis. *Eur J Vasc Endovasc Surg* 2010; **39**:112.

103. Bush RL, Lin PH, Bates JT, et al. Pharmacomechanical thrombectomy for treatment of symptomatic lower extremity deep venous thrombosis: safety and feasibility study. *J Vasc Surg* 2004; **40**:965.

104. Kim HS, Patra A, Paxton BE, et al. Adjunctive percutaneous mechanical thrombectomy for lower extremity deep venous thrombosis. *J Vasc Interv Radiol* 2006;**17**:1099.

105. Comerota AJ, Aldridge SC, Cohen G, et al. A strategy of aggressive regional therapy for acute iliofemoral venous thrombosis with contemporary venous thrombectomy or catheter-directed thrombolysis. *J Vasc Surg* 1994;**20**:244.

106. Kahn SR. The post-thrombotic syndrome: progress and pitfalls. *Br J Haematol* 2006;**134**:357.

107. Neglen P, Thrasher TL, Raju S. Venous outflow obstruction: an underestimated contributor to chronic venous disease. *J Vasc Surg* 2003;**38**:879.

108. Strandness Jr DE, Langlois Y, Cramer M, et al. Long-term sequelae of acute venous thrombosis. *JAMA* 1983;**250**:1289.

109. Kahn SR, Shrier I, Julian JA, et al. Determinants and time course of the postthrombotic syndrome after acute deep venous thrombosis. *Ann Intern Med* 2008;**149**:698.

110. Tran NT, Meissner MH. The epidemiology, pathophysiology, and natural history of chronic venous disease. *Semin Vasc Surg* 2002;**15**:5.

111. Raju S, Negien P. Clinical practice. Chronic venous insufficiency and varicose veins. *N Engl J Med* 2009;**360**:2319.

112. Gaitini D, Torem S, Pery M, et al. Image-directed Doppler ultrasound in the diagnosis of lower-limb venous insufficiency. *J Clin Ultrasound* 1994;**22**:291.

113. Baldt MM, Bohler K, Zontsich T, et al. Preoperative imaging of lower extremity varicose veins: color-coded duplex sonography or venography. *J Ultrasound Med* 1996;**15**:143.

114. Yang D, Sacco P. Reproducibility of air plethysmography for the evaluation of arterial and venous function of the lower leg. *Clin Physiol Funct Imaging* 2002;**22**:379.

115. Eklof B, Rutherford RB, Bergan JJ, et al. Revision of the CEAP classification for chronic venous disorders. Consensus statement. *J Vasc Surg* 2004;**40**:1248.

116. Delis KT, Bjarnason H, Wennberg PW, et al. Successful iliac vein and inferior vena cava stenting ameliorates venous claudication and improves venous outflow, calf muscle pump function, and clinical status in post-thrombotic syndrome. *Ann Surg* 2007;**245**:130.

117. Neglin P, Hollis KC, Olivier J, et al. Stenting of venous outflow in chronic venous disease: long-term stent-related outcome, clinical, and hemodynamic results. *J Vasc Surg* 2007;**46**:979.

118. Raju S, Neglen P. Percutaneous recanalization of total occlusions of the iliac vein. *J Vasc Surg* 2009;**50**:360.

119. Koelbel T, Lindh M, Akesson M, et al. Chronic iliac vein occlusion: midterms results of endovascular recanalization. *J Endovasc Ther* 2009;**16**:483.

120. Barwell JR, Davies CE, Deacon J, et al. Comparison of surgery and compression with compression alone in chronic venous ulceration (ESCHAR study): randomised controlled trial. *Lancet* 2004;**363**:1854.

121. Eklof BG, Kistner RL, Masuda EM. Venous bypass and valve reconstruction: long-term efficacy. *Vasc Med* 1998;**3**:157.

122. Meissner MH, Gloviczki P, Bergan J, et al. Primary chronic venous disorders. *J Vasc Surg* 2007;**46**:54S.

123. Travers JP, Brookes CE, Evans J, et al. Assessment of wall structure and composition of varicose veins with reference to collagen, elastin, and smooth muscle elements. *Eur J Vasc Endovasc Surg* 1996;**11**:230.

124. Kouri B. Current evaluation and treatment of lower extremity varicose veins. *Am J Med* 2009;**122**:513.

125. Evans CJ, Fowkes FG, Ruckley CV, et al. Prevalence of varicose veins and chronic venous insufficiency in men and women in the general population: Edinburgh Vein Study. *J Epidemiol Community Health* 1999;**53**:149.

126. Bergan JJ, Kumins NH, Owens EL, et al. Surgical and endovascular treatment of lower extremity venous insufficiency. *J Vasc Interv Radiol* 2002;**13**:563.

127. Jung SC, Lee W, Chung JW, et al. Unusual causes of varicose veins in the lower extremities: CT venographic and Doppler US findings. *Radiographics* 2009;**29**:525.

128. Fischer R, Linde N, Duff C, et al. Late recurrent saphenofemoral junction reflux after ligation and stripping of the great saphenous vein. *J Vasc Surg* 2001;**34**:236.

129. van Rij AM, Jones GT, Hill GB, et al. Neovascularization and recurrent varicose veins: more histologic and ultrasound evidence. *J Vasc Surg* 2004;**40**:296.

130. Tenbrook JA Jr, Iafrati MD, O'Donnell Jr TF, et al. Systematic review of outcomes after surgical management of venous disease incorporating subfascial endoscopic perforator surgery. *J Vasc Surg* 2004;**39**:583.

131. Rautio TT, Perala JM, Wiik HT, et al. Endovenous obliteration with radiofrequency-resistive heating for greater saphenous vein insufficiency: a feasibility study. *J Vasc Interv Radiol* 2002;**13**:569.

132. Pichot O, Kabnick LS, Creton D, et al. Duplex ultrasound scan findings two years after great saphenous vein radiofrequency endovenous obliteration. *J Vasc Surg* 2004;**39**:189.

133. Min RJ, Khilnani N, Zimmet SE. Endovenous laser treatment of saphenous vein reflux: long-term results. *J Vasc Interv Radiol* 2003;**14**:991.

134. Weiss RA, Weiss MA. Controlled radiofrequency endovenous occlusion using a unique radiofrequency catheter under duplex guidance to eliminate saphenous varicose vein reflux: a 2-year follow-up. *Dermatol Surg* 2002;**28**:38.

135. Merchant RF, DePalma RG, Kabnick LS. Endovascular obliteration of venous reflux: a multicenter study. *J Vasc Surg* 2002;**35**:1190.

136. Merchant RF, Pichot O. Long term outcomes of endovenous radiofrequency obliteration of saphenous vein reflux as a treatment for superficial venous insufficiency. *J Vasc Surg* 2005;**42**:502.

137. Lurie F, Creton D, Eklof B, et al. Prospective randomized study of endovenous radiofrequency obliteration (closure) versus ligation and stripping in a selected patient population. (EVOLVeS Study): 2-year followup. *Eur J Vasc Endovasc Surg* 2005;**29**:67.

138. Proebstle TM, Gul D, Lehr HA, et al. Infrequent early recanalization of greater saphenous vein after endovenous laser treatment. *J Vasc Surg* 2003;**38**:511.

139. Perkowski P, Ravi R, Gowda RC, et al. Endovenous laser ablation of the saphenous vein for treatment of venous insufficiency and varicose veins: early results from a large single-center experienc. *J Endovasc Ther* 2004;**11**:132.

140. van den Bos R, Arends L, Kockaert M, et al. Endovenous therapies of lower extremity varicosities: a meta-analysis. *J Vasc Surg* 2009;**49**:230.

141. Nazarian GK, Bjarnason H, Dietz Jr CA, et al. Iliofemoral venous stenoses: effectiveness of treatment with metallic endovascular stents. *Radiology* 1996;**200**:193.

142. Binkert CA, Schoch E, Stuckmann G, et al. Treatment of pelvic venous spur (May Thurner syndrome) with self expanding metallic endoprostheses. *Cardiovasc Intervent Radiol* 1998;**21**:22.

143. Baron HC, Shams J, Wayne M. Iliac vein compression syndrome: a new method of treatment. *Am Surg* 2000;**66**:653.

144. Vorwerk D, Guenther RW, Wendt G, et al. Iliocaval stenosis and iliac venous thrombosis in retroperitoneal fibrosis: percutaneous treatment by use of hydrodynamic thrombectomy and stenting. *Cardiovasc Intervent Radiol* 1996;**19**:40.

145. Hurst DR, Forauer AR, Bloom JR, et al. Diagnosis and endovascular treatment of iliocaval compression syndrome. *J Vasc Surg* 2001;**34**:106.

146. Neglen P, Tackett TP Jr, Raju S. Venous stenting across the inguinal ligament. *J Vasc Surg* 2008;**48**:1255.

147. Oderich GS, Panneton JM, Hofer J, et al. Iatrogenic operative injuries of abdominal and pelvic veins: a potentially lethal complication. *J Vasc Surg* 2004;**39**:931.

148. Schneider JR, Alonzo MJ, Hahn D. Successful endovascular management of an acute iliac venous injury during lumbar discectomy and anterior spinal fusion. *J Vasc Surg* 2006;**44**:1353.

149. Gagne PJ, Cone JB, McFarland D, et al. Proximity penetrating extremity trauma: the role of duplex ultrasound in the detection of occult venous injuries. *J Trauma* 1995;**39**:1157.

150. Alcocer F, Aguilar J, Agraz S, et al. Early Palma procedure after iliac vein injury in abdominal penetrating trauma. *J Vasc Surg* 2008;**48**:745.

151. Tillman BW, Vaccaro PS, Starr JE, et al. Use of an endovascular occlusion balloon for control of unremitting venous hemorrhage. *J Vasc Surg* 2006;**43**:399.

152. Roche-Nagle G, Wooster D, Oreopoulos G. Popliteal vein aneurysm. *Am J Surg* 2010;**199**:e5.

153. Russell DA, Robinson GJ, Johnson BF. Popliteal venous aneurysm: a rare cause of recurrent pulmonary emboli and limb swelling. *Cardiovasc Intervent Radiol* 2008;**31**:1026.

16

Inferior Vena Cava

Karim Valji

INFERIOR VENACAVOGRAPHY

Inferior venacavography is performed through the right internal jugular (IJ) vein or either common femoral vein (CFV). The jugular route must be taken in patients with bilateral common femoral, iliac vein, or inferior vena cava (IVC) thrombosis. Real-time sonographic guidance is mandatory for IJ vein puncture and is helpful for access at the groin. In some patients, the CFV lies posterior or posteromedial to the common femoral artery. To avoid traversing the artery, a single-wall needle is slowly inserted through the skin toward the vein with continuous aspiration on the needle hub.

Number 4- or 5-French (Fr) pigtail (or similarly shaped) catheters are used for venacavography with the side holes placed at the common iliac vein confluence. Sizing catheters with radiopaque markers assist in determining caval diameter in patients undergoing IVC filter placement. When iodinated contrast must be avoided because of renal insufficiency or history of severe contrast allergy, CO_2 is used.[1] A typical injection rate with iodinated material is 15 mL/sec for 2 seconds. With CO_2 venography, rapid manual injection of 40 to 60 mL is necessary for adequate opacification. CO_2 venography is prohibited in patients with a documented right-to-left circulatory shunt.

ANATOMY

Development

The posterior cardinal veins drain the caudal aspect of the fetus during the first weeks of development.[2,3] By the seventh week of gestation, these vessels start to involute, and the subcardinal and supracardinal venous channels emerge (Fig. 16-1). In the middle of the abdomen, the paired systems fuse into a vascular sinus, the *subcardinal-supracardinal anastomosis*. The normally positioned right-sided IVC and the azygous and hemiazygous venous circulations arise from the subcardinal and supracardinal vessels.

Normal Anatomy (Online Case 11)

The *IVC* begins at the confluence of the common iliac veins, which corresponds to the L4-L5 level[2,4] (see Fig. 16-1 and Fig. 16-2). The left common iliac vein and iliocaval junction pass between the right common iliac artery and the spine at this site. The IVC ascends in the retroperitoneum to the right of the aorta. In the midabdomen, the IVC courses behind the head of the pancreas, the superior portion of the duodenum, and the portal vein. The vessel then runs in a groove on the posterior surface of the liver. As it traverses the diaphragm, it is enveloped by the pericardium and then enters the inferoposterior aspect of the right atrium (RA). The *eustachian valve* is located on the right lateral side of the IVC at its junction with the RA. Otherwise, the IVC has no valves. The *ascending lumbar veins* originate from the common iliac veins and run alongside the vertebral bodies (Fig. 16-3). Above the L2 level, they drain into the azygous system (see later discussion). Four pairs of *lumbar veins* connect the IVC with the bilateral ascending lumbar channels (Fig. 16-4).

The *renal veins* empty into the IVC about the L1-L2 level (see Figs. 16-2 and 16-4). Renal vein anomalies (e.g., multiple veins, circumaortic or retroaortic left renal vein) are seen in up to 30% of individuals[5] (Fig. 16-5; see also Figs. 10-8 and 10-9). The *right gonadal vein* enters the IVC just below the right renal vein, and the *left gonadal vein* enters the undersurface of the left renal vein lateral to the vertebral column (see Fig. 16-4). The *right adrenal vein* drains into the right posterior wall of the suprarenal IVC in a horizontal plane at about the T12 level (see Figs. 13-8 and 13-9). In contradistinction, the *left adrenal vein* joins the left renal vein in a vertical plane as a common trunk with the left inferior phrenic vein (see Fig. 16-4; see also Fig. 10-3).

The *right, middle,* and *left hepatic veins* converge at the upper IVC just below the diaphragm (see Fig. 12-4). In many individuals, more caudally positioned accessory hepatic veins drain portions of the right or caudate lobes of the liver. In about 3% of the population, blood from the right lobe of the liver empties primarily through a

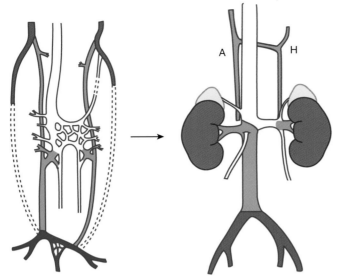

FIGURE 16-1 Embryologic development of the inferior vena cava. Shading indicates the posterior cardinal origin (dark), supracardinal origin (light), and subcardinal origin (white). *A,* Azygous vein; *H,* hemiazygous vein. *(Adapted from Lundell C, Kadir S. Inferior vena cava and spinal veins. In: Kadir S, ed: Atlas of normal and variant angiographic anatomy. Philadelphia: WB Saunders, 1991:187.)*

large *inferior right hepatic vein* that is situated on the IVC well below the other hepatic veins[6] (see Fig. 16-4).

The azygous venous system drains the posterior chest wall, esophagus, mediastinum, and pericardium. It also serves as an important collateral circulation for the IVC and tributaries when they become obstructed (Fig. 16-6). The *azygous vein* originates at the L1-L2 level as an indirect continuation of the right ascending lumbar veins. It then ascends through the abdomen and chest on the right side of the spine. At about the T4-T5 level, it arches anteriorly to join the back wall of the *superior vena cava (SVC).* The *hemiazygous vein* also begins at the L1-L2 level and runs on the left side of the spine. It crosses the midline to join the azygous vein at about the eighth thoracic vertebra. The *accessory hemiazygous vein,* which arises from the left brachiocephalic vein, joins the SVC just above the hemiazygous connection.

The mean transverse diameter of the infrarenal IVC in adults is about 19 mm.[5,7] Caval diameter usually decreases during inspiration or a Valsalva maneuver, and it usually increases during expiration.[8] On cross-sectional images, the IVC often appears elliptical rather than round in the transverse plane. Mild or moderate narrowing of the intrahepatic IVC is common (see Fig. 16-2B). Inflow defects at cavography caused by unopacified blood from the renal, hepatic, and contralateral iliac veins should not be confused with clot, which does not change appearance on sequential images (see Fig. 1-39). On the other hand, retrograde filling of the IVC (on contrast-enhanced computed tomography (CT)) or prominent filling of primary IVC branches (at cavography) is a sign of elevated right heart pressures from a variety of causes.[9]

Variant Anatomy (Online Cases 49 and 71)

The major IVC anomalies can be explained by errors in the normal fetal evolution of the major veins of the abdomen and pelvis[3,4,9-11] (see earlier and Fig. 16-1).

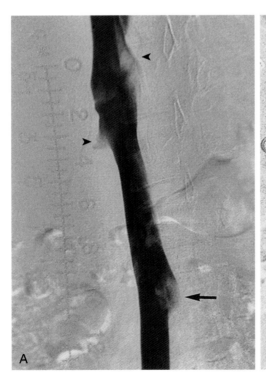

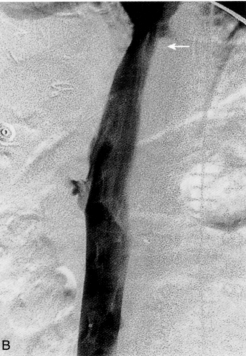

FIGURE 16-2 Normal frontal inferior venacavograms. **A,** Midabdominal inferior vena cava (IVC) with inflow defects from the left common iliac vein *(arrow)* and both renal veins *(arrowheads).* **B,** Upper abdominal IVC with mild compression of the intrahepatic segment below the right atrium *(white arrow).*

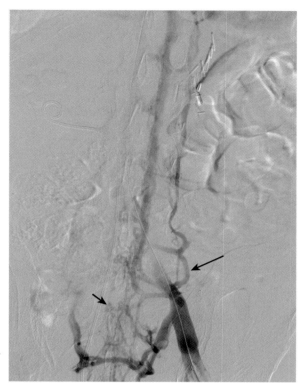

FIGURE 16-3   Ascending lumbar *(long arrow)* and vertebral *(short arrow)* venous system in a patient with complete inferior vena cava occlusion.

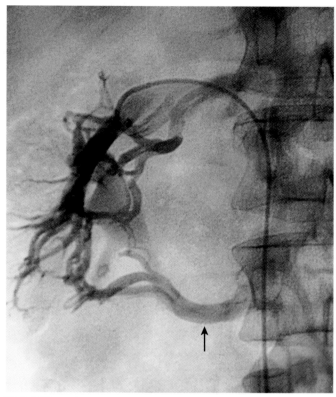

FIGURE 16-5   Multiple right renal veins communicate in the hilum. The accessory vein *(arrow)* was not suspected on the inferior venacavogram.

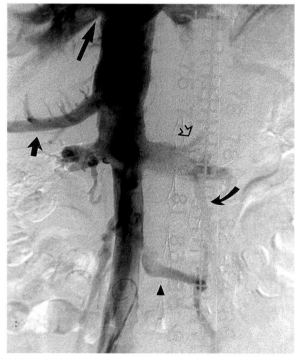

FIGURE 16-4   Inferior vena cava tributaries filling in a patient with elevated right-sided heart pressures. Notice the main hepatic vein confluence *(long arrow)*, anomalous inferior right hepatic vein *(short arrow)*, left gonadal vein *(curved arrow)*, left adrenal vein *(open arrow)*, and lumbar vein *(arrowhead)*.

Duplication of the IVC results from persistence of the inferior portion of the left supracardinal vein. The quoted prevalence of this anomaly varies from 0.2% to 3%.[4,12] Each iliac vein drains into its corresponding vena cava (Fig. 16-7). The left IVC usually joins the right IVC at the level of the left renal vein. The right and left common iliac veins sometimes communicate in the pelvis. At venacavography performed from the right femoral vein, IVC duplication may be suspected by the absence of an inflow defect from the left iliac vein and by the small caliber of the infrarenal IVC. However, it can go undetected on routine cavograms; if the initial study is suspicious, catheterization of the left iliac vein is advisable.

Left (transposed) IVC results from persistence of the inferior portion of the left supracardinal vein with involution of the inferior portion of the right supracardinal vein. In autopsy series, left IVC is found in 0.2% to 0.5% of cases; a similar frequency (0.2%) has been reported in imaging studies.[4,12] Usually, the left IVC joins the orthotopic IVC at or just inferior to the left renal vein (Fig. 16-8). Occasionally, it may join the azygous or hemiazygous system.[13] Very rarely, it connects with a left SVC, which ultimately drains into the coronary sinus.[14]

Interruption of the IVC with azygous or hemiazygous continuation occurs when the right subcardinal vein fails to

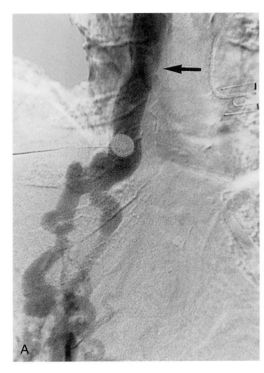 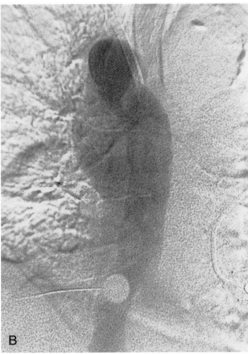

FIGURE 16-6 Ascending lumbar collaterals in a patient with complete inferior vena cava occlusion. Injection of the right iliac vein fills the ascending lumbar collaterals, which drain into the azygous vein (**A,** *arrow*) and then into the superior vena cava (**B**).

join the intrahepatic venous complex. IVC interruption is found in 0.6% of autopsy specimens but less often in imaging series.[4,10,15] In this situation, blood flows from the lower IVC into the azygous or hemiazygous vein and then into the heart (Fig. 16-9). The hepatic veins drain directly into the RA.[2] The anomaly often is associated with congenital heart disease and with abnormalities of the spleen (i.e., asplenia or polysplenia), cardiac position, and abdominal situs.[16,17]

Other exceedingly rare caval variants include double IVC with retroaortic right renal vein and hemiazygous continuation of the IVC, double IVC with retroaortic left renal vein and azygous continuation of the IVC, and absent infrarenal IVC with preserved suprarenal segment.[4]

Collateral Circulation

Several alternate pathways allow blood to return to the heart when there is severe stenosis or occlusion of the IVC.[18] The most common collateral route is the ascending lumbar venous plexus (see Fig. 16-3). These vessels also communicate freely with an extensive vertebral venous network. Blood flows cephalad through these veins into the azygous or hemiazygous systems and then into the SVC (see Fig. 16-6).

Blood from the pelvic veins also may bypass the IVC through periureteric and gonadal venous communications. The external iliac vein can also drain through the inferior epigastric vein; associated superficial abdominal wall vessels then merge with the internal thoracic and subclavian veins. Alternatively, blood may be redirected through the superficial epigastric and circumflex iliac veins into the lateral thoracic vein and then into the axillary vein. A systemic to portal venous pathway runs from the internal iliac veins through the hemorrhoidal plexus, then into the inferior mesenteric vein, and ultimately into the portal vein. Finally, superficial abdominal wall veins may communicate with paraumbilical veins that enter the left portal vein.

MAJOR DISORDERS

Inferior Vena Cava Filter Placement for Venous Thromboembolic Disease
(Online Cases 23, 49, and 71 and Video 16-1)

A filtering device is inserted into the IVC for only one reason: to prevent clinically relevant pulmonary embolism (PE).[19,20] However, IVC filters are not appropriate substitutes for standard medical therapy of venous thromboembolic disease (VTE) in patients who are reasonable candidates for anticoagulation (see later discussion and Chapter 15). In certain clinical situations, virtually every knowledgeable physician would support filter placement. Still, a substantial number of experts remain skeptical about their touted benefits (prevention of significant PE and associated reduction in mortality) and concerned about the associated risks (namely, the possible predisposition to deep vein thrombosis (DVT) and postthrombotic syndrome).[21,22]

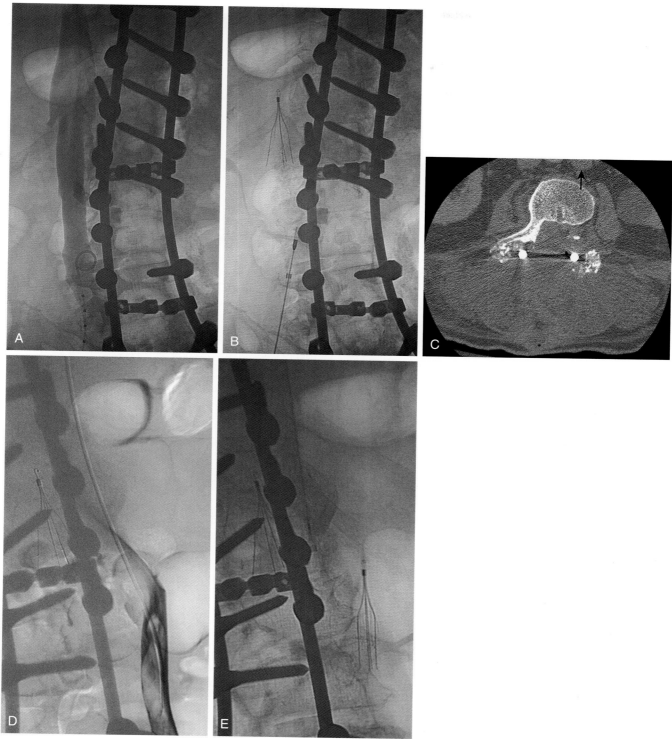

FIGURE 16-7 Duplicated inferior vena cava (IVC). **A,** Cavography prior to inferior vena cava filter placement did not suggest variant anatomy, so a single filter was placed **(B).** By serendipity, a colleague later noted IVC duplication at the edge of an image on a lumbar spine computed tomography study *(arrow)* **(C). D,** Left iliac venography confirms duplication and presence of large acute thrombus. **E,** From a jugular approach, a second Guenther tulip filter was placed in the duplicated moiety above the thrombus.

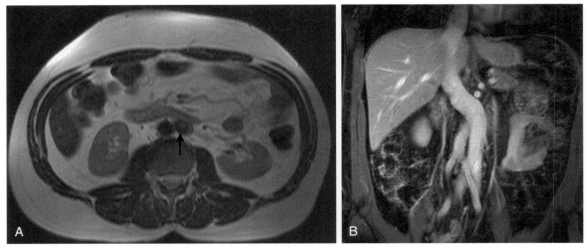

FIGURE 16-8   Left inferior vena cava (IVC). **A,** T1-weighted magnetic resonance image shows IVC *(arrow)* to the left of the aorta at the level of the kidneys. **B,** Coronal maximum intensity projection magnetic resonance angiogram shows the left IVC crossing the midline to join the orthotopic suprarenal IVC.

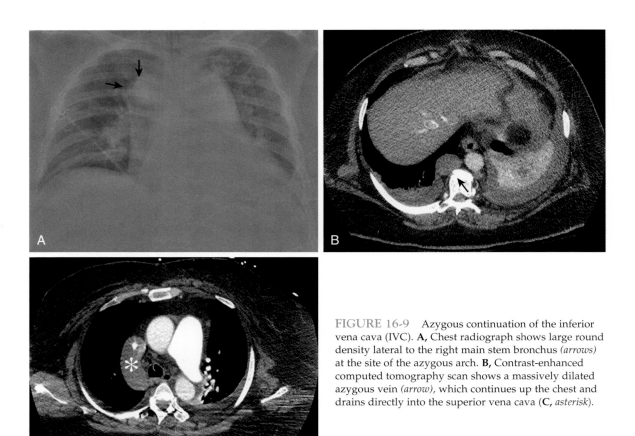

FIGURE 16-9   Azygous continuation of the inferior vena cava (IVC). **A,** Chest radiograph shows large round density lateral to the right main stem bronchus *(arrows)* at the site of the azygous arch. **B,** Contrast-enhanced computed tomography scan shows a massively dilated azygous vein *(arrow),* which continues up the chest and drains directly into the superior vena cava (**C,** *asterisk*).

Patient Selection

Box 16-1 outlines the indications for IVC filter insertion.[23-28] In the setting of documented VTE ("proximal" lower extremity DVT or PE), the widely accepted criteria are (1) a preexisting contraindication to anticoagulants (see Box 3-7), (2) a suboptimal response to therapeutic anticoagulation, and (3) a complication from anticoagulant medications. Relative contraindications include severe and uncorrectable coagulopathy, absence of a suitable access route to the IVC, and chronic thrombosis of the vena cava. Although some interventionalists are reluctant to place a filter in a septic patient, the risk of seeding a filter is probably more imagined than real.[23,29]

Placement of an IVC filter as an entirely prophylactic maneuver in patients at risk for VTE (particularly before major surgery or after major trauma) is extremely controversial. Certainly, DVT causes substantial morbidity and mortality in trauma populations; one large study cited a 27% overall incidence of DVT despite adequate prophylactic anticoagulation.[30] Both sides of the debate advance compelling arguments—substantial reductions in mortality from prophylactic insertion on the one hand, nonsignificant benefits and potential for exacerbating DVT on the other.[31-34] Notably, the most recent policy guidelines on this subject from the American College of Chest Physicians advise against prophylactic placement even when the risk for VTE is deemed high.[35]

In a small subset of patients, both permanent IVC filter insertion and lifelong anticoagulation are deemed necessary to adequately reduce the lifetime risk for PE (e.g., before surgical thromboendarterectomy for chronic thromboembolic pulmonary hypertension, see Chapter 14). The frequently cited PREPIC study (see later discussion) has led many physicians to infer that filter placement should generally be avoided unless long-term anticoagulation will be instituted (when safe) for as long as the filter remains in place[36]; however, there are persuasive arguments that refute this widely held view.[37]

The practice of deploying a temporary filter before lower extremity venous thrombolysis varies considerably.[38,39] One clinical study detected newly trapped clots during thrombolytic therapy in more than 50% of cases; another study failed to identify any such occurrences. Most interventionalists do not place filters routinely during this procedure, but instead reserve the device for high-risk situations (e.g., free-floating caval or iliac vein clot).

In rare circumstances, a *suprarenal* filter must be placed above the renal vein inflow[40] (Box 16-2). Finally, SVC filter placement is discussed in Chapter 17.

It is noteworthy that the anticipated growth in IVC filter placement procedures following the introduction of retrievable devices has been partly offset by concerns about the added risk for lower extremity DVT and consequent post-thrombotic syndrome.[41,42] The decision to implant a filter, even as a temporary measure, should be made carefully by the operator and patient. The ever-expanding indications for IVC filter insertion do not give license to referring physicians to request nor interventionalists to offer or agree to placement without solid evidence for the individual patient benefit.

BOX 16-1

INDICATIONS FOR INFERIOR VENA CAVA FILTER PLACEMENT

Widely Accepted Indications in Patients with Documented PE or "Proximal" DVT

- Contraindication to anticoagulation
- Complication of anticoagulation (e.g., bleeding, heparin-induced thrombocytopenia)
- Failure of anticoagulation (recurrent embolism or progression of DVT despite adequate treatment)
- Chronic pulmonary thromboembolism

Moderately Accepted Indications

- Massive pulmonary embolism with or without residual DVT
- Free-floating iliofemoral or inferior vena cava thrombus
- Severe cardiopulmonary disease
- Poor candidate for anticoagulation (e.g., high fall risk, medication compliance doubtful)
- Recurrent pulmonary embolism with filter in place

Controversial Indications (retrievable filter advisable)

- Prophylaxis
  - Severe trauma
    - Closed head injury (Glasgow coma scale >8)
    - Spinal cord injury with paraplegia/quadriplegia
    - Multiple long bone or pelvic fractures
  - Immobilized or intensive care unit patients
  - Multiple risk factors for venous thromboembolism in a preoperative patient
  - Open gastric bypass surgery in extreme obesity (BMI >55 kg/m²)
  - Advanced malignancy
- Prior to lower extremity deep venous thrombolysis
- Pregnancy with proximal DVT

BMI, body mass index; *DVT*, deep vein thrombosis; *PE*, pulmonary embolism.

Staging

Inferior venacavography is performed to guide filter selection and placement. Some of the required information may be obtained from prior cross-sectional imaging studies, thus allowing a more tailored angiographic study.

INFERIOR VENA CAVA DIAMETER AND LENGTH

About 1% to 2% of the general population has a *megacava*, whereby the transverse diameter exceeds 28 to 29 mm.[43,44] In this situation, only the Bird's nest filter (which expands to 40 mm) is guaranteed to remain in a stable position after release[45] (Fig. 16-10). Alternatively, standard filters (permanent or retrievable) can be inserted into each common iliac vein (Fig. 16-11). The Bird's nest filter system has a longer footprint than other devices (7 cm or greater); as such, the proposed infrarenal landing zone should be measured in advance.

LOCATION AND NUMBER OF RENAL VEINS

By convention, IVC filters are deployed with the most superior point immediately below the level of the renal veins. If the filter clots spontaneously (very unlikely) or becomes filled with emboli (much more likely), brisk blood flow from the renal veins will facilitate endogenous lysis of any clot at the top of the filter. Additionally, the lack of caval dead space above an occluded filter should minimize the likelihood of bilateral renal vein thrombosis. The position of the renal veins is identified by their inflow defects on the venacavogram (see Fig. 16-2). However, accessory renal veins are present in up to 25% to 30% of individuals (more frequently on the right than the left). These vessels are not always detected by venacavography alone. Appropriately performed CT or magnetic resonance imaging (MRI) may be helpful. If not, selective catheterization often is necessary to identify them[5] (Fig. 16-12). Accessory renal veins must be distinguished from lumbar veins or the right gonadal vein. In patients with multiple renal veins (circumaortic or otherwise), the filter is deployed with the apex below the inferiormost vein. This approach prevents the more superiorly located vessel from acting as a conduit for emboli in transit to the lung in case the more inferior portion of the IVC becomes occluded (Fig. 16-13).

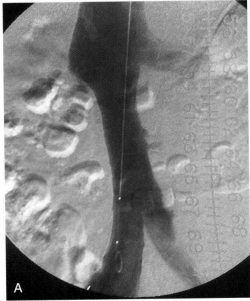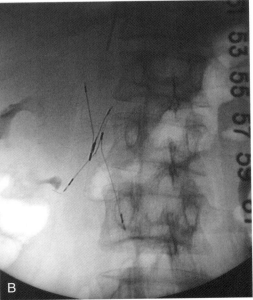

FIGURE 16-10   Megacava. **A,** Venacavogram shows caval diameter greater than 29 mm (based on catheter markers). **B,** A Bird's nest filter was inserted.

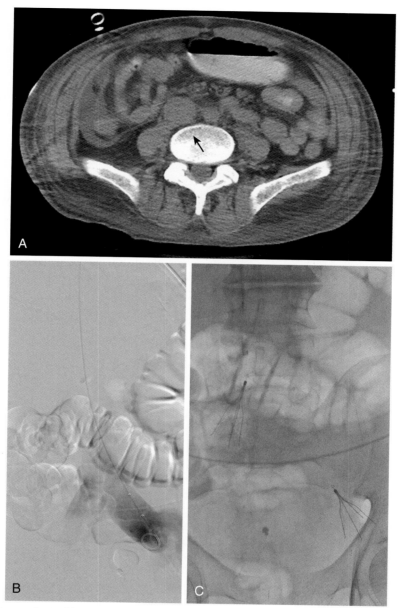

FIGURE 16-11 Megacava in a patient with temporary risk for venous thromboembolic disease. **A,** Preprocedure computed tomography scan showed huge inferior vena cava that measured more than 30 mm in diameter *(arrow)*. **B,** At left iliac venography from jugular approach, the left common iliac vein measures about 30 mm in diameter. **C,** Therefore, retrievable filters were placed in the right common iliac and left external iliac veins well above the inguinal ligament.

INFERIOR VENA CAVA ANOMALIES

Variants in IVC anatomy are sought (see earlier discussion). A duplicated IVC requires placement of filters in each moiety or suprarenal insertion of a single device (see Fig. 16-7).

INTRINSIC DISEASE

Filter location is influenced by the presence of intraluminal clot, chronic mural disease, or extrinsic compression. If caval thrombus is found, the filter is deposited just above the clot (when feasible) through the IJ vein (Fig. 16-14). Extension of clot into the IVC from tributaries may be a sign of occult malignancy (e.g., right gonadal vein thrombosis in ovarian neoplasms). Chronic total occlusion of the IVC possibly obviates the need for filter placement, although clots still can pass through enlarged collaterals. If suprarenal filter placement is required, it is critical to identify an appropriate landing site and to be certain that the nondiseased caval segment is long enough to accommodate the filter without extension into the RA (see Fig. 16-14).

FIGURE 16-12   Unsuspected circumaortic left renal vein in a patient requiring an inferior vena cava (IVC) filter. **A,** Digital cavogram identifies main left renal vein inflow without clear evidence for accessory veins. **B,** Selective injection of the renal vein shows a circumaortic moiety. The IVC filter apex was positioned below this vessel.

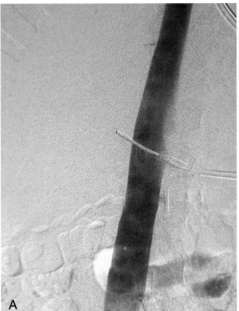
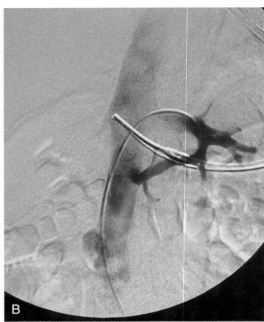

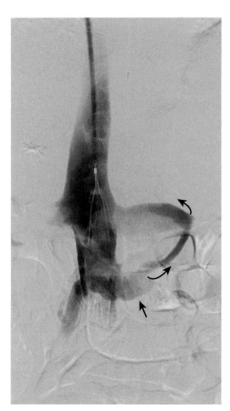

FIGURE 16-13   Improper placement of inferior vena cava filter in setting of circumaortic left renal vein. With the filter deposited above the circumaortic moiety *(straight arrow),* filter thrombosis could allow clots to pass through the renal sinus and to the lung (direction of *curved arrows*).

Device Selection

Before intraluminal IVC filtration devices were developed, operative caval interruption was achieved by ligation, stapling, plication, or clipping. However, subsequent IVC thrombosis was all too frequent.[46,47] The Greenfield filter was the first widely successful intraluminal device, placed initially by open surgery and beginning in 1984 by percutaneous means.[48,49]

At present, a variety of *permanent* IVC filters are commercially available[24] (Figs. 16-15 and 16-16 and Table 16-1). The critical properties of filters are clot-trapping efficiency, IVC and access vein occlusion rates, tendency for migration or embolization, mechanical integrity, and ease of placement. Despite decades of experimental and clinical studies comparing their relative merits (clot trapping ability vs. caval thrombosis rate), none of the currently used devices holds an unequivocal advantage.[20,24,50-55] Certain filters seem to possess superior clot-trapping ability compared with the others.[55-58] This attribute may be associated with higher rates of caval thrombosis, but it may make these devices more suitable for patients who cannot tolerate even small pulmonary emboli.

The more recently developed products that permit discontinuation of IVC filtration are termed *optional* filters, which fall into two categories.[59] *Convertible* IVC filters can be manipulated in situ to abolish their filtering capacity; none is currently commercially available in the United States. *Retrievable* IVC filters have the potential for complete removal. However, they are primarily approved by

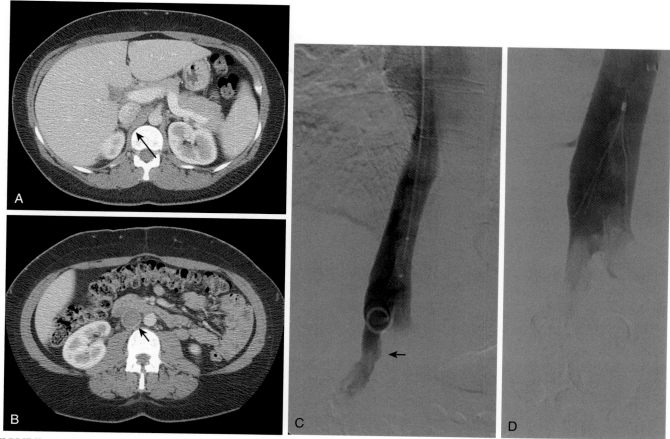

FIGURE 16-14 Suprarenal inferior vena cava filter. **A** and **B,** Contrast-enhanced computed tomography scans show caval thrombus *(short arrow)* at the level of the renal veins but a patent cava above *(long arrow)*. From a jugular approach, venacavography confirmed thrombus up to the level of the renal veins (**C,** *arrow*). **D,** A suprarenal retrievable Guenther tulip filter was inserted.

TABLE 16-1   Permanent Inferior Vena Cava Filters

Device/Manufacturer	Material	Sheath
Bird's nest (Cook, Inc.)	Stainless steel	12 Fr
Greenfield (Boston Scientific)	Stainless steel	12 Fr
Simon nitinol (Bard, Inc.)	Nitinol	7 Fr
TrapEase (Cordis Corp.)	Nitinol	6 Fr
Vena-Tech LP (B. Braun)	Phynox	7 Fr

American and European regulatory agencies for permanent placement.

Table 16-2 lists and Fig. 16-17 shows currently available *optional* IVC filter designs.[60,61] Again, none of these retrievable devices has emerged as clearly superior to the others. However, before selecting a particular filter, operators are cautioned to review the most recent data regarding postplacement filter migration and long-term integrity. Early versions of some optional filters had serious design flaws that required their removal from the market.

Box 16-3 outlines the typical scenarios that favor use of a retrievable filter.[62-64] For the most part, this group includes patients with a limited and fairly predictable period of increased risk for VTE. When risks factors for VTE resolve or when anticoagulation can be instituted safely, the filter may be removed. Certainly, a young, previously healthy individual who suffers major trauma and VTE is an ideal candidate for a retrievable device.[64,65] In fact, it might seem that having the option of filter removal is ideal for all patients. However, the evaluative period of optional filters is short compared with the decades-long experience with permanent devices. Thus, at present, if filter removal seems unlikely, a permanent device should be strongly considered.[66]

Insertion Technique

IVC filters usually are deployed from the right IJ vein or a CFV. The IJ approach has several advantages (Box 16-4). In the unusual circumstance in which both femoral and IJ veins are occluded or unavailable, an antecubital, upper arm, or external jugular vein route can be used.[67] Box 16-2 outlines indications for suprarenal IVC filter placement.[24,68-70] Suprarenal insertion is recommended in pregnant women to avoid compression of the device by the gravid uterus and to prevent PE if ovarian vein thrombosis develops.

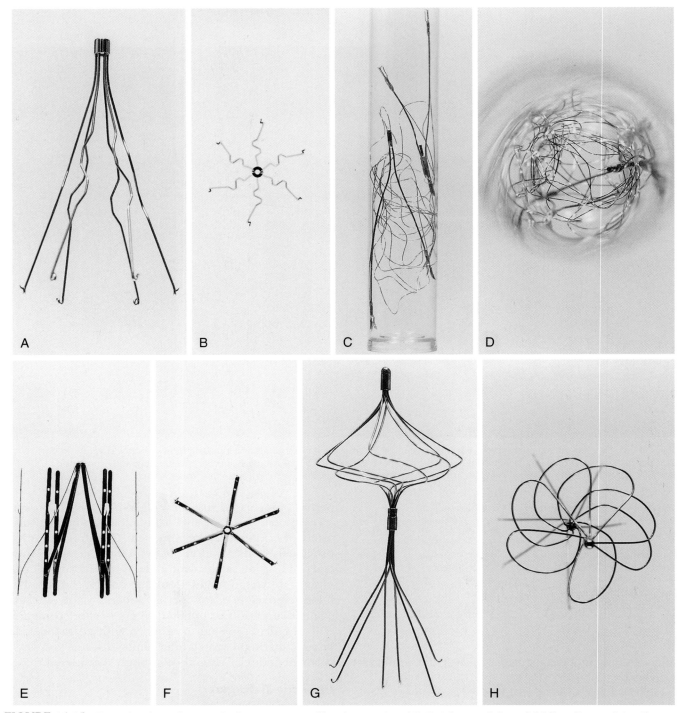

FIGURE 16-15   Frontal and aerial views of inferior vena cava filter designs. **A** and **B,** Stainless-steel Greenfield filter (Boston Scientific, Natick, Mass.). **C** and **D,** Bird's nest filter (Cook Inc., Bloomington, Ind.). **E** and **F,** Vena-Tech LGM filter (B. Braun, Evanston, Ill.). **G** and **H,** Simon nitinol filter (Bard, Inc., Tempe, Ariz.).

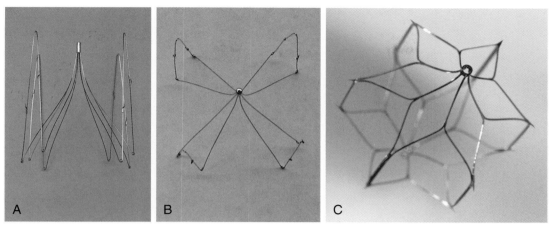

FIGURE 16-16 Frontal and aerial views of newer inferior vena cava filter designs. **A** and **B,** Low-profile Vena-Tech LP (**B,** Braun). **C,** TrapEase filter (Copyright Cordis Corp.)

TABLE 16-2   Optional Inferior Vena Cava Filters

Device/Manufacturer	Material	Sheath	Features
Guenther-Tulip (Cook, Inc.)	Conichrome	7 Fr (J)	Conical design, four hooked legs join at apex, four looped wires form tulip trap
		8.5 Fr (F)	
Celect (Cook, Inc.)	Conichrome	7 Fr (J)	Eight arms replace four looped wires for improved centering and retrievability
G2, G2X, Eclipse (Bard, Inc.)	Nitinol	7 Fr	Six arms, six legs diverge from apex, two filtering levels
			G2X can be removed without separate cone device, elastic hook lengthens retrieval period
OptEase (Cordis, Corp.)	Nitinol	6 Fr	Retrievable version of TrapEase device
			Requires femoral retrieval, hook at bottom
ALN (Implants Chirurgicaux)	SS alloy	7 Fr	Six upper legs with hooks
			Three lower legs facilitate device centering
Option (Angiotech)	Nitinol	6.5 Fr	Six radiating struts

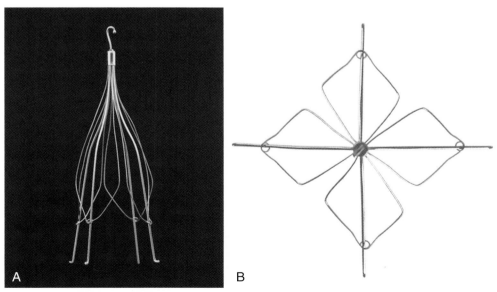

FIGURE 16-17 Retrievable inferior vena cava filters. **A** and **B,** Guenther-Tulip filter (Courtesy of Cook, Inc.).

Continued

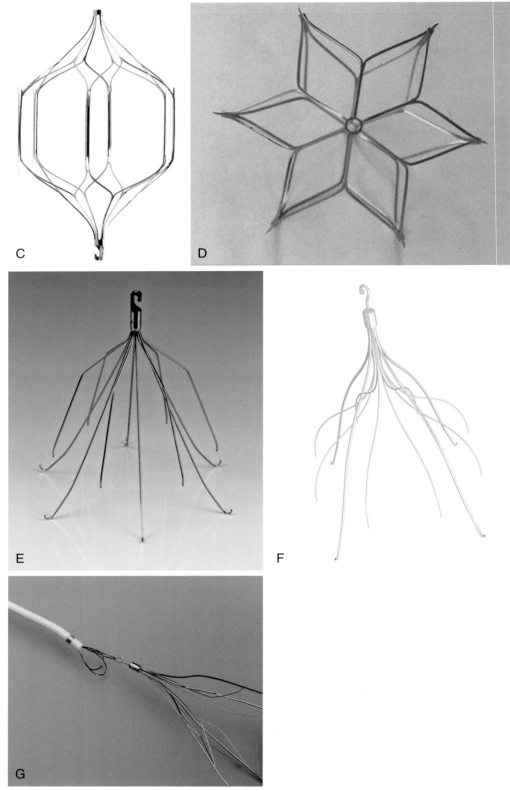

FIGURE 16-17, cont'd   **C** and **D,** OptEase filter (Copyright Cordis Corp., 2011). **E,** Eclipse filter (Courtesy of Bard, Inc.). **F,** Celect filter (Courtesy of Cook Medical, Inc.). **G,** Guenther tulip filter with tri-lobed snare around retrieval hook (Courtesy of Cook Medical, Inc).

Bedside placement of IVC filters with intravascular ultrasound guidance has become quite popular in some centers. This approach may be especially advantageous in unstable patients confined to the intensive care unit.[71-73] On occasion, however, the lack of fluoroscopic confirmation leads to malplacement of the device (e.g., in an iliac vein; Fig. 16-18).

The precise steps in filter deployment vary with each device. Several problems that may occur during deployment are common to multiple devices.

- Filter deploys more than 1 cm from intended position. If the filter is of a retrievable type (except the OptEase model), the device can be resheathed and repositioned if being inserted with a jugular vein approach.
- Filter is tilted more than 15 degrees off axis.[74-76] There is conflicting evidence regarding the *clinical* significance of major filter tilt with respect to clot trapping ability.[77,78] The major problem with filter asymmetry is that the retrieval process may be impeded or precluded if the retrieval hook becomes firmly embedded in the caval wall. As such, maneuvers to reposition the filter in line with the caval axis (both in frontal and lateral projections) are advocated by many experienced practitioners.
- Filter expansion is markedly asymmetric. The impact of leg asymmetry on recurrent PE is

---

BOX 16-3

FACTORS FAVORING RETRIEVABLE INFERIOR VENA CAVA FILTER PLACEMENT

- Young patient
- Prophylaxis after major trauma, in intensive care unit setting, or before high-risk operations
- During lower extremity deep vein thrombolysis, especially with inferior vena cava involvement
- During pregnancy

BOX 16-4

ADVANTAGES OF RIGHT INTERNAL JUGULAR APPROACH FOR INFERIOR VENA CAVA FILTER PLACEMENT

- Lower frequency of access site thrombosis
- Ability to reposition some retrievable devices if initial expansion is suboptimal
- Possibly better control of filter orientation
- Avoidance of failed opening and migration
- Necessary in presence of infrarenal inferior vena cava thrombus

---

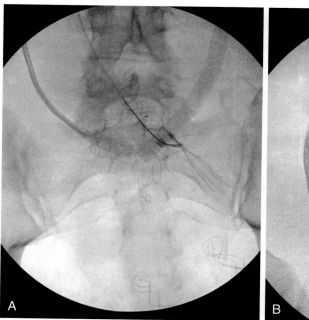
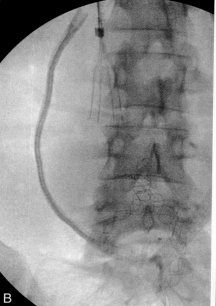
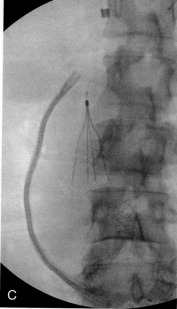

FIGURE 16-18 Malplacement of inferior vena cava (IVC) filter based on intravascular ultrasound guidance alone. Filter was inadvertently placed in the left iliac vein. The retrieval hook was captured with a snare device **(A)**, withdrawn into a guiding sheath **(B)**, and repositioned in the IVC **(C)**.

controversial.[78,79] However, some interventionalists attempt to improve the leg orientation or filter axis if it is grossly asymmetric, even though this practice is not recommended by the manufacturers or some experts.[24,80]

- Filter fails to open at all. If still attached to the delivery cable, it should be withdrawn into the sheath and removed. If not, the capture hook is carefully engaged with a snare device and the filter removed. Actual manipulation of an unexpanded filter poses some risk for central embolization to the heart.[81]

Results

Using fluoroscopic guidance, IVC filters (permanent or optional) can be placed successfully in almost every instance.[23,24,61,82-90] Technical "failures" are usually related to unsuspected caval disease that precludes or obviates the need for a filter.

It is disappointing that almost three decades after the first report of percutaneous placement of an IVC filter, there is not indisputable evidence for their efficacy and safety in preventing PE in certain populations. Only one well-recognized randomized study has addressed this issue.[91] The large multicenter PREPIC trial showed that permanent IVC filters significantly reduce the risk for PE in patients with documented "proximal" DVT without significant effect on mortality, but at the price of increased rates of leg DVT at 8 years.[21,36] Still, multiple large (though uncontrolled) clinical series show a fairly consistent 2% to 7% filter failure rate (i.e., new clinically significant PE after placement) among the various permanent and retrievable models.[75,92-98] The risk for subsequent fatal PE after an IVC filter is inserted is estimated at about 0.7%.[24] Suprarenal filter placement seems to be as effective and safe as infrarenal deployment.[40]

Recurrent pulmonary emboli have several causes, including device failure, propagation of thrombus above the filter, and embolization from other sources (e.g., upper extremity, gonadal or renal vein). Some patients may require anticoagulation or, rarely, placement of an additional filter.

Complications

Table 16-3 outlines immediate and long-term complications of IVC filter placement.[23,24,82-101] The major complication rate is about 0.3%. Less than 0.2% of patients die as a direct result of the procedure. Adverse outcomes are comparable with suprarenal and infrarenal placement.[40] Access site thrombosis is the most common untoward event after caval filter insertion (about 5% of cases with currently available sheath systems). However, it is rarely symptomatic.

TABLE 16-3   Complications from Inferior Vena Cava Filter Placement

Event	Frequency (%)
Access site thrombosis	0-6
Recurrent deep vein thrombosis	21
Inferior vena cava thrombosis	0-30
Inferior vena cava perforation (almost always inconsequential)	0-41
Filter migration (almost always inconsequential)	3-69
Filter embolization	<1
Filter fracture	2-10
Dislodgement or entrapment by catheters or guidewires	<1
Other complications	4-11
Bleeding, hematoma	
Pneumothorax	
Arteriovenous fistula	
Air embolism (to right heart chambers)	
Stroke (from paradoxical embolism of air or clot)	
Failed deployment	
IVC stenosis	
Infection	

A most concerning though hotly debated liability of IVC filters insertion is the reported excess risk of subsequent lower extremity post-thrombotic syndrome related to DVT (reported in 11% to 13% of procedures).[102] At the extreme end of the spectrum, complete IVC thrombosis is a serious and potentially life-threatening event (Fig. 16-19). The frequency of this occurrence falls in the 1% to 12% range.[95,103-105] There are conflicting data regarding the relative rates of filter thrombosis with the various devices.[97,106,107] In patients with profound or life-threatening symptoms from IVC thrombosis (e.g., phlegmasia cerulea dolens), catheter-directed thrombolysis may be indicated[108,109] (see Chapter 15).

Minor filter migration (<1 to 2 cm) is usually of little consequence. Significant permanent device migration after image-guided placement has been reported but is far less common than malplacement from inadequate or nonexistent imaging during insertion[110-112] (see Fig. 16-18). On the other hand, the very properties that allow retrievable filters to be removed make them more prone to movement. In fact, several early filter designs were removed from the market because of late occurrence of central embolization. Migration has been reported from cardiopulmonary resuscitation and inadvertent guidewire entrapment (see Fig. 18-21). It has been postulated that some cases of filter motion occur when a large embolus suddenly hits the filter, causing acute obstruction; the markedly elevated IVC pressure forces the filter to move centrally.[113,114]

Although embolization of all or part of an IVC filter to the heart or pulmonary artery is quite rare, the event is potentially lethal.[115-118] If an IVC filter becomes lodged in the heart, arrhythmias, tricuspid valve injury, pericardial

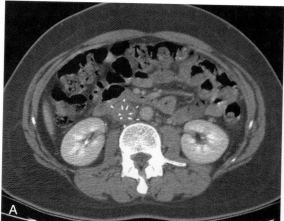
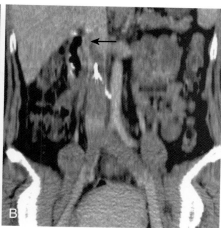

FIGURE 16-19   Inferior vena cava thrombosis after placement of a Recovery filter. **A,** Axial computed tomography (CT) angiogram shows thrombus within the cone of the filter. Note that some of the filter legs have penetrated the caval wall. **B,** Reformatted coronal CT image documents the thrombus, which extends above the filter (*arrow*).

tamponade, or acute myocardial infarction can result. Transvenous retrieval or repositioning has been performed successfully with a variety of techniques, including use of a large sheath system and looped guidewire or snare techniques[117,119-121] (see Chapter 18).

Filter fracture/fragmentation is more problematic with some retrievable models. This complication has been reported in about 2% to 4% of cases.[76,98] Penetration of the caval wall by device legs or hooks is very common but rarely consequential[101] (see Fig. 16-19). However, perforation into various neighboring structures (e.g., aorta, bowel, ureter, pancreas) can be problematic.[100,122,123]

Inferior Vena Cava Filter Retrieval (Video 16-2 and Online Case 38)

Patient Selection

A patient is considered for retrievable IVC filter removal when the risk for PE is low, either because underlying risk factors for VTE have resolved or because the patient is finally undergoing anticoagulant therapy. In addition, filter removal is advisable if the local standard-of-care demands lifelong anticoagulation by virtue of filter presence.[59,60] The following questions should be asked:

1. Is there no reason to expect progression of DVT since filter placement, new development of VTE, or near future return of risk factors for VTE?
2. If anticoagulation is underway, have appropriate therapeutic levels been achieved, patient tolerance confirmed, and no complications observed for at least 1 week (preferably 2 to 3 weeks)? For individuals receiving warfarin anticoagulation, an international normalized ratio (INR) should be obtained within several days of the planned procedure (typical target range is 2.0 to 3.0).
3. If the filter was placed for prophylactic reasons without a diagnosis of VTE, does a recent

duplex ultrasound (US) of the lower extremities exclude DVT?
4. Is the patient expected to live more than 6 months?

If the answer to any of these questions is "no," then the filter should *not* be removed at that time. Further clinical workup or medication adjustment is warranted.

Retrieval is safe even during therapeutic anticoagulation provided the INR does not exceed about 3.0.[124] The feasibility of filter removal is largely a function of dwell time and the presence of residual thrombus within the filter[125,126] (Table 16-4). If embolic protection is likely needed for longer than the accepted dwell time of the filter, the interventionalist can periodically capture the device and reposition it within the recovery sheath to a slightly different location in the IVC.[127] Some retrievable filters can be removed safely after much longer periods than recommended by the manufacturers, although the safety of this maneuver cannot be guaranteed.[65,82,128-130]

Technique

With the exception of the OptEase device, filter retrieval must be done through the IJ vein. Venacavography is necessary to identify thrombus within or extending above the filter. A pigtail (or similarly shaped) catheter

TABLE 16-4   Manufacturers' Guidelines for Inferior Vena Cava Filter Removal

Filter	Percentage of Thrombus Allowing Removal	Access Site
Guenther-Tulip/ Celect	<25% of cone	Jugular
G2, Eclipse	No recommendation	Jugular
Optease	No recommendation	Femoral

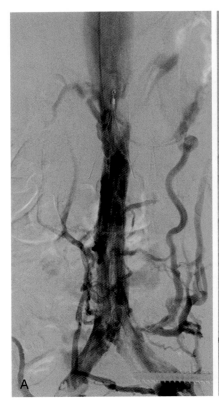
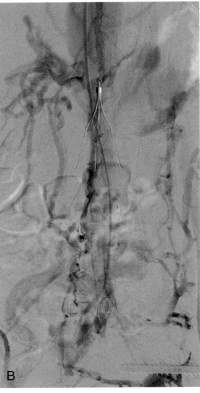

FIGURE 16-20 **A** and **B,** Inferior vena cava thrombosis after placement of a retrievable Guenther tulip filter

is carefully negotiated through the filter body with a guidewire.

- Small subcentimeter intrafilter thrombi are generally inconsequential if the patient is being anticoagulated. They should not interfere with removal. In an un-anticoagulated individual, however, even small clots may be harbingers of more dangerous peripheral thrombi; as such, the filter should remain in place for the time being.
- Large volumes of trapped or free-floating clot preclude removal, and the procedure should be abandoned (Figs. 16-20 and 16-21). The patient may be restudied in a month or so to see whether clot dissolution has been sufficient to make retrieval safe (Fig. 16-22). Another option is to place a second retrievable filter well above the thrombus-filled device to capture any clot that showers centrally during removal of the original filter. The second filter then may be retrieved.[131]
- If the clot burden is large and the patient is symptomatic, catheter-directed thrombolysis may be an option (see later discussion).

There are slight variations on the methods for filter capture and retrieval, but the common step is retrieval hook engagement with a snare device (e.g., Amplatz gooseneck snare, trilobed snare) advanced through a

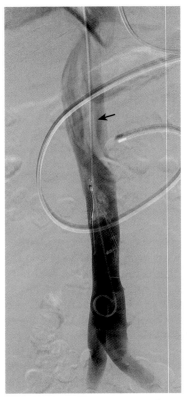

FIGURE 16-21 Trapped thrombus within inferior vena cava filter cone and extending above filter *(arrow).* Clearly this filter cannot be removed at this time, and the physician should consider placement of a second retrievable suprarenal device.

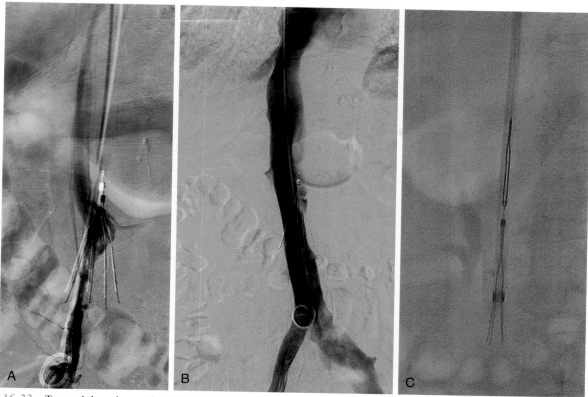

FIGURE 16-22   Trapped thrombus within IVC filter precludes removal **(A)**. Patient returned about 1 month later on anticoagulation, at which time complete clot lysis has occurred **(B)**. Nonetheless, the filter legs would not entirely release from the caval wall **(C)**, and the device was left in place permanently.

long 10- to 12-Fr sheath (see Fig. 16-17G). Once the snare is cinched down on the hook securely, the sheath is then slid over the filter, compressing the legs and disengaging the device from the caval wall. In most cases, retrieval is straightforward.

However, if the retrieval hook abuts or becomes embedded into the vascular wall, extraction may be quite challenging (Fig. 16-23). A variety of methods have been devised to remove stubborn filters[131-142] (Fig. 16-24 and Box 16-5). Even with extraordinary effort, capturing the filter apex and removing the filter may be impossible. Considerable force or complex manipulations may be needed to release some filters from the cava. In the process, however, the filter may become grossly distorted with the potential for caval thrombosis, gross filter leg perforation of vital structures, or embolization of filter fragments to the heart (Fig. 16-25).

Many interventionalist do not bother with postretrieval cavography unless the removal was difficult or the patient experienced severe pain. Most residual intimal flaps or adherent thrombi that are detected require no specific treatment. Frank IVC perforation with extravasation demands careful monitoring or direct treatment. The operator should examine the integrity of the device. Evidence of missing elements should prompt careful fluoroscopic examination over the abdomen and

chest to locate remaining filter fragments that may themselves require removal.

Results and Complications

Among published series, the removal rate for retrievable filters ranges from 78% to 100%.* The most common reasons for failure are the presence of substantial thrombus within the filter (precluding safe withdrawal), inability to engage the retrieval hook, and permanent incorporation into the IVC wall. Although filter retrieval becomes more challenging as the dwell time increases, some filters can be removed many months beyond the manufacturer's suggested period.[130,135,145,148]

IVC filter extraction is a remarkably safe procedure. Despite some almost heroic maneuvers used to retrieve stubborn filters, serious complications are extremely rare. Some early, creative methods of retrieval were associated with significant risk of partial caval thrombosis. With modifications of these techniques, most injuries to the caval wall are self-limited.[124,133,135] Still, the filter can become markedly distorted during an unsuccessful attempted withdrawal, which can predispose to IVC thrombosis, perforation of adjacent structures, or filter fragmentation.

*See references 61, 65, 82, 84-90, 101, 104, 107, 127, 130, 143-147.

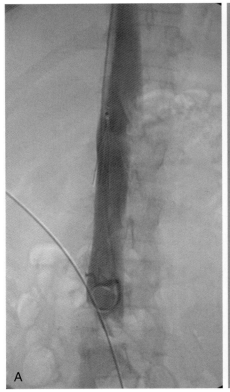
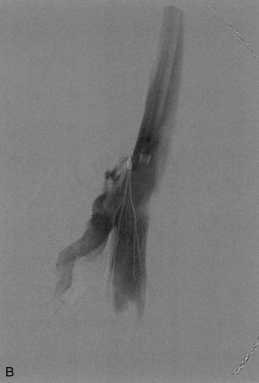

FIGURE 16-23 Unsuccessful removal of Guenther tulip filter. **A,** Initial frontal cavogram suggests that the retrieval hook is within the lumen. However, a steep oblique cavagram shows the hook imbedded in the caval wall **(B).** It could not be captured. More aggressive techniques might have allowed removal.

BOX 16-5

ADVANCED TECHNIQUES FOR INFERIOR VENA CAVA FILTER RETRIEVAL

- Loop-snare method
- Endobronchial or myocardial biopsy forceps tip dissection
- Curved sheath technique
- Balloon displacement
- Centering filter with stiff guidewire or tip-deflecting wire
- Guidewire shearing of tissue covering filter apex

BOX 16-6

CAUSES OF OBSTRUCTION OF THE INFERIOR VENA CAVA

- Thrombosis
  - Extension of iliac vein thrombus
  - Inferior vena cava filter or surgical interruption
  - Indwelling catheter
  - Trauma
  - Thrombophilic state
- Tumor extension
  - Intraluminal growth
  - Direct invasion
- Severe extrinsic compression
- Membranous webs
- Idiopathic causes

Inferior Vena Cava Thrombosis (Online Case 84)

Etiology and Clinical Features

There are numerous causes of total IVC occlusion[9,149-152] (Box 16-6). The most common reasons are propagation of clot from the iliac veins, indwelling IVC catheters, transvenous spread of tumor thrombus from abdominal or pelvic neoplasms, and thrombosis of IVC filters. In infants and children, IVC obstruction usually is caused by thrombosis from indwelling venous catheters, thrombophilic states, or intraabdominal tumors.[153] In contrast to the lower extremity and pelvic veins, apparently unprovoked *isolated* IVC thrombosis is rare.

If the collateral circulation has sufficient time to develop, caval occlusion may be clinically silent. Other-

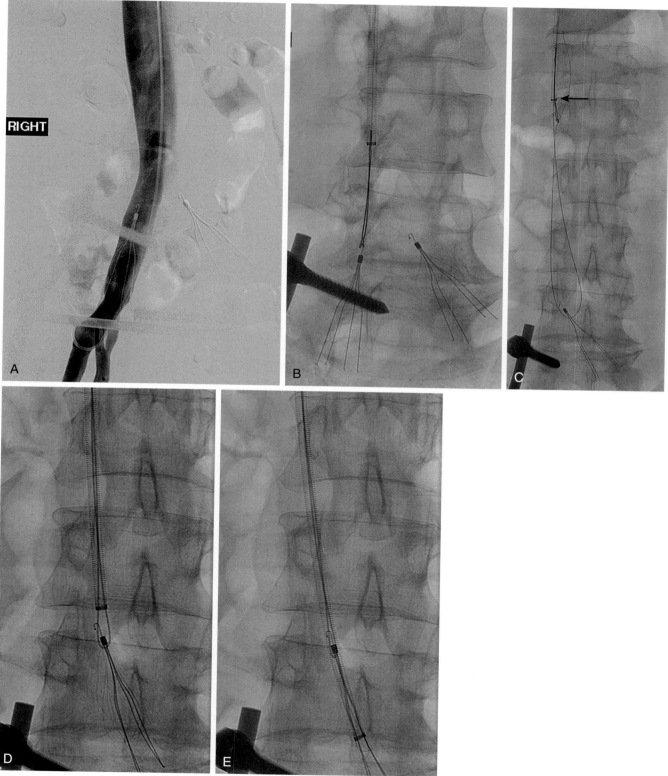

FIGURE 16-24   Loop snare technique for difficult inferior vena cava filter retrieval. **A,** Patient had required bilateral common iliac veins filters. **B,** The right-sided filter was easily snared and removed. The hook on the left-sided filter could not be engaged. Therefore, a guidewire was advanced around the embedded filter hook. The end of the wire loop was captured with a snare placed in tandem through the vascular sheath (**C,** *arrow*). The end of the wire was brought up through the sheath and out the body, allowing significant force to be applied to the filter apex. The sheath was passed down over the filter hook and onto the apex (**D),** and the device was pulled into the sheath (**E)** and ultimately out of the patient.

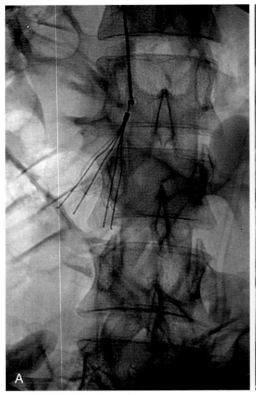

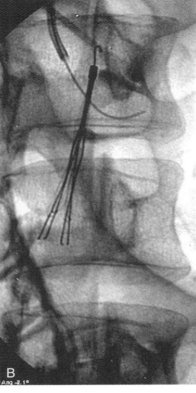

FIGURE 16-25 Unsuccessful removal of Guenther tulip filter. **A,** The retrieval hook was easily caught with a snare device. However, despite vigorous traction, the legs would not release. **B,** The filter became deformed but was left in the patient.

wise, patients develop bilateral leg edema, dilated superficial veins over the legs and abdomen, and subsequently skin changes resulting from chronic venous stasis. When the occlusion involves both renal veins, the nephrotic syndrome can occur. Acute IVC thrombosis associated with severe iliofemoral thrombosis may lead to the rare syndrome of *phlegmasia cerulea dolens*.[154] These patients suffer massive leg swelling, severe pain, cyanosis, and (ultimately) arterial ischemia (see Chapter 15). Despite aggressive treatment, a substantial number of cases ends in amputation, massive PE, or death.

Imaging

CROSS-SECTIONAL TECHNIQUES

IVC thrombosis is usually diagnosed by CT or MR angiography or by color Doppler sonography.[9,155,156] On contrast-enhanced CT, the IVC is enlarged, and collateral vessels may opacify. A low-density filling defect is seen (see Fig. 16-19). At first glance, heterogenous enhancement of the lumen (from mixing of unopacified blood) can mimic intraluminal clot in the early phases of dynamic CT scanning.[157] Intraluminal extension of tumor thrombus (typically from renal cell or hepatocellular carcinoma and typically heterogeneous in appearance) can mimic bland IVC thrombosis (see Fig. 10-33 and Fig. 16-26).

CATHETER ANGIOGRAPHY

A thrombus produces a discrete filling defect or abrupt shelf-like cut-off (see Fig. 16-26). In cases of complete or long-standing occlusion, the IVC does not opacify at all, and only collateral vessels are seen (see Fig. 16-3). The pattern of altered circulation depends on the level and extent of occlusion. In low IVC occlusion, the cava often remains patent at and above the entry of the renal veins. Venography from the IJ vein approach may be necessary to determine the upper extent of the obstruction.

Treatment

MEDICAL THERAPY

The major goals of treatment are to prevent PE, limit clot propagation that may cause renal vein and hepatic vein thrombosis, and potentially avoid the post-thrombotic syndrome (see Chapters 1 and 15). First-line management for IVC thrombosis is anticoagulation following the guidelines for lower extremity DVT.[158] However, this regimen is contraindicated in certain cases, including in patients with risk factors for bleeding from anticoagulants and those who have had a previous adverse reaction to heparin or warfarin. In such circumstances, placement of a suprarenal IVC filter may be appropriate (see earlier discussion).

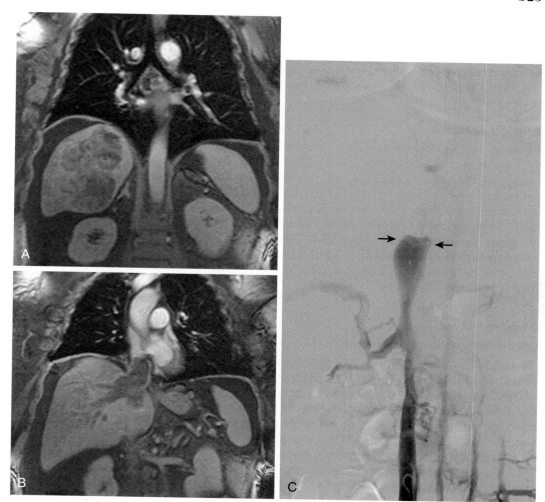

FIGURE 16-26 Extension of tumor thrombus from hepatocellular carcinoma into the inferior vena cava (IVC). Coronal images from gadolinium-enhanced magnetic resonance images show a huge heterogenous mass in the liver (**A**) with tumor thrombus expanding the hepatic veins and inferior vena cava up to the right atrium (**B**). **C,** Venacavography shows a shelflike occlusion of the suprarenal IVC *(arrows)* with prominent collateral circulation more inferiorly.

ENDOVASCULAR THERAPY

Catheter-directed thrombolysis has been used to treat acute IVC thrombosis from a variety of causes, including IVC filter occlusion, Budd-Chiari syndrome, nephrotic syndrome, indwelling central venous catheters, and spontaneous occurrences.[159-162] Thrombolysis should be considered in patients with severe symptoms and in those who fail to respond to anticoagulant therapy (see Chapters 3 and 15). Complete clot dissolution often requires prolonged infusions (>2 days), large doses of fibrinolytic agent, and adjunctive mechanical thrombectomy. The necessity for retrievable filter insertion before thrombolysis to prevent procedure-related PE is controversial (see earlier discussion).

Neoplasms (Online Case 57)

Etiology

Abdominal and pelvic tumors can affect the IVC by intraluminal extension, direct invasion through the caval wall, or extrinsic compression. Malignant neoplasms prone to transvenous spread are renal cell carcinoma (RCC), hepatocellular carcinoma, adrenal carcinoma, and some gynecologic and testicular neoplasms.[9] Very rarely, a benign neoplasm propagates into the vena cava (e.g., pheochromocytoma and angiomyolipoma). Tumors that typically invade the caval wall include pancreatic neoplasms and retroperitoneal sarcomas.

RCC has a propensity to involve the IVC, which happens in about 5% to 10% of cases.[163] Because RCC propagates entirely within the vascular lumen and leaves the wall intact, surgical resection of even widely advanced lesions is often feasible. Identification of renal vein or IVC invasion (Robson stage IIIA) is important in determining prognosis and guiding operative therapy. *Hepatocellular carcinoma* invades the IVC in about 10% to 26% of patients.[164] In end-stage cases, tumor thrombus will extend into the RA (see Fig. 16-26).

Primary malignancies of the IVC are rare. *Leiomyosarcoma* is the most common primary neoplasm to afflict the IVC, and the IVC is the most common vascular site for leiomyosarcoma.[165,166] These neoplasms may ultimately extend outside or into the lumen of the cava.[9] Extraluminal growth of vascular leiomyosarcoma happens in most cases; intraluminal extension alone is seen in about one fourth of patients. The segment from the renal veins to the hepatic veins is most frequently involved.[167]

Clinical Features

Luminal obstruction or extrinsic compression of the IVC by tumor is sometimes asymptomatic, but can cause leg swelling, distention of superficial veins, abdominal pain or bloating, and DVT. The Budd-Chiari syndrome may follow complete intrahepatic IVC occlusion. Although often largely silent until detected by imaging, leiomyosarcoma also may present with abdominal pain or a palpable abdominal mass. Classically, this extremely rare disease afflicts women in the fifth or sixth decade of life.[168]

Imaging

CROSS-SECTIONAL TECHNIQUES

CT and MRI are best for assessing patients with known or suspected IVC invasion from a malignancy.[169-171] Typical findings include caval enlargement, intraluminal filling defects, extension of tumor thrombus to the RA, and complete caval occlusion with opacification of collateral vessels (see Figs. 16-26 and 10-33). Occasionally, frank neovascularity within the tumor thrombus is apparent.

Leiomyosarcoma appears as an inhomogeneous enhancing mass replacing or filling the IVC (Fig. 16-27). MR findings are variable, with the mass typically showing intermediate signal intensity on T1-weighted sequences and increased signal on T2-weighted sequences. The lower one third of the vena cava is least often involved.[9,167,168] It is often impossible to differentiate primary caval leiomyosarcoma from the more common retroperitoneal leiomyosarcoma.

CATHETER ANGIOGRAPHY

Venacavography is almost never required for diagnosis, staging, or preoperative assessment of caval neoplasms. However, endovascular biopsy of suspected intraluminal IVC tumors is a valuable tool when the pathologic diagnosis is unknown[172,173] (see Fig. 10-37). Bleeding complications are less likely through an intraluminal route than a percutaneous approach.

Treatment

Radical surgery is favored in some patients with primary or secondary tumor, even when the disease has spread to the intrahepatic IVC.[174-177] Operative techniques include caval wall resection with patching or segmental caval resection with prosthetic grafting.

OTHER DISORDERS

Inferior Vena Cava Compression, Stenosis, and Obstruction

Focal or long-segment narrowing of the IVC is common[9] (Box 16-7). Normal extrinsic compression may be caused by the right common iliac artery (on the bifurcation),

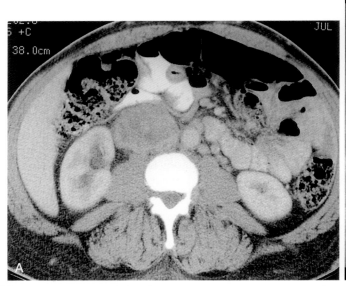
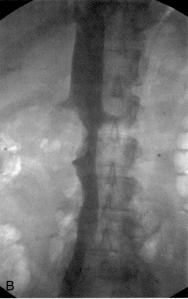

FIGURE 16-27　Leiomyosarcoma of the inferior vena cava (IVC) on contrast-enhanced computed tomography in one patient **(A)** and on venacavography in another **(B)**. In the latter case, the nonocclusive mural tumor mimics bland thrombus.

BOX 16-7

CAUSES OF NARROWING OF THE INFERIOR VENA CAVA

- Extrinsic compression
  - Right common iliac artery
  - Right renal artery
  - Vertebral column
  - Hepatic masses
  - Ascites
  - Hepatomegaly
  - Pregnancy
  - Retroperitoneal masses (e.g., tumor, hematoma)
  - Aortic ectasia or aneurysm
- After liver transplantation
- Wall thickening from resolved thrombotic disease
- Inferior vena cava filter
- Profound hypotension or hypovolemia ("flat IVC")
- Retroperitoneal fibrosis
- Functional obstruction (e.g., Valsalva maneuver)

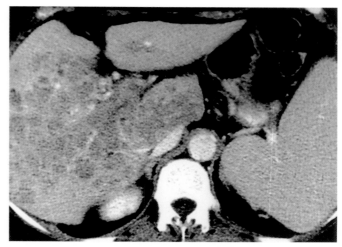

FIGURE 16-28 Massive hepatocellular carcinoma produces extrinsic compression of the intrahepatic inferior vena cava.

---

right renal artery (on the posterior cava), or the spine (see Fig. 15-6). The IVC can appear severely narrowed if the patient performs a vigorous Valsalva maneuver during imaging. The most frequent reason for pathologic extrinsic compression is liver disease (e.g., severe hepatomegaly, caudate lobe enlargement, hepatic masses, massive ascites) (Figs. 16-28 and 16-29). Large abdominal aortic aneurysms (AAA) also may efface the vena cava, and severe obstruction of the IVC by an AAA can lead to caval thrombosis.[178] Mural thickening from resolved thrombosis can leave mild or moderate caval narrowing. Focal caval obstruction in the setting of orthotopic liver transplantation is discussed in Chapter 12.

Intravascular stents are placed for certain IVC obstructions. Most often, stents are used for palliative relief of malignant IVC obstruction (e.g., hepatocellular carcinoma), after orthotopic liver transplantation, and for membranous IVC obstruction.[179-183] Gianturco Z-stents and Wallstents have been used (among others) for this purpose (Fig. 16-30 and see Fig. 12-39). Return of near normal caval blood flow is accomplished in the majority of cases; the IVC usually remains patent for the remainder of the patient's life. Placement of stents in the IVC, particularly near the heart, can be treacherous (Fig. 16-31). The major risk of IVC stent placement is immediate or delayed migration into the heart, which can have disastrous consequences. Therefore,

oversized stents (about 50% larger than measured nominal diameter) are routinely chosen.

Retroperitoneal Fibrosis

Retroperitoneal fibrosis is a rare, poorly understood chronic inflammatory disorder of the abdomen and pelvis. Genetic and autoimmune origins have been proposed; in a few cases, it is the result of tumor, infection, or chronic use of certain drugs, such as ergot derivatives.[184] The infiltrative fibrotic process often extends from the level of the kidneys into the pelvis. Symptomatic involvement of the IVC occurs in only 2% of cases.

CT or MRI reveals encasement of the IVC and iliac veins[185,186] (Fig. 16-32). In symptomatic patients, the cava may be completely obliterated. The inflammatory tissue often involves other central retroperitoneal structures, including the aorta, ureters, and small bowel.

Membranous Obstruction

Membranous obstruction of the IVC describes a related set of conditions in which a fibromuscular membrane develops within the IVC just below the RA (type 1) or a fibrous band completely replaces the intrahepatic IVC for a variable distance (type 2).[187] Central hepatic vein involvement is common. The etiology is unknown. Membranous IVC obstruction is most commonly seen in India, Japan, Korea, China, and South Africa. In those countries, it is the leading cause of *Budd-Chiari syndrome* (BCS), with a slowly progressive course rather than the fulminant disease of thrombotic BCS that is typical in Western nations.[188]

The diagnosis is made by cross-sectional imaging.[189,190] The radiographic appearance is variable, ranging from a discrete bandlike obstruction to long segment complete

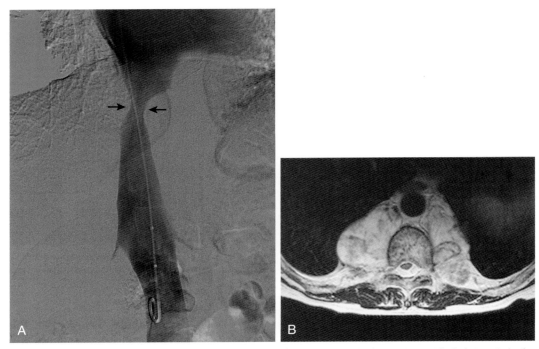

FIGURE 16-29   Extrinsic compression of the intrahepatic inferior vena cava (**A,** *arrows*). This patient with thalassemia had extramedullary hematopoiesis about the spine on T1-weighted magnetic resonance images **(B).** Note high signal intensity in the paraspinal masses and the vertebra.

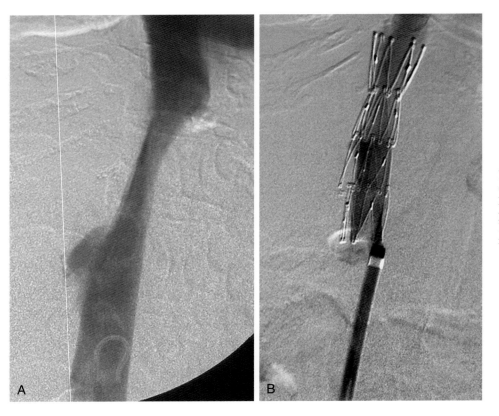

FIGURE 16-30   Inferior vena cava (IVC) stent placement. **A,** Intrahepatic IVC narrowing following liver transplant with a 14-mm Hg gradient. **B,** Widely patent vessel following placement of several Gianturco Z-stents.

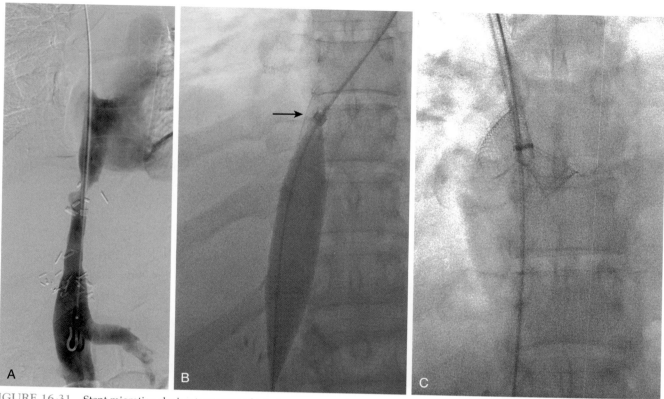

FIGURE 16-31 Stent migration during treatment of inferior vena cava (IVC) stenosis. **A,** Venacavography after liver transplant shows a significant intrahepatic stenosis. **B,** A Wallstent was placed at the site and dilated with a balloon. Movement of the upper end towards the right atrium is evident *(arrow).* After removing the balloon, the stent migrated completely into the heart but remained around the guidewire. **C,** The stent was ultimately snared and removed through the jugular vein.

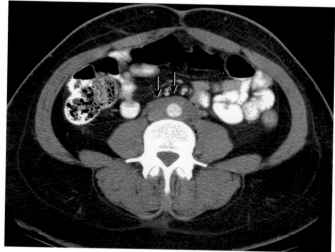

FIGURE 16-32 Retroperitoneal fibrosis involving the inferior vena cava (IVC) and aorta *(arrows).* The IVC is completely obliterated by the inflammatory mass.

caval obliteration. Intrahepatic and extrahepatic venous collaterals (e.g., portosystemic, superficial abdominal wall, azygous vein) are prominent features of this disease. Caudate lobe enlargement with associated extrinsic IVC compression is characteristic. There is an unfortunate association of this disorder with hepatocellular carcinoma in South African black and Japanese populations.[188]

Balloon angioplasty, stent placement, or catheter-directed thrombolysis are employed to recanalize the IVC in cases of partial or total obstruction.[191,192] The short-term results of these procedures have been excellent. Some patients are appropriate candidates for vascular decompression with a transjugular intrahepatic portosystemic shunt procedure. Surgical options include transcardiac membranectomy, decompression of the liver with a portosystemic shunt, or bypass procedure with a cavoatrial shunt or IVC to SVC graft.

Aortocaval Fistula

Aortocaval fistula is rare. Most cases result from erosion of an AAA into the IVC (untreated or after graft insertion); this event occurs in less than 1% of repaired AAAs. Less often, aortocaval fistula is a spontaneous event or secondary to infection or trauma (e.g., lumbar spine surgery).[193-195] The classic clinical triad is localized pain, a palpable aneurysm, and an abdominal bruit. The diagnosis is made by sonography, CT angiography, or MR angiography (see Fig. 7-12). The communication most frequently develops between the distal aorta and IVC. Stent grafts have been used to seal these connections.[196,197]

Trauma

Injury to the IVC may result from blunt or penetrating trauma to the abdomen or chest[198] (Fig. 16-33). Most patients who initially survive the event undergo immediate exploratory laparotomy because they are hemodynamically unstable or show evidence of bleeding on peritoneal lavage or imaging. With blunt abdominal trauma, the most common site of laceration is the retrohepatic portion of the IVC.

Aneurysms

Aneurysms of the IVC are exceedingly rare.[199-201] Many remain asymptomatic for years. They may only come to medical attention after complete thrombosis or PE. IVC aneurysm can mimic IVC occlusion from other causes. Surgical treatment requires partial or complete excision of the aneurysm.

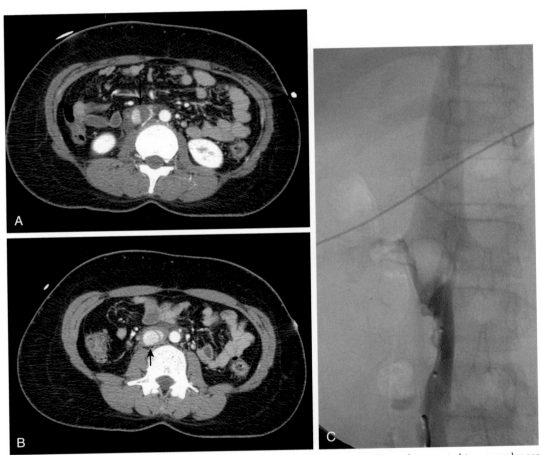

FIGURE 16-33   Inferior vena cava (IVC) disruption from motor vehicle crash. Contrast-enhanced computed tomography scans (**A** and **B**) show disruption of the IVC *(arrow).* The findings were confirmed at venacavography **(C).**

References

1. Dewald CL, Jensen CC, Park YH, et al. Vena cavography with CO_2 versus with iodinated contrast material for inferior vena cava filter placement: a prospective evaluation. *Radiology* 2000;**216**:752.

2. Gabella G, editor. Cardiovascular system. In: Williams PL, Bannister LH, Berry MM, et al, editors. *Gray's anatomy*, 38th ed. New York: Churchill Livingstone; 1995. p. 1600.

3. Collin P, editor. Embryology and development. In: Williams PL, Bannister LH, Berry MM, et al, editors. *Gray's Anatomy*. 38th ed. New York: Churchill Livingstone; 1995. p. 324.

4. Bass JE, Redwine MD, Kramer LA, et al. Spectrum of congenital anomalies of the inferior vena cava: cross-sectional imaging findings. *Radiographics* 2000;**20**:639.

5. Hicks ME, Malden ES, Vesely TM, et al. Prospective anatomic study of the inferior vena cava and renal veins: comparison of selective renal venography with cavography and relevance in filter placement. *J Vasc Interv Radiol* 1995;**6**:721.

6. LaBerge JM, Ring EJ, Gordon RL. Percutaneous intrahepatic portosystemic shunt created via a femoral vein approach. *Radiology* 1991;**181**:679.

7. Kaufman JA, Waltman AC, Rivitz SM, et al. Anatomical observations on the renal veins and inferior vena cava at magnetic resonance angiography. *Cardiovasc Intervent Radiol* 1995;**18**:153.

8. Grant E, Rendano F, Sevinc E, et al. Normal inferior vena cava: caliber changes observed by dynamic ultrasound. *AJR Am J Roentgenol* 1980;**135**:335.

9. Kandpal H, Sharma R, Gamangatti S, et al. Imaging the inferior vena cava: a road less traveled. *Radiographics* 2008;**28**:669.

10. Truty MJ, Bower TC. Congenital anomalies of the inferior vena cava and left renal vein: implications during open abdominal aortic aneurysm reconstruction. *Ann Vasc Surg* 2007;**21**:186.

11. Minniti S, Visentini S, Pracacci C. Congenital anomalies of the venae cavae: embryological origin, imaging features, and report of three new variants. *Eur Radiol* 2002;**12**:2040.

12. Trigaux JP, Vandroogenbroek S, De Wispelaere JF, et al. Congenital anomalies of the inferior vena cava and left renal vein: evaluation with spiral CT. *J Vasc Interv Radiol* 1998;**9**:339.

13. Munechika H, Cohan RH, Baker ME, et al. Hemiazgyous continuation of a left inferior vena cava: CT appearance. *J Comput Assist Tomogr* 1988;**12**:328.

14. Brickner ME, Eichhorn EJ, Netto D, et al. Left-sided inferior vena cava draining into the coronary sinus via persistent left superior vena cava: case report and review of the literature. *Cathet Cardiovasc Diagn* 1990;**20**:189.

15. Koc Z, Oguzkurt L. Interruption or congenital stenosis of the inferior vena cava: prevalence, imaging, and clinical findings. *Eur J Radiol* 2007;**62**:257.

16. Berg C, Geipel A, Smrcek J, et al. Prenatal diagnosis of cardiosplenic syndromes: a 10 year experience. *Ultrasound Obstet Gynecol* 2003;**22**:451.

17. Fulcher AS, Turner MA. Abdominal manifestations of situs anomalies in adults. *Radiographics* 2002;**22**:1439.

18. Kapur S, Paik E, Rezaei A, et al. Where there is blood, there is a way: unusual collateral vessels in superior and inferior vena cava obstruction. *Radiographics* 2010;**30**:67.

19. Kazmers A, Jacobs LA, Perkins AJ. Pulmonary embolism in Veterans Affairs Medical Centers: is vena cava interruption underutilized? *Am Surg* 1999;**65**:1171.

20. Athanasoulis CA, Kaufman JA, Halpern EF, et al. Inferior vena caval filters: review of a 26-year single-center clinical experience. *Radiology* 2000;**216**:54.

21. Decousus H, Leizorovicz A, Parent F, et al. A clinical trial of vena caval filters in the prevention of pulmonary embolism in patients with proximal deep-vein thrombosis. Prevention du Risque d'Embolie Pulmonaire par Interruption Cave Study Group. *N Engl J Med* 1998;**338**:409.

22. Girard P, Stern JB, Parent F. Medical literature and vena cava filters: so far so weak. *Chest* 2002;**122**:963.

23. Grassi CJ, Swan TL, Cardella JF, et al. Quality improvement guidelines for percutaneous permanent inferior vena cava filter placement for the prevention of pulmonary embolism. SIR Standards of Practice Committee. *J Vasc Interv Radiol* 2003;**14**:S271.

24. Kinney TB. Update on inferior vena cava filters. *J Vasc Interv Radiol* 2003;**14**:425.

25. Rosner MK, Kuklo TR, Tawk R, et al. Prophylactic placement of an inferior vena cava filter in high risk patients undergoing spinal recontruction. *Neurosurg Forum* 2004;**17**:E6.

26. Winchell RJ, Hoyt DB, Walsh JC, et al. Risk factors associated with pulmonary embolism despite routine prophylaxis: implications for improved protection. *J Trauma* 1994;**37**:600.

27. Gargiulo III NJ, Veith FJ, Lipsitz EC, et al. Experience with inferior vena cava filter placement in patients undergoing open gastric bypass surgery. *J Vasc Surg* 2006;**44**:1301.

28. Kucher N, Rossi E, DeRosa M, et al. Massive pulmonary embolism. *Circulation* 2006;**113**:577.

29. Greenfield LJ, Proctor MC. Vena caval filter use in patients with sepsis: results in 175 patients. *Arch Surg* 2003;**138**:1245.

30. Geerts WH, Code KI, Jay RM, et al. A prospective study of venous thromboembolism after major trauma. *N Engl J Med* 1994;**331**:1601.

31. Rogers F, Cipolle M, Velmahos G, et al. Practice management guidelines for the prevention of venous thromboembolism in trauma patients: the EAST practice management guidelines work group. *J Trauma* 2002;**53**:142.

32. Gorman PH, Qadri SF, Rao-Patel A. Prophylactic inferior vena cava (IVC) filter placement may increase the relative risk of deep venous thrombosis after acute spinal cord injury. *J Trauma* 2009;**66**:707.

33. McMurtry AL, Owings JT, Anderson JT, et al. Increased use of prophylactic vena cava filters in trauma patients failed to decrease overall incidence of pulmonary embolism. *Am J Coll Surg* 1999;**189**:314.

34. Velmahos GC, Kern J, Chan LS, et al. Prevention of venous thromboembolism after injury: an evidence-based report. *J Trauma* 2000;**49**:132.

35. Geerts WH, Bergqvist D, Pineo GF, et al. Prevention of venous thromboembolism: American College of Chest Physicians evidence-based clinical practice guidelines (8th edition). *Chest* 2008;**133**:381S.

36. PREPIC Study Group. Eight year follow-up of patients with permanent vena cava filters in the prevention of pulmonary embolism: the PREPIC (Prevention du Risque d'Embolic Pulmonaire par Interruption Cave) randomized study. *Circulation* 2005;**112**:416.

37. Ray CE Jr, Prochazka A. The need for anticoagulation following inferior vena cava filter placement: a systematic review. *Cardiovasc Intervent Radiol* 2008;**31**:316.

38. Protack CD, Bakken AM, Patel N, et al. Long-term outcomes of catheter directed thrombolysis for lower extremity deep venous thrombosis without prophylactic inferior vena cava filter placement. *J Vasc Surg* 2007;**45**:992.

39. Yamagami T, Yoshimatsu R, Matsumoto T, et al. Prophylactic implantation of inferior vena cava filter during endovascular therapies for deep venous thrombosis of the lower extremity: is it necessary? *Acta Radiol* 2008;**49**:391.

40. Kalva SP, Chlapoutaki C, Wicky S, et al. Suprarenal inferior vena cava filters: a 20-year single center experience. *J Vasc Interv Radiol* 2008;**19**:1041.

41. Hammond CJ, Bakshi DR, Currie RJ, et al. Audit of the use of IVC filters in the UK: experience from three centres over 12 years. *Clin Radiol* 2009;**64**:502.

42. Crowther MA. Inferior vena cava filters in the management of venous thromboembolism. *Am J Med* 2009;**120**:S13.

43. Danetz JS, McLafferty RB, Ayerdi J, et al. Selective venography versus nonselective venography before vena cava filter placement: evidence for more, not less. *J Vasc Surg* 2003;**38**:928.

44. Patil UD, Ragavan A, Nadaraj, et al. Helical CT angiography in evaluation of live kidney donors. *Nephrol Dial Transplant* 2001;**16**:1900.

45. Reed RA, Teitelbaum GP, Taylor FC, et al. Use of the Bird's nest filter in oversized inferior venae cavae. *J Vasc Interv Radiol* 1991;**2**:447.

46. Mansour M, Chang AE, Sindelar WF. Interruption of the inferior vena cava for the prevention of recurrent pulmonary embolism. *Am Surgeon* 1985;**51**:375.

47. Miles RM, Richardson RR, Wayne L, et al. Long term results with the serrated Teflon vena caval clip in the prevention of pulmonary embolism. *Ann Surg* 1969;**169**:881.

48. Greenfield LJ, McCrudy JR, Brown PP, et al. A new intracaval filter permitting continued flow and resolution of thrombi. *Surgery* 1973;**73**:599.

49. Tadavarthy SM, Castaneda-Zuniga W, Salomonowitz E, et al. Kimray-Greenfield vena cava filter: percutaneous introduction. *Radiology* 1984;**151**:525.

50. Katsamouris AA, Waltman AC, Delichatsios MA, et al. Inferior vena cava filters: in vitro comparison of clot trapping and flow dynamics. *Radiology* 1988;**166**:361.

51. Hammer FD, Rousseau HP, Joffre FG, et al. In vitro evaluation of vena cava filters. *J Vasc Interv Radiol* 1994;**5**:869.

52. Simon M, Rabkin DJ, Kleshinski S, et al. Comparative evaluation of clinically available inferior vena cava filters with an in vitro physiologic simulation of the vena cava. *Radiology* 1993;**189**:769.

53. Korbin CD, Reed RA, Taylor FC, et al. Comparison of filters in an oversized vena caval phantom: intracaval placement of a Bird's nest filter versus biiliac placement of Greenfield, Vena Tech-LGM, and Simon nitinol filters. *J Vasc Interv Radiol* 1992;**3**:559.

54. Joels CS, Sing RF, Heniford BT. Complications of inferior vena cava filters. *Am Surg* 2003;**69**:654.

55. Mahnken AH, Pfeffer J, Stanzel S, et al. In vitro evaluation of optionally retrievable and permanent IVC filters. *Invest Radiol* 2007;**42**:529.

56. Grassi CJ, Matsumoto AH, Teitelbaum GP. Vena caval occlusion after Simon nitinol filter placement: identification with MR imaging in patients with malignancy. *J Vasc Interv Radiol* 1992;**3**:535.

57. Lorch H, Dallmann A, Zwaan M, et al. Efficacy of permanent and retrievable vena cava filters: experimental studies and evaluation of a new device. *Cardiovasc Intervent Radiol* 2002;**25**:193.

58. Leask RL, Johnston KW, Ojha M. Hemodynamic effects of clot entrapment in the TrapEase inferior vena cava filter. *J Vasc Interv Radiol* 2004;**15**:485.

59. Kaufman JA, Kinney TB, Streiff MB, et al. Guidelines for the use of retrievable and convertible IVC filters: report from the Society of Interventional Radiology multidisciplinary consensus conference. *J Vasc Interv Radiol* 2006;**17**:449.

60. Keeling AN, Kinney TB, Lee MJ. Optional inferior vena caval filter: where are we now? *Eur Radiol* 2008;**18**:1556.

61. Asch MR. Initial experience in humans with a new retrievable inferior vena cava filter. *Radiology* 2002;**225**:835.

62. Wellons E, Rosenthal D, Schoborg T, et al. Renal cell carcinoma invading the inferior vena cava: use of a "temporary" vena cava filter to prevent tumor emboli during nephrectomy. *Urology* 2004;**63**:380.

63. Gosin JS, Graham AM, Ciocca RG, et al. Efficacy of prophylactic vena cava filters in high-risk trauma patients. *Ann Vasc Surg* 1997;**11**:100.

64. Hoff WS, Hoey BA, Wainwright GA, et al. Early experience with retrievable inferior vena cava filters in high-risk trauma patients. *J Am Coll Surg* 2004;**199**:869.

65. Morris CS, Rogers FB, Najarian KE, et al. Current trends in vena caval filtration with the introduction of a retrievable filter at a level I trauma center. *J Trauma* 2004;**57**:32.

66. Berczi V, Bottomley JR, Thomas SM, et al. Long-term retrievability of IVC filters: should we abandon permanent devices? *Cardiovasc Intervent Radiol* 2007;**30**:820.

67. Davison BD, Grassi CJ. TrapEase inferior vena cava filter placed via the basilic arm vein: a new antecubital access. *J Vasc Interv Radiol* 2002;**13**:107.

68. Streiff MB. Vena caval filters: a comprehensive review. *Blood* 2000;**95**:3669.

69. Matchett WJ, Jones MP, McFarland DR, et al. Suprarenal vena caval filter placement: follow-up of four filter types in 22 patients. *J Vasc Interv Radiol* 1998;**9**:588.

70. Greenfield LJ, Proctor MC. Suprarenal filter placement. *J Vasc Surg* 1998;**28**:432.

71. Spaniolas K, Velmahos GC, Kwolek C, et al. Bedside placement of removable vena cava filters guided by intravascular ultrasound in the critically injured. *World J Surg* 2008;**32**:1438.

72. Killingsworth CD, Taylor SM, Patterson MA, et al. Prospective implementation of an algorithm for bedside intravascular ultrasound-guided filter placement in critically ill patients. *J Vasc Surg* 2010;**51**:1215.

73. Rosenthal D, Wellons ED, Levitt AB, et al. Role of prophylactic temporary inferior vena cava filters placed at the ICU bedside under intravascular ultrasound guidance in patients with multiple trauma. *J Vasc Surg* 2004;**40**:958.

74. Rosenthal D, Kochupura PV, Wellons ED, et al. Guenther tulip and Celect IVC filters in multiple trauma patients. *J Endovasc Ther* 2009;**16**:494.

75. Sangwaiya MJ, Marentis TC, Walker TG, et al. Safety and effectiveness of the Celect inferior vena cava filter: preliminary results. *J Vasc Interv Radiol* 2009;**20**:1188.

76. Ziegler JW, Dietrich GJ, Cohen SA, et al. PROOF trial: protection from pulmonary embolism with the OptEase filter. *J Vasc Interv Radiol* 2008;**19**:1165.

77. Kinney TB, Rose SC, Weingarten KW, et al. IVC filter tilt and asymmetry: comparison of over-the-wire stainless-steel and titanium Greenfield IVC filters. *J Vasc Interv Radiol* 1997;**8**:1029.

78. Sag AA, Stavas JM, Burke CT, et al. Analysis of tilt of the Guenther tulip filter. *J Vasc Interv Radiol* 2008;**19**:669.

79. de Gregorio MA, Gamboa P, Gimeno MJ, et al. The Gunther Tulip retrievable filter: prolonged temporary filtration by repositioning within the inferior vena cava. *J Vasc Interv Radiol* 2003;**14**:1259.

80. Moore BS, Valji K, Roberts AC, et al. Transcatheter manipulation of asymmetrically opened titanium Greenfield filters. *J Vasc Interv Radiol* 1993;**4**:687.

81. Wang WY, Cooper SG, Eberhardt SC. Use of a nitinol gooseneck snare to open an incompletely expanded over-the-wire stainless steel Greenfield filter. *AJR Am J Roentgenol* 1999;**172**:499.

82. Millward SF, Oliva VL, Bell SD, et al. Guenther Tulip retrievable vena cava filter: results from the Registry of the Canadian Interventional Radiology Association. *J Vasc Interv Radiol* 2001;**12**:1053.

83. Offner PJ, Hawkes A, Madayag R, et al. The role of temporary inferior vena cava filters in critically ill surgical patients. *Arch Surg* 2003;**138**:591.

84. Imberti D, Bianchi M, Farina A, et al. Clinical experience with retrievable vena cava filters: results of a prospective observational multicenter study. *J Thromb Haemostat* 2005;**3**:1370.

85. Mismetti P, Rivron-Guillot K, Quenet S, et al. A prospective long-term study of 220 patients with a retrievable vena cava filter for secondary prevention of venous thromboembolism. *Chest* 2007;**131**:223.

86. Rosenthal D, Swischuk JL, Cohen SA, et al. OptEase retrievable inferior vena cava filter: initial multicenter experience. *Vascular* 2005;**13**:286.

87. Bovyn G, Gory P, Reynaud P, et al. The Tempofilter: a multicenter study of a new temporary caval filter implantable for up to six weeks. *Ann Vasc Surg* 1997;**11**:520.

88. Rosenthal D, Wellons ED, Lai KM, et al. Retrievable inferior vena cava filters: early clinical experience. *J Cardiovasc Surg* (Torino) 2005;**46**:163.

89. Schutzer R, Ascher E, Hingorani A, et al. Preliminary results of the new 6F TrapEase inferior vena cava filter. *Ann Vasc Surg* 2003;**17**:103.

90. Oliva VL, Szatmari F, Giroux MF, et al. The Jonas study: evaluation of the retrievability of the Cordis OptEase inferior vena cava filter. *J Vasc Interv Radiol* 2005;**16**:1439.

91. Young T, Tang H, Hughes R. Vena caval filters for the prevention of pulmonary embolism. *Cochrane Database Syst Rev* 2010; **17**:CD006212.

92. Ferris EJ, McCowan TC, Carver DK, et al. Percutaneous inferior vena caval filters: follow-up of seven designs in 320 patients. *Radiology* 1993;**188**:851.

93. Wojtowycz MM, Stoehr T, Crummy AB, et al. The Bird's nest inferior vena caval filter: review of a single-center experience. *J Vasc Interv Radiol* 1997;**8**:171.

94. Becker DM, Philbrick JT, Selby JB. Inferior vena cava filters: indications, safety, effectiveness. *Arch Intern Med* 1992; **152**:1985.

95. Neuerburg JM, Guenther RW, Vorwerk D, et al. Results of a multicenter study of the retrievable Tulip Vena Cava Filter: early clinical experience. *Cardiovasc Intervent Radiol* 1997;**20**:10.

96. Streiff MB. Vena caval filters: a review for intensive care specialists. *J Intensive Care Med* 2003;**18**:59.

97. Kim HS, Young MJ, Narayan AK, et al. A comparison of clinical outcomes with retrievable and permanent inferior vena cava filters. *J Vasc Interv Radiol* 2008;**19**:393.

98. Kalva SP, Wicky S, Waltman AC, et al. TrapEase vena cava filter: experience in 751 patients. *J Endovasc Ther* 2006;**13**:365.

99. Kinney TB, Rose SC, Lim GW, et al. Fatal paradoxic embolism occurring during IVC filter insertion in a patient with chronic pulmonary thromboembolic disease. *J Vasc Interv Radiol* 2001; **12**:770.

100. Putterman D, Niman D, Cohen G. Aortic pseudoaneurysm after penetration by a Simon nitinol inferior vena cava filter. *J Vasc Interv Radiol* 2005;**16**:535.

101. Oliva VL, Perrault P, Giroux MF, et al. Recovery G2 inferior vena cava filter: technical success and safety of retrieval. *J Vasc Interv Radiol* 2008;**19**:884.

102. Fox MA, Kahn SR. Postthrombotic syndrome in relation to vena cava filter placement: a systematic review. *J Vasc Interv Radiol* 2008;**19**:981.

103. LeBlanche AF, Benazzouz A, Reynaud P, et al. The VenaTech LP permanent caval filter: effectiveness and safety in the prevention of pulmonary embolism- a European multicenter study. *J Vasc Interv Radiol* 2008;**19**:509.

104. Pellerin O, Barral FG, Lions C, et al. Early and late retrieval of the ALN removable vena cava filter: results from a multicenter study. *Cardiovasc Intervent Radiol* 2008;**31**:889.

105. Crochet DP, Brunel P, Trogrlic S, et al. Long-term follow-up of Vena Tech-LGM filter: predictors and frequency of caval occlusion. *J Vasc Interv Radiol* 1999;**10**:137.

106. Harlal A, Ojha M, Johnston KW. Vena cava filter performance based on hemodynamics and reported thrombosis and pulmonary embolism patterns. *J Vasc Interv Radiol* 2007;**18**:103.

107. Onat L, Ganiyusufoglu AK, Mutlu A, et al. OptEase and TrapEase vena cava filters: a single-center experience in 258 patients. *Cardiovasc Intervent Radiol* 2009; **32**:992.

108. Sharafuddin MJ, Sun S, Hoballah JJ, et al. Endovascular management of venous thrombotic and occlusive disease of the lower extremities. *J Vasc Interv Radiol* 2003;**14**:405.

109. Vedantham S, Vesely TM, Parti N, et al. Endovascular recanalization of the thrombosed filter-bearing inferior vena cava. *J Vasc Interv Radiol* 2003;**14**:893.

110. Bochenek KM, Aruny JE, Tal MG. Right atrial migration and percutaneous retrieval of a Gunther Tulip inferior vena cava filter. *J Vasc Interv Radiol* 2003;**14**:1207.

111. Porcellini M, Stassano P, Musumeci A, et al. Intracardiac migration of nitinol TrapEase vena cava filter and paradoxical embolism. *Eur J Cardiothorac Surg* 2002;**22**:460.

112. LaPlante JS, Contractor FM, Kiproff PM, et al. Migration of the Simon nitinol vena cava filter to the chest. *AJR Am J Roentgenol* 1993;**160**:385.

113. Shmuter Z, Frederic FI, Gill JR. Fatal migration of vena caval filters. *Forensic Sci Med Pathol* 2008;**4**:116.

114. Galhotra S, Amesur NB, Zajko AB, et al. Migration of the Guenther tulip inferior vena cava filter to the chest. *J Vasc Interv Radiol* 2007;**18**:1581.

115. Friedell ML, Goldenkranz RJ, Parsonnet V, et al. Migration of a Greenfield filter to the pulmonary artery: a case report. *J Vasc Surg* 1986;**3**:929.

116. Rogoff PA, Hilgenberg AD, Miller SL, et al. Cephalic migration of the Bird's nest inferior vena caval filter: report of two cases. *Radiology* 1992;**184**:819.

117. Owens CA, Bui JT, Knuttinen MG, et al. Intracardiac migration of inferior vena cava filter: review of published data. *Chest* 2009; **136**:877.

118. Haddadian B, Shaikh F, Djelmami-Hani M, et al. Sudden cardiac death caused by migration of a TrapEase inferior vena cava filter: case report and review of the literature. *Clin Cardiol* 2008;**31**:84.

119. Malden ES, Darcy MD, Hicks ME, et al. Transvenous retrieval of misplaced stainless steel Greenfield filters. *J Vasc Interv Radiol* 1992;**3**:703.

120. Deutsch LS. Percutaneous removal of intracardiac Greenfield vena caval filter. *AJR Am J Roentgenol* 1988;**151**:677.

121. Owens CA, Bui JT, Knuttinen MG, et al. Endovascular retrieval of intracardiac inferior vena cava filters: a review of published techniques. *J Vasc Interv Radiol* 2009;**20**:1418.

122. Goldman HB, Hanna K, Dmochowski RR. Ureteral injury secondary to an inferior vena cava filter. *J Urol* 1996;**156**:1763.

123. Sadaf A, Rasuli P, Olivier A, et al. Significant caval penetration by the Celect inferior vena cava filter: attributable to filter design? *J Vasc Interv Radiol* 2007;**18**:1447.

124. Hoppe H, Kaufman JA, Barton RE, et al. Safety of inferior vena cava filter retrieval in anticoagulated patients. *Chest* 2007; **132**:31.

125. Kerlan RK Jr, Laberge JM, Wilson MW, et al. Residual thrombus within a retrievable IVC filter. *J Vasc Interv Radiol* 2005;**16**:555.

127. Tay KH, Martin ML, Fry PD, et al. Repeated Gunther Tulip inferior vena cava filter repositioning to prolong implantation time. *J Vasc Interv Radiol* 2002;**13**:509.

128. Binkert CA, Sasadeusz K, Stavropoulos SW. Retrievability of the recovery vena cava filter after dwell times longer than 180 days. *J Vasc Interv Radiol* 2006;**17**:299.

129. Reekers JA, Hoogeveen YL, Wijnands M, et al. Evaluation of the retrievability of the OptEase IVC filter in an animal model. *J Vasc Interv Radiol* 2004;**15**:261.

130. Terhaar OA, Lyon SM, Given MF, et al. Extended interval for retrieval of Gunther Tulip filters. *J Vasc Interv Radiol* 2004;**15**:1257.

131. Yavuz K, Geyik S, Barton RE, et al. Retrieval of a malpositioned vena cava filter with embolic protection with use of a second filter. *J Vasc Interv Radiol* 2005;**16**:531.

132. Hagspiel KD, Leung DA, Aladdin M, et al. Difficult retrieval of a Recovery IVC filter. *J Vasc Interv Radiol* 2004;**15**:645.

133. Doody O, Noe G, Given MF, et al. Assessment of snared-loop technique when standard retrieval of inferior vena cava filters fails. *Cardiovasc Intervent Radiol* 2009;**32**:145.

134. Kuo WT, Bostaph AS, Loh CT, et al. Retrieval of trapped Guenther tulip inferior vena cava filters: snare-over-guidewire loop technique. *J Vasc Interv Radiol* 2006;**17**:1845.

135. Kuo WT, Tong RT, Hwang GL, et al. High risk retrieval of adherent and chronically implanted IVC filters: techniques for removal and management of thrombotic complications. *J Vasc Interv Radiol* 2009;**20**:1548.

136. Stavropoulos SW, Dixon RG, Burke CT, et al. Embedded inferior vena cava filter removal: use of an endobronchial forceps. *J Vasc Interv Radiol* 2008;**19**:1297.

137. Van Ha TG, Vinokur O, Lorenz J, et al. Techniques used for difficult retrievals of the Guenther tulip inferior vena cava filter: experience in 32 patients. *J Vasc Interv Radiol* 2009;**20**:92.

138. Van Ha TG, Keblinskas D, Funaki B, et al. Removal of Guenther tulip vena cava filter through a femoral vein approach. *J Vasc Interv Radiol* 2005;**16**:391.

139. Hagspiel KD, Leung DA, Aladdin M, et al. Difficult retrieval of a Recovery IVC filter. *J Vasc Interv Radiol* 2004;**15**:645.

140. Contractor S, Bhagat N, Mahmood Y, et al. Retrieval of a tilted Guenther tulip filter with the superior hook embedded in the caval wall. *J Vasc Interv Radiol* 2007;**18**:1455.

141. Ullman JM. Technique for snaring an inaccessible Guenther tulip filter. *J Vasc Interv Radiol* 2006;**17**:1067.

142. Yamagami T, Kato T, Nishimura T. Successful retrieval of a Guenther tulip vena cava filter with the assistance of a curved sheath introducer. *J Vasc Interv Radiol* 2005;**16**:1760.

143. Stein PD, Alnas M, Skaf E, et al. Outcome and complications of retrievable inferior vena cava filters. *Am J Cardiol* 2004;**94**:1090.

144. Doody O, Given MF, Kavnoudias H, et al. Initial experience in 115 patients with the retrievable Cook Celect vena cava filter. *J Med Imaging Rad Oncol* 2009;**53**:64.

145. Looby S, Given MF, Geoghagen T, et al. Gunther tulip retrievable inferior vena caval filters: indications, efficacy, retrieval, and complications. *Cardiovasc Intervent Radiol* 2007;**30**:59.

146. Cantwell CP, Pennypacker J, Singh H, et al. Comparison of the recovery and G2 filter as retrievable inferior vena cava filters. *J Vasc Interv Radiol* 2009;**20**:1193.

147. Keller IS, Meier C, Pfiffner R, et al. Clinical comparison of two optional vena cava filters. *J Vasc Interv Radiol* 2007;**18**:505.

148. Marquess JS, Burke CT, Beecham AH, et al. Factors associated with failed retrieval of the Guenther tulip inferior vena cava filter. *J Vasc Interv Radiol* 2008;**19**:1321.

149. Joshi A, Carr J, Chrisman H, et al. Filter-related, thrombotic occlusion of the inferior vena cava treated with a Gianturco stent. *J Vasc Interv Radiol* 2003;**14**:381.

150. Kim HL, Zisman A, Han KR, et al. Prognostic significance of venous thrombus in renal cell carcinoma. Are renal vein and inferior vena cava involvement different? *J Urol* 2004;**171**:588.

151. Okuda K. Membranous obstruction of the inferior vena cava. *J Gastroenterol Hepatol* 2001;**16**:1179.

152. Kaushik S, Federle MP, Schur PH, et al. Abdominal thrombotic and ischemic manifestations of the antiphospholipid antibody syndrome: CT findings in 42 patients. *Radiology* 2001;**218**:768.

153. Hausler M, Hubner D, Delhaas T, et al. Long term complications of inferior vena cava thrombosis. *Arch Dis Child* 2001;**85**:228.

154. Gargiulo III NJ, O'Connor DJ, Veith FJ, et al. Long-term outcome of inferior vena cava filter placement in patients undergoing gastric bypass. *Ann Vasc Surg* 2010;**24**:946.

155. Sheth S, Fishman EK. Imaging of the inferior vena cava with MDCT. *AJR Am J Roentgenol* 2007;**189**:1243.

156. Lin J, Zhou KR, Chen ZW, et al. Vena cava 3D contrast enhanced MR venography: a pictorial review. *Cardiovasc Intervent Radiol* 2005;**28**:795.

157. Kaufman LB, Yeh BM, Breiman RS, et al. Inferior vena cava filling defects on CT and MRI. *AJR Am J Roentgenol* 2005;**185**:717.

158. Bates SM, Ginsberg JS. Treatment of deep-vein thrombosis. *New Engl J Med* 2004;**351**:268.

159. Rigatelli G, Cardaioli P, Roncon L, et al. Combined percutaneous aspiration thrombectomy and rheolytic thrombectomy in massive subacute vena cava thrombosis with IVC filter occlusion. *J Endovasc Ther* 2006;**13**:373.

160. Robinson DL, Teitelbaum GP. Phlegmasia cerulea dolens: treatment by pulse-spray and infusion thrombolysis. *AJR Am J Roentgenol* 1993;**160**:1288.

161. Ishiguchi T, Fukatsu H, Itoh S, et al. Budd-Chiari syndrome with long segmental inferior vena cava obstruction: treatment with thrombolysis, angioplasty, and intravascular stents. *J Vasc Interv Radiol* 1992;**3**:421.

162. Yan BP, Kiernan TJ, Gupta V, et al. Combined pharmacomechanical thrombectomy for acute inferior vena cava filter thrombosis. *Cardiovasc Revasc Med* 2008;**9**:36.

163. Wotkowicz C, Wszolek MF, Libertino JA. Resection of renal tumors invading the vena cava. *Urol Clin North Am* 2008;**35**:657.

164. Kanematsu M, Imaeda T, Minowa H, et al. Hepatocellular carcinoma with tumor thrombus in the inferior vena cava and right atrium. *Abdom Imaging* 1994;**19**:313.

165. Kieffer E, Alaoui M, Piette JC, et al. Leiomyosarcoma of the inferior vena cava: experience in 22 cases. *Ann Surg* 2006;**244**:289.

166. Hollenbeck ST, Grobmyer SR, Kent KC, et al. Surgical treatment and outcomes of patients with primary inferior vena cava leiomyosarcoma. *J Am Coll Surg* 2003;**197**:575.

167. Kyriazi MA, Stafyla VK, Chatzinikolaou I, et al. Surgical challenges in the treatment of leiomyosarcoma of the inferior vena cava: analysis of two cases and brief review of the literature. *Ann Vasc Surg* 2010;**24**:e13.

168. Jenkins S, Marshall GB, Gray R. Leiomyosarcoma of the inferior vena cava. *Can J Surg* 2005;**48**:252.

169. Hallscheidt PJ, Fink C, Haferkamp A, et al. Preoperative staging of renal cell carcinoma with inferior vena cava thrombus using multidetector CT and MRI: prospective study with histopathological correlation. *J Comput Assist Tomogr* 2005;**29**:64.

170. Sheth S, Scatarige JC, Horton KM, et al. Current concepts in the diagnosis and management of renal cell carcinoma: role of multidetector CT and three-dimensional CT. *Radiographics* 2001;**21**:S237.

171. Cuevas C, Raske M, Bush WH, et al. Imaging primary and secondary tumor thrombus of the inferior vena cava: multi-detector computed tomography and magnetic resonance imaging. *Curr Probl Diagn Radiol* 2006;**35**:90.

172. Fidias P, Fan CM, McGovern FJ, et al. Intracaval extension of germ cell carcinoma: diagnosis via endovascular biopsy and a review of the literature. *Eur Urol* 1997;**31**:376.

173. Armstrong PJ, Franklin DP. Pararenal vena cava leiomyosarcoma versus leiomyomatosis: difficult diagnosis. *J Vasc Surg* 2002;**36**:1256.

174. Hemming AW, Langham MR, Reed AI, et al. Resection of the inferior vena cava for hepatic malignancy. *Am Surg* 2001;**67**:1081.

175. Blute ML, Leibovich BC, Lohse CM, et al. The Mayo Clinic experience with surgical management, complications and outcome for patients with renal cell carcinoma and venous tumour thrombus. *BJU Int* 2004;**94**:33.

176. Ito H, Hornick JL, Bertagnolli MM, et al. Leiomyosarcoma of the inferior vena cava: survival after aggressive management. *Ann Surg Oncol* 2007;**14**:3534.

177. Cho SW, March JW, Geller DA, et al. Surgical management of leiomyosarcoma of the inferior vena cava. *J Gastrointest Surg* 2008;**12**:2141.

178. Myers PO, Kalangos A, Terraz S. Ruptured aortic aneurysm masquerading as phlegmasia cerulea. *Am J Emerg Med* 2008;**26**:1067.

179. Irving JD, Dondelinger RF, Reidy JF, et al. Gianturco self-expanding stents: clinical experience in the vena cava and large veins. *Cardiovasc Intervent Radiol* 1992;**15**:328.

180. Lee JM, Ko GY, Sung KB, et al. Long-term efficacy of stent placement for treating inferior vena cava stenosis following liver transplantation. *Liver Transpl* 2010;**16**:513.

181. Brountzos EN, Binkert CA, Panagiotou IE, et al. Clinical outcome after intrahepatic venous stent placement for malignant inferior vena cava syndrome. *Cardiovasc Intervent Radiol* 2004; **27**:129.

182. Razavi MK, Hansch EC, Kee ST, et al. Chronically occluded inferior venae cavae: endovascular treatment. *Radiology* 2000; **214**:133.

183. Borsa JJ, Daly CP, Fontaine AB, et al. Treatment of inferior vena cava anastomotic stenoses with the Wallstent endoprosthesis after orthotopic liver transplantation. *J Vasc Interv Radiol* 1999; **10**:17.

184. Rhee RY, Gloviczki P, Luthra HS, et al. Iliocaval complications of retroperitoneal fibrosis. *Am J Surg* 1994;**168**:179.

185. Vaglio A, Salvarani C, Buzio C. Retroperitoneal fibrosis. *Lancet* 2006;**367**:241.

186. Vorwerk D, Guenther RW, Wendt G, et al. Iliocaval stenosis and iliac vein thrombosis in retroperitoneal fibrosis: percutaneous treatment by use of hydrodynamic thrombectomy and stenting. *Cardiovasc Intervent Radiol* 1996;**19**:40.

187. Okuda K. Membranous obstruction of the inferior vena cava (obliterative hepatocavopathy, Okuda). *J Gastroenterol Hepatol* 2001;**16**:1179.

188. Kew MC, Hodkinson HJ. Membranous obstruction of the inferior vena cava and its causal relation to hepatocellular carcinoma. *Liver Int* 2006;**26**:1.

189. Kim TK, Chung JW, Han JK, et al. Hepatic changes in benign obstruction of the hepatic inferior vena cava: CT findings. *AJR Am J Roentgenol* 1999;**173**:1235.

190. Ciesek S, Rifai K, Bahr MJ, et al. Membranous Budd-Chiari syndrome in Caucasians. *Scan J Gastroenterol* 2010;**45**:226.

191. Zhang C, Fu L, Zhang G, et al. Ultrasonically guided inferior vena cava stent placement: experience in 83 cases. *J Vasc Interv Radiol* 1999;**10**:85.

192. Lee BB, Villavicencio L, Kim YW, et al. Primary Budd-Chiari syndrome: outcome of endovascular management for suprahepatic venous obstruction. *J Vasc Surg* 2006;**43**:101.

193. Torigian DA, Carpenter JP, Roberts DA. Mycotic aortocaval fistula: efficient evaluation by bolus-chase MR angiography. *J Magn Reson Imaging* 2002;**15**:195.

194. Schott III EE, Fitzgerald SW, McCarthy WJ, et al. Aortocaval fistula: diagnosis with MR angiography. *AJR Am J Roentgenol* 1997; **169**:59.

195. Waldrop Jr JL, Dart IV BW, Barker DE. Endovascular stent graft treatment of a traumatic aortocaval fistula. *Ann Vasc Surg* 2005;**19**:562.

196. Hetzel G, Gabriel P, Rompel O, et al. Aortocaval fistula after stent-graft repair. *J Endovasc Ther* 2006;**13**:117.

197. Kopp R, Weidenhagen R, Hoffmann R, et al. Immediate endovascular treatment of an aortoiliac aneurysm ruptured into the inferior vena cava. *Ann Vasc Surg* 2006;**20**:525.

198. Huerta S, Bui TD, Nguyen TH, et al. Predictors of mortality and management of patients with traumatic inferior vena cava injuries. *Am Surg* 2006;**72**:290.

199. Calligaro KD, Ahmad S, Dandora R, et al. Venous aneurysms: surgical indications and review of the literature. *Surgery* 1995; **117**:1.

200. Sullivan VV, Voris TK, Borlaza GS, et al. Incidental discovery of an inferior vena cava aneurysm. *Ann Vasc Surg* 2002;**16**:513.

201. Elliot A, Henn A, Pamuklar E, et al, Aneurysm of the inferior vena cava: case report. *Abdom Imaging* 2006;**31**:457.

17

Upper Extremity Veins and Superior Vena Cava

Karim Valji

ANATOMY

Development

In the embryo, the upper limb buds are drained by marginal veins.[1] The deep veins develop along with their corresponding arteries. The preaxial and postaxial portions of the marginal vein become the cephalic and basilic veins, respectively.

The central thoracic veins are formed from the precardinal (anterior) and common cardinal vessels[1] (Fig. 17-1). The upper segment of the precardinal vein becomes the internal jugular vein. The subclavian vein enters from the arm and joins the lower portion of the precardinal vein. An interprecardinal anastomosis connects the two precardinal veins and develops into the left brachiocephalic vein. The lower right precardinal vein becomes the upper superior vena cava. A remnant of the left precardinal vein becomes the left superior intercostal vein.

Normal Anatomy

The arms are drained by superficial and deep venous pathways. Numerous perforators connect these systems. Unlike the lower extremities, the superficial system is dominant. It arises from two complex venous plexuses on the dorsal and palmar surfaces of the hand.[2] The *cephalic* and *basilic veins* originate from the dorsal venous network and run on the radial and ulnar sides of the forearm, respectively. The median vein of the forearm drains the palmar venous plexus and joins the basilic vein near the elbow. The *median cubital vein* connects the basilic and cephalic veins at the elbow (Fig. 17-2). In the upper arm, the basilic vein lies medial to the biceps muscle and forms the axillary vein at the lateral border of the scapula (see Fig. 17-2). The cephalic vein runs superficial and lateral to the biceps muscle, into the deltopectoral groove, through the infraclavicular fossa, and onto the upper surface of the axillary vein (Fig. 17-3). The deep veins of the forearm follow the radial and ulnar arteries. They unite and then divide at the elbow to form paired *brachial veins*. These vessels run alongside the brachial artery and then join the basilic vein to become the axillary vein.

The *axillary vein* begins at the confluence of the brachial and basilic veins. Several branches of the brachial plexus course between the artery and vein in this region. At the lateral border of the first rib, the axillary vein becomes the *subclavian vein* (see Fig. 17-3). Several tributaries, including the *external jugular vein*, enter the subclavian vein. The vein runs in front of the anterior scalene muscle. At the medial edge of the anterior scalene muscle, the *internal jugular vein* joins the subclavian vein to form the brachiocephalic (innominate) vein.

The *right brachiocephalic vein* courses almost vertically in front of the right brachiocephalic artery. Tributaries include the right vertebral, internal thoracic (mammary), inferior thyroid, and first posterior intercostal veins. The *left brachiocephalic vein* (which is more than twice as long as the right) passes inferomedially in front of the left subclavian and left carotid arteries. Branches are comparable to those on the right with the addition of the *left superior intercostal* and *thymic veins*. In most cases, the former vessel is the continuation of the *accessory hemiazygous vein* (see Fig. 17-1). The major lymphatic ducts (including the *thoracic duct* on the left) enter the venous circulation near the junction of the left subclavian and jugular veins.

The brachiocephalic veins merge to form the *superior vena cava (SVC)*, which is valveless. The SVC enters the right atrium at about the level of the third costal cartilage. The *azygous vein* ascends from the abdomen into chest through the right crus of the diaphragm. It arches anteriorly to an opening in the back wall of the SVC above the right main stem bronchus (Fig. 17-4; see also Fig. 17-1). The main trunk of the azygous vein drains the right posterior and superior intercostal veins. The *hemiazygous vein*

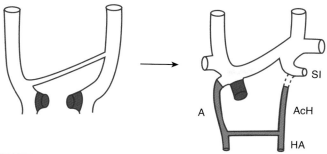

FIGURE 17-1 Embryologic development of the major thoracic veins. Shading indicates common cardinal vein origin *(dark)*, supracardinal vein origin *(light)*, and azygous line vein origin (white). *A*, azygous vein; *AcH*, accessory hemiazygous vein; *HA*, hemiazygous vein; *SI*, superior intercostal vein. *(Adapted from Collin P, ed. Embryology and development. In: Williams PL, Bannister LH, Berry MM, et al, eds. Gray's anatomy, 38th ed. London: Churchill Livingstone, 1995:327.)*

ascends to the left of the thoracic aorta. At about the T7-T8 level, it gives off a large branch to the azygous vein and then becomes the *accessory hemiazygous vein.*

Valves are present in the superficial and deep veins from the hand to the subclavian trunks. Changes in intrathoracic pressure during inspiration and expiration produce a corresponding increase or decrease in flow through the upper extremity veins, respectively. With rapid inspiration, the internal jugular and subclavian veins may even completely collapse. The Doppler ultrasound flow patterns in the subclavian, internal jugular, and axillary veins reflect both atrial and respiratory activity.

Variant Anatomy (Online Case 105)

The most common anomaly of the upper extremity veins is partial or complete duplication. Rare variants include separate drainage of the brachiocephalic veins into the right atrium and absence of the left brachiocephalic vein with blood return through the left superior intercostal vein.[3]

Persistent left SVC (duplication of the SVC) is an uncommon anomaly that results from persistence of the left precardinal vein, with or without a maldeveloped left brachiocephalic vein[3-5] (Fig. 17-5). It is found in less than 1% of the general population but is more frequent in patients with congenital heart disease. The left-sided moiety usually empties into the coronary sinus.

Isolated left SVC, which is a less common variant, occurs with persistence of the left precardinal vein and regression of the right precardinal vein.[6]

Variations in azygous and hemiazygous venous anatomy are frequent. In particular, the accessory hemiazygous vein may drain into the azygous, hemiazygous, or left brachiocephalic veins.[2]

Collateral Circulation

With axillosubclavian vein thrombosis, muscular and superficial veins around the shoulder and thorax are recruited as collateral pathways, which empty into the brachiocephalic, jugular, or azygous veins. With brachiocephalic vein occlusion, the principal collateral pathway

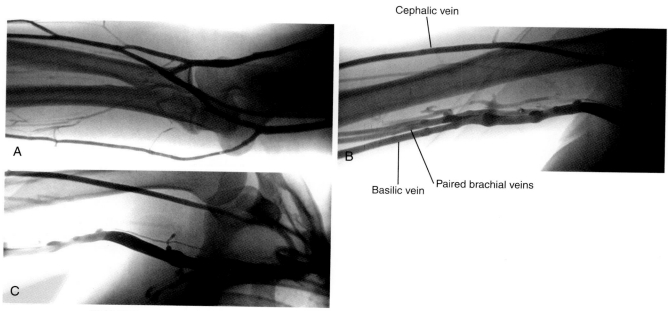

FIGURE 17-2 Venous anatomy of the right arm at the elbow **(A)**, upper arm **(B)**, and shoulder **(C)**.

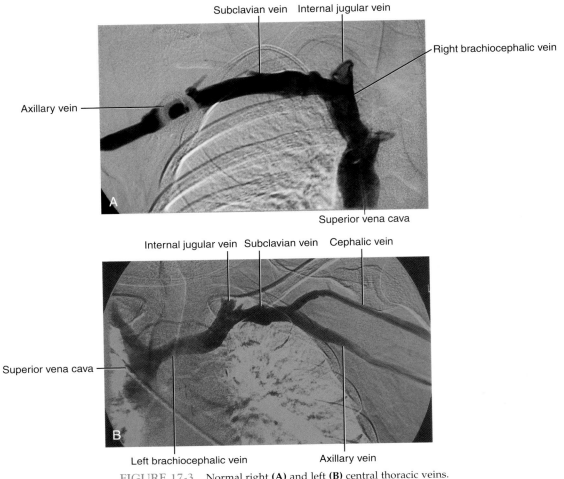

FIGURE 17-3   Normal right **(A)** and left **(B)** central thoracic veins.

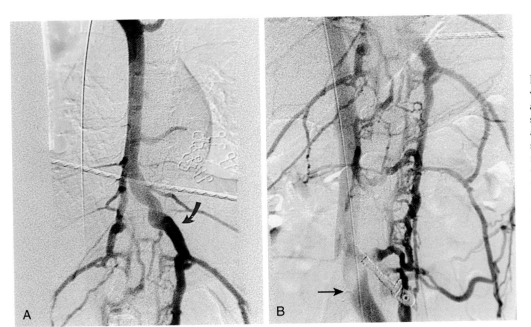

FIGURE 17-4   Azygous venous system in a patient with a low superior vena cava (SVC) stenosis. **A,** Injection of the azygous vein directly from the superior vena cava shows retrograde flow down the vein, with filling of the hemiazygous vein *(curved arrow)* and numerous lumbar collaterals. **B,** Late phase of the run with imaging over the mid-abdomen shows filling of the left iliac vein *(arrow)* and inferior vena cava through lumbar and vertebral collaterals.

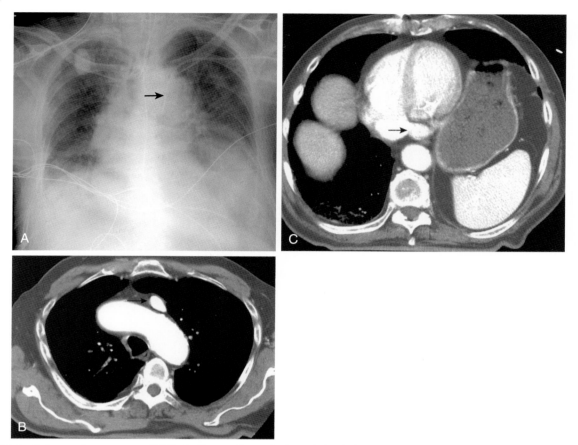

FIGURE 17-5   Left superior vena cava (SVC). **A,** Chest radiograph shows left subclavian central venous catheter passing to the left of the spine *(arrow).* **B,** Computed tomography angiogram shows left SVC *(arrow).* **C,** At a more inferior level, the left SVC enters the coronary sinus *(arrow).*

is up the ipsilateral jugular vein to the contralateral jugular or brachiocephalic veins via multiple head and neck channels (Fig. 17-6).

With partial or complete obstruction of the SVC, the major collateral routes are through the azygous-hemiazygous system, internal thoracic veins, lateral thoracic veins, and the vertebral venous plexus.[7,8] With *low* SVC obstruction below the azygous insertion, blood flows down the azygous and hemiazygous veins into the lumbar veins and into the iliac veins and inferior vena cava (IVC) (Fig. 17-7; see also Fig. 17-4). With *high* SVC obstruction above or at the azygous insertion, collateral flow is mainly through right and left superior intercostal branches and the left brachiocephalic vein and then into the azygous system (Fig. 17-8). If the obstruction engulfs the SVC and the brachiocephalic and azygous veins, drainage is through superficial chest wall, lateral thoracic, and internal thoracic veins into the iliac veins and IVC (Fig. 17-9).

MAJOR DISORDERS

Upper Extremity Venous Thrombosis (Online Case 51)

Etiology

Symptomatic venous thrombosis is much less common in the arm and chest than in the leg.[9] Box 17-1 outlines the major causes.[10-13] In many patients, prior or existing central venous devices of various types are the culprit. Subclavian vein catheters are much more prone to stenosis or occlusion than internal jugular vein lines.[10,14] In some populations, stenoses or complete occlusions (often asymptomatic) have been found in up to 50% of individuals with a history of subclavian vein catheters.[14-16] Most symptomatic patients have obstruction of the axillary or subclavian veins, with or without more central (brachiocephalic or SVC) occlusion. Hemodialysis catheters are especially

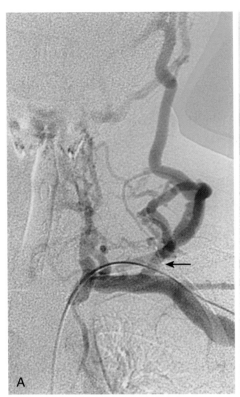

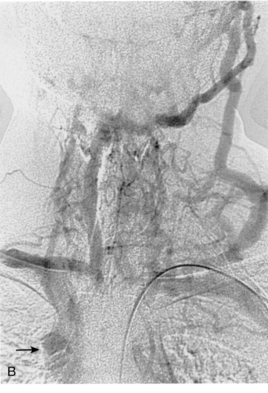

FIGURE 17-6   Left brachiocephalic vein occlusion. **A,** There is retrograde flow up the external jugular vein *(arrow)* and into small collateral channels. The left internal jugular vein was occluded. **B,** On delayed images, contrast flows into right-sided neck and thoracic veins and then into the superior vena cava *(arrow).*

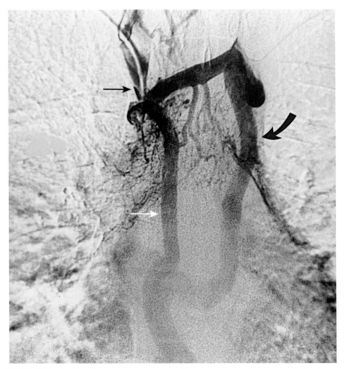

FIGURE 17-7   Superior vena cava obstruction with contrast injection into the central right brachiocephalic vein *(black straight arrow).* Contrast flows down the azygous vein *(white arrow)* and also up the left brachiocephalic vein into the accessory hemiazygous vein *(curved arrow).* Note the thymic tributaries on the undersurface of the left brachiocephalic vein.

problematic. Patients with end-stage kidney disease often require periodic placement of these large-caliber devices. Presence of a maturing or mature dialysis shunt in the arm only exacerbates the problem due to nonphysiologic high blood flow through the outflow veins.

Primary thrombosis (i.e., *spontaneous* or *"effort"* thrombosis), also known as *Paget-Schroetter disease,* accounts for about 20% of cases of upper extremity central venous occlusion.[17] In this venous form of the thoracic outlet syndrome, the subclavian or axillary vein is compressed by a musculoskeletal structure, most often between the first rib and subclavius tendon or the costoclavicular ligament. Unlike the subclavian artery, the vein runs in front of the anterior scalene muscle and is not trapped at this site. Chronic intimal injury (often exacerbated by strenuous shoulder activity) combined with slow flow or a hypercoagulable condition can lead to vessel thrombosis.

The natural history of acute upper extremity venous thrombosis is different from the comparable disease in the legs. It was notable in the European RIETE venous registry that co-incident symptomatic pulmonary embolism at presentation was much less common with upper extremity deep vein thrombosis (DVT) (9%) than with lower extremity DVT (29%).[9] Pulmonary embolism is ultimately detected in up to 35% of individuals

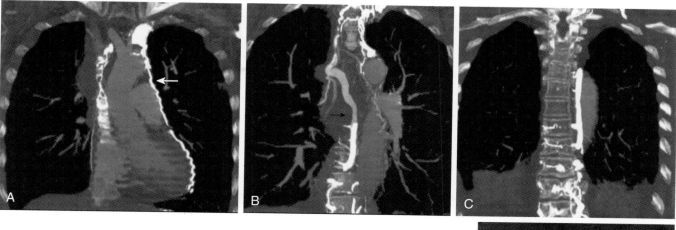

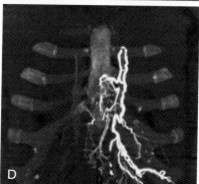

FIGURE 17-8 Collateral circulation with high superior vena cava (SVC) obstruction from Hodgkin disease on coronal reformatted computed tomography angiography. **A,** Note filling of the left subclavian vein and retrograde flow in the superior intercostal vein *(arrow)* and pericardiophrenic collateral. **B,** Retrograde filling of the azygous vein *(arrow)*. **C,** Retrograde filling of the accessory hemiazygous vein and paravertebral collaterals. **D,** Anterior chest wall collateral veins.

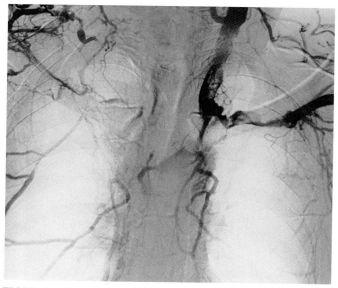

FIGURE 17-9 Occlusion of the superior vena cava and both brachiocephalic veins. Collateral circulation occurs primarily through superficial chest wall veins.

BOX 17-1

CAUSES OF UPPER EXTREMITY VENOUS THROMBOSIS

- Medical devices
  - Vascular access devices (prior or existing)
  - Transvenous cardiac pacemakers
  - Transvenous monitoring devices
- Extrinsic compression
  - Primary (spontaneous or effort thrombosis, Paget-Schroetter disease)
  - Secondary: malignancy/adenopathy
  - Thoracic masses
  - Fibrosing mediastinitis
- Thrombophilic state (see Boxes 1-4 and 1-5)
- Trauma/surgery
- Intravenous drug abuse
- Toxic agents (e.g., chemotherapeutic drugs)
- Heart failure
- Radiation therapy

with upper extremity or internal jugular DVT.[17-21] Even with anticoagulation, complete recanalization of thrombosed upper extremity veins is not the rule.[22] Rather, clots often organize over time, leaving a fibrotic lumen and scarred vein wall. Post-thrombotic syndrome with minor or severe functional disability follows in 7% to 46% of cases.[17,23,24]

Clinical Features

Some patients with acute venous thrombosis are completely asymptomatic. Others complain of arm swelling, pain, cyanosis, coolness, and distended superficial veins. These symptoms can mimic infection, lymphatic obstruction, or blunt trauma. With chronic venous occlusion, arm fatigue after exercise may be experienced. In less than 5% of patients (most of whom have an underlying malignancy), widespread venous thrombosis leads to the syndrome of phlegmasia cerulea dolens and arterial insufficiency.[25,26] The typical patient with Paget-Schroetter disease is a young person complaining of the sudden onset of arm swelling and pain. A history of vigorous physical activity (e.g., weight lifting) can often be elicited.

Imaging

CROSS-SECTIONAL TECHNIQUES

Color Doppler sonography is the first-line imaging tool for detecting axillosubclavian and central venous stenosis and thrombosis.[27,28] Even though ultrasound is simple and safe to perform, the sensitivity and specificity of ultrasound in this setting (82% in one contemporary study) are less than desirable.[29] The clavicle and sternum hide most of the central brachiocephalic veins and the SVC from direct visualization. When ultrasound is negative or equivocal and clinical suspicion remains high, catheter or magnetic resonance/computed tomography (MR/CT) venography should be done.

A thorough examination includes study of the accessible portions of the axillary, subclavian, brachiocephalic, and internal jugular veins; peripheral upper arm veins are occasionally interrogated. Color Doppler imaging detects stenoses, occlusions, and collateral channels, and Doppler waveform analysis is added to identify physiologic signs of more central obstruction. Normally, a triphasic atrial waveform with superimposed respiratory variation is present (Fig. 17-10). Absent or monophasic waveforms or asymmetry between sides may be a clue to central obstruction.[30] The subclavian vein dilates with a Valsalva maneuver and collapses with rapid inspiration (i.e., sniff test). Indwelling venous catheters do not seem to alter the accuracy of the technique.[31]

Signs of venous thrombosis include an intraluminal filling defect, absent flow, or an abnormal Doppler tracing (Fig. 17-11). The latter finding can be confirmed with contrast venography. Thrombosis can be missed for several reasons.

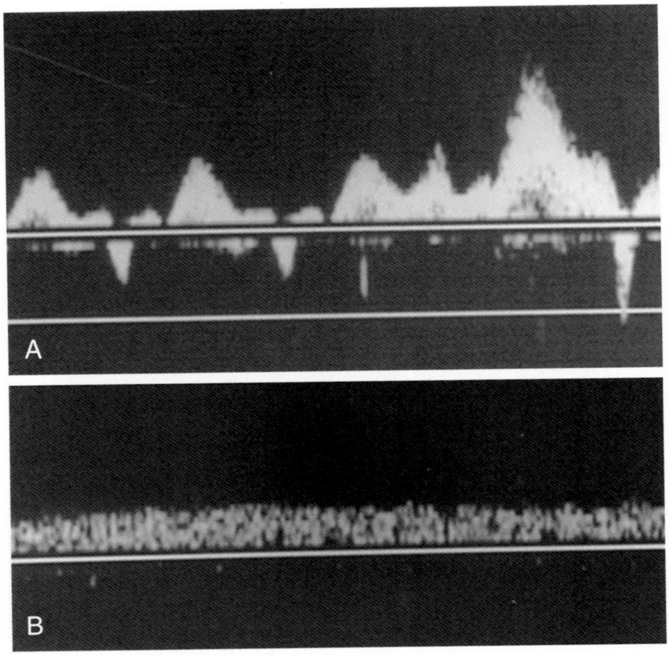

FIGURE 17-10   Duplex sonography of the subclavian veins. **A,** Normal spectral tracing with reflected atrial activity and superimposed respiratory variation. **B,** Abnormal flat tracing suggests a more central occlusion. In this case, the brachiocephalic vein was occluded.

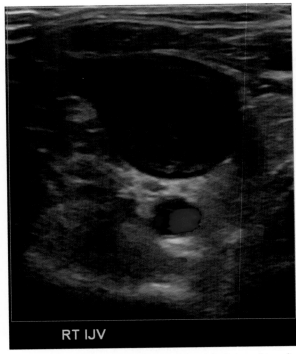

FIGURE 17-11   Partial thrombosis of the right internal jugular vein is identified by color Doppler sonography.

- Nonocclusive thrombus
- Short-segment occlusion
- Central occlusions
- Collateral channels mistaken for normal vessels

Because duplex sonography is simple to perform, fairly accurate, and relatively inexpensive, more complex cross-sectional techniques (MR or CT venography) are typically reserved for equivocal cases, for global mapping of the status of upper extremity veins, or for identifying potential vascular access sites in patients with extensive venous disease.[32-37]

CATHETER VENOGRAPHY

Venography is used to confirm the diagnosis or plan endovascular or surgical treatment of venous thrombosis of the upper extremity. In the acute stage, intraluminal filling defects may be seen (Fig. 17-12). In the subacute or chronic stages, long-segment scarring or stenosis is sometimes evident. Otherwise, the clotted vessels do not opacify and multiple collateral channels fill (see Fig. 17-6). If the brachiocephalic vein or SVC is difficult to visualize from a peripheral arm injection because of slow flow in the arm veins or washout from the internal jugular vein, a catheter should be placed centrally for more direct venography.

Treatment

MEDICAL THERAPY

The standard first-line therapy for upper extremity venous thrombosis is anticoagulation[38] (see treatment of documented pulmonary embolism in Chapter 14). Anticoagulants limit clot propagation and enable recruitment of collateral vessels. Most patients respond well to this approach without further intervention.[17] Those with

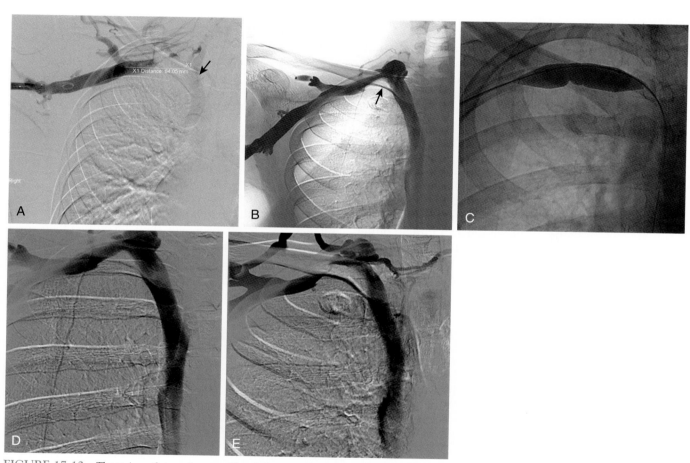

FIGURE 17-12   Thoracic outlet syndrome with subclavian vein thrombosis. **A,** Right basilic venography shows the basilic and axillary veins are patent. There is abrupt occlusion of the mid portion of the right subclavian vein. Of note, collateral circulation beyond this point is sparse. Faint opacification of the right brachiocephalic vein is observed *(arrow).* The occlusion was crossed with a guidewire. Tissue plasminogen activator was infused at 1 mg/hr overnight through a multiside hole catheter. Complete resolution of clot with normal antegrade blood flow has been accomplished **(B).** There is mural or extrinsic narrowing of the central right subclavian vein *(arrow).* In this case, the site of extrinsic compression was dilated with a 14-mm × 4-cm angioplasty balloon **(C).** Patient underwent surgical release of the costoclavicular space and first rib resection. Six-month follow-up venography reveals excellent flow through the central veins with only minimal residual narrowing **(D).** However, with extreme arm abduction, near-occlusive compression of the subclavian vein occurs **(E).**

indwelling central venous devices may require catheter removal or long-term anticoagulation.

ENDOVASCULAR AND OPERATIVE THERAPY

More aggressive transcatheter interventions are appropriate for:

- Poor response to medical treatment with severe persistent symptoms
- Suspected spontaneous (effort) thrombosis
- Widespread venous occlusion (phlegmasia cerulea dolens)

For acute venous thrombosis (less than 10 to 14 days), enzymatic fibrinolysis with or without adjunctive mechanical thrombectomy devices are favored.[38] If a central venous catheter or device is present, it is preferable to remove it. However, patients who are dependent on such catheters may have them left in place. Although systemic infusion can be used, the preferred method is catheter-directed local thrombolysis (see Fig. 17-12) (see Chapter 3 for technical details). Access is usually gained through an ipsilateral basilic or brachial vein. If necessary, the common femoral or internal jugular vein may be used. The patient and operator should understand that complete therapy may require several days of infusion and relatively large doses of fibrinolytic agents. Mechanical thrombectomy devices often serve as adjuncts to chemical lysis.[39]

Patients are vigorously anticoagulated during the procedure and often require long-term anticoagulation. Underlying stenoses are treated with balloon angioplasty. The role of stents in this setting is controversial.[40-42] They are generally avoided in thoracic outlet syndrome, although some reports claim good long-term results after stent placement.[43] Stents are used very judiciously in other cases. The drawbacks of stents in the upper extremity and torso include deformity and rethrombosis from extrinsic compression, in-stent restenosis, stent migration, shortening or fracture, and "jailing" of important tributaries such as the internal jugular vein.[44]

Short-term results of thrombolysis with or without mechanical thrombectomy devices are excellent in about 75% to 85% of cases; thrombolysis is clearly superior to anticoagulation alone for reestablishing flow in fresh occlusions.[43,45-47] Late reocclusion is a common problem, particularly when the underlying cause of thrombosis (e.g., indwelling catheter, thrombophilic state, extrinsic compression) is not eliminated. However, the evidence is weak with respect to the long-term benefit of catheter-directed thrombolysis compared with therapeutic anticoagulation for prevention of upper extremity post-thrombotic syndrome.[47]

For subacute and chronic venous thrombosis (more than 10 to 14 days), primary angioplasty with or without stent placement is recommended (Fig. 17-13). Given their general unresponsiveness to fibrinolytic agents, clinical benefit from thrombolysis in this situation is low compared with the risks entailed. Chronic organized occlusions can be difficult to cross. If antegrade traversal is impossible, retrograde entry from the common femoral vein may be successful. When standard guidewires and catheters fail, the back end of a hydrophilic wire can be tried. Finally, "sharp recanalization" with the catheter and stylet from a transjugular intrahepatic portosystemic shunt set may be fruitful.[48,49] These latter maneuvers should be done knowing the risks of entering major arteries nearby. If a cosmetically satisfying result is obtained from angioplasty alone, some interventionalists will then recommend at least short-term anticoagulation. In many instances, however, intravascular stent placement is deemed necessary to maintain patency.[50]

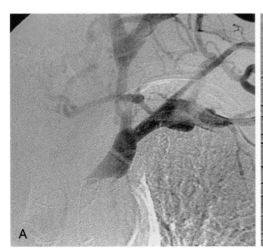
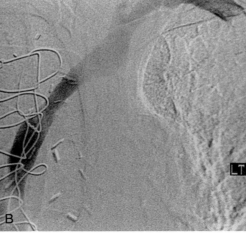

FIGURE 17-13   Chronic left brachiocephalic vein occlusion with collateral filling **(A)** was treated with a 12-mm angioplasty balloon **(B).** Many such cases require additional stent placement.

For primary axillosubclavian thrombosis (venous thoracic outlet syndrome), an integrated approach that combines catheter-directed therapy with surgery is now thoroughly embraced by many experts (see Fig. 17-12). The standard algorithm includes the following features[43,51-57]:

- Immediate anticoagulation
- Prompt catheter-directed thrombolysis as initial treatment (for *acute* occlusion)
- Angioplasty if flow-limiting obstruction is found; stents should be avoided
- A course of anticoagulation with warfarin (Coumadin)
- Medical therapy if no extrinsic compression is detected after thrombolysis
- Immediate or delayed surgical decompression (e.g., first rib resection and subclavius tendon release with patch venoplasty, bypass, or external venolysis) for axillary or subclavian vein compression detected after thrombolysis
- Angioplasty (with or without stent placement) or surgery for residual postoperative stenoses

SUPERIOR VENA CAVA FILTER PLACEMENT

Patients who cannot tolerate anticoagulation (see Box 3-7) and have progression of venous thrombosis or clinically significant pulmonary embolism are candidates for filter insertion into the SVC[38,58-60] (Fig. 17-14). Details of device selection and insertion are given in Chapter 16. The selected filter must be oriented with the apex toward the heart. For example, the jugular version of asymmetric filters must be used from the femoral approach. Superior venacavography is done to ensure proper positioning and adequate caval length to accommodate the device.

In the United States, SVC filter placement currently represents an off-label use of these devices. Long-term follow-up is limited. Nonetheless, there is some evidence to support the intervention (prevention of pulmonary embolism, low frequency of filter migration or SVC thrombosis.)[61] Still, there is a very small but real risk for potentially devastating complications from strut perforation into adjacent structures, including pericardial tamponade, bleeding from aortic laceration, and tension pneumothorax.[61-63] These events do not occur with inferior vena cava (IVC) filters.

Upper Extremity Venous Stenoses (Online Case 93 and Video 17-1)

Etiology and Clinical Features

Mild extrinsic compression of the axillosubclavian veins can be identified in 10% to 50% of the normal population on imaging studies when provocative arm maneuvers are performed.[64,65] The most common causes for pathologic venous stenosis are prior or existing central venous catheters or pacemaker wires, intimal hyperplasia related to

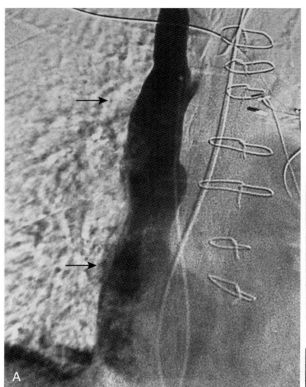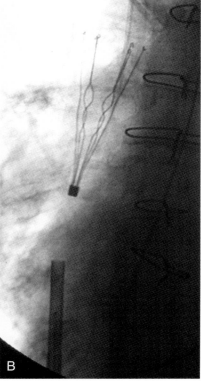

FIGURE 17-14 Superior vena cava (SVC) filter in a patient with recurrent pulmonary embolism from upper extremity venous thrombosis. **A,** SVC diameter and length *(arrows)* are outlined. **B,** After filter placement from a femoral approach using the jugular version of the Greenfield filter.

ipsilateral hemodialysis access, and extrinsic compression by musculoskeletal structures[66,67] (Box 17-2 and Fig. 17-15). Because stenoses develop slowly and the collateral circulation often is adequate, many patients tolerate these lesions as long as the vessel does not become completely occluded. A small percentage of individuals becomes symptomatic from the existing stenosis or subsequent thrombosis.

BOX 17-2

CAUSES OF UPPER EXTREMITY VENOUS NARROWING

- Vascular access devices (prior or existing)
- Extrinsic compression
  - Musculoskeletal structures
  - Neoplasm/adenopathy
- Intimal hyperplasia
  - Outflow veins of dialysis grafts
- Trauma/surgery
- Radiation therapy
- Vasospasm

Problematic upper extremity vein stenosis occurs most notably in patients with arm hemodialysis grafts or fistulas. About 50% of dialysis patients with prior subclavian vein catheters develop significant obstructions, which are attributed to direct vein injury, venous turbulence and supraphysiologic blood flow, and catheter motion within the vessel.[10,15] Extrinsic compression also can be identified in a substantial number of dialysis patients without a history of indwelling catheters.[68] The increased flow from the arm graft or fistula exaggerates the pressure gradient (and therefore the significance) of even moderate downstream stenoses. Although these lesions are most common near the venous anastomosis and at sites of prior temporary catheters, they may occur at any place in the outflow veins.

Many patients have arm swelling, pain, and superficial varicosities. Hemodialysis graft dysfunction is common, including elevated venous pressures at dialysis, poor shunt flow, or eventual graft thrombosis.

Imaging

CROSS-SECTIONAL TECHNIQUES

Stenoses of the central upper extremity veins are detected by color Doppler sonography or MR or CT venography. However, some patients require catheter venography prior to endovascular or surgical treatment.

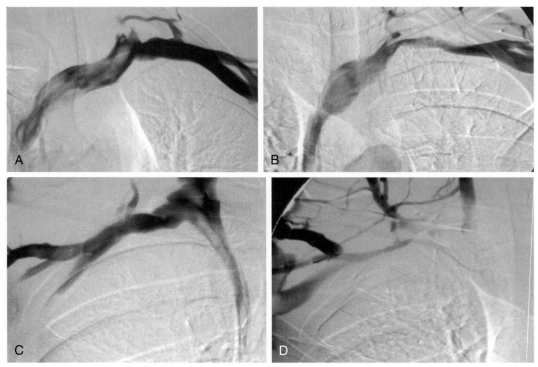

FIGURE 17-15   Extrinsic compression of both subclavian veins from thoracic outlet syndrome. **A,** Patent left subclavian vein (SCV). Lucency in the vessel is due to inflow from the unopacified internal jugular vein. **B,** With arm in abduction, there is mild narrowing of the left SCV with few collaterals. **C,** Right SCV in neutral position. **D,** With arm in abduction, near-complete occlusion of the right SCV is seen with exuberant filling of collateral channels.

Provocative maneuvers may be required to uncover the obstruction.[65,69]

CATHETER VENOGRAPHY

Upper extremity venous stenoses usually are smooth and focal (Fig. 17-16). It may be difficult to differentiate extrinsic compression (caused by musculoskeletal structures or tumor) from intrinsic mural disease (see Fig. 17-15). Several conditions can mimic fixed obstruction, including vasospasm from catheter or guidewire manipulation or trauma (Fig. 17-17) and external compression from an overlying surgical drape or compression between the humerus and ribs in arm adduction (Fig. 17-18).

The presence of an extensive collateral network around a stenosis is an indicator of hemodynamic significance. Moderate stenoses can be assessed by measuring a focal pressure gradient (>3 to 5 mm Hg) across the lesion (Fig. 17-19).

Treatment

ENDOVASCULAR THERAPY

Balloon angioplasty is the first-line therapy for hemodynamically significant venous stenoses. Obstructions can be approached directly from an antecubital or upper arm vein, a common femoral vein, or through a dialysis graft,

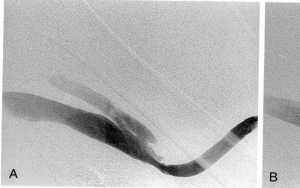
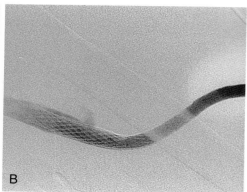

FIGURE 17-16 **A,** Smooth recurrent focal stenosis at the venous anastomosis of a left upper arm hemodialysis graft. **B,** The stenosis is relieved with a Wallstent.

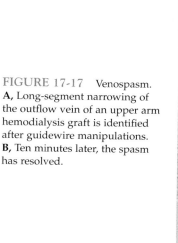

FIGURE 17-17 Venospasm. **A,** Long-segment narrowing of the outflow vein of an upper arm hemodialysis graft is identified after guidewire manipulations. **B,** Ten minutes later, the spasm has resolved.

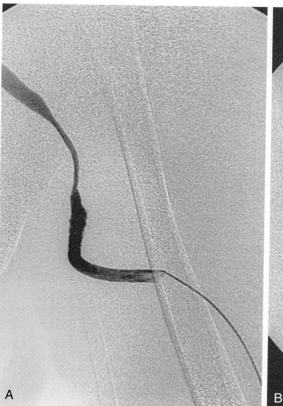
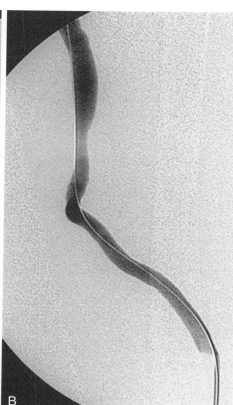

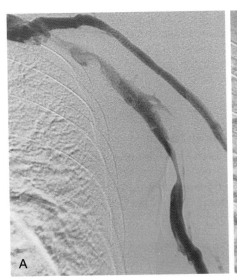

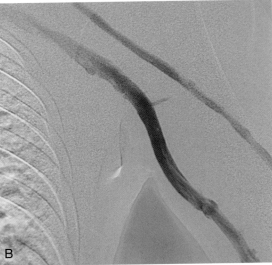

FIGURE 17-18 External compression of the left basilic vein. **A,** Narrowing of the vein is seen with the initial contrast injection. **B,** After releasing the overlying surgical drape and abducting the arm, the compression is resolved.

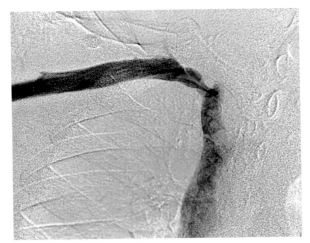

FIGURE 17-19 Nonsignificant right brachiocephalic vein stenosis. No collateral vessels are seen, and the pressure gradient was 2 mm Hg.

if present. Typically, the axillary and subclavian veins require at least 10- to 12-mm angioplasty balloons, and the brachiocephalic vein 12- to 14-mm balloons (Fig. 17-20). It is prudent to start with an undersized balloon if the adjacent normal vessel looks small. Multiple, prolonged inflations and high-pressure balloons (e.g., 30 atm) may be needed to open the vein fully. For completely resistant lesions, cutting balloons can be used to weaken the vein wall, making it more amenable to standard angioplasty. Patients usually experience mild discomfort during balloon inflation. Severe pain is a sign of overdilation or vein rupture.

The results of balloon angioplasty in this setting have been mixed. In central upper extremity stenoses, technical success (<30% residual stenosis) is achieved in about 75% to 90% of cases.[70,71] However, 6- and 12-month primary patency is often less than 30%.[72-74] In the setting of central venous stenosis downstream from a hemodialysis access,

primary and primary assisted access patency at 6 months were 46% and 77%, respectively, in one recent report.[71] Thus repeated dilations allow respectable primary assisted patency rates that approach surgical results and may extend the useful life of dialysis grafts. Complications (including vein rupture) occur in less than 10% of cases, and most are minor. Vein rupture is managed with repeat prolonged balloon inflation or placement of a bare stent, if necessary.

Intravascular stents are reserved for cases of failed angioplasty (elastic stenoses, acute vein rupture, or rapid restenosis) because they do not provide substantial benefit over "plain old" balloon angioplasty in routine cases[73] (Fig. 17-21). Stents should not be placed within very fibrotic lesions that cannot be fully dilated with a balloon. Stents are avoided in patients with obstructions from thoracic outlet syndrome. Stent selection is critical; balloon expandable devices with high plastic deformity are not appropriate. Self-expanding nitinol stents and the Wallstent are favored by many interventionists (see Fig. 17-16). The covered Flair stent graft may be even more durable than bare devices.[76] If possible, the stent should not be placed across the internal jugular vein orifice. Nominal stent diameter should be about 1-2 mm greater than the largest target vessel diameter to prevent stent migration. The patient and referring physician should understand that the device may interfere with future placement of central venous catheters if inserted over the internal jugular vein orifice.

In some series, primary patency rates have surpassed those with angioplasty alone (e.g., 50% at 6 months).[77] One study found comparable long-term results with surgical bypass and angioplasty plus stenting.[78] However, others report dismal results for angioplasty or stenting of central venous stenoses, with a 6-month primary patency rate of less than 31%

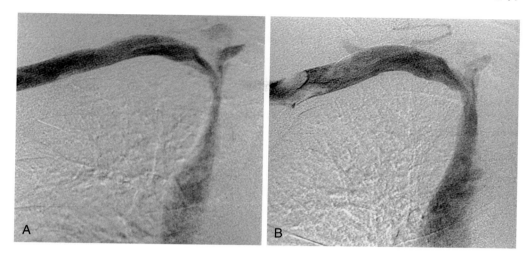

FIGURE 17-20 Angioplasty of a central venous stenosis. **A,** The brachiocephalic vein has a tight stenosis. **B,** After angioplasty with a 12-mm balloon, the lumen is widened.

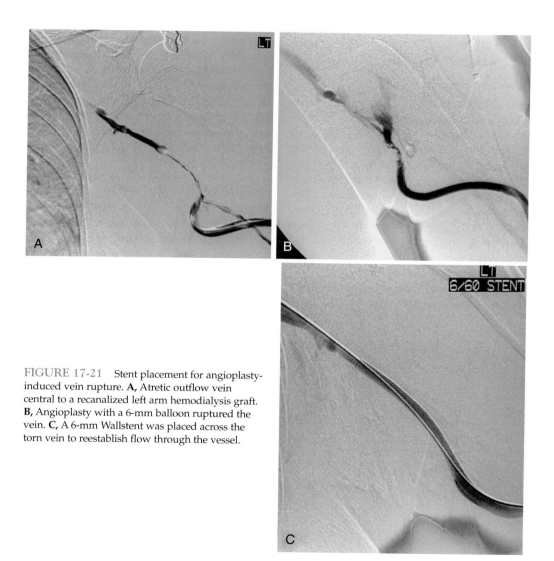

FIGURE 17-21 Stent placement for angioplasty-induced vein rupture. **A,** Atretic outflow vein central to a recanalized left arm hemodialysis graft. **B,** Angioplasty with a 6-mm balloon ruptured the vein. **C,** A 6-mm Wallstent was placed across the torn vein to reestablish flow through the vessel.

for central and peripheral lesions.[79] Stent restenosis may be relieved with balloon angioplasty, with or without placement of additional stents (Fig. 17-22). Primary assisted patency rates with angioplasty are excellent in most series. Periodic maintenance of these lesions should be anticipated. Complications of stent placement include vein rupture and stent migration, which can be disastrous (Fig. 17-23).

SURGICAL THERAPY

For brachiocephalic vein occlusions, direct bypass with prosthetic material or jugular-jugular bypass may be performed. For central subclavian vein occlusions, internal jugular to subclavian vein transposition is effective. For peripheral subclavian and axillary venous occlusions, direct axillary-jugular bypass is advocated. Although these operations are feasible, they are rarely ever done.

Superior Vena Cava Obstruction (Online Cases 12 and 39)

Etiology and Clinical Features

Obstruction of the SVC is the result of luminal disease (thrombus or tumor), extrinsic compression (tumor or adenopathy), or mural disease (intimal hyperplasia or tumor invasion). The lesion may be stenotic or frankly occlusive. A variety of underlying diseases is responsible[80,81] (Box 17-3). Bilateral brachiocephalic vein obstruction causes almost equivalent hemodynamic dysfunction. In older series, infection or malignancy (particularly lung cancer) were responsible in at least 90% of cases. However, indwelling vascular devices (e.g., infusion catheters, pacemaker wires) are an increasingly common cause of SVC stenosis.

Fibrosing mediastinitis is a localized or diffuse infiltrative disease of the mediastinum that may be idiopathic or caused by chronic infection such as histoplasmosis.[82] The SVC is affected in more than one third of cases; the pulmonary artery and bronchi also may be involved (see Chapter 14).

Significant SVC or bilateral brachiocephalic vein stenosis or obstruction can lead to the *superior vena cava syndrome*. This condition is marked by facial and neck swelling, bilateral arm swelling, cyanosis, distention of superficial veins, shortness of breath, hoarseness, and headache. Left untreated, severe laryngeal edema or cerebral congestion with altered mental status and, eventually, coma can ensue. Thus, SVC syndrome may be life-threatening.

Imaging

CROSS-SECTIONAL TECHNIQUES

Although sonography cannot directly evaluate the SVC, alterations in spectral waveform from both subclavian veins (e.g., lack of normal reflected atrial activity and respiratory phasicity or response to provocative maneuvers) should raise suspicion. CT and MR angiography are extremely effective in the diagnosis of SVC obstruction.[33,83] Findings include intraluminal defects, nonopacification of the vessel, extrinsic compression or mass invasion, and presence of collateral channels (Fig. 17-24; see also Fig. 17-8). The latter finding usually is associated with symptomatic disease.

CATHETER VENOGRAPHY

Catheter venography is reserved for cases in which cross-sectional studies are equivocal or transcatheter treatment is being considered. The SVC can be imaged from one or both antecubital veins, the internal jugular vein, or the femoral vein. Stenoses caused by indwelling or prior devices usually are long and smooth. Extrinsic masses efface the lumen (see Fig. 17-24). Collateral

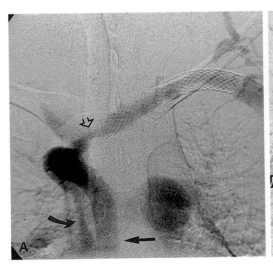

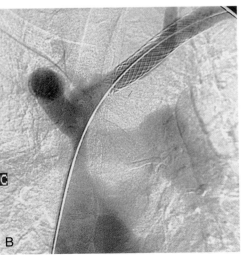

FIGURE 17-22   Left subclavian and brachiocephalic vein stent restenosis in a patient with a left arm hemodialysis graft. **A,** There is narrowing of the lumen of the subclavian vein and at the mouth of the brachiocephalic vein stent *(open arrow).* A tight superior vena cava stenosis *(curved arrow)* causes retrograde flow into a dilated azygous vein *(arrow).* **B,** The left brachiocephalic vein and superior vena cava are opened after balloon angioplasty.

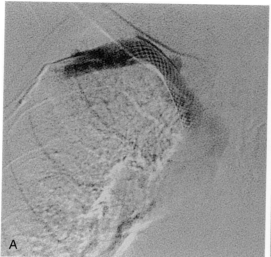

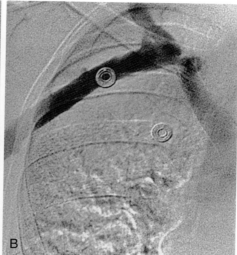

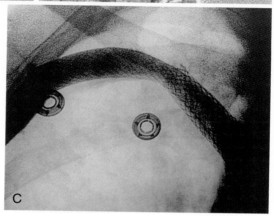

FIGURE 17-23   Malposition and migration of a venous stent. **A,** A Wallstent was inadequately positioned across a right subclavian vein stenosis. **B,** One month later, the stent has migrated to the superior vena cava. **C,** A second Wallstent was placed in the subclavian vein to help secure the malpositioned stent and treat the residual stenosis.

BOX 17-3

CAUSES OF SUPERIOR VENA CAVA STENOSIS OR OCCLUSION

- Medical devices
  - Central venous catheters
  - Pacemakers
- Malignancy
  - Lung cancer
  - Mediastinal tumor (e.g., lymphoma, metastases)
  - Primary leiomyosarcoma
- Inflammation
  - Fibrosing mediastinitis
  - Infection (e.g., tuberculosis)
- Trauma/surgery
- Thrombophilic state
- Radiation therapy
- Intimal injury: chemotherapeutic agents
- Aortic or brachiocephalic artery aneurysm

vessels fill when contrast is injected above the obstruction. Associated narrowing of the brachiocephalic (and, occasionally, the internal jugular) vein is common.

Treatment

MEDICAL THERAPY

For malignant obstructions with severe SVC syndrome, urgent chemotherapy and/or radiotherapy is used to treat the underlying cause of disease. Intravenous corticosteroids and diuretics also have a role to play. Patients may notice transient worsening of symptoms with the onset of radiation therapy as the tumor swells. Anticoagulation is given to limit clot progression.

ENDOVASCULAR THERAPY

Catheter-directed therapy should be considered when medical therapy fails for moderate to severe SVC syndrome, severe arm swelling, or for maintenance of dialysis access function. Most patients with causative malignancy die of their underlying disease; the purpose of catheter-based treatment is short-term palliation of

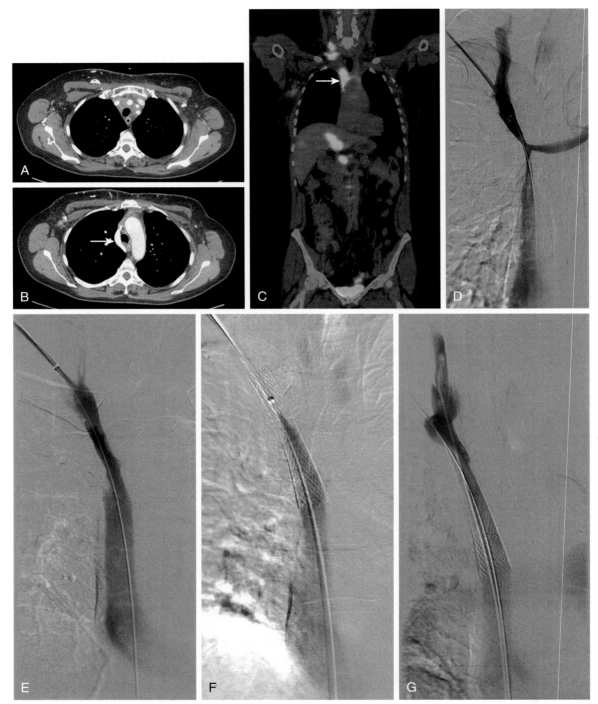

FIGURE 17-24   Superior vena cava (SVC) syndrome in a patient with lung cancer. **A** and **B,** Computed tomography (CT) scans show soft tissue in the mediastinum surrounding the central veins with an enlarged azygous arch *(arrow)* serving as a collateral. **C,** Coronal fluorodeoxyglucose positron emission tomography image shows intense uptake in the region of suspected mediastinal disease *(arrow)* and elsewhere in the body. **D,** Central venography shows the extrinsic malignant disease encasing the brachiocephalic vein–SVC confluence. **E,** Balloon angioplasty only partially improved flow down the jugular vein. **F,** Wallstent was inserted into the stenosis, but the stent slipped forward and is now precariously positioned in the SVC **(G).**

symptoms. On the other hand, long-term patency is the goal in patients with benign SVC obstruction.

For benign SVC stenoses, balloon angioplasty is sometimes sufficient. However, some experts maintain that stent placement is now the treatment of choice in most cases, with durable symptom relief achieved in more than 90% of cases.[84-89]

For benign SVC occlusions and difficult stenoses, stents are preferable. Thrombolysis precedes angioplasty if acute or subacute clot is present in the vena cava or central thoracic veins. Otherwise, angioplasty and stent insertion may be used alone. Stents may be placed safely over pacemaker wires.[90] Central venous catheters may

be repositioned and then reinserted after the stent is deployed.[91]

For malignant SVC obstructions, stents are virtually always used[92-94] (see Fig. 17-24 and Fig. 17-25). In SVC syndrome, inline flow from one internal jugular vein is usually sufficient to relieve symptoms. Stents can be placed through venous access from above or below the occlusion. If the obstruction can be traversed only from above, a snare placed from the femoral vein can be used to capture the guidewire. The procedure is then continued from the groin. The stenosis often is predilated with an angioplasty balloon to ensure it opens and to delineate its length. Heparin is given during the procedure.

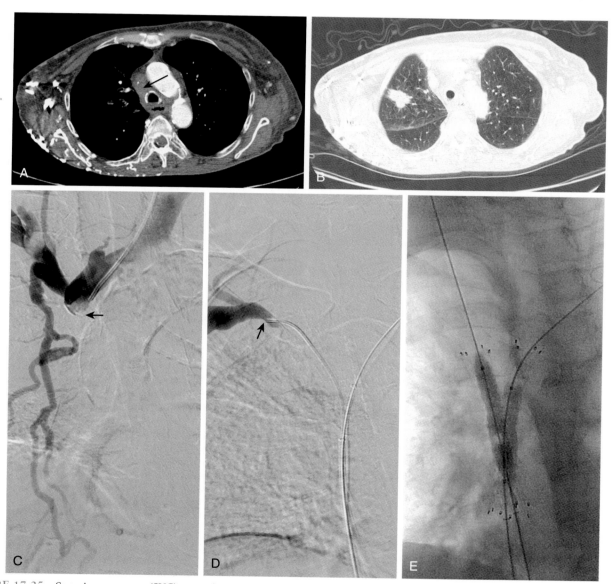

FIGURE 17-25 Superior vena cava (SVC) stent placement. **A,** Computed tomography scan shows soft tissue density in the right mediastinum encasing the SVC *(arrow)* due to spread from lung cancer **(B). C,** Left jugular vein access was used for central venography, which shows complete SVC occlusion *(arrow).* **D,** The occlusion was crossed. With additional right femoral vein access, the occlusion was crossed again to provide access to the right brachiocephalic vein *(arrow).* **E,** Finally, dual kissing stents were deployed across both brachiocephalic veins into the SVC.

A variety of different devices has been used for this purpose, including Wallstents, nitinol stents, Gianturco Z-stent, and Palmaz stents. Large stent, diameters (>16 mm) are required; stents are purposely oversized to ensure that they remain well secured to the SVC wall after deployment. If the occlusion involves the confluence of the brachiocephalic veins, stents may be extended into one vessel across the ostium of the other. Alternatively, a Y-shaped stent configuration may be created by laying stents into each brachiocephalic vein (see Fig. 17-25).

Benign SVC obstructions can be relieved in almost every case, with dramatic and rapid relief of symptoms.[84-89] In one large series comparing percutaneous and open surgical repair, 3-year primary patency rates were essentially identical (44%).[84] Still, assisted primary patency was much better in stented patients, who also had much lower 30-day mortality.

For malignant obstructions, partial or complete response is observed in 87% to 97% of individuals.[86,87,95-98] Most patients with malignant disease die of the underlying disease with a patent stent. Major complications are rare and include early or late stent thrombosis. Immediate or delayed stent migration is a particular problem when placing SVC stents (see Fig. 17-24). This event can be catastrophic if cardiac rupture or malignant arrhythmia ensues. The operator should choose a stent of sufficient length and avoid laying most of it central to the stenosis. He or she must be thoroughly familiar with techniques to capture and remove errant stent devices (e.g., direct snaring, balloon or guidewire-assisted snaring, or redeployment).[99,100]

A rare but devastating complication of SVC balloon angioplasty or stent placement is immediate or delayed massive bleeding into the mediastinum or pericardium.[101-104] Hemorrhage may occur from venous rupture at delivery (more likely with a fragile wall in malignant obstructions) or puncture by the ends of the stent through the caval wall or into the aorta. Appropriately sized covered stents should be on hand to seal these leaks if it becomes necessary.

SURGICAL THERAPY

Operations rarely are indicated for SVC obstruction unless endovascular means are unsuccessful. Bypass grafting can be performed with autologous vein or synthetic material. Venous transposition is possible.[105]

OTHER DISORDERS

Trauma

Traumatic injuries to the central thoracic veins may be criminal, iatrogenic, or accidental.[106] Iatrogenic injuries related to catheterization are discussed previously.

Significant venous trauma that requires specific therapy is far less common than arterial injury, and venography is rarely indicated. Color Doppler sonography is an excellent tool for screening this population. Unsuspected venous trauma often is detected during surgery for an associated arterial injury. The injured vein is then treated by direct repair, bypass grafting, or ligation. Balloon catheter tamponade or stent-graft insertion for life-threatening large thoracic vein trauma also has been described.[107-109]

Neoplasms

Almost all tumors that affect the SVC arise from the lung or mediastinum. Primary tumors of the SVC are an unusual cause of SVC syndrome.[110,111] Most are *leiomyosarcomas*. The diagnosis is usually made by CT or MR imaging, and transvenous biopsy may be performed to confirm the diagnosis.

Aneurysms

Aneurysms of upper extremity and thoracic veins are rare.[112-114] The most common site is the internal jugular vein. Congenital *jugular vein phlebectasia* is another unusual cause for enlargement of this vessel.[115] The diagnosis is made by color Doppler sonography. Because of the great propensity for thrombus formation and pulmonary embolism, venous reconstruction is advisable.

References

1. Collin P, editor. Embryology and development. In: Williams PL, Bannister LH, Berry MM, et al, editors. *Gray's Anatomy.* 38th ed. New York: Churchill Livingstone; 1995. p. 327.
2. Gabella G, editor. Cardiovascular system. In: Williams PL, Bannister LH, Berry MM, et al, editors. *Gray's Anatomy.* 38th ed. New York: Churchill Livingstone; 1995. p. 1589.
3. White CS, Baffa JM, Haney PJ, et al. MR imaging of congenital anomalies of the thoracic veins. *Radiographics* 1997;**17**:595.
4. Burney K, Young H, Barnard SA, et al. CT appearance of congenital and acquired abnormalities of the superior vena cava. *Clin Radiol* 2007;**62**:837.
5. Goyal SK, Punnam SR, Verma G, et al. Persistent left superior vena cava: a case report and review of literature. *Cardiovasc Ultrasound* 2008;**10**:50.
6. Gonzalez-Juanatey C, Testa A, Vidan J, et al. Persistent left superior vena cava draining into the coronary sinus: report of 10 cases and literature review. *Clin Cardiol* 2004;**27**:515.
7. Kim HC, Chung JW, Yoon CJ, et al. Collateral pathways in thoracic central venous obstruction: three-dimensional display using direct spiral computed tomography venography. *J Comput Assist Tomogr* 2004;**28**:24.
8. Bashist B, Parisi A, Frager DH, et al. Abdominal CT findings when the superior vena cava, brachiocephalic vein, or subclavian vein is obstructed. *AJR Am J Roentgenol* 1996;**167**:1457.
9. Munoz FJ, Mismetti P, Poggio R, et al. Clinical outcomes of patients with upper-extremity deep vein thrombosis. Results from the RIETE Registry. *Chest* 2008;**133**:143.

10. Trerotola SO, Kuhn-Fulton J, Johnson MS, et al. Tunneled infusion catheters: increased incidence of symptomatic venous thrombosis after subclavian versus internal jugular venous access. *Radiology* 2000;**217**:89.

11. Meissner MH. Axillary-subclavian venous thrombosis. *Rev Cardiovasc Med* 2002;**3**:S76.

12. Martinelli I, Battaglioli T, Bucciarelli P, et al. Risk factors and recurrence rate of primary deep vein thrombosis of the upper extremities. *Circulation* 2004;**110**:566.

13. Joffe HV, Kucher N, Tapson VF, et al. Upper extremity deep vein thrombosis: a prospective registry of 592 patients. *Circulation* 2004;**110**:1605.

14. Balestreri L, De Cicco M, Matovic M, et al. Central venous catheter-related thrombosis in clinically asymptomatic oncologic patients: a phlebographic study. *Eur J Radiol* 1995;**20**:108.

15. Schillinger F, Schillinger D, Montagnac R, et al. Postcatheterisation vein stenosis in haemodialysis: comparative angiographic study of 50 subclavian and 50 internal jugular accesses. *Nephrol Dial Transplant* 1991;**6**:722.

16. Horne MK, May DJ, Alexander HR, et al. Venographic surveillance of tunneled venous access devices in adult oncology patients. *Ann Surg Oncol* 1995;**2**:174.

17. Sajid MS, Ahmed N, Desai M, et al. Upper limb deep vein thrombosis: a literature review to streamline the protocols for management. *Acta Haematol* 2007;**118**:10.

18. Mustafa S, Stein PD, Otten TR, et al. Upper extremity deep venous thrombosis. *Chest* 2003;**123**:1953.

19. Hingorani A, Ascher E, Lorenson E, et al. Upper extremity deep venous thrombosis and its impact on morbidity and mortality rates in a hospital-based population. *J Vasc Surg* 1997;**26**:853.

20. Monreal M, Raventos A, Lerma R, et al. Pulmonary embolism in patients with upper extremity DVT associated to (sic) venous central lines—a prospective study. *Thromb Haemost* 1994;**72**:548.

21. Sheikh MA, Topoulos AP, Deitcher SR. Isolated internal jugular vein thrombosis: risk factors and natural history. *Vasc Med* 2002;**7**:177.

22. Persson LM, Arnhjort T, Larfars G, et al. Hemodynamic and morphologic evaluation of sequelae of primary upper extremity deep venous thromboses treated with anticoagulation. *J Vasc Surg* 2006;**43**:1230.

23. Sharafuddin MJ, Sun S, Hoballah JJ. Endovascular management of venous thrombotic disease of the upper torso and extremities. *J Vasc Interv Radiol* 2002;**13**:975.

24. Elman EE, Kahn SR. The post-thrombotic syndrome after upper extremity deep venous thrombosis in adults: a systematic review. *Thromb Res* 2006;**117**:609.

25. Kammen BF, Soulen MC. Phlegmasia cerulea dolens of the upper extremity. *J Vasc Interv Radiol* 1995;**6**:283.

26. Bedri MI, Khosravi AH, Lifchez SD. Upper extremity compartment syndrome in the setting of deep venous thrombosis and phlegmasia cerulea dolens: case report. *J Hand Surg Am* 2009;**34**:1859.

27. Weber TM, Lockhart ME, Robbin ML. Upper extremity venous Doppler ultrasound. *Radiol Clin North Am* 2007;**45**:513.

28. Chin EE, Zimmerman PT, Grant EG. Sonographic evaluation of upper extremity deep venous thrombosis. *J Ultrasound Med* 2005;**24**:829.

29. Baarslag HJ, van Beek EJ, Koopman MM, et al. Prospective study of color duplex ultrasonography compared with contrast venography in patients suspected of having deep venous thrombosis of the upper extremities. *Ann Intern Med* 2002;**136**:865.

30. Rose SC, Kinney TB, Bundens WP, et al. Doppler analysis of transmitted atrial waveforms, respiratory variation, and flow symmetry for detection of thoracic central veno-occlusive disease missed by sonographic imaging. *Radiology* 1997;**205**(P):499.

31. Burbidge SJ, Finlay DE, Letourneau JG, et al. Effects of central venous catheter placement on upper extremity duplex US findings. *J Vasc Interv Radiol* 1993;**4**:399.

32. Charon JP, Milne W, Sheppard DG, et al. Evaluation of MR angiographic technique in the assessment of thoracic outlet syndrome. *Clin Radiol* 2004;**59**:588.

33. Kim HC, Chung JW, Yoon CJ, et al. Collateral pathways in thoracic central venous obstruction: three-dimensional display using direct spiral computed tomography venography. *J Comput Assist Tomogr* 2004;**28**:24.

34. Lawler LP, Corl FM, Fishman EK. Multi-detector row and volume-rendered CT of the normal and accessory flow pathways of the thoracic systemic and pulmonary veins. *Radiographics* 2002;**22**:S45.

35. Kim CY, Mirza RA, Bryant JA, et al. Central veins of the chest: evaluation with time-resolved MR angiography. *Radiology* 2008;**247**:558.

36. Oxtoby JW, Widjaja E, Gibson KM, et al. 3D gadolinium-enhanced MRI venography: evaluation of central chest veins and impact on patient management. *Clin Radiol* 2001;**56**:887.

37. Demondion X, Herbinet P, van Sint Jan S, et al. Imaging assessment of thoracic outlet syndrome. *Radiographics* 2006;**26**:1735.

38. Kearon C, Kahn SR, Agnelli G, et al. Antithrombotic therapy for venous thromboembolic disease: American College of Chest Physicians Evidence-based Clinical Practice Guidelines (8th ed.). *Chest* 2008;**133**:454S.

39. Kasirajan K, Gray B, Ouriel K. Percutaneous AngioJet thrombectomy in the management of extensive deep venous thrombosis. *J Vasc Interv Radiol* 2001;**12**:179.

40. Hall LD, Murray JD, Boswell GE. Venous stent placement as an adjunct to the staged multimodal treatment of Paget-Schroetter syndrome. *J Vasc Interv Radiol* 1995;**6**:565.

41. Meier GH, Pollak JS, Rosenblatt M, et al. Initial experience with venous stents in exertional axillary-subclavian vein thrombosis. *J Vasc Surg* 1996;**24**:974.

42. Urschel HC Jr, Patel AN. Paget-Schroetter syndrome therapy: failure of intravenous stents. *Ann Thorac Surg* 2003;**75**:1693.

43. Kreienberg PB, Chang BB, Darling III RC, et al. Long-term results in patients treated with thrombolysis, thoracic inlet decompression, and subclavian vein stenting for Paget-Schroetter syndrome. *J Vasc Surg* 2001;**33**(2 Suppl.):S100.

44. Verstandig AG, Bloom AI, Sasson T, et al. Shortening and migration of Wallstents after stenting of central venous stenoses in hemodialysis patients. *Cardiovasc Intervent Radiol* 2003;**26**:58.

45. Chang R, Horne III MK, Mayo DJ, et al. Pulse-spray treatment of subclavian and jugular venous thrombi with recombinant tissue plasminogen activator. *J Vasc Interv Radiol* 1996;**7**:845.

46. Rutherford RB. Primary subclavian-axillary vein thrombosis: the relative roles of thrombolysis, percutaneous angioplasty, stents, and surgery. *Semin Vasc Surg* 1998;**11**:91.

47. Vik A, Holme PA, Singh K, et al. Catheter-directed thrombolysis for treatment of deep venous thrombosis in the upper extremities. *Cardiovasc Intervent Radiol* 2009;**32**:980.

48. Farrell T, Lang EV, Barnhart W. Sharp recanalization of central venous occlusions. *J Vasc Interv Radiol* 1999;**10**:149.

49. Athreya S, Scott P, Annamalai G, et al. Sharp recanalization of central venous occlusions: a useful technique for haemodialysis line insertion. *Br J Radiol* 2009;**82**:105.

50. Ozyer U, Harman A, Yildirim E, et al. Long-term results of angioplasty and stent placement for treatment of central venous obstructions in 126 hemodialysis patients: a 10-year single-center experience. *AJR Am J Roentgenol* 2009;**193**:1672.

51. Molina JE, Hunter DW, Dietz CA. Protocols for Paget-Schroetter syndrome and late treatment of chronic subclavian vein obstruction. *Ann Thorac Surg* 2009;**87**:416.

52. Lee JT, Karwowski JK, Harris EJ, et al. Long-term thrombotic recurrence after nonoperative management of Paget-Schroetter syndrome. *J Vasc Surg* 2006;**43**:1236.

53. Caparrelli DJ, Freischlag J. A unified approach to axillosubclavian venous thrombosis in a single hospital admission. *Semin Vasc Surg* 2005;**18**:153.

54. Melby SJ, Vedantham S, Narra VR, et al. Comprehensive surgical management of the competitive athlete with effort thrombosis of the subclavian vein (Paget-Schroetter syndrome). *J Vasc Surg* 2008; **47**:809.

55. Thomas IH, Zierler BK. An integrative review of outcomes in patients with acute primary upper extremity deep venous thrombosis following no treatment or treatment with anticoagulation, thrombolyis , or surgical algorithms. *Vasc Endovascular Surg* 2005; **39**:163.

56. Schneider DB, Dimuzio PJ, Martin ND, et al. Combination treatment of venous thoracic outlet syndrome: open surgical decompression and intraoperative angioplasty. *J Vasc Surg* 2004;**40**:599.

57. Landry GJ, Liem TK. Endovascular management of Paget-Schroetter syndrome. *Vascular* 2007;**15**:290.

58. Murphy KD. Superior vena cava filters. *Tech Vasc Interv Radiol* 2004;**7**:105.

59. Spence LD, Gironta MG, Malde HM, et al. Acute upper extremity deep venous thrombosis: safety and effectiveness of superior vena caval filters. *Radiology* 1999;**210**:53.

60. Ascher E, Hingorani A, Tsemekhin B, et al. Lessons learned from a 6-year clinical experience with superior vena caval Greenfield filters. *J Vasc Surg* 2000;**32**:881.

61. Usoh F, Hingorani A, Ascher E, et al. Long-term follow-up for superior vena cava filter placement. *Ann Vasc Surg* 2009;**23**:350.

62. Cousins GR, DeAnda Jr A. Images in cardiothoracic surgery. Superior vena cava filter erosion into the ascending aorta. *Ann Thorac Surg* 2006;**81**:1907.

63. Bhatt SP, Nanda S, Turki MA. Tension pneumothorax: a complication of superior vena cava filter insertion. *Ann Thorac Surg* 2008; **85**:1813.

64. Rayan GM, Jensen C. Thoracic outlet syndrome: provocative examination maneuvers in a typical population. *J Shoulder Elbow Surg* 1995;**4**:113.

65. Longley DG, Yedlicka JW, Molina EJ, et al. Thoracic outlet syndrome: evaluation of the subclavian vessels by color duplex sonography. *AJR Am J Roentgenol* 1992;**158**:623.

66. Yevzlin AS. Hemodialysis catheter-associated central venous stenosis. *Semin Dial* 2008;**21**:522.

67. Agarwal AK. Central vein stenosis: current concepts. *Adv Chronic Kidney Dis* 2009;**16**:360.

68. Itkin M, Kraus MJ, Trerotola SO. Extrinsic compression of the left innominate vein in hemodialysis patients. *J Vasc Interv Radiol* 2004;**15**:51.

69. Demondion X, Boutry N, Drizenko A, et al. Thoracic outlet: anatomic correlation with MR imaging. *AJR Am J Roentgenol* 2000; **175**:417.

70. Criado E, Marston WA, Jaques PF, et al. Proximal venous outflow obstruction in patients with upper extremity arteriovenous dialysis access. *Ann Vasc Surg* 1994;**8**:530.

71. Nael K, Kee ST, Solomon H, et al. Endovascular management of central thoracic veno-occlusive diseases in hemodialysis patients: a single institutional experience in 69 consecutive patients. *J Vasc Interv Radiol* 2009;**20**:46.

72. Beathard GA. Percutaneous transvenous angioplasty in the treatment of vascular access stenosis. *Kidney Int* 1992;**42**:1390.

73. Bakken AM, Protack CD, Saad WE, et al. Long-term outcomes of primary angioplasty and primary stenting of central venous stenosis in hemodialysis patients. *J Vasc Surg* 2007;**45**:776.

74. Kovalik EC, Newman GE, Suhocki P, et al. Correction of central venous stenoses: use of angioplasty and vascular Wallstents. *Kidney Int* 1994; **45**:1177.

75. Bjarnason H, Hunter DW, Crain MR, et al. Collapse of a Palmaz stent in the subclavian vein. *AJR Am J Roentgenol* 1993;**160**:1123.

76. Haskal Z, Trerotola S, Dolmatch B, et al. Stent graft versus balloon angioplasty for failing dialysis-access grafts. *New Engl J Med* 2010; **362**:494.

77. Vorwerk D, Guenther RW, Mann H, et al. Venous stenosis and occlusion in hemodialysis shunts: follow-up results of stent placement in 65 patients. *Radiology* 1995;**195**:140.

78. Bhatia DS, Money SR, Ochsner JL, et al. Comparison of surgical bypass and percutaneous balloon dilatation with primary stent placement in the treatment of central venous obstruction in the dialysis patient: one-year follow-up. *Ann Vasc Surg* 1996;**10**:452.

79. Quinn SF, Schuman ES, Demlow TA, et al. Percutaneous transluminal angioplasty versus endovascular stent placement in the treatment of venous stenoses in patients undergoing hemodialysis: intermediate results. *J Vasc Interv Radiol* 1995;**6**:851.

80. Wilson LD, Detterbeck FC, Yahalom J. Clinical practice. Superior vena cava syndrome with malignant causes. *N Engl J Med* 2007; **356**:1862.

81. Cheng S. Superior vena cava syndrome: a contemporary review of a historic disease. *Cardiol Rev* 2009;**17**:16.

82. Devaraj A, Griffin N, Nicholson AG, et al. Computed tomography findings in fibrosing mediastinitis. *Clin Radiol* 2007;**62**:781.

83. Sheth S, Ebert MD, Fishman EK. Superior vena cava obstruction evaluation with MDCT. *AJR Am J Roentgenol* 2010;**194**:W336.

84. Rizvi AZ, Kaira M, Bjarnason H, et al. Benign superior vena cava syndrome: stenting is now the first line treatment. *J Vasc Surg* 2008;**47**:372.

85. Sheikh MA, Fernandez Jr BB, Gray BH, et al. Endovascular stenting of nonmalignant superior vena cava syndrome. *Catheter Cardiovasc Interv* 2005;**65**:405.

86. Barshes NR, Annambhotla S, El Sayed HF, et al. Percutaneous stenting of superior vena cava syndrome: treatment outcomes in patients with benign and malignant disease. *Vascular* 2007; **15**:314.

87. Ganeshan A, Hon LQ, Warakaulle DR, et al. Superior vena caval stenting for SVC obstruction: current status. *Eur J Radiol* 2009; **71**:343.

88. Petersen BD, Uchida BT. Long-term results of treatment of benign central venous obstructions unrelated to dialysis with expandable Z stents. *J Vasc Interv Radiol* 1999;**10**:757.

89. Qanadli SD, El Hajjam M, Mignon F, et al. Subacute and chronic benign superior vena cava obstructions: endovascular treatment with self-expanding metallic stents. *AJR Am J Roentgenol* 1999;**173**:159.

90. Slonim SM, Semba CP, Sze DY, et al. Placement of SVC stents over pacemaker wires for the treatment of SVC syndrome. *J Vasc Interv Radiol* 2000;**11**:215.

91. Stockx L, Raat H, Donck J, et al. Repositioning and leaving in situ the central venous catheter during percutaneous treatment of associated superior vena cava syndrome: a report of eight cases. *Cardiovasc Intervent Radiol* 1999;**22**:224.

92. Furui S, Sawada S, Kuramoto K, et al. Gianturco stent placement in malignant caval obstruction: analysis of factors for predicting the outcome. *Radiology* 1995;**195**:147.

93. Gross CM, Kraemer J, Waigand J, et al. Stent implantation in patients with superior vena cava syndrome. *AJR Am J Roentgenol* 1997;**169**:429.

94. Kishi K, Sonomura T, Mitsuzane K, et al. Self-expandable metallic stent therapy for superior vena cava syndrome: clinical observations. *Radiology* 1993;**189**:531.

95. Kee ST, Kinoshita L, Razavi MK, et al. Superior vena cava syndrome: treatment with catheter-directed thrombolysis and endovascular stent placement. *Radiology* 1998;**206**:187.

95. Nguyen NP, Borok TL, Welsh J, et al. Safety and effectiveness of vascular endoprothesis for malignant superior vena cava syndrome. *Thorax* 2009;**64**:174.

96. Lanciego C, Chacon JL, Julian A, et al. Stenting as first option for endovascular treatment of malignant superior vena cava syndrome. *AJR Am J Roentgenol* 2001;**177**:585.

97. Lanciego C, Pangua C, Chacon JI, et al. Endovascular stenting as the first step in the overall management of malignant superior vena cava syndrome. *AJR Am J Roentgenol* 2009;**193**:549.

98. Nagata T, Makutani S, Uchida H, et al. Follow-up results of 71 patients undergoing metallic stent placement for the treatment of malignant obstruction of the superior vena cava. *Cardiovasc Intervent Radiol* 2007;**30**:959.

99. Warren MJ, Sen S, Marcus N. Management of migration of a SVC Wallstent into the right atrium. *Cardiovasc Intervent Radiol* 2008; **31**:1262.

100. Taylor JD, Lehmann ED, Belli AM, et al. Strategies for the management of SVC stent migration into the right atrium. *Cardiovasc Intervent Radiol* 2007;**30**:1003.

101. Smith SL, Manhire AR, Clark DM. Delayed spontaneous superior vena cava perforation associated with a SVC Wallstent. *Cardiovasc Intervent Radiol* 2001;**24**:286.

102. Martin M, Baumgartner I, Kolb M, et al. Fatal pericardial tamponade after Wallstent implantation for malignant superior vena cava syndrome. *J Endovasc Ther* 2002;**9**:680.

103. Recto MR, Bousamra M, Yeh Jr T. Late superior vena cava perforation and aortic laceration after stenting to treat superior vena cava syndrome secondary to fibrosing mediastinitis. *J Invasive Cardiol* 2002;**14**:624.

104. Brown KT, Getrajdman GI. Balloon dilation of the superior vena cava (SVC) resulting in SVC rupture and pericardial tamponade: a case report and brief review. *Cardiovasc Intervent Radiol* 2005;**28**:372.

105. Moore Jr WM, Hollier LH, Pickett TK. Superior vena cava and central venous reconstruction. *Surgery* 1991;**110**:35.

106. Kang TL, Dudick C, Ashiku S, et al. Blunt rupture of the subclavian-innominate venous junction: case report and review of literature. *J Trauma* 2009;**66**:1728.

107. DiGiacomo JC, Rotondo MF, Schwab CW. Transcutaneous balloon catheter tamponade for definitive control of subclavian venous injuries: case reports. *J Trauma* 1994;**37**:111.

108. Azizzadeh A, Pham MT, Estrera AL, et al. Endovascular repair of an iatrogenic superior vena caval injury: a case report. *J Vasc Surg* 2007;**46**:569.

109. Anaya-Ayala JE, Charlton-Ouw KM, Kaiser CL, et al. Successful emergency endovascular treatment for superior vena cava injury. *Ann Vasc Surg* 2009;**23**:139.

110. Spaggiari L, Regnard JF, Nottin R, et al. Leiomyosarcoma of the superior vena cava. *Ann Thorac Surg* 1996;**62**:274.

111. Tovar-Martin E, Tovar-Pardo AE, Marini M, et al. Intraluminal leiomyosarcoma of the superior vena cava: a cause of superior vena cava syndrome. *J Cardiovasc Surg* (Torino) 1997;**38**:33.

112. Calligaro KD, Ahmad S, Dandora R, et al. Venous aneurysms: surgical indications and review of the literature. *Surgery* 1995; **117**:1.

113. Kersting S, Roessel T, Hinterseher I, et al. Isolated aneurysm of the internal jugular vein. *Vasa* 2008;**37**:371.

114. Goddziuk K, Czekajska-Chehab E, Wrona A, et al. Saccular aneurysm of the superior vena cava detected by computed tomography and successfully treated with surgery. *Ann Thorac Surg* 2004; **78**:e94.

115. Haney JC, Shortell CK, McCann RL, et al. Congenital jugular vein phlebectasia: a case report and review of the literature. *Ann Vasc Surg* 2008;**22**:681.

MISCELLANEOUS VASCULAR INTERVENTIONS

18

Vascular Access Placement and Foreign Body Retrieval

Karim Valji

The demand for long-term central venous catheters (CVCs) has increased dramatically over the past several decades. CVCs are used for infusion of drugs (e.g., antibiotics, chemotherapeutic agents), administration of blood products, blood sampling, hyperalimentation, and dialysis and apheresis. In the past, CVCs were placed exclusively by surgeons in the operating room. Interventional radiologists have now assumed the major role in the insertion of these devices.[1] In some hospitals, vascular access placement is the most commonly performed procedure in the interventional radiology suite.

Image-guided placement of a CVC has several advantages over purely operative insertion.[2,3] The risk of immediate complications such as pneumothorax, arterial puncture, and catheter malposition is almost completely eliminated. Precise positioning of the catheter tip is almost guaranteed. Finally, imaging is critical when placing catheters through occluded thoracic or neck veins or outside the chest (e.g., into the inferior vena cava [IVC]).

ACCESS PLANNING

Devices

Tunneled, cuffed external infusion catheters are made of silicone or polyurethane-based material. They are manufactured with one, two, or three lumens in diameters from 3 to 12.5 French (Fr) (Fig. 18-1). These devices are inserted into a large vein and then travel through a subcutaneous tunnel before exiting the skin. A Dacron cuff embedded on the shaft incites a fibrotic reaction that ultimately secures the catheter in place and impedes the spread of infection from the skin exit site to the circulation. Infusion catheters have endholes or side valves (e.g., *Groshong type*). The valve design is intended to allow fluid injection and (possibly) blood aspiration but prevent blood or air from entering the catheter when it is not in use (Fig. 18-2). In theory, the risks of catheter occlusion and air embolism

are reduced. Although valved catheters require less frequent flushing, they actually confer no benefit in terms of catheter dysfunction or vascular thrombosis.[4-6] Some CVCs have a silver ion–impregnated cuff or silver coating that is meant to serve as an instant antimicrobial barrier; however, the value of this feature has been challenged.[7,8] On the other hand, metaanalysis of existing literature supports the value of anti-infective agents incorporated into the inside and outside of the catheter body in reducing device-related bloodstream infections (BSI).[9]

Tunneled hemodialysis and apheresis catheters are short, large-bore (typically 13.5 to 14.5 Fr), dual-lumen devices capable of handling high flow rates (e.g., 300 to 500 mL/min) (Fig. 18-3). These catheters have staggered or nonstaggered endholes or split lumens and are manufactured in preset lengths. From the right internal jugular (IJ) vein, 19- to 23-cm tip-to-cuff devices are usually appropriate. From the left IJ, 23- to 28-cm devices are often necessary. Tunneled hemodialysis catheters must be distinguished from nontunneled temporary catheters (usually placed by nephrologists) intended for several sessions of acute, emergent dialysis. No single catheter type has been proven to be most effective. Still, there is some evidence that split and symmetric tip catheters (e.g., Palindrome type) have a longer functional lifespan than the traditional staggered tip devices.[10-14] In principle, separation of the uptake and return lumens is necessary to prevent recirculation, which can significantly diminish the efficiency of dialysis.[15] Even so, the symmetrically tipped Palindrome catheter is reported to achieve the lowest recirculation rates among the various catheter models that are available.[14]

Implantable ports are constructed from a variety of materials, including titanium and plastic (Fig. 18-4). A silicone or polyurethane catheter is connected to a reservoir with a silicon window that is accessed through the skin using a noncoring (Huber) needle. The entire system is buried in the subcutaneous tissue of the chest or arm (or even the thigh or abdomen). These devices are available in single- and double-lumen configurations.

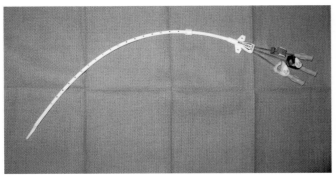

FIGURE 18-1 Triple-lumen tunneled external infusion catheter. Dacron cuff is mounted on the proximal portion of the catheter shaft. *(Courtesy of Bard Access Systems, Salt Lake City, Utah.)*

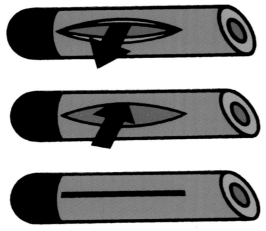

FIGURE 18-2 Side slits in catheter allow aspiration of blood or infusion of fluids but prevent blood from entering the catheter when not in use. *(Courtesy of Bard Access Systems, Salt Lake City, Utah.)*

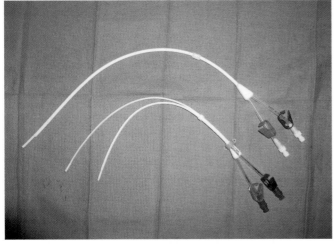

FIGURE 18-3 Hemodialysis catheters. *Top,* 13.5-Fr catheter with staggered lumens (proximal endhole is the arterial lumen). *(Courtesy of Bard Access Systems, Salt Lake City, Utah.)* Bottom, Split dialysis catheter. *(Courtesy of Medcomp, Harleysville, Pa.)*

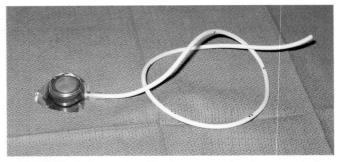

FIGURE 18-4 Implantable chest port with catheter attached.

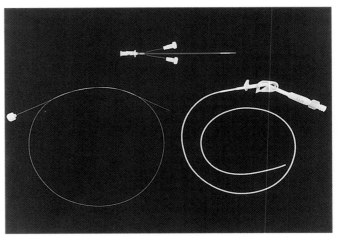

FIGURE 18-5 Single-lumen peripherally inserted central catheter *(right)* with inner stiffening guidewire *(left)* and peel-away sheath and dilator *(top). (Courtesy of Cook, Inc., Bloomington, Ind.)*

Ports provide central venous access without the need for an external catheter. Small ports are designed for children, patients with minimal subcutaneous fat, or arm placement. So-called power ports are suitable for rapid intravenous (IV) contrast injection during computed tomography (CT) examinations. It is purported that the overall frequency of device and BSI is lower with ports than external tunneled CVCs, but not every study has confirmed this tenet.[16,17]

Peripherally inserted central catheters (PICCs) are essentially long IV lines placed from a peripheral arm vein (or occasionally the IJ) into the central venous system (Fig. 18-5). Single-, double-, and triple-lumen configurations are available in sizes from 3.0 to 7.0 Fr. Some of the designs (Power type) are capable of handling the high flow rates demanded with injection of contrast material for CT scanning.

Device Selection

The selection of the most appropriate catheter in an individual case should be made jointly by the referring physician, interventionalist, and patient. Several factors

TABLE 18-1   Guidelines for Access Device Selection

Device	Purpose or Situation
External, tunneled catheter	Continuous use
	Multiple, simultaneous uses
	Patient preference
Implantable port	Intermittent use
	Immunocompromised patient
	Patient preference
High-flow tunneled catheter	Hemodialysis
	Apheresis
PICC	Short-term use (<2–3 mo)
	Infrequent blood drawing
	(lifetime risk for dialysis is low)

PICC, *peripherally inserted central catheter.*

are considered, including intended purpose, frequency and duration of use, underlying risk factors for infection or venous thrombosis, and patient preference for an external or implanted device (Table 18-1). Tunneled infusion catheters and implantable ports are only appropriate when the anticipated duration of need for continuous or periodic vascular access is more than several weeks. Whereas the risk of device-related infections is probably lower with chest ports, the consequences of infectious and other port site complications are more problematic. Finally, it is wise for the operator to personally confirm the device request just before placement to avoid an egregious implantation error due to miscommunication or an acute change in patient's condition.

VENOUS ACCESS

Access Route

CVCs are usually inserted through the IJV (tunneled catheters and ports) or upper arm vein (PICCs). The right IJV is preferred over the left because long-term catheter function is better and device-induced venous disease is less common.[4] The subclavian vein should be avoided if at all possible; symptomatic or asymptomatic stenosis or thrombosis is much more likely to occur with this route.[18-20] It is standard teaching to avoid placement on the side of the body that has undergone (or will undergo) mastectomy, radiation therapy, or axillary lymph node dissection, which may compromise lymphatic or venous limb drainage or wound healing.

If an occluded central vein can be recanalized or simply traversed with a guidewire (from the neck or the groin), catheter insertion still may be feasible.[21] Some practitioners will attempt to place a vascular access device into an external jugular vein or enlarged collateral veins (e.g., intercostal vein).[21,22] If no central thoracic vein is available, most operators will then turn to the common femoral vein. Practically, this situation occurs in patients requiring long-term hemodialysis. However, thrombotic, stenotic, and infectious complications are greatest with tunneled femoral catheters, which are prone to dysfunction and retraction.[23-25] As a last resort, central venous access is obtained directly into the IVC through a translumbar or transhepatic approach.[26-28]

Patient Preparation

With the notable exception of PICCs, vascular access insertion in an interventional suite demands the same aseptic environment as is found in an operating room. All procedures begin with antibacterial cleaning of surfaces that may come in contact with the patient, wide surgical preparation of the operating field, surgical scrub by all operators, and maintenance of strict sterile technique during the case. Some interventionalists give prophylactic antibiotics (e.g., 1 g of cephazolin IV) within 1 hour of placement of tunneled catheters or ports, even though the benefit of this step is questionable. Bacteremia or sepsis is a contraindication to placement of tunneled catheters and implantable ports.[29] Coagulation parameters should be checked and corrected before the procedure (see Chapter 2). One recent study suggested that the standard coagulation thresholds for vascular interventional procedures may be relaxed with tunneled CVC placement (e.g., acceptable with platelet count greater than 25,000/mm^3 or international normalized ratio less than 2.0).[30]

Venous Entry (Videos 18-1 and 18-2)

Doppler ultrasound spectral analysis of the IJs normally shows a triphasic waveform with respiratory variation. Dampening of the waveform suggests a central obstruction that may complicate or preclude device insertion. Sonographic guidance into the IJ is mandatory; this step unequivocally reduces the risk of inadvertent arterial puncture or pneumothorax and the number of needle passes required for venous entry.[31] A site on the neck just above the clavicle is selected. The vessel is visualized with the transducer in a transverse plane while the needle is advanced from the side or from above (Fig. 18-6). The transverse orientation ensures that the carotid artery is constantly observed during needle insertion. Skin entry lateral to vein puncture results in a more favorable subcutaneous catheter pathway from the chest to the vessel. One group of investigators described a method for single puncture entry into the IJ directly from the intended catheter exit site using a curved needle.[32]

Some interventionalists prefer to access the vein with a 21-gauge micropuncture needle, 0.018-inch guidewire, and transitional 4- or 5-Fr dilator. The needle is advanced through the skin with real-time sonographic

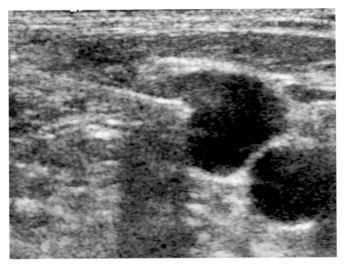

FIGURE 18-6   Right internal jugular vein entry under sonographic guidance in the transverse plane. Needle enters from a lateral approach; carotid artery is medial to the vein.

guidance. Weak blood return signals luminal entry. Sometimes, aspiration is required to confirm an intravascular location. Alternatively, continuous suction is applied to a saline-filled syringe and tubing connected to the needle until blood returns. If the needle coapts and then punctures the front and back walls of the vein, blood return occurs with needle withdrawal. The microwire is advanced down the jugular vein into the superior vena cava (SVC). Changes in needle angle or patient respiratory phase may be needed to redirect the wire if it passes up the jugular vein or into the subclavian or brachiocephalic vein. After the transitional dilator is placed, a standard guidewire is advanced into the right atrium or (preferably) IVC. If there is resistance to guidewire passage, contrast injection may show a central venous obstruction.

In the rare situation when a subclavian vein approach is necessary, the axillary vein is punctured lateral to the ribs in the subcoracoid region. This entry site almost completely eliminates the possibility of pneumothorax. It also ensures that the catheter is well within the subclavian vein as it passes through the costoclavicular space. If the catheter is extravascular at that site, chronic compression may occur and lead to catheter erosion and fracture ("pinch-off" syndrome)[33,34] (Fig. 18-7). The axillary vein lies just inferior to the axillary artery (Fig. 18-8). The ultrasound transducer is oriented parallel to the vessel while the needle is advanced with real-time imaging.

For *upper arm vein puncture* (PICCs and arm ports), the basilic vein is preferred, followed by the brachial and cephalic veins. Venospasm is particularly problematic with the latter route. It is helpful to place a tourniquet around the upper arm to distend the vein before puncture. The vein is entered with a 21-gauge needle from a micropuncture set or a 21- to 22-gauge sheath needle. Care must be taken to avoid puncturing the brachial artery. Because the veins are small and tend to go into spasm, it is wise to start peripherally on the vein and avoid a double wall puncture. After blood is aspirated, a 0.018-inch guidewire is inserted. If the guidewire does not advance despite needle adjustment, a more central site on the vein is used. Sometimes, the guidewire hangs up because it has entered a small collateral channel. In this case, contrast injection may outline the more direct route to the central circulation.

For *common femoral vein insertion*, sonographic guidance is most helpful although many practitioners still

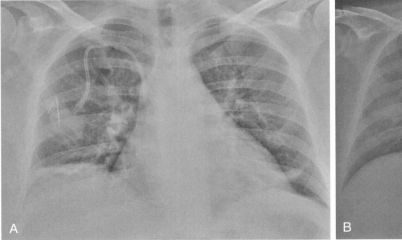
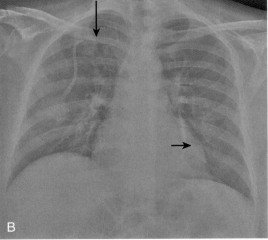

FIGURE 18-7   Pinch-off syndrome. **A,** Surgically placed right subclavian vein port. **B,** Some months later, port was no longer functional. Chest radiograph shows catheter fracture at site of "pinch off" in the costoclavicular space *(long arrow)*. The distal catheter fragment has embolized to the left pulmonary artery *(short arrow)*.

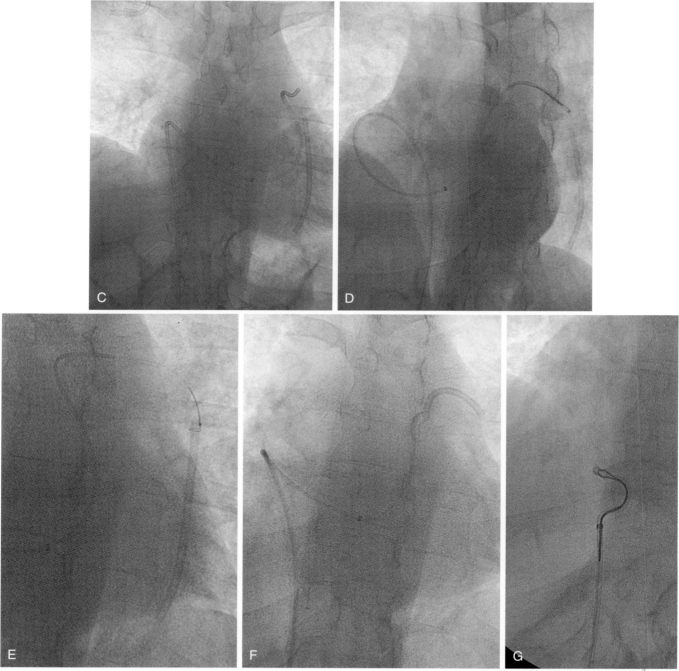

FIGURE 18-7, cont'd **C,** From a femoral vein approach, an Omniflush catheter has been advanced into the left pulmonary artery. **D,** The catheter was exchanged for the guiding catheter and gooseneck snare. **E,** The upper free end of the catheter fragment was snared with the retrieval device. The fragment was then pulled out of the heart **(F)** and into the large-caliber vascular sheath **(G)** for removal from the body.

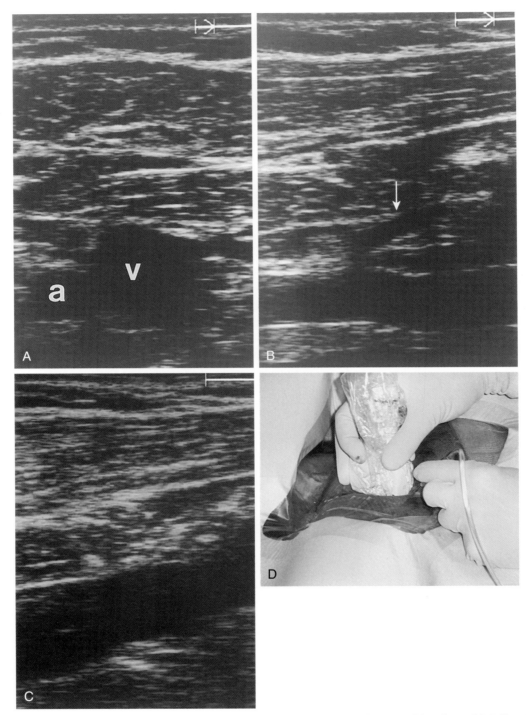

FIGURE 18-8   Axillary vein entry. **A,** Sagittal sonogram shows the relationship between the artery *(a)* and vein *(v)*. **B,** Longitudinal image of the axillary-subclavian artery with a side branch *(arrow)*. **C,** Longitudinal image of the axillary vein. **D,** Micropuncture needle is inserted under sonographic guidance with constant aspiration on the saline-filled tubing and syringe.

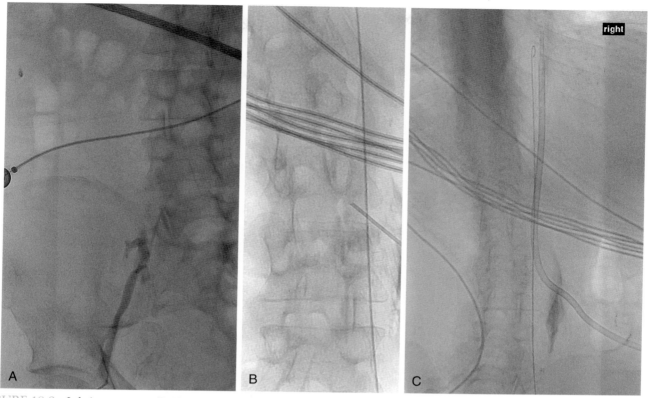

FIGURE 18-9   Inferior vena cava (IVC) vascular access placement. **A,** A guidewire is being placed in the IVC from the right common femoral vein through a diseased iliac system. **B,** With the patient prone, a 20-gauge, 15-cm Chiba needle is directed toward the guidewire from the right flank. **C,** The 55-cm tip to cuff dialysis catheter is in place with the tip near the cavoatrial junction.

use the laterally located femoral artery pulse as a landmark. Catheters are tunneled laterally onto the thigh or lower abdomen (see later discussion).

IVC puncture may be required if all potential access sites in the chest, arms, and groin are exhausted.[22,27,28,35] Prior CT scans are reviewed to identify any obstacles or contraindications to the intended route. Initially, a sheath, guidewire, or catheter may be placed into the IVC from the groin, although this step is not mandatory (Fig. 18-9). Bony landmarks alone may be used for caval entry. The patient is then placed prone on the interventional table. A skin site is chosen on the right flank above the iliac crest just lateral to the vertebral column. It is critical to plan a cephalic track into the IVC to avoid a sharp right angle turn as the needle enters the vessel, which can make sheath and catheter insertion exceedingly difficult. A long, 18- to 20-gauge needle is then advanced toward the catheter/wire in the IVC or toward the right lateral aspect of the spine in the calculated position of the IVC from prior imaging studies. Biplane fluoroscopy or frequent tube angulation is necessary to avoid overshooting the vena cava. Once blood is aspirated and contrast injection confirms the location, the remainder of the procedure is similar to catheter placement from other access routes. A stiff guidewire is necessary for placement of the peel-away sheath.

Transhepatic venous access is necessary for individuals whose only patent central vein is the suprarenal IVC. Even though this route is feasible in most cases, long-term catheter function is a serious problem.[26,28] Finally, transrenal venous entry into the IVC has been described for patients with end-stage renal disease who require tunneled dialysis catheters.[36]

Catheter Tip Position (Video 18-3)

The manufacturers of most vascular access devices instruct the operator to place the catheter tip in the SVC or at the cavoatrial junction. However, the long-term failure rate of CVCs placed with the tip at these locations at the termination of the procedure is significant. Most CVCs migrate 3 to 4 cm upward from the supine to standing position; PICCs move about 2 cm caudally when the arm is adducted after placement.[37-39] Although not widely understood nor even accepted outside the interventional radiology community, it is now standard of practice to position the catheter tip in the *upper to mid-right atrium* with the patient supine.[40,41] At this location, the catheter endholes will rarely become obstructed by a fibrin sheath because the tip hangs freely in the right atrium rather than plastered against the caval wall (Fig. 18-10). Several nonrandomized clinical studies lend credence to

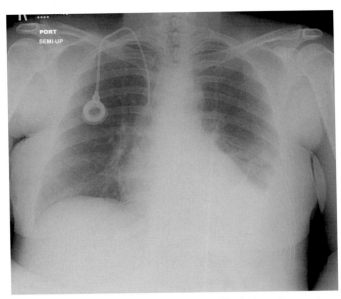

FIGURE 18-10 Implantable chest port with tip in an incorrect position in the superior vena cava.

this approach.[4,42-45] Because all of these devices are composed of soft polyurethane or silicone material, atrial dysrhythmias are quite rare (and easily managed by slight catheter withdrawal) and cardiac perforation is essentially reportable[46-48] (see later discussion).

To this end, the intravascular catheter length can be estimated by placing the tip of the guidewire in the upper to mid right atrium. The wire is clamped at the access catheter hub, and the exposed hub length is subtracted from the clamped guidewire length.

- If the catheter can be cut to size (e.g., PICCs, tunneled infusion catheters, port catheters), the shaft is trimmed appropriately after having been tunneled from the exit site to the venotomy.
- If the catheter cannot be cut to size because of the tip configuration (e.g., hemodialysis and apheresis catheter, Groshong catheters), an appropriately sized device is chosen based on the measured intravascular length and the desired tunnel distance.

DEVICE PLACEMENT

Tunneled Infusion Catheters (Video 18-4)

The subcutaneous tunnel should be about 7 to 10 cm long. A skin exit site is chosen on the anterior chest wall below the clavicle, away from the axilla and breast tissue. In female patients, a medial location is usually preferred to avoid interference with clothing or bra straps. The exit site and subcutaneous tissues along the planned tunnel track are infiltrated with 1% lidocaine. A stab incision is made just large enough to accommodate the catheter and cuff to ensure a snug fit in the track. The catheter is pulled through the tunnel with a tunneling device until the cuff is near the vein entry site. Before the completion of the case, the Dacron retention cuff is repositioned about 2 cm from the skin exit site to allow for easier removal. The catheter should form a gentle curve as it enters the vein.

The access vein is dilated to accommodate the delivery sheath. In some patients, serial dilation, a stiff guidewire, or both may be necessary to advance the sheath through the subcutaneous tissues. Central vein or right atrial laceration by the dilator or guidewire can occur if this step is not monitored under fluoroscopy. To avoid air embolism, the guidewire and inner dilator are removed while the sheath is gently pinched and patient suspends respiration. For some devices, valved sheaths are available to minimize air entrapment. The catheter is immediately inserted into the sheath and then advanced into the right atrium.

If the catheter does not pass easily because the sheath has kinked, the sheath is partially peeled back until it lies in the straight portion of the vein, and the catheter is then readvanced. Alternatively, a hydrophilic guidewire is advanced into the SVC through the catheter, which is then advanced over the wire. If the catheter tip enters the internal jugular, azygous, or contralateral brachiocephalic vein, it may be directed into the SVC by buckling it with a guidewire, withdrawing the sheath slightly and readvancing the catheter, or advancing the catheter over a guidewire.

The sheath is peeled away while the catheter is fixed in position at the venous entry site. The catheter is then withdrawn at the skin exit site until the tip is in the desired location in the upper to mid-right atrium. Traditionally, the catheter lumens are flushed with heparin solution. The device is secured to the skin to avoid early dislodgment before the Dacron cuff becomes incorporated into the subcutaneous tissues.

Hemodialysis and Apheresis Catheters

Up to 50% of chronic hemodialysis patients develop vein stenoses or frank occlusions after placement of temporary or tunneled venous catheters through the subclavian or axillary vein route.[18-20,49] In addition to causing disabling symptoms, these obstructions can interfere with the construction of future hemodialysis access. For this reason, CVC in patients on chronic hemodialysis must be placed in the right (or left) IJ whenever possible.

From an accessible site on the chest wall, the catheter is tunneled over the clavicle. Generous dissection of the subcutaneous tissues at the venotomy site and a somewhat low IJ puncture can prevent kinking of the catheter as it makes a turn out of the vein and toward the chest. For catheters with staggered lumens, the arterial lumen (proximal port) is positioned with the endhole away from the right atrial wall for optimal function. The catheter tip should be readjusted if rapid aspiration of blood is not possible after placement. Some dialysis units prefer to fill catheters with high-dose heparin (1000 or 5000 units/mL) to prevent thrombosis. Others opt for citrate solution to avoid the possibility of inadvertent injection of the anticoagulant.

Implantable Ports (Video 18-5)

Ports may be placed in the chest or arm (or even the thigh), depending on the patient's lifestyle and preference.[50-54] Chest ports are easiest to access. The intended port site must have enough subcutaneous fat to accommodate the device easily and avoid wound dehiscence or skin breakdown. Of note, port incision dehiscence is also a concern in patients who have received bevacizumab therapy within 10 days of insertion.[55] However, a port can be difficult to access if there is too much surrounding adipose tissue or if it is poorly supported by underlying bone. Ideally, the port septum should be about 0.5 to 2 cm below the skin surface. The operator should avoid placement in breast tissue or the axilla.

After venous access is obtained (see earlier discussion), a 3- to 5-cm transverse incision is made on the anterior chest wall using a No. 10 or 15 blade after infiltration with 1% or 2% lidocaine with epinephrine. Bleeding from small arterial branches always stops with manual compression or brief occlusion with a small hemostat. A pocket is created inferior to the incision using sharp and blunt dissection. The pocket should be large enough to accommodate the port and allow easy closure of the wound. Some interventionalists (but not most) place two stay sutures from eyelets in the port base through the anterior fascial plane to secure it in place after insertion into the pocket.[54]

The catheter is tunneled through the subcutaneous track and then connected securely to the port hub, usually with a retention sleeve. The port is placed in the pocket well below the incision. At the neck, the catheter is cut to size based on measured intravascular length (see earlier) and then inserted into the vein using a peel-away sheath. The catheter tip should land in the upper to mid right atrium. Under fluoroscopy, the entire course of the catheter is examined for kinks. The device is accessed with a noncoring (Huber) needle and flushed with heparin lock solution (100 units/mL). The incision may be closed with interrupted absorbable sutures in the subcutaneous layer to approximate tissues and continuous absorbable suture in the subcuticular layer. Some operators favor closure with Dermabond skin adhesive. Steri-Strips and a sterile dressing are placed over the incision. The venotomy may be closed with Dermabond, Steri-Strips, or suture material.

Arm ports are inserted above the elbow in a similar fashion. The tunnel can be very short, allowing the catheter to be pulled from the skin incision to the venotomy site using forceps rather than a tunneling device. Care must be taken to avoid damaging the brachial artery during placement.

Peripherally Inserted Central Catheters (Video 18-6)

PICCs are suitable for patients who need short-term central vascular access (typically for antibiotics, chemotherapy, or hyperalimentation for up to 4 to 6 weeks).[56-59] However, PICCs must be *strictly* avoided in patients expected to require hemodialysis in the future lest potential access sites become obliterated. It is more cost-effective for PICCs to be placed at the bedside by specially trained nurses than by physicians in the IR suite.[60] However, tip malposition is more frequent (about 10%) without fluoroscopic guidance.[61] Radiologic placement is indicated when bedside insertion is unsuccessful or unavailable. The dilator or sheath is inserted into the accessed vein. The catheter is cut to size and inserted through the peel-away sheath with the accompanying stylet to assist with catheter passage. It is then advanced into the upper right atrium and flushed with heparin lock solution. The hub is secured to the skin with suture material or an adhesive appliance.

ACCESS MANAGEMENT

Catheter and Exit Site Care (Video 18-7)

Meticulous catheter and exit site care is the key to limiting CVC-related infectious complications. Patient or caregiver education is done before and after device placement by a specially trained nurse. Protocols for catheter and wound care and for catheter flushing vary somewhat among institutions. A sterile gauze or occlusive plastic dressing is kept over the fresh incision or exit site; in trials of dialysis catheters, rates of exit site and BSI are similar for both coverings.[62] The incision must be kept completely dry for at least 3 days. Various sorts of topical antiinfectives are also popular. For dialysis catheters, mupirocin (and possibly Neosporin or povidone-iodine) ointment may reduce catheter-related infections.[62]

The exit site, incision, and tunnel track are examined daily by the patient or caregiver for signs of infection, catheter withdrawal, catheter fracture, wound dehiscence, or skin breakdown. The site also should be examined by a physician or nurse within 5 to 7 days of placement. By tradition, CVCs are flushed with heparin solution weekly and after each use to maintain patency. Some dialysis centers prefer trisodium citrate solution for its antimicrobial and anticoagulant activity.[63] Groshong catheters may be filled with saline and require less frequent flushing. In randomized trials, the use of antimicrobial catheter "lock" significantly diminishes the incidence of BSIs.[64,65]

Device Removal (Video 18-8)

To remove tunneled catheters, the exit site is sterilized and the tunnel track anesthetized. In many cases, firm steady traction will release the entire catheter. Retention of the polyester cuff is not associated with an increased risk of subsequent infection.[66] Otherwise, blunt and sharp dissection are used to separate the device from the subcutaneous tissues. If the cuff is far from the skin exit site, it is sometimes necessary to perform a cutdown over the cuff to release the catheter. The smaller caliber infusion catheters may fracture if excessive force is applied to remove them. If the catheter breaks, it may be possible to extricate the buried segment with a forceps under fluoroscopy. Otherwise, intravascular retrieval will be necessary (see later discussion).

To remove implanted ports, an incision is made over the original scar after local anesthesia is applied. Using sharp and blunt dissection, the port and catheter hub are separated from the surrounding tissue. The fibrous capsule around the port is incised with a dissecting scissors or scalpel to release the device. The stay sutures (if present) are cut, and the port and attached catheter are removed. The incision is closed in an iden-tical manner to port placement. If there is any evidence of actual pocket or tunnel infection, the wound is packed with iodoform gauze and allowed to heal by secondary intention.

COMPLICATIONS

Immediate Complications

The overall adverse event rate for CVC placement is about 4% to 7%.[29,53,58,67,68] Immediate complications occur less frequently with image-guided placement than without[2,49-54,69] (Table 18-2 and Fig. 18-11). With the exception of venous thrombosis, procedure-related complication rates generally are lower for PICCs and peripheral ports than for devices placed in the chest or neck. However, median nerve injury is a remote risk unique to catheter insertions in arm veins.[70]

TABLE 18-2   Early Complications from Image-Guided Vascular Access Placement

Event	Frequency (%)
Pneumothorax	0-1
Arterial puncture	1-2
Hemorrhage or hematoma	0-2
Air embolism	1
Catheter malposition	0
Venous perforation	<1

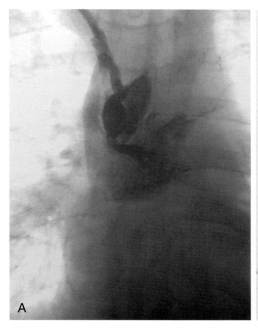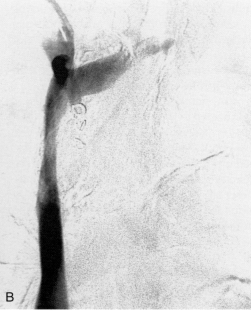

FIGURE 18-11   Superior vena cava (SVC) rupture during hemodialysis catheter placement. **A,** Contrast injection shows extravasation outside the SVC. **B,** Several large stainless-steel coils were used to close the leak. Subsequently, a tunneled catheter was placed into the SVC.

Air embolism can occur during the interval between removing the dilator and peeling away the sheath. If this untoward event is suspected, the chest is immediately examined with fluoroscopy. Conventional teaching recommends placing the patient in the left lateral decubitus position to keep the air in the right heart chambers and prevent "air lock." In reality, the air bolus almost always has already traveled to the pulmonary artery by the time the embolism is recognized. Supplemental oxygen and IV fluids are given, and the patient is carefully monitored. Air embolism is almost always self-limited, but fatal events have been reported.[71]

Persistent blood oozing from the skin exit site is an occasional problem. Prolonged manual pressure usually resolves the bleeding. Coagulation parameters should be checked and corrected if necessary. In patients with renal failure, normal hemostasis may be affected by platelet dysfunction. If necessary, Gelfoam pledgets or collagen sealant inserted into the tunnel may be helpful. Silver nitrate can be applied (to the subcutaneous tissue only) to achieve hemostasis. Some practitioners favor temporary placement of a purse-string suture at the site.[72]

Fatalities during vascular access placement have been reported from laceration of the central veins or heart by the tip of the dilator or guidewire.[73] This catastrophe is avoided by advancing the sheath or dilator with careful fluoroscopic monitoring.

Late Complications

The primary late complications of CVC placement are infection, catheter occlusion or malfunction, venous thrombosis, and catheter migration* (Table 18-3). Overall, the frequency of infections and catheter-related thrombosis is substantially higher for tunneled hemodialysis catheters than for small-bore infusion catheters.

Infections

Box 18-1 outlines the spectrum of infectious complications related to CVCs. The published rates of device-related infections vary from 0.6% to 27%.[76] There is incontrovertible evidence that BSIs are more common with nontunneled CVCs (both infusion and dialysis) than with tunneled or implanted devices. The incidence of infections after image-guided radiologic placement is comparable to (and perhaps better than) surgical placement.[2,3,52] Bacteremia and ascending infections usually are related to the biofilm that forms on all intravascular devices. This reactive coating provides a relative sanctuary for microorganisms.[77]

*See references 2, 4, 49, 51-53, 68, 69, 74-76.

TABLE 18-3 Late Complications from Image-Guided Vascular Access Placement

Event	Frequency (%)
Catheter occlusion	1-10
Catheter or device migration	0-3
Catheter dislodgment	2-9
Catheter fracture	1-9 (PICC)
Wound dehiscence	1
Port inversion	<1
Central venous thrombosis	0-10 (0.1-0.3/1000 catheter days)
Peripheral vein thrombosis (PICCs)	1-38
Local infection	1-7
Catheter-related bacteremia	1-4
Bloodstream infections (BSI)	
PICCs	2.1/1000 catheter days
Tunneled infusion catheters	1.6/1000 catheter days
Tunneled dialysis catheters	3/1000 catheter days
Implanted ports	0.1/1000 catheter days

BOX 18-1

INFECTIOUS COMPLICATIONS OF CENTRAL VENOUS CATHETERS

- Bacteremia (bloodstream infections, BSI)
- Exit site infection
- Port pocket infection
- Subcutaneous tunnel infection
- Septic thrombophlebitis
- Osteomyelitis
- Endocarditis
- Septic shock

There are well-established criteria for diagnosing catheter-related BSI. Fever alone is not usually sufficient. As a rule, two positive blood cultures (one obtained from a peripheral vein) are required. The offending organism is typically coagulase-negative *Staphylococcus* or *Staphylococcus aureus*.[77,78] In patients with fever and positive blood cultures, it is often difficult to determine whether the device itself is responsible for bacteremia. But left untreated, catheter-related bacteremia can lead to endocarditis, osteomyelitis, or septic shock.

The management of catheter-related infections depends largely on the site of infection, the offending organism, and the patient's underlying immunologic state. In stable patients, catheter salvage is often attempted in cases of uncomplicated skin infection or fever from unknown source.[78,79] Initial treatment involves broad-spectrum IV antibiotics or antibiotic lock and local wound care. Skin and blood cultures are obtained to guide ongoing antibiotic therapy. If the patient responds to treatment, the device is left in place or exchanged over a guidewire for a new catheter (see later discussion). Catheter removal is necessary if these measures fail or if one of the following conditions exist:

- Tunnel infections, port pocket infections, septic thrombophlebitis, osteomyelitis, or endocarditis[79]
- Unstable condition or sepsis
- Isolation of certain microorganisms[77] listed in Box 18-2
- Markedly compromised immune system

Even though it is accepted practice to culture the catheter tip upon retrieval, the impact of this step on patient management is questionable.[80] After removing an infected port, the pocket is irrigated and packed with iodoform gauze. The packing is changed every few days and the wound allowed to heal by secondary intention.

The timing for reinsertion of a new tunneled catheter in a patient with catheter-related BSI is very controversial.[77] Ideally, the interventionalist should wait until the entire course of antibiotics has been given, but such delay is often impractical. At the very least, the patient should become afebrile, have a normal white blood cell count and negative blood cultures, and have received at least 2 days of IV antibiotic therapy.

Catheter Malfunction (Video 18-9)

Catheter malfunction is a vexing problem in patients with central venous access devices. The best approach is prevention: position the catheter tip in the upper or mid right atrium. Malfunction can occur for several reasons:

- Fibrin "sleeve" or clot occluding the endhole
- Catheter malposition or migration
- Catheter kinks
- Catheter tip abutting or eroding into the vessel wall
- Catheter fracture

Material obstruction of the catheter endholes occurs by two mechanisms. A clot may form at the catheter tip. More commonly, however, a slick "fibrin sheath" composed of fibrin, albumin, lipoproteins, and coagulation factors covers the structure within hours after placement and continues to accumulate over 5 to 7 days.[63] If bacteria colonize this surface, a biofilm is produced through which antimicrobial agents are relatively resistant. If the catheter tip apposes a vein wall, this coating matures into a dense "sleeve" including collagen and smooth muscles cells. The sleeve can eventually obstruct the catheter endhole[81] (Fig. 18-12). Fluid usually

---

BOX 18-2

ORGANISMS THAT GENERALLY REQUIRE CENTRAL VENOUS CATHETER REMOVAL

- *Staphylococcus aureus*
- *Acinetobacter baumannii*
- *Agrobacterium* species
- *Aspergillus* species
- *Bacillus* species
- *Candida* species
- *Corynebacterium jeikeium*
- *Malassezia furfur*
- *Mycobacterium* species
- *Pseudomonas aeruginosa*
- Other *Pseudomonas* species
- *Stenotrophomonas* species
- Other gram-negative rods

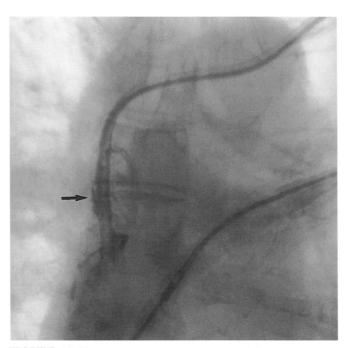

FIGURE 18-12   Fibrin sheath. Contrast injected through the catheter lumen runs back along the catheter shaft *(arrow)* rather than exiting the catheter freely.

can be injected, but blood cannot be aspirated. Hemodialysis catheter dysfunction often is signaled by diminished blood flow rates or inefficient dialysis. Catheters obstructed by thrombus or a fibrin sheath can be managed in several ways.

- Low-dose fibrinolytic agent. The catheter lumens are filled with 2 mg of Cathflo Activase (alteplase), reteplase, or tenecteplase. The solution is left to dwell for up to 90 minutes, after which aspiration is attempted. If unsuccessful, the maneuver should be repeated. This technique temporarily salvages about 90% of catheters, but the results are often not lasting.[82-84]
- High-dose fibrinolytic agent. If a large thrombus is detected at the catheter tip by echocardiography, CT, or venography, prolonged infusion of a thrombolytic agent may be warranted to dissolve the clot and prevent pulmonary embolism (see Chapter 3).
- Catheter exchange. The malfunctioning catheter is exchanged over a guidewire for a new catheter using the existing tunnel and venous entry site.[85] Some interventionalists use a large-caliber (e.g., 12-mm) angioplasty balloon to disrupt the fibrin sheath in the SVC. Catheter exchange is not acceptable if there is active infection at the skin exit site.
- Fibrin sheath stripping was once a popular method for salvaging dysfunctional vascular access devices.[85-87] However, it is clearly inferior to catheter exchange (with or without balloon disruption of the fibrin sheath).[63,85,86,89,90] Catheter replacement is also advocated in this setting by the National Kidney Foundation Dialysis Outcomes Quality Initiative.[91] For these reasons, the fibrin stripping technique has been largely abandoned.

Venous Thrombosis

Venous thrombosis (either partial or complete) can cause disabling arm or head and neck symptoms (e.g., SVC syndrome) and occasionally interferes with vascular access function[92,93] (Fig. 18-13). Up to two thirds of patients with an underlying malignancy develop venous thrombosis from CVCs.[79,94]

Peripheral thrombophlebitis is a clinical diagnosis that usually demands catheter removal. The diagnosis of *central* venous thrombosis is usually made by duplex sonography. The initial treatment is anticoagulation with low-molecular weight heparin compounds, or heparin followed by warfarin.[95] If anticoagulants are continued and the patient's symptoms improve,

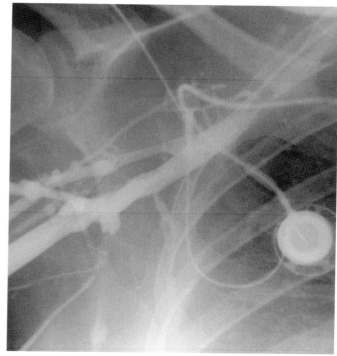

FIGURE 18-13   Right subclavian vein thrombosis from an indwelling vascular access device.

the catheter can often be left in place[4] Catheter-directed thrombolysis is used for severe or persistent symptoms despite anticoagulation. If symptoms fail to improve within several days or there is evidence for septic thrombophlebitis, the device should be removed.

To prevent catheter-related thrombosis and associated device malfunction, (1) prefer placement in a jugular vein and avoid the subclavian and femoral veins and (2) properly position the catheter tip. Whereas some investigators advocate routine use of prophylactic anticoagulation for higher risk patients (e.g., daily low-dose warfarin 1 mg or a low molecular weight heparin such as enoxaparin), the preponderance of evidence does not support this opinion.[4,79,96-102]

Catheter Misplacement
(Online Cases 61 and 86)

Catheter migration can occur despite correct initial positioning. The catheter tip may end up in a variety of places, most often the brachiocephalic, internal jugular, or azygous vein. Rarely, the catheter tip erodes through the vein wall and becomes extravascular.[103] This scenario occurs most often when the tip of a left-sided catheter abuts the right lateral wall of the SVC. Catheters that are placed or migrate into the low right atrium may have inadequate flow or induce cardiac dysrhythmias. Malpositioned catheters are detected by poor function or as an incidental finding on chest radiography. The catheter should not be used until an intravascular location is confirmed.

Catheters can be repositioned in several ways.[104] If the tip of an arm PICC or port migrates to or ends up in the IJ vein, brisk injection of saline through a 1- or 3-mL syringe may propel the catheter into its proper location. A guidewire can be inserted into one lumen of an external catheter and advanced until the catheter buckles into the SVC. Rarely, it is necessary to advance a pigtail catheter (with or without a tip-deflecting wire) from the femoral vein, engage the catheter shaft, and pull it back into the right atrium (Fig. 18-14).

For catheter malposition with ports, the internal jugular or common femoral vein is accessed. From this position, the catheter can be repositioned (Fig. 18-15). If the port catheter is too long, the tip is snared and withdrawn through a sheath inserted in the ipsilateral jugular vein. A short segment of the catheter is cut off, and the catheter end is then reinserted and positioned properly in the upper right atrium.

If the catheter falls out, it should be replaced immediately if the tract is mature and clean by probing the subcutaneous tunnel with a guidewire or catheter.[105] Finally, kits are available to repair the external portion of some damaged or fractured catheters.

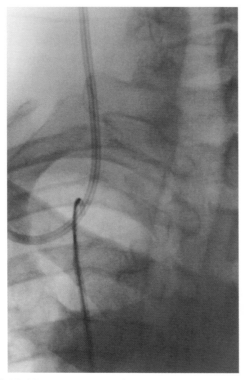

FIGURE 18-14 Repositioning of a central venous catheter. The catheter had spontaneously migrated from the superior vena cava to the right internal jugular vein. A pigtail catheter and tip-deflecting wire were used to engage the catheter and pull it back into the vena cava.

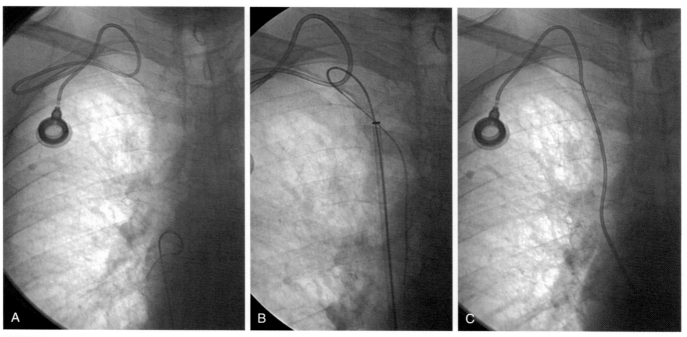

FIGURE 18-15 Spontaneous displacement of right chest port catheter. **A,** Chest radiograph shows that the right internal jugular vein catheter has migrated back into the right subclavian vein. **B,** Through a long vascular sheath placed in the right femoral vein, a pigtail type catheter and guidewire are used to loop the port catheter. Withdrawal of the pigtail catheter allowed the port catheter to prolapse back down the superior vena cava into proper position **(C).**

INTRAVASCULAR FOREIGN BODY RETRIEVAL (ONLINE CASE 26)

Sources

A wide variety of objects can become lodged in the vascular system, including catheter and guidewire fragments, coils and Amplatzer occluding devices, stents, balloon fragments, IVC filters or fragments, and bullets.[106-108] The ultimate destination of a foreign body depends on its shape, size, and stiffness, and on the hemodynamics of the local circulation. In some cases, catheter fracture (e.g., from pinch-off syndrome) is detected days to years after the actual event (see Fig. 18-7). Guidewires may become entrapped within IVC filters, usually during blind central venous catheter insertion into a neck or chest vein.

Potential complications of intravascular foreign bodies include clot formation and embolization, sepsis, cardiac dysrhythmias, and vascular or heart perforation with ensuing hemorrhage or cardiac tamponade. When feasible, intravascular foreign bodies should be retrieved by percutaneous means to prevent untoward consequences.[109] In most cases, long device dwell time itself is not a reason to avoid attempting removal.[110]

Technique

Several devices are available for endovascular retrieval. However, the most popular and versatile devices are the Amplatz nitinol gooseneck snare (Microvena) and the trilobed En Snare (Merit Medical).[111] The former system (Fig. 18-16) is available in a wide range of loop diameters and catheter sizes (standard, 5 to 35 mm, 4 to 6 Fr; micro, 2 to 7 mm, 3 Fr). The latter system (Fig. 18-17) is made in both standard (6 to 45 mm, 6 to 7 Fr) and mini sizes (2 to 8 mm, 3.2 Fr). An 8- to 10-Fr (or larger) vascular sheath is inserted in the common femoral or internal jugular vein. The sheath should be large enough to accommodate the collapsed foreign body and snare to minimize trauma to the access vein as the object is removed.

The guiding catheter provided with the kit is advanced through the vascular sheath up to the foreign body; the snare is inserted and exposed, and then manipulated around a free end (or loop) of the fragment (Fig. 18-18; see also Fig. 18-7). Often, both ends of the fragment abut the vein wall. In this case, the midsection of the fragment is engaged with a pigtail (or other) catheter. The pigtail is withdrawn at the access site to reposition the fragment and free one of the ends. After the fragment is snared (preferably near the tip), the wire loop is cinched around it tightly by withdrawing the snare wire while holding the guiding catheter stationary. The object then is pulled through the IVC or SVC into the sheath and out of the body. A *loop-snare technique* is also effective when simpler maneuvers do not work (see Fig. 16-24). Alternatively, an endomyocardial biopsy forceps device (Ceres Medical Systems) is used to directly grab the fragment without the need for a free end. Larger foreign bodies (e.g., IVC filters, stents) may require more

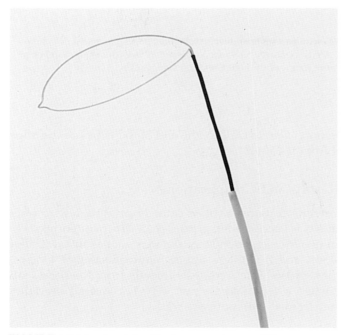

FIGURE 18-16 Amplatz nitinol gooseneck snare (Microvena, White Bear Lake, Minn.) with outer 6-Fr guiding catheter.

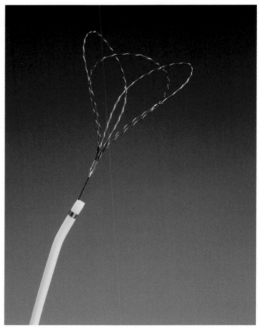

FIGURE 18-17 EnSnare trilobed retrieval device. (*Courtesy of Merit Medical.*)

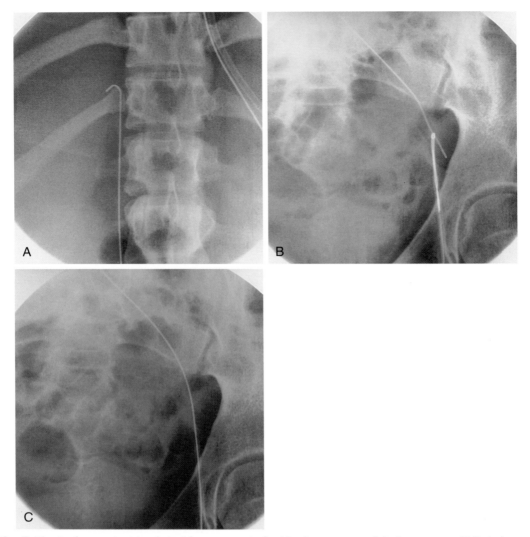

FIGURE 18-18   Guidewire fragment retrieval. **A,** A long segment of guidewire was severed during attempted blind placement of a central venous access device. The wire became lodged in the inferior vena cava. **B,** A nitinol gooseneck snare was inserted from the left femoral vein and used to grab the free end of the guidewire. **C,** The guidewire and snare are removed through a femoral vein sheath.

complex and creative maneuvers for removal[107,111-113] (Figs. 18-19 and 18-20). In some instances, the device must be withdrawn into the common femoral or internal jugular vein and removed through a simple surgical cut-down.

There are several ways to approach guidewires that have become trapped within IVC filters.[114,115] If the guidewire is still exiting the skin, a sheath may be placed over the wire and advanced into the IVC (Fig. 18-21). Gentle pressure may allow the wire to become dislodged from the catheter, both of which are then removed. Otherwise, a loop snare is introduced from the

femoral vein to capture the end of the wire and dislodge it from the filter.

Results and Complications

Percutaneous retrieval of catheter and guidewire fragments is successful in greater than 95% of attempts.[106,110] In many cases, even large devices such as intravascular stents and IVC filters can be removed safely.[116] One review of IVC filter removals (mostly from the heart) calculated a 69% success rate.[116,117] The overall mortality rate from all attempts was 6%.

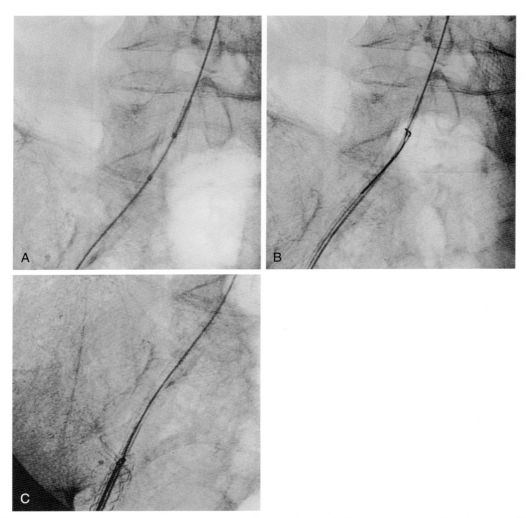

FIGURE 18-19 Retrieval of a Palmaz stent. **A,** Stent has slipped off an angioplasty balloon during renal artery treatment. **B,** A nitinol snare was placed around the lower end of the collapsed stent after the angioplasty balloon was removed. **C,** The stent was pulled into an 8-Fr sheath and removed.

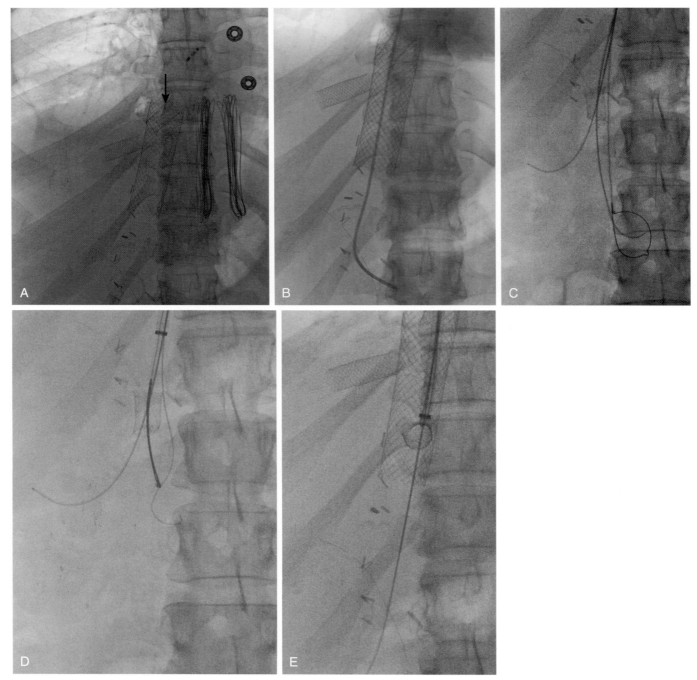

FIGURE 18-20   Retrieval of unstable Wallstent. Following orthotopic liver transplantation, hepatic confluence and inferior vena cava (IVC) stenosis had prompted placement of single IVC and dual hepatic vein Wallstents in Y-configuration. **A,** At the time of routine transjugular liver biopsy several months later, the central hepatic vein stent was noted to have migrated into the IVC *(arrow).* **B,** From the right jugular vein, a wire and then angled catheter were advanced through the barrel of the malpositioned stent. Manipulations caused the stent to move caudally. Through a 12-Fr vascular sheath, a gooseneck snare was advanced alongside the stent. **C,** The end of the guidewire running through the stent was captured with the snare. **D,** Both wires exiting the sheath at the neck were pulled, causing the stent to collapse and then be pulled into the sheath **(E).**

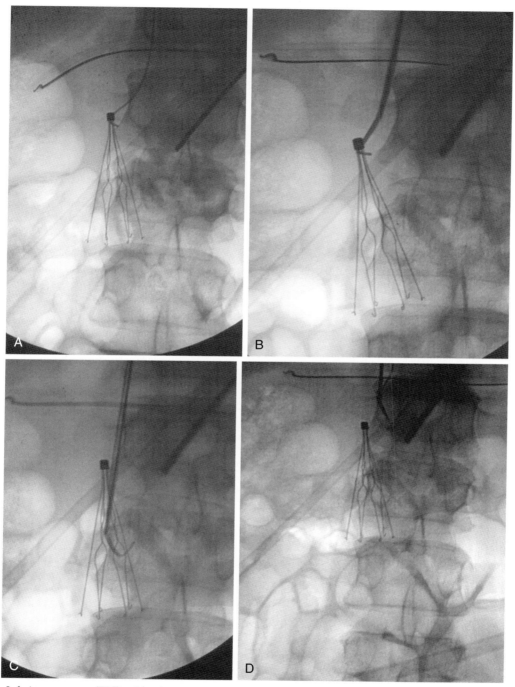

FIGURE 18-21   Inferior vena cava (IVC) guidewire entrapment. **A,** During bedside placement of a central venous line, the house officer felt resistance upon guidewire withdrawal from the subclavian vein. Subsequent image at fluoroscopy shows guidewire trapped in the legs of a Greenfield filter. **B,** A 5-Fr catheter was advanced over the wire into the IVC. **C,** A long vascular sheath was introduced over the catheter for stability. **D,** After advancing the entire system down off the filter neck, the guidewire was dislodged and ultimately removed.

References

1. Reeves AR, Seshadri R, Trerotola SO. Recent trends in central venous catheter placement: a comparison of interventional radiology with other specialties. *J Vasc Interv Radiol* 2001;**12**:1211.

2. McBride KD, Fisher R, Warnock N, et al. A comparative analysis of radiological and surgical placement of central venous catheters. *Cardiovasc Intervent Radiol* 1997;**20**:17.

3. Nosher JL, Shami MM, Siegel RL, et al. Tunneled central venous access catheter placement in the pediatric population: comparison of radiologic and surgical results. *Radiology* 1994;**192**:265.

4. Debourdeau P, Kassab Chahmi D, LeGal G, et al. 2008 SOR guidelines for the prevention and treatment of thrombosis associated with central venous catheters in patients with cancer: report from the working group. *Ann Oncol* 2009;**20**:1459.

5. Pasquale MD, Campbell JM, Magnant CM. Groshong versus Hickman catheters. *Surg Gynecol Obstet* 1992;**174**:408.

6. Biffi R, De Braud F, Orsi F, et al. A randomized, prospective trial of central venous ports connected to standard open-ended or Groshong catheters in adult oncology patients. *Cancer* 2001;**92**:1204.

7. Maki DG, Cobb L, Garman JK, et al. An attachable silver-impregnated cuff for prevention of infection with central venous catheters: a prospective randomized multicenter trial. *Am J Med* 1988;**85**:307.

8. Trerotola SO, Johnson MS, Shah H, et al. Tunneled hemodialysis catheters: use of a silver-coated catheter for prevention of infection—a randomized study. *Radiology* 1998;**207**:491.

9. Hockenhull JC, Dwan K, Boland A, et al. The clinical effectiveness and cost-effectiveness of central venous catheter treated with anti-infective agents in preventing bloodstream infections: a systematic review and economic evaluation. *Health Technol Assess* 2008;**12**:1.

10. Spector M, Mojibian H, Eliseo D, et al. Clinical outcome of the Tal Palindrome chronic hemodialysis catheter: single institution experience. *J Vasc Interv Radiol* 2008;**19**:1434.

11. Trerotola SO, Kraus M, Shah H, et al. Randomized comparison of split tip versus step tip high-flow hemodialysis catheters. *Kidney Int* 2002; **62**:282.

12. Richard III HM, Hastings GS, Boyd-Kranis RL, et al. A randomized, prospective evaluation of the Tesio, Ash split, and Opti-flow hemodialysis catheters. *J Vasc Interv Radiol* 2001;**12**:431.

13. Tal MG. Comparison of recirculation percentage of the Palindrome catheter and standard hemodialysis catheters in a swine model. *J Vasc Interv Radiol* 2005;**16**:1237.

14. Ash SR. Advances in tunneled central venous catheters for dialysis: design and performance. *Semin Dialysis* 2008;**21**:504.

15. Senecal L, Saint-Sauveur E, Leblanc M. Blood flow and recirculation rates in tunneled hemodialysis catheters. *ASAIO J* 2004;**50**:94.

16. Keung Y-K, Watkins K, Chen S-C, et al. Comparative study of infectious complications of different types of chronic central venous access devices. *Cancer* 1994;**73**:2832.

17. Mueller BU, Skelton J, Callender DPE, et al. A prospective randomized trial comparing the infectious and noninfectious complications of an externalized catheter versus a subcutaneously implanted device in cancer patients. *J Clin Oncol* 1992;**10**:1943.

18. Wilkin TD, Kraus MA, Lane KA, et al. Internal jugular vein thrombosis associated with hemodialysis catheters. *Radiology* 2003; **228**:697.

19. Trerotola SO, Kuhn-Fulton J, Johnson MS, et al. Tunneled infusion catheters: increased incidence of symptomatic venous thrombosis after subclavian versus internal jugular venous access. *Radiology* 2000; **217**:89.

20. Schillinger F, Schillinger D, Montagnac R, et al. Post catheterisation vein stenosis in haemodialysis: comparative angiographic study of 50 subclavian and 50 internal jugular accesses. *Nephrol Dial Transplant* 1991;**6**:722.

21. Funaki B, Zaleski GX, Leef JA, et al. Radiologic placement of tunneled hemodialysis catheters in occluded neck, chest, or small

22. thyrocervical collateral veins in central venous occlusion. *Radiology* 2001;**218**:471.

22. Weeks SM. Unconventional venous access. *Tech Vasc Interv Radiol* 2002;**5**:114.

23. Hamilton HC, Foxcroft DR. Central venous access sites for prevention of venous thrombosis, stenosis, and infection requiring long-term intravenous therapy. *Cochrane Database Syst Rev* 2007; **18**:CD004084.

24. Falk A. Use of the femoral vein as insertion site for tunneled hemodialysis catheters. *J Vasc Interv Radiol* 2007;**18**:217.

25. Contreras G, Liu PY, Elzinga L, et al. A multicenter, prospective randomized comparative evaluation of dual- versus triple-lumen catheters for hemodialysis and apheresis in 485 patients. *Am J Kidney Dis* 2003;**42**:315.

26. Smith TP, Ryan JM, Reddan DN. Transhepatic catheter access for hemodialysis. *Radiology* 2004;**232**:246.

27. Rajan DK, Croteau DL, Sturza SG, et al. Translumbar placement of inferior vena caval catheters: a solution for challenging hemodialysis access. *Radiographics* 1998;**18**:1155.

28. Stavropoulos SW, Pan JJ, Clark TWI, et al. Percutaneous transhepatic venous access for hemodialysis. *J Vasc Interv Radiol* 2003; **14**:1187.

29. Lewis CA, Allen TE, Burke DR, et al. Quality improvement guidelines for central venous access. *J Vasc Interv Radiol* 2003;**14**:S231.

30. Haas B, Chittams JL, Trerotola SO. Large-bore tunneled central venous catheter insertion in patients with coagulopathy. *J Vasc Interv Radiol* 2010;**21**:212.

31. Gordon AC, Saliken JC, Johns D, et al. US-guided puncture of the internal jugular vein: complications and anatomic considerations. *J Vasc Interv Radiol* 1998;**9**:333.

32. Contractor SG, Phatak TD, Klyde D, et al. Single-incision technique for tunneled central venous access. *J Vasc Interv Radiol* 2009; **20**:1052.

33. Diaz ML, Villanueva A, Herraiz MJ, et al. Computed tomographic appearance of chest ports and catheters: a pictorial review for noninterventional radiologists. *Curr Probl Diagn Radiol* 2009;**38**:99.

34. Mirza B, Vanek VW, Kupensky DT. Pinch-off syndrome: case report and collective review of the literature. *Am Surg* 2004;**70**:635.

35. Elduayen B, Martinez-Cuesta A, Vivas I, et al. Central venous catheter placement in the inferior vena cava via the direct translumbar approach. *Eur Radiol* 2000;**10**:450.

36. Murthy R, Arbabzadeh M, Lund G, et al. Percutaneous transrenal hemodialysis catheter insertion. *J Vasc Interv Radiol* 2002;**13**:1043.

37. Nazarian GK, Bjarnason H, Dietz Jr CA, et al. Changes in tunneled catheter tip position when a patient is upright. *J Vasc Interv Radiol* 1997;**8**:437.

38. Kowalski CM, Kaufman JA, Rivitz SM, et al. Migration of central venous catheters: implications for initial catheter tip positioning. *J Vasc Interv Radiol* 1997;**8**:443.

39. Forauer AR, Alonzo M. Change in peripherally inserted central catheter tip position with abduction and adduction of the upper extremity. *J Vasc Interv Radiol* 2000;**11**:1315.

40. Schutz JC, Patel AA, Clark TW, et al. Relationship between chest port catheter tip position and port malfunction after interventional radiologic placement. *J Vasc Interv Radiol* 2004;**15**:581.

41. Vesely TM. Central venous catheter tip position: a continuing controversy. *J Vasc Interv Radiol* 2003;**14**:527.

42. Luciani A, Clement O, Halimi P, et al. Catheter-related upper extremity deep venous thrombosis in cancer patients: a prospective study based on Doppler US. *Radiology* 2001;**220**:655.

43. Eastridge BJ, Lefor AT. Complications of indwelling venous access devices in cancer patients. *J Clin Oncol* 1995;**13**:233.

44. Cadman A, Lawrance JA, Fitzsimmons L, et al. To clot or not to clot? That is the question in central venous catheters. *Clin Radiol* 2004;**59**:349.

19

Hemodialysis Access

Erik Ray, Anne C. Roberts

ACCESS CONSTRUCTION

The ideal hemodialysis access is an endogenous fistula created by surgical anastomosis of an artery and vein. The updated National Kidney Foundation Kidney Dialysis Outcomes Quality Initiative (NKF-KDOQI) and clinical practice guidelines have set a goal of primary arteriovenous fistula construction in at least 65% of all new patients with kidney failure, with ultimately 65% of hemodialysis patients having a native fistula.[1] Arteriovenous (AV) accesses are placed as far distally in the upper extremity as possible to preserve proximal sites for future access. Ideal access is within the upper extremity and preferentially within the nondominant arm if opportunities exist.

- The *radiocephalic (Brescia-Cimino) fistula* is a side-to-side anastomosis of the radial artery and the cephalic vein at the wrist (Figs. 19-1 and 19-2); it is the first choice for a permanent access.[1]
- A *brachiocephalic fistula* also can be constructed between the brachial artery and the cephalic vein[1] (see Fig. 19-1). This access is more likely to result in arm swelling or distal ischemia than a more peripheral fistula.
- The *transposed brachiobasilic fistula* involves lateral rotation and superficialization of the basilic vein to allow easy cannulation (see Fig. 19-1).
- Less common forms include connections between the brachial artery and a median antecubital vein *(brachiomedian antecubital fistula),* and between the femoral artery and saphenous vein.[2]

Although an autologous arteriovenous fistula (AVF) is the ideal hemodialysis access, it may be difficult or impossible to create successfully in a significant number of patients. Failures are particularly common in older and diabetic patients. Still, with careful evalua-tion even these high-risk patients may be suitable for a fistula.[3] The reported failure rates range from 10% to 65%, but the usual figure in modern practice is about 15% to 25%.[3-8]

Because a fistula requires 3 to 4 months to mature, it should be created well in advance of the anticipated need for dialysis.[1,9] The veins in the arm must not have been damaged by previous venipunctures. Fistulas are ready for use when the blood flow is greater than 600 mL/min, vein diameter is at least 0.6 cm, depth under skin is less than 0.6 cm, and there are discernible vein margins under the skin.[1] In one postoperative study, fistulas with a diameter of at least 4 mm and a blood flow greater than 500 mL/min had a 95% likelihood of success for dialysis.[10] If an endogenous fistula can be constructed and matures properly, it should have excellent long-term patency.

A *synthetic graft* is the alternative to an endogenous fistula. These grafts are commonly made of polytetrafluoroethylene (PTFE). They may be placed in the forearm in a straight configuration from the radial artery to a brachial vein, but a looped configuration from the brachial artery to a brachial vein (Fig. 19-3) usually is preferred.[1] Grafts also may be constructed in the upper arm, usually in a looped configuration from the brachial or axillary artery to a high arm vein. If all possible sites in the arm and chest are exhausted, a loop graft can be placed in the thigh from the common femoral artery to the common femoral vein.

PTFE grafts may be used much earlier than native fistulas, usually within 14 days of placement.[1] However, they do not have the longevity that can be achieved with an endogenous fistula. Primary patency rate at 1 year is reported to be approximately 40%.[4,11] Secondary patency rate ranges from 60% to 90%.[1,12] The most common reason for failure is development of a stenosis in the outflow vein, leading to thrombosis of the graft.[1]

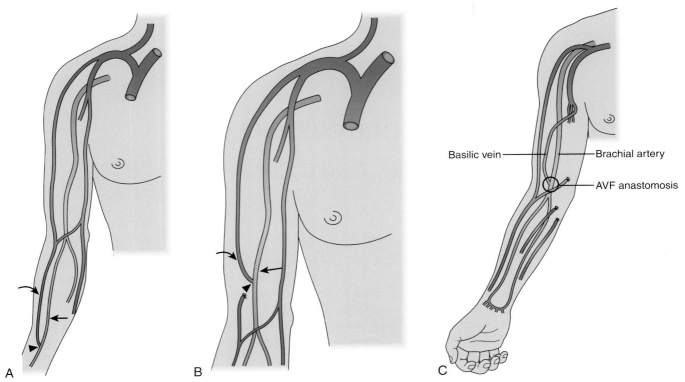

Basilic vein —————————— Brachial artery

————— AVF anastomosis

A   B   C

FIGURE 19-1   Hemodialysis access. **A,** Endogenous radiocephalic arteriovenous fistula. Note the inflow radial artery *(arrow)*, arteriovenous anastomosis *(arrowhead)*, and outflow cephalic vein *(curved arrow)*. **B,** Endogenous brachiocephalic fistula. Note the inflow brachial artery *(arrow)*, arteriovenous anastomosis *(arrowhead),* and outflow cephalic vein *(curved arrow)*. **C,** Endogenous transposed brachiobasilic fistula. Note the inflow brachial artery, arteriovenous anastomosis, and the transposed basilic vein.

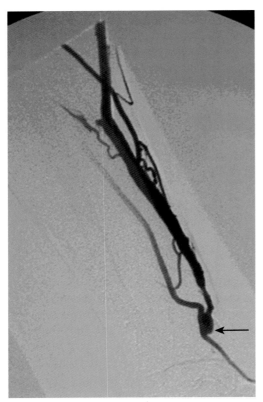

FIGURE 19-2   Normal radiocephalic dialysis fistula with arteriovenous anastomosis at wrist *(arrow)*.

MAJOR DISORDERS

Immature or Failing Dialysis Access (Online Cases 60 and 72)

Etiology

It is crucial to extend the functional life of each access for as long as possible, because the sites available for dialysis fistulas are limited and patients are dependent on dialysis for survival.

Some dialysis AVFs fail to become usable for dialysis. Causes of an *immature fistula* are outlined in Box 19-1. Ultrasound may be very helpful in evaluating the dysfunctional access and identifying the source of the problem. On physical examination, it may be possible to determine the etiology based on the pulse or thrill within or caliber of the outflow vein(s). Multiple small veins with a palpable thrill may be present instead of a single dominant vein. In other cases, the fistula may have developed but may have decreased flow and appear flat, suggesting a problem in the juxtaanastomotic region. If the vein is dilated in one area but then becomes flat further up the arm, an outflow problem is indicated.

Mature but failing arteriovenous fistulas may have multiple, tandem stenoses at various points in the access

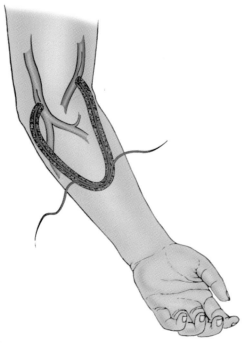

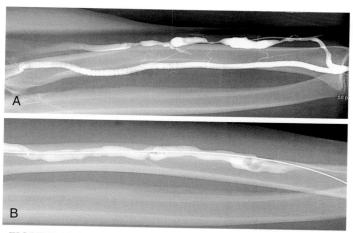

FIGURE 19-4   Endogenous radiocephalic arteriovenous fistula. **A,** Multiple outflow stenoses. **B,** Improvement after using a 6-mm angioplasty balloon.

FIGURE 19-3   Synthetic loop graft from the distal brachial artery to the cephalic vein. Crossed catheters are in place for pulse-spray thrombolysis. *(From Valji K. Pharmacomechanical thrombolysis of thrombosed hemodialysis access grafts. Semin Dialysis 1998;11:374.)*

circuit. The clinical consequences include large collateral veins, arm swelling, and inefficient dialysis from high venous pressure and low flow (Fig. 19-4). Synthetic dialysis grafts most often fail because of a venous anastomotic stenosis. In both types of access, veins that are subjected to the high flows, high pressures, vibratory and stretching effects, compliance mismatch, and turbulence are prone to develop stenoses from neointimal hyperplasia.[13-15] Regardless of the cause, the venous stenoses progressively worsen until blood flow is markedly reduced and thrombosis occurs. These venous lesions often recur (again and again) at the same site.

BOX 19-1

CAUSES OF IMMATURE DIALYSIS FISTULAS

- Juxtaanastomotic ("swing point") stenosis
- Damaged target veins
- Poor arterial inflow
- Central venous outflow obstruction
- Large collateral veins

Surveillance and Imaging

The NKF-KDOQI guidelines recommend an organized monitoring program to identify access in jeopardy of thrombosis by regular assessment of several clinical and functional dialysis parameters.[1] Proper clinical evaluation should be performed at least monthly and consists of inspection, physical examination, and auscultation of the fistula or graft. Although there continues to be controversy regarding the benefit of vascular access surveillance, surveillance can be performed in a number of direct and indirect methods. Direct monitoring may include intra-access flow, static venous dialysis pressure, and dynamic venous pressure.[1,9,16-19] Other studies that are used to detect arteriovenous graft stenosis include measurement of access recirculation, decreases in the measured amount of hemodialysis delivered, or elevated negative arterial pre-pump pressures that hinder blood flow.[1,20-22] Normal flow in a graft should be in excess of 800 to 1000 mL/min, and if flows decrease to less than 400 to 600 mL/min, risk of failure is increased.[1,23,24] Clinical indicators include changes in the physical characteristics of the graft thrill, difficulty with needle placement, prolonged bleeding after needle removal, swelling of the arm, or, ultimately, clotting of the graft.[1,25-27]

Persistent abnormalities in any of these parameters suggest graft dysfunction and should prompt venographic evaluation of the graft. Venography can be performed easily after dialysis through the indwelling needles or can be performed at a separate session, usually before dialysis. If a stenosis is discovered at the time of the venogram, angioplasty can be performed immediately. Early correction of venous stenoses reduces thrombosis rates. In a number of studies, a 50% to 90% decrease in the thrombosis rate can occur when monitoring is instituted[28,29] and prolongs access viability.[1,9,17,30,31]

Surveillance for AVFs depends on many of the same methods as those used for grafts. Physical examination is very helpful and may be even more informative than with grafts.[32] Ultrasound can be used both preoperatively to increase the rate of successful fistula placements[33] and to evaluate fistula maturation.[34] The other measures of graft function (recirculation, increased static venous pressures, decreased flow rates) are also evidence of fistula malfunction, but the thresholds for abnormality are not well established. As a result of the low resistance and presence of the collateral veins, a venous stenosis causes a reduction in blood flow in a fistula without the corresponding increase in access pressure.[35]

Endovascular Therapy

PATIENT SELECTION

The results of both percutaneous and surgical repair of failing dialysis access are disappointing. Several studies have reported comparable primary patency rates at 6 months (less than 25%) and 12 months.[29,30] The NKF-KDOQI advises that each dialysis center determine which procedure is best for an individual patient based on local expertise. Surgical revision is held to a higher standard than percutaneous transluminal angioplasty, because surgical revision usually extends the access further up the extremity by the use of a jump graft.[1]

Although angioplasty is plagued with the same problems with recurrent stenosis as surgery, it does have some advantages. Patients accept percutaneous balloon angioplasty better than they do a surgical procedure. The angioplasty procedure avoids using a site further up the venous outflow, leaving it available for subsequent revision when it becomes necessary. The graft is immediately available for dialysis, avoiding the need for temporary dialysis catheters. Redilations allow easy and safe graft salvage for months or years.[25] New data also demonstrate promising results with stent grafts at graft-related stenoses.[36] Percutaneous revision of venous anastomotic stenoses within a prosthetic hemodialysis graft with the use of a stent graft appears to provide superior long-term patency than standard balloon angioplasty.

TECHNIQUE

Dialysis graft/fistula venography should include a complete evaluation of the circuit from the inflow artery to the superior vena cava. Access is usually done by palpation in the direction of suspected disease. Evaluation of fistulas can be more complicated. A variety of techniques can be used to help with a difficult access. Real-time ultrasound guidance is extremely helpful. A tourniquet can be used to impede outflow and increase the size of the target veins. If direct fistula access fails, the brachial artery is punctured with a micropuncture needle central to the anastomosis.

The 3-French (Fr) inner dilator of the micropuncture set allows diagnostic angiography and minimizes the risk for complications.[37-41] Direct arterial access also allows evaluation of the palmar arch and antegrade or retrograde filling of the distal segment of the artery feeding the fistula.[37] After the diagnostic study has been performed, the fistula can be cannulated by a retrograde approach.[37]

Venous stenoses in fistulas are seen with both immature and mature accesses. Turmel-Rodrigues and colleagues[42] think these venous stenoses must be dilated to at least 5 mm to obtain adequate flows.[42] However, in a poorly developed fistula, it may be important to perform serial dilations, starting with undersized balloons (3 to 4 mm) to avoid rupturing a small, fragile vein. If the vein is not well developed, dilation with a small balloon during one procedure and a repeat evaluation in 1 to 3 weeks with dilation using a larger balloon may allow for development of the venous outflow and maturation of the fistula (see discussion below). One of the more common sites of stenosis in a brachiocephalic fistula involves the cephalic arch region with a 39% prevalence of stenosis.[43,44] This region is less problematic with a radiocephalic fistula with an overall prevalence of 2%.[43] Traditional angioplasty results within this region have been disappointing, with primary patency at 3, 6, and 12 months at 96%, 83%, and 75%, respectively.[44] These outcomes have been in part due to the resistant nature of the stenosis, early restenosis, high vein rupture rates, and other anatomic and hemodynamic considerations.[45]

As many as 30% of native fistulas never mature to enable cannulation and allow for successful hemodialysis.[46-49] If a fistula fails to mature over the first 1 to 3 months, early fistulography can enable identification of an underlying stenosis for endovascular treatment (Fig. 19-5). The initial salvage rate of nonmaturing AVFs ranges in the literature from 74% to 97%.[50-57] Numerous techniques have been used to improve fistula function, including venous and arterial angioplasty, stent placement, thrombectomy, venous branch ligation, and fistula superficialization.[58-59] In an effort to increase the number of primary fistulas and expedite the use of a functional AVF, two new techniques have emerged, which include primary balloon angioplasty during fistula creation (in selected patients with small veins) and "balloon-assisted maturation" of immature AVFs by angioplasty.[60,61] These techniques allow use of small or suboptimal veins to create functioning fistulas within 2 months and increase overall functional AVF rates to 90%.[60,61]

Venous anastomotic stenoses are the most common reason for malfunction of dialysis grafts. They usually occur in the vein within a few centimeters of the graft-vein anastomosis (Figs. 19-6 and 19-7). At times, multiple venous channels may overlap and conceal important stenosis. Several oblique views may be required

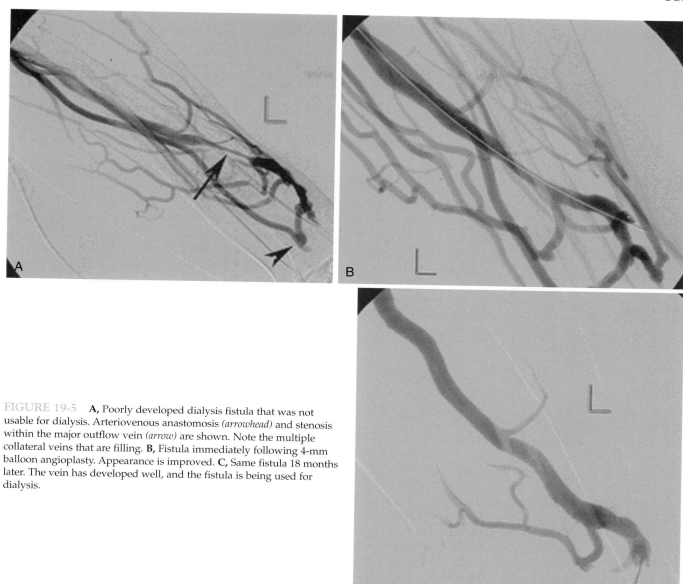

FIGURE 19-5 **A,** Poorly developed dialysis fistula that was not usable for dialysis. Arteriovenous anastomosis *(arrowhead)* and stenosis within the major outflow vein *(arrow)* are shown. Note the multiple collateral veins that are filling. **B,** Fistula immediately following 4-mm balloon angioplasty. Appearance is improved. **C,** Same fistula 18 months later. The vein has developed well, and the fistula is being used for dialysis.

to visualize the narrowing. NKF-KDOQI guidelines recommend treating stenoses greater than 50% only when there are concomitant clinical abnormalities and flow-rate reduction or pressure changes. After the stenosis is found, it is dilated with an appropriately sized angioplasty balloon catheter. Balloon diameter is generally 1 mm larger than the graft or 10% to 20% oversized compared to the adjacent normal vein. In the forearm and near the elbow, a 6- or 7-mm balloon typically is used initially. On occasion, veins may require 5- to 8-mm balloons. High-pressure balloons (burst pressures 20 to 30 mm Hg) often are required to dilate these lesions. Very high pressures (>20 atm) are more frequently needed in

native fistulas.[62] Some data may suggest longer inflation times are associated with less residual stenosis.[62]

If the stenosis does not yield to balloon dilation (*resistant stenosis*), repeated inflations may be required to open the vessel. Multiple, prolonged inflations (e.g., 5 minutes) are thought to be useful in resistant lesions. *Cutting balloons* have been used for extremely resistant stenoses[63-67] (Fig. 19-8). The devices have multiple microblades embedded in the balloon that incise the fibrotic vein wall and allow successful angioplasty to follow. There is no evidence that cutting balloons are superior to standard balloons for simple stenoses.[68] However, improved 6-month primary patency rates are noted for truly resistant lesions.[69]

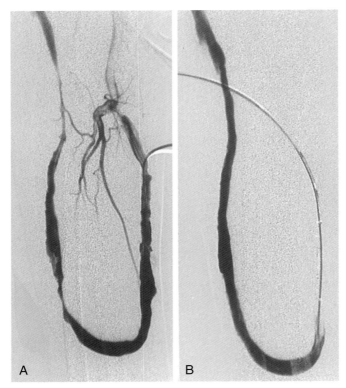

FIGURE 19-6   Venous anastomotic and intragraft stenoses.
A, Initial fistulogram through a catheter placed in the arterial limb
of the graft shows both lesions responsible for elevated venous
pressures at dialysis. **B,** After angioplasty with a 7-mm balloon, the
stenoses are relieved.

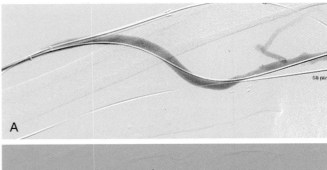

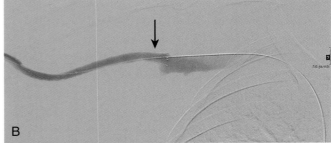

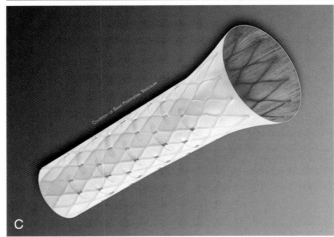

FIGURE 19-7   Primary treatment of venous stenosis with the
use of a stent graft within a right upper extremity graft. **A,** Stenosis
involving the venous anastomosis. **B,** Treatment of the lesion with
7-mm Flair stents *(arrow),* with flaired component extending into the
right axillary vein. **C,** Flair stent. *(Courtesy of Bard Peripheral Vascular.)*

In other cases, the balloon may completely inflate, but
the stenosis remains at angiography following the inflation *(elastic stenosis).* Multiple (usually two) cycles of
prolonged angioplasty (e.g., 5 minutes) can be effective
for treatment of elastic stenoses. If the patient has minimal to no pain with the initial angioplasty, a larger balloon can be used. Cutting balloons have also been used
to correct the elastic recoil. Regardless of the method, the
goal of angioplasty is less than 30% residual stenosis
after treatment, restoration of the thrill in the access, and
successful dialysis.[70]

Stent placement has been used for venous stenoses, but
the use of stents should be very selective. Indications for
metal stents include surgically inaccessible stenoses that
fail angioplasty, postangioplasty vein rupture not responsive to repeat balloon inflation, elastic recoil, and frequent
or exuberant restenosis[1] (Fig. 19-9). Stents may improve
the immediate results of angioplasty, but their long-term
benefit often is less favorable. Intimal hyperplasia commonly develops within the stent as well as at the ends of
the stent. Veins that could be used for a new access should
not be stented because that intervention limits potential
revision. The safety of stent insertion at sites of bending
or motion (e.g., the elbow joint) is debatable.

There are promising data concerning the use of stent
grafts within dysfunctional grafts and fistulas (see Figs.
19-7 and 19-9). A covered stent may prevent or limit restenosis related to intimal hyperplasia.[71] In a limited retrospective study, stent graft placement in dysfunctional
autogenous hemodialysis fistulas was effective in preserving function and preventing access abandonment
with patency exceeding angioplasty and uncovered
stents.[72] The new Flair (Bard Peripheral Vascular, Tempe,
Ariz.) stent graft is designed to optimize flow when the
graft and outflow vein have a diameter mismatch (see
Fig. 19-7). The device is covered with ePTFE and includes
a 4-mm flared end that extends into the outflow vein
for improved flow dynamics. A recent randomized trial

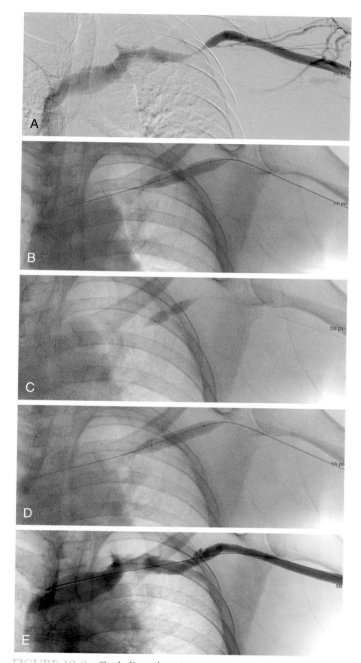

FIGURE 19-8   Cephalic arch resistant stenosis in a patient with a left upper extremity brachiocephalic fistula. **A,** Tight stenosis at the cephalic arch. **B,** Stenosis was resistant to 10-mm high pressure balloon angioplasty. **C,** An 8-mm cutting balloon in place in the lesion. The lesion can now be dilated. **D,** Successful relief of stenosis with a high-pressure 10-mm angioplasty balloon. **E,** No evidence of stenosis remains.

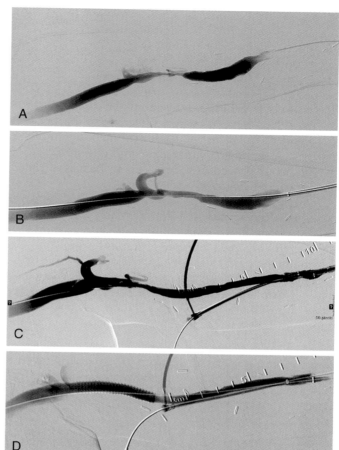

FIGURE 19-9   Elastic stenosis within upper extremity fistula treated with covered stent for salvage. **A,** Tight stenosis at basilic vein transposition swing point. **B,** Stenosis treated with angioplasty but elastic recoil is evident. **C,** Patient presents 6 weeks later with clotted fistula due to stenosis. After thrombus is removed, recurrent elastic stenosis remains. **D,** Successful treatment with a Viabahn covered stent. *(Courtesy of W.L. Gore and Associates, Flagstaff, Ariz.)*

noted significantly better long term patency and freedom from repeat interventions than standard balloon angioplasty.[36] Covered stents also allow rapid treatment of an acute venous rupture after angioplasty if balloon tamponade fails. [50,73-76]

Typically, a bare metal stent diameter 10% to 20% larger than the diameter of the blood vessel at the site of deployment is chosen, ideally with extension into normal adjacent vein being less than 10 mm. Technical considerations for stent grafts are slightly different, with only minor stent diameter oversizing (about 10%) recommended to avoid graft material infolding.

Arterial stenoses have been reported as being responsible for graft dysfunction in up to 28% of cases, although some series have noted an incidence of less than 15%.[77-80] Construction of the dialysis access creates a low-resistance/high-flow circuit that may unmask a significant arterial inflow stenosis.[77,80] The inflow artery and arterial anastomosis are visualized by direct injection at this site, manually compressing the mid-portion of the graft during injection, or inflating a balloon catheter with the end hole directed toward the anastomosis.

Several projections may be required to adequately delineate the arterial inflow. If a significant arterial stenosis is identified, angioplasty usually is indicated. The lesion often can be reached through the access. Otherwise, a direct brachial (or common femoral) arterial puncture is necessary. In some cases, the arterial lesion is in the inflow vessels, so arteriography should be considered during the evaluation of a dysfunctional access, particularly if the patient has recurring graft dysfunction without an evident cause.[77,81] Measuring flow and pressures during percutaneous procedures may lead to increased detection of arterial stenoses.[77]

Intragraft stenoses are relatively uncommon. These stenoses usually respond well to angioplasty (see Fig. 19-6). Balloon sizing in the graft should take into account that these grafts are most commonly 6 mm in diameter. Occasionally the grafts also are tapered at the arterial anastomosis (4 to 6 mm or 4 to 7 mm). In most cases a balloon that is 1 mm larger than the graft diameter is an appropriate size. If there is graft degeneration, it is particularly important that a larger balloon not be used because the graft can rupture.

Central venous stenoses are an important, although less frequent, problem with hemodialysis grafts. Stenosis of the subclavian and brachiocephalic veins usually is caused by venous injury from prior dialysis catheters (Fig. 19-10). The importance of these obstructions is their potential to compromise future dialysis access sites and to cause significant arm swelling. Outflow stenoses should be treated with angioplasty only if they are considered to be responsible for graft dysfunction (see Fig. 19-10). If the lesion is not causing symptoms, it should be left alone. Angioplasty of symptomatic central venous stenoses greater than 50% have been associated with more rapid stenosis progression of the lesion.[82] If a patient has a thrombosed graft, the most likely culprit is a stenosis at the venous anastomosis. Unless the outflow is thrombosed up to the level of the central vein, a central venous obstruction alone is probably not responsible for thrombosis. Near the shoulder and in the central veins, 10- to 12-mm balloons (or larger) may be necessary. The results of stent placement are not markedly better than those of balloon angioplasty in the central veins.[83] The NKF-KDOQI and

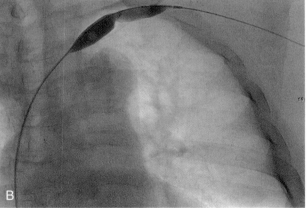

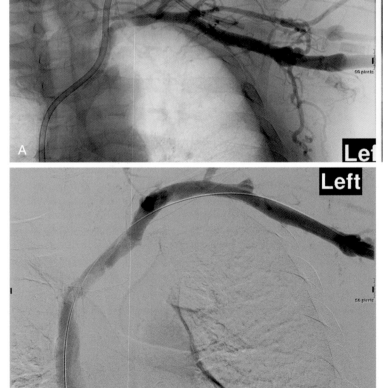

FIGURE 19-10   Treatment of central venous occlusion with angioplasty for dysfunctional left upper extremity fistula. **A,** Occlusion of the left brachiocephalic vein from a left internal jugular central venous catheter with neck collaterals in a patient with a left upper extremity fistula. **B,** Successful angioplasty with a 12-mm balloon from a right groin approach. **C,** The stenosis is improved, and collateral circulation has resolved.

Society of Interventional Radiology guidelines recommend transluminal angioplasty as the preferred treatment for central vein stenosis, and stent placement is indicated only with elastic lesions, when stenosis recurs within 3 months, or with occluded vessels[1,84] (Fig. 19-11). The stent needs to be carefully oversized to avoid migration.[85-88] Balloon-expandable stents must be avoided at sites subject to extrinsic compression (e.g., subclavian vein running through the costoclavicular space). Stents should not be placed across the internal jugular or contralateral innominate veins, which may be needed for future dialysis catheters.

RESULTS

Published series of nonthrombosed PTFE arteriovenous grafts have a reported 6-month primary (unassisted) patency of 40% to 50% after angioplasty.[89-94] Repeated angioplasty enabled a primary assisted patency of 68% at 1 year and 51% at 2 years in one study. The secondary patency rate (allowing for intercurrent thrombolysis and angioplasty) was 82% at 1 year and 65% at 2 years in the same study. Although these patency rates seem low, they are comparable to results of operative treatment. Based on such reports, NKF-KDOQI endorses secondary patency rates after endovascular treatment for dysfunction of at least 70% at 1 year, 60% at 2 years, and 50% at 3 years.[1] Primary unassisted patency (time from one intervention to any other intervention to maintain patency) following angioplasty of failing grafts should approach 50% at 6 months.[1] The role of stent grafts for treatment of venous anastomotic graft stenoses has shown promise, with recent data demonstrating 6-month treatment site and total access circuit patency of 51% and 38% in the stent graft group and 23% and 20% in the balloon angioplasty group, respectively.[36] In addition, freedom from subsequent interventions at 6 months was significantly greater in the stent graft group than in the balloon angioplasty group (32% vs. 16%). Longer-term data are unavailable, but stent grafts may have an important impact on future management of access grafts.

Clinical results for dialysis AVFs are variable. The initial salvage of nonmaturing AVFs ranges from 74% to 97% in the literature.[50-57] One study of dysfunctional fistulas had a primary, assisted primary, and secondary patency rates in 53 dysfunctional fistulas after intervention at 3 months of 84% ± 5%, 88% ± 5%, and 90% ± 4%, respectively. At 6 months, the patency rates were 55% ± 8%, 80% ± 6%, and 82% ± 6%. At 12 months the rates were 26% ± 11%, 80% ± 6%, and 82% ± 6%.[95] Turmel-Rodrigues reported a primary patency rate of 39% and a secondary patency rate of 79% at 12 months in dysfunctional forearm fistulas, and a rate of 57% in patients with upper arm fistulas.[96] Others have reported a 1-year secondary patency rate of 64% and a 2-year secondary patency rate of 53%, with fewer procedures to keep the fistulas functioning in comparison with grafts.[4]

In one report of 20 dialysis patients treated with stents in the central veins, primary patency rates of 90% at 1 month, 67% at 3 months, 42% at 6 months, and 25% at 1 year were noted. Assisted primary patency (additional angioplasty, stenting, or both) were 88% at 3 months, 62% at 6 months, and 47% at 1 year in that series.[97] Another study of 22 patients with a mix of stent devices showed primary patency rates after 3, 6, 9, and 12 months of 82%, 73%, 56%, and 43%, respectively. The primary assisted patency rates at the same time periods

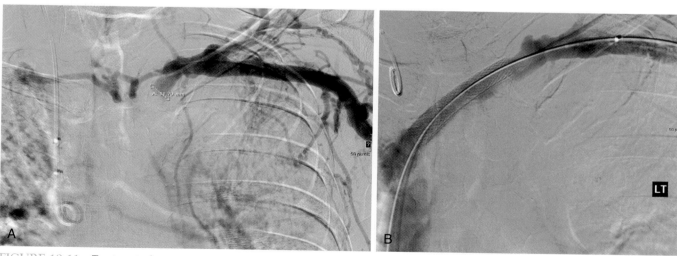

FIGURE 19-11 Treatment of recurrent central venous occlusion with stenting. **A,** Occlusion of the left brachiocephalic vein with neck collaterals in a patient with a left upper extremity fistula. **B,** Successful stenting with 14-mm Wallstent with improved patency. (*Courtesy of Boston Scientific, Natick, Mass.*)

was 91%, 90%, 88%, and 83%, respectively.[98] For salvage of angioplasty-induced vein rupture, the reported primary patency rates in one study were 52% at 60 days, 26% at 6 months, and 11% at 1 year.[99] Nitinol stents may have slightly more advantageous characteristics, which provide superior long-term patency when compared with other materials.[100] One study using Wallstents for graft-related venous stenoses reported a primary patency rate of 46% at 6 months, compared with another study revealing primary graft patency rates of 77% at 3 months and 51% at 6 months with a Smart nitinol stent.[101,102] In another investigation, the mean primary graft patency after percutaneous transluminal balloon angioplasty was 5.6 months compared with 8.2 months after Smart stent treatment.[103] Studies have shown no advantage of Wallstent placement for recurring peripheral venous stenoses compared with successful angioplasty.[104]

COMPLICATIONS

Complications from endovascular treatment of dysfunctional dialysis access are uncommon. Most complications entail minor, self-limited bleeding or hematoma formation. Occasionally, damage to the veins may occur, including rupture. Ruptures appear to be somewhat more common in autologous fistulas. The significance of the vein rupture depends on the extent of the leak. Because the angioplasty balloon should already be in place, the balloon can be placed across the rupture to seal the leak (Fig. 19-12). If prolonged balloon inflation (5 to 10 minutes) does not seal the rupture after two or three attempts, a bare or covered stent should be considered[50] (Fig. 19-13). If stenting is not an option or ineffective, the operator may be forced to control the rupture by manual compression of the access to achieve thrombosis. Vascular rupture should occur only in 2% to 4% of cases, and perforation requiring blood transfusion, emergent surgery, or limb-threatening ischemia should occur in fewer than 0.5% of cases.[84]

Surgical Therapy

Several surgical options are available for treatment of obstructions that fail to respond to percutaneous interventions, including revision with patch grafting, a jump graft with extension of the graft farther up along the venous outflows, or complete graft replacement.[105,106] Revision is preferred over a new graft when feasible. Replacement has the disadvantage of exhausting access sites much more rapidly. The 1-year primary patency rate after surgical revision is as low as 25%, with a secondary patency rate reported at 60% to 70%.[106,107] Most grafts require multiple additional procedures to maintain patency.

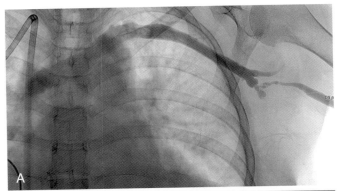

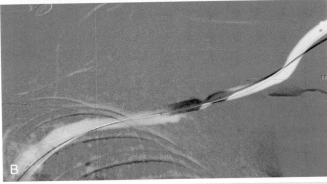

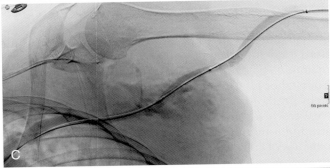

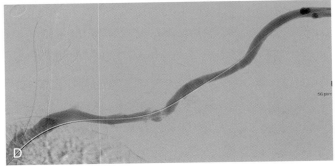

FIGURE 19-12   Immature left upper extremity fistula with angioplasty induced rupture treated with balloon tamponade. **A,** Tight stenosis within the left axillary vein. **B,** Stenosis relieved with angioplasty using an 8-mm balloon. **C,** Active extravasation after angioplasty. **D,** After two rounds of prolonged (e.g., 5 to 10 minutes) balloon inflation, no evidence of residual stenosis or extravasation is seen.

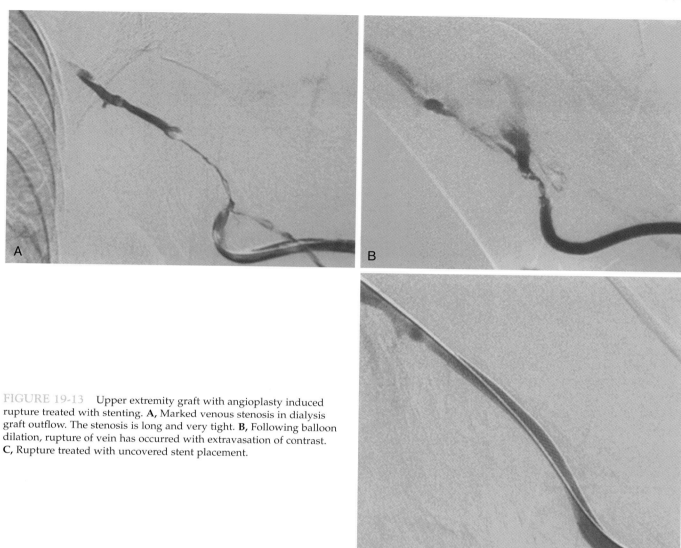

FIGURE 19-13   Upper extremity graft with angioplasty induced rupture treated with stenting. **A,** Marked venous stenosis in dialysis graft outflow. The stenosis is long and very tight. **B,** Following balloon dilation, rupture of vein has occurred with extravasation of contrast. **C,** Rupture treated with uncovered stent placement.

Thrombosed Dialysis Fistulas and Grafts

Etiology

In most cases, graft thrombosis occurs because of progressive stenosis in the graft circuit (usually at the venous end). The goal of graft or fistula surveillance is to identify and repair lesions that threaten access patency. It is much easier and less expensive to correct a venous stenosis than to have to declot the graft/fistula and then correct the venous stenosis that caused the thrombosis. Occasionally, dialysis access will clot because of hypotension, graft infection, trauma, or a hypercoagulable state.

Endovascular Therapy

PATIENT SELECTION

Virtually all patients with clotted dialysis access are candidates for percutaneous therapy. Unique characteristics of dialysis grafts make them particularly suitable for this approach. They are easy to access because of their superficial location, they contain fresh clot (usually not more than 48 to 72 hours old), and they are a closed system with only a single inflow and (sometimes) outflow. The criteria for rejecting patients for pharmacologic graft thrombolysis are similar to those for other thrombolysis procedures. If pharmacologic therapy is not appropriate, mechanical thrombolysis can be used. Absolute contraindications to pharmacologic therapy include recent cerebrovascular process/disease/procedure (tumor, recent stoke, trauma, surgery) or active gastrointestinal bleeding. Relative contraindications include major surgery or organ biopsy within 2 weeks, recent serious trauma, preexisting uncorrectable coagulation defects, uncontrolled severe hypertension, and pregnancy.

Dialysis graft infection is an important contraindication to any type of thrombolysis. Lysis of infected clot can precipitate bacteremia and lethal sepsis. Determining whether a graft is infected can be difficult.[108] Classic signs of infection (i.e., redness, tenderness, warmth, swelling, and fever) may be subtle or absent in patients with chronic renal failure. Definite signs of infection, such as a purulent discharge or skin breakdown over the graft, are rare. Needle aspirates of graft clot or fluid collections around the graft can be sent for Gram stain and culture.[109] Infection of the graft requires treatment with antibiotics and referral for surgical removal.

Small pulmonary emboli are produced during most percutaneous dialysis graft declotting procedures.[110-112] Although most patients tolerate these emboli, patients with significant pulmonary hypertension or severe underlying lung disease may not. A known right-to-left cardiac shunt (which could result in embolic stroke) is a strict contraindication to any type of lysis procedure.

Grafts that fail within days to several weeks of placement usually have a technical problem responsible for thrombosis. Although the graft may not be salvageable with percutaneous therapy, thrombolysis or simple contrast injection of the venous anastomosis and outflow veins may help guide surgical revision. Although some risk of hemorrhage from the anastomoses exists, manual compression usually controls such bleeding.

PULSE-SPRAY THROMBOLYSIS

There are several methods for administering thrombolytic agents into dialysis grafts. One of the techniques described relatively early in experience of treating dialysis grafts with thrombolysis was pulse-spray pharmacomechanical thrombolysis (PSPMT). Although perhaps supplanted by more recently described thrombolytic approaches, PSPMT remains a good technique, particularly for those who are just gaining experience in graft thrombolysis. If another thrombolytic approach is ineffective, this method can be used to salvage the situation.

Several catheter systems are suitable for PSPMT (e.g., Unifuse catheter). These devices have multiple side holes or slits over lengths of 5 to 40 cm. A tip-occluding wire is used to obstruct the catheter endhole. All of the devices allow a high-pressure fluid spray to be delivered into the substance of the clot. To lyse the entire clot and treat the arterial and venous ends of the grafts, a crossed catheter technique is used[78,113,114] (Fig. 19-14). A single-wall, 18-gauge

needle or micropuncture needle (Cook, Inc., Bloomington, Ind.) is used to access the graft. The first puncture is made toward the venous anastomosis. Puncturing the graft sometimes is difficult because of scar tissue from repeated dialysis needle puncture. It is helpful to hold the graft firmly between the thumb and fingers of one hand while puncturing the graft with the needle held in the other hand. When the needle passes through the graft material, usually there is a "popping" sensation or loss of resistance, although if scar has developed, this sensation may be diminished. There usually is little or no blood return when a thrombosed graft is entered. When the needle is in the graft, a guidewire normally passes easily. If the patient complains of pain with the guidewire passage or the wire fails to follow the course of the access, the guidewire probably is extraluminal. The needle is removed and a sheath placed. A guidewire is then advanced beyond the venous anastomosis and into the venous outflow. If the guidewire and catheter cannot be manipulated into the venous outflow, the procedure should be terminated. Attempting thrombolysis in the face of an impassable venous obstruction leads to bleeding when inflow is reestablished. In this situation, the patient is referred for thrombectomy and surgical revision of the venous anastomosis.

A small amount of contrast is injected through the catheter, and the catheter is withdrawn until the venous end of the thrombus is identified. The length of the thrombosed segment, from the venous end of the clot to the entrance site into the graft, is determined. A pulse-spray catheter with appropriate length of side holes is placed into the graft.

The arterial end of the graft is approached in a similar manner. The needle is placed into the graft a short distance away from the venous end of the graft and directed toward the arterial end. A pulse-spray catheter is positioned with the end hole just beyond the arterial anastomosis. It is important to manipulate guidewires and catheters gently at the arterial end of the graft. Forceful, vigorous motion of the wire or injection of contrast may dislodge clot into the feeding artery.

The most commonly used thrombolytic in the United States for dialysis grafts is recombinant tissue-type plasminogen activator (t-PA) 2 mg dissolved in 5 to 10 mL of normal saline.[115-117] *Reteplase* (a genetically altered version of t-PA) is also effective, typically in a dose of 1 to 3 units in 5 to 10 mL of saline.[118] Patients also receive 3000 to 5000 units of IV heparin. The thrombolytic solution is divided equally between two syringes. Aliquots of 0.2 to 0.3 mL of solution are injected into each catheter over about 10 minutes. Forceful injection enhances the diffusion of the thrombolytic agent into the clot and produces some mechanical disruption of the clot matrix, increasing the surface area exposed to the thrombolytic agent.[119] One dose of thrombolytic solution is sufficient

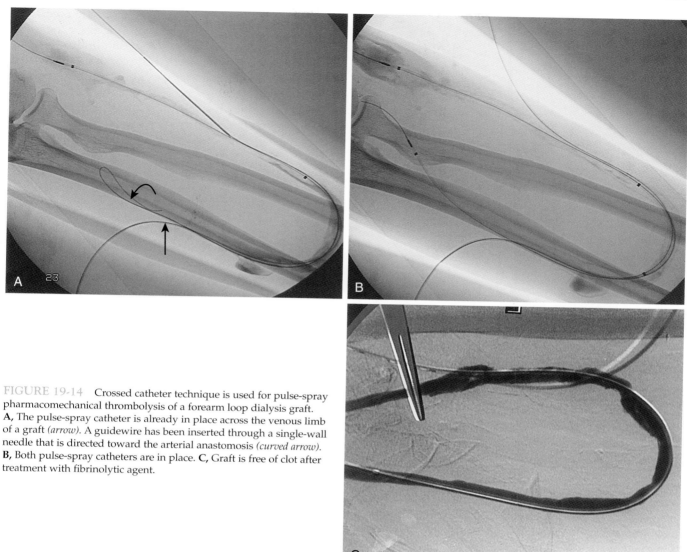

FIGURE 19-14   Crossed catheter technique is used for pulse-spray pharmacomechanical thrombolysis of a forearm loop dialysis graft. **A,** The pulse-spray catheter is already in place across the venous limb of a graft *(arrow)*. A guidewire has been inserted through a single-wall needle that is directed toward the arterial anastomosis *(curved arrow).* **B,** Both pulse-spray catheters are in place. **C,** Graft is free of clot after treatment with fibrinolytic agent.

to treat most hemodialysis grafts. The graft may have only a weak pulse despite near-complete lysis because of resistant clot at the arterial end. Small to moderate volumes of residual clot at other sites do not require further thrombolytic therapy. Large amounts of residual clot may indicate incomplete treatment of the entire clot, insufficient heparinization, or infected thrombus resistant to thrombolytic agents.

Contrast injection through the venous catheter withdrawn below the anastomosis demonstrates a stenosis in most cases. The venous stenosis is treated with balloon angioplasty to provide graft outflow before graft inflow is addressed. In many cases, a lysis-resistant clot remains at the arterial anastomosis (Fig. 19-15). This arterial "plug" is probably composed of densely packed layers of

platelets and fibrin.[120,121] Because these plugs are relatively resistant to thrombolysis, further thrombolytic treatment is of little value. Mechanical dislodgment and maceration of the plug is much more effective. Thrombectomy is performed using compliant balloons that can exert force and traction on the plug as it is pulled out of the arterial anastomosis (Fig. 19-16). These balloons include an 8.5-mm occlusion balloon catheter (Boston Scientific, Watertown, Mass.) or an over-the-wire Fogarty balloon catheter (Baxter, Irvine, Calif.). Maceration with a dilation balloon at the arterial anastomosis is avoided because of the risk of arterial embolization or injury. It is important to avoid overinflation of the balloon in the native artery. If the balloon is overexpanded, the balloon may rupture or damage to the artery may result. Two or

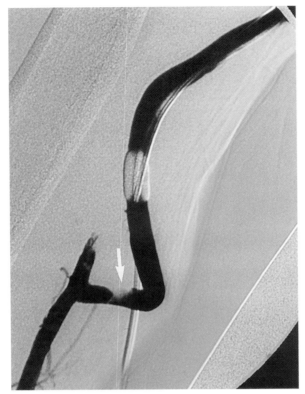

FIGURE 19-15 Lysis-resistant "plug" on the graft side of the arterial anastomosis *(arrow)*. Contrast has been injected into the proximal graft and feeding radial artery after inflating the occlusion balloon.

three passes may be necessary to completely remove the clot. When the plug is displaced from the anastomosis, it may become trapped in the graft, usually at the site where the catheters enters the graft. In this situation, an angioplasty balloon is used to fragment the clot. Any other residual clot in the graft also is macerated with an angioplasty balloon.

After flow has been established, the entire graft circuit from the arterial inflow to the superior vena cava is studied with venography for other obstructions. If the patient is going to dialysis immediately, short 7-Fr dialysis sheaths are placed. Otherwise, an activated clotting time is obtained to assess the patient's anticoagulation status before removing the catheters.

LYSE AND WAIT METHOD

The "lysis and wait" technique was first described by Cynamon and colleagues.[122,123] An Angiocath or micropuncture set is inserted into the arterial end of the graft by means of ultrasound or palpation. The graft is manually compressed at the arterial and venous anastomoses while the thrombolytic mixture (t-PA 2 mg in 5 to 10 mL normal saline) is slowly infused over 1 minute.[115,116,123] This portion of the procedure can be accomplished in a

holding area, thus requiring little or no interventional radiology (IR) room time and avoiding the expense of an infusion catheter.[119] After about 30 minutes, the patient is transferred to the IR suite, and the declotting procedure is continued with venography, angioplasty of the venous stenosis, and mobilization of the arterial plug as described for the pulse-spray technique. The "lysis and go" variation is very similar, but the thrombolytic agent is injected when the patient is in the IR suite, and the patient is prepped and draped and the procedure started without any waiting period.

MECHANICAL THROMBECTOMY

Multiple mechanical thrombectomy devices are approved by the U.S. Food and Drug Administration for treating dialysis grafts, including the AngioJet infusion system, Arrow-Trerotola Percutaneous Thrombectomy Device (PTD), Akonya Eliminator, Castaneda Over the Wire Brush, Helix Clot Buster Thrombectomy (Amplatz Device), Oasis Thrombectomy System, Prolumen, Thrombex PMT, and X-Sizer Catheter System. Thrombectomy devices have a variety of methods for removal of clot. Some cause clot fragmentation by producing a vortex created by a high-speed rotating impeller or basket.[124] Others work by Venturi effect, in which thrombus is sucked into the aperture of the device and macerated by high local shear forces. The fragments are removed through an exhaust lumen.[124] Heparin (3000 to 5000 units in most cases) is commonly infused through the sheath before the thrombectomy device is placed.[125] If it is not given through the sheath, it should be given intravenously.

The approach to using these devices is similar to that for pulse-spray thrombolysis. Vascular sheaths of appropriate size are required. Some operators do not open the venous stenosis until after performing the thrombectomy, whereas others perform angioplasty at the venous end to allow outflow and to decrease the risk of increased pressure, which itself could lead to arterial emboli.[125] Contrast can be injected through the sheath to visualize the clot. After the clot is removed from the venous end, the venous stenosis is dilated. After the venous angioplasty, the venous end of the graft is punctured in the direction of the arterial end. The thrombectomy device is then advanced to clear the clot at the arterial end. An occlusion balloon is placed to dislodge the arterial plug. Following this maneuver, the graft is assessed with contrast to determine whether the procedure is complete or whether other areas require therapy (Fig. 19-17).

Some operators prefer to use a single puncture at the apex of a loop graft as the access point and then direct the sheath toward the limb of the graft that requires treatment. Other operators pull the arterial plug back into the graft early in the procedure, before treating the

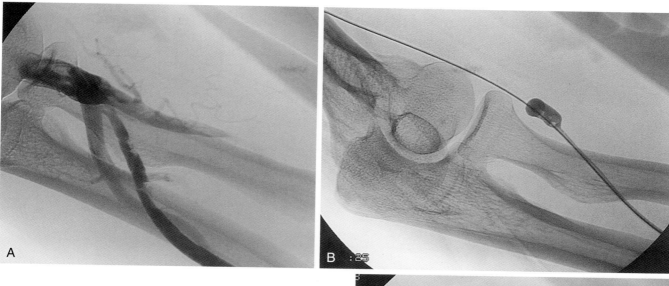

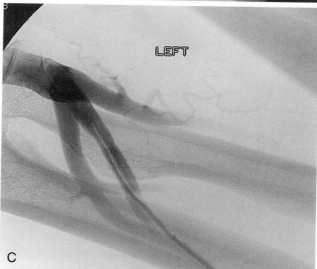

FIGURE 19-16   Treatment of arterial plug. **A,** Arterial end of the graft after pulse-spray thrombolysis shows residual clot. **B,** An occlusion balloon has been inflated in the inflow artery and then pulled into the graft to dislodge the thrombus. **C,** The arterial anastomosis is widely patent.

venous stenosis, so the plug can be fragmented by the mechanical device.[125]

ARTERIOVENOUS FISTULA THROMBOSIS

AVF thrombolysis is much more challenging than graft thrombolysis.[126-128] Ultrasound is used to confirm that the fistula is truly thrombosed rather than harboring a stenosis that results in poor flow and subsequent flattening of the fistula (see earlier discussion). Depending on the anatomy, fistulas may be accessed using antegrade and/or retrograde approach. As with dialysis grafts, pulse-spray, "lyse and wait," and mechanical devices have been used.[126,129-132] Direct thromboaspiration of the fistula may be successful.[91] This method can be performed with 7- or 8-Fr, thin-walled aspiration catheters and a 20-mL syringe to provide the aspiration suction.[124,133]

RESULTS

All three methods of treatment are similarly effective for clotted dialysis grafts, with initial clinical success (i.e., ability to undergo at least one session of dialysis) of greater than 90% with a NKF-KDOQI clinical success rate goal of 85%.* The overall procedure time is usually less than 2 hours. The different mechanical thrombectomy devices seem to be relatively comparable in their reported success rates; they all remove clot, and differences may be largely a function of operator experience.[125,134,135] The technical success results are comparable between devices, and pharmacologic thrombolysis and patency rates at 1, 3, and 6 months also are comparable.[116,134-140]

Long-term primary patency of thrombosed dialysis grafts is relatively poor whether grafts are treated by PSPMT, mechanical devices, or surgical thrombectomy and

*See references 1, 78, 84, 96, 108, 109, 113, 115-118, 132-140.

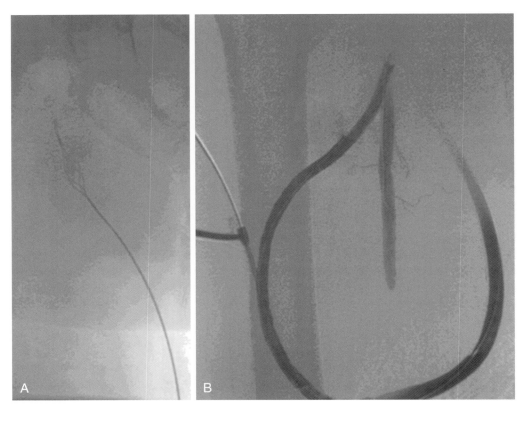

FIGURE 19-17   **A,** Arrow-Trerotola device in a looped graft in thigh. **B,** Following activation of the device, the graft is largely free of clot.

revision. For enzymatic thrombolysis, the primary patency rate at 1 year is 11% to 26% and secondary patency rate at 1 year is 51% to 69%.[114] Studies directly comparing surgical thrombectomy with thrombolysis and angioplasty demonstrate similar patency rates. However, reocclusion rates are similar following multiple declotting procedures, regardless of the technique used, so continual percutaneous managements should be undertaken to preserve each graft for as long as possible.[132] Even if grafts rethrombose early (within 2 months), aggressive retreatment of these grafts, commonly using a larger angioplasty balloon, or occasionally stent placement allowed salvage of the grafts without significantly decreased patency rates.[141]

Endovascular treatment of thrombosed dialysis fistulas is quite effective, with technical success rates for declotting fistulas ranging from 75% to 100%. Primary patency rates are reported to be 36% to 70% and 18% to 60% at 3 and 6 months, respectively, with 60% to 80% assisted primary patency rates at 6 months.[126,142-146] Declotting of fistulas may involve multiple modalities such as thrombolytics, thromboaspiration, mechanical thrombectomy, and angioplasty.

COMPLICATIONS

Major and minor complications of thrombolysis for dialysis access occur in about 1% and 10% of cases, respectively.[84] Most complications involve perigraft bleeding, arterial embolization, and vein rupture from angioplasty.[147] The complication rates for most of the mechanical devices are similar. Bleeding from previous needle punctures is seen occasionally, particularly when the venous outflow stenosis is not treated before flow is reestablished. In this situation, pressure is applied to the bleeding site, and the venous outflow is opened expeditiously.

Embolization into the arterial system occurs in up to 10% of procedures.[84] Further thrombolysis of these emboli (which usually arise from the arterial plug) is often ineffective, and mechanical removal is required when clots are symptomatic or arterial supply to the hand is compromised. After determining the location of the embolus, a wire is placed past the arterial anastomosis and past the embolus. An occlusion balloon catheter is placed from the graft into the artery beyond the clot, and the clot is pulled back into the graft. If the graft is patent, the "back-bleeding" technique can be tried.[148] The graft must first be patent. A balloon catheter is placed into the arterial inflow, just above the anastomosis, on the upstream side. The balloon is inflated, and the patient exercises the hand for about 1 minute. The balloon is deflated and an arteriogram is performed to evaluate the results. A successful procedure dislodges the embolus from its position in the artery below the anastomosis and into the graft.[149]

Small pulmonary emboli are produced with all percutaneous declotting techniques.[109-111,139,150,151] Symptomatic pulmonary embolism is rare. However, fatal pulmonary embolism has been reported after mechanical thrombectomy in which the entire clot burden of a graft was delivered to the lungs.[140,150]

OTHER DISORDERS

Ischemia and Steal Syndrome

Dialysis fistulas/grafts create a low-resistance circuit between the arterial and venous systems. Most patients tolerate this physiology without difficulty, but some patients may develop distal limb ischemia. The incidence of ischemic complications ranges between 1% and 10%.[152-154] The most common cause is high resistance in the arterial bed beyond the arteriovenous anastomosis, with shunting of blood into the graft. A "steal" from the ulnar artery through the palmar arches causes reversed flow in the distal radial artery, shunting of blood away from the peripheral tissues, and resulting hand ischemia (Fig. 19-18). This situation is most common in patients with coexisting small vessel disease such as diabetes, vasculitis, or peripheral vascular disease.[154] In these patients, even mild degrees of arterial

flow reversal may result in a clinically significant steal. A second cause for distal ischemia is occlusive disease in the inflow arteries.[81] The combination of decreased inflow and shunting of blood through the graft leads to ischemic hand symptoms.

A patient with dialysis graft-related ischemia has a cool, pale extremity. Trophic changes of the skin and nails or muscle wasting may develop. The patient may complain of numbness, tingling, impairment of motor function, or pain on exertion of the hand. The symptoms often are worse during dialysis.[152] In more severe cases, numbness and pain progress, with diminished sensation, muscle and nerve paralysis, ischemic ulcers, and progressive dry gangrene of one or more affected digits.[152]

The diagnosis of ischemia can be made in several ways, including digital plethysmography, pulse oximetry, and segmental pressure measurements.[154] A significant decrease in blood pressure along the extremity indicates an obstruction in the arterial circulation at this site. Pulse volume recordings documenting digital pressures less than 50 mm Hg and augmentation of the pulse wave with fistula compression are diagnostic of vascular steal.[152,154] Digital pulse oximetry also has proven useful in diagnosing vascular access–associated steal. Oxygen saturations are low, but they rise to normal levels when the fistula is compressed.[152] Angiography can be performed to identify

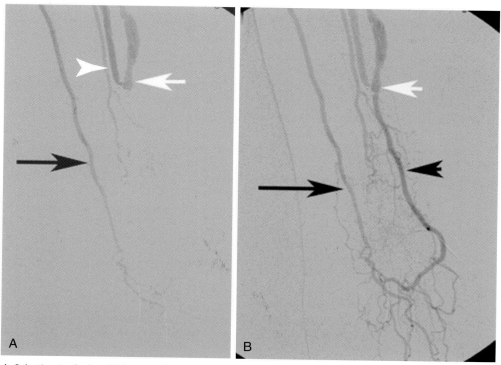

FIGURE 19-18   **A,** Injection in the brachial artery demonstrates filling of the ulnar artery *(black arrow),* and filling of the radial artery *(arrowhead)* that directly supplies the dialysis access *(white arrow).* **B,** Later in the injection, the distal radial artery *(arrowhead)* shows marked filling in a retrograde fashion from the palmar arch.

proximal or distal arterial obstruction that may be responsible for ischemia.

Angioplasty may be performed for arterial stenoses proximal to the arteriovenous access. This procedure may augment blood flow to the peripheral tissues with relief of pain and healing of ulcers.[81,154] Operative intervention may be required in patients with symptomatic vascular insufficiency. In forearm grafts, ligation of the radial artery immediately distal to the fistula abolishes the steal and may improve flow to the hand. Coil embolization of the radial artery distal to the graft can accomplish the same function as surgical ligation.[153,155] Fistula banding reduces steal through the graft but may jeopardize graft patency.[154] In severe cases, graft takedown is required.

Venous Hypertension

Obstruction of dialysis access venous outflow may lead to retrograde, high-pressure flow through collateral veins and result in venous hypertension. This situation is most common with upper arm fistulas when there is occlusion of central veins. Patients suffering from venous hypertension have edema, cyanotic discoloration, and, with long-standing hypertension, pigmentation changes of the skin.[156] Dilated, tortuous collateral veins are observed in the extremity and often across the chest. Swelling of the extremity causes pain and impaired function and may lead to ischemic ulceration.[156]

Patients should be evaluated before graft placement if they have preexisting arm edema, collateral vein development, history of subclavian vein catheters or pacemaker placement, or trauma to the extremity.[157] Imaging is done with duplex ultrasound or magnetic resonance imaging.[158,159] If symptoms of venous hypertension occur after access creation, a venogram should be performed. If there is a central venous stenosis or occlusion, angioplasty and possibly stenting (for an occlusion) should be attempted. In many cases, angioplasty resolves the arm swelling at least for 3 to 6 months, then repeated angioplasty can be performed, which can prolong the use of the access sometimes for years.[25]

Aneurysms and Pseudoaneurysms

Aneurysms and pseudoaneurysms are detected as pulsatile masses within synthetic dialysis grafts or arteriovenous fistulas. Aneurysms in fistulas occur from repeated dialysis needle puncture at the same site or venous hypertension from associated venous stenosis. Pseudoaneurysms in grafts result from graft degeneration at sites when repeated punctures have been made and occur in 2% to 10% of dialysis accesses.[160] When these pseudoaneurysms become large, they may compromise graft function.

Surgical intervention is warranted in the setting of skin breakdown, rapid expansion, massive dilation,

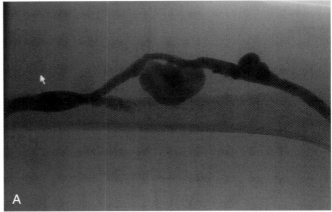

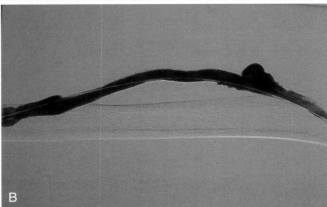

FIGURE 19-19   **A,** Angiogram shows a large graft pseudoaneurysm. **B,** The lesion was repaired by off label placement of a covered Flair stent. *(Courtesy of Dr. Carr, Boise, Idaho.)*

spontaneous bleeding, or infection. Surgery usually involves resection of the pseudoaneurysm and interposition or bypass grafting around the lesion. More recently, stent grafts have been used to treat patients with pseudoaneurysms of aging, degenerating dialysis grafts and aneurysms of AVFs[73,160-162] (Fig. 19-19). In one of the largest series, Vesely[162] used Viabahn stent graft placement for graft-related pseudoaneurysms with reported primary patency of 71% at 3 months and 20% at 6 months.

References

1. III. NKF-K/DOQI Clinical Practice Guidelines for Vascular Access: update 2000. *Am J Kidney Dis* 2001;**37**:S137.
2. Chin AI, Chang W, Fitzgerald JT, et al. Intra-access blood flow in patients with newly created upper-arm arteriovenous native fistulae for hemodialysis access. *Am J Kidney Dis* 2004;**44**:850.
3. Lok CE, Bhola C, Croxford R, Richardson RM. Reducing vascular access morbidity: a comparative trial of two vascular access monitoring strategies. *Nephrol Dial Transplant* 2003;**18**:1174.
4. Perera GB, Mueller MP, Kubaska SM, et al. Superiority of autogenous arteriovenous hemodialysis access: maintenance of function with fewer secondary interventions. *Ann Vasc Surg* 2004;**18**:66.

5. Allon M, Lockhart ME, Lilly RZ, et al. Effect of preoperative sonographic mapping on vascular access outcomes in hemodialysis patients. *Kidney Int* 2001;**60**:2013.

6. Dixon BS, Novak L, Fangman J. Hemodialysis vascular access survival: The upper arm native arteriovenous fistula. *Am J Kidney Dis* 2002;**39**:92.

7. Gibson KD, Caps MT, Kohler TR, et al. Assessment of a policy to reduce placement of prosthetic hemodialysis access. *Kidney Int* 2001;**59**:2335.

8. Miller A, Holzenbein TJ, Gottlieb MN, et al. Strategies to increase the use of autogenous arteriovenous fistula in end-stage renal disease. *Ann Vasc Surg* 1997;**11**:397.

9. D'Cunha PT, Besarab A. Vascular access for hemodialysis: 2004 and beyond. *Curr Opin Nephrol Hypertens* 2004;**13**:623.

10. Robbin ML, Chamberlain NE, Lockhart ME, et al. Hemodialysis arteriovenous fistula maturity: US evaluation. *Radiology* 2002;**225**:59.

11. Huber TS, Buhler AG, Seeger JM. Evidence-based data for the hemodialysis access surgeon. *Semin Dial* 2004;**17**:217.

12. Huber TS, Carter JW, Carter RL, Seeger JM. Patency of autogenous and polytetrafluoroethylene upper extremity arteriovenous hemodialysis accesses: a systematic review. *J Vasc Surg* 2003;**38**:1005.

13. Fillinger M, Reinitz E, Schwartz R, et al. Graft geometry and venous intimal-medial hyperplasia in arteriovenous loop grafts. *J Vasc Surg* 1990;**11**:556.

14. Windus DW. Permanent vascular access: a nephrologist's view. *Am J Kidney Dis* 1993;**21**:457.

15. Malchesky P, Koshino I, Pennza P, et al. Analysis of the segmental venous stenosis in blood access. *Trans Amer Soc Artif Int Organs* 1975;**21**:310.

16. Sullivan KL, Besarab A, Bonn J, et al. Hemodynamics of failing dialysis grafts. *Radiology* 1993;**186**:867.

17. Schwarz C, Mitterbauer C, Boczula M, et al. Flow monitoring: performance characteristics of ultrasound dilution versus color Doppler ultrasound compared with fistulography. *Am J Kidney Dis* 2003;**42**:539.

18. Roberts A, Valji K. Screening and assessment of dialysis graft function. *Tech Vasc Interv Radiol* 1999;**2**:186.

19. Besarab A, Lubkowski T, Frinak S, et al. Detection of access strictures and outlet stenoses in vascular accesses. Which test is best? *ASAIO J* 1997;**43**:M543.

20. Basile C, Ruggieri G, Vernaglione L, et al. A comparison of methods for the measurement of hemodialysis access recirculation. *J Nephrol* 2003;**16**:908.

21. Lopot F, Nejedly B, Valek M. Vascular access monitoring: methods and procedures—something to standardize? *Blood Purif* 2005;**23**:36.

22. Lopot F, Nejedly B, Sulkova S, Blaha J. Comparison of different techniques of hemodialysis vascular access flow evaluation. *Int J Artif Organs* 2003;**26**:1056.

23. Rittgers SE, Garcia-Valdez C, McCormick J, et al. Noninvasive blood flow measurement in expanded polytetrafluoroethylene grafts for hemodialysis access. *J Vasc Surg* 1986;**3**:635.

24. Shackleton C, Tailor DC, Buckle AR, et al. Predicting failure in polytetrafluoroethylene vascular access grafts for hemodialysis: a pilot study. *Can J Surg* 1987;**30**:442.

25. Ziegler TW, Safa A, Amarillis K, et al. Prolonging the life of difficult hemodialysis access using thrombolysis, angiography and angioplasty. *Adv Renal Replace Ther* 1995;**2**:52.

26. Beathard GA. Physical examination of AV grafts. *Semin Dial* 1996;**5**:74.

27. Trerotola SO, Scheel PJ Jr, Powe NR, et al. Screening for dialysis access graft malfunction: comparison of physical examination with US. *J Vasc Interv Radiol* 1996;**7**:15.

28. Schwab SJ, Raymond JR, Saeed M, et al. Prevention of hemodialysis fistula thrombosis. Early detection of venous stenoses. *Kidney Int* 1989;**36**:707.

29. Besarab A, Lubkowski T, Frinak S, et al. Detecting vascular access dysfunction. *ASAIO J* 1997;**43**:M539.

30. McCarley P, Wingard RL, Shyr Y, et al. Vascular access blood flow monitoring reduces access morbidity and costs. *Kidney Int* 2001;**60**:1164.

31. Cayco AV, Abu-Alfa AK, Mahnensmith RL, Perazella MA. Reduction in arteriovenous graft impairment: results of a vascular access surveillance protocol. *Am J Kidney Dis* 1998;**32**:302.

32. Campos RP, Chula DC, Perreto S, et al. Accuracy of physical examination and intra-access pressure in the detection of stenosis in hemodialysis arteriovenous fistula. *Semin Dial* 2008;**21**:269.

33. Robbin ML, Gallichio MH, Deierhoi MH, et al. US vascular mapping before hemodialysis access placement. *Radiology* 2000;**217**:83.

34. Robbin ML, Chamberlain NE, Lockhart ME, et al. Hemodialysis arteriovenous fistula maturity: US evaluation. *Radiology* 2002;**225**:59.

35. Polkinghorne KR, Kerr PG. Predicting vascular access failure: a collective review. *Nephrology* (Carlton) 2002;**7**:170.

36. Haskal Z, Trerotola S, Dolmatch B, et al. Stent graft versus balloon angioplasty for failing dialysis-access grafts. *New Engl J Med* 2010;**362**:494.

37. Turmel-Rodrigues L, Mouton A, Birmele B, et al. Salvage of immature forearm fistulas for haemodialysis by interventional radiology. *Nephrol Dial Transplant* 2001;**16**:2365.

38. Manninen HI, Kaukanen E, Makinen K, et al. Endovascular salvage of nonmaturing autogenous hemodialysis fistulas: comparison with endovascular therapy of failing mature fistulas. *J Vasc Interv Radiol* 2008;**19**:870.

39. Lui KW, Yeow KM, Wan YL, et al. Ultrasound guided puncture of the brachial artery for haemodialysis fistula angiography. *Nephrol Dial Transplant*. 2001;**16**:98.

40. Bucker A, Vorwerk D, Gunther RW. Transbrachial fine-needle arteriography with special focus on haemodialysis shunt imaging. *Nephrol Dial Transplant* 1995;**10**:838.

41. Wu CC, Wen SC, Chen MK, et al. Radial artery approach for endovascular salvage of occluded autogenous radial-cephalic fistulae. *Nephrol Dial Transplant* 2009;**24**:2497.

42. Turmel-Rodrigues L, Mouton A, Birmele B, et al. Salvage of immature forearm fistulas for haemodialysis by interventional radiology. *Nephrol Dial Transplant* 2001;**16**:2365.

43. Turmel-Rodrigues L, Pengloan J, Baudin S, et al. Treatment of stenosis and thrombosis in haemodialysis fistulas and grafts by interventional radiology. *Nephrol Dial Transplant* 2000;**15**:2029.

44. Rajan DK, Clark TW, Patel NK, et al. Prevalence and treatment of cephalic arch stenosis in dysfunctional autogenous hemodialysis fistulas. *J Vasc Interv Radiol* 2003;**14**:567.

45. Kian K, Asif A. Cephalic arch stenosis. *Semin Dial* 2008;**21**:78.

46. Kinnaert P, Vereerstraeten P, Toussaint C, et al. Nine years' experience with internal arteriovenous fistulas for haemodialysis: a study of some factors influencing the results. *Br J Surg* 1977;**64**:242.

47. Miller PE, Tolwani A, Luscy CP, et al. Predictors of adequacy of arteriovenous fistulas in hemodialysis patients. *Kidney Int* 1999;**56**:275.

48. Rodriguez JA, Armadans L, Ferrer E, et al. The function of permanent vascular access. *Nephrol Dial Transplant* 2000;**15**:402.

49. Miller CD, Robbin ML, Allon M. Gender differences in outcomes of arteriovenous fistulas in hemodialysis patients. *Kidney Int* 2003;**63**:346.

50. Turmel-Rodriguez L, Mouton A, Birmele B, et al. Salvage of immature forearm fistulas for haemodialysis by interventional radiology. *Nephrol Dial Transplant* 2001;**16**:2365.

51. Beathard GA, Arnold P, Jackson J, et al. Aggressive treatment of early fistula failure. *Kidney Int* 2003;**64**:1487.

52. Shin SW, Do YS, Choo SW, et al. Salvage of immature arteriovenous fistulas with percutaneous transluminal angioplasty. *Cardiovasc Intervent Radiol* 2005;**28**:434.

53. Nassar GM, Nguyen B, Rhee E, et al. Endovascular treatment of the "failing to mature" arteriovenous fistula. *Clin J Am Soc Nephrol* 2006;**1**:275.

54. Song HH, Won YD, Kim YO, et al. Salvaging and maintaining no-maturing Brescia-Cimino haemodialysis fistulae by percutaneous intervention. *Clin Radiology* 2006;**61**:404.

55. Natario A, Turmel-Rodrigues L, Fodil-Cherif M, et al. Endovascular treatment of immature, dysfunctional and thrombosed forearm autogenous ulnar-basilics and radio-basilic fistulas for dialysis. *Nephrol Dial Transplant* 2010;**25**:532.

56. Clark TW, Cohen RA, Kwak A, et al. Salvage of nonmaturing native fistulas by using angioplasty. *Radiology* 2007;**242**:286.

57. Manninen HI, Kaukanen E, Maekinen K, et al. Endovascular salvage of nonmaturing autogenous hemodialysis fistulas: comparison with endovascular therapy of failing mature fistulas. *J Vasc Interv Radiol* 2008;**19**:870.

58. Falk A. Maintenance and salvage of arteriovenous fistulas. *J Vasc Interv Radiol* 2006;**17**:807.

59. Berman SS, Gentile AT. Impact of secondary procedures in autogenous arteriovenous fistula maturation and maintenance. *J Vasc Surg* 2001;**34**:866.

60. Miller GA, Schur I, Song M. Balloon angioplasty maturation of arteriovenous fistulae: a new technique to facilitate placement and utilization of primary arteriovenous fistulae. *Vascular* 2005;**13**:S80.

61. De Marco Garcia LP, Davila-Santini LR, Feng Q, et al. Primary balloon angioplasty plus balloon angioplasty maturation to upgrade small-caliber veins (<3 mm) for arteriovenous fistulas. *J Vasc Surg* 2010;**52**:139.

62. Trerotola SO, Kwak A, Clark TW, et al. Prospective study of balloon inflation pressures and other technical aspects of hemodialysis access angioplasty. *J Vasc Interv Radiol* 2005;**16**:1613.

63. Sreenarasimhaiah VP, Margassery SK, Martin KJ, Bander SJ. Cutting balloon angioplasty for resistant venous anastomotic stenoses. *Semin Dial* 2004;**17**:523.

64. Vorwerk D, Adam G, Muller-Leisse C, Guenther RW. Hemodialysis fistulas and grafts: use of cutting balloons to dilate venous stenoses. *Radiology* 1996;**201**:864.

65. Bittl JA, Feldman RL. Cutting balloon angioplasty for undilatable venous stenoses causing dialysis graft failure. *Catheter Cardiovasc Interv* 2003;**58**:524.

66. Song HH, Kim KT, Chung SK, et al. Cutting balloon angioplasty for resistant venous stenoses of Brescia-Cimino fistulas. *J Vasc Interv Radiol* 2004;**15**:1463.

67. Singer-Jordan J, Papura S. Cutting balloon angioplasty for primary treatment of hemodialysis fistula venous stenoses: preliminary results. *J Vasc Interv Radiol* 2005;**16**:25.

68. Vesely TM, Siegal JB. Use of the peripheral cutting balloon to treat hemodialysis-related stenoses. *J Vasc Interv Radiol* 2005;**16**;1593.

69. Wu CC, Lin MC, Pu S, et al. Comparison of cutting balloon versus high pressure balloon angioplasty for resistant venous stenoses of native hemodialysis fistulas. *J Vasc Interv Radiol* 2008;**19**:877.

70. Trerotola SO, Ponce P, Stavropoulos SW, et al. Physical examination versus normalized pressure ratio for predicting outcomes of hemodialysis access interventions. *J Vasc Interv Radiol* 2003;**11**:1387.

71. Sapoval MR, Turmel-Rodrigues LA, Raynaud AC, et al. Cragg covered stents in hemodialysis access- initial and mid-term results. *J Vasc Interv Radiol* 1996;**7**:335.

72. Bent CL, Rajan DK, Tan K, et al. Effectiveness of stent-graft placement for salvage of dysfunctional arteriovenous hemodialysis fistulas. *J Vasc Interv Radiol* 2010;**21**:496.

73. Silas AM, Bettmann MA. Utility of covered stents for revision of aging failing synthetic hemodialysis grafts: a report of three cases. *Cardiovasc Intervent Radiol* 2003;**26**:550.

74. Lin PH, Johnson CK, Pullium JK, et al. Transluminal stent graft repair with Wallgraft endoprosthesis in a porcine arteriovenous graft pseudoaneurysm model. *J Vasc Surg* 2003;**37**:175.

75. Quinn SF, Kim J, Sheley RC. Transluminally placed endovascular grafts for venous lesions in patients on hemodialysis. *Cardiovasc Intervent Radiol* 2003;**26**:365.

76. Vesely TM. Role of stents and stent grafts in management of hemodialysis access complications. *Semin Vasc Surg* 2007;**20**:175.

77. Khan FA, Vesely TM. Arterial problems associated with dysfunctional hemodialysis grafts: evaluation of patients at high risk for arterial disease. *J Vasc Interv Radiol* 2002;**13**:1109.

78. Roberts AC, Valji K, Bookstein JJ, Hye RJ. Pulse-spray pharmacomechanical thrombolysis for treatment of thrombosed dialysis access grafts. *Am J Surg* 1993;**166**:221.

79. Saeed M, Newman GE, McCann RL, et al. Stenoses in dialysis fistulas: treatment with percutaneous angioplasty. *Radiology* 1987;**164**:693.

80. Huber TS, Seeger JM. Approach to patients with "complex" hemodialysis access problems. *Semin Dial* 2003;**16**:22.

81. Guerra A, Raynaud A, Beyssen B, et al. Arterial percutaneous angioplasty in upper limbs with vascular access devices for haemodialysis. *Nephrol Dial Transplant* 2002;**17**:843.

82. Levit RD, Cohen RM, Kwak A, et al. Asymptomatic central venous stenosis in hemodialysis patients. *Radiology* 2006;**238**:1051.

83. Bakken AM, Protack CD, Saad WE, et al. Long-term outcomes of primary angioplasty and primary stenting of central venous stenosis in hemodialysis patients. *J Vasc Surg* 2007;**45**:776.

84. Aruny JE, Lewis CA, Cardella JF, et al. Quality improvement guidelines for percutaneous management of the thrombosed or dysfunctional dialysis access. *J Vasc Interv Radiol* 2003;**14**:S247.

85. Verstandig AG, Bloom AI, Sasson T, et al. Shortening and migration of Wallstents after stenting of central venous stenoses in hemodialysis patients. *Cardiovasc Intervent Radiol* 2003;**26**:58.

86. Sharma AK, Sinha S, Bakran A. Migration of intra-vascular metallic stent into pulmonary artery. *Nephrol Dial Transplant* 2002;**17**:511.

87. Fernandez-Juarez G, Letosa RM, Mirete JO. Pulmonary migration of a vascular stent. *Nephrol Dial Transplant* 1999;**14**:250.

88. Yao L, Veytsman AM, Dhamee MS. Images in anesthesia: a right atrial foreign body. *Can J Anaesth* 2004;**51**:173.

89. Kanterman RY, Vesely TM, Pilgram TK, et al. Dialysis access grafts: Anatomic location of venous stenosis and results of angioplasty. *Radiology* 1995;**195**:135.

90. Beathard GA. Percutaneous transvenous angioplasty in the treatment of vascular access stenosis. *Kidney Int* 1992;**42**:1390.

91. Turmel-Rodrigues L, Pengloan J, Baudin S, et al. Treatment of stenosis and thrombosis in haemodialysis fistulas and grafts by interventional radiology. *Nephrol Dial Transplant* 2000;**15**:2029.

92. Lilly RZ, Carlton D, Barker J, et al. Predictors of arteriovenous graft patency after radiologic intervention in hemodialysis patients. *Am J Kidney Dis* 2001;**37**:945.

93. Beathard GA. Percutaneous angioplasty for the treatment of venous stenosis: A nephrologist's view. *Semin Dial* 1995;**8**:166.

94. Katz SG, Kohl RD. The percutaneous treatment of angioaccess graft complications. *Am J Surg* 1995;**170**:238.

95. Clark TW, Hirsch DA, Jindal KJ, et al. Outcome and prognostic factors of restenosis after percutaneous treatment of native hemodialysis fistulas. *J Vasc Interv Radiol* 2002;**13**:51.

96. Turmel-Rodrigues L, Pengloan J, Baudin S, et al. Treatment of stenosis and thrombosis in haemodialysis fistulas and grafts by interventional radiology. *J Vasc Interv Radiol* 2002;**13**:51.

97. Vesely TM, Hovsepian DM, Pilgram TK, et al. Upper extremity central venous obstruction in hemodialysis patients: treatment with Wallstents. *Radiology* 1997;**204**:343.

98. Maskova J, Komarkova J, Kivanek J, et al. Endovascular treatment of central vein stenoses and/or occlusions in hemodialysis patients. *Cardiovasc Intervent Radiol* 2003;**26**:27.

99. Funaki B, Szymski GX, Leef JA, et al. Wallstent deployment to salvage dialysis graft thrombolysis complicated by venous rupture: early and intermediate results. *AJR Am J Roentgenol* 1997;**169**:1435.

100. Clark TW. Nitinol stents in hemodialysis access. *J Vasc Interv Radiol* 2004;**15**:1037.

101. Vogel PM, Parise C. SMART stent for salvage of hemodialysis access graft. *J Vasc Interv Rad* 2004;**15**:1051.

102. Gray RJ, Horton KM, Dolmatch BL, et al. Use of Wallstents for hemodialysis access-related venous stenoses and occlusions untreatable with balloon angioplasty. *Radiology* 1995;**195**:479.

103. Vogel PM, Parise C. Comparison of SMART stent placement for arteriovenous graft salvage versus successful graft PTA. *J Vasc Interv Radiol* 2005;**16**:1619.

104. Hoffer EK, Shahnaz S, Herskowitz MM, et al. Prospective randomized trial of a metallic intravascular stent in hemodialysis graft maintenance. *J Vasc Interv Radiol* 1997;**8**:965.

105. Bitar G, Yang S, Badosa F. Balloon versus patch angioplasty as an adjuvant treatment to surgical thrombectomy of hemodialysis grafts. *Am J Surg* 1997;**174**:140.

106. Marston WA, Criado E, Jaques PF, et al. Prospective randomized comparison of surgical versus endovascular management of thrombosed dialysis access grafts. *J Vasc Surg* 1997;**26**:373.

107. Marston WA, Beathard GA. Surgical management of thrombosed dialysis access grafts. *Am J Kidney Dis* 1998;**32**:168.

108. Davis GB, Dowd CF, Bookstein JJ, et al. Thrombosed dialysis grafts: efficacy of intrathrombic deposition of concentrated urokinase, clot maceration, and angioplasty. *AJR Am J Roentgenol* 1987;**149**:177.

109. Valji K, Roberts A, Bookstein J. Thrombosed hemodialysis access grafts: management with pulse-spray thrombolysis and balloon angioplasty. In: Strandness D, Van Breda A, editors. *Vascular Diseases: Surgical and Interventional Therapy.* New York: Churchill Livingstone; 1994. p. 1087.

110. Kinney TB, Valji K, Rose SC, et al. Pulmonary embolism from pulse-spray pharmacomechanical thrombolysis of clotted hemodialysis grafts: urokinase versus heparinized saline. *J Vasc Interv Radiol* 2000;**11**:1143.

111. Smits HF, Van Rijk PP, Van Isselt JW, et al. Pulmonary embolism after thrombolysis of hemodialysis grafts. *J Am Soc Nephrol* 1997;**8**:1458.

112. Petronis JD, Regan F, Briefel G, et al. Ventilation-perfusion scintigraphic evaluation of pulmonary clot burden after percutaneous thrombolysis of clotted hemodialysis access grafts. *Am J Kidney Dis* 1999;**34**:207.

113. Bookstein J, Fellmeth B, Roberts A, et al. Pulsed-spray pharmacomechanical thrombolysis: preliminary clinical results. *AJR Am J Roentgenol* 1989;**152**:1097.

114. Valji K, Bookstein JJ, Roberts AC, Davis GB. Pharmacomechanical thrombolysis and angioplasty in the management of clotted hemodialysis grafts: early and late clinical results. *Radiology* 1991;**178**:243.

115. Falk A, Mitty H, Guller J, et al. Thrombolysis of clotted hemodialysis grafts with tissue-type plasminogen activator. *J Vasc Interv Radiol* 2001;**12**:305.

116. Vogel PM, Bansal V, Marshall MW. Thrombosed hemodialysis grafts: lyse and wait with tissue plasminogen activator or urokinase compared to mechanical thrombolysis with the Arrow-Trerotola Percutaneous Thrombolytic Device. *J Vasc Interv Radiol* 2001;**12**:1157.

117. Sofocleous CT, Hinrichs CR, Weiss SH, et al. Alteplase for hemodialysis access graft thrombolysis. *J Vasc Interv Radiol* 2002;**13**:775.

118. Falk A, Guller J, Nowakowski FS, et al. Reteplase in the treatment of thrombosed hemodialysis grafts. *J Vasc Interv Radiol* 2001; **12**:1257.

119. Roberts AC, Silberzweig JE. Hemodialysis access management. In: Bakal CW, Silberzweig JE, Cynamon J, Sprayregen S, editors. *Vascular and Interventional Radiology: Principles and Practice.* New York: Thieme; 2002. p. 459.

120. Etheredge E, Haid S, Maeser M, et al. Salvage operations for malfunctioning polytetrafluoroethylene hemodialysis access grafts. *Surgery* 1983;**94**:464.

121. Winkler TA, Trerotola SO, Davidson DD, Milgrom ML. Study of thrombus from thrombosed hemodialysis access grafts. *Radiology* 1995;**197**:461.

122. Cynamon J, Lakritz PS, Wahl SI, et al. Hemodialysis graft declotting: description of the "lyse and wait" technique. *J Vasc Interv Radiol* 1997;**8**:825.

123. Cynamon J, Pierpont CE. Thrombolysis for the treatment of thrombosed hemodialysis access grafts. *Rev Cardiovasc Med* 2002; **3**(Suppl. 2):S84.

124. Morgan R, Belli AM. Percutaneous thrombectomy: a review. *Eur Radiol* 2002;**12**:205.

125. Vesely TM. Techniques for using mechanical thrombectomy devices to treat thrombosed hemodialysis grafts. *Tech Vasc Interv Radiol* 1999;**2**:208.

126. Rajan DK, Clark TW, Simons ME, et al. Procedural success and patency after percutaneous treatment of thrombosed autogenous arteriovenous dialysis fistulas. *J Vasc Interv Radiol* 2002;**13**:1211.

127. Kumpe DA, Cohen MA. Angioplasty/thrombolytic treatment of failing and failed hemodialysis access sites: comparison with surgical treatment. *Prog Cardiovasc Dis* 1992;**34**:263.

128. Zaleski GX, Funaki B, Kenney S, et al. Angioplasty and bolus urokinase infusion for the restoration of function in thrombosed Brescia-Cimino dialysis fistulas. *J Vasc Interv Radiol* 1999;**10**:129.

129. Pattynama PM, van Baalen J, Verburgh CA, et al. Revascularization of occluded haemodialysis fistulae with the Hydrolyser thrombectomy catheter: description of the technique and report of six cases. *Nephrol Dial Transplant* 1995;**10**:1224.

130. Rocek M, Peregrin JH, Lasovickova J, et al. Mechanical thrombolysis of thrombosed hemodialysis native fistulas with use of the Arrow-Trerotola percutaneous thrombolytic device: our preliminary experience. *J Vasc Interv Radiol* 2000;**11**:1153.

131. Overbosch EH, Pattynama PM, Aarts HJ, et al. Occluded hemodialysis shunts: Dutch multicenter experience with the hydrolyser catheter. *Radiology* 1996;**201**:485.

132. Mansilla AV, Toombs BD, Vaughn WK, Zeledon JI. Patency and life-spans of failing hemodialysis grafts in patients undergoing repeated percutaneous de-clotting. *Tex Heart Inst J* 2001;**28**:249.

133. Turmel-Rodrigues L, Sapoval M, Pengloan J, et al. Manual thromboaspiration and dilation of thrombosed dialysis access: mid-term results of a simple concept. *J Vasc Interv Radiol* 1997;**8**:813.

134. Gibbens DT, Triolo J, Yu T, et al. Contemporary treatment of thrombosed hemodialysis grafts. *Tech Vasc Interv Radiol* 2001;**4**:122.

135. Smits HF, Smits JH, Wust AF, et al. Percutaneous thrombolysis of thrombosed haemodialysis access grafts: comparison of three mechanical devices. *Nephrol Dial Transplant* 2002;**17**:467.

136. Sofocleous CT, Cooper SG, Schur I, et al. Retrospective comparison of the Amplatz thrombectomy device with modified pulse-spray pharmacomechanical thrombolysis in the treatment of thrombosed hemodialysis access grafts. *Radiology* 1999;**213**:561.

137. Barth KH, Gosnell MR, Palestrant AM, et al. Hydrodynamic thrombectomy system versus pulse-spray thrombolysis for thrombosed hemodialysis grafts: a multicenter prospective randomized comparison. *Radiology* 2000;**217**:678.

138. Trerotola SO, Vesely TM, Lund GB, et al. Treatment of thrombosed hemodialysis access grafts: Arrow-Trerotola percutaneous thrombolytic device versus pulse-spray thrombolysis. Arrow-Trerotola Percutaneous Thrombolytic Device Clinical Trial. *Radiology* 1998;**206**:403.

139. Beathard GA, Welch BR, Maidment HJ. Mechanical thrombolysis for the treatment of thrombosed hemodialysis access grafts. *Radiology* 1996;**200**:711.

140. Soulen MC, Zaetta JM, Amygdalos MA, et al. Mechanical declotting of thrombosed dialysis grafts: experience in 86 cases. *J Vasc Interv Radiol* 1997;**8**:563.

141. Murray SP, Kinney TB, Valji K, et al. Early rethrombosis of clotted hemodialysis grafts: graft salvage achieved with an aggressive approach. *AJR Am J Roentgenol* 2000;**175**:529.

142. Turmel-Rodrigues L, Pengloan J, Rodrigue H, et al. Treatment of failed native arteriovenous fistulae for hemodialysis by interventional radiology. *Kidney Int* 2000;**57**:1124.

143. Haage P, Vorwerk D, Wildberger JE, et al. Percutaneous treatment of thrombosed primary arteriovenous hemodialysis access fistulae. *Kidney Int* 2000;**57**:1169.

144. Bent CL, Sahni VA, Matson MB. The radiological management of thrombosed arteriovenous dialysis fistula. *Clin Radiol* 2011;**66**:1.

145. Liang HL, Pan HB, Chung HM, et al. Restoration of thrombosed Brescia-Cimino dialysis. *Radiology* 2002;**223**:339.

146. Shatsky JB, Berns JS, Clark TW, et al. Single-center experience with the Arrow-Trerotola Percutaneous Thrombectomy Device in the management of thrombosed native dialysis fistulas. *J Vasc Interv Radiol* 2005;**16**:1605.

147. Sofocleous CT, Schur I, Koh E, et al. Percutaneous treatment of complications occurring during hemodialysis graft recanalization. *Eur J Radiol* 2003;**47**:237.

148. Tretotola SO, Johnson MS, Shah H, Namyslowski J. Backbleeding technique for treatment of arterial emboli resulting from dialysis graft thrombolysis. *J Vasc Interv Radiol* 1998;**9**:141.

149. Beathard GA. Management of complications of endovascular dialysis access procedures. *Semin Dial* 2003;**16**:309.

150. Swan TL, Smyth SH, Ruffenach SJ, et al. Pulmonary embolism following hemodialysis access thrombolysis/thrombectomy. *J Vasc Interv Radiol* 1995;**6**:683.

151. Trerotola SO, Johnson MS, Schauwecker DS, et al. Pulmonary emboli from pulse-spray and mechanical thrombolysis: evaluation with an animal dialysis-graft model. *Radiology* 1996;**200**:169.

152. Miles AM. Upper limb ischemia after vascular access surgery: differential diagnosis and management. *Semin Dial* 2000;**13**:312.

153. Morsy AH, Kulbaski M, Chen C, et al. Incidence and characteristics of patients with hand ischemia after a hemodialysis access procedure. *J Surg Res* 1998;**74**:8.

154. Tordoir JH, Dammers R, van der Sande FM. Upper extremity ischemia and hemodialysis vascular access. *Eur J Vasc Endovasc Surg* 2004;**27**:1.

155. Valji K, Hye RJ, Roberts AC, et al. Hand ischemia in patients with hemodialysis access grafts: angiographic diagnosis and treatment. *Radiology* 1995;**196**:697.

156. Neville RF, Abularrage CJ, White PW, Sidawy AN. Venous hypertension associated with arteriovenous hemodialysis access. *Semin Vasc Surg* 2004;**17**:50.

157. Teruya TH, Abou-Zamzam Jr AM, Limm W, et al. Symptomatic subclavian vein stenosis and occlusion in hemodialysis patients with transvenous pacemakers. *Ann Vasc Surg* 2003;**17**:526.

158. Paksoy Y, Gormus N, Tercan MA. Three-dimensional contrast-enhanced magnetic resonance angiography (3-D CE-MRA) in the evaluation of hemodialysis access complications, and the condition of central veins in patients who are candidates for hemodialysis access. *J Nephrol* 2004;**17**:57.

159. Laissy JP, Menegazzo D, Debray MP, et al. Failing arteriovenous hemodialysis fistulas: assessment with magnetic resonance angiography. *Invest Radiol* 1999;**34**:218.

160. Najibi S, Bush RL, Terramani TT, et al. Covered stent exclusion of dialysis access pseudoaneurysms. *J Surg Res* 2002;**106**:15.

161. Ryan JM, Dumbleton SA, Doherty J, Smith TP. Technical innovation. Using a covered stent (Wallgraft) to treat pseudoaneurysms of dialysis grafts and fistulas. *AJR Am J Roentgenol* 2003;**180**:1067.

162. Vesely TM. Use of stent grafts to repair hemodialysis graft-related pseudoaneurysms. *J Vasc Interv Radiol* 2005;**16**:1301.

Neurointerventions

Tony P. Smith

ANATOMIC AND TECHNICAL CONSIDERATIONS

Multiple sources describe the angiographic anatomy of the cerebrovascular system[1,2] (Fig. 20-1). Interestingly, large portions of the anterior (carotid) and posterior (vertebrobasilar) circulations supply areas of the brain in which little is understood regarding functionality. In effect, one may occlude a large vessel as seen by angiography, resulting in essentially no clinical neurologic change. Alternatively very small vessels may supply highly important areas where vessel occlusion may manifest as major neurologic deficits. In addition, whenever an artery is occluded, the clinical neurologic result not only depends upon the functionality and degree of cerebral tissue supplied, but also the presence and degree of collateral circulation. These collaterals can at times be troublesome, particularly during external carotid embolization, where they may supply the intracranial circulation[3] (Table 20-1).

Diagnostic angiography of the brachiocephalic vessels is performed using 4- or 5-French (Fr) catheters. These catheters have 0.038-inch lumens, which accommodate microcatheters, even of the larger lumen and higher flow variety. However, once the microcatheter is in place, contrast injections through the diagnostic catheter for angiographic runs or subtracted fluoroscopy are very limited. For that reason, most embolization procedures use a guiding catheter, with 6 Fr being the most common. This device easily accommodates a microcatheter while reserving ample guiding catheter lumen for contrast injections, permitting angiographic runs and high-quality subtracted fluoroscopic imaging. The latter is an integral part of extracranial and intracranial catheterizations. Just as for the peripheral circulation, guiding catheters come in a variety of shapes and microcatheters in a variety of sizes. The microcatheter should be sized appropriately for the intended embolic agent.

As in the peripheral circulation, all embolic agents are carefully chosen based on the disease process, and are individualized for a particular patient and his or her unique clinical situation. Coils and particles of various sizes are the most often used. Pushable standard coils (0.035 and 0.038 inch) are used to occlude large vessels such as the vertebral or carotid arteries, as well as larger branches of the external carotid artery (ECA). However, most neurointerventionalists are more comfortable with the precision and safety of electrolytically or mechanically detached coils.[4] Now that detachable balloons are no longer available in the United States, occlusive plugs are gaining favor for rapid occlusion of large vessels.[5] Particulate agents (polyvinyl alcohol [PVA] and gelatin microspheres) are used for small artery occlusion, such as in epistaxis or preoperative tumor embolization.[6] If the operator can place the microcatheter close to the tumor bed, particles of very small size (e.g., 50 to 100 microns) are appropriate. However, larger particles are also used if there is particular concern for nontarget embolization, especially of neural tissue or skin. Liquid agents such as cyanoacrylate, ethylene vinyl copolymer (Onyx Liquid Embolic System, eV3 Neurovascular, Irvine, Calif.), and sclerosants are more commonly used extracranially for facial arteriovenous malformations.[7]

Angioplasty and stenting of the extracranial and intracranial vessels has gained popularity. Stent placement at the carotid artery bifurcation is performed today through a variety of 6-Fr, 90-cm long sheaths, permitting insertion of stents up to 10 mm in diameter. Angioplasty of smaller arteries such as the intracranial vessels is usually performed via 6-Fr guiding catheters using coronary artery balloons and either specialized self-expanding intracranial stents or balloon-expandable coronary stents, all of which track over 0.014-inch guidewires.

Angioplasty and stenting of the extracranial internal carotid artery is carried out using embolic protection devices to prevent embolization to the intracranial circulation. Embolic protection involves either deployment of a filter beyond (above) the lesion or inflation of

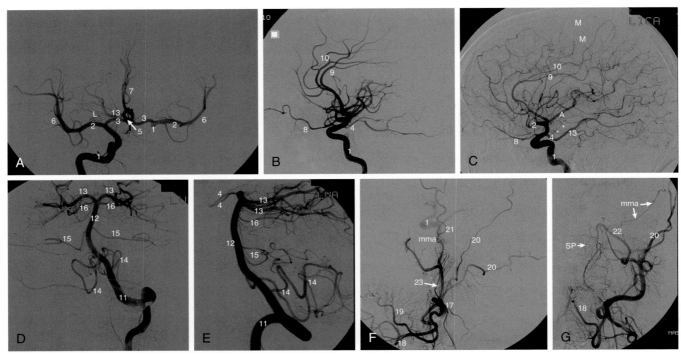

FIGURE 20-1   Normal craniofacial arterial distribution. Arteries: *1,* internal carotid artery; *2,* middle cerebral artery (M1); *3,* anterior cerebral artery (A1); *4,* posterior communicating artery; *5,* anterior communicating artery; *6,* M2 branches of the middle cerebral circulation; *7,* A2 branches of the anterior cerebral circulation; *8,* ophthalmic artery; *9,* pericallosal artery; *10,* callosomarginal artery; *11,* vertebral artery; *12,* basilar artery; *13,* posterior cerebral (P1) artery; *14,* posterior inferior cerebellar artery (PICA); *15,* anterior inferior cerebellar artery (AICA); *16,* superior cerebellar artery; *17,* external carotid artery; *18,* facial artery; *19,* lingual artery; *20,* occipital artery; *21,* superficial temporal artery (STA); *22,* internal maxillary artery (IMax); *23,* ascending pharyngeal artery; *A,* angular artery; *M,* motor cortex; *mma,* middle meningeal artery; *SP,* sphenopalantine artery; **,* anterior choroidal artery. **A,** Early phase of a right internal carotid artery angiogram in an anterior-posterior projection. Note the filling of the anterior communicating artery *(5),* which allows flow from the right to the left anterior (carotid) distributions. There is a very small amount of back-filling into the left distal intracranial carotid artery *(1).* The left internal carotid artery in this patient was normal by angiography. The lenticulostriate arteries *(L),* although small, provide important blood supply to the internal capsule. The patient has a patent posterior communicating artery giving supply to the posterior cerebral circulation *(13)* on the right. **B,** Early phase of a right internal carotid artery angiogram in a lateral projection. Posterior communicating artery *(4)* supplying the posterior cerebral artery is well seen. The ophthalmic artery *(8)* is best seen on the lateral projection. **C,** Later phase of a right internal carotid artery angiogram in a lateral projection. This is a different patient than in **B.** The posterior cerebral artery *(13)* has a complete origin from the carotid artery, although its first portion is often referred to as the posterior communicating artery *(4).* The double asterisks *(**)* represent the anterior choroidal artery, which in its proximal portion supplies the anterior limb of the internal capsule. The motor cortex in the posterior frontal lobe is estimated to be at the area marked by *M.* **D,** Left vertebral artery angiogram in the frontal view. The patient does not have a right vertebral artery. Therefore the left posterior inferior cerebellar artery (PICA) *(14)* supplies the right PICA *(14)* as well. **E,** Left vertebral artery angiogram in the lateral view. Note the bilateral posterior communicating arteries *(4).* **F,** Left external carotid artery injection in the lateral view. A small amount of reflux of contrast material is seen in the internal carotid artery *(1).* Note that most of the vessels of the external carotid artery distribution are better seen on the lateral projection. This is an early phase injection and the normal, small middle meningeal artery *(mma)* is faintly visualized. **G,** Left external carotid artery injection in the frontal view. Branches of the distal internal maxillary artery *(22)* and portions of the occipital artery are seen well in the frontal view. The delicate sphenopalantine *(SP)* artery branches are seen. These are the branches targeted in patients undergoing embolization for epistaxis.

proximal/distal endovascular balloon devices during the revascularization process. Filters consist of a basket mounted on a special 0.014-inch guidewire (Fig. 20-2). The mesh is calibrated to be small enough to trap emboli but large enough to permit normal blood flow through the basket. The device serves as the guide for balloon and stent placement. The filter is gently guided through the lesion and deployed in a normal, relatively straight segment of the internal carotid artery above the lesion. Once angioplasty and stenting is completed, angiography is performed to determine whether embolic material has been captured. If present, removal by suctioning is required, and specialized catheters are available to perform this task. Once the distal protection device is angiographically free of debris, it is collapsed and removed using a special catheter specific to each device. Although distal protection is now standard of practice and required by many payers in the United States, the data supporting this approach are controversial.[8]

TABLE 20-1   Summary of Major Extracranial and Intracranial Anastomoses

EXTRACRANIAL			INTRACRANIAL	
Major Artery	Location	Branch	Branch	Artery
Internal maxillary artery	Proximal	MMA	Orbital branches, anterior branch (anterior falcine artery)	Ophthalmic artery
			Cavernous branches	ILT
			Petrous branch	CN VII supply
		AMA	Artery of foramen ovale	ILT
	Distal	Vidian artery		Petrous ICA
		Artery of foramen rotundum		ILT
		Anterior deep temporal artery		Ophthalmic artery
Superficial temporal artery	Frontal branch		Supraorbital branch	Ophthalmic artery
Ascending pharyngeal artery	Pharyngeal trunk	Superior pharyngeal artery	Carotid branch (foramen lacerum)	Lateral clival artery
	Neuromeningeal trunk	Odontoid arch		Vertebral artery (C1)
		Hypoglossal and jugular branch		Meningohypophyseal trunk of ICA
Posterior auricular-occipital artery	Stylomastoid branch			CN VII supply
Occipital artery	Muscular branches			Vertebral artery (C1-C2)
Ascending and deep cervical arteries				Vertebral artery (C3-C7)

From Geibprasert S, Pongpech S, Armstrong D, et al. Dangerous extracranial-intracranial anastomoses and supply to the cranial nerves: vessels the neurointerventionalist needs to know. AJNR Am J Neuroradiol 2009;30:1460.

AMA, *accessory meningeal artery;* CN, *cranial nerve;* ICA, *internal carotid artery;* ILT, *inferolateral trunk;* MMA, *middle meningeal artery.*

Table provides the major extracranial artery and the location along its course where an extracranial branch potentially anastomoses with an intracranial branch supplying an important intracranial artery.

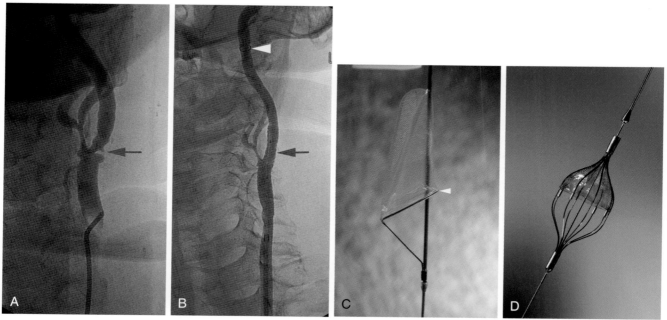

FIGURE 20-2   Cervical carotid artery angioplasty and stenting in a 74-year-old man with occluded right internal carotid artery and prior left cerebral transient ischemic attack. **A,** Anteroposterior view of left carotid bifurcation demonstrates a 60% narrowing of the proximal internal carotid artery *(arrow)* with ulceration and narrowing of the proximal external carotid artery as well. **B,** Anterior posterior angiogram of the left carotid bifurcation after angioplasty and stent placement. No residual stenosis is noted at the proximal internal carotid artery *(arrow).* Note the distal protection device *(arrowhead)* in a relatively straight segment of the internal carotid artery. **C,** Filter-Wire EZ distal protection device used in the patient shown in **B.** Note that the protection device is part of the guidewire and the mesh is radiolucent but fixed to a radiopaque ring inferiorly *(arrowhead).* **D,** Angioguard Emboli Capture Guidewire. Note that there are a number of designs for distal protection devices. (**C,** *Courtesy of Boston Scientific, Natick, Mass., with permission.* **D,** *Courtesy of Cordis, Miami Lakes, Fla., with permission.*)

EXTRACRANIAL ATHEROSCLEROTIC DISEASE

Etiology and Natural History

Atherosclerotic disease of the extracranial and intracranial carotid and vertebral arteries and their branches clearly place patients at risk for embolic stroke. The long-term natural history of arterial stenoses at the origins of the great vessels is essentially unknown as opposed to the carotid bifurcation where up to 60% of asymptomatic patients with a greater than 75% stenosis have symptoms within 1 year of diagnosis.[9]

Clinical Features

Treatment of atherosclerotic lesions in these vessels demands that the patient's symptoms correspond to the vascular territory supplied by the particular vessel (vertebrobasilar or carotid system). A thorough and unbiased neurologic examination must be performed and documented before any intervention is undertaken. Although carotid bruits have limited value for the diagnosis of carotid artery stenosis, they are good markers of generalized atherosclerosis, and their absence may constitute sufficient screening of the asymptomatic patient.[10] Because detection of a bruit depends on blood flow, it may actually disappear in the setting of a critical stenosis.

Imaging

Diagnostic imaging entails magnetic resonance (MR) or computed tomography (CT) angiography and sonography limited to the cervical common carotid artery (CCA) and internal carotid artery (ICA). Catheter angiography is usually reserved for patients who require some intervention. Rarely, a catheter angiogram is necessary to confirm or clarify findings in a patient not destined for direct treatment. As a general rule, symptomatic carotid artery stenoses greater than 50% of the lumen diameter and asymptomatic lesions of greater than 70% are considered for surgical or endovascular treatment.[11-13]

Treatment

Medical Therapy

Current medical therapy alone may be as good as surgery in asymptomatic patients with carotid bifurcation disease. This approach is estimated to be at least three to eight times more cost-effective than direct intervention in the prevention of stroke.[14]

Before endovascular or open repair, symptomatic patients with atherosclerotic disease should receive anticoagulation and/or antiplatelet agents until the time of intervention. Heparin is used until the time of surgery or intervention if the patient has symptoms, usually with a weight-based dose targeting a maximum prothrombin time of 60 to 80 seconds. Antiplatelet agents, in particular aspirin (325 mg/day) and clopidogrel (75 mg/day), are given for at least 5 days to patients before endovascular intervention. Antiplatelet agents are avoided preoperatively due to the possibility of bleeding at the operative site.

Surgical Therapy

Fortunately, the sites of typical disease in the extracranial carotid artery are readily accessible to the surgeon for carotid endarterectomy (CEA). The indications for CEA are based on the degree of arterial stenosis, presence of associated symptoms, and suitability for surgery. Current evidence to support CEA comes largely from two randomized trials: the North American Symptomatic Carotid Endarterectomy Trial (NASCET) and the Asymptomatic Carotid Atherosclerosis Study (ACAS).[11,12] NASCET proved that, compared with available medical therapy, CEA significantly reduced the risk for stroke in symptomatic patients. However, the surgical results were much more modest for asymptomatic patients, reducing the risk for stroke from 2% to 1% per year.

On the other hand, primary operative repair of lesions at the origins of the great vessels requires thoracotomy. Surgical exposure of the vertebral artery is difficult, in that the vessel is housed throughout its cervical course within the transverse foramina of the cervical spine. Disease at these sites requiring direct treatment is best managed by endovascular means, with surgical extraanatomic bypass grafting as a last resort.

Endovascular Therapy

Reports of successful balloon angioplasty for atherosclerotic disease of the brachiocephalic arteries, including the internal carotid artery, were first reported in the 1980s.[15] Balloon dilation continued to gain in popularity at anatomic sites that were surgically less accessible, including the subclavian and vertebral arteries. However, little was done endovascularly for carotid artery bifurcation disease because of fears, perceived and real, that an irregular lumen or abrupt closure would be the angioplasty result.[16,17] With the introduction of stents in the mid-1990s, these perceived problems were largely solved, with the pressing issue becoming the outcome differences between surgery and stenting.[18]

PATIENT SELECTION AND PREPARATION

Angioplasty and stenting of the cervical carotid artery has been the subject of extensive study. Until recently these procedures were restricted to patients who were considered at high-risk for surgery.[19] However, there is now approval from the U.S. Food and Drug Administration for all patients with significant cervical carotid artery stenoses regardless of symptomatology or suitability for surgery (Box 20-1). For the great vessel origins and the extracranial vertebral artery, endovascular techniques are often preferred over operation.

Before angioplasty and stenting of the cephalic vessels, antiplatelet and anticoagulation therapy is essential. Experimental and clinical data from animal models and human coronary intervention suggest that aspirin and clopidogrel (Plavix) have a synergistic effect on inhibition of platelet aggregation, antithrombotic activity, and prevention of myointimal proliferation.[20,21] Therefore patients receive a dual antiplatelet regimen consisting of aspirin (81 or 325 mg daily) and clopidogrel (75 mg daily). This treatment is started at least 5 days before the procedure or given as a loading dose of aspirin (325 to 700 mg) and clopidogrel (300 to 600 mg) early on the day of the procedure. This combination therapy is maintained for 1 month after stenting; one antiplatelet agent (usually aspirin) is continued without interruption indefinitely. For the procedure itself, heparin (or a direct thrombin inhibitor in allergic patients) is administered to achieve an activated clotting time of at least twice what is normal (e.g., 250 to 300 seconds.)

Contraindications specific to carotid and vertebral artery stenting are relative and include inability to tolerate antiplatelet therapy and recent stroke. The latter exclusion criterion is based on experience with CEA, where revascularizing the inflow to areas of acutely infarcted cerebral tissue may result in intracranial hemorrhage.[22]

TECHNIQUE AND RESULTS

Endovascular treatment of the *origins of the great vessels* often focuses upon the left subclavian artery, the common location for lesions resulting in subclavian steal syndrome (see later discussion). However, the same principles hold for the origins and proximal regions of the right brachiocephalic and left common carotid arteries. Although the latter two treatment sites are often grouped in publications with the left subclavian artery, their outflow into the internal carotid arteries entails added risks from embolic events.

Arterial access can be either transfemoral or via a retrograde arm approach. It is thought that the arm access enhances success in crossing total occlusions due to the proximity of the access site to the lesion as well as a more stable access via the distal subclavian artery rather than the aorta.

Atherosclerotic lesions involving the great vessels often occur at or near their origins and are therefore most often treated using stents.[23,24] Angioplasty alone may be undertaken in the midportions of these vessels but lesions located at the carotid bifurcation are currently relegated to stenting. Balloon-expandable stents are often preferred to allow accurate device placement at the origin of the vessel (Fig. 20-3). Fortunately, balloon-expandable stents are generally not subject to extrinsic compression and collapse at these locations deep in the chest. Self-expandable systems are a reasonable alternative, particularly if vessel tortuosity or variations in vessel diameter are encountered. The use of distal protection devices for proximal great vessel angioplasty is based on operator preference. The results of great vessel angioplasty for atherosclerotic lesions are excellent.[25-27] Primary technical success ranges from 93% to 99% with cerebral ischemic complications ranging from 2% to 3%. Long-term patency ranges from 93% at 1 year to 79% at 5 years.

The term *subclavian steal* is used when a significant stenosis or occlusion of the subclavian artery proximal to the vertebral artery origin occurs (Fig. 20-4). Blood from

---

BOX 20-1

HIGH-RISK CRITERIA FOR CAROTID ENDARTERECTOMY

Constitutional

- Clinically significant cardiac disease
  - Multivessel coronary artery disease, severe angina, LVEF 30% or less, heart failure, need for open heart surgery
- Severe pulmonary disease
  - FEV_1 <50%
- Age >80 years

Anatomic

- Anatomically high bifurcation
- Unable to position neck for surgery
  - Severe cervical spinal disease, cervical spine fixation
- Prior carotid endarterectomy
- Contralateral carotid occlusion
- Recurrent stenosis after endarterectomy
- Contralateral laryngeal nerve palsy
- Previous radical neck surgery
- Radiation therapy to the neck

From Yadav JS, Wholey MH, Kuntz RE, et al. Protected carotid-artery stenting versus endarterectomy in high-risk patients. *N Engl J Med* 2004;**351**:1493.
FEV₁, forced expiratory volume in 1 second; *LVEF*, left ventricular ejection fraction.
All risks are relative and somewhat dependent on the particular patient and surgeon.

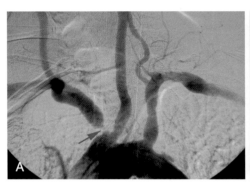
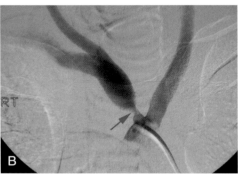
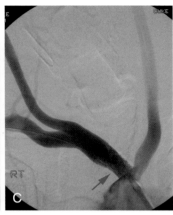

FIGURE 20-3 Great vessel angioplasty and stenting in a 75-year-old man with new onset blurred vision and transient ischemic attack. **A,** Angiogram of aortic arch demonstrates a common origin of the left common carotid artery with the right brachiocephalic artery. There is a short segment 75% stenosis *(arrow)* involving the proximal brachiocephalic artery immediately distal to the origin of the left common carotid artery. **B,** Angiogram via the introducer sheath confirms stenosis of proximal right brachiocephalic *(arrow)*. **C,** Angiogram via the introducer sheath following angioplasty and balloon-expandable stent (9 mm) placement *(arrow)* shows an excellent radiographic result. To avoid theoretical embolic complications from stent protrusion into the carotid artery, the stent was placed at the origin of the right brachiocephalic artery without extending into the left common carotid artery. This was not ideal in that the atherosclerotic disease extended by angiography to the origin of the brachiocephalic artery and could predispose to restenosis at the brachiocephalic origin.

the contralateral vertebral artery is "stolen" from the posterior fossa via the basilar artery then coursing down the ipsilateral vertebral artery to supply the arm. However, simple reversal of blood flow in a vertebral artery has been found in 6% of patients undergoing carotid ultrasound, far more often on the left than the right side (82%).[28] The diagnosis of *subclavian steal syndrome* is reserved for patients who are symptomatic from resulting posterior fossa ischemia, typically complaining of

dizziness or ataxia. Angioplasty and stenting have achieved widespread acceptance as the procedure of choice in this situation. Technical success exceeds 95% for stenotic lesions; for total obstructions, success rates fall to 65% to 85%, largely from failure to traverse the occlusion.[15-17] The 5-year clinical patency rates range between 82% and 89%.[29,30] Protection devices are rarely used in the vertebral artery during subclavian artery angioplasty and stenting based on the concept that the

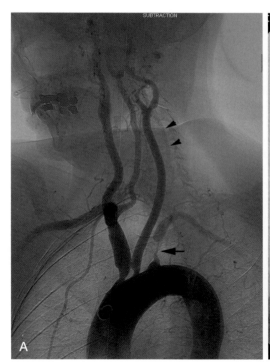
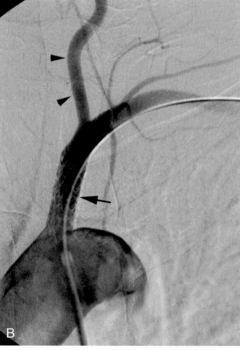

FIGURE 20-4 Subclavian steal syndrome treated by angioplasty and stenting in a 72-year-old female with gait disturbance and reversal of flow in left vertebral artery by prior imaging studies. **A,** Arch aortogram in a left anterior oblique projection demonstrates high-grade stenosis of the left subclavian artery *(arrow)*. Note the reversal of flow in the left vertebral artery *(arrowheads)*. **B,** Left subclavian angiogram following placement of a 7- × 24-mm balloon-expandable stent *(arrow)*. There is antegrade flow in the left vertebral artery *(arrowheads)*. Note that the stent extends just down into the aorta.

brain is protected from microemboli by the flow reversal in the ipsilateral vertebral artery.[31] Nonetheless, strokes have been reported.[30] Stenting across the vertebral artery origin has been undertaken, particularly when symptoms consist of arm claudication and the ipsilateral vertebral artery is the nondominant vertebral vessel.

Cervical vertebral artery atherosclerotic disease is prevalent in patients with peripheral arterial disease. However, the diagnosis is often difficult owing to the relative vagueness of symptoms. It may even be difficult to determine whether patient complaints are related to a vertebral artery stenosis or occlusion if the contralateral vertebral artery is patent or the ipsilateral collateral circulation is abundant. Once a connection is made between symptoms and vertebral artery obstruction, angioplasty itself is straightforward and produces acceptable results. Angioplasty with stent placement is performed for lesions at the orifice of the vertebral artery but angioplasty alone may be otherwise applied through the extracranial vertebral artery (Fig. 20-5). Procedural and clinical success has been reported to be 100% and 90.5%, respectively, with 79.3% of individuals remaining symptom-free at 1 year.[32] Only one small randomized study of vertebral artery angioplasty has been carried out, which included 16 patients with vertebral artery disease, eight treated with medical therapy and eight by endovascular stenting.[33] At a mean of nearly 5 years, neither group had strokes referable to the vertebral artery distribution. A Cochrane database review in 2005 identified 173 reports of vertebral artery stenting and found a 30-day major stroke and death rate of 3.2% and a 30-day transient ischemia and nondisabling stroke rate of 3.2%.[34]

The published results for angioplasty and stenting of the *carotid artery bifurcation* are mixed.[19,35-39] Table 20-2 presents the six clinical trials in which carotid artery stenting (CAS) was randomized to carotid endarterectomy (CEA).[19,35-39] The studies varied widely in terms of inclusion criteria, symptoms, endpoints, qualifications of the operators, and standardization of techniques. Out of five studies, three found that CAS was not inferior to CEA while two found CAS inferior. Thus far, the best study comparing CAS with CEA in surgically suitable patients is the Carotid Revascularization Endarterectomy versus Stenting Trial (CREST) published in 2010.[35] This randomized trial included 2502 patients, both symptomatic and asymptomatic, followed for a median of 2 years after treatment for the primary endpoints of stroke, myocardial infarction, and death. There was overall no difference between the two groups. However, in the 30-day periprocedural period, stroke occurred more often in the stenting group (CEA 2.3% vs. CAS 4.1%) whereas myocardial infarction was greater in the surgery group (2.3% vs. 1.1%) (see Table 20-2). The estimated 4-year rates for the primary endpoints were equivalent.

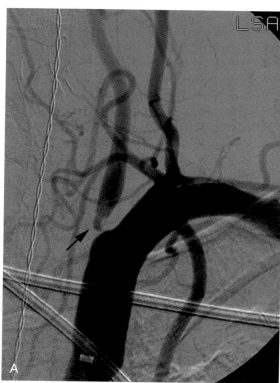
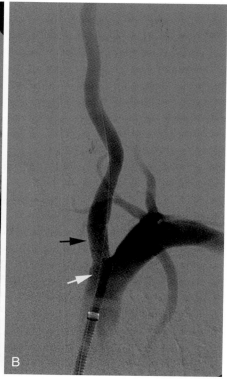

FIGURE 20-5 Proximal vertebral artery stenting in a 57-year-old man with history of left vertebral artery stenosis and questionable symptoms referable to the posterior fossa. **A,** Left subclavian angiogram demonstrates a greater than 90% stenosis of the proximal left vertebral artery at its origin *(arrow)*. **B,** Angioplasty and stenting was performed with 5- × 12-mm balloon-expandable stent with an excellent radiographic result *(black arrow)*. Because this is a lesion at the orifice of the vertebral artery, a small amount of stent was allowed to extend into the left subclavian artery *(white arrow)*.

TABLE 20-2   Comparison of Studies Randomizing Surgical Carotid Endarterectomy to Carotid Artery Stenting

Study	SAPPHIRE	SPACE	EVA-3S	CAVATAS	ICSS	CREST
Year published	2004	2006	2006	2009	2010	2010
Total no. patients randomized	334	1183	527	504	1710	2522
Symptomatic patients	28.8%	100%	100%	97%	100%	53%
Patients receiving CEA	167	595	262	253	858	1240
Patients receiving CAS	167	605	265	251	855	1262
Procedures using a DPD	95.6%	Not provided	91.9%	0%	80%	96.1%
Primary endpoint of study	Cumulative death, stroke, or MI at 30 days or death or ipsilateral stroke 31 days to 1 yr	Ipsilateral stroke or death within 30 days	Any stroke or death within 30 days	Death or disabling stroke within 30 days or any stroke lasting more than 7 days or death within 30 days	Any stroke, MI, or death within 120 days	Any stroke, death, or MI in peri-procedural 30-day period or ipsilateral stroke within 4 yr
CEA stroke	7.90%	5.14%	2.70%	8.00%	4.10%	2.30%
CAS stroke	6.20%	6.51%	8.80%	8.00%	7.70%	4.10%
CEA MI	7.50%	NA	0.80%	1.00%	0.47%	2.30%
CAS MI	3.00%	NA	0.40%	0.00%	0.35%	1.10%
CEA death	13.50%	0.86%	1.20%	2.00%	0.80%	0.30%
CAS death	7.40%	0.67%	0.80%	3.00%	2.00%	0.70%
Author's conclusions	Among patients with severe carotid artery stenosis and coexisting conditions, CAS with the use of an emboli-protection device is not inferior to CEA.	Failed to show noninferiority of CAS compared with CEA.	In patients with symptomatic carotid stenosis of 60% or more, the rates of death and stroke at 1 and 6 mo were lower with endarterectomy than with stenting.	Endovascular treatment had similar major risks and effectiveness at prevention of stroke during 3 yr compared with carotid surgery but with wide confidence intervals.	CEA should remain treatment of choice in those suitable for surgery.	No difference in outcome but higher periprocedural risk of MI with CEA and stroke with CAS.

CAVATAS, *Carotid and Vertebral Artery Transluminal Angioplasty Study*; CAS, *carotid artery stenting*; CEA, *carotid endarterectomy*; CREST, *Carotid Revascularization Endarterectomy versus Stenting Trial*; DPD, *distal protection device*; EVA-3S, *Endarterectomy versus Angioplasty in Patients with Symptomatic Severe Carotid Stenosis trial*; ICSS, *International Carotid Stenting Study*; MI, *myocardial infarction*; SAPPHIRE, *Stenting and Angioplasty with Protection in Patients at High Risk for Endarterectomy trial*; SPACE, *Stent-Supported Percutaneous Angioplasty of the Carotid Artery versus Endarterectomy trial.*

COMPLICATIONS

Stroke is the most dreaded complication when treating any vessel supplying cerebral tissue. For the carotid artery bifurcation, ischemic stroke ranges from 4.1% to 8.8% in the perioperative period for carotid artery stenting (see Table 20-2). Other complications, however, may occur. Hypotension and bradycardia following carotid artery stenting have been reported in up to 35% of patients because of stretching of the baroreceptors located in the carotid sinus.[40] These receptors operate through the autonomic nervous system and are an extremely important regulatory mechanism in the short-term control of blood pressure and heart rate. After CAS, stretching of these baroreceptors by the stent may induce dysfunction leading to hemodynamic instability.[41] For this reason,

patients undergoing CAS are often pretreated with atropine (up to 1 mg) and the interventional team must be ready to treat hypotension and bradycardia aggressively. Such cardiovascular changes may be very short-lived (minutes), or alternatively, vasopressive agents may be necessary until the baroreceptors autoregulate back to baseline. Patients older than 80 years have a greater incidence of neurologic symptoms following CAS than do the same aged-patients after CEA. These elderly individuals may have a greater propensity for symptomatic emboli in the face of a lessened cerebral reserve.[42]

The hyperperfusion syndrome is a rare but potentially lethal complication after endovascular or open carotid revascularization. It has been defined as a neurologic deficit or seizure ipsilateral to the treated carotid artery related to chronic ischemia rather than cerebral embolism. Complete recovery is the rule in mild cases, but disability and death can occur in more severe cases.

INTRACRANIAL ATHEROSCLEROTIC DISEASE

Natural History

Atherosclerosis of the major intracranial arteries accounts for an estimated 8% to 10% of ischemic strokes in the United States.[43] Furthermore, among patients with a 70% to 99% stenosis and symptoms (transient ischemic attacks or stroke), a second ischemic event occurs within 1 year in the territory of the symptomatic artery in 11% of individuals.[44] Although the actual prevalence of intracranial atherosclerotic disease is largely unknown, it is more common in African Americans and Hispanics, as well as patients with insulin-resistant diabetes and those with hypercholesterolemia and inflammation.[45,46]

Treatment

Medical and Surgical Therapy

Surgery for intracranial atherosclerosis was evaluated in the 1985 external carotid to internal carotid bypass study, which concluded that bypass failed to reduce the risk of ischemic stroke compared with medical therapy.[47] Although interest has revived recently, surgery is largely reserved for patients who have failed medical therapy and who are not candidates for or have failed endovascular interventions.

Based for the most part on the failure of surgical bypass, medical therapy for intracranial atherosclerosis has focused on the use of warfarin. However, the results of the Warfarin-Aspirin Symptomatic Intracranial Disease study (WASID) demonstrated that warfarin was associated with significantly higher rates of adverse events and provided no benefit over aspirin.[48] Antiplatelet agents, including aspirin and clopidogrel, are currently the primary drugs used in the medical treatment of intracranial atherosclerotic disease.

Endovascular Therapy

Endovascular therapy for intracranial atherosclerosis has been limited to symptomatic patients with greater than 50% stenosis who have failed medical therapy and asymptomatic patients with stenoses who are counseled regarding the therapeutic options and a wish to proceed with recanalization.[49] To lessen the likelihood of vessel perforation, intracranial endovascular therapy should be limited to the major proximal vessels (intracranial carotid and vertebral, basilar, M1, and rarely P1; see Fig. 20-1). Autopsy data have noted that the distribution of intracranial atherosclerotic disease largely involves these same vessels.[50]

Intracranial angioplasty procedures are typically (though not universally) performed with general anesthesia. The therapeutic options are angioplasty alone or angioplasty with stenting. It is usually easier to negotiate the tortuous vertebral and carotid vessels with a balloon alone; advancing a stent through these pathways can be quite difficult. Stenting has thus far not been shown to be superior to angioplasty alone and are thus usually grouped together in publications.[51] Angioplasty alone carries the fears of an intimal dissection, some advocating that the occurrence of a significant intimal flap can be limited by slow, prolonged balloon inflations (approximately 2 minutes) as opposed to quick, sudden inflations.[52] Stents can be either of the self-expanding or balloon-expandable variety (Figs. 20-6 and 20-7). Balloon-expandable stents are for the most part coronary stents used in an off-label fashion. A single self-expanding stent (Wingspan Stent System, Boston Scientific, Natick, Mass.) has a human device exemption from the

FIGURE 20-6 Middle cerebral artery (M1) angioplasty and stenting in a 42-year-old woman with a several-month history of right middle cerebral artery distribution stroke. **A,** Anteroposterior intracranial view demonstrates a focal high-grade stenosis (>90%) of the proximal right middle cerebral artery (arrow). Angioplasty was performed to 2.5 mm and a self-expanding 2.5- × 15-mm stent was placed. **B,** Angiography following angioplasty and stent placement shows an excellent radiographic result (arrow).

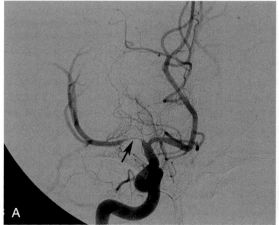
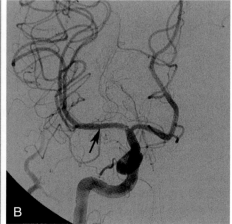

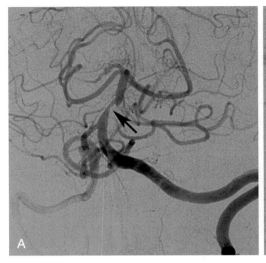
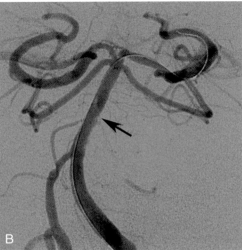

FIGURE 20-7 Basilar artery angioplasty and stenting in a 54-year-old man with a 3-month history of posterior circulation stroke. **A,** Left vertebral angiogram demonstrates an 80% to 90% stenosis of the midbasilar artery *(arrow).* Angioplasty and stenting was performed using a 3- × 13-mm balloon-expandable coronary drug-eluting stent. **B,** Angiography following angioplasty and stent placement shows an excellent radiographic result *(arrow).*

U.S. Food and Drug Administration (FDA) for intracranial use (see Fig. 20-6).

Data regarding intracranial angioplasty and stenting are now being published.[53] A systematic outcomes review in 2009 identified 31 studies reporting on 1177 procedures, performed mostly (98%) in symptomatic patients with high-grade (mean 79%) intracranial stenoses.[54] There was a high technical success rate (median 96%) with periprocedural minor or major stroke and death rates ranging from 0% to 50% (median 7.7%). Periprocedural complications were significantly higher in the posterior versus the anterior circulation, but did not differ between patients treated with balloon-mounted versus self-expanding stents. However, restenosis greater than 50% at a mean of 8.7 months occurred more frequently after the use of self-expanding stents.

Two multicenter prospective nonrandomized patient registries have been conducted by product manufacturers resulting in human device exemption status from the FDA: the Stenting of Symptomatic Atherosclerotic Lesions in the Vertebral or Intracranial Artery (SSYLVIA) study and the Wingspan stent system with Gateway PTA Dilation Catheter (Boston Scientific, Fremont, Calif.).[55,56] The SSYLVIA trial used the Neurolink System, a self-expanding stent (then Guidant, Menlo Park, Calif.), and found an overall symptomatic restenosis rate of 13.7% with an initial procedural success rate of 85.5%.[55] The Wingspan study had a procedural success rate of 98%, although a 7.5% greater than 50% restenosis rate at 6 months.[56] The Wingspan self-expanding stent is available under a human device exemption; the Neurolink stent is not currently available. A randomized study between the Wingspan stent and best medical therapy was undertaken in the Stenting and Aggressive Medical Management for Preventing Recurrent Stroke and Intracranial Stenosis trial (SAMMPRIS). This large study compared medical to endovascular therapy in symptomatic patients with a 70% to 99% stenosis of a major intracranial artery. The study was recently stopped due to a high rate of complications in the stenting group. Publication of the data is pending at this writing.

Complications of intracranial angioplasty include stroke from intimal dissection or distal embolization. Intracranial arteries are very thin-walled structures. Vessel perforation is a particular risk of angioplasty at these sites with increasing likelihood at more distal locations. Careful guidewire placement during lesion traversal is essential, taking care to avoid migration of the wire tip into small vessels. Balloon and stent sizing must be carefully calculated to avoid overdistention of the artery during angioplasty. There is little chance for rescue of an acutely perforated intracranial vessel.

ACUTE STROKE

Etiology and Natural History

By definition, stroke refers to a fixed neurologic deficit of greater than 24 hours duration. The estimated incidence of stroke in the United States is approximately 795,000 per year. Stroke is the third leading cause of death in the United States and the leading cause of long-term disability.[57] Eighty-three percent of strokes are ischemic and related to large artery atherosclerosis, thromboembolism, small vessel occlusion, or other causes.[58] The remaining 17% of cases are hemorrhagic (about 10% intracerebral and 7% subarachnoid).

Stroke is the clinical situation that follows neurologic cell death because of decreased blood flow. However, acute stroke has a large component of fluctuating ischemia. The *ischemic penumbra* refers to the region of threatened tissue adjacent to the core of evolving infarction. It is thought that this area has a limited and variable interval of viability and is potentially salvageable by the quick restoration of blood flow. The primary goal of acute stroke treatment is preventing frank infarction in this fragile region.

Clinical Features

The patient should be expediently evaluated by the neurologic stroke team for findings of ischemic stroke (Fig. 20-8). A complete history is obtained, sometimes from a family member. The presence of contraindications to the administration of intravenous thrombolytic

therapy is determined (Box 20-2). A key item in the history is the exact time of symptom onset (or time the patient was last known to be in his usual state of health).

The physical examination should determine vital signs, the National Institutes of Health Stroke Scale (NIHSS), and likely vascular territory and etiology of stroke if possible. The NIHSS evaluates neurologic impairment on a scale of 1 to 42, with higher scores (21 to 42) indicating severe neurologic impairment (www. ninds.gov/disorders/stroke/strokescales). Laboratory studies should include coagulation parameters and blood glucose levels, because profound hypoglycemia or hyperglycemia can mimic stroke.

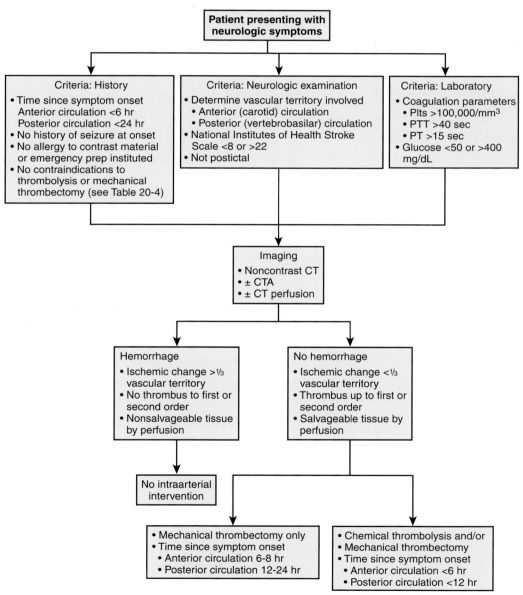

FIGURE 20-8 Flow chart of the workup of stroke. Evaluation and treatment flow diagram for patients presenting with acute stroke symptoms.

BOX 20-2

INTRAVENOUS RECOMBINANT TISSUE PLASMINOGEN ACTIVATOR FOR ACUTE ISCHEMIC STROKE*

Contraindications to Administration

Recombinant tissue plasminogen activator (t-PA) therapy in patients with acute ischemic stroke is contraindicated in the following situations because of an increased risk of bleeding, which could result in significant disability or death:

- Evidence of intracranial hemorrhage on pretreatment evaluation
- Suspicion of subarachnoid hemorrhage on pretreatment evaluation
- Recent (within 3 months) intracranial or intraspinal surgery, serious head trauma, or previous stroke
- History of intracranial hemorrhage
- Uncontrolled hypertension at time of treatment (e.g., >185 mm Hg systolic or >110 mm Hg diastolic)
- Seizure at the onset of stroke
- Active internal bleeding
- Intracranial neoplasm, arteriovenous malformation, or aneurysm
- Known bleeding diathesis including but not limited to:
  - Current use of oral anticoagulants (e.g., warfarin sodium) or an international normalized ratio (INR) >1.7 or a prothrombin time (PT) >15 seconds
  - Administration of heparin within 48 hours preceding the onset of stroke and elevated activated partial thromboplastin time (aPTT) at presentation
  - Platelet count <100,000/mm^3

Risks for the administration of intravenous t-PA may be increased and should be weighed against the benefits in the following situations:

- Severe neurologic deficits (National Institutes of Health Stroke Scale [NIHSS] >22) at presentation
- Early signs of infarct on computed tomography

The administration of intravenous t-PA is not recommended in the following cases:

- Acute ischemic stroke more than 3 hours after symptom onset[†]
- Minor neurologic deficits or rapidly improving symptoms

Generally Accepted Guidelines for Administration

Indications
- Neurologic symptoms must be significant: isolated aphasia or hemianopsia, or NIHSS >4.
- Neurologic symptoms must be concordant with the vascular territory of ischemia.
- Patients with anterior circulation occlusion are eligible for intraarterial t-PA if thrombolysis within 6 hours, and eligible for mechanical thrombolysis if revascularization is possible within 8 hours of symptom onset.
- Patients with basilar artery occlusion are eligible for intraarterial t-PA if thrombolysis within 12, and eligible for mechanical thrombolysis if revascularization is possible within 24 hours of symptom onset.
- Mechanical thrombolysis is possible only for proximal M2, M1, A1, P1, ICA, basilar, and vertebral arteries. More distal occlusion can be treated with intraarterial t-PA.

Contraindications
- Any acute intracranial hemorrhage.
- Parenchymal hypodensity by CT of greater than one third of the affected vascular territory
- Any mass effect with significant midline shift or central nervous system lesion with high likelihood of hemorrhage (e.g., brain tumors except small meningioma, vascular malformation, aneurysm, significant head trauma)
- Intracranial tumor except small meningioma

Relative Contraindications
- Rapidly improving neurologic examination (NIHSS <4)
- Seizures at the time of presentation (if residual neurologic deficits due to postictal state)
- Baseline NIHSS >22
- Recent intracranial or spinal surgery, head trauma, or stroke within the past 90 days
- Stroke within the past 60 days
- Recent surgery/trauma (>15 days)
- Baseline INR >1.7, aPTT >1.5 × normal, platelets <100 K
- Glucose <50 or >400 mg/dL
- Systolic blood pressure >180 mm Hg and diastolic blood pressure >100 mm Hg

*From package insert for alteplase (Acitvase; Genetech, Inc., South San Francisco, Calif.).
[†]Only the time from symptom onset for the administration of intravenous t-PA is greatly different than the intraarterial administration.

Imaging

Prompt CT examination is critical. A noncontrast head CT is obtained to identify intracerebral or subarachnoid hemorrhage or other etiologies to account for the presenting symptoms (e.g., intracranial tumor). To some extent, the CT images quantify the extent of cerebral infarction. Secondary signs include the hyperdense middle cerebral artery sign, which correlates relatively well with artery occlusion especially in younger patients (Fig. 20-9). The location and extent of early ischemic changes can influence a patient's qualification for intraarterial (IA) thrombolytic therapy as noted later. In many centers, noncontrast CT imaging is followed by CT angiography to verify and localize large-vessel occlusions and assess the aortic arch, and carotid and vertebral arteries. In some centers, a CT perfusion study is coupled with CT angiography. Perfusion imaging enables a determination of estimated tissue at risk, that is, the ischemic penumbra, which can be potentially salvaged with reperfusion techniques. Data supporting the value of perfusion imaging in clinical

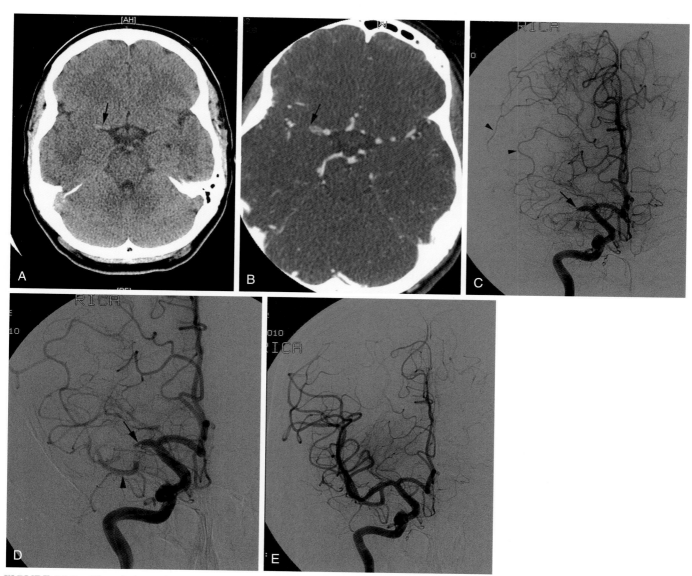

FIGURE 20-9 Thrombolysis of acute stroke in a 16-year-old male patient with acute onset of dense left hemiparesis approximately 4 hours before the procedure. **A,** Noncontrast computed tomography (CT) demonstrates dense left middle cerebral artery *(arrow)*. **B,** CT angiography demonstrates thrombus within the right M1 segment *(arrow)* with preservation of distal perfusion to into branches. **C,** Right internal carotid angiogram and anterior posterior projection demonstrates occlusion of the right middle cerebral artery *(arrow)* with pial collaterals from the anterior cerebral artery *(arrowheads)*. **D,** Angiogram after microcatheter *(arrow)* has been placed into thrombus and infusion of rtPA has begun. There is now some antegrade flow within the middle cerebral artery *(arrowhead)*. **E,** Final angiogram following the infusion of 25 mg of rtPA into the right middle cerebral artery. There is antegrade flow in the vessel with an excellent radiographic result.

decision-making is still lacking. MR imaging (MRI) has many features that make it attractive as an initial imaging tool, but it is often too time-consuming to obtain in the acute setting.

Treatment

Medical Therapy

The cornerstone of modern medical therapy for acute stroke is administration of intravenous (IV) recombinant tissue plasminogen activator (t-PA) (see Fig. 20-8). The standard protocol for t-PA administration is based on the pivotal National Institute of Neurological Disorders and Stroke (NINDS) study published in 1995, which compared IV t-PA with placebo administered within 3 hours of the onset of stroke symptoms.[59] This trial found a statistically significant reduction in the degree of long-term disability for the group treated with IV t-PA. Importantly, although there were more symptomatic hemorrhages in the t-PA group, the benefit from thrombolytic therapy was not offset with any increase in mortality. The biggest obstacle for the administration of IV t-PA is timing. Many patients do not arrive at the hospital within 3 hours of symptom onset, and even when they do, a comprehensive effort is required to evaluate a patient, make a treatment decision, and then expediently administer t-PA. Practically speaking, a patient must present to the hospital well before 3 hours of symptom onset to qualify for IV t-PA treatment. Recent studies, most notably the European Cooperative Acute Stroke Study, suggest that the therapeutic window for safe, effective intravenous thrombolysis in acute stroke may be extended up to 4.5 hours following symptom onset, albeit in a very select patient population.[60]

Endovascular Therapy

PATIENT SELECTION

If IV t-PA administration is not an option, endovascular intervention should be considered. Recanalization can be accomplished by chemical thrombolysis with IA infusion of a thrombolytic agent, mechanical thrombectomy, or both.

Because the fibrinolytic agent is delivered directly into the thrombus, the effective dose is much lower than with systemic administration. Based on animal studies and limited human data, a therapeutic window of 6 hours for reperfusion of anterior cerebral (carotid distribution) ischemia with IA delivery is the threshold used by most stroke centers. This 6-hour limit has been chosen as a realistic time interval that will maximize both patient safety and chances of success.

Without direct treatment, outcomes for vertebrobasilar stroke are often dismal, with an 80% rate of death or significant disability.[61,62] Stroke in this circulation is less likely to be thromboembolic in nature and is more often associated with intracranial atherosclerotic disease.[63] As such, angioplasty and sometimes stent placement is often necessary after thrombolysis (Fig. 20-10). For that reason as well as a lessened rate of hemorrhagic complications following IA thrombolysis in the posterior circulation, the window for the administration of thrombolytic agents is usually increased to 12 hours from symptom onset.[64]

As with thrombolysis in the peripheral system, there are controversies regarding protocols (drug, dose, infusion duration) for the application of IA thrombolytic agents in acute stroke. In the United States, the most commonly used agent is t-PA, although much of the data are based on prior reported experience with urokinase.[64,65] Although there is widespread agreement

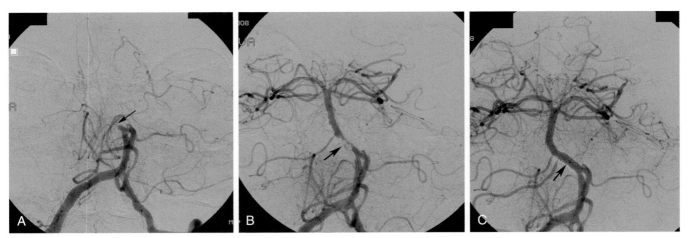

FIGURE 20-10   Basilar thrombolysis and angioplasty with stent placement in a 56-year-old man who was admitted to the stroke service with evidence of posterior fossa ischemia. The patient's neurologic examination acutely deteriorated. **A,** Right vertebral artery angiogram shows complete occlusion of the proximal basilar artery *(arrow)*. **B,** Following thrombolysis, residual stenosis *(arrow)* was noted, which reoccluded and was again opened with additional recombinant tissue plasminogen activator (total dose 10 mg). **C,** Angioplasty and stenting with a 3- × 9-mm coronary stent produced an excellent radiographic result *(arrow)*.

on which patients are eligible for IV t-PA, the indications for IA therapy vary from institution to institution and even among interventionists within the same institution. Some practitioners reserve IA therapy for patients not eligible for IV therapy; others routinely give eligible patients lower bridging doses of IV t-PA to transition to IA therapy; still others proceed with IA therapy even after full-dose IV t-PA has been given in clinically refractory patients.

Technique

Although subject to some controversy, stroke interventions are probably best performed under the more controlled conditions of general anesthesia. The use of heparin in stroke thrombolysis is controversial, because there is an increased risk of intracranial hemorrhage.[64] Diagnostic angiography is performed initially to evaluate areas of occlusion and degree of collateral flow, and as a map for thrombolytic therapy. Through a 6-Fr guiding catheter, a microcatheter is placed either against or into the thrombus, and the thrombolytic agent is slowly

injected (see Fig. 20-9). Multiple injections can be performed until the thrombus is dissolved, a predetermined maximum dose of agent is administered, or a predetermined time allotted for revascularization expires. Doses for t-PA vary among interventionists but it is typically injected in small increments (1 to 5 mg) with frequent angiography to assess for recanalization. Predetermined maximum doses vary among operators but were reported in a safety and efficacy analysis to range from 20 to 60 mg.[66]

Mechanical thrombus disruption or removal is considered when chemical thrombolysis is failing or as a therapeutic option when the patient presents too late from symptom onset to be considered for IA thrombolysis (see Fig. 20-8). Although the time frame varies considerably, a window of up to 8 hours in the anterior circulation and 24 hours in the posterior circulation is used for mechanical thrombus removal. However, few data are available to substantiate these intervals. Several specialized mechanical thrombus removal systems are approved by the FDA for intracerebral use (Fig. 20-11). The Merci mechanical

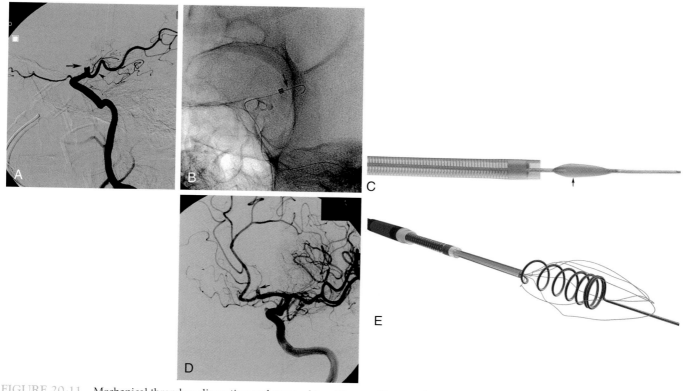

FIGURE 20-11 Mechanical thrombus disruption and removal in a 62-year-old man who recently underwent coronary bypass surgery and during his postoperative course became acutely hemiplegic on the right side and aphasic. **A,** Lateral angiogram of the left internal carotid artery demonstrates occlusion of the internal carotid artery *(arrow)* just above the take-off of the posterior communicating artery *(arrowhead).* Following the administration of 20 mg of recombinant tissue plasminogen activator (t-PA) in divided doses, forward flow could not be established in the distal internal carotid artery. **B,** The Penumbra stroke system was placed into the distal internal carotid artery and middle cerebral arteries *(arrow).* **C,** Image of Penumbra System demonstrating catheter and separation *(arrow).* **D,** Postangiogram of the left internal carotid artery demonstrates flow in the distal internal carotid artery and into the middle cerebral artery and anterior (A1) artery. There is occlusion of the left A2 vessel *(arrow),* and a microcatheter was placed in this location and additional t-PA was given but this did not open. **E,** Merci Retriever demonstrating the platinum wire as well as suture material that served to remove thrombus. *(C, Courtesy of Penumbra, Alameda, Calif., with permission.* **E,** *Courtesy of Concentric Medial, Mountain View, Calif., with permission.)*

thrombolysis device (Concentric Medical, Mountain View, Calif.) consists of a microwire and suture which grasps the thrombus for removal via a large lumen balloon catheter (see Fig. 20-11E). The device and the microcatheter are withdrawn together through the balloon catheter to remove intact clot. The Penumbra Stroke System (Penumbra, Alameda, Calif.) consists of a specialized microcatheter with a distal tip that separates from the catheter lumen (see Fig. 20-11C). Thrombus is then removed using controlled suction provided by a specialized pump.

Results

Despite relatively widespread use, evidence for the value of endovascular treatment of acute stroke consists of small series, case reports, and manufacturer sponsored studies.[67] The best published study to date is the Prolyse in Acute Cerebral Thromboembolism trial (PROACT).[64] In this investigation, patients with middle cerebral artery thrombus were randomized to receive recombinant pro-urokinase (rproUK), a non–FDA-approved agent similar to urokinase or heparin. In the initial phase of the trial (often termed *PROACT I*), 26 patients were treated with rproUK and 14 with placebo. Both recanalization and intracranial hemorrhage were greater in the rproUK group. All patients in the rproUK group who had hemorrhage had early CT changes (five patients) of greater than 33% of the middle cerebral artery territory. Such a pattern on CT has become a relative contraindication for thrombolysis. It was also noted that hemorrhage was associated with higher heparin doses. The second phase of the study (often termed *PROACT II*) enrolled 180 patients who received either rproUK plus low-dose heparin or low-dose heparin alone.[64] The results of this study showed long-term benefit (slight or no neurologic impairment) in 40% of patients in the thrombolysis group versus 25% with the heparin group.

Another randomized study, the Middle Cerebral Artery Embolism Local Fibrinolytic Intervention Trial (MELT) randomized 114 patients to receive urokinase versus heparin alone.[65] The results showed improved functional outcomes in the thrombolysis group compared with controls. The study, however, was discontinued upon the approval of IV t-PA in Japan. No randomized trials have been completed for posterior circulation IA thrombolytic therapy. The one study that was initiated was terminated due to slow recruitment of patients and ultimately the removal of urokinase from the market.[68] Metaanalyses of existing reports that encompassed 344 patients treated with IA thrombolysis found death or neurologic dependency in 76%, essentially equal to those receiving IV t-PA. There were, however, better recanalization rates with IA administration.[69]

Data on mechanical removal devices is principally based on manufacturer-sponsored publications. The Merci device was initially studied in a 30-patient phase I multicenter trial, in which successful recanalization with the retriever alone was achieved in 43% of patients and with additional IA t-PA in 64%.[70] The Mechanical Embolus Removal in Cerebral Ischemia (MERCI) trial, which was a prospective single-arm trial of 164 patients, demonstrated recanalization in 55% of the vessels with the device alone. The initial Penumbra trial consisted of 20 patients treated within 8 hours of symptom onset and produced recanalization in all treated cases.[71] This study was followed by a larger prospective single-arm multicenter trial (the Penumbra Stroke Trial) conducted at 24 international centers that enrolled 125 patients and found partial or complete recanalization in 82% of patients.[72]

Complications

The most dreaded complication of endovascular stroke therapy is significant intracranial bleeding, which occurs in about 15% of cases.[64] Keep in mind, to some degree hemorrhage is part of the evolution of stroke, occurring in 43% of patients absent any intervention and is dependent upon a number of factors including degree of neurologic deficit, size of the infarct, and an embolic etiology.[73] Intraprocedure hemorrhage is suggested by sudden hemodynamic fluctuation due to increased intracranial pressure and proven by extravasation of contrast on the cerebral angiogram. Alternatively, newer flat panel angiographic systems allow for CT scanning of sufficient quality to detect hemorrhage. If bleeding is suspected, thrombolytic infusion should be discontinued immediately and anticoagulation reversed.

PREOPERATIVE TUMOR EMBOLIZATION

Etiology and Clinical Features

Meningiomas are thought to arise from arachnoidal cap cells, which reside in the arachnoid layer covering the surface of the brain and thus may arise in a variety of locations.[74] They may be entirely asymptomatic or present with headaches or neurologic deficits. In the head and neck region, the normal paraganglia are associated with the parasympathetic nervous system and *paragangliomas* arise from these parasympathetic sites.[75] Patients with cervical paragangliomas typically develop a painless, slowly enlarging mass in the lateral aspect of the neck. Tinnitus and hearing loss are earliest symptoms of tympanicum and jugulare tumors. The pathophysiology of *juvenile angiofibromas* is incompletely understood with various theories as to even its site of origin including originating from nonchromaffin paraganglionic cells of the terminal branches of the maxillary artery, accounting for their dense hypervascularity and arterial supply.[76] Juvenile nasopharyngeal angiofibroma presents clinically as a nasal mass and, when symptomatic, usually causes epistaxis.

Imaging

Imaging with CT or MRI is critical to the diagnosis and treatment planning for these tumors. In particular, they assess the degree of vascularity and therefore the need for preoperative embolization. Doppler sonography of the neck is the usual first imaging step for suspected cervical paragangliomas. Digital subtraction angiography is necessary to characterize the vascular anatomy and flow dynamics before preoperative embolotherapy. Meningiomas derive their blood supply from meningeal arteries and classically display a "starburst" appearance in the capillary phase of the study.[74]

Treatment

In theory, preoperative embolization of vascular head and neck tumors renders them smaller, softer, less vascular, and therefore easier to manipulate and remove surgically. Thus embolotherapy may shorten operative time, reduce blood loss, enable more precise tumor resection, and lessen the potential for surrounding tissue injury from retraction and manipulation.[77] The goal of preoperative embolization is obliteration of the capillary bed as thoroughly as possible while still preserving normal tissue (including the brain, cranial nerves, and skin). Proximal embolization of the feeding artery alone affords little advantage to surgical ligation at the time of surgery. Embolization is almost universally performed with particles, most often PVA, via a microcatheter inserted directly into the arterial supply to the tumor

(Table 20-3). Particle size depends on position of the microcatheter relative to the tumor and presence of arteriovenous shunting. The closer the microcatheter to the tumor, the less potential for nontarget embolization, and smaller particles (<150 μm) can be used to more effectively obliterate the tumor capillary bed.[78] There are, however, reports of increased complications related to small particles, mostly consisting of postembolization hemorrhage.[79] In addition, large particles (up to 750 μm) may need to be used if the microcatheter is well proximal in the feeding vessel or if large arteriovenous shunts are present, although the latter are relatively unusual. Embolization is ideally carried out until stasis or near stasis of blood flow.

Meningiomas

Meningiomas are the most common benign brain tumors in adults and are therefore encountered relatively often in neurosurgical practice. Angiography is only used for diagnosis if noninvasive studies are equivocal.[79] In most situations, therefore, patients with meningiomas only present to the neurointerventionalist for preoperative embolization (Fig. 20-12).

The timing of meningioma or other tumor surgical resection relative to preoperative embolization is controversial. The classic teaching has been to perform surgery as soon as possible following embolization, usually within 24 hours, to prevent excessive tumor swelling and revascularization.[80] However, recent studies have found that this swelling is easily controlled and the greatest degree of tumor softening at surgery occurs

TABLE 20-3   Arterial Supply from the External Carotid Artery to Tumors and Epistaxis

	Arterial Blood Supply	**Embolic Agents**
Meningioma	MMA (most common) Accessory MA branches IMax-ethmoidal branches Occipital artery (tumor posterior) STA (tumor superior/falcine)	Particles <150 μm if microcatheter tip close to tumor; otherwise particles 250 μm and larger
Paraganglioma		
Cervical carotid body/vagal	Ascending pharyngeal Facial Thyroidal Lingual	Particles <150 μm if microcatheter tip close to tumor; otherwise particles 250 μm and larger, especially if A-V shunting
Temporal jugular/tympanic	Ascending pharyngeal Distal internal maxillary Posterior auricular Occipital	Particles <150 μm if microcatheter tip close to tumor; otherwise particles 250 μm and larger, especially if A-V shunting
Juvenile angiofibroma and epistaxis	Distal internal maxillary Facial	Particles >250 μm, even larger if bilateral supply being embolized Especially worrisome for skin necrosis

Important to assess venous anatomy, particularly relative to the dural sinus for meningioma and the jugular veins for paragangliomas, which will affect the surgical approach.

Many of these may also have supply from vertebral and intracranial arteries. For juvenile angiofibroma, arterial supply may vary significantly if prior surgery has been undertaken.

Smith TP. Embolization in the external carotid artery. J Vas Interv Radiol 2006;**17**:1897.

IMax, *internal maxillary;* MA, *meningeal artery;* MMA, *middle meningeal artery;* STA, *superficial temporal artery.*

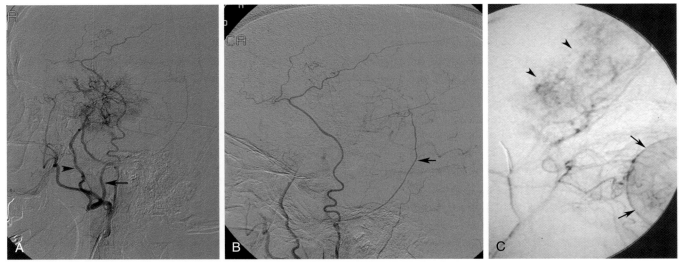

FIGURE 20-12   Embolization of meningioma. A 72-year-old male with large right sphenoid meningioma for preoperative embolization. **A,** Injection of the internal maxillary artery demonstrates supply to the meningioma mostly from the middle meningeal artery *(arrow)* and an accessory meningeal artery *(arrowhead)*. Note the sunburst pattern of the meningioma. **B,** Following particle embolization of both meningeal arteries, there is an excellent radiographic result. Only a small amount of tumor blush is noted from a small posterior meningeal supply *(arrow)*. **C,** Lateral view of angiogram after particle embolization of the middle meningeal artery in a different patient with a meningioma *(arrowheads)*. Note the prominent choroidal blush *(arrows)* demonstrating supply to the orbital contents. Embolization of this vessel runs a very high risk of causing ipsilateral blindness. Angiography of the middle meningeal artery should always include the orbit on at least one lateral view to rule out the presence of the choroidal blush. *(From Smith TP. Embolization in the external carotid artery.* J Vas Interv Radiol *2006;17:1897, with permission.)*

between 7 and 9 days following embolization.[80,81] There was no significant correlation between interval from embolotherapy and operative blood loss or procedure-related complications.[81] Therefore the interventionalist can perform the embolization procedure at any time within 7 days of surgery and still achieve the desired results.

Since its first description in 1973, preoperative embolization for meningiomas has been controversial.[82] It is not clear whether the procedure actually reduces operative blood loss sufficiently to outweigh the potential for complications. Some historical series describe decreased blood loss and reduced number of blood transfusions with preoperative embolization.[83] Unfortunately, no randomized trials are available to properly answer the question.

Major complications from meningioma embolization include neurologic deficits and tumor hemorrhage. Neurologic deficits (including cranial nerve palsy, blindness and stroke) occur in up to 3% of patients.[84] The most feared cranial nerve palsy is attributed to the facial ganglia after middle meningeal artery (MMA) embolization proximal to the facial canal. Blindness most often originates from MMA embolization when a meningolacrimal variant supplying the ophthalmic/central retinal artery is not recognized (see Fig. 20-12C). Stroke can occur when there is a failure to recognize extracranial to intracranial

collateral blood supply (see Table 20-1). Postembolization hemorrhage is reported in up to 5% of patients.[79]

Given the relative paucity of data supporting the technique, most experts recommend preoperative meningioma embolization only for highly vascular tumors as assessed by cross-sectional imaging, in particular those at the skull base.[77] In surgery at the cranial base, the feeding vessel is often not approachable operatively until the majority of the tumor has been resected. In this situation, preoperative embolization is thought to be highly useful.

Paragangliomas

Paragangliomas of the head and neck are neoplasms derived from neural crest cells and occur along the paraganglion pathway.[85] They are typically at four locations from which they derive their names: *carotid body tumors, jugular bulb (jugulare), tympanic plexus (tympanicum)*, and *vagal nerve (vagale)*. The carotid body tumor is the most common and characteristic due to its splaying of the common carotid bifurcation (Fig. 20-13). Paragangliomas are notoriously hypervascular lesions and may be multifocal in up to 22% of patients.[86] Diagnostic angiography of these tumors should include ICA injection with venous phase imaging. Venous phase imaging is particularly important with jugulare tumors to assess the extent of intravenous involvement. ICA angiography is

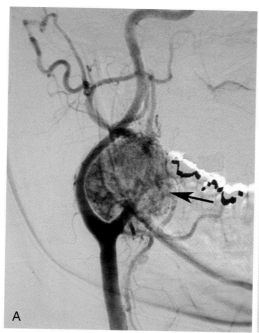
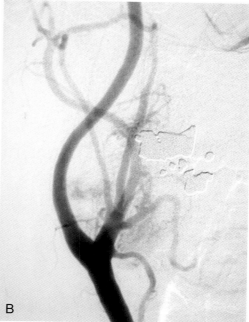

FIGURE 20-13 Embolization of carotid body tumor in a 59-year-old man with a right carotid body paraganglioma. **A,** Right common carotid artery angiogram demonstrates a hypervascular mass *(arrow),* which splays the carotid bifurcation. **B,** Postembolization angiogram demonstrates only minimal residual flow to the carotid body tumor.

particularly useful when cross-sectional imaging suggests vessel encasement by tumor and as such may necessitate surgical vessel sacrifice. In such instances, a formal test occlusion of the ICA should be considered.

The ascending pharyngeal artery provides a unique link among paragangliomas in all four regions and therefore has been called the "artery of the paraganglioma"[87] (see Table 20-3). Other potential feeding vessels are the stylomastoid artery, MMA, internal maxillary artery, and cavernous ICA. When tumors are located at the skull base, one must search carefully for intracranial extension, which may be associated with blood supply coursing intracranially.

As with meningiomas, there is controversy as to whether paraganglioma embolotherapy is necessary before surgical resection. Embolization may reduce tumor size by as much as 25%, simplify tumor manipulation during surgery, and theoretically decrease surgical blood loss.[88] The value of preoperative embolization is fairly well accepted for all but the carotid body tumors.[89,90] Some experts contend that carotid body tumors are easily and safely removed without preoperative embolization whereas others have shown in small, retrospective series that, depending on tumor size, embolization aids surgical resection.[91]

The most devastating complication of paraganglioma embolization is neurologic deficit, which is quite rare. In one series in which 53 paragangliomas were embolized in 47 individuals, six patients (13%) suffered complications (four cranial nerve weakness, one transient paresis, one asymptomatic traumatic vessel dissection).[92]

Juvenile Nasopharyngeal Angiofibroma

Juvenile nasopharyngeal angiofibroma (JNA) is a benign though locally aggressive tumor that is most common in adolescent males.[93] JNA most often presents with epistaxis, which itself is an indication for intervention. Surgery remains the definitive treatment although endoscopic measures are making inroads.[94] Preoperative embolization has become widespread since its introduction in 1979.[95] The blood supply to JNAs initially originates from the ipsilateral internal maxillary artery[96] (Fig. 20-14). As the tumor grows, other arteries contribute to the blood supply. As with other tumors, PVA appears to be the embolic agent of choice.

There are conflicting reports on the value of preoperative embolization for JNA with respect to operative times and blood loss.[97,98] As with ECA branch embolization for other reasons, neurologic deficits are the most worrisome complication. Blindness is particularly of concern due to ethmoidal feeding vessels to the ophthalmic artery.[98]

EPISTAXIS

Etiology and Clinical Features

Epistaxis has an approximate 60% lifetime incidence worldwide. However, in the vast majority of patients, bleeding stops spontaneously. Medical treatment is necessary in less than 10% of patients.[99] Epistaxis originates from one of two sites: anteriorly from predominately the anterior septum or posteriorly within

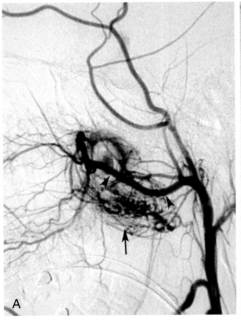
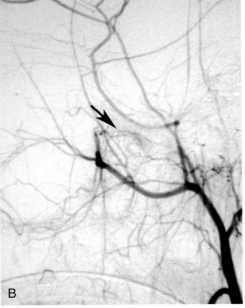

FIGURE 20-14 Embolization of juvenile nasopharyngeal angiofibroma in a 13-year-old boy with epistaxis and known nasal juvenile angiofibroma. **A,** Lateral external carotid angiography demonstrates hypervascular mass *(arrow)* in the nasal cavity bed solely from the internal maxillary artery *(arrowheads).* **B,** Postembolization images demonstrate an excellent result with only minimal residual hypervascularity *(arrow).*

the nasal cavity. There are myriad causes of epistaxis. Management and prognosis are influenced by the etiology of the condition (Box 20-3). However, approximately 80% of cases of epistaxis are idiopathic.[100]

Imaging

Endoscopic evaluation is the first-line diagnostic tool. The suspected etiology will guide the choice of imaging modality[101] (see Box 20-3). Thus imaging needs to be tailored to the individual patient. Nearly all patients with benign or malignant sinonasal neoplasms present with unilateral or at least asymmetric symptoms and therefore any recurrent unilateral epistaxis warrants radiographic studies, such as computed tomography or magnetic resonance imaging.[102]

Treatment

Medical and Surgical Therapy

The vast majority of nasal bleeding arises from the anterior cavity and can be controlled by local compression (pinching of the ala). When this maneuver fails, alternative therapies include topical vasoconstrictors, chemical or electrocautery, anterior nasal packing, and finally endoscopic ligation of the anterior ethmoidal artery. Embolotherapy for anterior epistaxis is rarely necessary due to the success of local therapies.

Posterior epistaxis occurs in the minority of cases (5%) but is more difficult to control.[103] Aggressive formal packing or balloon placement are temporizing measures for posterior epistaxis. The now widespread use of endoscopes has allowed identification of bleeding sites, more directed local therapies, and even arterial ligations

---

BOX 20-3

COMMON ETIOLOGIES OF EPISTAXIS

Local Causes

- Facial trauma
- Digital trauma
- Foreign body
- Septal perforation
- Benign nasal polyps
- Sinus neoplasm
- Nasopharyngeal neoplasm
- Nasal hemangioma
- Mucosal drying
- Substance inhalation

Systemic Causes

- Hereditary hemorrhagic telangiectasia
- Leukemia
- Coagulation disorders
- Blood dyscrasias
- Anticoagulant medications
- Hepatic disease
- Uremia
- Vitamin K deficiency
- Upper respiratory infection

From Upile T, Jerjes W, Sipaul F, et al. A change in UK epistaxis management. *Eur Arch Otorhinolaryngol* 2008;**265**:1349.

reserving open surgical ligation of the sphenopalatine and ethmoidal arteries for when other measures fail.

Endovascular Therapy

Less than 1% of patients presenting with epistaxis require embolization or surgery.[104] Embolotherapy should be considered for intractable epistaxis that is refractory to several trials of nasal packing and endoscopic therapy. Embolization is an excellent therapeutic choice for posterior epistaxis, and in some centers takes an early and prominent role in its treatment. The choice between surgery and embolotherapy is often based on local expertise.

The anatomy of the arteries usually responsible for epistaxis is complex and involves both external and internal carotid artery branches. The *sphenopalatine* and *greater palatine branches* from the *internal maxillary artery* are the usual sources (Fig. 20-15). Less often, bleeding occurs from the facial artery branch of the ECA (in particular its small labial branch) or the anterior and posterior ethmoidal branches of the ophthalmic artery arising from the ICA.

Complete diagnostic angiography is essential in the evaluation of the patient with epistaxis. Full ECA angiography is imperative as bleeding can originate from unsuspected sites such as the accessory meningeal artery.[105] In addition, angiography may demonstrate the etiology for bleeding (e.g., tumor blush, vascular malformation, traumatic pseudoaneurysm.) The ECA gives rise to important extracranial to intracranial collaterals, particularly when the ICA is occluded (Fig. 20-16). Visualization of the ICA distribution is therefore critical, not only to identify occlusions with reconstitution from ECA collaterals but also because epistaxis may be caused by ICA disease itself (e.g., aneurysms.) During angiography, the actual bleeding site is rarely visualized particularly in idiopathic epistaxis and when nasal packing is in place.

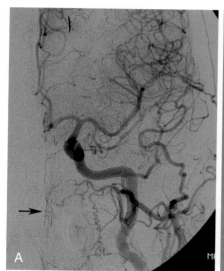
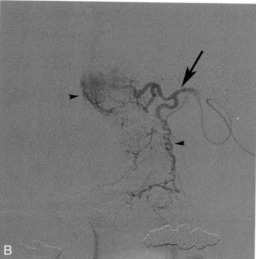
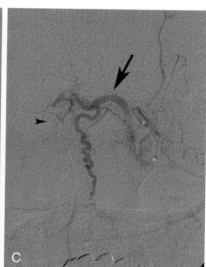
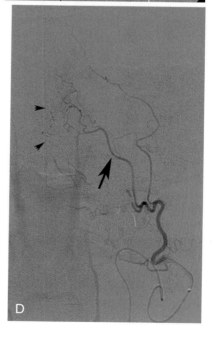

FIGURE 20-15 Epistaxis embolization in a 74-year-old woman with history of persistent left epistaxis. **A,** Left common carotid angiogram in the frontal view demonstrates a normal internal carotid artery and a nasal mucosal blush from the external carotid artery *(arrow)*. **B,** Angiogram via the microcatheter of the distal internal maxillary/sphenopalatine artery *(arrow)* showing intense nasal mucosal blush *(arrowheads)*. **C,** Postembolization angiogram via the microcatheter of the distal internal maxillary/sphenopalatine artery *(arrow)* showing significant decrease in the nasal mucosal blush *(arrowhead)*. **D,** Lateral view of the alar branch *(arrow)* of left facial artery showing supply to the nasal mucosa. If epistaxis is confined to the left side, this artery should be embolized as well.

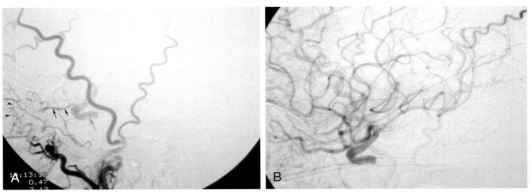

FIGURE 20-16 Lateral view of a common carotid injection in which the internal carotid artery is occluded. **A,** Early intracranial views demonstrate filling of the ophthalmic artery *(arrows)* via ethmoidal collaterals *(arrowheads).* Flow in the ophthalmic artery is retrograde and fills the internal carotid artery *(gray arrow).* **B,** Later view demonstrates complete filling of the intracranial internal carotid artery supply via retrograde flow from the ophthalmic artery. *(From Smith TP. Embolization in the external carotid artery.* J Vas Interv Radiol *2006;17:1900, with permission.)*

Embolization is most often performed via a guiding catheter (usually 6 Fr) placed in the proximal ECA with a microcatheter advanced into the vessel to be embolized, usually the internal maxillary artery. The most popular embolic agent is PVA, 150 to 250 μm in diameter, but size ranges from 50 to 750 μm have been used.[6] Proximal embolic agents (coils) have been used safely and effectively for treatment of epistaxis but are not generally recommended because rebleeding may occur from collateral circulation that develops beyond the occluded site.

If no bleeding or abnormality is seen, empirical embolization may be indicated. As a rule, the bilateral internal maxillary arteries are treated when the side of hemorrhage is clinically unknown, or the ipsilateral internal maxillary artery and facial artery are treated when the side of hemorrhage is known (see Table 20-3). In general, at least one internal maxillary artery is embolized in virtually all patients and the facial artery in about 27% to 48% of patients.[6] Embolization of the facial artery must be performed with great care, particularly with respect to particle size. Particles should lodge distal enough to control hemorrhage yet proximal enough to preserve the distal supply of the terminal alar artery supplying the skin of the nasal ala.

Smith[6] reviewed the literature for epistaxis embolization from 1994 to 2006 and since that time three additional studies have been reported.[106-108] Series size ranged from 12 to 107 patients. Primary success rates averaged 87% and ranged from 75% to 100% with recurrence rates, following successful embolization, ranging up to 25%. There were 23 (3%) major complications consisting of 15 strokes, two cases of monocular blindness, four cases of skin sloughing, one asymptomatic ICA dissection, and one postprocedure myocardial infarction. In addition, patients often complained of facial pain and numbness and a degree of trismus, all self-limited. Fukutsuji and coworkers[106] described minor complications consisting of local pain, headache, numbness or edema occurring in 13 of 22 (59%) patients; however, none of these symptoms persisted for more than 1 week. Interestingly, there is still some disagreement as to the utility of embolotherapy for epistaxis. Direct comparison of surgery and transcatheter embolization in a randomized prospective form has not been undertaken. Santaolalla and colleagues[107] retrospectively reviewed 28 patients with intractable posterior epistaxis treated by embolization and 28 unembolized control patients and found no significant differences in outcomes between the two groups.

HEAD AND NECK TRAUMA

Etiology and Clinical Features

The mechanisms for neurovascular arterial trauma include criminal or accidental blunt or penetrating injuries, iatrogenic causes (e.g., surgery, biopsy, endovascular procedures, central venous line placement), and radiation therapy. The head and neck has an extensive vascular supply, which is advantageous for endovascular treatment because the rich collateral network helps prevent postembolic ischemic injury. The common and internal carotid arteries are closely associated with the jugular veins, and the vertebral arteries are surrounded by an extensive venous network. Therefore injury to the carotid or vertebral artery with concomitant venous injury predisposes to arteriovenous fistula formation.

When symptomatic, patients present with external bleeding, an expanding or pulsatile mass, or neurologic symptoms. When asymptomatic, vascular injury is usually detected on imaging studies obtained to identify bony or parenchymal trauma.

Imaging

Whereas sonography can delineate some vascular abnormalities in the neck (e.g., intimal dissections of the carotid arteries, arteriovenous fistulas, major vessel occlusions), its primary role is evaluation of very unstable patients who cannot be readily moved. CT (including CT angiography) is the principal imaging modality for head and neck trauma. It provides excellent images of the bony structures, including the face, cranium, and spine, and can readily delineate arterial injuries. Catheter angiography is usually reserved for patients who are clinically unstable and have a high clinical suspicion for an arterial injury, for difficulty with diagnosis, or as a prerequisite to intervention. In evaluating the trauma patient, complete, "four vessel" angiography is recommended if the patient's clinical situation allows. This study includes both carotids and both vertebral arteries, and demonstrates the suspected areas of abnormality, while also excluding other areas of injury and defining potential collateral supply if vessel sacrifice (occlusion) should become necessary. The typical angiographic findings are vasospasm, intimal disruption or dissection, extravasation, pseudoaneurysm, arteriovenous fistula, and vessel occlusion.

Treatment

Surgical Therapy

Based on the ease and suitability for surgical repair, carotid artery injuries are categorized by location:

- Zone 1, from the origins of the great vessels inferiorly to the thoracic outlet
- Zone 2, from the thoracic outlet to the angle of the mandible
- Zone 3, superior to the angle of the mandible

Classically, zone 2 lesions are managed with surgical repair although endovascular means have also been applied. Zones 1 and 3 are most often approached by endovascular techniques. Injuries to branches of the ECA are not easily reached by surgical exposure and are better treated by endovascular means.[109] Surgical ligation of the proximal ECA trunk is not usually performed in deference to endovascular therapy.

Endovascular Therapy

Intimal dissection may occur spontaneously, from blunt or penetrating trauma, or catheterization procedures. Dissection is most worrisome in the extracranial carotid and vertebral arteries due to the possible associated neurologic ischemic events. Treatment of these dissections must be highly individualized to a particular patient and their symptoms. Patients with extensive traumatic injuries cannot be systemically anticoagulated particularly for long intervals; medical therapy alone is often a poor option. Endovascular stenting using either bare metal or covered devices has been shown in small series to be quite effective in these patients, even for complete occlusions[82] (Fig. 20-17). In a recent literature

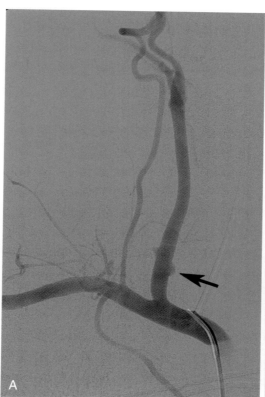
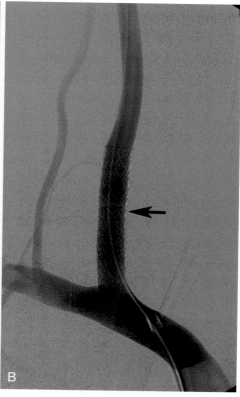

FIGURE 20-17 Stent grafting of right common carotid artery injury in a 43-year-old woman with gunshot wound to right chest and neck. **A,** Right brachiocephalic angiogram in an anteroposterior projection demonstrates irregularity of the proximal right common carotid artery *(arrow)*. **B,** After stent grafting of the right common carotid artery following placement of a covered balloon-expandable stent (8 × 38 mm) demonstrates an excellent radiographic result *(arrow)*.

review of spontaneous and traumatic carotid artery dissections, endovascular techniques had a 100% technical success rate, 100% 1-year patency, and led to complete neurologic recovery or the absence of new ischemic complications in 87% of patients.[110] Intimal injury during endovascular procedures can be treated by either medical therapy or stenting. It is an attractive option to place a stent because there is already a catheter in place, but the decision to do so should be made based on the individual case, taking into account the reason for the initial catheterization.

Penetrating injury, blunt injury, and radiation damage to the carotid ("carotid blowout syndrome" [CBS]) or vertebral artery may present with arterial disruption manifested as extravasation, pseudoaneurysm, and/or arteriovenous fistula. Extravasation presents with frank hemorrhage outside the body, often via the nose (epistaxis) or mouth or via a wound site. Pseudoaneurysm may cause extravasation or present as a pulsatile mass. Although it is tempting to simply coil an acute pseudoaneurysm, this is often unsuccessful in that there is no definable wall to hold the coil pack. Extravasation and pseudoaneurysms are for the most part treated in the same manner using one of two approaches: vessel occlusion or stenting. Covered stents are usually the first choice for the common and internal carotid and vertebral arteries if they can be negotiated to the site of hemorrhage (see Fig. 20-17). As with atherosclerotic disease, self-expanding stents are preferred for the cervical region, whereas either self- or balloon-expandable stents are perfectly acceptable for arteries within the chest, above the mandible, and for the vertebral artery.

Alternatively, vessel occlusion for arterial disruption is an attractive option, because it is quick and effective. However, the patient must be able to tolerate occlusion of the artery without neurologic compromise (Box 20-4). This approach is more problematic with the internal carotid or vertebral artery. It is safe to state that occlusion of the vertebral artery in the neck is very well tolerated when the contralateral vertebral artery supplying the basilar artery is normal. Even when the contralateral vertebral artery is absent or diminutive, proximal occlusion is usually well tolerated because there is collateral supply from branches of the ipsilateral external carotid and subclavian arteries. Occlusion of the common carotid artery is usually well tolerated when the ipsilateral ECA is normal in face of a normal contralateral external carotid system.

Intentional occlusion of the internal carotid artery demands patency of the circle of Willis so that flow from the anterior and posterior communicating arteries is sufficient to support the ipsilateral cerebral hemisphere. Given adequate time in an awake and alert patient who may receive full anticoagulation, *test occlusion* of the vessel before permanent occlusion is ideal (Fig. 20-18). The test occlusion is usually performed with a compliant balloon at the proposed site of permanent occlusion.

BOX 20-4

TEST OCCLUSION PROTOCOL

Diagnostic angiography to determine:
- Site of injury
- Extent of collateral flow
  - Carotid compression while injecting contralateral carotid to assess flow from anterior communicating artery
  - Carotid compression while injecting ipsilateral carotid to assess flow from posterior communicating artery
- Integrity of carotid bifurcation or integrity of contralateral vertebral artery

Anticoagulate the patient fully (activated clotting time of at least 2× baseline, preferably over 300 seconds)

Balloon placement
- Balloon is ideally a soft occlusion balloon, angioplasty balloon sized well to vessel also acceptable
- Heparin (or alternative if heparin allergic) saline slowly flushed through the wire lumen during occlusion
- Common carotid artery
  - At anticipated occlusion site, just above or below site of injury
- Internal carotid artery
  - Just above bifurcation
- Vertebral artery
  - At anticipated occlusion site, just above or below site of injury

Examination of patient
- Clinical examination
- Test occlusion for 20 to 30 minutes
- Neurologic examination performed at least every 5 minutes
- Additional testing for integrity of collateral flow
  - Single photo emission computed tomography (SPECT)
  - Electroencephalography (EEG)

There is rarely time for additional testing in an acute trauma situation.

Total time of balloon inflation is 20 to 30 minutes if the patient is tolerating occlusion well. If the patient develops a neurologic deficit, the balloon is immediately deflated to restore flow. If the patient tolerates test occlusion well, the vessel can then be sacrificed. Complications of test occlusion are in the range of 3%, including vessel injury and ischemic events. Permanent neurologic complications occur in less than 1% of cases (0.4%).[111] If there is no time to devote to a test occlusion and no other therapies are reasonable, the decision to perform

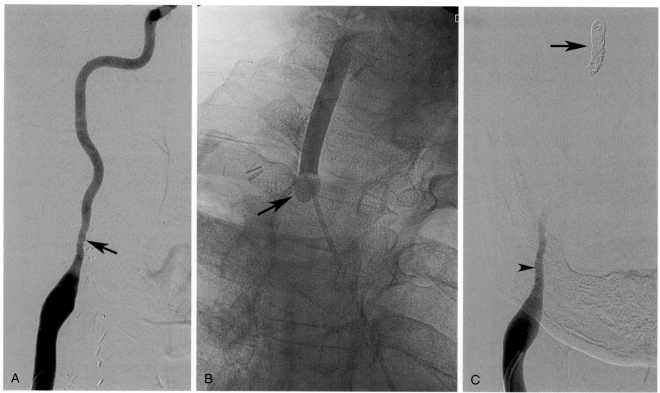

FIGURE 20-18   Test occlusion and carotid artery occlusion in a 56-year-old man with a history of recurrent vocal cord squamous cell carcinoma that involves the right internal carotid artery. He is scheduled for additional surgery that may include carotid artery resection. For preoperative test occlusion and endovascular carotid artery occlusion. **A,** Right common carotid angiogram demonstrates narrowing of the distal common and proximal internal carotid artery *(arrow)* with occlusion of the external carotid artery. **B,** Occlusion balloon *(arrow)* placed in proximal common carotid artery for 20 minutes. Neurologic examination was normal. Patient also had a normal single photon emission computed tomogram following clinical test occlusion, whose results were normal. **C,** Internal carotid artery was occluded in the high cervical region using coils *(arrow).* Carotid artery shows no flow after occlusion *(arrowhead).* Carotid artery was occluded distally at the request of the referring surgeon.

carotid artery occlusion can be based solely on the degree of collateral flow as assessed at angiography.

Vessel occlusion is performed using coils or vascular plugs. Occlusions of the ICA can be performed just proximal to the site of injury, although proximal and distal deployment is ideal, particularly when an arteriovenous fistula is noted. For the vertebral artery, proximal and distal occlusion should be undertaken to prevent the later formation of an arteriovenous fistula (Fig. 20-19). If a fistula forms distal to the site of occlusion, subsequent embolotherapy may require difficult or treacherous negotiation through collaterals or the contralateral vertebral artery coursing across the basilar and down the ipsilateral vertebral artery. Following vessel occlusion, it is essential to monitor the patient closely and administer appropriate medical therapy to control blood pressure, and maintain hydration and gradual increase in activity.

Carotid blowout syndrome describes rupture of the carotid artery as a complication of aggressive surgery and radiation therapy for carcinoma of the neck. These treatments can result in poor wound healing, eventual exposure of the carotid artery, and minor sentinel to frank life-threatening hemorrhage (about 50% and 60%, respectively). A recent literature review found patients with CBS typically have a history of radiotherapy (89%), nodal metastasis (69%), and neck dissection (63%).[112] This disease usually occurs proximal to the carotid bifurcation and is commonly associated with soft tissue necrosis in the neck (55%) and mucocutaneous fistulas (40%). More than 90% of patients with CBS are treated with endovascular therapy (Fig. 20-20); surgical ligation is rarely indicated. Endovascular treatment consists of covered stent placement or occlusion of the carotid artery. The morbidity and mortality rates of patients with CBS are significant.

Although the internal carotid and vertebral arteries are commonly injured in penetrating trauma, the ECA is the most common artery when one includes individual branch injuries[113] (Fig. 20-21). Major vessel injury occurs even more often with blunt trauma. Branches of the ECA may be occluded but not require intervention. Trauma may present as pseudoaneurysm, extravasation (including epistaxis), and/or arteriovenous fistula formation. The standard endovascular therapy for trauma to the ECA is proximal vessel occlusion, most often with coils.

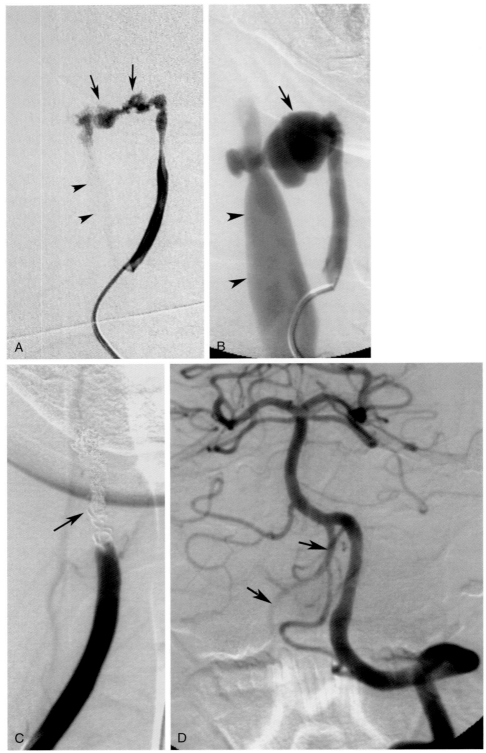

FIGURE 20-19   Right vertebral artery to jugular vein fistula with vessel occlusion in an 18-year-old patient with a self-inflicted gunshot wound to neck. **A,** Right anterior oblique angiogram of right vertebral artery shows arterial occlusion just above a relatively small fistula to the jugular vein *(arrows).* The jugular vein is very lightly opacified *(arrowheads).* Given the patient's condition and diminutive size of the arteriovenous fistula with vertebral artery occlusion, endovascular therapy was not performed. **B,** Follow-up right vertebral artery angiography shows enlarged arteriovenous fistula *(arrow)* to the jugular vein *(arrowheads)* with continued vertebral artery occlusion distal to the fistula. Left vertebral artery angiogram demonstrated a normal left vertebral artery without retrograde flow down the right vertebral to the fistula site. **C,** Right vertebral artery occlusion. Microcatheter was advanced above the fistula site in the right vertebral artery and coiling was performed above and below the fistula *(arrow).* **D,** Left vertebral arteriography after coiling of right vertebral artery fistula site, confirming no-flow down the right vertebral artery *(arrows)* to supply the arteriovenous fistula. Minimal contrast opacification of distal right vertebral artery *(arrow)* is normal with more proximal occlusion.

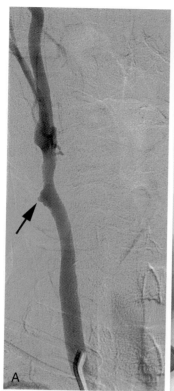
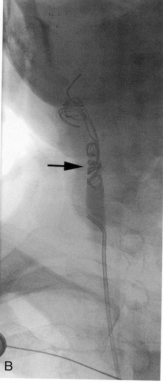

FIGURE 20-20   Right common carotid artery blowout in a 49-year-old man with a history of squamous cell carcinoma of the right neck. The patient has undergone radiation and surgery, and currently has an open wound and massive extravasation. **A,** Right common carotid angiogram demonstrates a narrowing and irregularity *(arrow)* at the site of the patient's extravasation. Because the situation was emergent, occlusion was performed based on intracranial collateral flow. **B,** Angiogram of the right common carotid artery following complete occlusion of the vessel using coils *(arrow).*

Due to the possibility of delayed arteriovenous fistula formation, the site of injury should be occluded both proximally and distally if possible.

There is a relative paucity of data regarding endovascular treatment of ECA trauma, particularly when compared with ICA injury. The existing small series demonstrate excellent results from endovascular arterial occlusive therapy.[114] These small series also include intractable oronasal bleeding from severe craniofacial injuries treated by endovascular means.[115]

SPONTANEOUS CAROTID ARTERY DISSECTION

Spontaneous dissection can occur in the carotid or vertebral artery. Treatment for cervical vertebral artery dissection follows that for the carotid artery, but there is a greater tendency for intracranial extension. Spontaneous dissection of the internal carotid artery is associated with a number of predisposing factors.[116] The most common presenting symptom is neck pain, sometimes with headache. Patients may have Horner syndrome or central neurologic symptoms. Sonography may be the initial imaging study for suspected spontaneous carotid dissection, but CT or MRI is preferable.[117] Angiography is rarely needed unless coupled with endovascular therapy.

In most centers, the treatment for spontaneous carotid dissection is anticoagulation to reduce the risk for distal embolization and allow the intimal injury to heal (Fig. 20-22). Recanalization of the vessel depends to a degree on whether it was initially stenosed or occluded;

FIGURE 20-21   External carotid artery (ECA) embolization for trauma in a 14-year-old female patient who suffered a gunshot wound. **A,** Lateral view of the right common carotid artery injection demonstrating injury including both the internal and external carotid arteries. The internal carotid artery was occluded several days earlier *(arrowheads).* The current view demonstrates the injury to the ECA just superior to the facial artery *(arrow).* **B,** The external carotid artery was occluded just above the facial artery with coils *(arrows).* Note that the injury site was occluded both above and below by the coils to prevent late development of an arteriovenous fistula via retrograde flow. *(From Smith TP. Embolization in the external carotid artery. J Vas Interv Radiol 2006;17:1909, with permission.)*

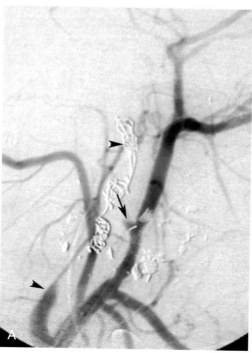
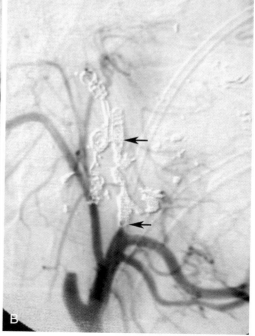

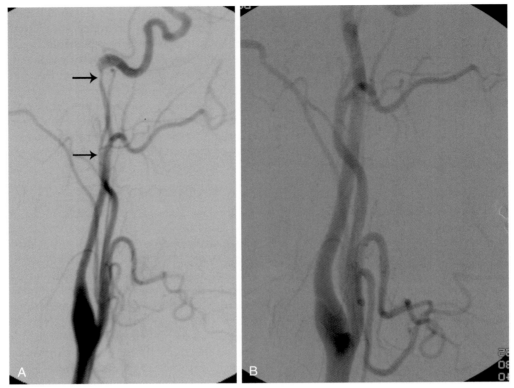

FIGURE 20-22　Spontaneous carotid artery dissection in a 44-year-old man with headache and left-sided Horner syndrome for 3 weeks. **A,** Right common carotid angiogram shows dissection of right internal carotid artery extending to base of skull *(arrows)*. **B,** Right common carotid angiogram shows dissection of right internal carotid artery completely healed following 15 months of medical therapy consisting of both warfarin and antiplatelet agents.

long-term symptoms are unusual (about 1%).[118] More invasive therapies are usually undertaken when medical therapy fails. Primary surgical repair for spontaneous internal carotid dissection is rarely performed because the procedure is difficult and the distal extent of the dissection is often buried in the skull base. The better surgical option is ICA bypass. The most attractive endovascular option has been stenting the dissected segment with the goal to close the flap and restore true lumen patency. Since this approach is only taken for patients who fail medical therapy, the numbers of reported cases is relatively small. Nonetheless, results have been excellent.[110]

References

1. Arteries of the head and neck. In: Uflacker R. *Atlas of vascular anatomy: an angiographic approach.* 2nd ed. Philadelphia: Lippincott Williams and Wilkins; 2007.
2. Krishnaswamy A, Klein JP, Kapadia SR. Clinical cerebrovascular anatomy. *Catheter Cardiovasc Interv* 2010;**75**:530.
3. Geibprasert S, Pongpech S, Armstrong D, et al. Dangerous extracranial-intracranial anastomoses and supply to the cranial nerves: vessels the neurointerventionalist needs to know. *AJNR Am J Neuroradiol* 2009;**30**:1459.
4. Barr JD, Lemley TJ. Endovascular arterial occlusion accomplished using microcoils deployed with and without proximal flow arrest: results in 19 patients. *Am J Neuroradiol* 1999;**20**:1452.
5. Ong CK, Lam DV, Ong MT, et al. Neuroapplication of Amplatzer vascular plug for therapeutic sacrifice of major craniocerebral arteries: an initial clinical experience. *Ann Acad Med Singapore* 2009;**38**:763.
6. Smith TP. Embolization in the external carotid artery. *J Vas Interv Radiol* 2006;**17**:1897.
7. Lee BB, Do YS, Yakes W, Kim DI, Mattassi R, Hyon WS. Management of arteriovenous malformations: a multidisciplinary approach. *J Vasc Surg* 2004;**39**:590.
8. Vos JA, van den Berg JC, Ernst SM, et al. Carotid angioplasty and stent placement: comparison of transcranial Doppler US data and clinical outcome with and without filtering cerebral protection devices in 509 patients. *Radiology* 2005;**234**:493.
9. O'Holleran LW, Kennelly MM, McClurken M, et al. Natural history of asymptomatic carotid plaque. *Am J Surg* 1987;**144**:659.
10. Lanzino G, Rabinstein AA, Brown Jr RD. Treatment of carotid artery stenosis: medical therapy, surgery, or stenting? *Mayo Clin Proc* 2009;**84**:362.
11. North American Symptomatic Carotid Endarterectomy Trial Collaborators. Beneficial effect of carotid endarterectomy in patients with high-grade carotid stenosis. *N Engl J Med* 1991;**325**:445.
12. Executive Committee for the Asymptomatic Carotid Atherosclerosis Study. Endarterectomy for asymptomatic carotid artery stenosis. *JAMA* 1995;**273**:1421.
13. Higashida RT, Meyers PM, Phatouros, et al. Reporting standards for carotid artery angioplasty and stent placement. *J Vasc Interv Radiol* 2009;**20**:S349.
14. Abbott AL. Medical (nonsurgical) intervention alone is now best for prevention of stroke associated with asymptomatic severe carotid stenosis: results of a systematic review and analysis. *Stroke* 2009;**40**:e573.

15. Kachel R, Endert G, Basche S, Grossmann K, Glaser FH. Percutaneous transluminal angioplasty (dilatation) of carotid, vertebral, and innominate artery stenoses. *Cardiovasc Intervent Radiol* 1987;**10**:142.

16. Motarjeme A, Keifer JW, Zuska AJ. Percutaneous transluminal angioplasty of the brachiocephalic arteries. *AJR Am J Roentgenol* 1982;**138**:457.

17. Brown MM, Butler P, Gibbs J, Swash M, Waterston J. Feasibility of percutaneous angioplasty for carotid artery stenosis. *J Neurol Neurosurg Psychiatry* 1990;**53**:238.

18. Roubin GS, Yadav S, Iyer SS, Vitek J. Carotid stent-supported angioplasty: a neurovascular intervention to prevent stroke. *Am J Cardiol* 1996;**78**(Suppl. lA):8.

19. Yadav JS, Wholey MH, Kuntz RE, et al. Protected carotid-artery stenting versus endarterectomy in high-risk patients. *N Engl J Med* 2004;**351**:1493.

20. Makkar RR, Eigler NL, Kaul S et al. Effects of clopidogrel, aspirin and combined therapy in a porcine ex vivo model of high-shear induced stent thrombosis, *Eur Heart J* 1998;**98**:1538.

21. Pham SV, Pham PC, Pham PM, Miller JM, Pham PT, Pham PA. Antithrombotic strategies in patients undergoing percutaneous coronary intervention for acute coronary syndrome. *Drug Des Devel Ther* 2010;**4**:203.

22. Ferrero E, Ferri M, Viazzo A, et al. Early carotid surgery in patients after acute ischemic stroke: is it safe? A retrospective analysis in a single center between early and delayed/deferred carotid surgery on 285 patients. *Ann Vasc Surg* 2010;**24**:890.

23. Schillinger M, Haumer M, Schillinger S, et al. Risk stratification for subclavian artery angioplasty: is there an increased rate of restenosis after stent implantation? *J Endovasc Ther* 2001;**8**:550.

24. Przewlocki T, Kablak-Ziembicka A, Pieniazek P, et al. Determinants of immediate and long-term results of subclavian and innominate artery angioplasty. *Catheter Cardiovasc Interv* 2006;**67**:519.

25. Paukovits TM, Lukacs L, Berczi V, et al. Percutaneous endovascular treatment of innominate artery lesions: a single-centre experience on 77 lesions. *Eur J Vasc Endovasc Surg* 2010;**40**:35.

26. Paukovits TM, Haász J, Molnár A, et al. Transfemoral endovascular treatment of proximal common carotid artery lesions: A single-center experience on 153 lesions. *J Vasc Surg* 2008;**48**:80.

27. Chio Jr FL, Liu MW, Khan MA. Effectiveness of elective stenting of common carotid artery lesions in preventing stroke. *Am J Cardiol* 2003;**92**:1135.

28. Labropoulos N, Nandivada P, Bekelis K. Prevalence and impact of the subclavian steal syndrome. *Ann Surg* 2010;**252**:166.

29. Wang KQ, Wang ZG, Yang BZ, et al. Long-term results of endovascular therapy for proximal subclavian arterial obstructive lesions. *Chin Med J (Engl)* 2010;**123**:45.

30. De Vries JP, Jager LC, Van den Berg JC, et al. Durability of percutaneous transluminal angioplasty for obstructive lesions of proximal subclavian artery: long-term results. *J Vasc Surg* 2005;**41**:19.

31. Henry M, Amor M, Henry I, Ethevenot G, Tzvetanov K, Chati Z. Percutaneous transluminal angioplasty of the subclavian arteries. *J Endovasc Surg* 1999;**6**:33.

32. Jenkins JS, Patel SN, White CJ, et al. Endovascular stenting for vertebral artery stenosis. *J Am Coll Cardiol* 2010;**55**:538.

33. Brown MM, Rogers J, Bland JM. Endovascular versus surgical treatment in patients with carotid stenosis in the Carotid and Vertebral Artery Transluminal Angioplasty Study (CAVATAS): a randomized trial. *Lancet* 2001;**357**:1729.

34. Coward LJ, Featherstone RL, Brown MM. Percutaneous transluminal angioplasty and stenting for vertebral artery stenosis. *Cochrane Database Syst Rev* 2005 Apr 18;**2**:CD000516.

35. Brott TG, Hobson RW, Howard G, et al. Stenting versus endarterectomy for the treatment of carotid-artery stenosis. *N Engl J Med* 2010;**363**:11.

36. Ringleb PA, Allenberg J, Buckmann H, et al. 30 day results from the SPACE trial of stent-protected angioplasty versus carotid endarterectomy in symptomatic patients: randomized non-inferiority trial. *Lancet* 2006;**368**:1239.

37. Mas JL, Chatellier G, Beyssen B, et al. Endarterectomy versus stenting in patients with symptomatic severe carotid stenosis. *N Engl J Med* 2006;**355**:1660.

38. International Carotid Stenting Study Investigators. Carotid artery stenting compared with endarterectomy in patients with symptomatic carotid stenosis (International Carotid Stenting Study): an interim analysis of a randomized controlled trial. *Lancet* 2010;**375**:985.

39. Ederle J, Bonati LH, Dobson J et al. Endovascular treatment with angioplasty or stenting versus endarterectomy in patients with carotid artery stenosis in the Carotid And Vertebral Artery Transluminal Angioplasty Study (CAVATAS): long-term follow-up of a randomized trial. *Lancet Neurol* 2009;**8**:898.

40. Park BD, Divinagracia T, Madej O, et al. Predictors of clinically significant postprocedural hypotension after carotid endarterectomy and carotid angioplasty with stenting. *J Vasc Surg* 2009;**50**:526.

41. Yakhou L, Constant I, Merle JC, Laude D, Becquemin J-P, Duvaldestin P. Noninvasive investigation of autonomic activity after carotid stenting or carotid endarterectomy. *J Vasc Surg* 2006;**44**:472.

42. Hobson RW, Howard VJ, Roubin GS, et al. for the CREST Investigators. Carotid artery stenting is associated with increased complications in octogenarians: 30-day stroke and death rates in the CREST lead-in phase. *J Vasc Surg* 2004;**40**:1106.

43. Wityk RJ, Lehman D, Klag M, Coresh J, Ahn H, Litt B. Race and sex differences in the distribution of cerebral atherosclerosis. *Stroke* 1996;**27**:1974.

44. Kasner SE, Chimowitz MI, Lynn MJ, et al.: Predictors of ischemic stroke in the territory of a symptomatic intracranial arterial stenosis. *Circulation* 2006;**113**:555.

45. Sacco RL, Kargman DE, Gu Q, Zamanillo MC. Race-ethnicity and determinates of intracranial atherosclerotic cerebral infarction: the Northern Manhattan Stroke Study. *Stroke* 1995;**26**:14.

46. White H, Boden-Albala B, Wang C, et al. Ischemic stroke subtype incidence among whites, blacks, and Hispanics: the Northern Manhattan Study. *Circulation* 2005;**111**:1327.

47. The EC-IC Bypass Study Group. Failure of extracranial-intracranial arterial bypass to reduce the risk of ischemic stroke. *N Engl J Med* 1985;**313**:1191.

48. Chimowitz MI, Lynn MJ, Howlett-Smith H, et al. Comparison of warfarin and aspirin for symptomatic intracranial arterial stenosis. *N Engl J Med* 2005;**352**:1305.

49. Higashida RT, Meyers PM, Connors JJ, et al. Intracranial angioplasty and stenting for cerebral atherosclerosis: a position statement of the American Society of Interventional and Therapeutic Neuroradiology, Society of Interventional Radiology, and the American Society of Neuroradiology. *J Vasc Interv Radiol* 2005;**16**:1281.

50. Baker AB, Iannone A. Cerebrovascular disease: a study of etiologic mechanisms. *Neurology* 1961;**11**:23.

51. Higashida RT, Meyers PM, Connors JJ, et al. Intracranial angioplasty and stenting for cerebral atherosclerosis: a position statement of the American Society of Interventional and Therapeutic Neuroradiology, Society of Interventional Radiology, and the American Society of Neuroradiology. *J Vasc Interv Radiol* 2009;**20**:S312.

52. Connors JJ, Wojak JC. Percutaneous transluminal angioplasty for intracranial atherosclerotic lesions: evolution of technique and short-term results. *J Neurosurg* 1999;**91**:415.

53. Lanfranconi S, Bersano A, Branca V, et al. Stenting for the treatment of high-grade intracranial stenoses. *J Neurol* epub July 2010;**257**:1899.

54. Groschel K, Schnaudigel S, Pilgram SM, Wasser K, Kastrup A. A systematic review on outcome after stenting for intracranial atherosclerosis. *Stroke* 2009;**40**:e340.

55. SSYLVIA Study Investigators. Stenting of Symptomatic Atherosclerotic Lesions in the Vertebral or Intracranial Arteries (SSYLVIA): study results. *Stroke* 2004;**35**:1388.

56. Fiorella D, Levy EI, Turk AS, et al. US multicenter experience with the Wingspan stent system for the treatment of intracranial atheromatous disease: periprocedural results. *Stroke* 2007;**38**:881.

57. Roger VL, Go AS, Lloyd-Jones DM, et al. Heart disease and stroke statistics—2011 update. A report from the American Heart Association. *Circulation* 2011;**123**:e240.

58. Adams HP, Bendixen BH, Kappelle LJ, et al. Classification of subtype of acute ischemic stroke: definitions for use in a multicenter clinical trial—TOAST, trial of Org 10172 in acute stroke treatment. *Stroke* 1993;**24**:35.

59. The National Institute of Neurological Disorders and Stroke rt-PA Stroke Study Group. Tissue plasminogen activator for acute ischemic stroke. *N Engl J Med* 1995;**333**:1581.

60. Hacke, M. Kaste and E. Bluhmki et al. Thrombolysis with alteplase 3 to 4.5 hours after acute ischemic stroke, *N Engl J Med* 2008; **359**:1317.

61. Weimar C, Goertler M, Harms L, et al. Distribution and outcome of symptomatic stenoses and occlusions in patients with acute cerebral ischemia. *Arch Neurol* 2006;**63**:1287.

62. Schonewille WJ, Wijman CAC, Michel P, et al. Treatment and outcomes of acute basilar artery occlusion in the Basilar Artery International Cooperation Study (BASICS): a prospective registry study. *Lancet Neurol* 2009;**8**:724.

63. Eckert B, Kucinski T, Pfeiffer G, Groden C, Zeumer H. Endovascular therapy of acute vertebrobasilar occlusion: early treatment onset as the most important factor. *Cerebrovasc Dis* 2002;**14**:42.

64. Del Zoppo GJ, Higashida RT, Furlan AJ, et al. PROACT: a phase II randomized trial of recombinant pro-urokinase by direct arterial delivery in acute middle cerebral artery stroke. *Stroke* 1998;**29**:4.

65. Ogawa A, Mori E, Minematsu K, et al. Randomized trial of intra-arterial infusion of urokinase within 6 hours of middle cerebral artery stroke: the middle cerebral artery embolism local fibrinolytic intervention trial (MELT) Japan. *Stroke* 2007;**38**:2633.

66. Lisboa RC, Jovanovic BD, Alberts MJ. Analysis of the safety and efficacy of intra-arterial thrombolytic therapy in ischemic stroke. *Stroke* 2002;**33**:2866.

67. Nogueira RG, Yoo AJ, Buonanno FS, et al. Endovascular approaches to acute stroke, part 2: a comprehensive review of studies and trials. *AJNR Am J Neuroradiol* 2009;**30**:859.

68. Ducrocq X, Bracard S, Taillandier L, et al. Comparison of intravenous and intra-arterial urokinase thrombolysis for acute ischaemic stroke. *J Neuroradiol* 2005;**32**:26.

69. Lindsberg PJ, Mattle HP. Therapy of basilar artery occlusion: a systematic analysis comparing intra-arterial and intravenous thrombolysis. *Stroke* 2006;**37**:922.

70. Gobin YP, Starkman S, Duckwiler GR, et al. MERCI 1: a phase 1 study of Mechanical Embolus Removal in Cerebral Ischemia. *Stroke* 2004;**35**:2848.

71. Bose A, Henkes H, Alfke K, et al. The Penumbra System: a mechanical device for the treatment of acute stroke due to thromboembolism. *AJNR Am J Neuroradiol* 2008;**29**:1409.

72. Penumbra Pivotal Stroke Trial Investigators. The Penumbra pivotal stroke trial: safety and effectiveness of a new generation of mechanical devices for clot removal in intracranial large vessel occlusive disease. *Stroke* 2009;**40**:2761.

73. Hornig CR, Dorndorf W, Agnoli AL. Hemorrhagic cerebral infarction: a prospective study. *Stroke* 1986;**17**:179.

74. Murtagh R, Linden C. Neuroimaging of intracranial meningiomas. *Neurosurg Clin N Am* 1994;**5**:217.

75. Wieneke JA, Smith A. Paraganglioma: carotid body tumor. *Head Neck Pathol* 2009;**3**:303.

76. Schick B, Urbschat S. New aspects of pathogenesis of juvenile angiofibroma. *Hosp Med* 2004;**65**:269.

77. Englehard HH. Progress in the diagnosis and treatment of patients with meningiomas. Part 1: diagnostic imaging, preoperative embolization. *Surg Neurol* 2001;**55**:89.

78. Wakhloo AK, Juengling FD, Van Velthoven V, et al. Extended preoperative polyvinyl alcohol microembolization of intracranial meningiomas: assessment of two embolization techniques. *AJNR Am J Neuroradiol* 1993;**14**:571.

79. Carli DMF, Sluzewski M, Beute GN, van Rooij WJ. Complications of particle embolization of meningiomas: frequency, risk factors, and outcome. *AJNR* 2010;**31**:152.

80. Rosen CL, Ammerman JM, Sekhar et al. Outcome analysis of preoperative embolization in cranial base surgery. *Acta Neurochir* 2002;**144**:1157.

81. Kai Y, Hamada J, Morioka M, Yano S, Todaka T, Ushio Y. Appropriate interval between embolization and surgery in patients with meningioma. *AJNR* 2002;**23**:139.

82. Manelfe C, Guiraud B, David J, et al. Embolization by catheterization of intracranial meningiomas. *Rev Neurol (Paris)* 1973;**128**:339.

83. Dean BL, Flom RA, Wallace RC, et al. Efficacy of endovascular treatment of meningiomas: evaluation with matched samples. *AJNR* 1994;**15**:1675.

84. Probst EN, Grayscale U, Westphalia M, Zimmer H. Preoperative embolization of intracranial meningiomas with a fibrin glue preparation. *AJNR* 1999;**20**:1695.

85. Rao AB, Koeller KK, Adair CF. Paragangliomas of the head and neck: radiologic-pathologic correlation. *Radiographics* 1999; **19**:1605.

86. Netterville JL. Vagal paragangliomas: a review of 46 patients treated during a 20-year period. *Arch Otolarnygol Head Neck Surg* 1988;**124**:1133.

87. Lasjaunias P, Berenstein A. Temporal and Cervical tumors. In: *Surgical neuroangiography: endovascular treatment of craniofacial lesions.* Berlin: Springer-Verlag; 1987. p. 127.

88. Lui D, Ma X, Li B, Zhang J. Clinical study of preoperative angiography and embolization of hypervascular neoplasms in the oral and maxillofacial region. *Oral Surg Oral Med Oral Pathol Radiol Endod* 2006;**101**:102.

89. Bakoyianna KC, Georgopoulos SE, Klonaris CN, et al. Surgical treatment of carotid body tumors without embolization. *Int Angiol* 2006;**25**:40.

90. Karaman E, Yilmaz M, Isildak H, et al. Management of jugular paragangliomas in otolaryngology practice. *J Craniofac Surg* 2010; **21**:117.

91. Zeitler DM, Glick J, Har-El G. Preoperative embolization in carotid body tumor surgery: is it required? *Ann Otol Rhinol Laryngol* 2010; **119**:279.

92. Perskey MS, Setton A, Niimi Y, et al. Combined endovascular and surgical treatment of head and neck paragangliomas: a team approach. *Head Neck* 2002;**24**:423.

93. Thompson LDR, Fanburgh-Smith JC. Nasopharyngeal angiofibroma. In: Barnes L, Eveson JW, Reichart P, et al, editors. *World Health Organization Classification of Tumours: pathology & genetics head and neck tumours,* 1st ed. Lyon: IARC Press; 2005. pp. 102.

94. Midilli R, Karci B, Akyildiz S. Juvenile nasopharyngeal angiofibroma: analysis of 42 cases and important aspects of endoscopic approach. *Int J Pediatr Otorhinolaryngol* 2009;**73**:401.

95. Roberson GH, Price AC, Davis JM, et al. Therapeutic embolization of juvenile angiofibroma. *AJR Am J Roentgenol* 1979;**133**:657.

96. Gaillard AL, Anastácio VM, Piatto VB, et al. A seven-year experience with patients with juvenile nasopharyngeal angiofibroma. *Braz J Otorhinolaryngol* 2010;**76**:245.

97. Mohammadi M, Saedi B, Basam A. Effect of embolisation on endoscopic resection of angiofibroma. *J Laryngol Otol* 2010;**124**:631.

98. Önceri M, Gumus K, Cil B, Eldem B. A rare complication of embolization in juvenile nasopharyngeal angiofibroma. *Int J Ped Otorhinolaryngol* 2005;**69**:423.

99. Small M, Murray JA, Maran AG. A study of patients with epistaxis requiring admission to hospital. *Health Bull (Edinb)* 1982;**40**:20.

100. Pope LER, Hobbs CGL. Epistaxis: an update on current management. *Postgrad Med J* 2005;**81**:309.

101. Upile T, Jerjes W, Sipaul F, et al. A change in UK epistaxis management. *Eur Arch Otorhinolaryngol* 2008;**265**:1349.

102. Schlosser RJ. Epistaxis. *N Engl J Med* 2009;**360**:784.

103. Viducich RA, Blanda MP, et al. Posterior epistaxis: clinical features and acute complications. *Ann Emerg Med* 1995;**25**:592.

104. Kotecha B, Fowler S, Harkness R, et al. Management of epistaxis: a national survey. *Ann R Coll Surg Engl* 1996;**78**:444.

105. Duncan IC, Dos Santos C. Accessory meningeal arterial supply to the posterior nasal cavity: another reason for failed endovascular treatment of epistaxis. *Cardiovasc Intervent Radiol* 2003;**26**:488.

106. Fukutsuji K, Nishiike S, Aihara T, et al. Superselective angiographic embolization for intractable epistaxis. *Acta Otolaryngol* 2008;**128**:556.

107. Santaolalla F, Araluce I, Zabala A, et al. Efficacy of selective percutaneous embolization for the treatment of intractable posterior epistaxis in juvenile nasopharyngeal angiofibroma (JNA). *Acta Otolaryngol* 2009;**129**:1456.

108. Sadri M, Midwinter K, Ahmed A, et al. Assessment of safety and efficacy of arterial embolisation in the management of intractable epistaxis. *Eur Arch Otorhinolaryngol* 2006;**263**:560.

109. Mangla S, Sclafani SJA. External carotid arterial injury. *Injury* 2008;**39**:1249.

110. Donas KP, Mayer D, Guber I, et al. Endovascular repair of extracranial carotid artery dissection: current status and level of evidence. *J Vasc Interv Radiol* 2008;**19**:1693.

111. Mathis JM, Barr JD, Horton JA. Therapeutic occlusion of major vessels, test occlusion and techniques. *Neurosurg Clinic NA* 1994;**5**:393.

112. Powitzky R, Vasan N, Krempl G, et al. Carotid blowout in patients with head and neck cancer. *Ann Otol Rhinol Laryngol* 2010;**119**:476.

113. Sclafani AP, Sclafani SJ. Angiography and transcatheter arterial embolization of vascular injuries of the face and neck. *Laryngoscope* 1996;**106**(2 Pt. 1):168.

114. Bynoe RP, Kerwin AJ, Parker III HH, et al. Maxillofacial injuries and life-threatening hemorrhage: treatment with transcatheter arterial embolization. *J Trauma* 2003;**55**:74.

115. Komiyama M, Nishikawa M, Kan M, et al. Endovascular treatment of intractable oronasal bleeding associated with severe craniofacial injury. *J Trauma* 1998;**44**:330.

116. Agostoni E, Aliprandi, A, Longoni M. Dissection of the epiaortic and intracranial arteries. *Neurol Sci* 2010;**31**(Suppl. 1):S123.

117. Provenzale JM, Sarikaya B. Comparison of test performance characteristics of MRI, MR angiography, and CT angiography in the diagnosis of carotid and vertebral artery dissection: a review of the medical literature. *AJR* 2009;**193**:1167.

118. Kim Y-K, Schulman S. Cervical artery dissection: Pathology, epidemiology and management. *Thromb Res* 2009;**123**:810.

119. Herault JP, Peyrou V, Savi P, Bernat A, Herbert JM. Effect of SR121566A, a potent GP IIb-IIIa antagonist on platelet-mediated thrombin generation in vitro and in vivo. *Thromb Haemost* 1998;**79**(2):383.

NONVASCULAR AND ONCOLOGIC INTERVENTIONS

21

Gastrointestinal Interventions

Sandeep Vaidya, Gerant Rivera-Sanfeliz, Gregory Lim

ESOPHAGUS

Esophageal Strictures

Etiology

Peptic disease is the most common cause of benign esophageal strictures[1,2] (Box 21-1). Benign nonpeptic esophageal strictures are rare in routine clinical practice.

Esophageal strictures can be divided into two groups: simple and complex. *Simple strictures* are short (<2 cm), focal, not angulated, and permit passage of an endoscope. *Complex strictures* may be angulated, long (>2 cm), irregular, or have a severely narrowed lumen. These strictures are often refractory to dilation therapy. Strictures caused by surgical anastomoses, radiation therapy, caustic ingestion, and photodynamic therapy constitute most of these refractory lesions.

Carcinoma of the esophagus is notoriously difficult to manage; approximately 60% of patients may only receive palliative treatment. Even among those cases that appear curable, many cases will recur and face a 5-year survival of approximately 20%.[3] After surgical resection, almost 20% to 30% of patients have dysphagia secondary to recurrence of the disease or anastomotic strictures.[4]

Esophageal Stricture Dilation

PATIENT SELECTION

Esophageal dilation is contraindicated in the setting of recent or acute esophageal perforation, bleeding diathesis, severely compromised pulmonary function or airway obstruction, severe or unstable cardiac disease, or in patients with large thoracic aortic aneurysms.

TECHNIQUE

Although most of these procedures can be performed under endoscopic guidance, fluoroscopy is instrumental in the setting of complex strictures because it aids not only in crossing the stricture but also in monitoring the actual dilatation. Several authors report reduced complication rates and improved therapeutic results when fluoroscopy is used.[5,6] Very proximal esophageal lesions are difficult to cross with an endoscope and in these situations fluoroscopy becomes the only practical means of guidance.

Three general types of dilators are in use: mercury- or tungsten-filled bougies, over-the-wire polyvinyl dilators, and balloon catheters. The dilators and bougies range in size from 15 to 60 French (Fr) (5 to 20 mm), including Safe-Guide over-the-wire dilators, Weight-Right mercury-/tungsten-filled dilators/bougies, and Quantum TTC dilators. Esophageal dilatation balloons range in size from 8 to 18 mm in diameter and are available from various manufacturers (e.g., Boston Scientific, Cook Inc., ConMed, Medovations Inc.). These noncompliant balloons are similar to angioplasty balloons but are slightly less supple. The bougie-type dilators exert more radial and longitudinal force compared with the other two types. Except in instances in which longitudinal forces should be avoided, no clear advantage has been demonstrated among the dilator types.[7]

After moderate resistance is encountered during dilation therapy with Savary-type dilators, no greater than three consecutive dilators should be used in a single session.[8] There are no objective data to guide balloon therapy; therefore, a conservative approach to dilation is usually undertaken to reduce the chances of perforation. Multiple dilation sessions frequently are required to achieve a luminal diameter of at least 12 mm.

RESULTS

For benign strictures, balloon dilation is technically successful in 90% of cases. Clinical success is achieved in approximately 70% of patients at 2-year follow-up. The results are not as favorable for radiation strictures, and malignant strictures only show transient results.[9,10] External compression of the esophagus rarely responds to dilation.

> ## BOX 21-1
>
> ## CAUSES OF BENIGN ESOPHAGEAL STRICTURES
>
> - Peptic ulcer disease
> - Esophageal intramural pseudodiverticulosis
> - Caustic ingestion
> - Eosinophilic esophagitis
> - Schatzki (-Gary) ring
> - Incomplete esophageal atresia (with or without repair)
> - Heterotopic gastric mucosa
> - Mucosal pemphigoid
> - Spondylotic induced stenosis
> - Epiphrenic diverticulum
> - Radiation therapy
> - Extrinsic compression
> - Tracheostomy
>
> Adapted from Vetter S, Jakobs R, Weickert U. [Benign non-peptic esophageal stenosis: causes, treatment and outcome in routine clinical practice]. *Dtsch Med Wochenschr* 2010;**135**:1061.

Although initial dilation typically results in symptomatic relief, recurrence of the stricture with return of symptoms is common. In the setting of peptic stricture, approximately 30% to 60% of patients require repeat dilations within a year.[8] Several studies have attempted to identify prognostic factors associated with increased need for multiple dilations. Patients with peptic strictures who experienced weight loss or lacked symptoms of heartburn were more likely to require multiple sessions; however, the severity of the initial stenosis or the type and size of dilator used did not have an impact on recurrence.[11]

Malignant esophageal stricture dilation is both safe and effective.[12,13] This intervention is performed either as an adjunct to endoscopic staging of esophageal tumors or as a temporary palliative treatment before surgery, placement of self-expanding stents, or laser photoablation.

COMPLICATIONS

Several early studies demonstrated a high complication rate associated with aggressive dilation of malignant esophageal strictures.[14,15] The most serious complication following dilation is esophageal perforation. The reported rate is 0.1% to 0.4%.[16,17] As expected, complex strictures have an increased risk for rupture. Contained esophageal perforations usually can be managed nonoperatively but occasionally may require surgical rescue.[18-20]

Mild bleeding is common following dilation and usually is self-limited. Severe bleeding occurs in 0.4% of patients.[21] Inadvertent passage of the dilator into the trachea is a rare event. Unusual complications including discitis and epidural abscess have been described after both dilatation and stenting.[21]

Esophageal Stricture Stent Placement

PATIENT SELECTION

Laser therapy, radiation therapy, and placement of plastic stents have been used for palliation of aggressive esophageal strictures. Laser therapy offers effective palliation with a low rate of complications. However, it is not suitable for extrinsic compression, is difficult to perform if the narrowed region is long and tortuous, and requires repeated treatments with expensive equipment that is not readily available.[22] Radiation therapy achieves palliation of dysphagia in less than 40% of patients and may take up to 2 months until dysphagia is relieved.[23]

Although rigid *plastic* stents are inexpensive and readily available, complications, (including perforation (8%), stent migration, tumor overgrowth, and bleeding) are not infrequent.[24] Other treatments, such as steroid injection, hyperbaric therapy, and radial incision, have been used for tenacious strictures with sporadic success.

The indications for *metallic* stent placement in the esophagus include the following:

- Palliative treatment of malignant dysphagia
- Palliation of malignant esophageal fistulas or perforations
- Benign refractory strictures in poor surgical candidates

The indications for permanent esophageal stenting in patients with *benign* strictures have not been established. Some strictures, especially those caused by radiation or caustic ingestion, recur commonly after dilation and may benefit from stenting. Stents have been occasionally used in treatment of such resistant benign lesions.[25] Plastic self-expanding stents are more commonly used in esophageal strictures because of their ease of placement and retrieval, and the limited local tissue reaction. More recently, biodegradable stents have been employed to manage benign esophageal stenosis.[26]

Recently, stents have been used for leaks and fistulas, with the potential benefits being healing without diversion or reconstruction and early return to an oral diet. Most commonly, covered stents are employed although bare stents can also be used in cases of small leaks or minute tears or fistulas.[27,28]

TECHNIQUE

The stents approved by the U.S. Food and Drug Administration are the covered/uncovered Wallstent (Boston Scientific, Natick, Mass.), covered Gianturco-Rosch Z-stent (Cook Inc., Bloomington, Ind.), and covered/uncovered Ultraflex stents (Boston Scientific). The Wallstent has excellent radiopacity, has the highest radial force (more appropriate for extrinsic compression), and is easy to deploy (Fig. 21-1). However, it foreshortens during deployment, which must be taken into consideration when choosing the length of the stent. The Z-stent has good radiopacity, minimal shortening, and can accommodate an antireflux valve. The latter consists of a pressure sensitive "windsock type" valve created by extending the polyurethane covering over the edge at the esophageal end of the stent or a silicone membrane with a slit-type valve opening. The downside is that it lacks flexibility, requires a bulky sheath (up to 31 Fr), and is difficult to deploy. Greater stent shortening, poor radiopacity, and an unprotected delivery system make the Ultraflex stent deployment more difficult to insert than the Wallstent. The lower radial force and greater flexibility of the Ultraflex probably are responsible for less chest pain and better patient tolerance. It is the preferred stent for high esophageal lesions. Ultraflex has been shown to be equal in performance to Choostent.[29,30] Newer stent designs include the SX-ELLA (Ella CS), which is fully covered to resist tissue ingrowth and has an antimigration ring to withstand migration, and the controlled release Evolution stent (Cook Medical, Limerick, Ireland).[31]

Stents should never be placed across the superior esophageal sphincter (C5-C6 level) because of aspiration risk and patient discomfort.[32] Crossing the gastroesophageal junction with the stent should also be avoided to prevent reflux.[32] A transoral route is used commonly. Predilation is performed to facilitate rapid stent expansion and removal of the delivery system. If a fistula is present or suspected, dilation is avoided because of fear of enlarging the abnormal communication. After deployment, the stent should cover the lesion and have a safety margin of at least 2 cm of normal esophagus at each end. In an ideally positioned stent, the esophageal stricture produces a waist at the center of the stent.

Esophageal stent placement may compress the trachea and precipitate respiratory distress. When significant airway compression is present, tracheobronchial stent placement should be performed first.[32]

After stent placement, patients need to modify their diets to prevent large boluses of food from becoming impacted within the stent. If a stent without a valve is used to cross the distal esophageal sphincter, the

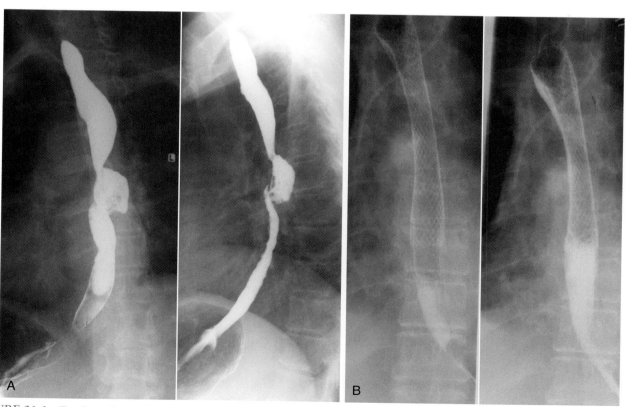

FIGURE 21-1   Esophageal stent placement for malignant stricture. **A,** Esophagogram shows narrowing of the midesophagus secondary to an excavating esophageal carcinoma. **B,** Widely patent esophagus following deployment of covered Wallstent.

patient is placed on antireflux measures that include elevation of the head of the bed and pharmacologic acid suppression therapy.

RESULTS

Esophageal stent placement is technically successful in 97% to 100% of cases.[33] Overall procedure-related morbidity and mortality with self-expanding metallic stents are low.[34-38] Dysphagia is relieved in 90% of patients who undergo esophageal stent placement.[39] Successful closure of tracheoesophageal or bronchoesophageal fistulas can be achieved in 70% to 100% of patients.[40] Treatment failure occurs more frequently when the esophagus is dilated, preventing stent-wall apposition, and when the fistula is in proximity to the superior esophageal sphincter. Overall, the reintervention rate is 25%.[32]

COMPLICATIONS

Adverse events related to esophageal stent placement are uncommon. Major complications include bleeding (up to 6%), aspiration pneumonia, tracheal compressions, perforations, and tracheoesophageal fistulas (up to 8%). Minor complications include chest pain/discomfort, tumor in-growth or overgrowth, stent migration (up to 35%), gastroesophageal reflux, hiccups, foreign body sensation, failure in stent expansion, granulation tissue formation, and food bolus obstruction (4% to 18%).[41,42] Vocal cord paralysis and stent fracture have also been reported.[43,44] The mortality rate associated with esophageal stent placement is approximately 0.5% to 2%.[39]

The most common complication seen with covered stents is migration, whereas the most common complication seen in uncovered stents is tumor in-growth (Fig. 21-2). Ileus and perforation have been reported with stent migration.[45] To minimize migration, changes in stent design have been implemented that include covering inside the metal mesh (exoskeleton), uncovered segments at both ends (longer proximally), and larger proximal diameter (cone-shaped stent). A device with some of these modifications is the Flamingo stent (Boston Scientific).

STOMACH

Enteral Nutrition and Decompression

Background

Malnutrition is a common problem affecting up to 40% of hospitalized patients, increasing their morbidity and mortality.[46] Nutritional support can be given either enterally or parenterally. Parenteral nutrition is costly and has high risks of complications, including sepsis, hepatic dysfunction, metabolic disturbances, catheter-associated vein thrombosis, and intestinal mucosal atrophy.[47] Several studies have shown that enteral feeding has lower complication rates when compared with its parenteral counterpart.[48,49]

Enteral feeding requires a functioning gut and can be provided in the short term via nasogastric or nasojejunal tubes. In the long term, however, these tubes have high complication rates, including mechanical problems, local erosions and aspiration pneumonia. Patients with chronic

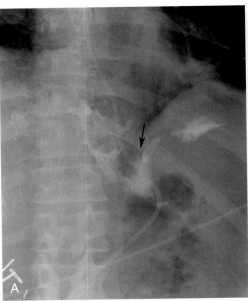
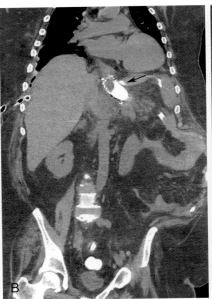
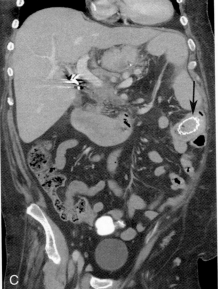

FIGURE 21-2   Stent migration in the esophagus. **A,** Swallow study showing leak at the gastroesophageal junction *(black arrow).* **B,** First follow-up computed tomography (CT) scan after an esophageal stent was placed to seal the leak shows good device position *(black arrow).* **C,** Patient developed abdominal pain 6 months after stent placement. Reformatted coronal CT scan reveals that the stent has migrated *(black arrow).*

swallowing disorders or obstruction to swallowing, or those who are unable to ingest food because of head trauma or stroke, or those with anorexia resulting from underlying diseases such as cancer require more permanent access by placement of a gastrostomy, gastrojejunostomy, or jejunostomy.

Minimally invasive gastrostomy can be performed using endoscopic (percutaneous endoscopic gastrostomy [PEG]) or fluoroscopic (percutaneous gastrostomy [PG]) guidance. The advantage of PG over PEG is that endoscopy is avoided, which is a significant advantage in patients with an esophageal or pharyngeal obstruction. In addition, sedation requirements are less during PG. Wollman and colleagues published a comparison of surgical, endoscopic, and fluoroscopic techniques for gastrostomies that included a metaanalysis of the literature.[50] Their conclusion was that PG is associated with a higher success rate than is PEG and with less morbidity than either PEG or surgery. More recently, Hoffer and colleagues performed a prospective, randomized comparison and concluded that percutaneous gastrojejunostomy had a higher success rate and fewer complications, whereas PEG took less time, cost less, and required less tube maintenance.[51]

Percutaneous Gastrostomy (Online Video 21-1)

PATIENT SELECTION

The major indication for PG as a means of nutritional support are listed in Box 21-2. PG also may be used for gastrointestinal decompression. This indication is more common in patients with carcinomatosis causing chronic intestinal obstruction. Less common indications include craniofacial abnormalities and impaired intestinal absorption, requiring slow infusions of alimental diet into the small bowel via a gastrojejunostomy or jejunostomy.[52] Absolute contraindications to PG include uncorrectable coagulopathy and unsatisfactory anatomy (Box 21-3 and Fig. 21-3), such as an overlying colon or left lobe of liver or the entire gastric lumen located above the costal margin even after air insufflation.

The presence of a ventriculoperitoneal (VP) shunt was considered a contraindication, but this notion has been challenged. One study found a 9% VP shunt infection

---

BOX 21-2

INDICATIONS FOR PERCUTANEOUS GASTROSTOMY OR GASTROJEJUNOSTOMY

Gastrostomy

- Head and neck tumors or malignant esophageal tumors
- Swallowing impairment due to cerebrovascular accident or neuromuscular disorder
- Nutritional supplementation for chronic illness or extensive surgery

Gastrojejunostomy

- Severe gastroesophageal reflux and recurrent aspiration
- Functional or organic gastric outlet obstruction

BOX 21-3

CONTRAINDICATIONS TO PERCUTANEOUS GASTROSTOMY

Absolute Contraindications

- Uncorrectable coagulopathy
- Life expectancy less than 1 week
- Imminent abdominal surgery
- Unsatisfactory anatomy

Relative Contraindications

- Massive ascites
- Abdominal varices
- Prior gastric surgery
- Inflammatory, neoplastic, or infectious involvement of the gastric wall
- Severe gastroesophageal reflux
- Ventriculoperitoneal shunt

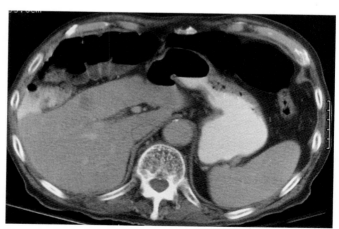

FIGURE 21-3   Colon interposition between the stomach and abdominal wall precludes placement of a percutaneous gastrostomy.

rate 1 month after PEG placement.[53] Another study found that PEGs placed between 1 and 2 weeks after shunt placement caused no infections.[54] Finally, Taylor and colleagues performed 16 shunts in 13 patients requiring gastrostomies (half before and half after PEG) and found a 50% shunt infection rate overall.[55] They concluded that the development of infection was not related to the sequence or interval between shunt and gastrostomy placement and recommended avoiding simultaneous placement in the acute phase of a patient's hospital admission. These are small series that include only PEG procedures, limiting our ability to reach conclusions or extrapolating these results toward the safety of PG in conjunction with VP shunt placement.

Placing PG or percutaneous gastrojejunostomy (PGJ) in patients with short life expectancies is debated in the medical literature. The mortality rate after PG is highly dependent on the patient's underlying conditions (e.g., advanced age, malignancy, diabetes mellitus, and pulmonary disease).[56,57] It is estimated that the cost of hospital visits for tube dislodgment or malfunction is almost $11 million per annum in the United States.[58] Some argue that if no physiologic benefit is expected or if the improvement in physiologic status has no effect on quality of life (e.g., permanent vegetative state), then there is no obligation to offer or perform this intervention.[59] The issue is controversial and depends on the philosophy of the institution, the physician in charge, the individual who inserts the tube, and the wishes of the patient and the family.

DEVICE SELECTION

There is a wide variety of gastrostomy and gastrojejunostomy tubes that differ in both size and retention mechanisms. No single gastrostomy catheter is appropriate for all patients (Fig. 21-4). The various types of gastrostomy options range from the simple pigtail configuration, such as the Deutsch gastrostomy (Cook Inc.), to balloon-retained devices such as the MIC tube (Kimberly Clark). "Button" gastrostomy tubes are popular for children. They lie flush with abdominal wall and have a very short external stem, making them much more cosmetically acceptable. However, with the increasing frequency of long-term gastrostomy placement in adults who are otherwise mobile, these are being used more often in adults as well.[60]

Radiologically placed tubes tend to be smaller (12 to 16 Fr) and therefore are more prone to occlusions, especially when pill fragments are administered. During initial placement, the pigtail variety is often selected because of its ease of placement; however, as mentioned, they are smaller and have greater propensity to occlude.

Endoscopic tubes have better retention systems, including large internal bolsters or bulbs that prevent dislodgment, a common scenario with the radiologically

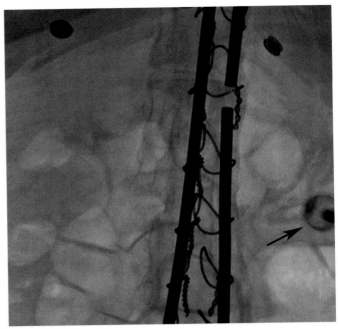

FIGURE 21-4   Balloon-type (MIC) gastrostomy tube. *Arrow* indicates retention balloon.

placed tubes regardless of the type of retention device. They are also of a larger diameter compared with the initially placed percutaneous tubes, which makes for less chance of occlusion. The MIC tube (Kimberly Clark) is a silicone transparent tube with an internal balloon and an external ring flange commonly used in open or laparoscopic or endoscopic gastrostomy procedures. The advantage of balloon retention is that, if needed, a wire exchange can be done easily after deflating the balloon. Some interventionalists place the MIC tube as the primary percutaneous tube; however, this is a more involved procedure than using the more commonly placed Deutsch tube.

Another variety of endoscopic and laparoscopic tubes have an internal bolster/flange ("mushroom") that provides the most secure retention but at the same time is the most challenging to exchange.

TECHNIQUE

A fasting period of 8 hours is required before the procedure (Fig. 21-5). Any available cross-sectional imaging studies should be evaluated to determine suitability and best site for PG placement. Knowledge of any prior abdominal surgery is critical. Barium frequently is administered the day before for colonic opacification, and ultrasound is used to delineate the liver contour. A nasogastric tube is inserted and used for stomach insufflations during the procedure (Fig. 21-6). A small, 4-Fr angiographic catheter will suffice. Glucagon 1 mg intravenously will close the pylorus and

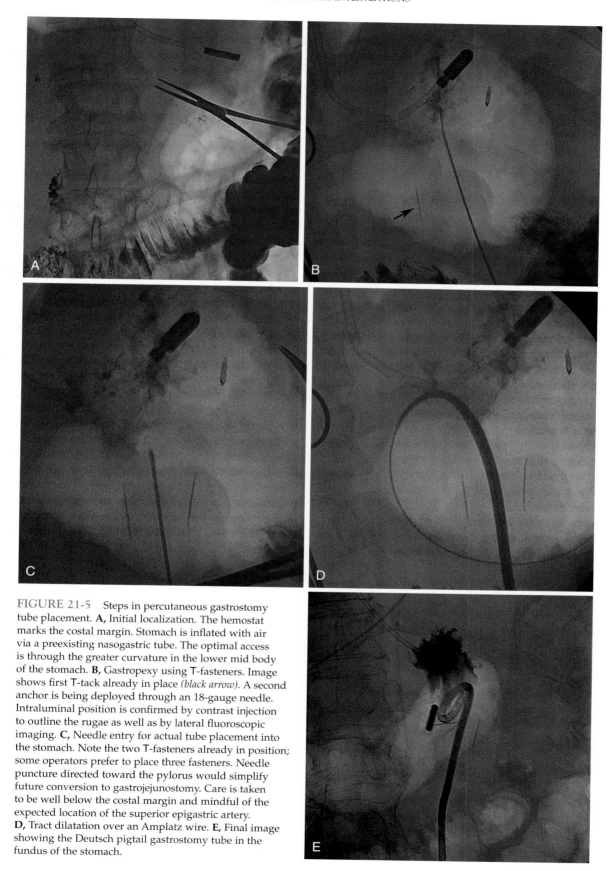

FIGURE 21-5   Steps in percutaneous gastrostomy tube placement. **A,** Initial localization. The hemostat marks the costal margin. Stomach is inflated with air via a preexisting nasogastric tube. The optimal access is through the greater curvature in the lower mid body of the stomach. **B,** Gastropexy using T-fasteners. Image shows first T-tack already in place *(black arrow).* A second anchor is being deployed through an 18-gauge needle. Intraluminal position is confirmed by contrast injection to outline the rugae as well as by lateral fluoroscopic imaging. **C,** Needle entry for actual tube placement into the stomach. Note the two T-fasteners already in position; some operators prefer to place three fasteners. Needle puncture directed toward the pylorus would simplify future conversion to gastrojejunostomy. Care is taken to be well below the costal margin and mindful of the expected location of the superior epigastric artery. **D,** Tract dilatation over an Amplatz wire. **E,** Final image showing the Deutsch pigtail gastrostomy tube in the fundus of the stomach.

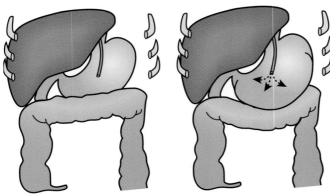

FIGURE 21-6   Insufflation of the stomach provides a larger target for puncture and displaces the transverse colon inferiorly.

help retain injected air in the stomach; however, it may increase the difficulty in crossing the pylorus when placing a gastrojejunostomy tube. Patients with prior gastric resection, upper abdomen interventions, esophageal obstruction, or a nondistensible stomach due to carcinomatosis may require computed tomography (CT) to assist in stomach identification and puncture (Fig. 21-7). Prophylactic antibiotics (e.g., cephazolin 1 g intravenously) are given by some interventionalists based on PEG studies.[61]

All stomach punctures are made in the subxiphoid/upper abdomen with care taken to avoid the superior epigastric artery that runs beneath the rectus abdominis muscle as well as the gastric and gastroepiploic arteries located along the lesser and greater curvatures of the stomach, respectively.

Gastropexy is done by most interventionalists using T-fasteners. T-fasteners are 1-cm metallic spring bars that have a monofilament suture attached at their midportion, forming a T configuration. This step is meant to adhere the anterior gastric wall to the abdominal wall, thus isolating the tube from the peritoneal cavity. Gastropexy is intended to minimize the risk of peritoneal leakage, prevent tube migration into the peritoneal cavity, and tamponade gastric bleeding (Fig. 21-8). The need for gastropexy is most crucial during the first week after insertion; thereafter, a fibrous tract develops around the catheter between the outside and the gastric lumen.[62] Gastropexy also helps during the tube placement as it prevents the stomach wall from being pushed away during tube advancement. Finally, this maneuver should facilitate later insertion of larger tubes and simplify access to the gastric tract in cases of inadvertent tube dislodgment.

Most operators place two or three T-fasteners about 1 to 2 cm from the intended catheter exit site. With the stomach inflated with air and using direct fluoroscopy, the mid to lower segment of the gastric body is punctured with each T-fastener–loaded 18-gauge needle. As the needle is advanced, tenting of the anterior gastric wall can often be visualized at fluoroscopy just before the lumen is entered. Contrast injection will outline the gastric rugae; lateral fluoroscopy can also be used to confirm an intraluminal location. The fastener is deployed by pushing it through the needle with a guidewire or pressing the spring-loaded mechanism on the needle. If the fastener does not deploy, the assembly can be removed en bloc as long as the fastener has not exited the needle. If the fastener lodges within the abdominal wall, reasonably gentle attempts can be made to retrieve it. If retrieval is unsuccessful, it can be left in place and the suture string cut at the skin. Its retention is as benign

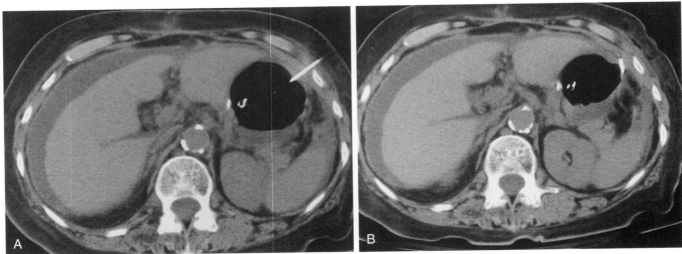

FIGURE 21-7   Placement of a needle (A) and T-fastener (B) for percutaneous gastrostomy under computed tomography guidance in a patient with prior partial gastrectomy.

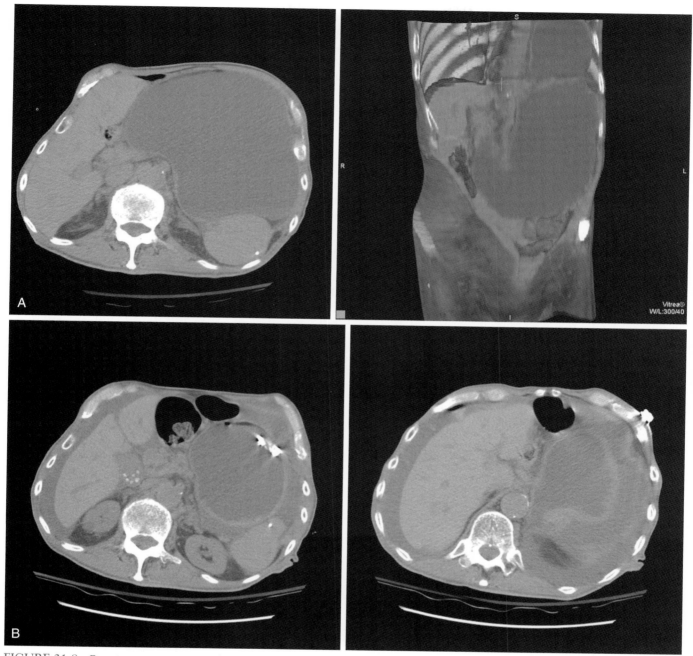

FIGURE 21-8 Percutaneous gastrostomy for gastric outlet obstruction without T-fasteners. **A,** Axial *(left)* and coronal *(right)* computed tomography (CT) images show gastric outlet obstruction. **B,** Axial CT images 12 hours after non–T-fastener gastrostomy show peritoneal leakage and associated inflammation.

as an internal surgical staple. The operator may choose to give intravenous antibiotics to cover skin flora in this situation.

Dewald and colleagues compared over 700 gastropexy and nongastropexy gastrostomies and concluded that no risk was added with gastropexy.[63] Thornton and colleagues performed a randomized comparison of gastrostomies with and without T-fasteners and concluded that fasteners should be used routinely based on a 10%

incidence of serious technical complications in the nongastropexy group that included four catheters that migrated into the peritoneal cavity.[64] However, they also noted a 10% incidence of pain and 13% incidence of skin excoriation at the T-fastener sites. Until recently, all T-fasteners had nonabsorbable sutures, which necessitated follow-up for cutting these sutures so as not to form local stitch abscesses. With the advent of new designs that incorporate absorbable sutures, there may be no need to ever cut the strings. However, there are few data to support the actual benefit of these new materials.

The procedure is performed under fluoroscopic guidance using an over-the-guidewire technique. Most interventionalists prefer to place the tube with a retrograde ("push") technique, although antegrade ("pull") techniques are favored by other practitioners. Indications for the pull method include insertion in patients who are at high risk for pulling out the gastrostomy, who may desire a button device in the future, or who need a very large-bore tube.[65] This technique requires retrograde catheterization of the esophagus followed by exteriorizing the wire through the mouth and delivering the catheter using an antegrade technique typical of PEG placement. However, the method poses a potentially increased risk for stomal infections due to passage of the tube through the oral cavity.[66]

Large-bore tubes can be inserted with standard push radiologic technique by dilating the tract with a 10-mm diameter × 12-cm-long balloon, inserting a 24- to 26-Fr peel-away sheath, followed by delivery of a 20- to 24-Fr MIC-type gastrostomy catheter.[67] In one report, investigators used a three-point T-fastener gastropexy in all of their 109 gastrostomies and concluded that percutaneous large-bore catheter placement is safe and has the same technical success and morbidity and mortality rates when compared with surgically or endoscopically placed tubes, as well as small-bore tubes placed under fluoroscopic guidance.

POSTPROCEDURE CARE

Patients remain fasting for the following 24 hours. They are observed for 4 hours for abdominal pain, distention, and bleeding. The catheter is placed to gravity drainage or to low intermittent suction for 24 hours to decompress the stomach and monitor for bleeding complications. Twenty-four hours later, tube feeding can start gradually if there are no signs of peritonitis (fever, abdominal pain, tenderness) and there are good bowel sounds. Tolerance and progression can be assessed using residual volume measurements every 6 hours, with full nutrition generally achieved within 48 hours. However, results from various randomized clinical trials indicate earlier feeding (<3 hours) may be safe for endoscopically placed devices.[68] T-fasteners are cut in 7 to 10 days. Catheter care instructions are given to the patient and caregivers, including information about tube feedings, catheter maintenance, and how to recognize signs and symptoms that may herald complications.

RESULTS

Technical success rate for PG is 95% to 100% and the procedure-related mortality rate varies between 0% and 3.2%.[52] A metaanalysis of the literature reported a technical success of 95% for PEG and 100% for surgical gastrostomies.[50] Technical "failure" results from lack of safe access route, most commonly from overlying transverse colon. Other reasons for inability to insert at PG include massive ascites, gastric cancer, peritoneal carcinomatosis, overlying open abdominal wound, and previous gastric surgery.

COMPLICATIONS

A small pneumoperitoneum immediately after the procedure is normal. Complications are uncommon. A recent metaanalysis reported a 5.9% overall complication rate and a 0.3% mortality rate for PG.[50] By contrast, PEG was associated with a 9.4% complication rate, whereas surgery was associated with a complication rate of 19.9%.

Peritonitis is a rare but serious complication following gastrostomy and may follow leakage or inadvertent infusion of the nutrient into the peritoneal cavity. Early detection, discontinuation of feedings, and antibiotics can control a minor leak. Contrast studies through the tube may fail to show the defect, but an enlarging pneumoperitoneum is considered to be a reliable sign of intraperitoneal leakage.[52]

Aspiration pneumonia secondary to gastroesophageal reflux has long been considered a major cause of morbidity and mortality in patients with feeding gastrostomies. Gastrostomies affect gastric emptying and, theoretically, may increase the risk for aspiration.[69] However, Olson and colleagues found no causal relationship between gastrostomy tube placement and gastroesophageal reflux.[70] They recommend PGJ placement only in patients with preexisting moderate to severe reflux or who are at high risk for aspiration pneumonia.

Bleeding following PG placement usually is self-limited but can be significant in patients with an underlying coagulopathy. If bleeding persists, direct arterial injury should be suspected. Other etiologies include gastritis or gastric ulceration.

In some instances, the tube may get pulled in along with the flange/bumper due to peristalsis, resulting in the flange/bumper digging into the skin and subcutaneous tissue. The so-called "buried bumper" can result in secondary infection of the skin and subcutaneous tissue. In this case, the infection can be deeper and hence more serious than a simple skin site infection. Buried bumper syndrome is a potentially serious complication of percutaneous gastrostomy tube placement.[71]

Wound infections after PG are not uncommon and occur within days to months following tube placement. They are treated with local care and antibiotics. In this respect, PG differs from PEG, in which the latter has a higher frequency of skin infections because the tube is contaminated by oral flora as it is passed through the mouth and oropharynx on its way to the stomach.[72-74] Overall PG and PEG seem to have similar 30-day and 1-year mortality rates.

Tube malfunction or dislodgment is treated with tube replacement, which should be accomplished within a day or so before the track has closed. To prevent frequent occlusion, vigorous tube flushing must be performed after each use, particularly when dealing with small-bore gastrostomies.

Percutaneous Transgastric Jejunostomy and Gastrojejunostomy

Some interventionalists prefer jejunal placement of feeding tubes, citing the high prevalence of pulmonary aspiration in chronically ill patients and the fact that gastrostomies adversely affect gastric emptying, which may increase the risk of aspiration even further.[69] Primary placement is often done using the pigtail retention tube (e.g., 14-Fr Shetty catheter, Cook Inc.). The pigtail catheter is sometimes exchanged for a balloon-retention catheter at a later date (Fig. 21-9).

PATIENT SELECTION

PGJ is preferred in some circumstances. If direct jejunal feeding is required due to gastric pathology, a transgastric jejunostomy (with jejunal endhole only) will suffice. When gastric decompression needs to occur in addition to jejunal feeding, the tube configuration is a coaxial one with the gastric portion or hub having the decompressive holes in the stomach while the jejunal feeding portion resides beyond the ligament of Treitz.

There are marked differences between gastrostomy and gastrojejunostomy feedings. Gastric feedings can be given in boluses and prepared at home with a blender; patient tolerance is excellent. Jejunal feedings, on the other hand, require nutrient solutions prepared in a pharmacy and delivered by a pump; patient tolerance is variable. Tolerance to enteral nutrition may be improved by tailoring the solution's volume, rate, and concentration to the individual's condition.

TECHNIQUE

The gastric puncture should be directed toward the pylorus. Direct puncture into the antrum should be avoided to prevent potential impairment of gastric emptying function. Placement of the transgastric jejunostomy is relatively straightforward unless there is gastric outlet obstruction. In that case, some degree of manipulation may be needed with shaped catheters and a wire to cross the pylorus and achieve a suitable position.

Placing a fresh large-bore dual-lumen gastrojejunostomy tube can be fraught with problems. More commonly, a gastrostomy tube is placed and then converted to a dual-lumen balloon retention gastrojejunostomy tube after 2 to 4 weeks when the track is mature[62] (Figs. 21-10 and 21-11). If a transgastric jejunostomy tube is indicated, the interventionalist is limited to the Marx-Cope device (Cook Inc.), which is a 16-Fr pigtail catheter with a side port for a 5-Fr jejunal tube. The gastric portion is inserted in the regular manner. The jejunal portion is then manipulated through this tube, exiting the side port and then crossing the pylorus (see Figs. 21-10 and 21-11). The jejunal limb is prone to occlusion due to its small caliber.

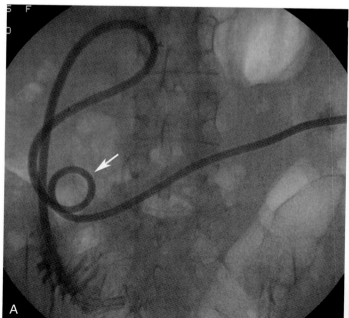
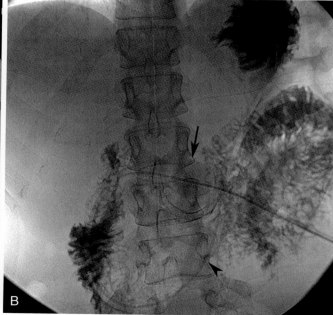

FIGURE 21-9 Transgastric balloon retention jejunostomy tubes. **A,** Primary placed 14-Fr Shetty gastrojejunostomy tube. *Arrow* indicates retention loop, which is ideally positioned beyond the pylorus. The distal catheter should lie beyond the ligament of Treitz. **B,** Later replacement with a balloon-retained *(arrow)* transgastric jejunostomy tube.

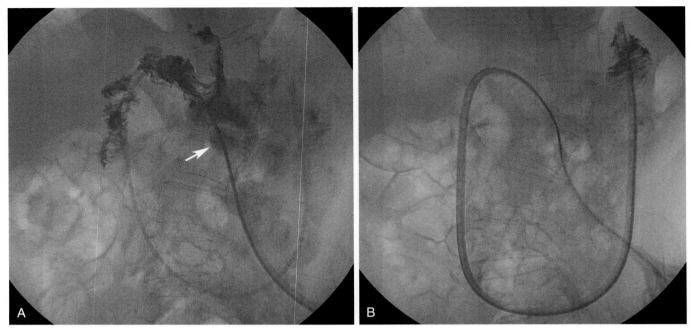

FIGURE 21-10   Balloon-retained dual-lumen gastrojejunostomy tube. This device is usually inserted after primary gastrostomy tube placement. *Arrow* indicates the retention balloon. Gastric port injection **(A)** and jejunal portion injection **(B)**.

Gastroduodenal Obstructions

Stent Placement

PATIENT SELECTION

Gastric outlet and duodenal obstruction in patients with inoperable cancer cause inability to tolerate food, vomiting, and cachexia. As a palliative tool, self-expanding metallic stents provide prompt relief for patients with these conditions.[75] Endoscopic and/or percutaneous treatment is preferable to surgery due to their lower morbidity and mortality, shorter hospitalization, and rapidity of symptom relief. Furthermore, percutaneous enteral stenting can be performed under conscious sedation, eliminating the risk of general anesthesia.

TECHNIQUE

The Wallstent was the most commonly used device. However, with advances in stent technology, self-expanding nitinol stents are slowly becoming popular. Tumor ingrowth of the uncovered stent has not been of significant clinical concern because of the limited life expectancy of these patients.

A "big cup" nitinol stent has been designed for treatment of patients with gastric outlet obstruction resulting from gastric cancer.[76] This new stent is composed of a proximal big cup segment (20 mm in length and 48 to 55 mm in diameter), a middle segment (60 mm in length and 20 mm in diameter) covered by a polyethylene membrane, and a distal spherical segment (20 mm in length and 28 mm in diameter). Half of the proximal big cup segment is also covered by a polyethylene membrane that acts as an antireflux mechanism.[76]

Duodenal stents can be covered or uncovered. Nitinol stents have almost completely replaced other materials because of their marked flexibility and excellent radial force. Complications related to duodenal self-expanding metallic stents are recurrence of gastric outlet obstruction symptoms due to stent clogging (tissue ingrowth/overgrowth and food impaction) and stent migration.[77]

JEJUNUM

Enteral Feeding and Decompression

In critically ill adults and children, feeding by enteral tube is preferred over parenteral nutrition when the gastrointestinal tract is functional. Enteral feeding also prevents atrophy of intestinal villi and prevents or minimizes translocation of bacteria from the gastrointestinal tract to the bloodstream.

Percutaneous Jejunostomy

PATIENT SELECTION

Patients with history of chronic aspiration, gastric or esophageal surgery, or abnormal stomach position may not be suitable candidates for PG/PGJ and may require

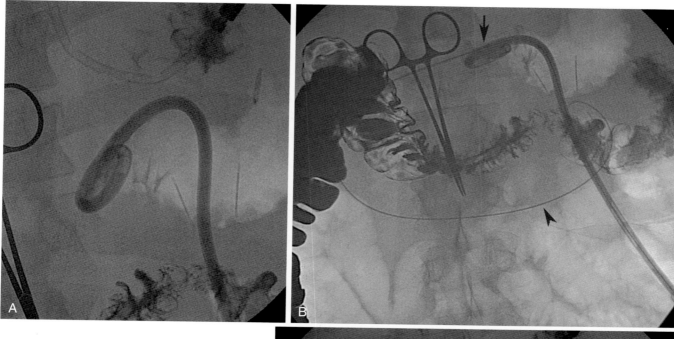

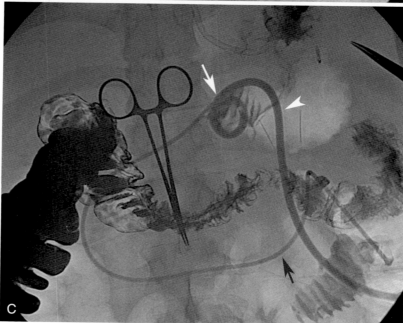

FIGURE 21-11   Percutaneous placement of a dual-lumen Marx-Cope gastrojejunostomy tube. This tube is appropriate for patients who need gastric decompression and jejunal feeding. **A,** Gastric portion is placed percutaneously in the usual manner. **B,** Jejunum is cannulated through the gastric portion. The wire *(arrowhead)* exits through a specially demarcated sidehole *(arrow).* The wire is manipulated into the jejunum. **C,** Final configuration after the distal jejunal portion *(black arrow)* has been placed over the wire through the gastric portion *(white arrowhead).* The jejunal portion exits the retention loop from the designated side opening *(white arrow).*

a jejunostomy (Box 21-4). Jejunostomy can be performed using surgical, endoscopic, laparoscopic, or percutaneous means.

Surgical jejunostomy is constructed in one of three ways: Witzel jejunostomy, Roux-en-Y jejunostomy, and needle catheter jejunostomy.[46] The needle catheter method is used most frequently and involves the placement of a thin tube into the jejunum via a seromuscular tunnel. Created by using a shallow needle path into the bowel wall, this step is akin to a subcutaneous tunnel that helps maintain catheter position and acts as an

---

BOX 21-4

INDICATIONS FOR PERCUTANEOUS JEJUNOSTOMY

- Chronic aspiration
- Previous gastric surgery or resection
- Abnormal stomach position
- Duodenal or gastric outlet obstruction

antileak mechanism. Some surgeons may additionally invaginate about 2 cm of the tube on the bowel wall and anchor it to the serosa with sutures. However, this makes it much more difficult to replace percutaneously, if necessary, using the Seldinger technique. The outer end of the tube is exteriorized through the abdominal wall at a site distant from the laparotomy incision. However, surgical jejunostomy can be associated with significant morbidity and mortality.[78] In addition, patients usually are poor surgical candidates because of chronic illness, debilitated state, or poor nutritional status.

Direct percutaneous endoscopic jejunostomy can be performed in patients who have had gastric surgery with a gastroscope; otherwise, a long enteroscope is needed to reach the first 2 feet of jejunum.[79] In addition to access issues, it may be difficult to transilluminate the abdominal wall through a deeply seated or easily mobile bowel. The failure rate can be as high as 14%, and the procedure can be complicated by colonic perforation or abdominal wall abscess.[79]

Laparoscopic jejunostomy requires general anesthesia, absence of significant intraabdominal adhesions, and a skilled operator. In two series, there was a conversion rate to open surgery of 8% to 12.5% and a serious complication rate (including volvulus) of 11% to 25%.[80,81]

TECHNIQUE

Percutaneous jejunostomy (PJ) can be performed de novo or through a previous jejunostomy site. Gray and colleagues were first to describe this approach. Several technical reports have since confirmed its feasibility and safety for feeding, decompression, and the management of bilioenteric anastomotic strictures.[82,83] PJ is more challenging than PG because of mobility and easy compressibility of the jejunum. Technical success rates vary between 85% and 95%, with most of the failures resulting from difficulty in puncturing the bowel loop and loss of access during dilatation for tube placement.[84-88]

Fluoroscopy in frontal and lateral projections is routinely used for guidance. CT fluoroscopy (or even ultrasound) guidance recently has been suggested to facilitate the visualization and catheterization of mobile, anteriorly positioned, unopacified, or nondistended bowel.[84,87,89-91]

Most interventionalists agree that appropriate bowel distention and the use of T-fasteners are two important factors for the technical success of percutaneous jejunostomy.[92] Bowel distention can be achieved with a nasogastric or nasoduodenal tube. A 5-Fr catheter is usually placed into the proximal jejunum, either from the nose or through an existing PG, and is used for jejunal inflation using either saline or, more commonly, air. A catheter with an occlusion balloon may be used to increase the intraluminal pressure and provide a target for the needle puncture. A suitable bowel loop that is close to the abdominal wall is selected for access. Occasionally, it may be necessary to decompress overlying large bowel loops. Access is gained using a 21-gauge needle, and stay fasteners are delivered. Intraluminal positioning can be confirmed by gentle contrast injection. The tract is then dilated and a 10- or 12-Fr pigtail catheter is placed.[84,87,90]

Care should be taken not to create torsion during deployment of the locking tube, and emphasis should be placed on correctly sizing the diameter of the catheter loop with the target segment of jejunum. Feeding can be started 24 hours following the intervention.

A dislodged surgical jejunostomy can be replaced percutaneously. Success is more likely if attempted less than 10 days after dislodgment or removal of the tube and when the original tube was in place for more than 4 weeks for the tract to mature. Hietmiller and colleagues recommend marking the jejunopexy site at surgery with radiopaque markers to assist visualization if re-access is needed.[93]

RESULTS AND COMPLICATIONS

With experience, the technical success rate of percutaneous jejunostomy approaches 95%. Minor complications included localized pain, infection at the insertion site, and tube occlusion.[87,90] Major complications include pericatheter leakage and peritonitis or abdominal abscess formation. Data reported by van Overhagen and colleagues[91] as well as Yang and associates[88] showed that peritonitis occurred in about 13% of cases, all of which were managed nonoperatively. A 30-day mortality of 5% to 17% has been reported.[87,88,91]

The jejunostomy tube can be subsequently upsized if needed. With proper management, these catheters will function for long periods of time. Richard and coworkers calculated a primary patency of 95% from a large series with mean follow-up of 285 days.[86]

Nasojejunal Tube Placement

Nasojejunal (NJ) tubes are used for temporary nutritional support in patients at risk of aspiration pneumonia, patients intolerant of gastric feeding, patients with recurrent emesis or severe reflux, and patients who have undergone major surgery or sustained severe trauma.[94] NJ tubes can be placed at the bedside, with fluoroscopic guidance, or via endoscopy.[95]

Care is taken to anesthetize the nasopharynx and oropharynx with Cetacaine (benzocaine; tetracaine) spray and Xylocaine (lidocaine) jelly, which is injected into the selected nostril. Using fluoroscopic guidance, a long diagnostic catheter (4- or 5-Fr Kumpe or vertebral) and guidewire are manipulated through the pylorus past the ligament of Treitz. An exchange-length guidewire is advanced and an NJ tube (Cook, Inc.) is delivered over the guidewire.

The pylorus usually is the most difficult site to traverse when placing an NJ tube. Injecting air admixed with contrast through the catheter may facilitate manipulations as well as stimulate peristalsis. Mucosal and skin erosion around the nostril caused by prolonged NJ intubation can be minimized by careful tube fixation and keeping the skin dry.

COLON

Functional and Mechanical Obstruction

Etiology

Cecal dilation can result from functional obstruction *(Ogilvie syndrome)* or mechanical obstruction from distal colonic carcinoma or volvulus.[96] The risk for colonic perforation increases when the cecal diameter exceeds 12 cm and when the distention has been present for several days.[97] In the event of perforation, the mortality rate approaches 40%.[97]

Between 10% and 30% of patients with colorectal carcinoma have large bowel obstruction at the time of presentation.[98] Emergency colectomy carries a high morbidity (50%) and mortality (23%) rate in poor surgical candidates.[99]

Percutaneous Cecostomy

PATIENT SELECTION

Percutaneous cecostomy (PC) is an alternative to open or laparoscopic surgical cecostomy for decompression of sustained cecal dilation. PC has been used as colonic access for the administration of antegrade enemas in children with chronic fecal incontinence and adults with neurogenic bowel disease.[100-102] PC also has been described using various endoscopic techniques.[103]

Contraindications to PC include severe bowel ischemia, perforation, or an uncorrectable coagulopathy.

TECHNIQUE

The technique is similar to placement of a gastrostomy, and T-fasteners are used. Both transperitoneal and retroperitoneal approaches are practiced. The retroperitoneal route is considered safer. In the unlikely event that spillage of feces occurs, this event would contaminate the retroperitoneum but not the peritoneal cavity. However, the retroperitoneal route is technically more difficult because of the presence of the iliac bone, presence of interposed mesentery, or the possibility of peritoneum wrapping around the posterior aspect of the cecum.[104,105] Initial access with CT may facilitate the retroperitoneal approach; the remainder of the case is then done with fluoroscopy. A CT fluoroscopy unit is ideal for this situation (Fig. 21-12). Access is gained using an 18-gauge needle in a similar fashion

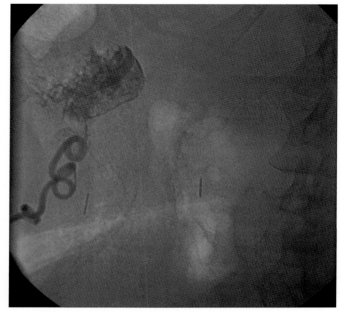

FIGURE 21-12 Chait cecostomy tube. Note the numerous loops designed to prevent expulsion.

to percutaneous gastrostomy. Two or three T-fasteners are deployed in the colonic lumen. Intraluminal position of the needle is confirmed by gentle contrast injection. If needed, a cross-table lateral fluoroscopic view can be obtained to confirm the location. Once the T-fasteners are in place, the cecum is repunctured with an 18-gauge needle. A long, stiff guidewire that will accommodate the device is advanced well into the lumen. The tract is dilated, and a Chait cecostomy tube loaded onto the wire. The catheter is constructed as a tightly wound coil at its distal end that anchors the tube in the lumen.

RESULTS

Technical success rate is close to 100%. Clinical success rate is close to 89% for patients with benign causes of obstruction.[96,104,106] In patients with a malignant etiology of obstruction, cecostomy is adequate as a temporizing method; definite treatment is needed in the long term.

COMPLICATIONS

The reported complication rate is about 60%, but most of these are minor.[102] Severe complications are rare and consist of sepsis and peritonitis from spillage of contents into the peritoneum.[102]

Minor complications include pericatheter leak, superficial wound infection, tube occlusion, skin excoriation, premature tube dislodgment, colocutaneous fistula, and ventral hernia. Catheter obstruction is avoided by frequent flushing.

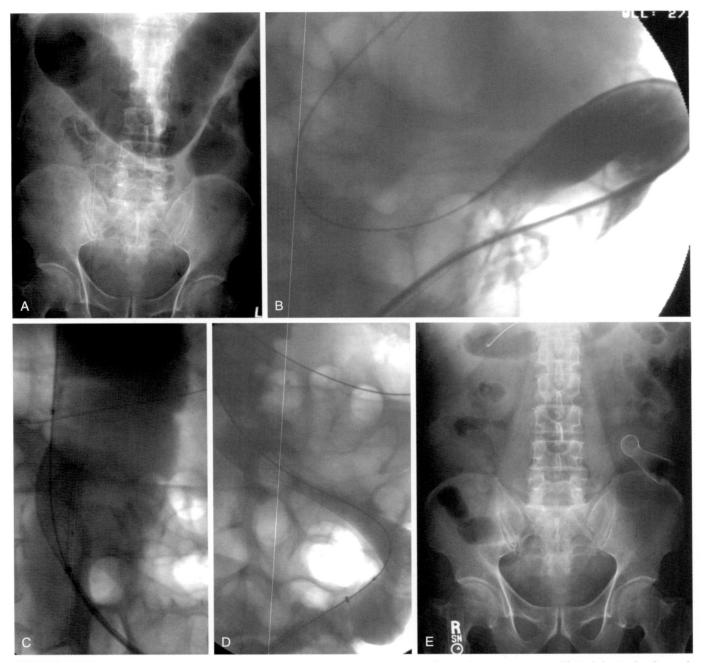

FIGURE 21-13   Colonic stent placement for temporary decompression in preparation for single stage surgery. **A,** Plain abdominal radiograph shows large bowel dilation secondary to obstructing distal descending colon carcinoma. **B,** Guidewires and catheters are manipulated across the obstruction. **C,** Deployment of Wallstent is initiated. **D,** Deployment is completed. **E,** Abdominal film 12 hours after the procedure shows successful relief of obstruction. The stent was not dilated with a balloon.

Colonic Stent Placement

PATIENT SELECTION

Stents can be placed across the obstruction in poor surgical candidates for palliative treatment of unresectable colonic malignancy or for temporary colonic decompression to allow bowel cleansing in preparation for single-stage colonic surgery.[107,108] Patients who benefit most are those at high risk for operation and candidates for laparoscopic resection, because emergency surgery can be avoided in more than 90% of these cases.[109] Stents are placed rectally or via an existing cecostomy or colostomy.[110] Despite concerns of tumor seeding following colorectal stent placement, no difference exists in long-term survival between patients who undergo stent placement followed by elective resection and those undergoing emergency bowel resection.[109]

TECHNIQUE

Stent placement is accomplished using fluoroscopy with the patient in a lateral or oblique position (Fig. 21-13). Uncovered stents are used due to high rates of migration with covered devices.[109] Available stents include the enteral Wallstent, Gianturco-Rosch Z-stent, and Ultraflex stent. The use of a long sheath facilitates catheter manipulations. The lesion should not undergo pre-stent or post-stent dilation because of the risk for perforation.[111] The ends of the stent are placed in bowel segments that are straight to avoid kinks. An abdominal radiograph is obtained at 24 hours to assess for stent expansion, position, and success of decompression.

RESULTS

The technical success rate is 78% to 100%, and the clinical success rate is 84% to 100%.[112-115] The complication rate has been reported to be from 14% to 42%, with most complications being minor.[112-115] Severe complications are rare and consist of migration, perforation, and sepsis.

COMPLICATIONS

Perforation may result from catheter manipulations and balloon dilation or late erosion of the colonic wall by the ends of the stent. Tenesmus and incontinence can occur when stents are placed in the rectum.

Early migration is often due to selection of undersized stents, fully covered stents, or stents with weak radial force. Late stent migration is usually attributed to shrinkage of the tumors following adjuvant chemotherapy. Reobstruction follows tumor ingrowth or overgrowth or fecal impaction within the stent lumen. Dietary restrictions and stool softeners are frequently employed to minimize the risk of stent obstruction.

References

1. Antoniou D, Soutis M, Christopoulos-Geroulanos G. Anastomotic strictures following esophageal atresia repair: a 20-year experience with endoscopic balloon dilatation. *J Pediatr Gastroenterol Nutr* 2010;**51**:464.
2. Serhal L, Gottrand F, Sfeir R, et al. Anastomotic stricture after surgical repair of esophageal atresia: frequency, risk factors, and efficacy of esophageal bougie dilatations. *J Pediatr Surg* 2010;**45**:1459.
3. Urba S, Orringer M, Turrisi A, et al. Randomized trial of preoperative chemoradiation versus surgery alone in patients with locoregional esophageal carcinoma. *J Clin Oncol* 2001;**19**:305.
4. Earlam R, Cunha-Melo J. Malignant oesophageal strictures: a review of techniques for palliative intubation. *Br J Surg* 1982;**69**:61.
5. Broor S, Raju G, Bose P, et al. Long term results of endoscopic dilatation for corrosive oesophageal strictures. *Gut* 1993;**34**:1498.
6. McClave S, Brady P, Wright R, et al. Does fluoroscopic guidance for Maloney esophageal dilation impact on the clinical endpoint of therapy: relief of dysphagia and achievement of luminal patency. *Gastrointest Endosc* 1996;**43**:93.
7. Yamamoto H, Hughes RJ, Schroeder K, Viggiano T, DiMagno E. Treatment of benign esophageal stricture by Eder-Puestow or balloon dilators: a comparison between randomized and prospective nonrandomized trials. *Mayo Clin Proc* 1992;**67**:228.
8. Lew R, Kochman M. A review of endoscopic methods of esophageal dilation. *J Clin Gastroenterol* 2002;**35**:117.
9. McLean G, Cooper G, Hartz W, et al. Radiologically guided balloon dilation of gastrointestinal strictures. Part I. Technique and factors influencing procedural success. *Radiology* 1987;**165**:35.
10. McLean G, Cooper G, Hartz W, et al. Radiologically guided balloon dilation of gastrointestinal strictures. Part II. Results of long-term follow-up. *Radiology* 1987;**165**:41.
11. Agnew S, Pandya S, Reynolds R, Preiksaitis H. Predictors for frequent esophageal dilations of benign peptic strictures. *Dig Dis Sci* 1996;**41**:931.
12. Pfau P, Ginsberg G, Lew R, et al. Esophageal dilation for endosonographic evaluation of malignant esophageal strictures is safe and effective. *Am J Gastroenterol* 2000;**95**:2813.
13. Wallace M, Hawes R, Sahai A, et al. Dilation of malignant esophageal stenosis to allow EUS guided fine-needle aspiration: safety and effect on patient management. *Gastrointest Endosc* 2000;**51**:309.
14. Catalano M, Van Dam J, Sivak MJ. Malignant esophageal strictures: staging accuracy of endoscopic ultrasonography. *Gastrointest Endosc* 1995;**41**:535.
15. Roubein L. Endoscopic ultrasonography and the malignant esophageal stricture: implications and complications. *Gastrointest Endosc* 1995;**41**:613.
16. Hernandez L, Jacobson J, Harris M, Hernandez L. Comparison among the perforation rates of Maloney, balloon, and Savary dilation of esophageal strictures. *Gastrointest Endosc* 2000;**51**:460.
17. Karnak I, Tanyel F, Büyükpamukçu N, Hiçsünmez A. Esophageal perforations encountered during the dilation of caustic esophageal strictures. *J Cardiovasc Surg (Torino)* 1998;**39**:373.
18. Dellon E, Cullen N, Madanick R, et al. Outcomes of a combined antegrade and retrograde approach for dilatation of radiation-induced esophageal strictures (with video). *Gastrointest Endosc* 2010;**71**:1122.
19. Hu H, Shin J, Kim J, et al. Fluoroscopically guided balloon dilation for pharyngoesophageal stricture after radiation therapy in patients with head and neck cancer. *AJR Am J Roentgenol* 2010;**194**:1131.
20. Goguen L, Norris C, Jaklitsch M, et al. Combined antegrade and retrograde esophageal dilation for head and neck cancer-related complete esophageal stenosis. *Laryngoscope* 2010;**120**:261.

21. Silvis S, Nebel O, Rogers G, et al. Endoscopic complications. Results of the 1974 American Society for Gastrointestinal Endoscopy Survey. *JAMA* 1976;**235**:928.

22. Mason R, Bright N, McColl I. Palliation of malignant dysphagia with laser therapy: predictability of results. *Br J Surg* 1991;**78**:1346.

23. Wagner HJ, Stinner B, Schwerk WB, et al. Nitinol prostheses for the treatment of inoperable malignant esophageal obstruction. *J Vasc Interv Radiol* 1994;**5**:899.

24. Ogilvie A, Dronfield M, Ferguson R, Atkinson M. Palliative intubation of oesophagogastric neoplasms at fibreoptic endoscopy. *Gut* 1982;**23**:1060.

25. Schembre D. Advances in esophageal stenting: the evolution of fully covered stents for malignant and benign disease. *Adv Ther* 2010;**27**:413.

26. Güitrón-Cantú A, Adalid-Martínez R, Gutiérrez-Bermúdez J, et al. [Foreign body reaction of a biodegradable esophageal stent. A case report]. *Rev Gastroenterol Mex* 2010;**75**:203.

27. Chak A, Singh R, Linden P. Covered stents for the treatment of life-threatening cervical esophageal anastomotic leaks. *J Thorac Cardiovasc Surg* 2011;**141**:843.

28. Blackmon S, Santora R, Schwarz P, et al. Utility of removable esophageal covered self-expanding metal stents for leak and fistula management. *Ann Thorac Surg* 2010;**89**:931.

29. Bona D, Laface L, Bonavina L, et al. Covered nitinol stents for the treatment of esophageal strictures and leaks. *World J Gastroenterol* 2011;**141**:843.

30. Bona D, Laface L, Siboni S, et al. [Self-expanding oesophageal stents: comparison of Ultraflex and Choostent]. *Chir Ital* 2009;**61**:641.

31. Uitdehaag M, Siersema P, Spaander M, et al. A new fully covered stent with antimigration properties for the palliation of malignant dysphagia: a prospective cohort study. *Gastrointest Endosc* 2010;**71**:600.

32. Therasse E, Oliva V, Lafontaine E, et al. Balloon dilation and stent placement for esophageal lesions: indications, methods, and results. *Radiographics* 2003;**23**:89.

33. Acunaş B, Poyanlí A, Rozanes I. Intervention in gastrointestinal tract: the treatment of esophageal, gastroduodenal and colorectal obstructions with metallic stents. *Eur J Radiol* 2002;**42**:240.

34. Song H, Lee D, Seo T, et al. Retrievable covered nitinol stents: experiences in 108 patients with malignant esophageal strictures. *J Vasc Interv Radiol* 2002;**13**:285.

35. Cwikiel W, Tranberg K, Cwikiel M, Lillo-Gil R. Malignant dysphagia: palliation with esophageal stents–long-term results in 100 patients. *Radiology* 1998;**207**:513.

36. Park H, Do Y, Suh S, et al. Upper gastrointestinal tract malignant obstruction: initial results of palliation with a flexible covered stent. *Radiology* 1999;**210**:865.

37. Poyanli A, Sencer S, Rozanes I, Acuna B. Palliative treatment of inoperable malignant esophageal strictures with conically shaped covered self-expanding stents. *Acta Radiol* 2001;**42**:166.

38. Sabharwal T, Hamady M, Chui S, et al. A randomised prospective comparison of the Flamingo Wallstent and Ultraflex stent for palliation of dysphagia associated with lower third oesophageal carcinoma. *Gut* 2003;**52**:922.

39. Baron T. Expandable metal stents for the treatment of cancerous obstruction of the gastrointestinal tract. *N Engl J Med* 2001;**344**:1681.

40. Morgan R, Adam A. Use of metallic stents and balloons in the esophagus and gastrointestinal tract. *J Vasc Interv Radiol* 2001;**12**:283.

41. Turkyilmaz A, Eroglu A, Aydin Y, et al. Complications of metallic stent placement in malignant esophageal stricture and their management. *Surg Laparosc Endosc Percutan Tech* 2010;**20**:10.

42. Wang M, Sze D, Wang Z, et al. Delayed complications after esophageal stent placement for treatment of malignant esophageal obstructions and esophagorespiratory fistulas. *J Vasc Interv Radiol* 2001;**12**:465.

43. Gellad Z, Hampton D, Tebbit C, et al. Bilateral vocal cord paralysis following stent placement for proximal esophageal stricture. *Endoscopy* 2008;**40**(Suppl. 2):E150.

44. Wadsworth C, East J, Hoare J. Early covered-stent fracture after placement for a benign esophageal stricture. *Gastrointest Endosc* 2010;**72**:1260.

45. Bay J, Penninga L. [Small bowel ileus caused by migration of oesophageal stent]. *Ugeskr Laeger* 2010;**172**:2234.

46. Pearce C, Duncan H. Enteral feeding. Nasogastric, nasojejunal, percutaneous endoscopic gastrostomy, or jejunostomy: its indications and limitations. *Postgrad Med J* 2002;**78**:198.

47. Waitzberg D, Plopper C, Terra R. Access routes for nutritional therapy. *World J Surg* 2000;**24**:1468.

48. Kudsk K, Croce M, Fabian T, et al. Enteral versus parenteral feeding. Effects on septic morbidity after blunt and penetrating abdominal trauma. *Ann Surg* 1992;**215**:503.

49. Moore F, Feliciano D, Andrassy R, et al. Early enteral feeding, compared with parenteral, reduces postoperative septic complications. The results of a meta-analysis. *Ann Surg* 1992;**216**:172.

50. Wollman B, D'Agostino H, Walus-Wigle J, et al. Radiologic, endoscopic, and surgical gastrostomy: an institutional evaluation and meta-analysis of the literature. *Radiology* 1995;**197**:699.

51. Hoffer E, Cosgrove J, Levin D, et al. Radiologic gastrojejunostomy and percutaneous endoscopic gastrostomy: a prospective, randomized comparison. *J Vasc Interv Radiol* 1999;**10**:413.

52. Ozmen M, Akhan O. Percutaneous radiologic gastrostomy. *Eur J Radiol* 2002;**43**:186.

53. Sane S, Towbin A, Bergey E, et al. Percutaneous gastrostomy tube placement in patients with ventriculoperitoneal shunts. *Pediatr Radiol* 1998;**28**:521.

54. Graham S, Flowers J, Scott T, et al. Safety of percutaneous endoscopic gastrostomy in patients with a ventriculoperitoneal shunt. *Neurosurgery* 1993;**32**:932.

55. Taylor A, Carroll T, Jakubowski J, O'Reilly G. Percutaneous endoscopic gastrostomy in patients with ventriculoperitoneal shunts. *Br J Surg* 2001;**88**:724.

56. Taylor C, Larson D, Ballard D, et al. Predictors of outcome after percutaneous endoscopic gastrostomy: a community-based study. *Mayo Clin Proc* 1992;**67**:1042.

57. Stuart S, Tiley Er, Boland J. Feeding gastrostomy: a critical review of its indications and mortality rate. *South Med J* 1993;**86**:169.

58. Odom S, Barone J, Docimo S, et al. Emergency department visits by demented patients with malfunctioning feeding tubes. *Surg Endosc* 2003;**17**:651.

59. Angus F, Burakoff R. The percutaneous endoscopic gastrostomy tube. medical and ethical issues in placement. *Am J Gastroenterol* 2003;**98**:272.

60. Lyon S, Haslam P, Duke D, et al. De novo placement of button gastrostomy catheters in an adult population: experience in 53 patients. *J Vasc Interv Radiol* 2003;**14**:1283.

61. Ahmad I, Mouncher A, Abdoolah A, et al. Antibiotic prophylaxis for percutaneous endoscopic gastrostomy—a prospective, randomised, double-blind trial. *Aliment Pharmacol Ther* 2003;**18**:209.

62. vanSonnenberg E, Wittich G, Brown L, et al. Percutaneous gastrostomy and gastroenterostomy: 1. Techniques derived from laboratory evaluation. *AJR Am J Roentgenol* 1986;**146**:577.

63. Dewald C, Hiette P, Sewall L, et al. Percutaneous gastrostomy and gastrojejunostomy with gastropexy: experience in 701 procedures. *Radiology* 1999;**211**:651.

64. Thornton F, Fotheringham T, Haslam P, et al. Percutaneous radiologic gastrostomy with and without T-fastener gastropexy: a randomized comparison study. *Cardiovasc Intervent Radiol* 2002;**25**:467.

65. Clark J, Pugash R, Pantalone R. Radiologic peroral gastrostomy. *J Vasc Interv Radiol* 1999;**10**:927.

66. Pitton M, Herber S, Düber C. Fluoroscopy-guided pull-through gastrostomy. *Cardiovasc Intervent Radiol* 2008;**31**:142.

67. Giuliano A, Yoon H, Lomis N, Miller F. Fluoroscopically guided percutaneous placement of large-bore gastrostomy and gastrojejunostomy tubes: review of 109 cases. *J Vasc Interv Radiol* 2000;**11**:239.

68. Szary N, Arif M, Matteson M, et al. Enteral feeding within three hours after percutaneous endoscopic gastrostomy placement: a meta-analysis. *J Clin Gastroenterol* 2011;**45**:e34.

69. Ho C, Yeung E. Percutaneous gastrostomy and transgastric jejunostomy. *AJR Am J Roentgenol* 1992;**158**:251.

70. Olson D, Krubsack A, Stewart E. Percutaneous enteral alimentation: gastrostomy versus gastrojejunostomy. *Radiology* 1993;**187**:105.

71. Piskac P, Wasiková S, Hnízdil L, et al. [Buried bumper syndrome (BBS) as a complication of percutaneous endoscopic gastrostomy]. *Rozhl Chir* 2010;**89**:298.

72. Jain N, Larson D, Schroeder K, et al. Antibiotic prophylaxis for percutaneous endoscopic gastrostomy. A prospective, randomized, double-blind clinical trial. *Ann Intern Med* 1987;**107**:824.

73. Leeds J, McAlindon M, Grant J, et al. Survival analysis after gastrostomy: a single-centre, observational study comparing radiological and endoscopic insertion. *Eur J Gastroenterol Hepatol* 2010;**22**:591.

74. Galaski A, Peng W, Ellis M, et al. Gastrostomy tube placement by radiological versus endoscopic methods in an acute care setting: a retrospective review of frequency, indications, complications and outcomes. *Can J Gastroenterol* 2009;**23**:109.

75. Park K, Do Y, Kang W, et al. Malignant obstruction of gastric outlet and duodenum: palliation with flexible covered metallic stents. *Radiology* 2001;**219**:679.

76. Shi D, Liao S, Geng J. A newly designed big cup nitinol stent for gastric outlet obstruction. *World J Gastroenterol* 2010;**16**:4206.

77. Boškoski I, Tringali A, Familiari P, et al. Self-expandable metallic stents for malignant gastric outlet obstruction. *Adv Ther* 2010.;**27**:691.

78. Tapia J, Murguia R, Garcia G, et al. Jejunostomy: techniques, indications, and complications. *World J Surg* 1999;**23**:596.

79. Mellert J, Naruhn M, Grund K, Becker H. Direct endoscopic percutaneous jejunostomy (EPJ). Clinical results. *Surg Endosc* 1994;**8**:867; discussion 869.

80. Duh Q, Senokozlieff-Englehart A, Siperstein A, et al. Prospective evaluation of the safety and efficacy of laparoscopic jejunostomy. *West J Med* 1995;**162**:117.

81. Hotokezaka M, Adams R, Miller A, et al. Laparoscopic percutaneous jejunostomy for long term enteral access. *Surg Endosc* 1996;**10**:1008.

82. Gray R, Ho C, Yee A, et al. Direct percutaneous jejunostomy. *AJR Am J Roentgenol* 1987;**149**:931.

83. Perry L, Stokes K, Lewis W, et al. Biliary intervention by means of percutaneous puncture of the antecolic jejunal loop. *Radiology* 1995;**195**:163.

84. Shin JH, Park AW. Updates on Percutaneous Radiologic Gastrostomy/Gastrojejunostomy and Jejunostomy. *Gut Liver* 2010;**4**:S25.

85. Cope C, Davis AG, Baum RA, et al. Direct percutaneous jejunostomy: techniques and applications–ten years experience. *Radiology* 1998;**209**:747.

86. Richard HM, Widlus DM, Malloy PC. Percutaneous fluoroscopically guided jejunostomy placement. *J Trauma* 2008;**65**:1072.

87. Hu HT, Shin JH, Song HY, et al. Fluoroscopically guided percutaneous jejunostomy with use of a 21-gauge needle: a prospective study in 51 patients. *J Vasc Interv Radiol* 2009;**20**:1583.

88. Yang ZQ, Shin JH, Song HY, et al. Fluoroscopically guided percutaneous jejunostomy: outcomes in 25 consecutive patients. *Clin Radiol* 2007;**62**:1061; discussion 1066.

89. Davies R, Kew J, West G. Percutaneous jejunostomy using CT fluoroscopy. *AJR Am J Roentgenol* 2001;**176**:808.

90. Sparrow P, David E, Pugash R. Direct percutaneous jejunostomy–an underutilized interventional technique? *Cardiovasc Intervent Radiol* 2008;**31**:336.

91. van Overhagen H, Ludviksson MA, Laméris JS, et al. US and fluoroscopic-guided percutaneous jejunostomy: experience in 49 patients. *J Vasc Interv Radiol* 2000;**11**:101.

92. Ryan JM, Hahn PF, Boland GW, et al. Percutaneous gastrostomy with T-fastener gastropexy: results of 316 consecutive procedures. *Radiology* 1997;**203**:496.

93. Heitmiller R, Venbrux A, Osterman F. Percutaneous replacement jejunostomy. *Ann Thorac Surg* 1992;**53**:711.

94. Jabbar A, McClave S. Pre-pyloric versus post-pyloric feeding. *Clin Nutr* 2005;**24**:719.

95. Phipps L, Weber M, Ginder B, et al. A randomized controlled trial comparing three different techniques of nasojejunal feeding tube placement in critically ill children. *JPEN J Parenter Enteral Nutr* 2005;**29**:420.

96. Benacci J, Wolff B. Cecostomy. Therapeutic indications and results. *Dis Colon Rectum* 1995;**38**:530.

97. Saunders M, Kimmey M. Colonic pseudo-obstruction: the dilated colon in the ICU. *Semin Gastrointest Dis* 2003;**14**:20.

98. Deans G, Krukowski Z, Irwin S. Malignant obstruction of the left colon. *Br J Surg* 1994;**81**:1270.

99. Buechter K, Boustany C, Caillouette R, Cohn IJ. Surgical management of the acutely obstructed colon. A review of 127 cases. *Am J Surg* 1988;**156**:163.

100. Teichman J, Zabihi N, Kraus S, et al. Long-term results for Malone antegrade continence enema for adults with neurogenic bowel disease. *Urology* 2003;**61**:502.

101. Uno Y. Introducer method of percutaneous endoscopic cecostomy and antegrade continence enema by use of the Chait Trapdoor cecostomy catheter in patients with adult neurogenic bowel. *Gastrointest Endosc* 2006;**63**:666.

102. Chait P, Shlomovitz E, Connolly B, et al. Percutaneous cecostomy: updates in technique and patient care. *Radiology* 2003;**227**:246.

103. Ramage JJ, Baron T. Percutaneous endoscopic cecostomy: a case series. *Gastrointest Endosc* 2003;**57**:752.

104. vanSonnenberg E, Varney R, Casola G, et al. Percutaneous cecostomy for Ogilvie syndrome: laboratory observations and clinical experience. *Radiology* 1990;**175**:679.

105. Vanek V, Al-Salti M. Acute pseudo-obstruction of the colon (Ogilvie's syndrome). An analysis of 400 cases. *Dis Colon Rectum* 1986;**29**:203.

106. Morrison M, Lee M, Stafford S, et al. Percutaneous cecostomy: controlled transperitoneal approach. *Radiology* 1990;**176**:574.

107. Mainar A, Tejero E, Maynar M, et al. Colorectal obstruction: treatment with metallic stents. *Radiology* 1996;**198**:761.

108. Binkert C, Ledermann H, Jost R, et al. Acute colonic obstruction: clinical aspects and cost-effectiveness of preoperative and palliative treatment with self-expanding metallic stents—a preliminary report. *Radiology* 1998;**206**:199.

109. Bonin E, Baron T. Update on the indications and use of colonic stents. *Curr Gastroenterol Rep* 2010;**12**:374.

110. Gómez Herrero H, Paúl Díaz L, Pinto Pabón I, Lobato Fernández R. Placement of a colonic stent by percutaneous colostomy in a case of malignant stenosis. *Cardiovasc Intervent Radiol* 2001;**24**:67.

111. Canon C, Baron T, Morgan D, et al. Treatment of colonic obstruction with expandable metal stents: radiologic features. *AJR Am J Roentgenol* 1997;**168**:199.

112. Choo I, Do Y, Suh S, et al. Malignant colorectal obstruction: treatment with a flexible covered stent. *Radiology* 1998;**206**:415.

113. Camúñez F, Echenagusia A, Simó G, et al. Malignant colorectal obstruction treated by means of self-expanding metallic stents: effectiveness before surgery and in palliation. *Radiology* 2000;**216**:492.

114. Baron T, Dean P, Yates Mr, et al. Expandable metal stents for the treatment of colonic obstruction: techniques and outcomes. *Gastrointest Endosc* 1998;**47**:277.

115. de Gregorio M, Mainar A, Tejero E, et al. Acute colorectal obstruction: stent placement for palliative treatment—results of a multicenter study. *Radiology* 1998;**209**:117.

116. Vetter S, Jakobs R, Weickert U. [Benign non-peptic esophageal stenosis: causes, treatment and outcome in routine clinical practice]. *Dtsch Med Wochenschr* 2010;**135**:1061.

Biliary System

Steven C. Rose

Percutaneous invasive procedures involving the biliary system are designed to prove, characterize, and treat suspected biliary obstruction and, occasionally, biliary leaks. Huard provided the initial description of transhepatic cholangiography (THC) in 1937.[1] Remolar and coworkers first described external percutaneous biliary drainage (PBD) in 1956.[2] Nevertheless, these procedures did not become widely accepted until the late 1970s, when skinny-needle puncture techniques and coaxial exchange systems were developed to minimize the incidence of serious procedure-related hemorrhagic complications. Since their development in the late 1980s, endoscopic retrograde cholangiopancreatography (ERCP) and subsequently transendoscopic biliary drainage have diminished the need for THC and PBD. Percutaneous therapy continues to have a role in patients with anatomy unfavorable to endoscopic procedures and in institutions without skilled interventional endoscopists.[3]

NORMAL ANATOMY

The bile ducts of the posterior and anterior segments of the right hepatic lobe join near the porta hepatis to form the main right hepatic duct. The bile ducts of the medial and lateral segments of the left hepatic lobe merge to become the left main hepatic duct.[4] The right posterior and right anterior segmental bile ducts join the left main hepatic duct directly in about 25% and 6% of individuals, respectively. The right and left main hepatic ducts coalesce in the hilum to form the common hepatic duct. At the porta hepatis, the bile ducts run anterior to the hepatic artery and portal vein. The gallbladder empties into the cystic duct, which is joined by the common hepatic duct to become the common bile duct (CBD), which travels within the hepatoduodenal ligament to drain through the sphincter of Oddi into the duodenum. A number of potential aberrant communications exists between the biliary tree and the gallbladder. The complex relationship between the biliary ductal system and the Couinaud hepatic segmental nomenclature has been described by Gazelle and colleagues.[5]

TRANSHEPATIC CHOLANGIOGRAPHY

Patient Selection and Preparation

Given the widespread use of advanced cross-sectional imaging and ERCP, nearly all patients have THC in conjunction with PBD. The primary indication for THC is to confirm, localize, and characterize obstructive disease of the biliary system in patients with symptoms of pruritus or cholangitis who are not amenable to ERCP.[6] Increasingly, magnetic resonance (MR) cholangiography is being used to image the biliary system noninvasively.[7,8] Occasionally, THC and PBD are used as part of the nonoperative management of patients with biliary leaks from bile duct injuries.

In addition to establishing the presence of biliary obstruction, cholangiography can localize the obstruction and frequently suggests the benign or malignant cause of the stricture. However, the cholangiographic appearance may be misleading. The final diagnosis rests on tissue analysis. In patients who are candidates for operative resection and biliary-enteric decompression, the tissue diagnosis usually is made from the operative specimen. In cases managed nonoperatively, the transhepatic access is a convenient route for obtaining the necessary material.

The relative benefits and risks of THC are weighed against those of endoscopic and operative diagnostic methods. Primary factors in the selection of patients include the suspected anatomic level, cause of biliary obstruction, and the availability of highly skilled practitioners.

Most distal (periampullary) bile duct obstructions are managed endoscopically. Middle (extrahepatic and extrapancreatic) CBD lesions typically undergo operative resection with creation of a biliary-enteric anastomosis. Proximal (hilar) hepatic duct and intrahepatic bile duct strictures usually are treated with percutaneous techniques.

Bacterial overgrowth is common with biliary obstruction, particularly when caused by malignancy. Infectious complications are one of the common sources of fatal and major nonfatal complications. Biliary colonization with enteric organisms should be assumed in all patients with obstructive jaundice, whether evidence of suppurative cholangitis exists or not. Antibiotic prophylaxis is therefore routinely recommended.[9-12] An antibiotic with appropriate coverage for gram-negative bacteria should be administered parenterally approximately 1 hour before the procedure to obtain adequate periprocedural blood levels.

The liver is a highly vascular organ, and the targeted bile ducts course adjacent to hepatic arteries and portal veins, which may be inadvertently injured. Coagulation factors (i.e., prothrombin time, partial thromboplastin time, platelet count, and, occasionally, the bleeding time) should be assessed and corrected if possible.[13,14] A severe uncorrectable coagulopathy is a contraindication to the procedure. Massive, circumferential ascites impedes effective tamponade of blood or bile in addition to increasing the difficulty of catheter manipulation and the likelihood of accidental catheter dislodgment. These patients should have an alternative procedure or undergo paracentesis immediately before the transhepatic intervention. Uncooperative patients are also at high risk for bleeding complications for several reasons and should undergo an alternative procedure or receive general anesthesia.

Transhepatic biliary drainage procedures are significantly more painful than most diagnostic and interventional vascular procedures. Pain management should be liberal, particularly because multistaged procedures are common. Abundant local anesthesia and heavy conscious sedation, appropriately trained personnel, and monitoring equipment are essential. Frequently, assistance from anesthesia personnel is advisable and may include monitored analgesia (e.g., propofol and nitrous oxide) or general anesthesia.[15] Intercostal nerve blocks can help with body wall pain. Most operators have found celiac plexus blocks to be cumbersome and ineffective.[16]

Technique

Skinny-needle (21 to 22 gauge) access into the intrahepatic bile ducts is the essence of THC and the first step of PBD. Access into the biliary system is gained through the right intrahepatic bile ducts using a low right intercostal approach or through the left intrahepatic bile ducts using an anterior subxiphoid entry (Fig. 22-1). The right-sided approach often is preferred, because most interventional

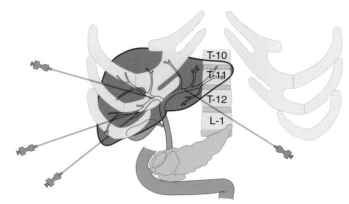

FIGURE 22-1 Routes for percutaneous biliary access. Left-sided access is subcostal from the anterior abdomen. Right-sided access is subcostal or low intercostal from the right mid-axillary line, directed toward the 11th thoracic vertebral body.

radiologists are comfortable with the technique, the operator's hands are not in the fluoroscopic field during guidewire and catheter manipulation, and the right lobe contains most of the hepatic parenchyma. Disadvantages include pain related to irritation of the rib periosteum, risk for crossing the parietal pleura (leading to bilothorax, empyema, and, rarely, pneumothorax), occasionally unfavorable angles for manipulation of catheters into the CBD, and the palmate-type (i.e., like a maple leaf), right-sided biliary branching pattern. This anatomic feature is more likely to result in isolated biliary segments in the setting of invasive hilar malignancy (Fig. 22-2).

Advantages to the left-sided approach include the ability to use ultrasound guidance to find a suitable bile duct while avoiding the adjacent vascular structures, the usually favorable angles for catheterization between the left-sided bile ducts and the CBD, and the more pinnate (i.e., like a feather) branching pattern typical of the left-sided bile duct (see Fig. 22-2), which is less likely to result in segmental isolation with invasive malignancy. Subxiphoid catheters avoid the pleura completely, usually are less uncomfortable than intercostal catheters, and are easier for the patient to flush. Disadvantages of left-sided access include increased radiation exposure to the radiologist's hands and less experience by many interventional radiologists with this sometimes challenging technique. In patients with hilar malignancy that has resulted in isolation of right and left bile ducts, right- and left-sided biliary procedures should be planned, particularly when there is evidence of suppurative cholangitis.

Right-sided access involves placement of a skinny needle into the right-sided bile ducts from a low intercostal approach along the right mid-axillary line (see Fig. 22-1). The needle should enter below the 10th rib to avoid the parietal pleural reflection, although a

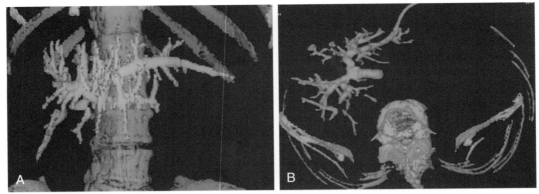

FIGURE 22-2   Biliary branching pattern. Shaded surface display of a spiral computed tomography cholangiogram performed through an indwelling left-sided percutaneous biliary drainage catheter in a patient with pancreatic adenocarcinoma. **A,** Right anterior oblique view displays the pinnate-type (feather-like), left-sided branching pattern. **B,** Inferior view depicts palmate-type (maple leaf–like), right-sided branching pattern.

more cephalad entry point frequently is required by the position of the inferior margin of the right lobe of the liver or the anticipated location of the porta hepatis. Fluoroscopy is used to assess the costophrenic sulcus during full inspiration to guarantee that the lung does not cross the projected access route. The needle is passed over the superior aspect of a given rib to minimize the risk for injury to the intercostal arteries. Under fluoroscopic guidance, the needle is then directed along a plane parallel to the tabletop and aimed toward the 11th thoracic vertebral body. If the same access may be used for biliary drainage, the needle pass should stop

at approximately the right midclavicular line to avoid inadvertent puncture of left-side bile ducts, through which it would be nearly impossible to negotiate a guidewire or catheter toward the CBD.

The needle stylet is removed, and a small-volume syringe (e.g., 1 to 5 mL) with 60% strength contrast medium is attached. Small aliquots (e.g., 0.1 to 0.2 mL) of contrast material are delivered while the needle tip is slowly retracted under fluoroscopy. If the contrast material remains as a smudge at the needle tip, the tip is located in the liver parenchyma, and it should continue to be withdrawn. If contrast medium enters a tubular structure but

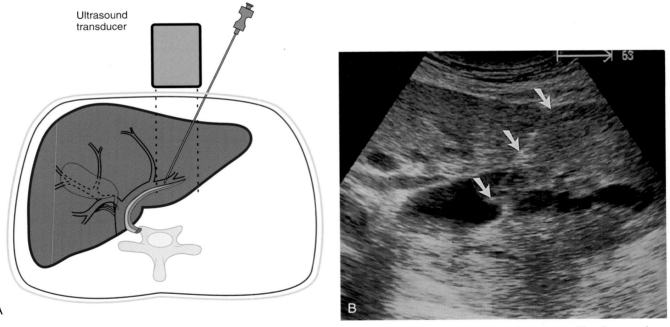

FIGURE 22-3   Sonographic guidance for left-sided transhepatic cholangiography and percutaneous biliary drainage. **A,** The ultrasound probe has a transverse orientation along the axis of the left-sided bile duct and adjacent hepatic artery and portal vein. The skinny needle courses along the sonographic imaging plane to selectively enter the bile duct. **B,** The transverse sonogram depicts the needle course (arrows) through the liver and into the dilated left-sided bile duct.

then flows readily away, the needle tip probably resides within a vascular structure and withdrawal is continued. If contrast material fills a tubular structure and remains in the region of the needle tip, the tip probably is within the biliary system. Injection of an additional 5 to 10 mL should confirm the intrabiliary location and determine the ductal diameter and relationship to the porta hepatis and obstructive lesions.

Left-sided access originates from the left subcostal aspect of the epigastrium. Sonographic guidance permits direct visualization of the skinny needle as it is directed into an acceptable left bile duct while minimizing the likelihood of traversing the adjacent left hepatic artery or left portal vein branch (Fig. 22-3). Aspirated bile should be sent for routine Gram stain, culture, and sensitivity tests; if infectious complications arise, informed choices can be made regarding antimicrobial therapy.

If a diagnostic THC is to be performed without subsequent PBD, removal of 5 to 10 mL of bile alternating with instillation of 5 to 10 mL of contrast material permits diagnostic cholangiographic images while minimizing the risk of bacteremia and possible gram-negative sepsis. If a biliary leak is suspected, full-strength (60%) contrast material is warranted to visualize the fistula. However, if intraluminal filling defects (e.g., stones) or disease with subtle bile duct wall abnormalities (e.g., sclerosing cholangitis) is suspected, 60% contrast medium should be diluted by one half with normal saline solution. The biliary system should be aspirated before removal of the skinny needle if drainage is not planned.

Imaging Findings

Most pathologic processes of the biliary tree are manifested in a few forms[17-23]

- Abnormally small-caliber bile ducts or occlusion of the bile ducts (Table 22-1; Figs 22-4 through 22-11)

Text continued on p. 664

TABLE 22-1 Narrowing or Occlusion of the Biliary Ducts

Disease or Cause	Suggestive Findings
Pseudostricture due to positional underfilling of contrast material (see Fig. 22-4)	Supine: narrow proximal (hilar) CBD and nonopacified left bile ducts
	Prone: narrow distal CBD and nonopacified right bile ducts
	Eliminated by positional changes
Pseudocalculus due to mucosal prolapse (see Fig. 22-5)	Distal CBD meniscus
	Mimics stone or polyp
	Intermittently disappears as sphincter opens
Cholangiocarcinoma (see Fig. 22-6)	Usually located near or associated with hilum
	Usually occlusive
	Usually abrupt margin
	Nodular surface
Pancreatic or ampullary carcinoma (see Fig. 22-7)	Located at distal CBD
	Fixed lesion
	"Rat tail" appearance
	Usually occulsive
Extrinsic adenopathy	Usually hilar or suprapancreatic CBD
	Nonspecific
	May have smooth surface
Fibrosis (see Fig. 22-8)	Located at biliary-enteric or biliary-biliary anastomosis, site of injury, papilla, or in proximity to stones
	Usually short segment
	Usually smooth
Sclerosing cholangitis (see Fig. 22-9)	Multifocal strictures
	Intrahepatic and extrahepatic
	May have diffuse narrowing
	Often mural diverticular outpouching
Ischemic or AIDS-related cholangitis (see Fig. 22-10)	Ischemic or chemotoxic structures
	Similar to sclerosing cholangitis, papillary stenosis, or both
	Patients with liver transplant or liver malignancy and transcatheter chemoinfusion or chemoembolization
	Multifocal, diffuse intrahepatic strictures
	May have anastomotic stricture
	May have associated sloughed debris, leaks
Recurrent pyogenic cholangitis (Oriental cholangitis) (see Fig. 22-11)	Multiple intrahepaic strictures
	Upstream dilation, especially left lobe
	Usually associated with innumerable stones

AIDS, *acquired immunodeficiency syndrome*; CBD, *common bile duct.*

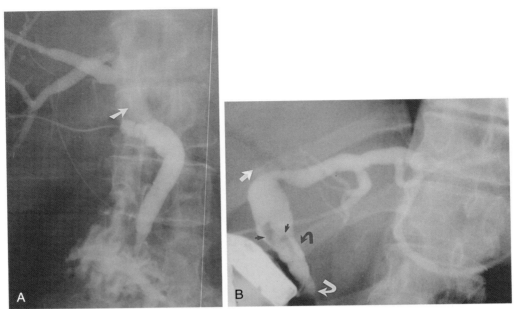

FIGURE 22-4 Artifactual nonopacification of bile ducts caused by underfilling with contrast material, which has a higher specific gravity than bile. **A,** T-tube cholangiogram in a supine patient. The nondependent common hepatic duct *(arrow)* appears narrow, and the left-sided bile ducts did not fill at all. **B,** Endoscopic retrograde cholangiopancreatography in a nearly prone patient. The nondependent distal common bile duct appears narrow (between *curved arrows*). Right-sided ducts *(straight white arrow)* are not opacified. The irregular filling defect *(small black arrows)* in the distal common bile duct is viscous bile.

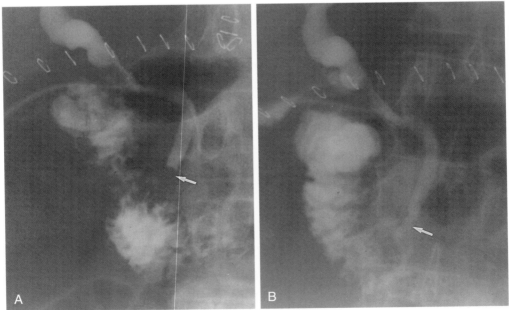

FIGURE 22-5 Mucosal prolapse. **A,** A polypoid filling defect is identified in the distal common bile duct *(arrow)*. **B,** A few minutes later, the sphincter has opened *(arrow)*.

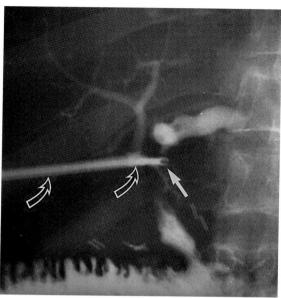

FIGURE 22-6 Cholangiographically guided transluminal biopsy of hilar cholangiocarcinoma using a myocardial biopsy forceps *(straight arrow)* introduced through a vascular-type percutaneous transhepatic sheath *(curved arrows)*.

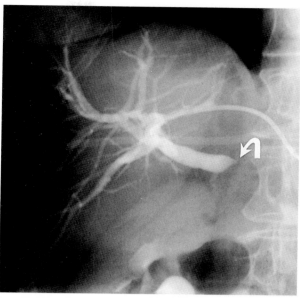

FIGURE 22-7 Malignant stricture in the common bile duct caused by pancreatic carcinoma. The stricture has a "rat-tail" or beaked appearance *(curved arrow)*, typical of malignant periampullary strictures.

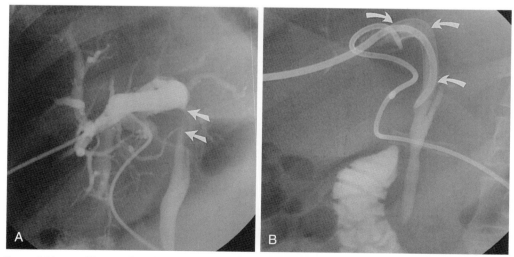

FIGURE 22-8 Expandable metallic stent for a benign tuberculous stricture. Contrast-enhanced computed tomography scan showed dilation of intrahepatic bile ducts bilaterally. The extrahepatic bile ducts were normal. **A,** Left anterior oblique view of a cholangiogram performed through a bilateral percutaneous biliary drainage catheter defined a near-occlusive eccentric stricture *(arrows)* of the hilar portion of the common bile duct, which had been retracted posteriorly, presumably because of fibrosis. **B,** After attempted percutaneous cholangioplasty, which failed because of elastic recoil, an 8-mm-diameter, 40-mm–long Wallstent *(arrows)* was deployed successfully. The left anterior oblique view documented excellent stent position and expansion.

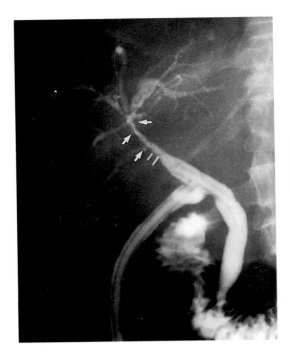

FIGURE 22-9   Sclerosing cholangitis. Cholangiogram through an indwelling T-tube shows multiple strictures of intrahepatic and extrahepatic bile ducts. Scattered normal segments of intrahepatic bile ducts are seen upstream from the strictures; otherwise, intrahepatic ducts are of small caliber. Subtle diverticula (arrows) of the strictured common hepatic duct are detected, and the surgical clips are from a cholecystectomy.

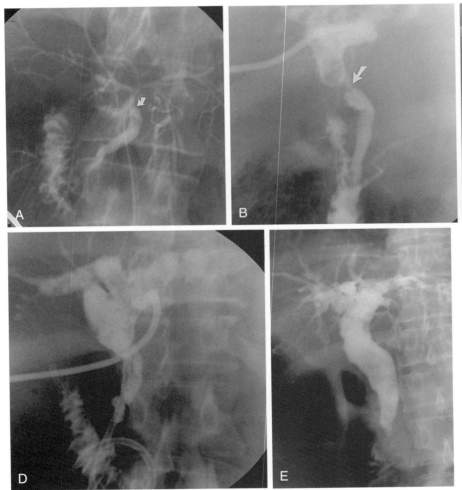

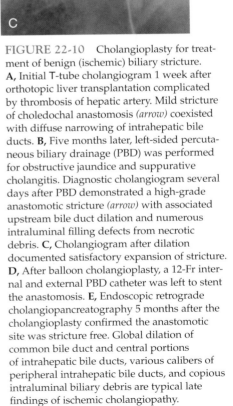

FIGURE 22-10   Cholangioplasty for treatment of benign (ischemic) biliary stricture. **A,** Initial T-tube cholangiogram 1 week after orthotopic liver transplantation complicated by thrombosis of hepatic artery. Mild stricture of choledochal anastomosis (arrow) coexisted with diffuse narrowing of intrahepatic bile ducts. **B,** Five months later, left-sided percutaneous biliary drainage (PBD) was performed for obstructive jaundice and suppurative cholangitis. Diagnostic cholangiogram several days after PBD demonstrated a high-grade anastomotic stricture (arrow) with associated upstream bile duct dilation and numerous intraluminal filling defects from necrotic debris. **C,** Cholangiogram after dilation documented satisfactory expansion of stricture. **D,** After balloon cholangioplasty, a 12-Fr internal and external PBD catheter was left to stent the anastomosis. **E,** Endoscopic retrograde cholangiopancreatography 5 months after the cholangioplasty confirmed the anastomotic site was stricture free. Global dilation of common bile duct and central portions of intrahepatic bile ducts, various calibers of peripheral intrahepatic bile ducts, and copious intraluminal biliary debris are typical late findings of ischemic cholangiopathy.

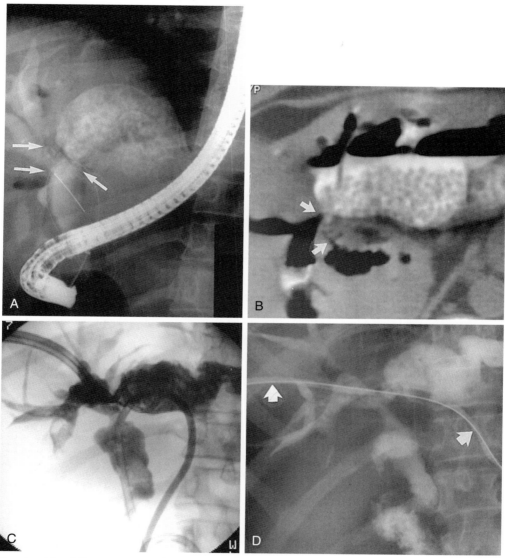

FIGURE 22-11   Staged multimodality management of complex biliary disease (recurrent pyogenic cholangitis). **A,** Endoscopic retrograde cholangio-pancreatography (ERCP) demonstrated multiple hilar biliary strictures *(arrows),* dilation of multiple intrahepatic bile ducts, and innumerable biliary calculi located within a massively dilated left bile duct. Pneumobilia resulted from prior endoscopic papillotomy. **B,** Magnified view of the abdominal computed tomography scan after the ERCP confirmed the hilar biliary strictures *(arrows),* bile duct dilation, and calculi. **C,** After bilateral biliary drainage, balloon cholangioplasty of the hilar biliary strictures, multiple sessions of basket retrieval of pigmented biliary calculi, and oral administration of ursodeoxycholic acid, the cholangiogram demonstrated improvement in the hilar biliary luminal diameter, partial resolution of the intrahepatic bile duct dilation, and near-complete removal of the calculi. **D,** After successful transluminal therapy, the bilateral percutaneous biliary drainage catheters have been converted to a long-term indwelling Silastic U-tube *(arrows)* to preserve transhepatic biliary access. *(Courtesy of Thomas Kinney, MD, and Horacio D'Agostino, MD, University of California, San Diego, Medical Center.)*

TABLE 22-2   Dilated Biliary Ducts

Disease or Cause	Suggestive Findings
Obstruction (see Figs. 22-7 and 22-8)	Diffuse, though may disproportionately affect extrahepatic or left lobe ducts Upstream from obstructing structure (stricture, stone)
Prior obstruction	History of treated obstruction Contrast material flows to bowel May need manometry to distinguish from true obstruction
Choledochal cysts	
Type I (80%-90%) (see Fig. 22-12)	Extrahepatic CBD Fusiform, single
Type II (2%) (see Fig. 22-13)	Extrahepatic CBD Saccular or diverticular, single
Type III (1%-5%)	Intraduodenal, single Choledochocele
Type IV	Multiple cysts Usually intrahepatic and extrahepatic
Type V (see Fig. 22-14)	Caroli disease Single or multiple Intrahepatic or extrahepatic bile ducts Associated with hepatic fibrosis, renal cysts, renal tubular ectasia
Late phase ischemic injury (see Fig. 22-10)	History of liver transplantation Central biliary ectasia with debris* Peripheral pruning of intrahepatic bile ducts
Denervation	History of liver transplantation Diffuse dilation May have sphincter of Oddi dysfunction
Oriental cholangiohepatitis (see Fig. 22-11)	Listed in Table 22-1

From Silverman SG, Coughin BF, Selzer SE, et al. Current use of screening laboratory tests before abdominal interventions: a survey of 603 radiologists. Radiology 1991;181:669.
CBD, common bile duct.

- Abnormally large-caliber bile ducts (Table 22-2; Figs. 22-12 through 22-14)
- Filling defects within the intraluminal contrast material (Table 22-3; Figs. 22-15 through 22-17)
- Extraluminal location of contrast material (Table 22-4; Fig. 22-18)

Biliary manometry is required occasionally to establish the presence of distal obstruction. The technique is modeled on the urodynamic Whitaker test.[24,25] A baseline biliary pressure is established through the THC needle or through an external PBD catheter. A resting biliary pressure that exceeds 15 cm H_2O is diagnostic for downstream obstruction. If the resting pressure is less than 15 cm H_2O, a saline infusion challenge is indicated. Saline mixed with dilute contrast material is infused through a suitable infusion pump, initially at a rate of 2 mL/min and then at 4, 8, and 10 mL/min. After 5 to 10 minutes of infusion at each rate, the biliary pressure is recorded. If the biliary pressure exceeds 20 cm H_2O at any point during saline infusion, a diagnosis of a significant downstream obstruction can be made. If the pressure does not exceed 20 cm H_2O despite a saline infusion rate of 10 mL/min, a significant downstream occlusion is excluded.

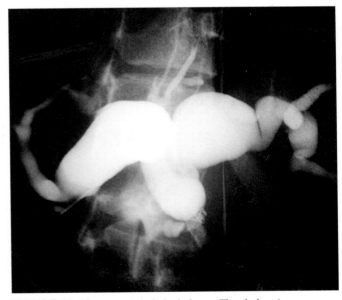

FIGURE 22-12   Type I choledochal cyst. The cholangiogram shows diffuse dilation of the common hepatic duct and central portions of both left and right intrahepatic ducts. The patient previously had undergone resection of the common bile duct (high risk for cholangiocarcinoma) with creation of choledochojejunostomy drainage.

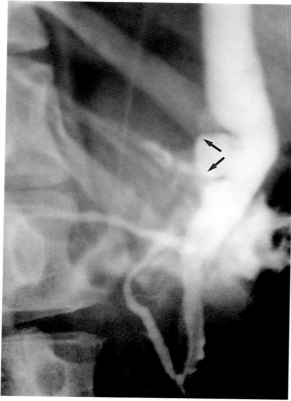

FIGURE 22-13   Type II choledochal cyst. Endoscopic retrograde cholangiopancreatography (with scope removed) shows a focal eccentric outpouching *(arrows)* in the suprapancreatic portion of the common bile duct.

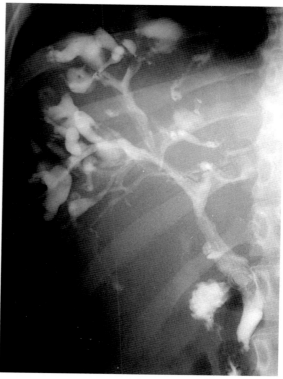

FIGURE 22-14   Caroli disease. The cholangiogram was performed by means of a right percutaneous biliary drainage catheter. Multiple intrahepatic segments of cystic dilation are evident. *(From Rose SC, Kumpe DA, Weil R III. Percutaneous biliary drainage in diffuse Caroli's disease. AJR Am J Roentgenol 1986;**147**:159. Copyright 1986, American Roentgen Ray Society.)*

TABLE 22-3   Biliary Duct Filling Defects

Disease or Cause	Suggestive Findings
Air bubbles (see Fig. 22-15)	Shape conforms to surrounding structures
	Shape changes with movement
	Fragmentation and coalescence
	May be able to be aspirated
	May be seen exiting catheter
	Usually move to nondependent bile ducts
Blood clot (see Fig. 22-16)	History of invasive procedure or injury
	Usually forms cast of bile duct
	Usually disappears or shrivels within 48 hr
Stones (see Fig. 22-17; see also Fig. 22-11)	Often faceted, smooth
	If mobile, often falls to dependent portion of bile duct
	Constant shape
	No fragmentation without manipulation
	No coalescence
	Single or multiple
	Frequently associated with strictures or gallstones
	May be impacted in distal common bile duct (meniscus) or cystic duct (Mirizzi syndrome with common hepatic duct obstruction)
Pseudocalculus	Listed in Table 22-1
Polypoid tumor	Eccentric, nonmobile
	Usually nodular surface
Debris (see Fig. 22-10)	Irregular, mobile
	Usually associated with sphincterotomy, biliary-enteric anastomosis, metallic expandable stent into bowel, or ischemic injury
Parasites	May appear curvilinear or wormlike
	May be associated with strictures or stones
	Others listed in Table 22-1

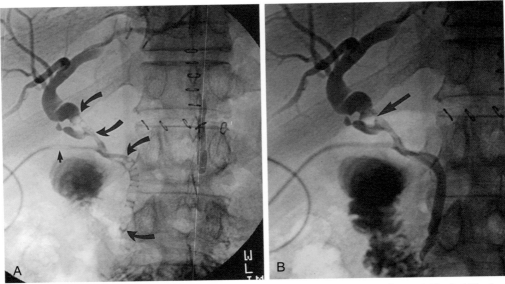

FIGURE 22-15   Air bubbles at cholangiography. **A,** An air bubble is seen within the T-tube *(small arrow)*. The bubble shape conforms to the wall of the common bile duct and to other bubbles (between *curved arrows*). **B,** Continued injection of contrast material expels the bubbles from the distal duct. The three bubbles in the common hepatic duct have coalesced into a single large bubble *(arrow)*.

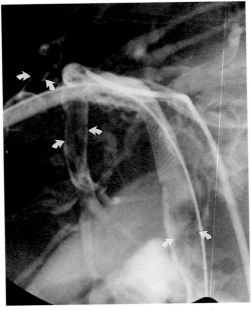

FIGURE 22-16   Intrabiliary blood clot. After deployment and expansion of a Wallstent for a tuberculous biliary stricture, a cast of the biliary system caused by the blood clot is evident *(arrows)*. A cholangiogram performed several days later showed spontaneous clearance of blood.

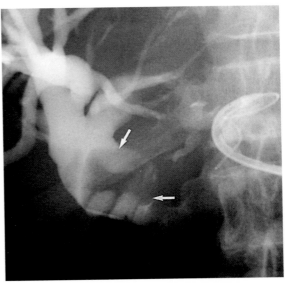

FIGURE 22-17   An impacted, large biliary stone is seen on a cholangiogram performed through the left percutaneous biliary drainage catheter. The stone *(arrows)* has a typical faceted surface and causes peripheral biliary dilation.

TABLE 22-4   Biliary Duct Leakage

Disease or Cause	Suggestive Findings
Elevated intraluminal pressure (obstruction) (see Fig. 22-18)	Downstream stricture Hepatic abscesses or suppurative cholangitis
Poor ductal wall integrity Bile duct injury Dehisced biliary anastomosis or cystic duct stump	History of right upper quadrant surgery or injury, hepatic artery thrombosis, or irradiation
Ischemia	Associated with bilomas, intrahepatic or extrahepatic abscesses, ascites, and fistulas to bowel, skin, or wounds
Radiation therapy	May be associated with downstream strictures

Aspirated bile may be collected for cytologic examination. Cytologic material also can be obtained using a miniature brush biopsy device mounted on a guidewire[26] (Fig. 22-19). The brush biopsy device is introduced through an angiographic catheter with the brush passed intraluminally to and fro across the stricture. The brush tip is then cut off and placed in a fixative solution. Another technique for obtaining cytologic material is fluoroscopically guided percutaneous skinny-needle aspiration (Fig. 22-20). Using the THC or PBD access, cholangiography is performed to localize the stricture. Through a second percutaneous approach (usually anterior subcostal), a skinny needle is advanced using fluoroscopic guidance to sample the identified stricture.

Higher diagnostic yields for proving benign or malignant disease come from histologic examination of larger tissue samples because cellular architecture can be evaluated. To accommodate the larger transluminal biopsy devices, a vascular access sheath is placed into the biliary system through the transhepatic route. The hemostatic valve permits passage of the device while contrast material is injected through the side arm port to guide the biopsy.

Currently available devices suitable for endoluminal biliary biopsy are flexible forceps developed for transvenous biopsy of the myocardium[27] (see Fig. 22-6). The flexible transjugular liver biopsy needle (Cook Inc., Bloomington, Ind.) should not be used because it is designed to penetrate several centimeters beyond the

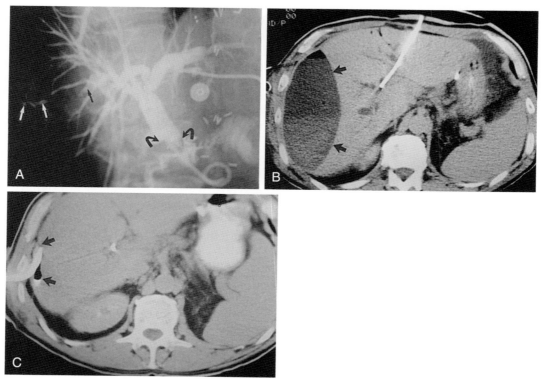

FIGURE 22-18   Biliary leak. **A,** Cholangiogram performed through the left internal-external drainage catheter shows extravasation of contrast *(straight arrows)* along a prior right-sided biliary drainage track and an obstructive stricture at the choledochojejunostomy anastomosis *(curved arrows).* **B,** A large subcapsular hepatic abscess *(arrows)* is identified by contrast-enhanced computed tomography (CT). Percutaneous drainage of the abscess was performed with initial return of thick, purulent material, which later converted to bile. **C,** Another CT scan 12 days later documents successful treatment of the abscess *(arrows)* by simultaneous diversion of bile through the left percutaneous biliary drainage catheter and drainage of the infected biloma. The biliary-enteric anastomotic stricture was treated with balloon cholangioplasty.

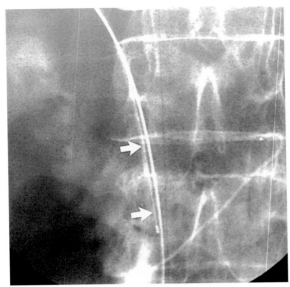

FIGURE 22-19   Transluminal brush biopsy of extrahepatic common bile duct cholangiocarcinoma. Brush biopsy *(arrows)* passes adjacent to the safety guidewire.

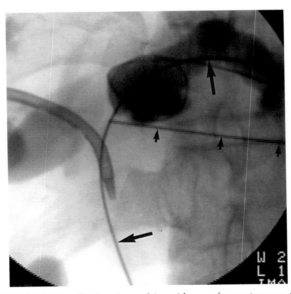

FIGURE 22-20   Cholangiographic guidance of percutaneous fine-needle aspiration biopsy of cholangiocarcinoma. A fine needle *(small arrows)* was advanced under fluoroscopic guidance until it struck the left-sided biliary safety guidewire *(large arrows)* within the strictured segment.

lumen and may injure the adjacent hepatic artery or portal vein, possibly in an intraperitoneal location.

Results and Complications

When the bile ducts are dilated, THC can be performed in almost every case.[6] With nondilated biliary systems, the success rates range from 60% to 96%, depending

on the number of passes that the operator is willing to make.[6,21,28-33] THC is extremely accurate (96%) in differentiating obstructive from hepatocellular causes of jaundice.[28] Bile duct dilation usually indicates biliary obstruction, although in certain diseases, such as sclerosing cholangitis and the cholangiopathy associated with hepatic arterial chemoinfusion therapy and hepatic arterial occlusive disease in liver transplant recipients, the bile ducts may not dilate significantly in response to downstream obstruction.[21,34,35] Alternatively, the cholangiographic appearance of the intrahepatic bile ducts may not reflect the biliary dynamics of an incompletely occlusive benign stricture (e.g., at a biliary-enteric anastomosis) or the physiologic response to an intervention (e.g., cholangioplasty or stent placement). In these occasional situations, biliary manometry may be helpful to establish the presence of downstream obstruction.[24,25] The major complications of transhepatic cholangiography are sepsis and bleeding. Serious complications occur in 2% to 8% of cases.[6,25-29]

Cytologic study performed on aspirated bile may identify cells shed by bile duct malignancy. Fluid obtained from the initial puncture probably has the highest yield. Harell and coworkers collected 20 mL of bilefor cytodiagnosis through THC, PBD, T-tube, or operative biliary duct aspiration in 27 patients with obstructive jaundice; malignant cells were detected in 7 of 15 patients who had malignant strictures, for a sensitivity of 47%, specificity of 100%, and accuracy of 58%.[35] Muro and colleagues[36] reported 34% sensitivity and 100% specificity for cytologic examination of bile obtained from PBD in patients with malignant strictures. Despite a relatively low sensitivity, a biliary cytologic study probably is worthwhile because it involves no additional risk, is relatively inexpensive, and may avoid more costly and invasive tests if results are positive for malignancy. The reported sensitivity of fluoroscopically guided skinny-needle aspiration ranges from 60% to 83%.[37,38] Savader and associates[39] found fluoroscopic intraductal brush biopsy to have a sensitivity of 26% and specificity of 96% for detection of malignancy. Although all of the cytologic techniques involve little risk, they are relatively insensitive in diagnosing biliary malignancy, particularly cholangiocarcinoma, and generally are of no use in excluding malignancy.

Although published reports are limited, diagnostic yields using biopsy devices seem higher than those for cytologic techniques, with sensitivities from 30% to 80% for patients who had prior negative skinny-needle aspiration or brush biopsy results.[26,27,35-39] Periprocedural morbidity is acceptably low (up to 10% of cases).

PERCUTANEOUS BILIARY DRAINAGE (ONLINE CASE 90)

Patient Selection

PBD is performed for decompression of symptomatic biliary obstruction or diversion of bile flow away from biliary leaks in patients whose anatomy (e.g., prior choledochojejunostomy) or disease location (e.g., porta hepatitis or intrahepatic bile ducts) is not favorable for endoscopic or operative drainage procedures.[3] In addition to the contraindications for THC (including severe uncorrectable coagulopathy and massive ascites), PBD is ineffective and therefore relatively contraindicated in patients with multifocal biliary obstruction due to hepatic metastases.

Technique

Initial transhepatic access into the biliary system is identical to the technique used for THC. If the skinny needle used for the THC has entered the biliary system in a suitable location, a 0.018-inch guidewire should be advanced sufficiently far enough into the system that the stainless steel mandrel is positioned within the bile ducts (Fig. 22-21). Features favorable for use of a biliary radical for PBD include a bile duct diameter adequate to accept

an 8- to 10-French (Fr) drain, a system with favorable angles of approach to the porta hepatis and CBD, and an entry point at least a couple of centimeters upstream from the biliary stricture or leak to allow a pigtail loop to form or accommodate several side holes of a drainage catheter.

If the initial biliary puncture is unsuitable, the biliary system can be opacified through the first needle to guide a second skinny needle into a more desirable location. Over the 0.018-inch guidewire, the skinny needle is replaced for a coaxial exchange set so that a 0.038-inch working guidewire can be advanced into the biliary system with the original 0.018-inch wire left as a safety guidewire. The access set can be removed and an angiographic catheter advanced over the working guidewire into the intrahepatic bile ducts.

In patients with evidence of suppurative cholangitis, manipulation (including contrast injection) should be minimized and an external-type PBD placed and left to gravity drainage. In uninfected patients, 5 to 15 minutes of gentle probing with the guidewire and catheter frequently is successful in traversing the stricture or leak to pass a guidewire into the bowel. If the obstructing lesion cannot be traversed safely at the initial sitting, a repeated attempt often is successful after 2 to 3 days of decompression. The transhepatic tract is then dilated using serial fascial dilators before advancement of the biliary drain.

FIGURE 22-21 Steps for converting transhepatic cholangiography into percutaneous biliary drainage. **A,** The 0.018-inch guidewire is advanced well into the biliary system through the skinny needle, which is then removed. **B,** Over the 0.018-inch guidewire, a coaxial exchange set is passed into the bile ducts. **C,** After removing the metal stiffening cannula and inner small-bore coaxial dilator, a 0.038-inch working guidewire and a 5-Fr angiographic catheter are introduced through the sheath and negotiated across the stricture (represented by a pancreatic head mass in these diagrams). **D,** After removal of the outer exchange system sheath, the 0.018-inch safety guidewire has been secured on the drape. Over the 0.038-inch heavy-duty working guidewire, an 8- to 12-Fr multiple-side-hole biliary drain is passed into an appropriate position.

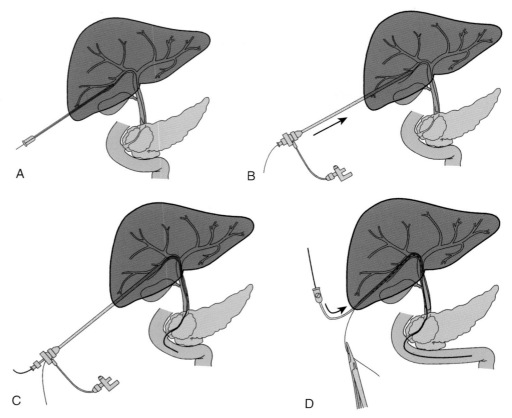

After the biliary drainage catheter is positioned, it is secured in two locations: intraabdominally, using the locking pigtail tip of the catheter looped within the dilated bile duct or bowel, and at the skin, using sutures or various adhesive devices to secure the catheter to the abdominal wall. The catheter is then attached to a drainage bag for at least overnight external-type decompression. The catheter and tubing of the drainage bag need to be fluid filled and the drainage bag placed in a more dependent position than the patient's bile ducts to allow siphonage to occur effectively. The drain should be flushed with approximately 10 mL of sterile saline solution two to three times daily and the biliary output recorded.

Selection of Biliary Drainage Route

Fundamentally, three types of biliary drainage exist: external, internal-external (universal), and internal. Each option has advantages and disadvantages. The choice of drainage mechanism should reflect the patient's clinical situation and lifestyle, the anatomy and pathology of the underlying stricture or leak, the patient's life expectancy, and planned adjunctive or operative therapy.

In external PBD, all catheter side holes are located upstream from the site of obstruction, usually along the inside curvature of the pigtail loop (Fig. 22-22). The catheter shaft passes out the abdominal wall. Bile, by necessity, must drain externally through the catheter lumen into a drain bag. *External drainage* using siphonage is the most effective transcatheter method for decompression of the biliary system and, therefore, is usually indicated in patients with evidence of suppurative cholangitis or severe liver dysfunction from long-standing biliary obstruction. An external PBD is flushed and exchanged easily. However, it is the least secure of the three drainage options, is a nuisance for the patient and caregivers because of the drain exiting the body and the required drainage bag, and is associated with the loss of biliary fluids, electrolytes, and bile salts. Serum fluid and electrolyte status need to be monitored and replaced as needed. In the malnourished patient, bile may be collected and administered orally to assist with fat and fat-soluble vitamin absorption.

Internal-external PBD involves a percutaneous transhepatic catheter that traverses the obstructive lesion and has side holes proximal and distal to the site of obstruction (Fig. 22-23). Frequently, a locking pigtail tip secures the downstream (central) portion within the bowel. When attached to a drainage bag, bile is handled by entering the upstream side holes and exiting by the transhepatic catheter shaft into a drainage bag. Alternatively, when the PBD catheter is capped, bile that enters the upstream side holes is diverted across the site of obstruction to be dumped into the downstream

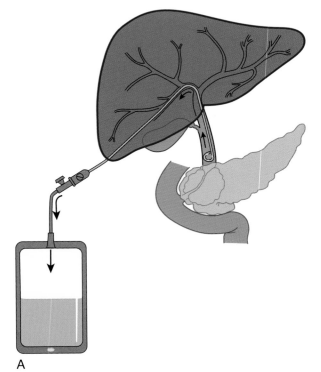

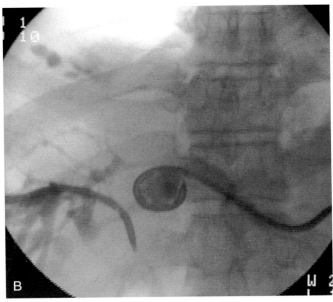

FIGURE 22-22   External-type biliary drainage. **A,** The catheter position relative to the site of obstruction and the mandatory external direction of bile flow into the attached bile bag are illustrated. **B,** Right and left external biliary drains in a patient with suppurative cholangitis caused by an obstructing hilar carcinoma (i.e., Klatskin tumor).

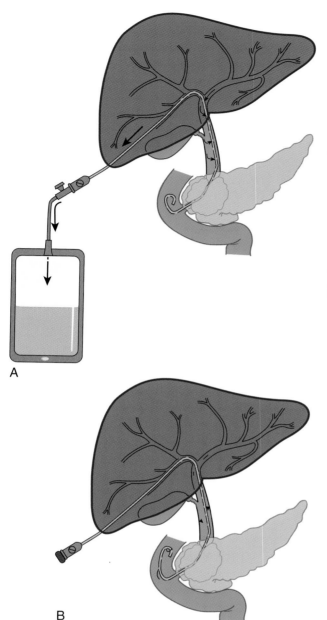

A

B

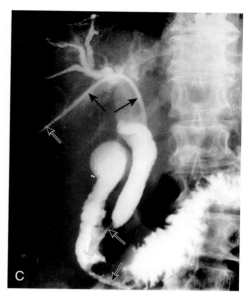

C

FIGURE 22-23 **A,** Internal-external percutaneous biliary drainage (PBD) with external drainage. Note the entrance of bile into the catheter side holes and delivery of bile into the dependent drainage bag. **B,** The internal-external PBD catheter has been capped so that bile is diverted into the duodenum. **C,** Cholangiogram performed through an internal-external PBD catheter *(arrows)* in a patient with ampullary carcinoma. Contrast fills the common bile duct and duodenum.

CBD or small bowel. Advantages of internal-external PBD include improved catheter security relative to external drainage, avoidance of a drainage bag, easy catheter exchange over a guidewire, and excellent access for adjunctive treatment of benign or malignant strictures. Disadvantages include frequent occlusion of the catheter by debris (usually mucus produced by the small bowel) and the catheter shaft exiting the body, which may be distasteful or limit some patients' lifestyles.

Internal PBD involves a conduit (i.e., plastic tube or expandable metallic stent) that traverses the obstructive

stricture and allows bile to flow directly into the bowel (Fig. 22-24). No drain exits the body wall. Advantages include a high degree of security (i.e., no catheter shaft to entangle passing objects or be grasped by delirious patients); physiologic use of biliary fluid, electrolytes, and bile salts; and optimized lifestyle (i.e., no exiting catheter, required flushing, or drainage bags). Significant disadvantages include the loss of access for adjunctive biliary intervention (i.e., any transcatheter adjuncts should be considered before conversion of internal-external drainage to complete internal-type drainage) and loss of ability to exchange occluded drainage systems altogether

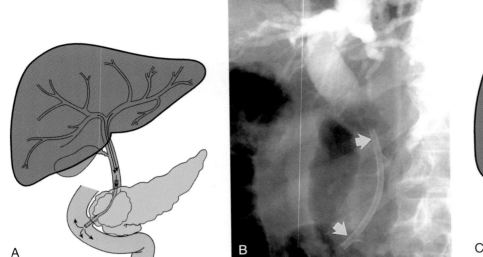

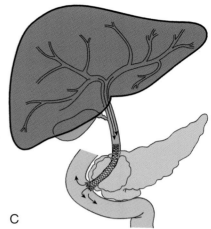

FIGURE 22-24   Internal-type biliary drainage. **A,** Bile flows from the common bile duct (CBD) through the plastic internal biliary endoprosthesis into the duodenum. **B,** Radiograph of an endoscopically placed 10-Fr plastic endoprosthesis *(arrows)* after the endoscope has been removed in a patient with CBD obstruction by pancreatic head adenocarcinoma. **C,** Expandable metallic stent for internal biliary drainage.

(i.e., expandable metallic stents) or dependency on transendoscopic exchange (i.e., plastic endoprostheses).

Results and Complications

Reported technical success for external and internal-external PBD ranges from 94% to 97% in patients with dilated bile ducts and approximately 70% in patients with nondilated bile ducts.[6,40-42] Complications may be minor or life threatening. Major periprocedure complications primarily are caused by hemorrhage (usually hemobilia) and infection (i.e., sepsis, suppurative cholangitis, or hepatic abscesses) and occur in 4% to 8% of cases.[6,40-45] Massive hemobilia may be caused by fistulous connections between the hepatic artery or portal vein branches and the biliary tree. Hepatic arterial injury is diagnosed with hepatic arteriography and treated with transcatheter embolization.[45] During arteriography, the biliary drain may need to be removed over a guidewire to identify the point of contrast extravasation. If no hepatic arterial injuries are identified, a portal vein injury is probable and is treated with placement of a second transhepatic biliary drain, followed by embolization of the initial transhepatic tract, usually with a combination of angiographic coils and large Gelfoam "torpedoes," cyanoacrylate glue, and Onyx liquid embolic material[46] (Fig. 22-25). An alternative technique involves obtaining ultrasound-guided access into the intrahepatic portal venous system, then selective embolization of the injured portal vein branch.

Procedure-related fatality is reported in 1% to 6% of patients who undergo PBD.[40-42] In patients with malignant strictures, however, fatal and major nonfatal complications are two to three times higher than in

patients with benign strictures, probably because of poorer overall health, longer duration of intubation, and the likelihood of bacterial colonization in patients with malignant biliary obstruction.[47]

Minor procedure-related complications occur in 20% to 30% of procedures. Delayed complications are probably a function of the type of PBD drainage, catheter hygiene, and duration of intubation. Complications include catheter occlusion, catheter dislodgment, and suppurative cholangitis.

TREATMENT OF BENIGN BILIARY STRICTURES

Patient Selection

Appropriate case selection for treatment of benign strictures centers on the likelihood of restenosis and the results of alternative methods. Most patients with periampullary benign strictures should undergo endoscopic sphincterotomy. Surgical biliary-enteric diversion provides better long-term patency than does cholangioplasty or placement of expandable metallic stents in patients with anastomotic or extrahepatic, extrapancreatic biliary strictures, particularly if the stricture has not been repaired previously and the surgeon is highly experienced. Because of the lack of viable surgical alternatives short of liver transplantation for treatment of intrahepatic biliary strictures, percutaneous treatment is warranted in patients with dominant strictures caused by sclerosing cholangitis, nonanastomotic strictures after liver transplantation, and other benign intrahepatic strictures.[48-53]

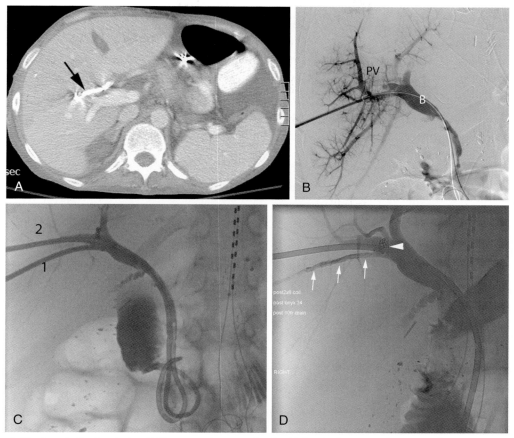

FIGURE 22-25 **A,** Track embolization to treat biliary-portal venous fistula. Abdominal computed tomography with original internal-external biliary drain *(arrow)* traversing branch of right portal vein. **B,** Cholangiogram through vascular sheath in transhepatic track opacifying both the biliary system *(B)* and the right portal vein *(PV).* **C,** After placement of a second internal-external biliary drain *(2)* prior to sacrificing original biliary drain *(1).* **D,** Cholangiogram through the second biliary drain. A metallic coil *(arrowhead)* placed into the track dislodged into the biliary system (subsequently passed into bowel). The track was then sealed with Onyx 34 *(arrows)* delivered through an angiographic catheter.

Techniques

Benign biliary strictures may be dilated with transluminal angioplasty balloons (i.e., balloon cholangioplasty)[52,53] (see Fig. 22-10). In addition to the transhepatic route, balloon dilation catheters may be introduced into the biliary system by an operatively placed T-tube, a Hutson-Russell loop (i.e., the Roux-en-Y bowel loop used to drain the biliary system is tacked to the anterior abdominal wall), or an endoscope. The densely fibrotic nature and propensity for elastic recoil of most benign biliary strictures frequently require higher dilation pressures (e.g., 10 to 15 atm), prolonged expansion (e.g., 2 to 20 minutes), and repeated balloon expansion.[53] Because cholangioplasty is significantly more painful than most interventional radiologic procedures, deep sedation or general anesthesia is required.[15] The relatively high likelihood of stricture recurrence suggests that the preservation of access to the biliary system (e.g., chronic indwelling PBD, T-tube) is prudent in many of these patients, particularly those with sclerosing cholangitis or recurrent pyogenic cholangitis,

to minimize discomfort and complications associated with reaccessing the biliary system for subsequent cholangioplasty and possible stone extraction (see Fig. 22-11).

Given the long life expectancy of most patients with benign biliary strictures, stent occlusion due to epithelial hyperplasia, mucinous debris, or calculi is a serious impediment to routine use of an expandable metallic stent.[3,50,54-59] In benign disease, expandable metallic biliary stents should be reserved for patients who are not operative candidates and in whom balloon dilation has failed (see Fig. 22-8), who have a limited life expectancy (e.g., obstructive cholangiopathy in a patient with advanced acquired immunodeficiency syndrome), or who have biliary strictures in a transplanted liver and require a bridge to liver retransplantation.[51,52] In such cases, use of expandable metallic stents with a relatively low metallic surface area (e.g., Gianturco-Rosch Z-stent [Cook Inc., Bloomington, Ind.] or Sentinol Biliary Self-Expanding Stent [Boston Scientific, Natick, Mass.]) may give longer primary patency than other types of stents.[52,57,58]

Recently introduced covered stents may hold promise for improved long-term patency compared with bare metallic stents or repeated balloon cholangioplasty. One surface of the stent is covered with a thin layer of fabric with very small pore size (approximately 1 μm) to minimize biliary epithelial ingrowth and adherence of debris.[60,61] Metallic wires provide radial expansion. Because these stents are covered with an impermeable membrane, particular care must be taken not to cover and potentially occlude the pancreatic duct (risk of pancreatitis), the cystic duct (risk of cholecystitis), or a bile duct branch (risk of biliary obstruction, cholangitis, and cholangitic abscesses). Long-term biostability of the fabric membrane is not known.

Results and Complications

After internal-external PBD has been established, the initial technical success rates for balloon cholangioplasty are typically high (88% to 100%). Complication rates vary widely (as high as 60%) and usually are caused by suppurative cholangitis.* Long-term patency rates depend on the location and cause of the stricture. Mueller and colleagues[64] reported 36-month clinical primary patency rates of 76% for iatrogenic strictures, 67% for biliary-enteric anastomotic strictures, and 42% for strictures caused by sclerosing cholangitis. For patients who have developed biliary strictures (usually intrahepatic) after liver transplantation, a 6-year secondary patency of 70% was by reported Zajko and colleagues.[53] However, Diamond and associates[51] observed recurrence in all patients. In patients with transplanted livers, primary patency is longer for nonanastomotic strictures than for anastomotic strictures.[20,53] Citron and Martin[68] reported primary clinical patency rates (mean follow-up, 32 months) of 100% for intrahepatic CBD strictures; 92% for extrahepatic, extrapancreatic CBD strictures; 33% for intrapancreatic strictures; and 75% for biliary-enteric anastomotic strictures. Cantwell[69] reported clinically significant restenosis rates following balloon cholangioplasty for treatment of benign postoperative biliary strictures of 48% at 5 years and 59% at 25 years. Restenosis rates were significantly higher in patients who underwent repeated dilations. Most investigators leave 10- to 14-Fr (3.3- to 4.7-mm) soft catheters across the cholangioplasty site for several weeks or months to act as a stent, although the need for postdilation catheter stenting is undocumented.

Reported technical success and clinical response for use of metallic expandable stents to treat benign biliary strictures approaches 100%.† The rate of major nonfatal complications is 5% to 18%, although only one procedure-related fatality occurred among 174 patients so treated.

*See references 15, 20, 48-50, 53, 62-69.
†See references 50-52, 56-58, 71, 72.

Primary patency rates range from 73% to 92% at 6 months, 66% to 75% at 12 months, 40% to 59% at 24 months, 22% to 38% at 48 months, and up to 9% at 60 months. Depending on the duration of follow-up, 13% to 60% of patients require reintervention, with resulting secondary patency rates of 69% to 88% at 3 to 5 years.[54] Because most patients with benign biliary strictures have life expectancies that far exceed the expected bare metallic stent patency, use of these bare stents has been judged to be inappropriate when alternative therapies are feasible.[3,57]

Recently, placement of covered bilary self-expanding metallic stents followed by stent retrieval after 2 to 6 weeks has been reported to result in a primary patency rate of 90.6% and a secondary patency rate of 97% with a mean clinical and imaging follow-up of 27.9 months.[73] These results are preliminary and need to be replicated by other centers.

TREATMENT OF MALIGNANT BILIARY STRICTURES (ONLINE CASE 16)

Patient and Stent Selection

Expandable metallic stents usually are indicated in long-term patients with malignant strictures, because the stent is likely to remain patent for a longer period (median patency, 6 to 8 months) than most patients' life expectancies (mean, 3.4 to 7.8 months, depending on tumor type)[3,54,72,73] (Fig. 22-26). Multiple investigators have found that metallic expandable stents remain patent longer, have lower complication rates, and require fewer repeat interventional procedures to maintain patency compared with plastic endoprostheses, particularly those delivered through the transhepatic route.[75-77] Metallic stents with a relatively tight lattice such as the Wallstent (Boston Scientific) or the Strecker nitinol stent (Boston Scientific), and stents that are significantly longer than the diseased segment provide optimized patency, because they resist tumor ingrowth through the stent struts and are less prone to tumor overgrowth beyond the ends of the stent. Covered stents such as the Viabil stent (WL Gore Inc., Flagstaff, Ariz.) may improve primary patency because the impermeable fabric prevents tumor ingrowth into the stent lumen.[60,61] Krokidis and colleagues[78] demonstrated less stent dysfunction and improved overall survival in patients with malignant extrahepatic bilary obstructions treated with covered Viabil stents compared to those treated with bare Wallstents.

Results and Complications

Reported initial technical success rates range from 75% to 100%.[56,72,79] Initial clinical relief of symptoms occurs in greater than 70% of patients.[56,72,74,79-86] Reported

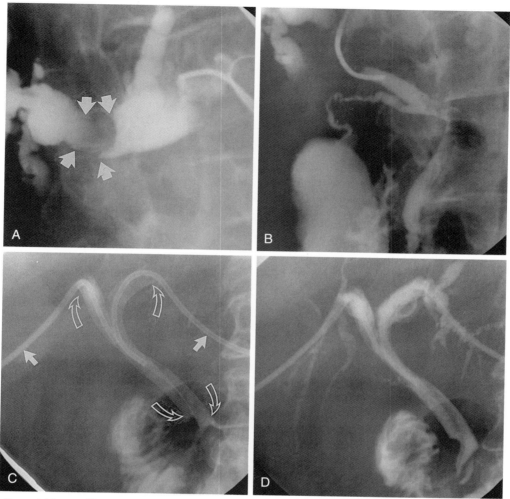

FIGURE 22-26 Expandable metallic stent for treatment of malignant stricture (hilar cholangiocarcinoma). Computed tomography (not shown) identified bilateral bile duct dilation. **A,** Transhepatic cholangiography through a left-sided approach documents hilar common bile duct (CBD) occlusion and mass *(arrows).* **B,** An angiographic catheter has been negotiated across the occlusive tumor into the CBD. **C,** Two 10-mm–diameter, 90-mm–long Wallstents *(curved arrows)* have been deployed from separate left- and right-sided biliary accesses to drain both biliary systems. Temporary external-type drainage catheters *(straight arrows)* have been left to provide overnight external biliary decompression to minimize the risk of cholangitis or sepsis and to provide transhepatic biliary access while the external drains are capped during a trial of internal drainage. The external biliary drains usually are removed after 1 to 2 days if internal drainage is successful. **D,** Cholangiogram performed through the external drains documents satisfactory stent placement and free drainage into the duodenum.

procedure-related fatality rates range up to 3%. Major nonfatal periprocedure complications range from 8% to 61% and are related primarily to the initial establishment of PBD rather than the additional deployment of a metallic stent.

Reported primary patency rates of bare stents range from 67% to 85% at 6 months, 50% to 55% at 1 year, and 10% to 37% at 2 years. Given the relatively short life expectancies of these patients, only about 7% to 29% of stents require reintervention. Thirty-day mortality rates are approximately 10% to 15%, and death results primarily from the underlying malignancy. Several investigators are studying coated and impregnated stents to preserve conduit patency.[60,61,87-89] Some investigators

report improved primary patency results at 6 months (76%, 77%) and 12 months (76%, 77%) using covered stents to treat malignant strictures, although mean survival remained short (146 days and 9.2 months).[60,61] The incidence of cholecystitis (12%) and branch duct obstruction (10%) was higher than expected with bare metallic stents. The cost of the covered stents is approximately two to three times that of most bare metallic stents, although total cost was equivalent in the Krokidis study.[78]

For percutaneous brachytherapy, the internal-external PBD catheters make ideal conduits for passage of iridium Ir-192 wires or seeds incorporated into a modified angiographic guidewire. This treatment is useful particularly for locally invasive Klatskin-type cholangiocarcinomas of the porta hepatis. A thin platinum shield absorbs beta particle emission, resulting in local intraductal delivery of pure gamma radiation. Brachytherapy may be combined with external beam irradiation. Although this treatment is not commonly used, several reports suggest modest survival improvement (i.e., 10 to 17 months vs. 2 to 8 months for historical controls treated with PBD and no irradiation).[90-94] Infectious and hemorrhagic complications are common in this group of patients with or without irradiation; however, ulceration of the gastrointestinal tract is an added risk of radiation therapy.[90] After irradiation, deployment of expandable metallic stents may provide improved biliary drainage with a lower rate of infectious complications and possibly longer survival.[57,94]

TREATMENT OF BILIARY STONES (ONLINE CASES 41 AND 63)

As an alternative to operative removal, endoscopic sphincterotomy followed by biliary stone extraction using wire retrieval baskets or occlusion balloons often is used in patients with retained CBD stones after cholecystectomy. It is used also for patients with choledocholithiasis and an intact gallbladder who are older than 65 years or are at high risk for operative CBD exploration. The procedure is associated with a high rate of technical success (i.e., successful sphincterotomy in approximately 95% in current series, with clearance of stones in approximately 85%).[95-102] The morbidity rate of approximately 4% to 16% is relatively low. Major complications usually are caused by hemorrhage from the sphincterotomy, pancreatitis, sepsis, or bowel perforation.

A mature T-tube sinus tract (at least 5 weeks old) can be used for stone extraction (Fig. 22-27). A guidewire is placed through the T-tube, and the T-tube is removed and replaced with a sheath, which is directed toward the stone. The guidewire is withdrawn and replaced with a wire basket (e.g., Wittich or Dormia Stone basket [Cook Inc.]). The expanded diameter of the basket varies and should be selected to match the diameter of the bile duct. The basket is opened by withdrawing a protective sheath. The stone is entrapped by spinning the basket, after which the sheath is gently snuggled down over the basket. Sufficiently small stones may be removed through the T-tube sinus tract. Otherwise, a balloon occlusion catheter can be used to deliver intrahepatic calculi into the CBD and then to push them into the bowel (see Fig. 22-27). At the end of the procedure, a drainage catheter is left in place to minimize the likelihood of sepsis, provide a route for follow-up cholangiography, and preserve access in case some stones remain. Technical success rates in experienced hands range from 77% to 97%, with major complications in 4% to 9% of cases and procedure-related fatality rates of 0 to 1%.[102-106] Percutaneous stone extraction through a T-tube

sinus tract may require multiple sessions, particularly if the stones are numerous, large, or impacted in intrahepatic bile ducts located peripheral to biliary strictures.

In patients with innumerable biliary calculi (e.g., recurrent pyogenic cholangitis), large stones (>1.5 cm diameter), or unfavorable anatomy (e.g., prior biliary-enteric drainage procedure), stone removal may be performed by a percutaneous transhepatic route (see Fig. 22-11). Although some cases may be managed with fluoroscopically guided techniques similar to those employed for stone extraction through a T-tube sinus tract, many of these patients have such a large stone burden or complex biliary anatomy (dilated and strictured) that percutaneous endoscopically guided lithotripsy techniques are required for successful therapy.[107-109]

Between 4 and 10 days after biliary drainage has been established and cholangitis or sepsis has been treated, the transhepatic tract is dilated to accommodate a large (e.g., 18-Fr) sheath. A small-bore endoscope (e.g., 15-Fr choledochoscope with a 6-Fr working channel) is advanced through the sheath into the biliary system, directed to the stones, and used to guide stone fragmentation with a suitable lithotriptor (e.g., electrohydraulic lithotriptor, ultrasonic lithotriptor, pulsed-dye laser). Care must be taken to avoid the surrounding bile duct walls or subjacent blood vessels.

Reported technical success for percutaneous transhepatic lithotripsy ranges from 93% to 100%, although complications can be substantial; procedure-related fatality rates are 0% to 4%, and nonfatal major morbidity rates are 0% to 24%.[107-112] Patients with large stones or innumerable stones are likely to have recurrent calculi even if the biliary tracts appear stone free, especially when strictures are present. Transhepatic endoscopy also has been used for staging and biopsy in patients with suspected cholangiocarcinoma, differentiation of cholangiographic masses or filling defects, removal of postoperative biliary foreign bodies (e.g., sutures or clips), guidance for cauterization of intraductal bleeding sites, and inspection of biliary-enteric anastomoses.*

BILIARY LEAKS

Biliary leaks usually result from biliary tract surgery. Other causes include hepatic surgery or invasive procedures, ischemia due to hepatic arterial occlusive disease (e.g., liver transplant recipients), downstream biliary obstruction, or penetrating injuries (see Fig. 22-18). Because bile can escape into the peritoneum or a localized space, the intrahepatic bile ducts usually are not dilated. The diagnosis and characterization of the biliary injury require cross-sectional imaging, preferably with computed tomography (CT), to assess for bilomas or abscesses, and cholangiography with or without endoscopy.

*See references 26, 39, 109, 110, 113, 114.

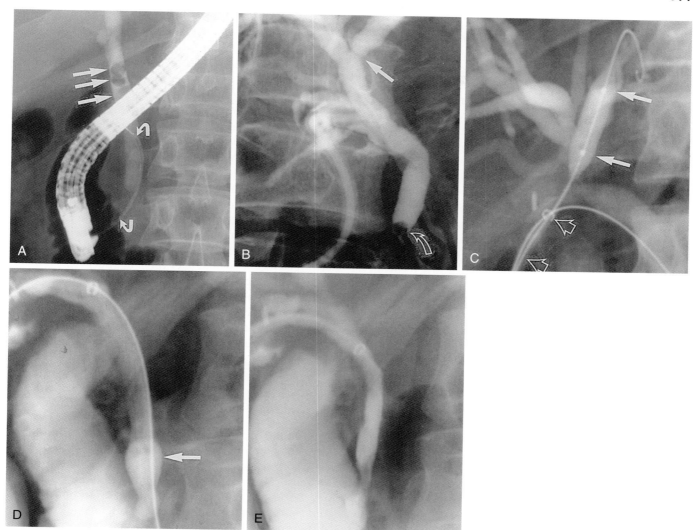

FIGURE 22-27 Endoscopic, operative, and percutaneous T-tube treatment of biliary calculi. **A,** Endoscopic retrograde cholangiopancreatography shows multiple common bile duct (CBD) and intrahepatic biliary stones *(straight arrows)*. The sphincterotome *(curved arrows)* was used to perform a papillotomy; multiple CBD calculi were removed using wire stone retrieval baskets and an occlusion balloon catheter. **B,** One week after an operative cholecystectomy for cholecystolithiasis and CBD exploration, the T-tube cholangiogram detected a retained 7-mm–diameter stone in the distal CBD *(curved arrow)* and a weblike stricture of the central left bile duct *(straight arrow)*. **C,** After passage of a heavy guidewire, the T-tube was replaced with a 12-Fr vascular-type sheath *(open arrows)*. A 10-mm × 4-cm balloon dilation catheter *(solid arrows)* was used to dilate the left bile duct stricture. **D,** An occlusion balloon *(arrow)* was used to push the stone into the CBD and through the papilla into the duodenum. **E,** A completion cholangiogram confirmed the stone's absence.

Nonoperative management of biliary fistulas includes certain features:

- Diversion of biliary flow through PBD or transendoscopically
- Placement of a catheter across the injured segments to preserve bile duct continuity
- Drainage of associated fluid collections (e.g., bilomas, abscesses)
- Relief of downstream obstruction, if present[115-120]

If downstream strictures are present, often they require operative decompression.[121] Although transcatheter embolization of biliary leaks has been described, the safety and effectiveness of this technique have yet to be proved.[122]

COMBINED PERCUTANEOUS, ENDOSCOPIC, AND OPERATIVE PROCEDURES

Percutaneous transhepatic access to the biliary system may be a useful adjunct to operative or transendoscopic procedures. Preoperative placement of a relatively stiff PBD catheter (e.g., Ring biliary drainage catheter [Cook Inc.]) through one or both intrahepatic duct systems and then into the duodenum may assist the surgeon during porta hepatis dissection in patients with biliary strictures who have had prior right upper quadrant surgery and in whom extensive adhesions have occurred. The time required for exposure of the bile ducts or vascular structures is reduced significantly.[123] PBD also may assist intraoperative placement of transhepatic Silastic biliary stents or U-tube drains (Silastic tubes placed across a stricture or anastomosis, one end externalized through the liver and the other end externalized through an enterotomy).

In patients in whom endoscopic drainage has failed because of inability of the endoscopist to cannulate the bile ducts, the so-called rendezvous procedure may be performed to permit endoscopic access into the biliary systems or to provide improved guidewire tension for delivery of transluminal devices across difficult strictures.[124,125] The rendezvous procedure is performed by passing a 300- to 400-cm guidewire and 5- to 6-Fr angiographic catheter percutaneously through the biliary system and into the small bowel. The endoscopist then can snare the guidewire easily and withdraw it through the mouth. The through-and-through "body floss" guidewire is threaded through the working channel of the interventional endoscope, and the desired transluminal device (e.g., endoprostheses and pusher catheter, expandable metallic stent delivery system) is passed over the guidewire retrograde into the desired location in the biliary system. After the guidewire is removed, the angiographic catheter may be used for antegrade cholangiography and as a safety drain in case of infectious complications or unexpected biliary obstruction.

The primary advantage of the rendezvous procedure is the ability to place a relatively large-bore drain (3.3 to 12 mm) with a small-caliber transhepatic route (1.7 to 2 mm). However, expandable metallic stents often can be placed more simply by a transhepatic approach. Rendezvous procedures now are used less frequently than in the past.

PERCUTANEOUS CHOLECYSTOSTOMY (ONLINE CASE 9)

Patient Selection

Most benign disease of the gallbladder is managed by operative cholecystectomy. During the late 1980s and early 1990s, several nonoperative techniques were developed as an alternative to open cholecystectomy for treatment of calculus cholecystitis, including percutaneous cholecystostomy with percutaneous lithotripsy or stone dissolution and extracorporeal shock wave lithothripsy.[126] The rapid growth of laparoscopic cholecystectomy during the early 1990s has largely rendered these techniques obsolete.

There are two major indications for percutaneous cholecystostomy.[6] The first is possible acalculous cholecystitis in critically ill patients with sepsis of unknown origin (Fig. 22-28). In septic patients, clinical features suggesting this diagnosis include abnormal liver function test results, right upper quadrant pain, and sonographic findings of a distended gallbladder, thickened gallbladder wall, intraluminal sludge or stones, pericholecystic fluid, or the presence of a sonographic Murphy's sign. Radionuclide studies are of little value, because most critically ill patients do not show radionuclide uptake by the gallbladder on hepatobiliary scintigraphy. The diagnosis is based on the clinical response to percutaneous cholecystostomy because neither the Gram stain nor the results of bile culture are helpful.[127]

The second indication is calculus cholecystitis in poor operative candidates (Fig. 22-29). In patients whose operative contraindication is temporary (e.g., acute myocardial infarction), percutaneous cholecystostomy permits drainage of the gallbladder so that cholecystectomy may be performed electively at a later time. In patients with a permanent contraindication to surgery (e.g., intractable congestive heart failure), the percutaneous cholecystostomy access route can be used to extract the gallstones using forceps, wire baskets, or various lithotriptors.[128] In approximately one half of patients, gallstones do not recur.[129]

Technique

Percutaneous cholecystostomy may be performed at the bedside under sonographic guidance in critically ill patients. When feasible, the procedure should be performed in an interventional radiology suite to permit manipulation of guidewires and catheters under fluoroscopy. In patients with distorted anatomy, CT may be necessary to obtain initial skinny-needle and guidewire access into the gallbladder.

Two percutaneous approaches may be used for cholecystostomy. In the *transhepatic approach*, a needle is directed from a subcostal or intercostal site in the right mid-axillary line toward the "bare area" of the gallbladder fossa, where the gallbladder is attached to the liver capsule. The primary advantages of this route are that the likelihood of bile spillage into the peritoneum is minimized and the gallbladder is relatively fixed to the liver, which facilitates puncture of the gallbladder wall. Disadvantages include the risk of hemorrhagic complications from transhepatic passage and the 90-degree angle with the long axis of the gallbladder, which makes catheter manipulations difficult.

In the *transperitoneal approach,* the needle is directed from the subcostal right anterior abdomen, beneath the liver margin into the fundus of the gallbladder along the long axis of the organ. This technique is safest in patients with a distended gallbladder, which is often adherent to the anterior abdominal wall (see Fig. 22-28). Advantages of transperitoneal access include avoidance of the hemorrhagic complications associated with the transhepatic route and pain from intercostal catheter passage

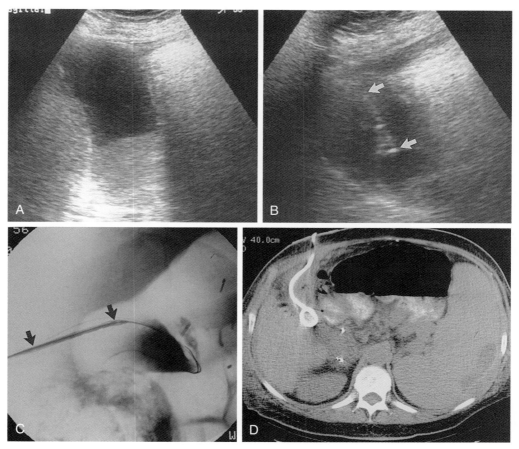

FIGURE 22-28 Percutaneous cholecystostomy in a critically ill postoperative patient with sepsis of unknown origin. **A,** The sonogram shows thickening of the gallbladder wall and intraluminal sludge. **B,** Sonographic guidance was used to puncture the gallbladder with a 22-gauge Chiba needle *(arrows)* through a transperitoneal route. **C,** Fluoroscopic guidance permitted the Seldinger technique to be used to introduce a 12-Fr locking pigtail catheter *(arrows).* **D,** Repeat computed tomography scan 3 days later confirmed the intracholecystic pigtail location adjacent to the cystic duct with adequate gallbladder decompression.

and the ease of intraluminal manipulation. Disadvantages include the risk of accidental perforation of bowel (especially the colon) and peritoneal spillage of bile if the gallbladder fundus is not adherent to the abdominal wall.[130] If the gallbladder fundus is mobile, the trocar technique rather than Seldinger technique may be used to minimize peritoneal spillage.[131]

Regardless of the access route, the percutaneous cholecystostomy drain should be left in place for at least 4 weeks to allow formation of a mature fibrinous sheath or sinus tract around the catheter shaft. The percutaneous cholecystostomy catheter should not be removed from patients with persistent gallstones, because they may obstruct normal drainage through the cystic duct. In patients without gallstones, cholecystography should be performed to ensure normal drainage through the cystic duct and CBD. When catheter removal is anticipated, it should be withdrawn over a guidewire and replaced with a suitably sized vascular access sheath.[132] Contrast material can be injected through the sheath side arm while the sheath is withdrawn along the tract. If contrast material remains only within the tract and gallbladder lumen, the sheath and guidewire can be removed safely. However, if leakage is seen (indicating an immature or incomplete track), a new catheter can be placed over the guidewire.

Results and Complications

Most percutaneous cholecystostomy catheters are placed at the bedside in the intensive care unit (ICU) with a transhepatic approach using ultrasound. Even in these suboptimal conditions, percutaneous cholecystostomy is technically successful in 93% to 100% of cases.[6,132-139] The procedure-related mortality rate is 0% to 2%, and the nonfatal complication rate is 0% to 12%.[6] One complication relatively unique to percutaneous cholecystostomy is intraprocedural vasovagal reaction, probably because of manipulation within the gallbladder.[140] Minimizing intracystic manipulation may prevent this reaction, which usually responds to fluid administration and intravenous atropine.

The likelihood of clinical response to percutaneous cholecystostomy drainage depends on the patient's clinical situation. Among critically ill patients in the ICU with sepsis of an unknown cause and an abnormal gallbladder sonogram, 39% to 63% become afebrile with normalization of leukocytosis and weaning from pressor drips within 24 to 72 hours. Among patients who respond, many have the drainage tube removed after recovery and avoid cholecystectomy altogether. Percutaneous cholecystostomy in this group is diagnostic and therapeutic.[136]

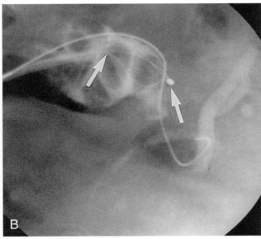

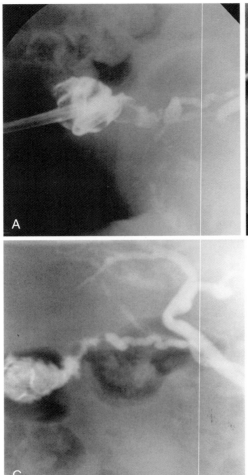

FIGURE 22-29 Percutaneous cholecystostomy for treatment of cholelithiasis and chronic cholecystitis in a 79-year-old patient with severe chronic obstructive pulmonary disease. **A,** Cholecystogram after percutaneous cholecystostomy documented multiple large gallstones. **B,** After multiple sessions of gallstone extraction using wirestone retrieval baskets *(arrows)* and transcatheter contact dissolution therapy using ethyl propionate, the gallstones were eliminated successfully. **C,** Termination cholecystogram documented complete removal of gallstones and satisfactory drainage through the cystic duct.

Most critically ill septic patients who fail to respond to percutaneous cholecystostomy die, usually of their underlying illnesses, but also commonly from biliary sepsis.[139] The diagnostic significance of a clinical failure of percutaneous cholecystostomy is less clear. It implies that sepsis originated from a different source or that the gallbladder is gangrenous.

Among stable patients with acute calculus cholecystitis and a contraindication to surgery, 93% respond clinically.[135,139] Many of these patients undergo a delayed, elective cholecystectomy, although a few are treated with stone removal and subsequent percutaneous cholecystostomy removal. A significant minority require lifelong intubation because of the critical nature of their underlying medical condition.[138-140]

ACKNOWLEDGMENT

We wish to express gratitude to Azniv Zeronian for her assistance in manuscript preparation.

References

1. Huard P, Do-Xuan-Hop. La ponction transhepatique des canaux biliares. *Bull Soc Med Chir Indochine* 1937;**15**:1090.
2. Remolar J, Katz S, Rybak B, et al. Percutaneous transhepatic cholangiography. *Gastroenterology* 1956;**31**:39.
3. Owens CA, Funaki BS, Ray Jr CE, et al. *Expert Panel on Interventional Radiology. ACR Appropriateness Criteria® Percutaneous Biliary Drainage in Benign and Malignant Biliary Obstruction.* American College of Radiology (ACR). www.guidline.gov/content.aspx?id=15731;2008:7.
4. Shlansky-Goldberg R, Weintraub J. Cholangiography. *Semin Roentgenol* 1997;**32**:150.
5. Gazelle GS, Lee MJ, Mueller PR. Cholangiographic segmental anatomy of the liver: implications for interventional radiology. *Semin Intervent Radiol* 1995;**12**:119.
6. Saad WEA, Wallace MJ, Wojak JC, Kundu S, Cardella JF. Quality Improvement Guidelines for Percuaneous Transhepatic Cholangiography, Biliary Drainage, and Percutaneous Cholecystostomy. *J Vasc Interv Radiol* 2010;**21**:789.
7. Lopera JE, Soto JA, Munera F. Malignant hilar and perihilar biliary obstruction: use of MR cholangiography to define the extent of biliary ductal involvement and plan percutaneous interventions. *Radiology* 2001;**220**:90.
8. Kaltenthaler EC, Walters SJ, Chilcott J, Blakeborough A, Vergel YB, Thomas S. *MRCP compared to diagnostic ERCP when biliary obstruction*

is suspected: a systematic review. BMC Medical Imaging doi:10.1186/1471-2342-6-9. www.biomedicalcentral.com/1471.2342/6/9;2006;6:9.

9. Venkatesan A, Kundu S, Sacks D, et al. Practice guideline for adult antibiotic prophylaxis during vascular and interventional radiology procedures. Written by the Standards of Practice Committee of the Society of Interventional Radiology and Endorsed by the Cardiovascular and Interventional Radiology Society of Europe and the Canadian Interventional Radiology Association. *J Vasc Interv Radiol* 2010;21:1611.

10. Spies JB, Rosen RJ, Lebowitz AS. Antibiotic prophylaxis in vascular and interventional radiology: a rational approach. *Radiology* 1988;166:381.

11. Clark CD, Picus D, Dunagan WC. Bloodstream infections after interventional procedures in the biliary tract. *Radiology* 1994;191:495.

12. McDermott, Schuster MG, Smith TP. Antibiotic prophylaxis in vascular and interventional radiology (review). *AJR Am J Roentgenol* 1997;169:31.

13. Mallory PC, Grassi CJ, Kundu S, et al. for the Standards of Practice Committee with Cardiovascular and Interventional Radiological Society of Europe (CIRSE). Endorsement consensus guidelines for periprocedural management of coagulation status and hemostasis risk in percutaneous image-guided interventions. *J Vasc Interv Radiol* 2009;20:S240.

14. Silverman SG, Coughin BF, Selzer SE, et al. Current use of screening laboratory tests before abdominal interventions: a survey of 603 radiologists. *Radiology* 1991;181:669.

15. Lee MJ, Mueller PR, Saini S, et al. Percutaneous dilatation of benign biliary strictures: single session therapy with general anesthesia. *AJR Am J Roentgenol* 1991;157:1263.

16. Savader SJ, Bourke DL, Venbrux AC, et al. Randomized double-blind clinical trial of celiac plexus block for percutaneous biliary drainage. *J Vasc Interv Radiol* 1993;4:539.

17. Eisenberg RL. Bile duct marking and obstruction. In: *Gastrointestinal radiology: a pattern approach*, 3rd ed. Philadelphia: Lippincott-Raven; 1996. p. 851.

18. Chartrand-Lefebre C, Dufresne M-P, Lafortune M, et al. Iatrogenic injury to the bile duct: a working classification for radiologists. *Radiology* 1994;193:523.

19. Majoie CB, Reeders JW, Sanders JB, et al. Primary sclerosing cholangitis: a modified classification of cholangiographic findings. *AJR Am J Roentgenol* 1991;157:495.

20. Ward EM, Kiely MJ, Maus TP, et al. Hilar biliary strictures after liver transplantation: cholangiography and percutaneous treatment. *Radiology* 1990;177:259.

21. Eisenberg RL. Cystic dilatation of the bile ducts. In: *Gastrointestinal radiology: a pattern approach.* 3rd ed. Philadelphia: Lippincott-Raven; 1996. p. 872.

22. Savader SJ, Benenati JF, Venbrux AC, et al. Choledochal cysts: classification and cholangiographic appearance. *AJR Am J Roentgenol* 1991;156:327.

23. Eisenberg RL. Filling defects in the bile ducts. In: *Gastrointestinal radiology: a pattern approach*, 3rd ed. Philadelphia: Lippincott-Raven; 1996. p. 837.

24. vanSonnenberg E, Ferrucci JT, Neff CC, et al. Biliary pressure: manometric and perfusion studies at percutaneous transhepatic cholangiography and percutaneous biliary drainage. *Radiology* 1983;148:41.

25. Savader SJ, Cameron JL, Pitt HA, et al. Biliary manometry versus clinical trial: value as predictors of success after treatment of biliary tract strictures. *J Vasc Inter Radiol* 1994;5:757.

26. Mendez Jr G, Russell E, Levi JV, et al. Percutaneous brush biopsy and internal drainage of biliary tree through endoprosthesis. *AJR Am J Roentgenol* 1980;134:653.

27. Kim D, Porter DH, Siegel JB, et al. Common bile duct biopsy with the Simpson atherectomy catheter. *AJR Am J Roentgenol* 1990;154:1213.

28. Pereiras Jr R, Chiprut RU, Greenward RA, et al. Percutaneous transhepatic cholangiography with a "skinny" needle: a rapid, simple, and accurate method in the diagnosis of cholestasis. *Ann Intern Med* 1977;86:562.

29. Okuda K, Tanikawa K, Emura T, et al. Nonsurgical percutaneous transhepatic cholangiography—diagnostic significance in medical problems of the liver. *Am J Dig Dis* 1974;19:21.

30. Redeker AG, Karvountzis GG, Richman RH, et al. Percutaneous transhepatic cholangiography: an improved technique. *JAMA* 1975; 231:386.

31. Harbin WP, Mueller PR, Ferrucci Jr JT. Transhepatic cholangiography—complications and use patterns of the fine needle technique: a multi-institutional survey. *Radiology* 1980;135:15.

32. Gold RP, Casarella WJ, Stern G, et al. Transhepatic cholangiography: the radiological method of choice in suspected obstructive jaundice. *Radiology* 1979;133:39.

33. Funaki B, Zaleski GX, Straus CA, et al. Percutaneous biliary drainage in patients with nondilated intrahepatic bile ducts. *AJR Am J Roentgenol* 1999;173:1541.

34. Shea Jr WJ, Demas BE, Goldberg HI, et al. Sclerosing cholangitis associated with hepatic arterial FUDR chemotherapy: radiographic-histologic correlation. *AJR Am J Roentgenol* 1986;146:717.

35. Harell GS, Anderson MF, Berry PF. Cytologic bile examination in the diagnosis of biliary duct neoplastic strictures. *AJR Am J Roentgenol* 1981;137:1123.

36. Muro A, Mueller PR, Ferrucci Jr JT, Taft PD. Bile cytology: a routine addition to percutaneous biliary drainage. *Radiology* 1983;149:846.

37. Hall-Craggs MA, Lees MR. Fine-needle aspiration biopsy: pancreatic and biliary tumors. *AJR Am J Roentgenol* 1986;147:399.

38. Teplick SK, Haskin PH, Kline TS, et al. Percutaneous pancreaticobiliary biopsies in 173 patients using primarily ultrasound or fluoroscopic guidance. *Cardiovasc Intervent Radiol* 1988;11:26.

39. Savader SJ, Prescott CA, Lund GB, et al. Intraductal biliary biopsy: comparison of three techniques. *J Vasc Interv Radiol* 1996;7:743.

40. Mueller PR, vanSonnenberg E, Ferrucci Jr JT. Percutaneous biliary drainage: technical and catheter-related problems in 200 procedures. *AJR Am J Roentgenol* 1982;138:17.

41. Hamlin JA, Friedman M, Stein MG, et al. Percutaneous biliary drainage: complications of 118 consecutive catheterizations. *Radiology* 1986;158:199.

42. McNicholas MM, Lee MJ, Dawson SL, et al. Complications of percutaneous biliary drainage and stricture dilatation. *Semin Intervent Radiol* 1994;11:242.

43. Carrasco CH, Zounoza J, Bechter WJ. Malignant biliary obstruction: complications of percutaneous biliary drainage. *Radiology* 1984; 152:343.

44. Yee AC, Ho C-S. Complications of percutaneous biliary drainage: benign vs malignant diseases. *AJR Am J Roentgenol* 1987;148:1207.

45. Fidelman N, Bloom AI, Kerlan Jr RK., et al. Hepatic arterial injuries after percutaneous biliary interventions in the era of laparscopic surgery and liver transplantation: experience with 930 patients. *Radiology* 2008;247:880.

46. Lyon SM, Terhaar O, Given MF, O'Dwyer HM, McGrath FP, Lee MJ. Percutaneous embolization of transhepatic tracks for biliary intervention. *Cardiovasc Intervent Radiol* 2006;29:1011.

47. Cohan RH, Illescas FF, Saeed M, et al. Infectious complications of percutaneous biliary drainage. *Invest Radiol* 1986;21:705.

48. May GR, Bender CE, LaRusso NF, et al. Nonoperative dilation of dominant strictures in primary sclerosing cholangitis. *AJR Am J Roentgenol* 1985;145:1061.

49. Skolkin MD, Alspaugh JP, Casarella WJ, et al. Sclerosing cholangitis: palliation with percutaneous cholangioplasty. *Radiology* 1989;170:199.

50. Rossi P, Salvatori FM, Bezzi M, et al. Percutaneous management of benign biliary strictures with balloon dilatation and self-expanding metallic stents. *Cardiovasc Intervent Radiol* 1990;13:231.

51. Diamond NG, Lee SP, Niblett RL, et al. Metallic stents for the treatment of intrahepatic biliary strictures after liver transplantation. *J Vasc Interv Radiol* 1995;6:755.

52. Culp WC, McCowan TC, Lieberman RP, et al. Biliary strictures in liver transplant recipients: treatment with metal stents. *Radiology* 1996;**199**:339.

53. Zajko AB, Sheng R, Zetti GM, et al. Transhepatic balloon dilation of biliary strictures in liver transplant patients: a 10-year experience. *J Vasc Interv Radiol* 1995;**6**:79.

54. Gabelmann A, Hamid H, Brambs H-J, Rieber A. Metallic stents in benign biliary strictures: long-term effectiveness and interventional management of stent occlusion. *AJR Am J Roentegenol* 2001;**177**:813.

55. Moreira AM, Carnevale FC, Tannuri U, Suzuki L, Gibelli N, Maksoud JG, Cerri GG. Long-term results of percutaneous bilioenteric anastomotic stricture treatment in liver-transplanted children. *Cardiovasc Intervent Radiol* 2010;**33**:90.

56. Tesdal IK, Adamus R, Poeckler C, et al. Therapy for biliary stenoses and occlusions with use of three different metallic stents: single center experience. *J Vasc Interv Radiol* 1997;**8**:869.

57. Coons H. Metallic stents for the treatment of biliary obstruction: a report of 100 cases. *Cardiovasc Intervent Radiol* 1992;**15**:367.

58. Hausegger KA, Kugler C, Uggowitzer M, et al. Benign biliary obstruction: is treatment with the Wallstent advisable? *Radiology* 1996;**200**:437.

59. Sirwiwardana HPP, Siriwardana AK. systematic appraisal of the role of metallic endobiliary stents in the treatment of benign bile duct stricture. *Ann Surg* 2005;**242**:10.

60. Schoder M, Rossi P, Uflacker R, et al. Malignant biliary obstruction: treatment with ePTFE-FEP-covered endoprostheses—initial technical and clinical experiences in a multicenter trial. *Radiology* 2002;**225**:35.

61. Bezzi M, Zolovkins A, Cantisani V, et al. New ePTFE/FEP-covered stent in the palliative treatment of malignant biliary obstruction. *J Vasc Intervent Radiol* 2002;**13**:581.

62. Salomonowitz E, Castaneda-Zuniga WR, Lund G, et al. Balloon dilation of benign biliary strictures. *Radiology* 1984;**151**:613.

63. Gallacher DJ, Kadir S, Kaufman SL, et al. Nonoperative management of benign postoperative biliary strictures. *Radiology* 1985;**156**:625.

64. Mueller PR, vanSonnenberg E, Ferrucci Jr JT, et al. Biliary stricture dilatation: multicenter review of clinical management in 73 patients. *Radiology* 1986;**160**:17.

65. Williams Jr HJ, Bender CE, May GR. Benign postoperative biliary strictures: dilation with fluoroscopic guidance. *Radiology* 1987;**163**:629.

66. Moore Jr AV, Illescas FF, Mills SR, et al. Percutaneous dilation of benign biliary strictures. *Radiology* 1987;**163**:625.

67. Gibson RN, Adam A, Yeung E, et al. Percutaneous techniques in benign hilar and intrahepatic strictures. *J Intervent Radiol* 1988;**3**:125.

68. Citron SJ, Martin LG. Benign biliary strictures: treatment with percutaneous cholangioplasty. *Radiology* 1991;**178**:339.

69. Cantwell CP, Pena CS, Gervais DA, Hahn PF, Dawson SL, Mueller PR. Thirty years' experience with balloon dilation of benign postoperative biliary strictures: long-term outcomes. *Radiology* 2008;**249**:1050.

70. Suman L, Civelli EM, Cozzi G, et al. Long-term results of balloon dilation of benign bile duct strictures. *Acta Radiologica* 2003;**44**:147.

71. Irving JD, Adam A, Dick R, et al. Gianturco expandable metallic biliary stents: results of a European clinical trial. *Radiology* 1989;**172**:321.

72. Rossi P, Bezzi M, Rossi M, et al. Metallic stents in malignant biliary observation: results of a multicenter European study of 240 patients. *J Vasc Interv Radiol* 1994;**5**:279.

73. Gwon DI, Shim HJ, Kwak BK. Retrievable biliary stent-graft in the treatment of benign biliary strictures. *J Vasc Interv Radiol* 2008;**19**:1328.

74. Boguth L, Tatalovic S, Antonucci F, et al. Malignant biliary obstruction: clinical and histopathologic correlation after treatment with self-expanding metal prostheses. *Radiology* 1994;**192**:669.

75. Knyrim K, Wagner HJ, Pausch J, et al. A prospective randomized controlled trial of metal stents for malignant obstruction of the common bile duct. *Endoscopy* 1993;**25**:207.

76. Wagner H-J, Knyrim K, Vakil N, et al. Plastic endoprostheses versus metal stents in the palliative treatment of malignant hilar biliary obstruction: a prospective and randomized trial. *Endoscopy* 1993;**25**:213.

77. Lammer J, Hausegger KA, Fluckiger F, et al. Common bile duct obstruction due to malignancy: treatment with plastic versus metal stents. *Radiology* 1996;**201**:167.

78. Krokidis M, Fanelli F, Orgera G, Bezzi M, Passariello R, Hatzidakis A. Pericutaneous treatment of malignant jaundice due to extrahepatic cholangiocarcinoma: covered viabil stent versus uncovered Wallstents. *Cardiovasc Intervent Radiol* 2010;**33**:97.

79. Lameris JS, Stoker J, Nijs HG. Malignant biliary obstruction: percutaneous use of expandable stents. *Radiology* 1991;**179**:703.

80. Lee MJ, Dawson SL, Mueller PR, et al. Palliation of malignant bile duct obstruction with metallic biliary endoprostheses: technique, results and complications. *J Vasc Interv Radiol* 1992;**3**:665.

81. Salomonowitz EK, Antonucci F, Heer M, et al. Biliary obstruction: treatment with self-expanding metal prostheses. *J Vasc Interv Radiol* 1992;**3**:365.

82. Gordon RL, Ring EJ, La Berge JM, et al. Malignant biliary obstruction: treatment with expandable metallic stents—follow-up of 50 consecutive patients. *Radiology* 1992;**182**:697.

83. Becker CD, Glattli A, Malbach R, et al. Percutaneous palliation of malignant obstructive jaundice with the Wallstent endoprosthesis: follow-up and reintervention in patients with hilar and non-hilar obstruction. *J Vasc Interv Radiol* 1993;**4**:597.

84. Pinol V, Castells A, Bordas JM, et al. Percutaneous self-expanding metal stents versus endoscopic polyethylene endoprostheses for treating malignant biliary obstruction: randomized clinical trial. *Radiology* 2002;**225**:27.

85. Lee BH, Choe DH, Lee JH, et al. Metallic stents in malignant biliary obstruction: prospective long-term clinical results. *AJR Am J Roentgenol* 1997;**168**:741.

86. Inal M, Akgul E, Aksungur E, et al. Percutaneous self-expanding uncovered metallic stents in malignant biliary obstruction. Complications, follow-up, and reinterventions in 154 patients. *Acta Radiologica* 2003;**44**:139.

87. Alvarado R, Palmaz JC, Garcia OJ, et al. Evaluation of polymer-coated balloon expandable stents in the bile ducts. *Radiology* 1989;**170**:975.

88. Miyayama S, Matsui O, Terayama N, et al. Covered Gianturco stents for malignant biliary obstruction: preliminary clinical evaluation. *J Vasc Interv Radiol* 1997;**8**:641.

89. Severini A, Mantero S, Tanzi MC, et al. In vivo study of polyurethane-coated Gianturco-Rosch biliary Z-stents. *Cardiovasc Intervent Radiol* 1999;**22**:510.

90. Hayes Jr JK, Sapozink MD, Miller FJ. Definitive radiation therapy in bile duct carcinoma. *Int J Radiat Oncol Biol Phys* 1988;**15**:735.

91. Nunnerly HB, Karani JB. Intraductal radiation. *Radiol Clin North Am* 1990;**28**:1237.

92. Fritz P, Brambs H-J, Schraube P, et al. Combined external beam radiotherapy and intraductal high dose rate brachytherapy on bile duct carcinomas. *Int J Radiat Oncol Biol Phys* 1994;**29**:855.

93. Montemaggi P, Costamagna G, Dobelbower RR, et al. Intraluminal brachytherapy in the treatment of pancreas and bile duct carcinoma. *Int J Radiat Oncol Biol Phys* 1995;**32**:437.

94. Kamada T, Saitou H, Takamura A, et al. The role of radiotherapy in the management of extrahepatic bile duct cancer: an analysis of 145 consecutive patients treated with intraluminal and/or external beam radiotherapy. *Int J Radiat Oncol Biol Phys* 1996;**34**:767.

95. Allen B, Shapiro H, Way LW. Management of recurrent and residual common duct stones. *Am J Surg* 1981;**142**:41.

96. Mee AS, Vallon AG, Croker JR, et al. Non-operative removal of bile duct stones by duodenoscopic sphincterotomy in the elderly. *Br Med J* 1981;**283**:521.

97. Passi RB, Raval B. Endoscopic papillotomy. *Surgery* 1982;**92**:581.
98. Escourrou J, Cordova JA, Lazordities F, et al. Early and late complications after endoscopic sphincterostomy for biliary lithiasis with and without the gallbladder "in situ." *Gut* 1984; **25**:598.
99. Leese T, Neo PT, Lemos JP, Carr-Locke DL. Successes, failures, early complications and their management following endoscopic sphincterostomy: results in 394 consecutive patients from a single centre. *Br J Surg* 1985;**72**:215.
100. Broughan TA, Sivak MV, Hermann RE. The management of retained and recurrent bile duct stones. *Surgery* 1985;**98**:746.
101. Vaira D, D'Anna L, Ainlesy C, et al. Endoscopic sphincterotomy in 1000 consecutive patients. *Lancet* 1989;**2**:431.
102. Nussinson E, Cairns SR, Vaira D, et al. A 10-year single centre experience of percutaneous and endoscopic extraction of bile duct stones with T-tube in situ. *Gut* 1991;**32**:1040.
103. Mazzariello RM. A fourteen-year experience with nonoperative instrument of retained bile duct stones. *World J Surg* 1978;**2**:447.
104. Burhenne HJ. Percutaneous extraction of the retained biliary tract stones: 661 patients. *AJR Am J Roentgenol* 1980;**134**:888.
105. Caprini JA, Thorpe CJ, Fotopoulos JP. Results of nonsurgical treatment of retained biliary calculi. *Surg Gynecol Obstet* 1980; **151**:630.
106. Mason R. Percutaneous extraction of retained gallstones via the T-tube track—British experience of 131 cases. *Clin Radiol* 1980; **31**:497.
107. Stokes KR, Falchuk KR, Clouse ME. Biliary duct stones: update in 54 cases after percutaneous transhepatic removal. *Radiology* 1988;**170**:999.
108. Picus D, Weyman PJ, Marx MV. Role of percutaneous intracorporeal electrohydraulic lithotripsy in the treatment of biliary tract calculi: works in progress. *Radiology* 1989;**170**:989.
109. Rossi P, Bezzi M, Fiocca F, et al. Percutaneous cholangioscopy. *Semin Intervent Radiol* 1996;**13**:185.
110. Venbrux AC, Robbins KV, Savader SJ, et al. Endoscopy as an adjunct to biliary radiologic intervention. *Radiology* 1991; **180**:355.
111. Bonnel DH, Liguory CE, Cornud FE, et al. Common bile duct and intrahepatic stones: results of transhepatic electrohydraulic lithotripsy in 50 patients. *Radiology* 1991;**180**:345.
112. Harris VJ, Sherman S, Trerotola SO, et al. Complex biliary stones: treatment with a small choledochoscope and laser lithotripsy. *Radiology* 1961;**199**:71.
113. Picus D. Percutaneous biliary endoscopy. *J Vasc Interv Radiol* 1995;**6**:303.
114. Guenther RW, Vorwerk D, Klose KJ, et al. Fine-caliber cholangioscopy. *Radiol Clin North Am* 1990;**28**:1171.
115. Kaufman SL, Kadir S, Mitchell SE, et al. Percutaneous transhepatic biliary drainage for bile leaks and fistulas. *AJR Am J Roentgenol* 1985;**144**:1055.
116. Liguory C, Vitale GC, Lefebre JF, et al. Endoscopic treatment of postoperative biliary fistulae. *Surgery* 1991;**110**:779.
117. Binmoeller KF, Katon RM, Shneidman R. Endoscopic management of postoperative biliary leaks: review of 77 cases and report of two cases with biloma formation. *Am J Gastroenterol* 1991;**86**:227.
118. Trerotola SO, Savader SJ, Lund GB, et al. Biliary tract complications following laparoscopic cholecystectomy: Imaging and intervention. *Radiology* 1992;**184**:195.
119. vanSonnenberg E, D'Agostino HB, Easter DW, et al. Complications of laparoscopic cholecystectomy: coordinated radiologic and surgical management in 21 patients. *Radiology* 1993; **188**:399.
120. Ernst O, Sergent G, Mizrahi D, et al. Biliary leaks: treatment by means of percutaneous transhepatic biliary drainage. *Radiology* 1999;**211**:345.
121. Zuidema GD, Cameron JL, Sitzmann JV, et al. Percutaneous transhepatic management of complex biliary problems. *Ann Surg* 1983;**197**:584.
122. Oliva VL, Nicolet V, Soulez G, et al. Bilomas developing after laparoscopic biliary surgery: percutaneous management with embolization of biliary leaks. *J Vasc Interv Radiol* 1997;**8**:469.
123. Crist DW, Kadir S, Cameron JL. The value of preoperatively placed percutaneous biliary catheters in reconstruction of the proximal part of the biliary tract. *Surg Gynecol Obstet* 1987; **165**:421.
124. Chespak LW, Ring EJ, Shapiro HA, et al. Multidisciplinary approach to complex endoscopic biliary intervention. *Radiology* 1989;**170**:995.
125. Gordon RL, Ring EJ. Combined radiologic and retrograde endoscopic and biliary interventions. *Radiol Clin North Am* 1990;**28**:1289.
126. Malone DE. Interventional radiologic alternatives to cholecystectomy. *Radiol Clin North Am* 1990;**28**:1145.
127. McGahan JP, Lindfors KK. Acute cholecystitis: diagnostic accuracy of percutaneous aspiration of the gallbladder. *Radiology* 1988; **167**:669.
128. Gillams A, Curtis SC, Donald J, et al. Technical considerations in 113 percutaneous cholecystolithostomies. *Radiology* 1992;**183**:163.
129. Gibney RG, Chow K, So CB, et al. Gallstone recurrence after cholecystolithostomy. *AJR Am J Roentgenol* 1989;**153**:287.
130. Warren LP, Kadir S, Dunnick NR. Percutaneous cholecystostomy: anatomic considerations. *Radiology* 1988;**168**:615.
131. Garber SJ, Mathieson JR, Cooperberg PL, et al. Percutaneous cholecystostomy: safety of the transperitoneal route. *J Vasc Interv Radiol* 1994;**5**:295.
132. D'Agostino HB, vanSonnenberg E, Sanchez RB, et al. Imaging of the percutaneous cholecystostomy tract: observations and utility. *Radiology* 1991;**181**:675.
133. Teplick SK, Harshfield DL, Brandon JC, et al. Percutaneous cholecystostomy in critically ill patients. *Gastrointest Radiol* 1991;**16**:154.
134. Lee MJ, Saini S, Brink JA, et al. Treatment of critically ill patients with sepsis of unknown cause: value of percutaneous cholecystostomy. *AJR Am J Roentgenol* 1991;**156**:1163.
135. de Manzoni G, Furlan F, Guglielmi A, et al. Acute cholecystitis: ultrasonographic staging and percutaneous cholecystostomy. *Eur J Radiol* 1992;**15**:175.
136. Browning PD, McGahan JP, Gerscovich EO. Percutaneous cholecystostomy for suspected acute cholecystitis in the hospitalized patient. *J Vasc Interv Radiol* 1993;**4**:531.
137. Lo LD, Vogelzang RL, Braun MA, et al. Percutaneous cholecystostomy for the diagnosis and treatment of acute calculous and acalculous cholecystitis. *J Vasc Interv Radiol* 1995;**6**:629.
138. Boland GW, Lee MJ, Leung J, Mueller PR. Percutaneous cholecystomy in critically ill patients: early response and final outcome in 82 patients. *AJR Am J Roentgenol* 1994;**163**:339.
139. England RE, McDermott VG, Smith TP, et al. Percutaneous cholecystostomy: who responds? *AJR Am J Roentgenol* 1997; **168**:1247.
140. van Sonnenberg E, D'Agostino HB, Goodacre BW, et al. Percutaneous gallbladder puncture and cholecystostomy: results, complications and caveats for safety. *Radiology* 1992;**183**:167.

Urologic and Genital Systems

Matthew Kogut, Todd L. Kooy, Steven B. Oglevie

Genitourinary interventional radiology has evolved with the advances in knowledge and technology. With vast improvements in the diagnostic capabilities of non-invasive imaging, purely diagnostic catheter-based imaging studies are performed infrequently. Although many of the genitourinary interventions have been performed for decades, the procedures have been refined with new equipment and continuous improvements in imaging guidance. Various percutaneous drainage procedures involving the urinary collecting system remain necessary tools for the interventionalist. However, collaboration with urologists, transplant surgeons, obstetricians, and gynecologists has also allowed us to hone advanced techniques and expand into new areas such as renal transplant interventions and transcervical sterilization via fallopian tube occlusion.

PERCUTANEOUS NEPHROSTOMY (ONLINE CASES 24 AND 36)

Anatomy

The kidneys are retroperitoneal organs surrounded by perinephric fat and enclosed by Gerota fascia. Their axes parallel the psoas muscle so that the upper pole is medial and slightly more posterior than the lower pole. During normal development, the kidney ascends and rotates medially about its vertical axis such that the renal hilum is directed anteromedially at an angle of approximately 30 degrees from the horizontal plane.

The main renal artery and vein lie anterior to the renal pelvis. However, a posterior branch of the renal artery courses behind the renal pelvis to supply the dorsal segments. A percutaneous nephrostomy (PCN) track extending directly into a calyx has the least chance of causing substantial arterial injury (Fig. 23-1). Punctures into an infundibulum or directly into the renal pelvis carry a higher risk of hemorrhagic complications, because larger arterial branches may be traversed. Direct

renal pelvic punctures also risk the formation of a urinoma after the tube is removed.

The calyces are usually arranged in anterior and posterior rows. At the upper and lower poles, fusion can result in compound calyces. During urography in the anteroposterior projection, classic teaching is that posterior calyces are located medially and seen en face, while anterior calyces are located more laterally and seen in profile. However, a recent evaluation of calyceal anatomy on computed tomography (CT) showed that this is not the case in the lower pole. Most lower poles have two to three calyces and the most posterior calyx was often more lateral.[1] However, normal variation occurs, which is why, with the patient in prone position, oblique imaging, ultrasound, or injection of air is recommended to identify posterior calyces. Discrimination between the anterior and posterior calyces is critical, because posterior calyces are strongly preferred for most PCN procedures.

Understanding the normal and variant relationships of the kidneys with surrounding structures is important for safe and successful placement of a PCN.[2] The descending colon lies in the anterior pararenal space, and its relationship to the left kidney is determined by the position of the lateroconal fascia. In approximately 10% of patients, the descending colon lies behind a horizontal line at the posterior edge of the left kidney. In about 1% of cases, the descending colon extends behind the left kidney.[3] Rarely, the ascending colon lies posterolateral to the right kidney and medial to the liver.

The pleura extends posteriorly down to the 12th vertebral body and then extends laterally, crossing the 12th, 11th, and 10th ribs. Although great normal variation occurs, about one half of the right kidney and one third of the left kidney lie above this posterior reflection of the pleura.

The liver is anterolateral to the upper pole of the right kidney. In some patients, a portion of the right lobe of the liver may extend posterolaterally to the upper pole of the kidney. The position of the spleen is more

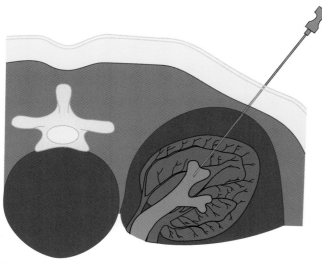

FIGURE 23-1 Posterolateral approach to posterior calyx for percutaneous nephrostomy. This approach is advantageous because it minimizes the risk of arterial injury and provides a straight vector for advancement of guidewires, dilators, and catheters into the renal pelvis. The track is lateral enough to avoid the paraspinal muscles but not so lateral as to risk colon perforation.

variable. It typically lies superolateral to the kidney but often is adjacent to the lateral margin and frequently may be posterolateral to the upper pole. Because of these variants of colonic, hepatic, and splenic anatomy, review of prior cross-sectional imaging studies is critical before PCN.

Patient Selection

The indications for PCN fall into four broad categories (Box 23-1). Each patient must be considered individually, because some have both indications for and contraindications to the procedure. The decision about whether to perform PCN depends on the details of the particular situation and on the other available options.

Relief of Urinary Obstruction

The most common indication for PCN is relief of urinary obstruction. Imaging studies should be performed to demonstrate dilated collecting systems, and they usually delineate the anatomic level of obstruction and the cause. The ureteral obstruction may be acute, as with obstructing ureteral calculi or traumatic ureteral injury. However, the obstruction may be long-standing, as with primary urothelial neoplasms, extrinsic compression, or direct invasion by retroperitoneal or pelvic malignancies.

In patients with bilateral obstruction or with obstruction of a solitary kidney, PCN is indicated for preservation of renal function. In some patients with widely disseminated malignances and very short life expectancies, decompression may not be indicated. Many oncologists believe a uremic death is a reasonably painless way for a terminal patient to die. This decision must be addressed individually and tailored to the desires of the patient and his or her family.

In patients with acute unilateral ureteral obstruction, decompression is justified to preserve renal function on the affected side. Long-standing obstruction is associated with an irreversible deterioration of renal function and parenchymal atrophy. Although the patient's serum blood urea nitrogen and creatinine levels usually do not become elevated with unilateral obstruction, the damage to the ipsilateral kidney is progressive and irreversible when not addressed promptly. Decompression with PCN may allow the cause of acute ureteral obstruction to be addressed on a more elective basis without risk of losing renal function.

In any patient with obstruction and suspicion of infection, emergent decompression is indicated. Infection may be suggested by fever, leukocytosis, flank pain, or sepsis. These patients must also be treated immediately with appropriate intravenous (IV) antibiotics and hemodynamic support as needed. The decompressive procedures in patients with pyonephrosis must be conducted and monitored with care, because the septic condition may be worsened with the intervention.

Patients with chronic unilateral hydroureteronephrosis due to malignancy do not necessarily require decompression unless infection is suspected. In the absence of malignant disease, kidneys with an estimated renographic glomerular filtration rate (GFR) of greater than 10 mL/min/1.73 m^2 will likely stabilize or improve renal function, while kidneys with worse function may not be worth salvage.[4] The finding of mild or moderate cortical atrophy on CT or ultrasound is not a reliable predictor of limited potential for functional recovery

after a PCN. In fact, decompressive PCN may be indicated to assess the recoverable function of a chronically occluded kidney.

Diversion of Urine

PCN is used to divert urine in cases of urinary leakage (Fig. 23-2). PCN, usually in combination with ureteral stent placement, allows most ureteral injuries to seal. The stent is thought to serve as a scaffold for ureteral healing. Percutaneous drainage of associated urinomas that accumulated before urinary diversion also may be performed. In cases of malignant or inflammatory fistulas, PCN is indicated to divert urine in conjunction with stent placement. PCN has been used also to divert urine and treat patients successfully with hemorrhagic cystitis.[5]

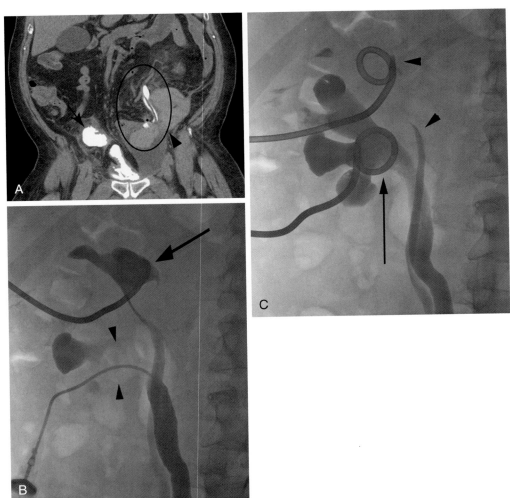

FIGURE 23-2   Decompression of a duplicated collecting system to assist in healing an anastomotic leak between the ureters and neobladder. **A,** Computed tomography shows the duplicated ureters near the anastomosis *(circle)* adjacent to dilute contrast seen in a large urinoma *(arrowhead).* The neobladder *(arrow)* opacified with contrast is partially seen. **B,** A percutaneous nephrostomy has already been placed into the upper pole moiety *(arrow).* Access has been gained to a posterior calyx *(arrowheads)* in the lower pole. The calyx is outlined by air, which was injected to confirm a posterior location. **C,** The upper moiety is now decompressed *(arrowheads).* The more inferior nephrostomy was injected with contrast to confirm appropriate location, with the pigtail now formed in the lower moiety renal pelvis *(arrow).*

Access for Diagnostic Interventions

Percutaneous access may be performed to permit antegrade pyelography. However, advances in diagnostic radiology dominated by CT and magnetic resonance (MR) urography have rendered this indication extremely rare.[6] Biopsies of urothelial lesions may be performed through nephrostomy access using brushes and forceps. Nephrostomy access may be used for diagnostic nephroscopy and ureteroscopy. Functional studies (e.g., Whitaker test) can be performed to determine the significance of urographically detected stenoses and to assess the results of interventions such as endopyelotomy or balloon ureteral dilation. This procedure is typically reserved for complicated cases in which nuclear scintigraphy or MR urography fail to give adequate physiologic information.[7] MR urography may become the "one-stop shop" for anatomic and functional information regarding the genitourinary system.

Access for Therapeutic Interventions

Ureteral strictures may be dilated percutaneously, and ureteral stents can also be placed. Foreign bodies (e.g., encrusted or occluded ureteral stents) may be retrieved through the nephrostomy access (Fig. 23-3). Stone therapy can be performed by chemodissolution or mechanical fragmentation and extraction. Antifungal agents may be infused directly through the nephrostomy tube to treat fungus balls in the upper urinary tract.[8,9] Nephroscopically guided operations can be performed, including resection of urothelial neoplasms and endopyelotomy. Intracavitary adjuvant chemotherapy can be administered through a nephrostomy in certain cases of transitional cell carcinoma.[10]

Access provided for stone treatment is one of the most common indications for PCN placement. By the age of 70 years, 11% of men and 5.6% of women will have a symptomatic urinary tract stone.[11] Although stones smaller than 5 mm often pass without intervention, stones between 5 and 10 mm have variable outcomes, and stones larger than 10 mm will not pass without intervention.[11] Many renal calculi can be managed successfully with extracorporeal shock wave lithotripsy (ESWL) or percutaneous nephrostolithotomy (PCNL), with success rates that rival open surgery but with significantly less morbidity, recovery time, and cost.

Planning the approach and entry site is the most critical step of the PCNL procedure and should be made by consultation between the urologist and interventional radiologist. The puncture site must allow the stone to be accessed and removed but not be made directly into the pelvis or infundibulum. This is one of the situations where occasionally supracostal access and/or access to an anterior calyx is optimal for future treatment (Fig. 23-4). If the initial puncture site is not ideal, it is better to make a new puncture in a more suitable position than to proceed with track dilation through which the stone cannot be removed. The best approach depends on several factors, the most important of which is the location of the stone burden.

Contraindications

Contraindications to PCN include uncorrectable coagulopathy and an uncooperative patient. If hyperkalemia is severe (i.e., potassium level greater than 7 mEq/L), hemodialysis should be performed to correct the electrolyte balance before the procedure.

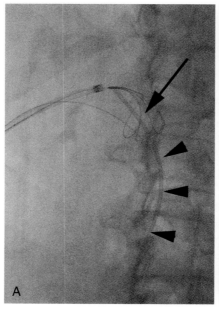 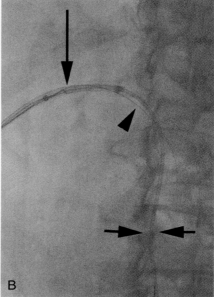

FIGURE 23-3   Percutaneous nephrostomy for retrieval of a broken internal ureteral stent. **A,** There is a sheath in position over a "safety" wire. A snare *(arrow)* has been placed around the proximal aspect of the broken stent *(arrowheads).* **B,** The snare *(long arrow)* is secured around the stent, which is being pulled out of the sheath. *Short arrows* mark the distal aspect of the stent and the *arrowhead* indicates the "safety" wire.

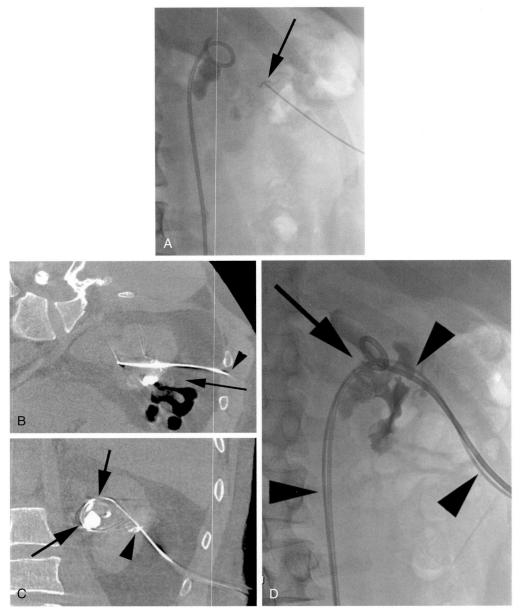

FIGURE 23-4   Access for percutaneous nephrolithotomy (PCNL). After consultation with the urologist, the best approach was deemed to be supracostal and lateral, targeting an anterior midpole calyx containing a stone. **A,** Initial fluoroscopic guided puncture directed at the midpole stone *(arrow).* **B,** A DynaCT was performed on the fluoroscopic table after initial puncture to confirm a safe approach into the calyx that avoided the colon. An *arrowhead* shows the supracostal approach and the *arrow* indicates the fat plane between the track and colon. **C,** Access was confirmed to be along the course of the stone *(arrowhead)* and a 0.018-inch wire *(arrows)* is coiled in the renal pelvis around the larger stone. **D,** Final spot image shows the nephrostomy pigtail formed in the superior aspect of the renal pelvis. A 5-Fr angled catheter *(arrowheads)* also traverses the stone down the ureter, terminating in the bladder. This ureteral catheter provides stable access for the urologist.

Surgical and Medical Alternatives

It usually is advantageous to initially consider a retrograde approach for renal drainage in patients with obstructive uropathy. PCN is typically reserved for patients in whom retrograde attempts are unsuccessful or not feasible. Although retrograde stents need routine changes and management, the patient will not have an external tube to manage. A "surgical" nephrostomy may be placed during open surgery directly into the renal pelvis, but this is rarely indicated because PCN can be performed safely and effectively in almost all patients (Fig. 23-5). Medical therapy for obstructive uropathy is limited. In some patients with widely disseminated malignancy or retroperitoneal fibrosis and obstructive uropathy, renal function may improve with the administration of corticosteroids.[12,13]

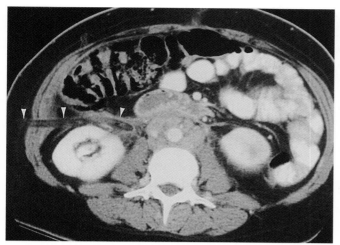

FIGURE 23-5   Surgical nephrostomy. A Foley catheter *(arrowheads)* directly enters the renal pelvis. Such open surgical nephrostomies are rarely indicated unless another open procedure is being performed at the same time.

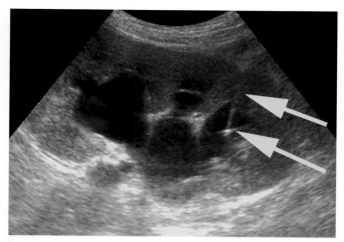

FIGURE 23-6   Ultrasound guidance used for initial puncture during decompressive nephrostomy. *Arrows* show the course of the needle into a dilated posterior lower pole calyx. Adjacent structures can be identified and avoided with ultrasound.

Technique

Preprocedure Care

Before the procedure, patients should be screened and treated for any coagulopathy. Review of any prior abdominal imaging is indicated to detect variant anatomy of colon, spleen, and liver, which should be considered when selecting the nephrostomy approach.

Prophylactic antibiotics should be administered intravenously before the procedure. The most common urinary tract pathogens are *Escherichia coli, Klebsiella, Enterococcus, Proteus,* and *Staphylococcus* species.[14] For prophylaxis in the absence of any overt infection, a third-generation cephalosporin or a fluoroquinolone is usually chosen. Ciprofloxacin is commonly used in both oral and IV forms. When infection exists, therapy is directed toward the isolated organisms. Another option for broad coverage would be ampicillin with gentamicin.[14,15]

Procedure

The patient is typically placed in the prone or oblique prone position on the interventional radiology (IR) table. In critically ill patients or pregnant patients who are unable to be placed prone, the procedure can be performed with the patient in a supine oblique position.

The initial puncture for PCN is performed with ultrasound, fluoroscopy, or very occasionally with CT imaging. Ultrasound is the optimum modality. A suitable calyx can be selected and entered with continuous sonographic guidance while avoiding surrounding organs (Fig. 23-6). Fluoroscopy can be used when renal function permits the IV administration of contrast material and results in satisfactory opacification of the collecting system. Fluoroscopy also may be used to puncture directly onto a radiopaque

calyceal calculus (see Fig. 23-4). If a retrograde ureteral catheter has been placed, it may be used to opacify the collecting system. CT guidance for puncture occasionally may be required in patients with congenital anomalies (i.e., horseshoe or pelvic kidneys) or issues with body habitus or positioning (e.g., severe scoliosis, morbid obesity) (Fig. 23-7).

Planning the puncture pathway is the most crucial step in PCN placement because poorly placed punctures are associated with higher complication rates and may preclude successful completion of subsequent interventions. For a simple decompressive nephrostomy, puncture of a lower pole calyx is satisfactory. This approach minimizes the risk of pleural complications. If ureteral stent placement is planned, puncture of an interpolar calyx is preferable to create a gentle curve down the ureter. However, ureteral stents usually can be placed from an inferior polar approach using stiff guidewires and sheaths. Access through an upper pole calyx is required occasionally for stone extraction. In this case, the track is occasionally intercostal, and pleural complications are more frequent.

The ideal skin entry site is at least 12 cm lateral to the midline but medial to the posterior axillary line. If the skin entry site is too medial, the paraspinal muscles are traversed, and subsequent interventions are rendered more difficult because the guidewire and catheter must abruptly turn medially on entering the calyx. A medially placed nephrostomy also is more painful for the supine patient. If the skin entry is too lateral, the risk of colonic perforation increases. However, this risk is typically very small, estimated at up to 3% when the expected path during placement of lower pole nephrostomy tube is simulated using multiplanar CT.[16]

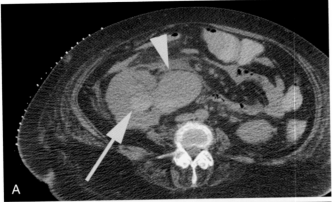

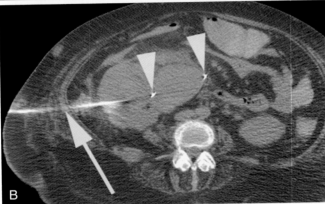

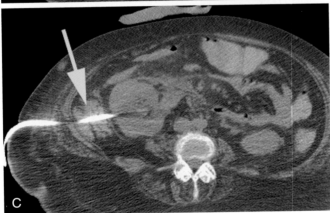

FIGURE 23-7   Computed tomography–guided placement of a percutaneous nephrostomy in an obese patient in the supine position. The patient would not tolerate a prone position. **A,** A grid is on the patient's skin. An *arrowhead* indicates the renal pelvis and the *arrow* is on the targeted dilated calyx. **B,** The needle *(arrow)* has been placed into the calyx and a 0.018-inch wire *(arrowheads)* is coiled in the renal pelvis. **C,** The nephrostomy is in place, and a small amount of hemorrhage *(arrow)* is seen along the track.

A posterolateral approach, with the needle angled about 30 to 40 degrees from vertical, directly into a posterior calyx is favored (see Fig. 23-1). This route follows the relatively avascular posterolateral plane of the kidney (i.e., Brödel line). Punctures generally should be made directly into a posterior calyx (see Fig. 23-1). This choice

provides a straight vector into the renal pelvis and minimizes the amount of renal parenchyma traversed by the nephrostomy track. Infundibular punctures or punctures directly into the renal pelvis should be avoided because large arteries may be traversed. Inadvertent puncture of anterior calyces makes subsequent interventions more difficult because of the tortuous pathway and increases the risk for significant arterial injury. Anterior calyces should be targeted only in the rare patient with an anterior calyceal stone (see Fig. 23-4). Oblique imaging and injection of air or carbon dioxide is helpful to determine whether a calyx punctured under fluoroscopy is posterior or anterior (Fig. 23-8).

When the collecting system has been entered with a 21- to 22-gauge needle, a sample of urine should be aspirated initially for cultures. If clinical suspicion for infection is high or the urine is cloudy, opacification of the collecting system must be performed gently after evacuating an equal amount of urine. Instillation of contrast by gravity may help prevent overdistention and worsening of sepsis. Likewise, subsequent manipulations that may have been planned should be minimized until the collecting system has been adequately decompressed and urine has cleared.

The initial puncture site is carefully scrutinized before dilation and catheter placement. If instillation of contrast or air reveals the initial puncture is not into a suitable posterior calyx, the needle should be left in place to opacify the system while a new needle is guided fluoroscopically into an appropriate calyx (Fig. 23-9). After the puncture is deemed satisfactory, a 0.018-inch guidewire is advanced into the renal pelvis and ideally down the ureter. A skin nick is made along the needle track. Blunt dissection of the subcutaneous tissue is performed. A coaxial access set, such as the Accustick set (Boston Scientific), is advanced under fluoroscopic guidance over the wire into the collecting system (see Fig. 23-8C). Urine can be aspirated and contrast injected through the sidearm of some access sets. The inner portions of the access set are removed. A 0.038-inch guidewire is advanced through the outer portion of the access set into the renal pelvis or ureter. In some access sets, the 0.018-inch wire can be left alongside the 0.038-inch wire as a "safety wire." An angled guiding catheter may help direct the guidewire down the ureter into a more secure position if necessary (Fig. 23-10).

The track is then dilated, and an 8- to 12-French (Fr) locking pigtail nephrostomy catheter is placed. The pigtail is formed and locked within the renal pelvis (see Fig. 23-8E). Care must be taken to avoid forming the pigtail in the ureter or in a calyceal infundibulum. The 8-Fr tubes are satisfactory in patients with clear urine. Larger tubes may be helpful in patients with grossly purulent urine or stone debris. Locking pigtail catheters

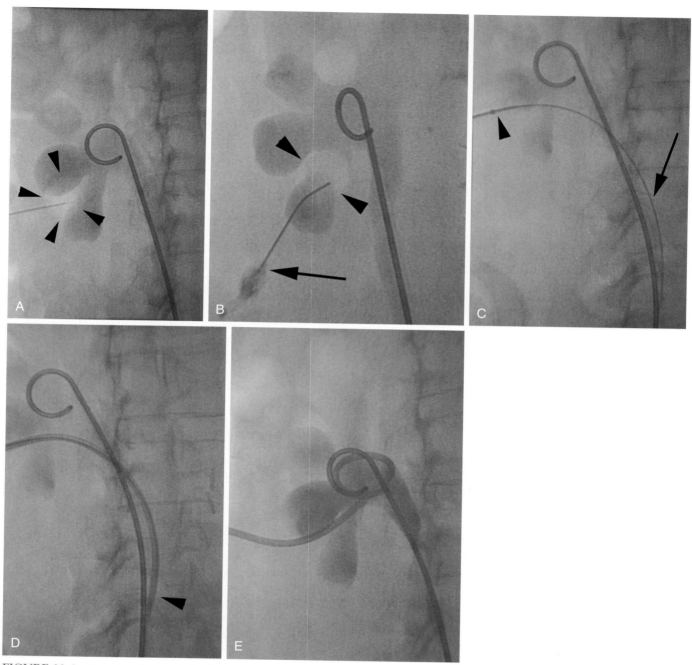

FIGURE 23-8 Stepwise placement of a decompressive nephrostomy. A retrograde stent is in position, which was not adequately decompressing the system. **A** and **B**, Two different obliquities show puncture of a posterior lower pole calyx, outlined by injected air *(arrowheads)*. The 22-gauge needle *(arrow)* has been connected to tubing for injection with continuous fluoroscopic observation. A 0.018-inch wire was advanced through the collecting system. **C**, The coaxial set *(arrowhead)* has been advanced over the 0.018-inch wire, which has been removed and a stiffer 0.035-inch wire *(arrow)* has been advanced down the ureter. **D**, The nephrostomy tube *(arrowhead)* has been advanced down the ureter over the wire. **E**, The nephrostomy tube has been partially withdrawn and the pigtail has been formed in the renal pelvis.

generally are preferred over other self-retaining catheters (e.g., Malecot, accordion, Foley). The nonpigtail catheters occasionally may be useful in collecting systems not capacious enough to accommodate a pigtail. In patients for whom access was provided for PCNL, a 5-Fr catheter is often left in the bladder alongside the nephros-tomy tube, giving the urologist a stable access for a stiff working wire as well as access to the renal pelvis from the nephrostomy tube.

The catheter is secured to the skin using adhesive dressings or suture. Adhesive dressings minimize cath-eter kinking and reduce the risk of catheter dislodgment.

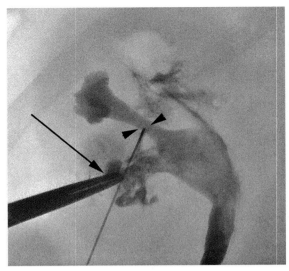

FIGURE 23-9 Initial puncture *(arrowheads)* was into an infundibulum. This needle was left in place to inject contrast/air to guide a second needle into a lower pole calyx. A needle driver *(arrow)* is placed on the patient to mark the proposed skin entrance site. A small amount of extravasation is seen.

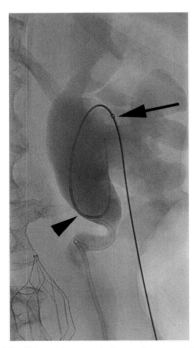

FIGURE 23-10 The patient needed a nephrostomy for treatment of a lower pole stone not well seen on this image. Urology requested superior pole access. The outer dilator of the coaxial set is at the access point in the posterior superior pole calyx, which is outlined by injected air *(arrow)*. Given the steep angle of entry to the renal pelvis, an angled catheter *(arrowhead)* was necessary to guide the 0.035-inch wire into a more stable position before placement of the nephrostomy.

After the track has matured, a simple dry dressing may be placed over the exit site. The catheter is left to gravity drainage with close monitoring of urine output. It typically requires irrigation only if blood clots occlude the tube.

Patients should be followed closely after the procedure for hemorrhagic or septic complications. In patients with bilateral obstructive uropathy undergoing PCN, dramatic fluid and electrolyte shifts may occur with postobstructive diuresis. In carefully selected patients, PCN may be performed safely as an outpatient procedure.[17] In this situation, however, the operator should have a low threshold for admitting the patient if there is any evidence of hemorrhage, sepsis, or severe pain during or after the procedure.

Catheter Maintenance

Chronic indwelling nephrostomy tubes usually should be exchanged every 3 to 6 months to prevent encrustation and occlusion. Some patients may require exchanges as often as every 6 weeks. It is better to err on the side of frequent catheter exchanges than to have the catheter occlude and have the patient develop sepsis or further deterioration of renal function due to obstruction. If the catheter is initially exchanged at 3 months and appears to be functioning well, the interval may be increased by 1 month at a time for up to 6 months.

Colonization with bacteria, fungi, or both invariably develops in patients with chronic indwelling nephrostomy tubes.[18] Asymptomatic bacteremia occurs frequently (about 10% of the time) during routine catheter exchanges; preprocedural antibiotics are not successful at preventing bacteremia.[19] Nonetheless, some operators routinely give antibiotics for tube exchanges, particularly when the tube has been functioning poorly. For patients with cardiac valvular disease, a full course of antibiotics should be administered before catheter exchange to minimize the risk of bacteremia. Despite therapeutic levels of antibiotics during catheter exchange, a septic reaction may still occur as a reaction to endotoxin released into the vascular system.

Patients with occluded catheters can present a challenge for catheter exchange. The pigtail catheter retention string initially should be secured so that it is not pushed down the catheter into an occlusive tangle with repeated attempts at guidewire passage. Hydrophilic guidewires are preferred for negotiating an occluded catheter. If the endhole cannot be passed, a side hole is acceptable. After the guidewire is through the catheter, the string is released to allow the loop to open. If no guidewire can be passed, a sheath may be passed over the catheter, after its hub has been cut off. The catheter can then be removed and replaced through the sheath.

Catheter dislodgment represents an urgent situation, because rapid tube replacement is required to maintain track patency. Tracks that have not had a tube replaced within 48 to 72 hours are difficult to renegotiate. All patients with PCN tubes should be educated about the urgency of this situation. After sterile preparation, the track is probed with an angled 5-Fr catheter. Contrast may be injected to define the track, and a hydrophilic wire and/or the angled catheter is then negotiated back into the collecting system.

Results

In patients with obstructed, dilated collecting systems, a decompressive PCN can be placed successfully in almost all cases. Technical success should be expected in greater than 95% of cases.[20,21] In nondilated collecting systems or complex stone cases, technical success may decrease to 85% or less.

The clinical response to PCN by patients with urosepsis often is dramatic. In one series of patients with gram-negative septicemia and urinary obstruction complicated by infection, PCN reduced mortality from 40% to 8%.[22] However, PCN in patients with pyonephrosis may exacerbate or precipitate septicemia as a result of bacteria entering the bloodstream through peripapillary veins from catheter manipulation or overdistention.[22,23]

In patients with fungal urinary infections, antifungal agents can be infused directly into the collecting system. This approach is advantageous because effective therapeutic levels can be achieved in the urinary tract without the associated systemic toxicity from IV administration. Fungus balls can be disrupted mechanically and extracted through the nephrostomy tract.[8,24]

In most patients with azotemia due to obstruction, PCN provides rapid improvement of renal function.[25] The procedure commonly is used as a temporizing measure to improve renal function while the underlying obstruction is addressed definitively. In patients with terminal malignancies and azotemia due to bilateral obstruction, unilateral PCN usually suffices to preserve renal function.[26] Bilateral drainage is indicated if pyonephrosis is suspected or unilateral drainage is unsatisfactory for restoring renal function. Unfortunately, the median survival rate of patients with advanced malignant urinary obstruction is 3 to 7 months.[27] Even with careful patient selection, 32% of patients are unable to achieve any improvement in quality of life after PCN.[28] After an open and frank discussion about the physical, emotional, and financial burdens associated with a drainage catheter, most patients and families opt for the drainage catheter as a means to extend life for as little as a few months.

Complications

The mortality rate for PCN is about 0.2%, which compares favorably with the mortality rate for surgical nephrostomy ($\leq$6%).[20] The major procedure-related complications are bleeding and sepsis. Hemorrhage requiring transfusion or other treatment occurs in 1% to 3% of patients undergoing PCN.[20] One series of 144 nephrostomies placed using combined CT and fluoroscopic guidance had no hemorrhagic or other major complications.[29] Most bleeding associated with PCN is transient and self-limited. It is not uncommon to have pink urine for several days after the procedure. If small clots block the catheter, the catheter should be irrigated with sterile saline.

Major arterial injury should be suspected when the urine remains grossly bloody after 3 to 5 days, when new clots are demonstrated in the collecting system on follow-up nephrostograms, or when there is a significant drop in hematocrit. These patients should undergo angiographic evaluation with embolization of injured vessels (Fig. 23-11). If the initial angiogram is negative, the nephrostomy may be removed over a guidewire to relieve the tamponading effect of the catheter, and the angiogram is repeated. If the drop in hematocrit is out of

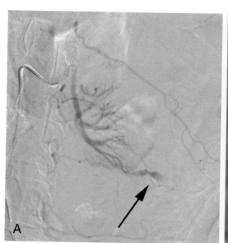
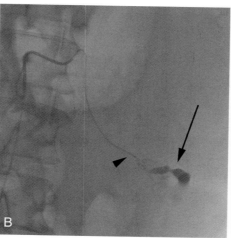
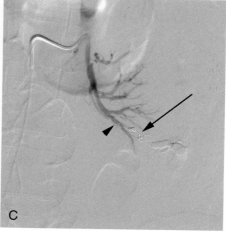

FIGURE 23-11 Arterial injury from percutaneous nephrostomy. The patient had persistent bright red hematuria after removal of a lower pole nephrostomy. **A,** Selective left renal artery angiography shows active extravasation *(arrow)* from a lower pole branch in the previous location of the nephrostomy tube. **B,** A 3-Fr microcatheter *(arrowhead)* has been advanced to the distal aspect of the offending branch and injection shows extravasation *(arrow).* **C,** Angiography from the microcatheter *(arrowhead)* after coil embolization *(arrow)* shows reflux into normal renal artery branches and occlusion of the previously bleeding lower pole branch.

proportion to the quantity of blood in the urine, the patient may have a retroperitoneal hematoma. Retroperitoneal hemorrhage is best evaluated with CT. Unsuspected retroperitoneal hematomas not requiring treatment have been reported in up to 13% of patients.[30] Significant hemorrhage usually is caused by laceration of lobar arteries. Pseudoaneurysm, arteriovenous fistula, arteriocaliceal fistula, or frank extravasation may be seen at arteriography. The risk of hemorrhage is minimized by using fine needles for puncture, using appropriate guidance, and avoiding puncture of the anteromedial renal vessels. The vast majority of these complications can be managed endovascularly.[31]

Although there is always concern for infection in patients with the need for urinary decompression, sepsis only occurs in approximately 1% to 3.6% of patients undergoing nephrostomy placement (the higher incidence seen in patients undergoing decompression for suspected infection).[32] Patients with infected urine or stones are at higher risk for PCN-related sepsis. For elective PCN for stone disease, antibiotic therapy ideally should be initiated and continued until the urine is clear. Diagnostic nephrostograms, ureteral catheterization, and stent placement should be delayed in patients with pyonephrosis until the urine has cleared.

Pleural complications include pneumothorax and empyema from infected urine entering the pleural space along the nephrostomy track. These complications are prevented by obtaining access beneath the 12th rib. One study showed that PCN tracks above the 12th rib traverse the pleura in 29% of cases on the right and 14% of cases on the left.[33] Pleural complications occur in only about 0.2% of decompressive nephrostomies.[21] When supracostal access is required for stone therapy, the risk of pleural complications increases to as much as 12%.[34,35] However, many pleural transgressions remain clinically silent.

Minor perforations of the collecting system occur in about 2% of patients. If a satisfactory drainage catheter is placed in the collecting system, these leaks usually heal spontaneously over the next 48 to 72 hours. The risk of urine leak as well as hemorrhage is increased with a direct renal pelvis puncture (Fig. 23-12). Urinomas requiring drainage are less common and occur rarely with standard 8- to 12-Fr PCN tubes. After removal of larger PCN catheters used for nephrostolithotomy, urinomas are more common. Other rare complications of PCN include air embolism and puncture of the colon, spleen, liver, and gallbladder.[36-39]

Catheter dislodgment is a relatively common occurrence. In a recent review of 283 patients with 325 nephrostomy tubes, there was an episode of complete dislodgment of the catheter in 16.6% of the patients. The vast majority of the tubes were replaced through the

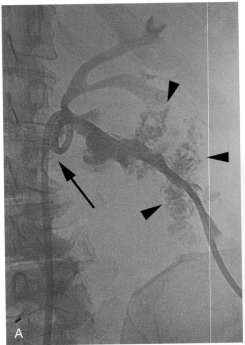
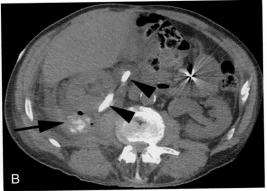

FIGURE 23-12   **A,** Nephroureteral catheter *(arrow)* was placed to treat a ureteral stricture. Injection of the catheter shows extravasation *(arrowheads)* extending from the pelvis and along the track. **B,** Computed tomography shows that the catheter *(arrowheads)* directly enters the renal pelvis. Extravasated contrast *(arrow)* is present in the perinephric space along the track.

preexisting track, with a limiting factor of track maturity. Successful replacement rates were 17%, 35%, and 97% in tracks less than 4 weeks old, less than 6 weeks old, and more than 6 weeks old, respectively.[40] Some patients have recurrent dislodgment of their tubes. One author describes a solution by placement of a renal "U-tube." This tube goes in one polar calyx and out the other pole with side holes within the collecting system.[41] Malecot catheters commonly used after nephrostomy track dilation may become difficult to extract if tissue bridges grow over the catheter flanges.[42] These devices should therefore be used with caution for long-term drainage. The entrapped catheters may be safely removed using endoscopic techniques to cut the anchoring tissue bridges.

URETERAL STENT PLACEMENT

Patient Selection

Ureteral stent placement is indicated for a broad variety of clinical problems (Box 23-2). PCN tube placement with antegrade stent placement usually is reserved for patients in whom retrograde attempts are unsuccessful or not feasible. For patients with nephroureteral obstruction, ureteral stents have distinct advantages over external drainage through a PCN tube. The drainage with stents is internalized, eliminating the need for external drainage tubing and collecting bags. The completely internalized ureteral stent is tolerated better by patients, and it decreases the risk of urosepsis from the inevitable colonization of external drainage catheters.[43,44] Ureteral stents also have several disadvantages. Stent malfunction may not be detected quickly and often requires sonography or cystography for diagnosis. Stent patency varies with the clinical situation. Stone-forming patients tend to develop rapid stent occlusion, and stent

exchange may be required as frequently as every 6 weeks. In general, stents should be exchanged at least every 6 months with transurethral cystoscopic or fluoroscopic guidance to prevent encrustation and occlusion. Stents may cause debilitating irritation of the bladder wall or trigone. Some patients prefer externally draining PCN tubes because function can be assessed easily and replacement is simple.

The nephroureteral (NU) stent is an alternative to externally draining PCN tubes and internally draining ureteral stents. This device differs from the standard double-J ureteral stent in that it has a retention loop positioned in the renal pelvis and a short segment of catheter extending out the nephrostomy track. The external segment of catheter may be capped to restore antegrade flow of urine from the renal pelvis, through the stent, and into the urinary bladder. The advantage of this device is that diagnosis of occlusion requires only a nephrostogram. If the patient develops flank pain or fever, she or he can open the catheter to external drainage until receiving medical attention. Likewise, catheter exchange over a guidewire is simple and does not require anesthesia, cystoscopy, or other transurethral interventions. These catheters are ideal for short-term ureteral stenting when it is advantageous to maintain access to the upper urinary tract for further evaluation with nephrostograms or a Whitaker test.

External PCN drainage is preferred over ureteral stents in several situations, particularly when there are contraindications to ureteral stent placement (Box 23-3). In the occasional patient with vesicocutaneous fistula due to advanced pelvic malignancy, diversion of urine with ureteral occlusion is beneficial to facilitate fistula closure and minimize tissue breakdown and nursing care requirements. Nephroureteral catheters are available with ureteral occlusion balloons to treat this difficult group of patients.

BOX 23-2

INDICATIONS FOR URETERAL STENT PLACEMENT

- Bypass ureteral obstructions
- Divert urinary stream to allow leaks to heal
- Maintain ureteral caliber after interventions
- Facilitate stone fragment passage during extracorporeal shock wave lithotripsy
- Provide palpable landmark for localization of the ureter at surgery

---

BOX 23-3

CONTRAINDICATIONS TO URETERAL STENT PLACEMENT

- Bladder outlet obstruction
- Spastic or noncompliant bladder
- Bladder fistula
- Incontinence
- Active hematuria
- Active infection

Technique

For antegrade stent placement, the ideal nephrostomy access should provide a reasonably straight vector down the ureter from an interpolar or upper pole calyx. However, with available guidewires, catheters, and sheaths, antegrade stents can be placed even from a lower pole access. Stent placement is facilitated by allowing the PCN track to mature for 1 to 2 weeks. Waiting allows access-related bleeding and hematuria to clear, decreasing the risk of stent occlusion from blood clots. Decompression via percutaneous drainage also reduces urothelial inflammation and edema. Once the system has been decompressed for several weeks, it is generally easier to negotiate the ureteral obstruction with a wire, catheter, and subsequently a stent.

Almost all ureteral strictures can be traversed with a curved catheter and an angled hydrophilic guidewire (Fig. 23-13). If the catheter buckles in the renal pelvis, a sheath may be advanced into the proximal ureter. When the guidewire has crossed the obstruction, a catheter should be advanced and injected to confirm its location in the bladder. Vigorous or overzealous manipulation of the hydrophilic guidewire may easily puncture the urothelium. A 4-5 Fr hydrophilic catheter usually follows the hydrophilic guidewire into the urinary bladder. The hydrophilic guidewire should then be exchanged for a stiff guidewire. If necessary, the stricture is dilated to allow the ureteral stent to pass freely to the bladder. Dilators may be used to dilate to 1 Fr size larger than the ureteral stent. Alternatively, a 3- to 4-mm angioplasty balloon may be used.

The appropriate stent length is determined by using a guidewire to measure the distance between the midbladder and the renal pelvis. Most patients require a 22- to 26-cm stent. If the stent is too long, it may irritate the bladder trigone. Ureteral stent placement can be placed either directly over the wire or through a peel-away sheath. For most cases, 6- to 8-Fr stents are preferred. Larger stents may cause ureteral ischemia and stricture formation but are used routinely when preservation of ureteral caliber is important, such as after stricture dilation. The stent is assembled with the inner stiffener and the pushing catheter.[45,46] It is advanced over the guidewire, through either a peel-away or standard sheath, and into the urinary bladder (Fig. 23-14). The upper end of the stent must be identified fluoroscopically and positioned well within the

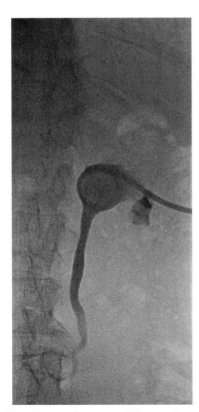

FIGURE 23-13   Ureteral obstruction following decompression with percutaneous nephrostomy. Approximately 2 weeks after percutaneous nephrostomy tube placement, antegrade nephrostogram shows high-grade stenosis of the low ureter.

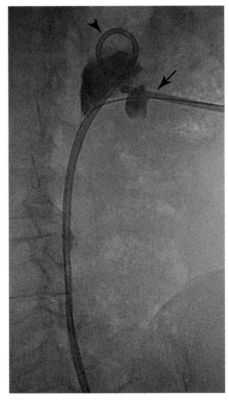

FIGURE 23-14   Double-J ureteral stent placement through preexisting percutaneous nephrostomy (PCN) tube track. A safety wire was placed through a sheath in the PCN tube track. A double-J ureteral stent *(arrowhead)* was placed over a stiff guidewire and the sheath *(arrow)* was left in to help form the retention loop in the renal pelvis.

collecting system, usually in the renal pelvis. The peel-away sheath is then removed. Holding the pushing catheter in place, the stiffener is removed. By gently pulling on the suture attached to the proximal end of the stent, it can be positioned in the renal pelvis and the pigtail configuration formed. This step usually requires withdrawal of the stiff guidewire, at least until only the floppy tip remains in the proximal end of the stent. When the proximal end of the stent is released, the guidewire may be advanced and coiled in the renal pelvis for subsequent nephrostomy placement. Alternatively, the nephrostomy may be placed over a safety guidewire introduced at the beginning of the procedure. The suture is cut and removed by pulling on one end while observing the stent fluoroscopically to ensure it remains in optimal position.

A nephrostomy tube usually is left in place, draining externally, for 24 hours (Fig. 23-15). After 2 hours, if hematuria has cleared, the PCN should be capped to force urine through the stent and prevent early stent occlusion with clot. If the patient subsequently develops flank pain or fever, the PCN can be opened to gravity drainage. An antegrade nephrostogram is performed the day after stent placement to confirm stent location and patency before nephrostomy removal. The nephrostomy should be removed under fluoroscopic observation, preferably over a wire to ensure that it does not become entangled in the ureteral stent or cause trauma as the tip of the loop drags against the track wall.

If there is great difficulty advancing catheters over the guidewire and through the stricture, the guidewire may be passed through the urethra to provide through-and-through access and facilitate catheter passage. A blunt Foley catheter lubricated with viscous lidocaine jelly is passed into the bladder. A guidewire then is advanced through the Foley catheter, which is exchanged for a short vascular sheath to protect the urethra during subsequent interventions. The ureteral guidewire may be captured in the bladder using a vascular snare and pulled out through the urethra to provide secure, through-and-through access.[47] With both ends of the wire held securely, a stent can be advanced through almost any stricture.

This technique also has proven useful for replacement of ureteral stents in women (Fig. 23-16). After capturing the free end of the stent in the urinary bladder, it is pulled through the urethra. As soon as the stent tip is brought out of the urethra, a guidewire is advanced up the stent into the renal pelvis. Stent replacement over the guidewire is then straightforward. This fluoroscopically guided technique is successful in up to 97% of cases.[48] It is simple and well tolerated by female patients because of the short urethra.

Patients with urinary diversions into an ileal conduit who develop obstruction may be treated with retrograde, antegrade, or combined placement of ureteral stents. If contrast refluxes from the conduit into the ureter, the

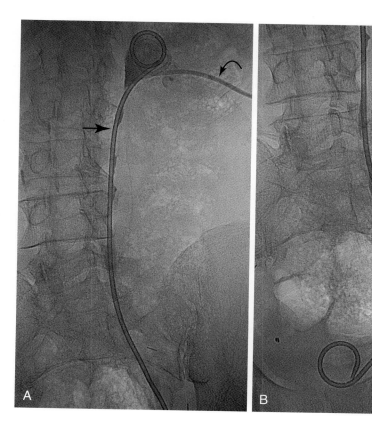

FIGURE 23-15 Double-J ureteral stent in a patient with ureteral obstruction from cervical carcinoma. **A,** Final placement with double-J stent *(arrow)* and low-profile percutaneous nephrostomy (PCN) *(curved arrow).* **B,** Appropriately placed double-J stent with the lower loop in the bladder.

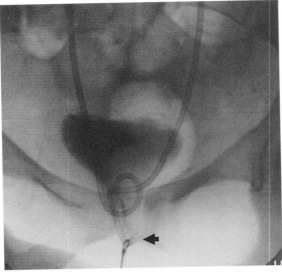

FIGURE 23-16   Fluoroscopically guided exchange of ureteral stents. The left stent has been snared (*arrow*) and is being withdrawn through a sheath placed in the urethra.

ureter may be fluoroscopically catheterized.[49] Alternatively, after decompressive PCN, antegrade catheterization of the occluded ureteroenteric anastomosis is usually simple. The guidewire then may be passed out the ileal loop and a locking pigtail catheter may be advanced retrograde into the renal pelvis (Fig. 23-17). The hub of the catheter is left free in the urinary collection bag. This approach minimizes the number of catheters and collection bags required for decompression.[50-52]

Results and Complications

Successful antegrade placement of ureteral stents can be achieved in greater than 80% of cases. The most frequent complication encountered with ureteral stents is occlusion due to encrustation. The rate at which encrustation develops is highly variable and depends on the degree of crystalloid supersaturation in the urine and on the presence of infection. Long-term stent patency varies from 2 to 18 months. Stent life may be optimized by

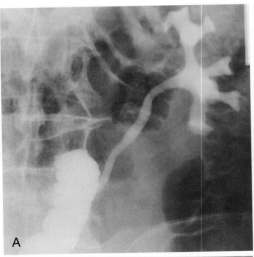

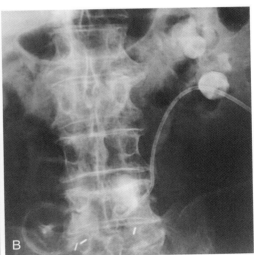

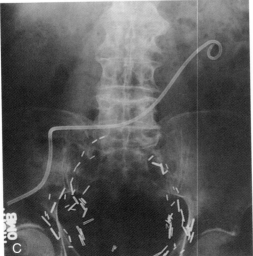

FIGURE 23-17   Conversion of a percutaneous nephrostomy (PCN) to a retrograde ureteral catheter in a patient with urinary diversion into an ileal loop. **A,** Initial loopogram shows reflux into the left ureter. **B,** The ureteroenteric anastomosis subsequently became strictured and a left PCN was performed. At that time, it was easy to cross the anastomotic obstruction and place a nephroureteral catheter. **C,** To simplify the drainage, a guidewire is passed out the loop, and a locking pigtail catheter is advanced retrograde up the ureter. The catheter hub is left free in the loop drainage bag.

encouraging patients to maintain a high fluid intake. Stents ideally should not be placed into bloody or infected collecting systems. Prophylactic antibiotics may prolong stent patency by minimizing the risk of infection and the associated acceleration of encrustation but increase the risk of infection with resistant organisms. Patients should be evaluated clinically at 3 months, and if stent occlusion is suspected, sonography or cystography should be performed. Stents should be routinely exchanged at least every 6 months.

Other complications of ureteral stent placement include stent migration and malpositioning, stent fracture, collecting system perforation, and urinary tract infection due to reflux and bladder irritation. Hematuria and erosive damage to the ureter can also occur. Bladder irritation often occurs if the stent is too long, especially when it pushes against the bladder trigone. Urinary urgency and frequency are common symptoms associated with bladder irritation from ureteral stents. Symptoms may be reduced with antispasmodics and usually resolve over several days. However, if symptoms of bladder irritation persist or are refractory to medical therapy, the stent may have to be removed or resized.

Mild hematuria is a relatively common complication of ureteral stents and is usually due to urothelial inflammation. A less common complication associated with more chronic placement of ureteral stents is erosion, either into the renal parenchyma or through the ureter, leading to urine leak. The stent can also erode into vascular structures, either in the renal parenchyma or along the course of the ureter, leading to hematuria. Hematuria can be mild to severe and intermittent to constant. Radiation exposure, pelvic surgery, ureteral ischemia, and iliac artery aneurysms are predisposing factors.[53] Management includes removal or repositioning of the stent, urinary diversion, and embolization as needed to control hemorrhage.

BENIGN URETERAL STRICTURE DILATION

Etiology

Ureteral stricture and obstruction are relatively common urologic problems that have many different etiologies (Box 23-4). Diagnostic and treatment options include PCN placement, antegrade nephrostogram and at times, ureteroplasty and ureteral stent placement. Ideally, the underlying abnormality can be corrected, but either ureteral stent or percutaneous drainage is often required for long term preservation of renal function.

Iatrogenic injuries to the ureter are very common with urologic procedures; almost half of all iatrogenic ureteral injuries result in strictures.[54] Stricture is generally due to ischemia and subsequent scarring of the ureter.

BOX 23-4

CAUSES OF URETERAL STRICTURES

Malignant Lesions

- Primary urothelial tumor
- Compression or invasion by retroperitoneal or pelvic malignancies

Benign Lesions

- Iatrogenic
- Urologic procedures
- Gynecologic or general surgical procedures
- Ureteroenteric anastomotic strictures
- Recurrent stone passage
- Penetrating trauma
- Radiation therapy
- Infection (e.g., tuberculosis, bilharziasis)
- Retroperitoneal fibrosis

Technique

Access to the renal collecting system for ureteroplasty is similar to that for any other purpose. Entry through the relatively avascular Brödel plane helps decrease the risk of bleeding and a posterior calyx is selected, taking care to optimize the angle of approach. A steep angle, either through a lower pole or upper pole calyx can make treatment much more challenging. Once the collecting system is accessed, a gentle nephrostogram is performed and guiding catheter or sheath placed into the proximal ureter (Fig. 23-18).

Through the guide catheter, the stenosis or occlusion is crossed with a hydrophilic wire and, if needed, a curved hydrophilic catheter. The guidewire is then exchanged for a stiff working wire. If there is difficulty advancing the catheter over the guidewire, the guidewire may be snared in the urinary bladder, affording through-and-through control, enabling the catheter (and later the balloon) to be more easily advanced over the wire. After confirming correct catheter placement in the bladder, a balloon should be advanced to the level of the stenosis and inflated (Fig. 23-19). Typical balloon sizes range from 4 to 10 mm in size and if there is scar or fibrosis, a high pressure or cutting balloon may be necessary.[55,56]

Once ureteroplasty has been performed, a nephro-ureteral (NU) stent is left across the lesion for at least 6 weeks to serve as a scaffold for urothelial healing.

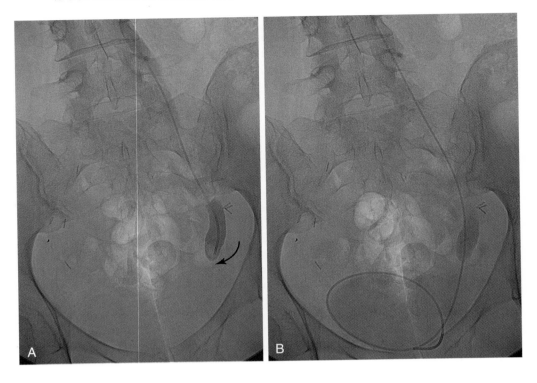

FIGURE 23-18 Ureteral dilatation and occlusion related to prior pelvic surgery. **A,** Following percutaneous access, wire and catheter are used to select the distal ureter. Contrast injection shows abrupt termination of the ureter *(curved arrow).* **B,** The obstruction has been crossed with a wire and catheter, which is looped in the bladder.

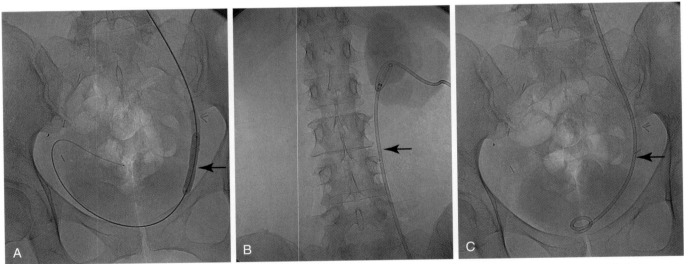

FIGURE 23-19 Treatment of ureteral occlusion related to prior pelvic surgery. **A,** The low ureteral stenosis has been crossed, initially with a glidewire and angled catheter. The glidewire has been exchanged for a stiff guidewire and an 8-mm balloon is inflated at the level of stenosis. **B** and **C,** Following ureteroplasty, a nephroureteral stent was placed (8 Fr) and will remain as a scaffold to urothelial healing for at least 6 weeks.

Stents of at least 8 to 10 Fr are generally used. If larger catheters are needed or desired, an internal-external biliary catheter with extra proximal side holes can be placed with the pigtail loop formed in the bladder. After 6 to 8 weeks, the NU stent is removed over a guidewire and an antegrade nephrostogram is performed. The Whitaker test may also be helpful if there is concern for residual obstruction (see later). If the ureter looks patent and there is flow across the lesion into the bladder, the NU stent can be replaced with a double-J ureteral stent and nephrostomy catheter or just a nephrostomy catheter. A trial of capping the nephrostomy tube is recommended before giving up percutaneous access. If initial trials fail, attempts should be made with either a larger balloon, a cutting balloon with a larger stent, or possibly with a cryoballoon[43,57,58] (Fig. 23-20).

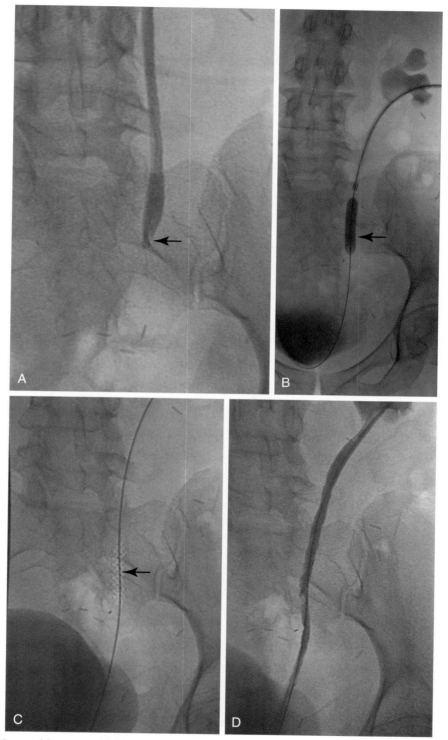

FIGURE 23-20   **A,** A 40-year-old woman with history of anorectal carcinoma and low anterior resection of the colon and rectum with adjuvant chemotherapy and external beam radiation to the pelvis. She developed ureteral obstruction following external beam radiation therapy. Despite a trial with double-J ureteral stents, she suffered from recurrent obstruction, urinary tract infection, and urosepsis. Initial image from antegrade nephrostogram shows occlusion of the ureter *(arrow).* **B,** Initial attempt at ureteroplasty performed with a conventional 8-mm balloon after ureteral obstruction was crossed with a glidewire and lesion predilated with a low-profile 4-mm balloon. **C,** After failing ureteroplasty with an 8-mm conventional balloon and cutting balloon, an attempt was made with a cryoplasty balloon *(arrow).* **D,** Final image from antegrade nephrostogram following ureteroplasty with 8-mm cryoballoon and 6 weeks of nephroureteral stent placement.

Results

Although the immediate technical success of ureteral dilation exceeds 90%, long-term patency is highly variable. In one series of multiple balloon dilation procedures on 28 benign strictures, long-term patency was maintained in only 18% of treated lesions.[55] Other investigators have identified groups of patients who respond more favorably. Lang and Glorioso[59] reported that 91% of strictures less than 3 months old responded to dilation, compared with 53% of older strictures. Strictures associated with ischemia or fibrosis responded in only 21%, whereas 70% of strictures without vascular compromise responded well. Other series found no such difference in outcome based on the interval between ureteral injury and treatment.[60]

Tuberculous strictures have been treated successfully in 75% of cases and probably close to 100% for strictures less than 1.5 cm long.[61] Strictures of ureteroenteric anastomoses have been treated successfully with balloon dilation in 50% and 70% of native and transplant kidneys, respectively.[62,63] Strictures related to ureterolithotomy, ureteral endoscopy, and gynecologic surgery responded in 100%, 71%, and 62% of cases, respectively, in one series.[64] However, strictures associated with radical hysterectomy or retroperitoneal fibrosis responded poorly (33% and 0%, respectively). Interpretation of this widely varying and often contradictory literature is difficult. Series with the most meticulous and rigorous follow-up also tend to report the lowest long-term patency.

SUPRAPUBIC BLADDER CATHETER PLACEMENT

Patient Selection

Suprapubic catheters are indicated for the treatment of patients with urinary retention who are unable to have a transurethral catheter placed or for whom transurethral placement is contraindicated.[65,66] It is also useful in patients with urethral injury requiring urinary diversion (often after pelvic trauma or surgery). These tubes also avoid the urethral trauma and subsequent urethral stricture formation associated with transurethral catheters. Additionally, suprapubic catheters are associated with increased patient satisfaction when compared to chronic indwelling transurethral catheters, and they do not directly interfere with sexual function. Voiding trials can be performed by clamping the catheter, while maintaining access to the bladder, and the suprapubic track can be used for percutaneous instrumentation of the bladder and ureter. Suprapubic catheters are also associated with lower rates of urinary tract infection than long-term indwelling transurethral catheters.[67,68] However, intermittent catheterization is still the preferred and safest means of managing chronic bladder dysfunction.

Historically, suprapubic catheter placement was performed by the urologist in the operating room under general anesthesia. More recently, urologists place smaller (8- to 12-Fr) catheters at the bedside, in clinic, or in surgery, without image guidance.[69] Larger bore catheters are generally thought to be superior for long-term management, and if placed by urology staff, are placed in the operating room under general anesthesia.[66] Using ultrasound or CT guidance allows safe placement of larger bore catheters with local anesthetic and conscious sedation, even in complicated cases.

The few contraindications to suprapubic catheter placement include bladder malignancy, abdominal wall infection, coagulopathy, and a nondistensible bladder.

Technique

Preprocedure antibiotic coverage should be based on the clinical scenario and presence or absence of infection and obstruction. If urine cultures are clear with no overt signs of urinary tract infection, a single preprocedural dose of a first-generation cephalosporin is recommended.

The bladder should be distended for suprapubic catheter placement. If necessary, fluid can be infused through a transurethral catheter and contrast can be used to improve visualization of the bladder with fluoroscopy. An appropriate entry site should be midline and low enough to avoid the peritoneal reflection and bowel. Placing the patient in Trendelenburg orientation may help move abdominal contents away from the suprapubic region. The entry site and catheter track are then anesthetized with lidocaine. A small incision is made in the anterior abdominal wall and a needle is advanced into the bladder (Fig. 23-21). Once placement is confirmed with ultrasound, CT, or fluoroscopy, a stiff wire is advanced into the bladder.

Serial dilatation of the track and a peel-away sheath are generally needed to introduce the catheter through the anterior abdominal wall.[66] Almost any type of percutaneous drain can be used. However, a Foley (with an end ole) is preferred by the urology service and is well tolerated, relatively safe from inadvertent removal (with a retention balloon), and inexpensive. In addition, it is the catheter with which most ancillary care providers are most comfortable working.

Small-bore (8- to 12-Fr) suprapubic catheters can be placed via a trochar technique as well as Seldinger technique. Larger suprapubic catheter placement (up to 18- to 20-Fr) can be performed percutaneously with image guidance, Seldinger technique, local anesthesia, and conscious sedation. It is particularly helpful to place them with image guidance in patients with complex bladder anatomy or in patients who have had prior bladder surgery, augmentation, or sphincter placement.

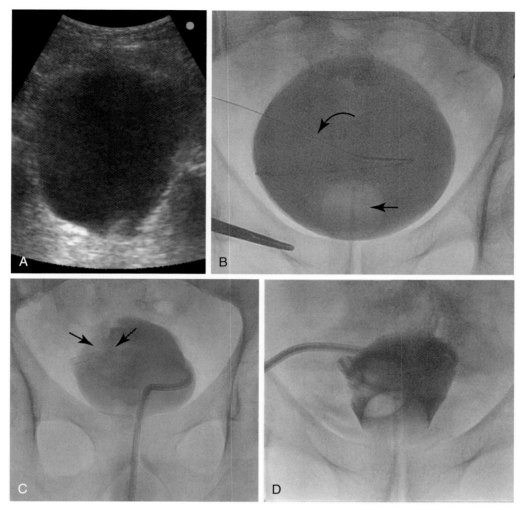

FIGURE 23-21 Suprapubic catheter placement. **A,** Typical ultrasound image of the bladder with moderate distention before suprapubic catheter placement. **B,** Transurethral Foley catheter placement *(arrow)* and distention of the bladder with contrast. The anterior bladder wall has been punctured and a guidewire is in place *(curved arrow).* **C,** Typical appearance following suprapubic catheter placement. A midline approach was used and the retention balloon is seen displacing contrast. **D,** A Council tip Foley catheter has been placed in the bladder from a suprapubic approach. A transurethral Foley is also in place, which allows bladder distention and improves visualization during suprapubic catheter placement.

Complications

Potential complications include bleeding, infection, and transperitoneal catheter placement with possible transcolonic or small bowel insertion.[70] The likelihood of adverse events is increased in patients with prior surgery, altered bladder anatomy, or adhesions.

URETERAL PERFUSION CHALLENGE (WHITAKER TEST)

Dilatation of the renal collecting system is a common finding in diagnostic radiology, and the differential diagnosis is large. Particularly in adults, most causes of hydronephrosis and ureteral dilatation are well evaluated with ultrasound, CT, or MR imaging (MRI). However, if no obvious obstructing lesion is identified, there are few options for differentiating obstructive from nonobstructive dilatation of the upper urinary tract (Box 23-5). Diuretic renography can be used in some cases, but in complex or equivocal cases, the ureteral perfusion challenge (Whitaker test) remains quite useful. This method has also been used to identify residual obstruction following surgical correction of obstruction.[71] The Whitaker test was developed and popularized by Robert Whitaker in the early 1970s.[72,73] It relies on serial pressure measurements in the renal pelvis and bladder during infusion of fluid into the upper collecting system to detect a pressure gradient across the ureteropelvic junction (UPJ), ureter, and ureterovesicular junction (UVJ).

Patient Selection

The Whitaker test is most useful in patients with persistent upper urinary tract dilatation with suspected obstruction and in patients following surgical or medical (chemotherapy) correction of obstruction (Fig. 23-22). It can be particularly useful for assessing potential upper urinary tract obstruction in the following circumstances: equivocal results from less invasive tests; suspected obstruction with poor kidney function; gross dilatation

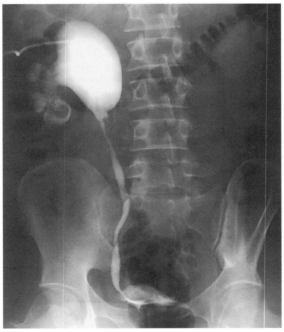

FIGURE 23-22   Positive ureteral perfusion challenge (Whitaker test) after pyeloplasty for ureteropelvic junction obstruction. The patient subsequently underwent endopyelotomy, which was followed by a normal perfusion challenge result and a good clinical outcome.

with a positive diuresis renogram.[71] Patients have generally already been evaluated with IV urography or radionuclide renography without a confident diagnosis being made. This procedure can also be helpful in a transplant kidney with suspected or poorly characterized obstruction. There are a few conditions that preclude the use of the ureteral perfusion challenge. Contraindications include uncorrectable coagulopathy, urinary tract infection, pregnancy, and inability to safely administer conscious sedation or general anesthesia.

Technique

The test uses a relatively simple apparatus. A small PCN tube or catheter is placed into the renal pelvis. A sample of urine from initial access should be sent for Gram stain and culture, even when infection is not suspected. Many patients with chronic obstruction and dilatation of the renal collecting system may be colonized and identification of an organism may be helpful for patient management.[74] Before ureteral perfusion is initiated, baseline manometry should be performed. If a large gradient is found at rest or the resting pressure within the kidney approaches 30 cm H_2O, no perfusion test is required and the test is considered positive for obstructive uropathy.

Although normal ureteral flow is only 0.25 to 0.5 mL/min, flow rates exceeding 10 mL/min have been recorded.[71,74] Infusion should thus be initiated at 10 mL/min for adults and 2 to 5 mL/min for children for up to 5 minutes, ideally through a power injector.[74] The infusate is dilute iodinated contrast material (about 50%), which allows fluoroscopic visualization of the dilated upper collecting system, the lower collecting system (often with a narrowed or stenotic segment), and the bladder. The perfusion pressure gradient is then measured serially in the kidney and in the bladder. If during infusion the pressure in the renal pelvis rises above 30 cm H_2O or continues to rise steadily, the exam is considered positive for obstructive uropathy.

Typically, the renal pelvis pressure is measured through a nephrostomy tube or antegrade percutaneous access. If a small-bore needle is used, it can introduce resistance to flow in the system and lead to a falsely elevated pressure is the renal pelvis. The bladder pressure can be measured via a Foley catheter or a suprapubic catheter. The bladder catheter should be left open to gravity to ensure that no urine is collecting in the bladder. Fluoroscopic confirmation of a nondistended bladder should be made before pressure measurement, because distention can lead to falsely elevated pressure readings in the bladder.

A pressure gradient less than 15 cm H_2O is considered normal. Pressure gradients between 15 and 22 cm H_2O are equivocal, and differences greater than 22 cm H_2O

indicate obstructive uropathy.[71] More recent reports claim that decreasing the pressure gradient threshold increases the sensitivity of the exam. These investigators have proposed using 12 cm H_2O gradient as the cutoff for normal, 12 to 18 cm H_2O as equivocal, and greater than 18 cm H_2O as indicative of obstructive uropathy.[74]

If the pressure gradient is initially equivocal, increasing the perfusion rate (up to 20 mL/min) can help resolve uncertainty and may unmask functional obstruction. When the test result is positive, spot films should be obtained to document the site of obstruction. If the challenge test result is negative or indeterminate, it may be helpful to repeat the study with the bladder distended, because some cases of obstruction are evident only after bladder filling. Likewise, repeating the challenge with the patient in different positions may produce a positive result.[75]

Results and Complications

The accuracy of the ureteral perfusion challenge has not been established, in part because there is no gold standard against which test results can be compared. Lupton and colleagues, in a study of 145 patients, found that 61 cases showed obstruction, 53 were unobstructed, 4 were equivocal, 17 showed abnormal peristalsis, and 10 described loin pain during the test.[71] They reported that the Whitaker test influenced patient management in 84% of cases and was accurate in diagnosing both obstructive and nonobstructive uropathy in 77% of cases.

Complications are, for the most part, related to percutaneous access to the upper collecting system and include pain, bleeding (retroperitoneal, parenchymal, or subcapsular hematoma), infection, sepsis, and damage or perforation of the collecting system with resultant urinoma. It is possible to rupture the collecting system during fluid infusion, making it important to limit perfusion pressures to approximately 30 cm H_2O.

HYSTEROSALPINGOGRAPHY AND FALLOPIAN TUBE RECANALIZATION

Of all causes of infertility, up to 45% have been attributed to the female partner. Between 10% and 35% of female infertility is due to tubal disease.[76,77] The leading cause of tubal disease is pelvic inflammatory disease (PID). Selective salpingography and fallopian tube recanalization can be used to treat proximal tubal occlusion and has been endorsed by the American Society for Reproductive Medicine as primary treatment of tubal occlusion when one or both tubes fail to fill at hysterosalpingography (HSG).[76,78] The proximal aspect (first 2 cm) of the fallopian tube is most amenable to recanalization. Recanalization of the more distal fallopian tube is more technically challenging

and is less likely to be associated with successful intrauterine pregnancy.[79]

The most common site of tubal occlusion is within the proximal, intramural portion of the fallopian tube, which is about 1 cm long and has a diameter of approximately 1 mm. Infection and subsequent inflammation or fibrosis are almost always responsible for tubal disease. Gonococcal and chlamydial salpingitis, postpartum endometritis, spasm, impacted mucus and debris, polyps and synechiae are all causes of proximal tubal occlusion. Fallopian tube occlusion in the isthmic, ampullary, or fimbriated portions of the tube usually is caused by previous pelvic infection or endometriosis.

Patient Selection

HSG and selective salpingography are indicated for evaluation and possible treatment of women thought to have infertility related to tubal occlusion, particularly in the isthmic portion of the tube. Recanalization should be attempted when bilateral proximal tubal occlusion is identified on hysterosalpingogram.

Technique

The procedure is generally performed on an outpatient basis and should be scheduled during the first 10 days of the menstrual cycle (i.e., follicular phase).[80] A pregnancy test should be performed on the day of the procedure, because pregnancy is one of the only absolute contraindications to the procedure. Prophylactic antibiotics (e.g., 100 mg of doxycycline, given twice daily) should be started on the day before the procedure and continued for 4 days afterward. The procedure is performed with sterile technique after standard scrubbing and draping of the perineum. IV conscious sedation usually is sufficient for patient comfort; paracervical anesthesia usually is not required.

A guiding catheter is inserted through the cervix under direct visualization. Commonly used catheters have an intrauterine retention balloon or a vacuum cup that is placed on the cervix. These devices provide a sterile conduit through which catheters and guidewires may be introduced. Conventional HSG should be performed with diluted water-soluble contrast to confirm proximal tubal occlusion and to localize the uterine cornua without obscuring the catheters. If HSG shows flow through the fallopian tubes, no further steps are taken (Fig. 23-23).

If the proximal tube is occluded, a 5-Fr catheter is advanced coaxially through the guiding catheter and used to selectively catheterize the tubal ostium. Full-strength contrast is then injected. If proximal tubal obstruction persists, efforts to clear the obstruction should be made (Fig. 23-24). A coaxial microcatheter system with

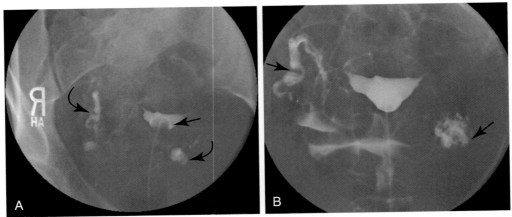

FIGURE 23-23   Normal hysterosalpingogram. **A,** Initial image from normal hysterosalpingogram shows balloon retention catheter *(straight arrow)* and flow through both fallopian tubes *(curved arrows)*, consistent with patent bilateral tubes. **B,** Later image shows further distension of the uterine cavity and contrast collecting in the peritoneum.

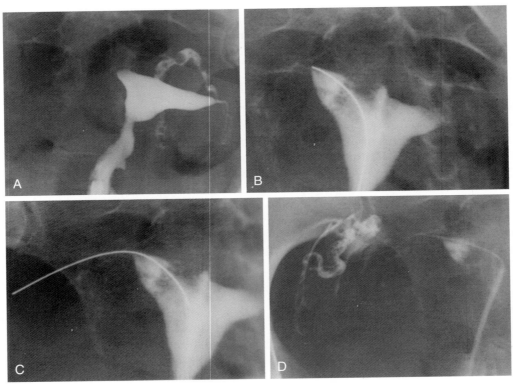

FIGURE 23-24   Fallopian tube recanalization. **A,** Hysterosalpingogram shows a left fallopian tube with intraperitoneal contrast spillage but no filling of the right tube. **B,** Selective right salpingography confirms occlusion of the right fallopian tube. **C,** A microcatheter and wire were manipulated across the occlusion. **D,** After removal of the microcatheter, repeat selective salpingography revealed patency of the right fallopian tube.

a 3-Fr catheter and a 0.018-inch or smaller guidewire is advanced through the 5-Fr outer catheter. When the microcatheter has been advanced beyond the obstruction, the guidewire is removed, and contrast is injected to check distal tubal patency. The microcatheter is then removed, and contrast is injected through the 5-Fr catheter to evaluate the tube. Recanalization is then performed on the other side, if necessary. A final HSG is obtained to confirm and document tubal patency.

A 0.035-inch hydrophilic guidewire placed directly through the 5-Fr catheter may cross the obstruction more easily and eliminate the need for microcatheters.[81] After successful guidewire traversal, the wire is removed, and distal tubal patency is confirmed by ostial injection through the 5-Fr catheter. The patient is observed for 30 to 60 minutes after the procedure and advised that vaginal spotting may occur for 3 days or less.

Instead of using a guide sheath or balloon catheter, a 5-Fr angle-tipped catheter can be advanced through the cervix with direct visual guidance. HSG can then be performed through the catheter. If the fallopian tube is obstructed, the catheter can be used to select the ostium and contrast injection performed. Ostial injection of contrast alone may clear the obstruction and result in fallopian tube visualization. However, if the tube does not fill following ostial injection, a glidewire or equivalent is advanced across the occluded segment. If the tube remains occluded, either a glidewire or microcatheter and wire can be used to attempt traversal of the tube. Once the occluded segment has been traversed, contrast injection should be performed to further delineate the fallopian tube anatomy.[82] At this point the tube may be patent and show only minimal persistent irregularity, which would be interpreted as successful recanalization. If the tube remains occluded proximally, opens proximally but remains occluded distally, or looks markedly irregular, the patient will require other solutions (e.g., surgical tube repair, in vitro fertilization).[83]

Results and Complications

Reporting standards for selective salpingography and fallopian tube recanalization have not been established, which makes comparison of techniques, success rates, and treatment strategies difficult.[76] No convincing evidence indicates that any one technique is superior. Technical success is high, with studies showing up to 73% success opening at least one fallopian tube.[76,84] Multiple studies have shown fertility rates as high as 20% to 34% following HSG and fallopian tube recanalization (in selected patients though to have tubal disease and occlusion per HSG).[76,84-86]

The rate of ectopic pregnancy is about 3% to 4%, which is comparable to the rate in the general population.[80,83] Fallopian tubes that require only minimal manipulation to reestablish patency are more likely to be associated with subsequent pregnancy than tubes requiring excessive guidewire and catheter manipulation. Some patients in the former category may have mucous plugs (which are flushed out by the initial selective contrast injection) without underlying mural disease. Although tubal disease does not preclude successful pregnancy, the pregnancy rates are higher when the tubes appear normal at salpingography. In one series, 95% of patients with tubal obstruction but normal tubes were successfully recanalized, and 45% became pregnant.[80]

If pregnancy has not occurred within 6 months of successful tubal recanalization, approximately 50% of evaluated patients are found to have reblockage of one or both fallopian tubes.[80] Repeat recanalization is possible, and pregnancies have resulted after the second or even third procedure.

Mild uterine cramping and vaginal bleeding are common after fallopian tube catheterization and should resolve within 2 to 3 days. Low-grade fevers may develop but infection is rare, especially with the use of prophylactic antibiotics. Tubal perforations occur in 2% to 5% of patients and usually require no additional treatment.[80] The radiation dose to the ovaries is generally less than 1 rad (10 mGy).[87]

STERILIZATION BY FALLOPIAN TUBE OCCLUSION

Permanent sterilization has been used as a means of contraception for many years. Historically, sterilization has been performed surgically, with either open or laparoscopic tubal ligation or vasectomy. Approximately 700,000 tubal ligations are performed each year in the United States and roughly half of them are performed separately from delivery (either vaginal or cesarean).[88] Transcervical approaches to sterilization have been developed as a minimally invasive alternative to surgical sterilization.[88,89]

Devices

Two hysteroscopic sterilization methods are currently available in the United States and approved by the FDA. The Essure Permanent Birth Control Systems (Conceptus, Inc.) method involves transcervical placement of a nickel titanium coil in the proximal fallopian tube. It measures 2 mm in diameter and is 4 cm long. It expands to fill the fallopian tube and induces an inflammatory response that over several weeks creates fibrosis and eventual scar. Because the device relies on fibrosis and scar formation, it cannot be relied on for contraception immediately after placement. A hysterosalpingogram is repeated 3 months after coil placement to confirm occlusion. Once bilateral occlusion is confirmed, the patient can discontinue other means of contraception.

The Adiana Permanent Contraception device (Hologic, Inc.) was introduced in 2002. In contrast to the Essure device, the Adiana system combines a low energy radiofrequency ablation with deposition of a polymer matrix in the proximal fallopian tube. It is designed to be performed with hysteroscopic guidance.

Patient Selection

Preprocedural evaluation should include a recent normal Pap smear, negative chlamydia and gonorrhea cultures, and negative pregnancy test. Contraindications to transcervical fallopian tube occlusion are the desire to maintain fertility, recent or current PID, prior tubal ligation, immunosuppression, nickel allergy, unexplained menometrorrhagia, pregnancy, and recent (<6 weeks) delivery or termination of pregnancy.[88,89]

Technique

The device can be placed with only moderate sedation and both fallopian tubes can be occluded in the same setting. Ideally the procedure is performed in the first 7 to 14 days following the patient's menstrual cycle (follicular phase). The patient is placed in a lithotomy position on the angiography table and the vulva and perineum are prepared and draped in a standard sterile fashion.[88] A sterile speculum is placed and the cervix is visualized, then prepped. Typically, a 12-Fr balloon catheter is placed and inflated to minimize contrast leakage from the cervix. A hysterosalpingogram is then performed. The fallopian tubes must be well visualized in order to proceed and visualization may require selective catheterization. Only if both tubes can be safely occluded should placement be performed, leading to the recommendation that the most difficult-appearing fallopian tube be addressed first.[88] The device has a 4.3-Fr outer diameter and once the fallopian tube is cannulated, the device is advanced until the third of four radiopaque markers is at the level of the tubal ostium. The coil is deployed and the process is repeated on the contralateral side.

Results

Successful placement of the Essure device has been reported in multiple studies to be 92% to 99%.[88,90]

The Essure device has been evaluated in the Essure phase II and pivotal trials.[88] Device placement was attempted in 745 patients between the two trials. Successful bilateral placement was performed in 88% of the phase 2 trial and 90% of the pivotal trial. Ninety-seven percent of women who had successful bilateral coil placement were able to rely on the device for primary birth control, and the device is effective in preventing pregnancy in 99.8% of cases. As of 2005, more than 50,000 Essure devices have been placed worldwide, most with hysteroscopic guidance.[91] Currently, device placement with fluoroscopic guidance is off-label.

A total of 770 women were enrolled in a trial using the Adiana system; 645 patients were actually treated.[92] Bilateral placement was achieved in 95% of patients. Evaluation with HSG was performed at 3 months to confirm tubal occlusion. Of the 645 women in the initial treatment group, 88% were able to rely on FTO for primary contraception, and based on pregnancy

rates in the first year of follow-up, there was a 1.07% failure rate.[91,92]

NONVASCULAR RENAL TRANSPLANT COMPLICATIONS

Approximately 18,000 kidney transplants were performed in the United States in 2009, as recorded by UNOS (United Network for Organ Sharing).[93] The most common nonvascular complications of kidney transplantation are perinephric fluid collections, obstruction, and ureteral stricture. Many perinephric fluid collections are asymptomatic and sometimes self-limited. Fluid collections associated with renal transplants include lymphoceles, urinomas, hematomas, seromas, and abscess. Ultrasound, CT, and MRI are used to detect and sometimes characterize these lesions.[94] However, aspiration and drainage are typically required for definitive diagnosis and treatment and percutaneous drainage for diagnosis and treatment is preferred over surgery in most patients.

All of these fluid collections can cause symptoms either from infection or mass effect. The most likely structures to be compressed are the ureter and the iliac vein. However, compression of the transplant renal vein, iliac artery and other pelvic veins has been reported. Ureteral compression can be associated with obstruction, and hydronephrosis and iliac vein compression can be associated with deep vein thrombosis and pulmonary embolism.[95,96]

Urinoma

Urinomas usually occur within the first several weeks of transplant and are associated with a urine leak. Urine leak following renal transplant is seen in up to 3% of cases with mean onset of 45 days.[97] Urine leaks are most common at the ureterobladder insertion and generally results from ureteral ischemia.[97] Diagnosis is typically made with a combination of imaging and aspiration or drain placement. Aspirated fluid should be sent for analysis and will show a high creatinine level. Ultrasound of urinomas typically shows an anechoic fluid collection with a paucity of septations and debris. The urine leak should be identified with either antegrade nephrostogram or retrograde nephrostogram/cystogram. Treatment should address the urine leak with ureteral stent placement, either from above via PCN or from below with double-J ureteral stent. A double-J ureteral stent is preferred for long-term stent placement due to the decreased incidence of infection in the immunocompromised transplant patient.[96] The urinoma often resolves once the leak has been addressed but if it persists or causes mass effect, a small-bore percutaneous drain is indicated.

Lymphocele

Lymphoceles are caused by leakage from damaged lymphatics in the pelvis or transplanted kidney. They are seen within weeks to years of surgery (usually within 1 to 2 months) and have been associated with up to 40% to 50% of kidney transplant patients.[96,98] Whereas they are often asymptomatic and resolve spontaneously, some cause graft dysfunction and loss.[99] Ultrasound and CT show hypoechoic fluid collections in the peritransplant region and may lead to outflow obstruction and hydronephrosis (Fig. 23-25). Analysis of the fluid will show creatinine content similar to serum. The gram stain and culture should be negative, and the cell count and differential may show few white blood cells with a predominance of lymphocytes.[98] First-line therapy consists of percutaneous drainage and (if necessary) sclerosis of the cavity with povidone-iodine, alcohol, doxycycline, or sotradecol.[100] Alternative treatment methods include open or laparoscopic marsupialization of the cavity.

Abscess

Any of the previously mentioned fluid collections can become infected and lead to abscess formation. In addition to mass effect, localized infection can extend to the kidney, and if severe, can lead to bacteremia. A peritransplant abscess usually presents with fever and pain. Imaging with ultrasound typically shows a mixed echogenicity cavity, often with septations and gas. Ultrasound can be used to place a percutaneous drain and, combined with IV antibiotics, is considered first-line therapy.[101]

Hematoma

Post kidney transplant hematomas are common and if small are typically asymptomatic. Larger hematomas can cause mass effect and are more likely to become infected, leading to abscess formation. Initial evaluation consists of ultrasound, usually showing an echogenic fluid collection with internal septations and debris. If there is no evidence of infection, aspiration and drainage should be avoided. If there is clinically significant mass effect or evidence of infection, a drainage catheter should be placed. Larger bore catheters (12- to 14-Fr) are often needed due to the thick, viscous nature of hematoma. If either an abscess or hematoma does not resolve with initial percutaneous drainage, intracavitary administration of 2 to 4 mg of tissue plasminogen activator (t-PA) can be used to help decrease overall viscosity and improve percutaneous drainage.[102]

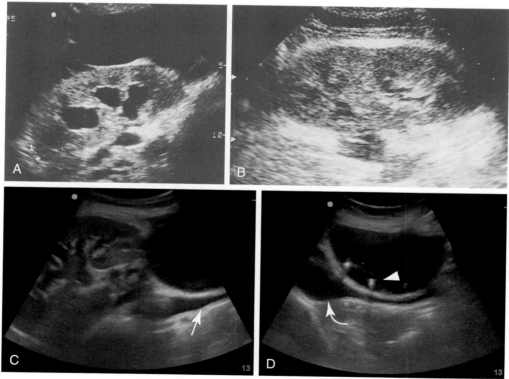

FIGURE 23-25 Renal transplant hydronephrosis due to extrinsic compression by a lymphocele. **A,** Initial ultrasound scan shows a large fluid collection superficial to the hydronephrotic transplant kidney. **B,** After percutaneous drainage and alcohol sclerosis of the lymphocele, ultrasound shows that hydronephrosis has resolved. **C,** A 69-year-old woman 6 weeks after a renal transplant complained of urinary frequency and had mildly elevated creatinine level. Initial ultrasound scan shows a large fluid collection *(arrow)* superficial to the hydronephrotic transplant kidney that after drainage was revealed to be a lymphocele. **D,** The lymphocele also compresses the bladder *(curved arrow)*. Percutaneous drain was placed for decompression *(arrowhead).*

t-PA administration will likely need to be repeated several times per day with regular flushing of the catheter to maximize percutaneous drainage.

Ureteral Obstruction

Ureteral obstruction in a transplant kidney may be difficult to distinguish from other causes of renal transplant dysfunction. Obstruction can result from multiple different etiologies, including blood clots, external compression, kinking, or frank anastomotic stricture (Figs. 23-26 and 23-27). Initial evaluation is done with ultrasound. Because the risk of PCN is low and the consequence of a delayed diagnosis of obstruction may be loss of the transplant, a low threshold for PCN as a diagnostic challenge is advocated.[103,104]

The transplant ureter is prone to ischemic injury and stenosis in part because of the disrupted blood flow during kidney harvest and transplant. The most common sites of stenosis are the distal ureter and the ureterovesical anastomosis. Extrinsic compression on the collecting system by hematoma, lymphocele, or urinoma can also produce an obstruction. If obstruction coexists with a fluid collection, percutaneous drainage of the fluid may relieve the collection and the obstruction (see Fig. 23-25).

When planning PCN of a kidney transplant, it is important to avoid entry into the peritoneum by making the needle entry lateral to the transplant and skin incision. Ultrasound is ideal for imaging guidance. An anterolateral upper or middle polar calyx should be selected to facilitate ureteral catheterization. Internalized stents are preferred over catheters that protrude externally to minimize the risk of infection in this immunocompromised group of patients. An antegrade nephrostogram is then done to evaluate the collecting system and ureter. The PCN access can also be used to traverse a ureteral stenosis or occlusion and dilate the stenotic lesion. Ureteral stents can also be placed from an antegrade access (Fig. 23-28).

Ureteral strictures are treated successfully with balloon dilation in about 60% to 70% of cases[103,104] (Fig. 23-29). However, the success of balloon dilation decreases with more chronic strictures and with longer stenoses.[96,103,104] In renal transplants with ureteral leakage, percutaneous treatment with nephroureteral stents is successful in 59% of cases.[104] However, surgical repair of post transplant urine leaks, especially in the early post transplant period, is still considered the gold standard of therapy.

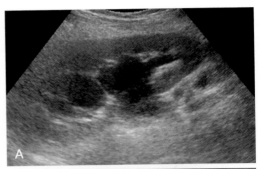

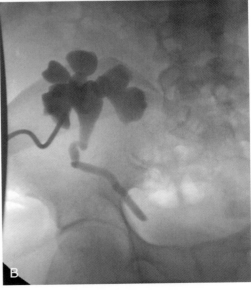

FIGURE 23-27   Outflow obstruction in a transplant kidney. **A,** Typical ultrasound image of left pelvic transplant kidney with moderate hydronephrosis. **B,** Antegrade nephrostogram performed after percutaneous nephrostomy tube placement shows a low ureteral obstruction at the ureterovesicular junction. There is also a mild stenosis in the midureter, likely representing a kink related to redundancy of the ureter.

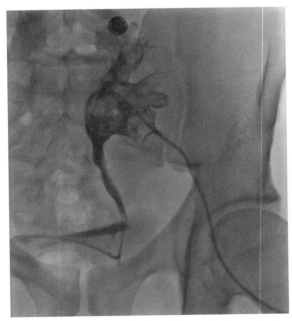

FIGURE 23-26   Transplant kidney 2 days after transplant with minimal urine output and small blood clots passing in urine. Antegrade nephrostomy catheter placed and antegrade nephrostogram performed, showing the entire renal collecting system filled with blood clot.

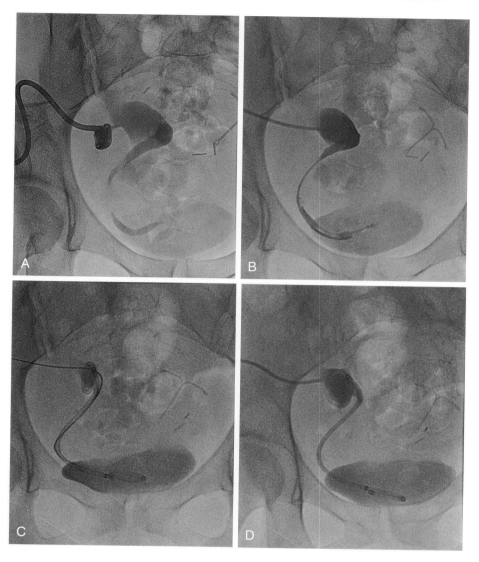

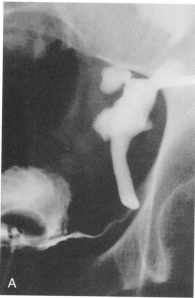

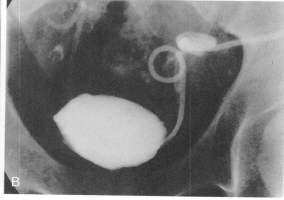

FIGURE 23-28 Transplant kidney ureteral stenosis and ureteral stent placement. **A,** Percutaneous nephrostomy (PCN) pulled back into a calyx of right pelvic transplant kidney. High-grade ureteral stenosis is present in the midureter, leading to hydronephrosis and renal compromise. **B,** The stenosis has been crossed with a wire and catheter. **C,** Double-J ureteral stent placed with safety wire in place. **D,** Double-J ureteral stent and PCN tube both in place. Once hematuria has cleared, capping trial of PCN will be performed and, if well tolerated, the PCN will be removed.

FIGURE 23-29 Treatment of an ischemic transplant ureteral stricture. **A,** The antegrade nephrostogram shows a stricture of the distal ureter 6 weeks after transplantation. **B,** The stricture was dilated with an 8-mm balloon, and a short ureteral stent was left in place for 8 weeks. The stent was then removed, and stricture has not recurred.

RENAL CYST ASPIRATION AND SCLEROSIS

Patient Selection

Cystic kidney lesions on imaging may represent a simple benign renal cyst, a complicated benign renal cyst, or a cystic malignancy. Cystic lesions are often classified with the Bosniak system.[105] Increased utilization combined with technologic advances in imaging have led to the increased diagnosis of cystic renal lesions. Some authors recommend a core biopsy of Bosniak category 3 lesions because of variability in the reported rates of malignancy in this subgroup.[106] However, lesions categorized into Bosniak category 1 or 2 are benign.[107] With continued advancements in multiphase, multidetector CT and MRI, diagnostic cyst puncture with cytologic evaluation and cystography is rarely necessary. However, cyst aspiration may be indicated in patients with recurrent urinary tract infections and concern for cyst infection.

Therapeutic cyst drainage with sclerosis is performed for renal cysts that may be responsible for pain, urinary tract obstruction, infection, or renin-dependent hypertension. Cyst sclerosis is performed to devitalize the secreting cuboidal epithelial cells lining the cyst cavity and prevent recurrence. Absolute alcohol (the most commonly used sclerosant) destroys the cyst epithelium within minutes and penetrates the cyst wall within 4 to 12 hours of exposure.[108] Other agents that have been used include sodium tetradecyl sulfate, glucose, phenol, Pantopaque, tetracycline, bismuth, and povidone-iodine.[109-111] Alternatives to cyst aspiration with sclerosis include percutaneous marsupialization or open and laparoscopic cyst unroofing.[109-111]

Technique

Renal cysts are aspirated easily using 21- or 22-gauge needles and sonographic guidance. Computed tomography occasionally is required for obese patients. The fluid in a benign simple cyst should be clear or slightly yellow. A small amount of blood that clears during the drainage usually indicates a traumatic tap. When malignancy is suspected, the entire volume of aspirated fluid is sent for cytologic analysis. Although this technique is reported to be quite sensitive, a negative result does not entirely exclude malignancy.[112]

A cystogram is performed after the cyst has been completely drained by replacing the aspirated volume with dilute contrast material. A simple benign cyst should have a perfectly smooth wall. Any wall irregularity suggests there may be a solid component, which should undergo biopsy.

Cyst sclerosis generally is performed through small pigtail catheters that tolerate absolute alcohol infusion. The cyst volume is estimated by calculations from imaging studies and by measuring the aspirated fluid volume. Dilute contrast then is injected using a volume that exceeds the anticipated volume of sclerosant to be administered. It is critical to confirm that all contrast remains in the cyst cavity and does not communicate with the collecting system or the vascular system or extravasate into the retroperitoneum. If extravasation is observed, the cystogram is repeated in several days to document closure from track maturation before proceeding with sclerosis. If communication with the collecting system or vascular system is seen, sclerosis should be withheld to avoid urothelial or vascular injury. Essentially all injected contrast material must be withdrawn easily to ensure that sclerosant is not sequestered.

Pain may be minimized by injection of lidocaine into the cyst immediately before cyst sclerosis. The proper volume of sclerosant is about 25% to 50% of the estimated cyst volume. Absolute alcohol is typically left within the cavity for 20 minutes.[108-110,113] However, some authors advocate leaving the alcohol in place for up to 2 hours.[114,115] Depending of the size of the cyst, positional maneuvers may be employed to distribute the alcohol around the walls of the cyst. The sclerosant then is aspirated completely. The catheter may be removed immediately or left in place to monitor output. If daily catheter output exceeds 10 mL, sclerosis may be repeated. Some authors treat cysts greater than 150 mL with two sessions of sclerotherapy in one sitting while leaving the catheter in place to give multiple treatments over several days in cysts larger than 500 mL.[113,116]

Results and Complications

False-negative results do occur when only cyst aspiration is performed for the exclusion of malignancy. The accuracy may be lower if the cyst is hemorrhagic or highly septate.[112] Track seeding along the needle pathway after fine-needle aspiration and/or biopsy of a cystic malignancy has rarely been reported.[117]

Aspirated renal cysts often recur (30% to 100% of procedures) because the cuboidal epithelium around the cavity rapidly produces fluid and refills the cyst.[108] For initial symptomatic improvement followed by recurrence of symptoms, cyst sclerosis should be considered. A recent study followed approximately 100 patients treated with a single session of alcohol sclerosis for more than 1 year; the cysts had an average volume reduction of 93%. Success rates were 90% for pain reduction and 83% for relief of hydronephrosis. Eight patients were also treated for hypertension with a normotensive status being achieved in seven of the eight patients. The largest amount of alcohol injected was 200 mL.[109]

Significant complications are very unusual.[109,110,116] Mild flank pain and occasionally microscopic hematuria occur.[110,116] Low grade fevers are usually self-limited.[116] Sclerosis of parapelvic cysts carries the additional theoretical risk of damage to the adjacent hilar structures. Pelvic-ureteric obstruction caused by sclerosis-induced fibrosis has been reported.[118]

Surgical alternatives to percutaneous cyst aspiration and sclerosis include open surgical cyst unroofing, laparoscopic cyst unroofing, and marsupialization of the cyst.[111] However, these techniques are much more expensive and usually involve general anesthesia. Most believe that surgical results are similar to percutaneous sclerotherapy; however, direct comparisons are very difficult due to the significant variations in technique.

TUBO-OVARIAN ABSCESS

In the United States, PID occurs in about 800,000 women per year, most of whom are younger than 25 years of age.[119] About one third of women hospitalized for PID develop a frank pelvic abscess. In premenopausal women, tubo-ovarian abscess (TOA) is commonly associated with PID. In post-menopausal women, TOA is more often the consequence of underlying malignancy or diverticulitis.[120] While mortality has improved markedly over the past several decades, morbidity remains high. Complications associated with TOA include ectopic pregnancy, infertility, thrombophlebitis, venous thrombosis, and chronic pelvic pain.[121]

Ultrasound is the ideal imaging modality for TOA diagnosis. Typical findings are thin-walled cystic pelvic masses with relatively uniform echogenicity in or adjacent to the ovaries. Air-fluid levels and septations are common. CT typically shows unilateral, multilocular, low-attenuation collections in the pelvis with thick, enhancing walls[122] (Fig. 23-30).

For many years, the standard therapy for TOA was broad-spectrum IV antibiotics and surgical drainage with washout when necessary. Percutaneous drainage is now the widely accepted first-line treatment when antimicrobial agents alone are not effective.[123] The only major (relative) contraindications to this method are pregnancy and pelvic neoplasm.

Catheters may be placed by a transabdominal, transgluteal, or transvaginal route.[121,123] When a transgluteal access is chosen, entry close to the sacrum and inferior to the pyriformis muscle is advisable to avoid major blood vessels and nerves.[124,125] Also, pericatheter pain is diminished when the tube runs below the pyriformis muscle. In one recent study of women with TOA, clinical response rates for drainage and antibiotics versus antibiotics alone were 100% and 58%, respectively.[126] All but one of the 19 patients in the latter group later responded to percutaneous drainage. Additionally, patients in the primary drainage group had shorter hospital stays and had faster resolution of fever. Dewitt and associates[121] noted that TOA greater than 8 cm in size were more likely to require percutaneous drainage. Based on experience in 58 patients, Goharkhay and colleagues[126] suggested a threshold of >150 mL for primary drainage rather than a trial of medical management.

RENAL ABSCESS

Renal and perirenal abscesses usually result from ascending infection (simple urinary tract infection or pyelonephritis) or hematogenous spread. Risk factors for renal abscess include immunocompromised state, diabetes, underlying urinary tract abnormality (e.g., stone, duplicated collecting system, vesicoureteral reflux, neurogenic bladder, polycystic kidney disease), or an obstructive mass (e.g., tumor, cyst, lymphocele, urinoma).[127] The

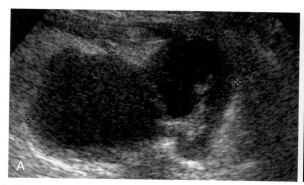
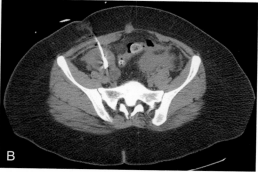

FIGURE 23-30 Tubo-ovarian abscess (TOA). **A,** Ultrasound shows a fluid collection adjacent to the right ovary consistent with TOA. The patient had a fever, elevated white cell count, pelvic pain, and a palpable pelvic mass on bimanual examination. **B,** Image following computed tomography–guided drain placement shows transabdominal percutaneous drain into the abscess. Purulent material (20 mL) was aspirated. Left pelvic collection was also drained percutaneously.

most common symptoms are fever and chills. Abdominal pain, flank pain, dysuria, and urinary frequency, while classically associated with renal infection, are less common. Abdominal pain and flank pain are present in less than 50% to 70% of cases and urinary tract symptoms in less than 30% of cases.[128,129] CT imaging is superior to ultrasound for characterizing the lesion and surrounding structures. Typical findings are thickening of the Gerota fascia, renal swelling or hypertrophy, decreased parenchymal attenuation, focal fluid or gas collection within the kidney, or frank necrosis.[130]

The most common organism isolated from renal abscesses is *Escherichia coli* (26.5%). Other organisms found in abscess cultures include *Klebsiella pneumoniae* (22.4%), *Staphylococcus aureus* (18.3%), *Proteus mirabilis* (18.3%), and *Streptococcus viridans* (6%).[131]

Some reports suggest that small (<3 to 5 cm) renal and perirenal abscesses will resolve with broad-spectrum IV antibiotics alone.[129,132] Indications for aspiration or drainage require a large, symptomatic focal fluid collection that does not respond (or is unlikely to respond) to medical therapy alone. Using ultrasound or CT guidance, a pigtail catheter is inserted directly into the collection. Incomplete drainage after several days may be improved by upsizing the catheter. If a urine leak is created or identified at any time, a PCN tube is placed to decompress the central collecting system and optimize flow away from the urine leak and abscess cavity.

Meng[131] reports a series of patients with renal and perinephric abscess. Lesions treated with antibiotics alone were all less than 3cm in size. Larger lesions were treated with antibiotics and percutaneous drainage (10 of 25 patients with mean abscess size 11 cm); four patients required eventual surgical exploration and nephrectomy due to persistent infection and poorly functioning kidney.

Surgical drainage or nephrectomy are infrequently needed for treatment of abscesses confined to the kidney (12%) but are much more common with perinephric abscess (48%) or with mixed renal and perinephric abscesses (50%).[132] Surgical drainage is also preferred with multiloculated and septated renal abscess in patients who are surgical candidates. Nephrectomy is generally reserved for treatment of patients with a renal abscess and a nonfunctional kidney.[130]

Complications associated with percutaneous drainage of renal and perirenal abscesses are infrequent. One small study of patients without underlying urinary tract abnormalities reported no complications and complete resolution of symptoms in all patients treated with antibiotics alone or in combination with either aspiration or percutaneous drainage.[128] No patients in this series required surgical drainage.

References

1. Eisner BH, Cloyd J, Stoller ML. Lower-pole fluoroscopy-guided percutaneous renal access: which calix is posterior. *J Endourol* 2009;**23**:10.
2. Goodwin WE, Casey WC, Woolf W. Percutaneous trocar (needle) nephrostomy in hydronephrosis. *JAMA* 1955;**157**:891.
3. Prassopoulos P, Gourtsoyiannis N, Cavouras D, et al. A study of the variation of colonic positioning in the pararenal space as shown by computed tomography. *Eur J Radiol* 1990;**10**:44.
4. Khalaf IM, Shokeir AA, El-Gyoushi FI, et al. Recoverability of renal function after treatment of adult patients with unilateral obstructive uropathy and normal contralateral kidney: a prospective study. *Urology* 2004;**64**:664.
5. Zagoria RJ, Hodge RG, Dyer RB, et al. Percutaneous nephrostomy for treatment of intractable hemorrhagic cystitis. *J Urol* 1993;**149**:1449.
6. Silverman SG, Leyendecker JR, Amis ES. What is the current role of CT urography and MR urography in evaluation of the urinary tract? *Radiology* 2009;**250**:2.
7. Riccabona M. Obstructive diseases of the urinary tract in children: lessons from the last 15 years. *Pediatr Radiol* 2010;**40**:6.
8. Bell DA, Rose SC, Starr NK, et al. Percutaneous nephrostomy for nonoperative management of fungal urinary tract infections. *J Vasc Interv Radiol* 1993;**4**:311.
9. Oliver SE, Walker RJ, Woods DJ. Fluconazole infused via a nephrostomy tube: a novel and effective route of delivery. *J Clin Pharm Ther* 1995;**20**:317.
10. Soderdahl DW, Fabrizio MD, Rahman NU, et al. Endoscopic treatment of upper tract transitional cell carcinoma. *Urol Oncol Semin Orig Invest* 2005;**23**:2.
11. Worcester EM, Coe FL. Clinical practice. Calcium kidney stones. *N Engl J Med* 2010;**363**:954.
12. Hamdy FC, Williams JL. Use of dexamethasone for ureteric obstruction in advanced prostate cancer: percutaneous nephrostomies can be avoided. *Br J Urol* 1995;**75**:782.
13. van Bommel EFH, Siemes C, Hak LE, et al. Long-term renal and patient outcome in idiopathic retroperitoneal fibrosis treated with prednisone. *Am J Kidney Dis* 2007;**49**:615.
14. DasGupta R, Grabe M. Preoperative antibiotics before endourologic surgery: current recommendations. *J Endourol* 2009;**23**:10.
15. Ryan JM, Ryan BM, Smith TP. Antibiotic prophylaxis in interventional radiology. *J Vasc Interv Radiol* 2004;**15**:547.
16. Tuttle D, Yeh B, Meng M, et al. Risk of injury to adjacent organs with lower-pole fluoroscopically guided percutaneous nephrostomy: evaluation with prone, supine, and multiplanar reformatted CT. *J Vasc Interv Radiol* 2005;**16**:1489.
17. Millward SF. Percutaneous nephrostomy: a practical approach. *J Vasc Interv Radiol* 2000;**11**:955.
18. Cronan JJ, Marcello A, Horn DL, et al. Antibiotics and nephrostomy tube care: preliminary observations: part I. Bacteriuria. *Radiology* 1989;**172**:1041.
19. Cronan JJ, Horn DL, Marcello A, et al. Antibiotics and nephrostomy tube care: preliminary observations: part II. Bacteremia. *Radiology* 1989;**172**:1043.
20. Ramchandani P, Cardella JF, Grassi CJ, et al. Quality improvement guidelines for percutaneous nephrostomy. *J Vasc Interv Radiol* 2003;**14**:S277.
21. Farrel TA, Hicks ME. A review of radiologically guided percutaneous nephrostomies in 303 patients. *J Vasc Interv Radiol* 1997;**8**:769.
22. Lang EK, Price ET. Redefinitions of indications for percutaneous nephrostomy. *Radiology* 1983;**147**:419.
23. Yoder IC, Pfister RC, Lindfors KK, et al. Pyonephrosis: imaging and intervention. *AJR Am J Roentgenol* 1983;**141**:735.
24. Shih MC, Leung DA, Roth JA, et al. Percutaneous extraction of bilateral renal mycetomas in premature infant using mechanical thrombectomy device. *Urology* 2005;**65**:1226.

25. Gadducci A, Madrigali A, Facchini V, et al. Percutaneous nephrostomy in patients with advanced or recurrent cervical cancer. *Clin Exp Obstet Gynecol* 1994;**21**:71.

26. Chapman ME, Reid JH. Use of percutaneous nephrostomy in malignant ureteric obstruction. *Br J Radiol* 1991;**64**:318.

27. Kouba EM, Wallen, Pruthi RS. Management of ureteral obstruction due to advanced malignancy: optimizing therapeutic and palliative outcomes. *J Urol* 2008;**180**:444.

28. Hoe JW, Tung KH, Tan EC. Reevaluation of indications for percutaneous nephrostomy and interventional uroradiologic procedures in pelvic malignancy. *Br J Radiol* 1993;**71**:469.

29. Barbaric ZL, Hall T, Cochran ST, et al. Percutaneous nephrostomy: placement under CT and fluoroscopy guidance. *AJR Am J Roentgenol* 1997;**169**:151.

30. Cronan JJ, Dorfman GS, Amis ES, et al. Retroperitoneal hemorrhage after percutaneous nephrostomy. *AJR Am J Roentgenol* 1985;**144**:801.

31. Richstone L, Reggio E, Ost MC, et al. Hemorrhage following percutaneous renal surgery: characterization of angiographic findings. *J Endourol* 2008;**22**:6.

32. Smith MT, Ryan J. Sepsis in the interventional radiology patient. *Tech Vasc Intervent Radiol* 2006;**9**:64.

33. Hopper KD, Yakes WF. The posterior intercostal approach for percutaneous renal procedures: risk of puncturing the lung, spleen, and liver as determined by CT. *AJR Am J Roentgenol* 1990;**154**:115.

34. Richenberg J, Kellet M, Records D. Three cases of thoracic complication of intercostal percutaneous nephrostolithotomy and a review of the literature. *J Vasc Interv Radiol* 1995;**10**:23.

35. Picus D, Weyman PJ, Clayman RV, et al. Intercostal space nephrostomy for percutaneous stone removal. *AJR Am J Roentgenol* 1986;**147**:393.

36. Miller GL, Summa J. Transcolonic placement of a percutaneous nephrostomy tube: recognition and treatment. *J Vasc Inter Radiol* 1997;**8**:401.

37. Reinberg Y, Moore LS, Lange PH. Splenic abscess as a complication of percutaneous nephrostomy. *Urology* 1989;**34**:274.

38. Martin E, Lujan M, Paez A, et al. Puncture of the gallbladder: an unusual cause of peritonitis complicating percutaneous nephrostomy. *Br J Urol* 1996;**77**:464.

39. Cadeddu JA, Arrindell D, Moore RG. Near fatal air embolism during percutaneous nephrostomy placement. *J Urol* 1997;**158**:1519.

40. Saad WEA, Virdee S, Davies MG, et al. Inadvertent discontinuation of percutaneous nephrostomy catheters in adult native kidneys: incidence and percutaneous management. *J Vasc Interv Radiol* 2006;**17**:1457.

41. Adamo R, Saad WEA, Brown DB. Management of nephrostomy drains and ureteral stents. *Tech Vasc Intervent Radiol* 2009;**12**:1669.

42. Sardina JI, Bolton DM, Stoller ML. Entrapped Malecot nephrostomy tube: etiology and management. *J Urol* 1995;**153**:1882.

43. Adamo R. Percutaneous ureteral interventions. *Tech Vasc Intervent Radiol* 2009;**12**:3.

44. Byun SS, Kim JH, Oh SJ. Simple retrograde balloon dilatation for treatment of ureteral strictures: etiology-based analysis. *Yonsei Med J* 2003;**44**:2.

45. D'Agostino R, Yucel EK. New method for simultaneous placement of antegrade ureteral stent and nephrostomy tube. *AJR Am J Roentgenol* 1994;**162**:879.

46. D'Agostino R, Goldberg RM. Percutaneous ureteral stents: a modified system to facilitate antegrade placement. *J Vasc Interv Radiol* 1996;**7**:427.

47. Kwok PC, Cheung JY. A radiological approach to the through and through technique for percutaneous passage of ureteric strictures. *Clin Radiol* 1996;**51**:879.

48. DeBaere T, Denys A, Pappas P, et al. Ureteral stents: exchange under fluoroscopic control as an effective alternative to cystoscopy. *Radiology* 1994;**190**:887.

49. Banner MP, Amendola MA, Pollack HM. Anastomosed ureters: fluoroscopically guided transconduit retrograde catheterization. *Radiology* 1989;**170**:45.

50. Cornud FE, Casanova JP, Bonnel DH, et al. Impassable ureteral strictures: management with percutaneous ureteroneocystostomy. *Radiology* 1991;**180**:451.

51. Lang EK. Percutaneous ureterocystostomy and ureteroneocystostomy. *Am J Roentgenol* 1988;**150**:1065.

52. Lingam K, Paterson PJ, Lingam MK, et al. Subcutaneous urinary diversion: an alternative to percutaneous nephrostomy. *J Urol* 1994;**152**:1.

53. Dyer R, Chen M, Zagoria R, et al. Complications of ureteral stent placement. *Radiographics* 2002;**22**:5.

54. Selzman AA, Spirnak JP. Iatrogenic ureteral injuries: a 20-year experience in treating 165 injuries. *J Urol* 1996;**155**:3.

55. Atar E, Bachar GN, Eitan M, et al. Peripheral cutting balloon in the management of resistant benign ureteral and biliary strictures: long-term results. *Diagn Interv Radiol* 2007;**13**:1.

56. Iezzi R, Di Stasi C, Simeone A. Bonomo L. Cutting-balloon angioplasty of resistant ureteral stenosis as bridge to stent insertion. *Eur J Radiol* 2009;**11**:2.

57. Heran MK, Bergen DC, MacNelly AE. The use of cryoplasty in a benign ureteric stricture. *Pediatr Radiol* 2010;**40**:11.

58. Hausegger KA, Portugaller HR. Percutaneous nephrostomy and antegrade ureteral stenting-technique, indications, complications. *Eur Radiol* 2006;**16**:2016.

59. Lang EK, Glorioso LW. Antegrade transluminal dilatation of benign ureteral strictures: long-term results. *Am J Roentgenol* 1988; **150**:1.

60. Modi A, Ritch C, Arend D, et al. Multicenter experience with metallic ureteral stents for malignant and chronic benign ureteral obstruction. *J Endourol* 2010;**24**:7.

61. Chang R, Marshall FF, Mitchell S. Percutaneous management of benign ureteral strictures and fistulas. *J Urol* 1987;**137**:1126.

62. Bierkens AF, Oosterhof GO, Meuleman EJ, Debruyne FM. Anterograde percutaneous treatment of ureterointestinal strictures following urinary diversion. *Eur Urol* 1996;**30**:3.

63. Benoit G, Alexandre L, Moukarzel M, et al. Percutaneous antegrade dilation of ureteral strictures in kidney transplants. *J Urol* 1993; **150**:37.

64. Van Arsdalen KN, Banner MP. The management of ureteral and anastomotic strictures. *Probl Urol* 1992;**6**:420.

65. Hilton P, Stanton SL. Suprapubic catheterization. *Br Med J* 1981;**282**:479.

66. Papanicolaou N, Pfister RC, Nocks BN. Percutaneous, large-bore, suprapubic cystostomy: technique and results. Alternative to cystoscopy. *AJR Am J Roentgenol* 1989;**152**:2.

67. McPhail MJ, Avu-Hilal M, Johnson CD. A meta-analysis comparing suprapubic and transurethral catheterization for bladder drainage after abdominal surgery. *Br J Surg* 2006;**93**:9.

68. Warren, J. Catheter-associated urinary tract infections. *Int J Antimicrob Ag* 2001;**17**:4.

69. Irby P III, Stoller M. Percutaneous suprapubic cystostomy. *J Endourol* 1993;**7**:2.

70. Wu CC, Su CT, Lin AC. Terminal ileum perforation from a misplaced percutaneous suprapubic cystostomy. *Eur J Emerg Med* 2007;**14**:2.

71. Lupton E, George N. The Whitaker test: 35 years on. *Br J Urol* 2010;**105**:1.

72. Whitaker RH. Methods of assessing obstruction in dilated ureters. *Br J Urol* 1973;**45**:15.

73. Whitaker RH. An evaluation of 170 diagnostic pressure flow studies of the upper urinary tract. *J Urol* 1979;**121**:602.

74. Jaffe R, Middleton A. Whitaker test: differentiation of obstructive from nonobstructive uropathy. *AJR Am J Roentgenol* 1980;**134**:9.

75. Ellis JH, Campo RP, Marx MV, et al. Positional variation in the Whitaker test. *Radiology* 1995;**197**:253.

76. Thurmond AS. Pregnancies after selective salpingography and tubal recanalization. *Radiology* 1994;**190**:11.

77. Woolcott R, Petchpud A, O'Donnell P, Stanger J. Differential impact on pregnancy rate of selective salpingography, tubal catheterization and wire-guided recanalization in the treatment of proximal fallopian tube obstruction. *Hum Reprod* 1995;**10**:6.

78. *Guidelines for practice.* Birmingham, Ala: American Fertility Society; September 1993.

79. Thurmond A. Selective salpingography and fallopian tube recanalization. *AJR Am J Roentgenol* 1991;**156**:1.

80. Thurmond AS, Rösch J. Nonsurgical fallopian tube recanalization for treatment of infertility. *Radiology* 1990;**174**:371.

81. Millward SF, Claman P, Leader A, Spence JE. Technical report: fallopian tube recanalization—a simplified technique. *Clin Radiol* 1994;**49**:496.

82. Thurmond A. Fallopian tube recanalization. *Semin Intervent Radiol* 2000;**17**:3.

83. Thurmond AS, Machan LS, Maubon AJ, et al. A review of selective salpingography and fallopian tube catheterization. *Radiographics* 2000;**20**:6.

84. Flood JT, Grow DR. Transcervical tubal cannulation: a review. *Obstet Gynecol Surv* 1993;**48**:768.

85. Darcy MD, McClennan BL, Picus D, et al. Transcervical salpingoplasty: current techniques and results. *Urol Radiol* 1991;**13**:74.

86. Verma A, Krarup K, Donuru A. Selective salpingography and fallopian tube catheterisation by guidewire. *J Obstet Gynecol* 2009;**29**:4.

87. Hedgpeth PL, Thurmond AS, Fry R. Radiographic fallopian tube recanalization: absorbed ovarian radiation dose. *Radiology* 1991;**180**:121.

88. McSwain H, Brodie M. Fallopian tube occlusion, an alternative to tubal ligation. *Tech Vasc Intervent Radiol* 2006;**9**:1.

89. Vancaillie TG, Anderson TA, Johns DA. A 12 month prospective evaluation of transcervical sterilization using implantable polymer matrices. *Obstet Gynecol* 2008;**112**:6.

90. Mino M, Arjona JE, Cordon J, et al. Success rate and patient satisfaction with the Essure sterilization in an outpatient setting: a prospective study of 857 women. *Br J Obstet Gynaecol* 2007;**114**:6.

91. Castano P, Adakunle L. Transcervical sterilization. *Semin Reprod Med* 2010;**28**:2.

92. Vancaillie TG, Anderson T, Alan, J. A 12 month prospective evaluation of transcervical sterilization using implantable polymer matrices. *Obstet Gynecol* 2008;**112**:6.

93. U.S. Department of Health and Human Services. http://optn.transplant.hrsa.gov/latestData/rptData.asp.

94. Friedewald SM, Molmenti EP, et al. Vascular and nonvascular complications of renal transplants: sonographic evaluation and correlation with other imaging modalities, surgery and pathology. *J Clin Ultrasound* 2005;**33**:3.

95. Dodd GD, Tublin ME, Shah A. Imaging of vascular complications associated with renal transplants. *AJR Am J Roentgenol* 1991;**157**:3.

96. Akbar S, Zafar S, Jafri H, et al. Complications of renal transplantation. *Radiographics* 2005;**25**:5.

97. Streeter EH, Little DM, Cranston DW, Morris PJ. The urological complications of renal transplantation: a series of 1535 patients. *Br J Urol Int* 2002;**90**:7.

98. Iwan-Zietek I, Zietek Z, et al. Minimally invasive methods for the treatment of lymphocele after kidney transplantation. *Transplant Proc* 2009;**41**:8.

99. Howard R. Perirenal transplant fluid collections. *Semin Intervent Radiol* 2004;**21**:4.

100. Johnson S, Berry R. Interventional radiological management of the complications of renal transplantation. *Semin Intervent Radiol* 2001;**18**:1.

101. Hedegard W, Saad Wael EA, Davies M. Management of vascular and nonvascular complications after renal transplantation. *Tech Vasc Intervent Radiol* 2009;**12**:4.

102. Beland M, Gervais B, Levis D, et al. Complex abdominal and pelvic abscesses: efficacy of adjunctive tissue-type plasminogen activator for drainage. *Radiology* 2008;**247**:2.

103. Benoit G, Alexandre L, Moukarzel M, et al. Percutaneous antegrade dilation of ureteral strictures in kidney transplants. *J Urol* 1993;**150**:34.

104. Fontaine AB, Nijjar A, Rangaraj R. Update on the use of percutaneous nephrostomy/balloon dilation for the treatment of renal transplant leak/obstruction. *J Vasc Intervent Radiol* 1997;**8**:4.

105. Bosniak MA. The current radiological approach to renal cysts. *Radiology* 1986;**158**:1.

106. Harisinghani MG, Maher MM, Gervais DA, et al. Incidence of malignancy in complex cystic renal masses (Bosniak category III): should imaging-guided biopsy precede surgery? *AJR Am J Roentgenol* 2003;**180**:3.

107. Curry NS, Cochran ST, Bissada NK. Cystic renal masses: accurate Bosniak classification requires adequate renal CT. *AJR Am J Roentgenol* 2000;**175**:2.

108. Bean WJ. Renal cysts: treatment with alcohol. *Radiology* 1981;**138**:2.

109. Akinci D, Akhan O, Ozmen M, et al. Long-term results of single-session percutaneous drainage and ethanol sclerotherapy in simple renal cysts. *Eur J Radiol* 2005;**54**:2.

110. Cho D, Ahn H, Kim S, et al. Sclerotherapy of renal cysts using acetic acid: a comparison with ethanol sclerotherapy. *Br J Radiol* 2008;**81**:946.

111. Okeke A, Mitchelmore A, Keeley Jr F. A comparison of aspiration and sclerotherapy with laparoscopic de-roofing in the management of symptomatic simple renal cysts. *Br J Urol* 2003;**92**:610.

112. Truong L, Todd T, Dhurandhar B, et al. Fine-needle aspiration of renal masses in adults: analysis of results and diagnostic problems in 108 cases. *Diagn Cytopathol* 1999;**20**:339.

113. Mohsen T, Gomha M. Treatment of symptomatic simple renal cysts by percutaneous aspiration and ethanol sclerotherapy. *BJU Int* 2005;**96**:1369.

114. Zerem E, Imamovic G. Symptomatic simple renal cyst: comparison of continuous negative-pressure catheter drainage and single-session alcohol sclerotherapy. *AJR Am J Roentgenol* 2008;**190**:1193.

115. Lin Y, Pan H, Liang H, et al. Single-session alcohol-retention sclerotherapy for simple renal cysts: comparison of 2-and 4-hr retention techniques. *AJR Am J Roentgenol* 2005;**185**:860.

116. Demir E, Alan C, Kilciler M, et al. Comparison of ethanol and sodium tetradecyl sulfate in the sclerotherapy of renal cyst. *J Endourol* 2007;**21**:1459.

117. Volpe A, Kachura J, Geddie W, et al. Techniques, safety and accuracy of sampling of renal tumors by fine needle aspiration and core biopsy. *J Urol* 2007;**178**:379.

118. Camacho MF, Bondhus MJ, Carrion HM, et al. Ureteropelvic junction obstruction resulting from percutaneous cyst puncture and intracystic isophendylate injection: an unusual complication. *J Urol* 1979;**124**:713.

119. Soper D. Pelvic Inflammatory Disease. *Obstet Gynecol* 2010;**16**:2.

120. Protopapas AG, Diakomanolis, ES, et al. Tubo-ovarian abscesses in postmenopausal women: gynecological malignancy until proven otherwise? *Eur J Obstet Gynecol Reprod Biol* 2004;**114**:2.

121. Dewitt J, Reining A, Allsworth JE, Peipert JF. Tuboovarian abscesses: is size associated with duration of hospitalization and complications? *Obstet Gynecol Int* 2010;**2010**:847041.

122. Hiller N, Sella T, Lev-Sagi A, et al. Computed tomographic features of tuboovarian abscess. *J Reprod Med* 2005;**50**:3.

123. McNeeley SG, Hendrix SL, Mazzoni MM, et al. Medically sound, cost-effective treatment for pelvic inflammatory disease and tuboovarian abscess. *Am J Obstet Gynecol* 1998;**178**:6.

124. Woo J, Millard S. Transgluteal approach for percutaneous drainage of deep pelvic abscesses: how to avoid injury to vital structures. *Radiology* 2004;**233**:1.

125. Harisinghani MG, Gervais DA, Maher MM, et al. Transgluteal approach for percutaneous drainage of deep pelvic abscesses: 154 cases. *Radiology* 2003;**228**:3.

126. Goharkhay N, Verma U, Maggiorotto F. Comparison of CT- or ultrasound-guided drainage with concomitant intravenous antibiotics vs. intravenous antibiotics alone in the management of tubo-ovarian abscesses. *Ultrasound Obstet Gynecol* 2007; **29**:1.

127. Yen DH, Hu SC, Tsai J, et al. Renal abscess: early diagnosis and treatment. *Am J Emerg Med* 1999;**17**:2.

128. Shu T, Green J, Orihuela E. Renal and perirenal abscesses in patients with otherwise anatomically normal urinary tracts. *J Urology* 2004;**172**:1.

129. Siegel JF, Smith A, Moldwin R. Minimally invasive treatment of renal abscess. *J Urol* 1996;**155**:1.

130. Kaplan DM, Rosenfield AT, Smith RC. Advances in the imaging of renal infection. Helical CT and modern coordinated imaging. *Infect Dis Clin North Am* 1997;**11**:681.

131. Meng M, Mario L, McAninch J. Current treatment and outcomes of perinephric abscesses. *J Urol* 2002;**168**:4.

132. Coelho RF, Schneider-Monteiro ED, Mesquita JL, et al. Renal and perinephric abscesses: analysis of 65 consecutive cases. *World J Surg* 2007;**31**:2.

Interventional Oncology

Eric J. Hohenwalter, David Sella, William Rilling

The number of patients diagnosed with cancer each year is growing. In 2002, there were 10.9 million new cases worldwide, 6.7 million deaths, and 24.6 million people alive with cancer (within 3 years of diagnosis).[1] The most commonly diagnosed cancers are lung, breast, and colorectal, and the most common causes of cancer death are lung, stomach, and liver cancer.[2] Primary liver cancer is the sixth most common cancer worldwide and the incidence of primary liver cancer is increasing. However, metastatic tumors to the liver are more common than primary tumors.[3] Significant improvements in chemotherapy and surgical options as well as the advancement of endovascular and image-guided treatments and the expanded role of interventional oncology have led to increased survival in these patients.

Several factors are important when determining the most effective therapy for a patient diagnosed with cancer. Previous treatment, extent of disease, and performance status are just a few of the important factors to consider when evaluating patients in clinic. In addition, the goals of therapy may vary widely from patient to patient, from curative, to tumor downstaging for surgery or transplantation, to palliative therapy. As with most solid organ tumors, the consideration of which patients will benefit from the available treatment options should be made by the careful assessment of a multidisciplinary team of physicians.

LIVER

Hepatocellular Carcinoma and Other Primary Liver Tumors (Online Cases 25, 58, 79, and 101)

There were an estimated 17,550 new cases and 15,420 deaths due to primary liver cancer in 2005 in the United States. These numbers yield an incidence of 5.4 per 100,000.[4] Hepatocellular carcinoma (HCC) accounts for the vast majority of primary liver cancer in the United States and around the world. Other less common primary liver cancers include cholangiocarcinoma, fibrolamellar carcinoma, hepatoblastoma, and angiosarcoma of the liver.

Etiology and Natural History

Hepatitis B virus (HBV) and hepatitis C virus (HCV) infections are the main risk factors for HCC.[5] Risk factors for viral hepatitis include contaminated blood transfusions, intravenous drug use, needle sharing, and unsafe sexual practice. HCC develops from HBV and HCV after a latency period of one to three decades.[6] Other risk factors for developing HCC include alcohol abuse, hemochromatosis, aflatoxin exposure, diabetes mellitus, and nonalcoholic fatty liver disease. Studies have demonstrated a dose-response relationship between alcohol consumption and the risk for HCC development.[7] As with alcohol, most risk factors are linked to HCC through the development of cirrhosis. However, up to one fourth of HCC cases arise in nonfibrotic livers.[8] If untreated, the 1-, 2-, and 3-year survival rates in patients with HCC is 54%, 40%, and 28%, respectively.[9]

Clinical Features

Patients with HCC often have symptoms related to their underlying liver disease as well as their malignancy. The prognosis of solid tumors is generally related to tumor stage at presentation and thus tumor stage ultimately guides treatment decisions. However, assessment of clinical outcome is particularly complex in HCC because the underlying liver function also affects prognosis. Historically, HCC was classified by the traditional TMN staging system based on pathologic findings without consideration of underlying liver function.[10] The Okuda Staging System takes tumor size and liver function into account; however it is unable to adequately stratify patients with early or intermediate stage disease[11] (Table 24-1). The Child-Pugh and the Model for End-stage Liver Disease (MELD) assessment classifications only consider liver function. The Barcelona Clinic Liver Cancer

TABLE 24-1 Okuda Staging System

Criteria	SCORE	
	0	1
Tumor size	<50% of liver	>50% of liver
Ascites	Absent	Present
Albumin (g/dL)	≥3.0	<3.0
Bilirubin (mg/dL)	<3.0	>3.0

Stage I, *score 0*; stage II, *score 1 or 2*; stage III, *score 3 or 4*.

(BCLC) staging system is based on the combination of data from several independent studies representing different disease stages and treatment strategies.[12-14] This classification scheme comprises four stages that match the best candidates for the best therapies and includes variables related to tumor stage, liver functional status, physical status, and cancer-related symptoms (Fig. 24-1).

Imaging

The tests used to diagnose and stage HCC include imaging, alpha-fetoprotein (AFP) serology, and biopsy. Optimal imaging depends on the clinical scenario and the

size of the lesion. Some form of imaging is required to evaluate the extent of disease.

ULTRASOUND

Ultrasound is an excellent and inexpensive screening tool for HCC diagnosis, but it is highly dependent on the operator. HCC usually appears as a round or oval mass with sharp boundaries. HCC may exhibit a hypoechoic, isoechoic, or hyperechoic appearance with respect to the surrounding liver parenchyma. A small hyperechoic HCC may be indistinguishable from hemangioma.[15] The reported sensitivity of conventional ultrasound in the detection of HCC ranges from 35% to 84%.[16] Using Doppler or power Doppler sonography to evaluate for hypervascularity or portal venous invasion can increase the accuracy in the detection of HCC; however, detection of smaller lesions (≤1 cm) remains problematic.

COMPUTED TOMOGRAPHY

Computed tomography (CT) is a common imaging modality used for detection and diagnosis of HCC. A three-phase technique including noncontrast, early arterial, and portal venous (PV) inflow imaging is standard of care.[17]

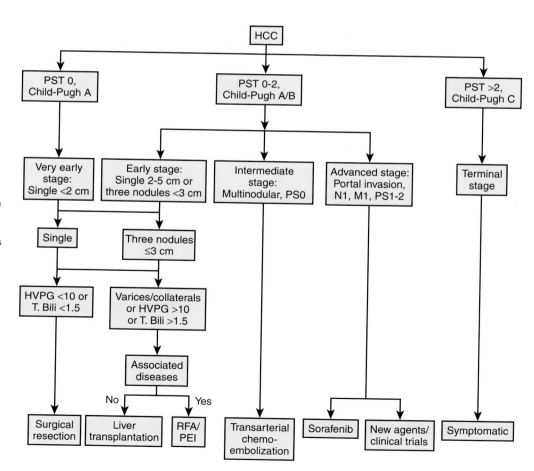

FIGURE 24-1 Barcelona Clinic Liver Cancer (BCLC) staging system. PS/PST refers to performance status, which is staged 0-4. N and M refer to nodal and metastatic staging. *HVPG* is the hepatic venous pressure gradient, a measure of portal pressure obtained through hepatic vein catheterization (via jugular or femoral vein). An HVPG of 10 or higher defines clinically significant portal hypertension, which is also indicated by the presence of varices or portosystemic collaterals on imaging studies. *HCC,* hepatocellular carcinoma; *RFA,* radiofrequency ablation; *PEI,* percutaneous ethanol injection. See www.hepatitis.va.gov/provider/guidelines/2009HCC-bclc-staging.

The value of adding delayed scans (e.g., 3 to 5 minutes after contrast injection) to depict pathologic tumor washout has been demonstrated.[18] HCC typically appears as a hypervascular lesion in the early arterial phase with washout to an isodense or hypodense appearance in the portovenous phase (Fig. 24-2). In addition to the number and size of lesions, patency of the portal vein and the presence of extrahepatic disease can be assessed. According to American Association for the Study of Liver Disease (AASLD) and European Association for the Study of the Liver (EASL) guidelines, hypervascularity with washout in the PV phase on two imaging examinations for small lesions (1 to 2 cm) or one imaging examination for larger lesions (>2 cm) is diagnostic of HCC. A biopsy is not necessary in these cases. However, for small lesions (<1 cm), it is difficult to distinguish between regenerative nodules and HCC. In addition, arteriovenous shunts may mimic small HCCs.[19]

MAGNETIC RESONANCE IMAGING

As with CT, hypervascularity with delayed washout in a cirrhotic liver are characteristics most consistent with HCC (Fig. 24-3). As with CT and ultrasound, the detection and characterization of lesions smaller than 1 cm remains problematic. However, with magnetic resonance imaging (MRI), the criteria for evaluation of focal lesions in cirrhotic liver can be expanded from vascularity alone to cellular density and tissue composition by means of precontrast sequences and diffusion-weighted MRI, to the presence of Kupffer cells by means of uptake of superparamagnetic particles of iron oxide and to the integrity of hepatocellular function and biliary excretion by means of hepatobiliary contrast agents.[20] Whereas the use of these agents is not standard practice, they may prove to increase the sensitivity and specificity of lesion detection and diagnosis of HCC with MRI, especially in

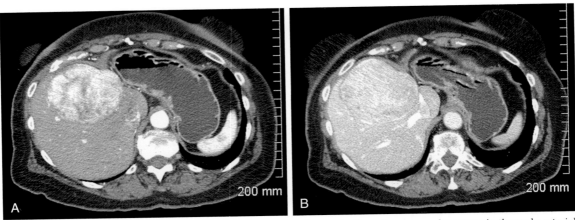

FIGURE 24-2   Hepatocellular carcinoma. Computed tomography scan demonstrating a hypervascular tumor in the early arterial phase **(A)** with subsequent washout on delayed imaging **(B)**.

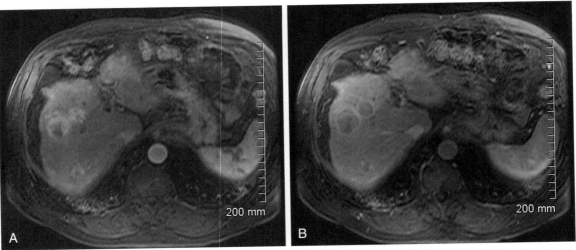

FIGURE 24-3   Hepatocellular carcinoma. Magnetic resonance imaging demonstrating hypervascular tumors in the early arterial phase **(A)** with subsequent washout on delayed imaging **(B)**.

the case of lesions that are less than 1 cm in size. Burrel and colleagues reported a sensitivity of 100% for lesions larger than 2 cm, 89% for lesions between 1 and 2 cm, and 34% for lesions smaller than 1 cm.[21]

Treatment

For patients diagnosed with HCC, there are many treatment options available that will potentially have a positive impact on survival.[22] To achieve the best outcome requires careful selection of candidates for each treatment option. Because this is a complicated disease process and there are multiple potentially beneficial therapies, patients with HCC should be referred to a multidisciplinary team of doctors, including hepatologists, oncologic surgeons, transplant surgeons, interventional radiologists, and medical oncologists, among others.

MEDICAL THERAPY

Historically, no systemic chemotherapy has improved survival in patients with advanced HCC.[23,24] However, sorafenib (Nexavar) is an oral tyrosine kinase inhibitor agent that has shown some survival benefit in patients with advanced HCC. Sorafenib inhibits tumor cell proliferation and angiogenesis. In a recent multicenter, phase III clinical trial with more than 600 patients, median survival in patients treated with sorafenib was nearly 3 months longer than those treated with placebo.[25] The most common side effects of sorafenib in the trial were diarrhea, weight loss, hand-foot skin reactions, and alopecia.

SURGICAL THERAPY

For treatment with curative intent, surgical resection (partial hepatectomy or liver transplantation) has been at the forefront of treatment options for patients with HCC (see Fig. 24-1). However, HCC often occurs in patients with cirrhosis, which increases the risks associated with operation. Advances in perioperative care, patient selection, and radiologic assessment have led to decreased morbidity and mortality associated with surgical resection.[26] Some of the most important factors in determining whether surgery is an option for patients with HCC include performance status, hepatic function and reserve, extent and location of tumor, and the presence of vascular invasion. Some of the surgical options include tumor excision, trisegmentectomy, and right or left hepatectomy.

To improve results following hepatectomy, portal vein embolization may be necessary. In cirrhotic patients in whom resections to remove more than two functional segments are planned, portal vein embolization should be considered as a preoperative adjunct to induce hypertrophy of the liver remnant.[27] Portal vein embolization is a technique used to occlude portal inflow to the portion of the liver that is going to be removed, inducing hypertrophy in the portion of the liver that will be left behind, known as the liver remnant, over a period of 3 to 4 weeks (Fig. 24-4). This technique increases the ability to resect the liver safely.[28]

Transplantation represents effective treatment for the underlying liver disease as well as the cancer. However, the surgical risks of graft failure and infection, the shortage of donor organs leading to a long waiting list, and the risks associated with lifelong immunosuppression therapy can be seen as disadvantages.[29] The most widely accepted Milan criteria include patients with a solitary tumor of 5 cm or less in diameter or patients with no more than three tumors, each 3 cm or less in diameter, and no invasion of major blood vessels, lymph nodes, or extrahepatic sites.[30] Using these criteria, 4-year survival rates of up to 85% have been reported. Slightly expanded thresholds such as the UCSF criteria (single lesion ≤6.5 cm or two lesions ≤4.5 cm with total tumor diameter ≤8 cm) have also shown favorable 1-and 5-year survival rates of 92.1% and 80.7%, respectively.

PERCUTANEOUS THERAPY

TRANSCATHETER ARTERIAL CHEMOEMBOLIZATION AND BLAND EMBOLIZATION Liver tumors, both primary and metastatic, receive their blood supply predominantly from the hepatic artery.[31] Because the normal liver has dual blood supply (75% portal vein, 25% hepatic artery), chemoembolization delivers localized treatment to tumors without significant damage to the adjacent parenchyma. Chemoembolization also delivers higher doses of chemotherapeutic agents to liver tumors than does systemic therapy. In addition, the embolization component of chemoembolization prolongs the dwell time of the chemotherapeutic agents within the liver, thereby limiting systemic toxicity.[32] Regarding transcatheter arterial chemoembolization (TACE), variations in protocol exist, including the chemotherapeutic used, use of lipiodol, and the type of embolic agent used to decrease blood flow. In the United States, doxorubicin, cisplatin, and mitomycin are the drugs most often used.[33] Our protocol for a standard chemoembolization is 50 mg doxorubicin, 10 mg mitomycin, and 100 mg cisplatin. Lipiodol is an iodized ester from poppyseed oil. When it is injected into the hepatic artery, it is cleared from normal hepatic tissue but accumulates in tumor cells because of the absence of Kupffer cells.[34]

Patient Selection Several factors are important when determining whether a nonoperable patient is an appropriate candidate for chemoembolization. In patients with advanced liver disease, treatment-induced liver failure may offset the antitumoral effect or survival benefit of the intervention.[35] Therefore some of the predictors of outcome are related to neoplastic burden:

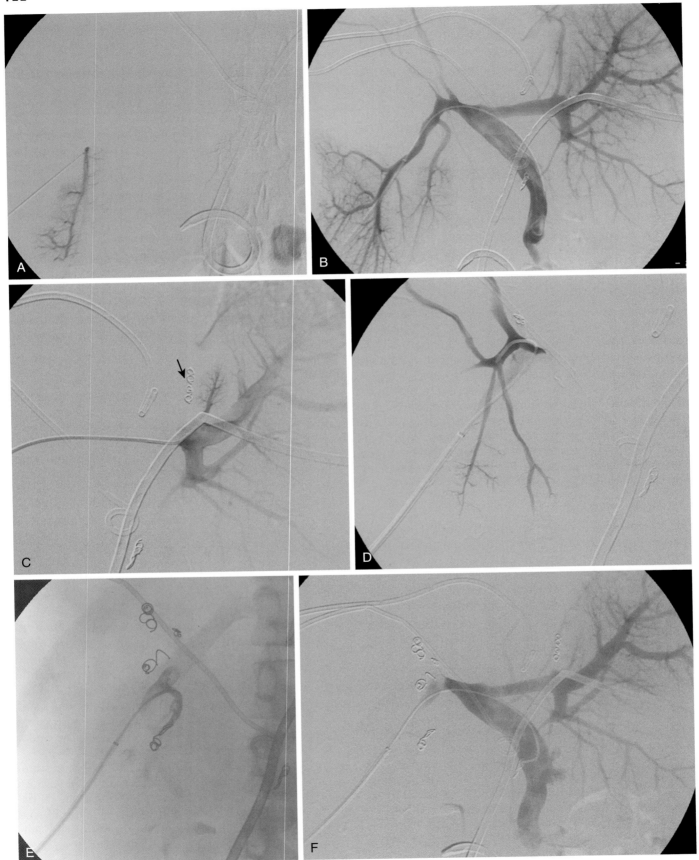

FIGURE 24-4   Portal vein embolization before right trisegmentectomy. **A,** Access is gained to a right portal vein branch with sonographic guidance. **B,** A vascular sheath has been placed, followed by portography, which shows distortion of right portal branches by tumor. **C,** Portal branches to segment IV have been embolized *(arrow)*. **D** and **E,** Right portal venous branches are engaged and then occluded. **F,** Final portogram shows complete obstruction of branches to liver segments IV-VIII.

tumor size, number of tumors or percentage of liver involved with tumor, and extent of vascular invasion, if present. The degree of liver dysfunction should also be evaluated. This can be accomplished with the MELD assessment. Exclusion criteria base on specific laboratory values have not been definitively established. In addition, the performance status of the patient is vital in determining whether a patient will be able to tolerate chemoembolization as a treatment for the liver tumor. Two scales of performance status include the Karnofsky index and the Eastern Cooperative Oncology Group (ECOG) toxicity and response criteria (Tables 24-2 and 24-3). The best candidates are patients with liver dominant disease (no significant extrahepatic disease), preserved liver function, and a performance status of ECOG 0 or 1.

In addition to prolonging survival and/or treating symptoms in unresectable patients, locoregional therapies have been shown to maintain patients on the transplant waiting list as well as downstage the disease in some patients.[36]

TABLE 24-2   Eastern Cooperative Oncology Group Performance Status

Grade	ECOG
0	Fully active, able to carry on all predisease performance without restriction
1	Restricted in physically strenuous activity but ambulatory and able to carry out work of a light or sedentary nature (e.g., light house work, office work)
2	Ambulatory and capable of all self-care but unable to carry out any work activities. Up and about more than 50% of waking hours
3	Capable of only limited self-care, confined to bed or chair more than 50% of waking hours
4	Completely disabled. Cannot carry on any self-care. Totally confined to bed or chair
5	Dead

TABLE 24-3   Karnovsky Performance Status Scale

100%	Normal, no complaints, no signs of disease
90%	Capable of normal activity, few symptoms or signs of disease
80%	Normal activity with some difficulty, some symptoms or signs
70%	Caring for self, not capable of normal activity or work
60%	Requiring some help, can take care of most personal requirements
50%	Requires help often, requires frequent medical care
40%	Disabled, requires special care and help
30%	Severely disabled, hospital admission indicated but no risk of death
20%	Very ill, urgently requiring admission, requires supportive measures or treatment
10%	Moribund, rapidly progressive fatal disease processes
0%	Death

Absolute contraindications for chemoembolization include intractable systemic infection and extensive extrahepatic disease. Relative contraindications include portal vein invasion, the presence of encephalopathy, and unrelieved biliary obstruction. Several studies have demonstrated the safety and effectiveness of TACE in patients with portal venous invasion when chemoembolization is performed in a subselective manner.[37,38] Other relative contraindications include uncorrectable coagulopathy, significant arteriovenous shunting, and significant renal insufficiency. These are relative contraindications because these may be correctable or the treatment regimen may be altered to accommodate the abnormality. For example, in the case of a patient with angiographically visible shunting within the tumor, a bland embolization could be performed before chemoembolization in order to reduce the shunt and ensure adequate treatment of the tumor.

Technique   Patients receive preprocedure hydration as well as antiemetics and steroids (Box 24-1). Preprocedure antibiotics are altered for the patient who has a compromised sphincter of Oddi from prior surgery or biliary stent placement. These individuals are at increased risk for infection and abscess formation following chemoembolization.[39,40] For these patients, we prescribe moxifloxacin 400 mg daily for 10 days before the procedure. Diagnostic arteriography of the celiac and superior mesenteric arteries is essential to identify the arterial supply to the tumor as well as aberrant vessels supplying the tumor or extrahepatic structures. The arteriogram should be carried out to the venous phase to evaluate the patency of the portal vein. A microcatheter is then used to selectively catheterize the tumor arteries. It is also important to evaluate and identify any arteriovenous shunting, which has been reported to occur in 31% to 63% of cases between second order branches[41] (Fig. 24-5).

BOX 24-1

TRANSCATHETER ARTERIAL CHEMOEMBOLIZATION: PREPROCEDURE MEDICATION REGIMEN

- Intravenous (IV) fluids, 100 to 150 mL/hr
- Cefazolin, 1 g IV
- Metronidazole, 500 mg IV
- Dexamethasone, 10 mg IV
- Ondansetron, 16 mg IV
- Diphenhydramine, 50 mg IV

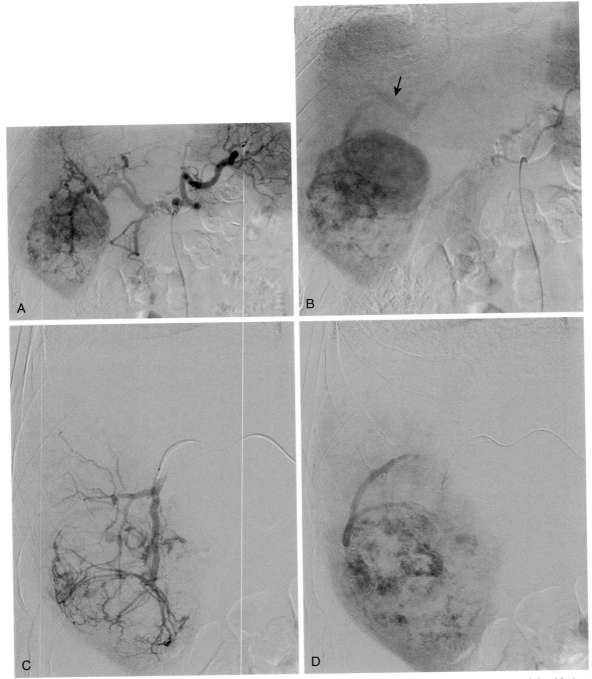

FIGURE 24-5 Hepatocellular carcinoma. **A** and **B,** Celiac arteriogram demonstrating lesion within the right hepatic lobe. Notice the early appearance of the portal vein *(arrow)*. **C** and **D,** Subselective arteriogram demonstrating arterial portal shunting within the tumor.

Practice patterns vary as to whether a superselective, segmental, or lobar approach is performed (Fig. 24-6). However, treatment of the entire liver in one session is associated with increased mortality.[42] It may be necessary to evaluate extrahepatic arterial supply to the tumor as well, such as the inferior phrenic artery. In a retrospective study of more than 2300 procedures, TACE through an extrahepatic collateral was considered in 25% of cases[43] (Fig. 24-7). A variety of TACE protocols exist and there is great variability in the amount and type of the chemotherapeutic agents used, type and amount of embolization agents, and sequencing of embolization.

Results   Chemoembolization has been shown to be a safe and effective treatment for selected patients with HCC. Two prospective, randomized trials demonstrating the survival benefits of chemoembolization in HCC have been published. A study by Lo and colleagues[44] compared patients treated with chemoembolization with those given supportive care and demonstrated improved survival at 1, 2, and 3 years. Another study by Llovet and colleagues compared chemoembolization and hepatic arterial embolization with supportive care and demonstrated a survival benefit in the embolization treatment groups.[45]

Complications   Postembolization syndrome is characterized by abdominal pain, fever, anorexia, nausea, and fatigue. The cause is not completely understood but several theories exist including distention of the liver capsule, tumor necrosis, and ischemia of liver parenchyma.[46] The severity of symptoms is variable. They may last as long as 10 days and may occasionally require an extended hospital admission. The postembolization syndrome occurs in up to 90% of patients following chemoembolization and for that reason is considered a side effect rather than a complication.[47]

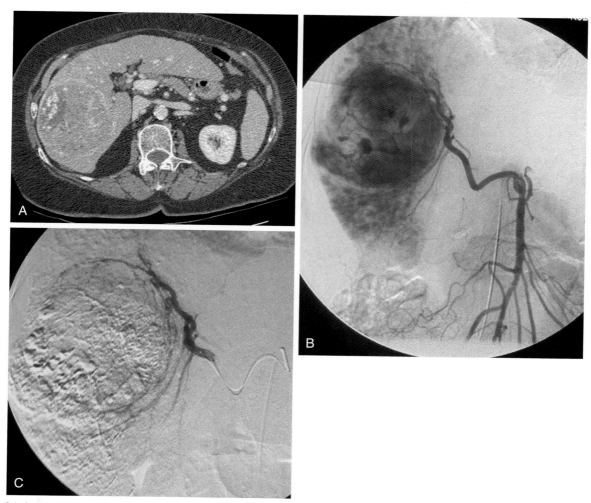

FIGURE 24-6   Hepatocellular carcinoma. **A,** Contrast computed tomography scan in the arterial phase reveals a large hypervascular mass in the right lobe of the liver with central puddling of contrast. **B,** Superior mesenteric arteriography with replaced right hepatic artery confirms a large vascular mass with displacement of vessels. **C,** Following chemoembolization, flow has been abolished and lipiodol has accumulated within the tumor.

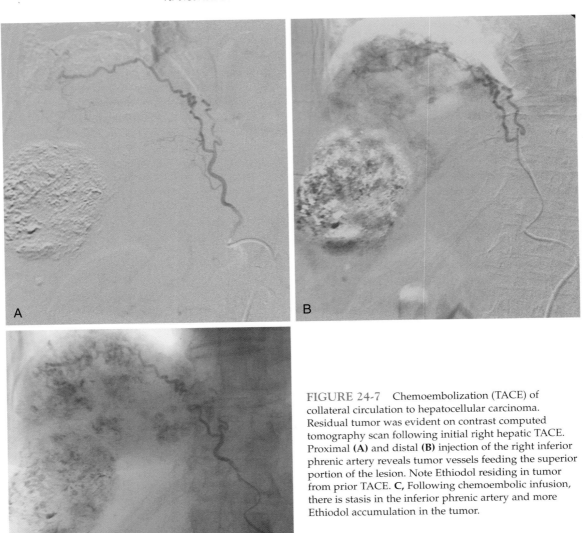

FIGURE 24-7   Chemoembolization (TACE) of collateral circulation to hepatocellular carcinoma. Residual tumor was evident on contrast computed tomography scan following initial right hepatic TACE. Proximal **(A)** and distal **(B)** injection of the right inferior phrenic artery reveals tumor vessels feeding the superior portion of the lesion. Note Ethiodol residing in tumor from prior TACE. **C,** Following chemoembolic infusion, there is stasis in the inferior phrenic artery and more Ethiodol accumulation in the tumor.

Nontarget embolization, bile duct injury, and hepatic failure are the potentially most severe complications following chemoembolization (Table 24-4). Nontarget embolization is defined as the inadvertent distribution of chemotherapeutic agents into unintended territories. Diagnostic arteriography prior to infusion of chemotherapeutic agents is vital to identify any extrahepatic arterial variants in the treatment region. Nontarget embolization of a gastric artery or the gastroduodenal artery can cause gastrointestinal ischemia. If TACE cannot be performed distal to the extrahepatic artery, embolization of the extrahepatic artery (with coils, if safe) can be effective in preventing complications related to nontarget embolization.[31] Hepatic failure is more likely to occur in patients with impaired hepatic function prior to treatment. Acute liver failure has been reported in up to 2.3% of patients following chemoembolization.[48] In contrast to normal hepatic parenchyma, intrahepatic bile ducts do not have dual blood supply. Rather, they are fed exclusively from hepatic arterial branches that give off a vascular plexus around the bile ducts.[49] Therefore, ischemic bile duct injury can occur following chemoembolization.

YTTRIUM-90 RADIOEMBOLIZATION   Normal hepatic parenchyma is very sensitive to tumoricidal radiation doses. External beam radiation has had a limited role, in that as doses greater than 35 Gy have been shown to cause the development of radiation-induced liver disease. Radioembolization is defined as the intraarterial delivery of radioisotope-labeled particles that become embedded in the tumor preferentially to surrounding parenchyma because of differences in vascular supply.[50] Yttrium-90 (^{90}Y) is a pure beta emitter and decays to ^{90}Zr

TABLE 24-4 Major Complications of Hepatic Arterial Chemoembolization

Major Complication	Reported Rate (%)	Suggested Threshold (%)
Liver failure	2.3	4
Postembolization syndrome requiring extended stay or readmission	4.6	10
Abscess with functional sphincter of Oddi	1.0	2
Abscess with biliary-enteric anastomosis/biliary stent/sphincterotomy	25.0	25
Surgical cholecystitis	1.0	1
Biloma requiring percutaneous drainage	1.0	2
Pulmonary arterial oil embolus	1.0	1
Gastrointestinal hemorrhage/ulceration	1.0	1
Iatrogenic dissection preventing treatment	1.0	1
Death	1.0	2

From Brown DB, Cardella JF, Sacks D, et al. Quality improvement guidelines for transhepatic arterial chemoembolization, embolization, and chemotherapeutic infusion for hepatic malignancy. J Vasc Interv Radiol 2006;17:225.

BOX 24-2

⁹⁰Y RADIOTHERAPY: PATIENT SELECTION

Indications

- Unresectable hepatic primary or metastatic cancer
- Liver-dominant tumor burden
- Life expectancy at least 3 months

Contraindications

- Pretreatment shunt demonstrating potential for ≥30 Gy radiation exposure to the lung or flow to the gastrointestinal tract that cannot be corrected by catheter embolization techniques
- Excessive tumor burden with limited hepatic reserve
- Elevated total bilirubin (>2 mg/dL) in the absence of a reversible cause

---

with a physical half-life of 64.2 hours. The energy has a mean tissue penetration of 2.5 mm and a maximum penetration of 11 mm. There are two commercially available agents: *SIR-Spheres* (Sirtex Medical Ltd, Lane Cove, Australia) and *TheraSphere* (MDS Nordion, Ottawa, Canada). The ⁹⁰Y is bound to either glass or resin microspheres and delivered into the hepatic arteries via a microcatheter. To optimize safety and efficacy, radiation dose planning and administration is modified on the basis of tumor and liver volumes. Flow dynamics cause the particles to travel preferentially to the tumor.

Patient Selection A Consensus Panel Report[51] that was published in 2007 provides detailed guidelines in regard to patient selection for radioembolization. A summary of some general patient selection criteria and contraindications are included in Box 24-2. Because a small amount of adjacent liver will be affected by the radiation, sufficient hepatic reserve is required. Parameters of adequate hepatic reserve include lack of ascites, normal synthetic liver function (e.g., albumin >3 g/dL) and normal total bilirubin (<2 mg/dL).[52] Performance status is also critical in patient selection and good candidates have a performance status of ECOG 0-2. An absolute contraindication to radioembolization is the predicted administration of a dose of at least 30 Gy to the lungs in a single treatment or greater than 50 Gy as a cumulative dose on multiple treatments[53] (see later discussion).

Technique Starting a ⁹⁰Y program is complicated. The treatment itself consists of two phases. In the first phase, patients undergo an angiogram to map the arterial system and embolize any vessels that would allow the microspheres to enter the gastrointestinal tract (i.e., skeletonize the hepatic circulation).[51] A superior mesenteric angiogram is performed to detect replaced or accessory hepatic arteries. In addition, the arteriogram is carried out to the venous phase to evaluate the status of the portal vein. A celiac arteriogram and subsequent selective hepatic angiography is performed to define the hepatic and tumoral anatomy and to evaluate for anatomic variants (Fig. 24-8). This step is critical in that the presence of unrecognized collateral vessels with consequent infusion of radioactive microspheres could lead to gastrointestinal ulceration, pancreatitis, and irradiation of other nontarget sites.[54] For this reason, aggressive prophylactic embolization of these aberrant vessels before therapy is essential. The gastroduodenal artery (GDA) is virtually always embolized to its origin with microcoils. Some of the relatively common vessels of interest include the right gastric, esophageal, accessory left gastric, falciform accessory phrenic, and supraduodenal or retroduodenal arteries. Once the arterial anatomy has been evaluated and the aberrant gastrointestinal supply, if present, is embolized, the degree of lung shunting through the tumor must be estimated. To this end, 5 mCi of ⁹⁹ᵐTc-labeled macroaggregated albumin particles is injected through the microcatheter into the desired liver distribution. Single photon emission computed tomography gamma imaging is done afterward to detect shunting of the albumin

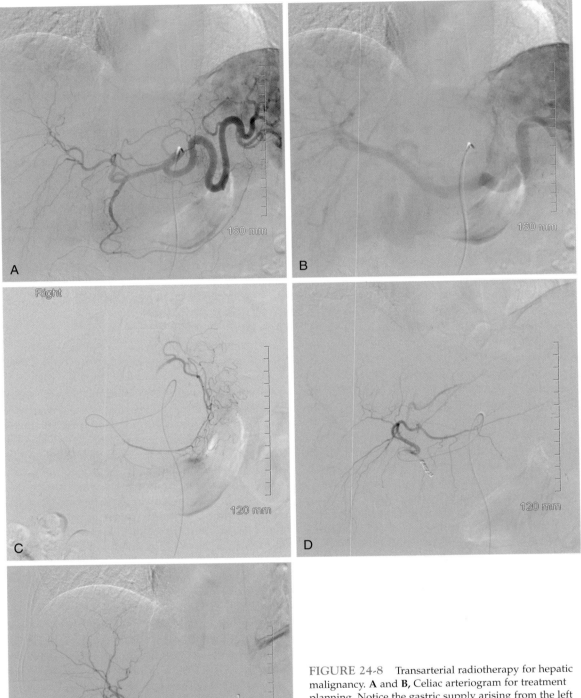

FIGURE 24-8 Transarterial radiotherapy for hepatic malignancy. **A** and **B,** Celiac arteriogram for treatment planning. Notice the gastric supply arising from the left hepatic artery **(C)** with subsequent coil embolization **(D). E,** Final selective right hepatic arteriogram prior to ^{90}Y infusion.

particles into the pulmonary or gastrointestinal vasculature. This information is then used to calculate an appropriate treatment dose.[51] Specific dosimetry calculations have been described previously and are beyond the scope of this text.[55]

The second phase is the delivery of the microspheres. Radiation safety is an important consideration in this procedure. [90]Y is a beta emitter; therefore, the primary concern is exposure to the eyes, skin, and hands.[51] If the delivery system becomes compromised, radioactive contamination is a concern and steps should be taken to prevent the spread of contamination.

The ^{90}Y infusion varies depending on the agent being used, the location of the catheter, and the vessel undergoing infusion. The delivery is dependent on blood flow through the hepatic artery distal to the catheter tip. Radiation monitoring must be used to establish when optimal delivery has been achieved. Typical surface radiation dose rates from the patient will be less than 1 mrem/hr after implantation. Therefore, standard biohazard precautions are sufficient to protect from exposure to others after they have been discharged.[51]

Results Several studies have demonstrated the therapeutic benefits of radioembolization for primary liver cancer in patients with advanced, unresectable disease.[56-59] Kooby and colleagues[60] have compared radioembolization to chemoembolization in a series of retrospectively studied patients and concluded that radioembolization and chemoembolization have similar effectiveness and safety profiles. Time to progression and survival benefit in general varies by initial tumor stage and liver function. In addition, Kulik and associates[61] concluded that radioembolization may have a role in downstaging patients to fall within Milan criteria for liver transplantation.

Complications As in chemoembolization, postembolization syndrome may develop following radioembolization treatment, although the symptoms are usually less severe. Fatigue, nausea, vomiting, anorexia, fever, abdominal pain, and cachexia have been reported.[62] Other potential complications include hepatic dysfunction, biliary injury, and gastrointestinal complications resulting from nontarget embolization. Altered hepatic function may predispose patients to the hepatotoxic effects of radioembolzation.[63] Kennedy and colleagues[64] observed radiation-induced liver disease (elevated liver enzymes, anicteric hepatomegaly, ascites) in 4% of patients after radioembolization with resin microspheres. The potential gastrointestinal complications result from the inadvertent spread of microspheres to the gastrointestinal tract, which results in ulceration. As mentioned previously, meticulous mapping, identification, and embolization of any potential gastrointestinal arterial supply arising from the treatment zone can prevent this untoward event. Radiation

pneumonitis is a theoretical concern with ^{90}Y treatment. Previous preclinical and clinical studies have demonstrated that as much as 30 Gy to the lungs can be tolerated with a single injection.[54]

PERCUTANEOUS ABLATION Tissue ablation as a form of treatment has gained increasing popularity over the past few decades. The development of improved devices and imaging modalities continue to push image-guided thermal ablation to the forefront of treatment in selected primary and secondary malignancies, medically inoperable patients, and as palliative treatment.[65] Tissue ablation generally falls under one of two categories: thermal ablation and chemical ablation. Thermal ablation includes technologies such as radiofrequency ablation, microwave ablation, cryoablation, laser ablation, and high-intensity focused ultrasound (HIFU). These techniques cause cell death by directly altering the temperature of the tumor. Chemical ablation involves infusing substances such as absolute ethanol into tumors, which directly produces necrosis.

Radiofrequency ablation (RFA) has the most substantial track record of the various thermal ablation technologies used in HCC. The goal is to create a zone of coagulative necrosis of 0.5 to 1 cm around a lesion to achieve a tumor-free margin.[65] Tumor recurrence is significantly reduced when a 1-cm tumor free margin is achieved with operative resection.[66] RFA involves the insertion of percutaneous straight or expandable electrodes directly into a tumor (Fig. 24-9). Delivery of high-frequency alternating current (200 to 1200 Hz) causes ionic agitation in the tissues, leading to frictional heat. Local tissue temperatures are increased to a targeted range of 60° to 100° C resulting in cellular protein denaturation, cell membrane dysfunction, and coagulative necrosis.[67] When temperatures greater than 100° C are reached, carbonization and charring usually occur, with less effective energy transmission and diminished volume of the ablation zone.[67] The applied current in RFA exits the body through grounding pads placed on the patient, generally at the thigh. Treatment of lesions in close proximity to high-flow vessels (>3 mm in diameter) requires consideration of the "heat sink effect." Temperature variations are limited by flowing blood, which carries the deposited heat away, essentially increasing the chance of tumor progression. There are several commercially available RFA devices, which use varied techniques to maximize the target ablation zone. Examples of a few RF devices include the Valleylab RF Ablation Generator, Boston Scientific LaVeen RF ablation system, and the Angiodynamics RITA medical system.

Cryoablation also utilizes percutaneously placed probes. Room temperature argon gas travels from an area of high pressure to the tip of the probe where it

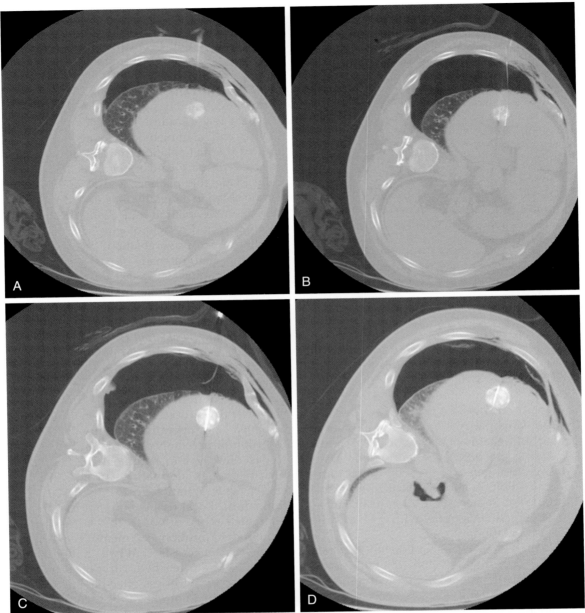

FIGURE 24-9   Radiofrequency (RF) ablation for hepatocellular carcinoma. **A,** A pneumothorax has been induced to allow transthoracic entry into the lesion in the dome of the liver. Ethiodol from prior chemoembolization demarcates the tumor. **B,** A second pass is required for central needle placement. **C,** An RF probe is advanced to the far end of the lesion. **D,** The tines are deployed, and ablation is begun.

meets an area of low pressure and is allowed to rapidly expand within the sealed probe tip (a closed-loop, gas expansion system).[68] The rapid expansion of the gas causes a temperature decrease (Joule-Thompson effect), which is transferred by conduction and convection to the probe tip, achieving a temperature of less than $-40°$ C within seconds. Temperatures of at least $-20°$ to $-40°$ C are required to cause cell death and adequate tumor-free margins, generally considered to be greater than 1 cm.[69] Cryoablation causes direct and indirect cell death by intracellular and extracellular ice crystal formation and small vessel thrombosis.[65]

When treating lesions near vessels larger than 3 mm in diameter, consider the "cold-sink" phenomenon, which is analogous to the heat sink that interferes with RFA (see earlier discussion). Cryoablation generally entails standard protocols of multiple freezing stages with periods of interspersed active thawing. The currently available cryotherapy systems in the United States use compressed argon gas for cooling, which requires storage of large pressurized containers. Advantages over RFA include the ability to use multiple simultaneous probes, the ability to actively monitor the cryoablation zone with multiple imaging modalities, and decreased intraprocedural pain.[70]

Microwave ablation involves the insertion of microwave-transmitting antennae into a tumor. The microwaves generate an oscillating electromagnetic field with a frequency greater than 900 MHz.[71] The weak unequal dipoles of surrounding water molecules orient with the field, the field oscillates, and the water molecules oscillate rapidly, producing friction and heat.[71] Advantages of microwave ablation over RFA include creation of a wider ablation zone with decreased charring, increased temperatures within a shorter time, less heat sink effect, and the ability to treat with multiple probes simultaneously. The ablation system requires a microwave generator, power distribution system (flexible coaxial cable), and microwave antennae. No prospective trials have compared microwave and RFA ablations.

Patient Selection and Technique The goal for any ablative therapy should be to obtain complete destruction of the tumor and some surrounding margin. Local ablation of tumors requires careful planning regardless of the method of destruction. The geometry produced by the ablation can be somewhat unpredictable and neglecting to ensure complete coverage can lead to treatment failure.[72] Therefore, tumor size and location are vital when treating patients with one of the ablative therapies in order to choose the appropriate probe size and number. Durable success of ablation and resultant improved survival depends on complete ablation of the tumor.[73] The likelihood of complete ablation decreases with increasing tumor size, and multiplicity of tumor compounds this consideration.[74]

Pretreatment imaging must accurately define the location of each lesion with respect to surrounding structures. As mentioned earlier, treatment of a lesion that is close to a major vessel may result in suboptimal results. In addition, ablation of lesions which are close to portions of the gastrointestinal tract, diaphragm, heart, and kidney may induce injury to the structure. Likewise, central lesions treated with ablation may be at increased risk for bile duct injuries. Various techniques have been used to protect adjacent structures during ablation, including the use of "hydrodissection" or the instillation of fluid (saline, D_5W). [73]

Results There are substantial data supporting the role of percutaneous RFA as an effective, safe, first-line therapy for cirrhotic patients with HCC smaller than 3 cm who are not candidates for surgical resection or liver transplantation.[75,76] In fact, recent studies have demonstrated 5-year survival rates ranging from 51% to 76% in Child's A patients.[77] These results have raised the question as to whether RFA should be first-line therapy for some patients with HCC smaller than 3 cm. A recent randomized controlled trial comparing resection versus ablation in patients with Child's A cirrhosis and solitary HCC smaller than 5 cm failed to show statistically significant differences in overall survival and disease-free survival between the two groups.[78] There are fewer data regarding the safety and efficacy of cryoablation and microwave ablation for HCC.[79] However, in retrospective analysis of 288 patients with HCC treated with percutaneous microwave ablation, 1-, 2-, 3-, and 5- year survival rates were 93%, 82%, 72%, and 51%, respectively.[80]

Complications Knowledge of the potential complications associated with percutaneous ablation is critical in assessing the risks of the procedure for each patient. Proper patient selection and technique will help limit the risk of procedural complications. An overall complication rate of 8.9% was observed in a meta-analysis of 82 independent reports with a total of 3670 patients.[81] The most common complications included hemorrhage, abscess, and biliary stricture. Another potential complication is *tumor lysis syndrome*, which has been described after both RFA and cryoablation of large tumor.[82,83] This is an uncommon systemic complication that may present with severe thrombocytopenia and hepatic or renal failure. Tumor lysis syndrome occurs more frequently with cryoablation than with the heat based methods, likely due to the mechanism of tissue destruction.[65]

Colorectal Liver Metastases

Etiology and Natural History

Colorectal cancer (CRC) is the third most common cancer in the United States, with nearly 147,000 new cases and approximately 50,000 deaths reported annually.[84] The liver is the major site of metastastic disease. Liver metastases from CRC are common and can be found in up to 80% of patients diagnosed with CRC.[85] Synchronous hepatic metastases may be identified in 10% to 20% of patients with colorectal cancer.[86] Without treatment, survival for patients with CRC and liver metastases is less than 1% at 5 years.[87]

Imaging

Ultrasound, CT, and MRI are all commonly used in the evaluation of hepatic metastases. The appearance can be quite variable, but in general, metastases appear similar to the gross morphology of the primary tumor.[88] Colorectal cancer metastases usually appear as hypovascular lesions on contrast-enhanced CT and MRI. Positron-emission tomography (PET) and PET-CT also play a crucial role in the diagnosis and staging of patients with colorectal metastases. Unlike HCC, there are no specific imaging criteria for metastatic lesions that allow confident diagnosis. Therefore, pathologic confirmation is usually necessary.

Treatment

Although liver metastases from CRC previously carried a dismal prognosis, advances in systemic therapy, interventional oncology, and surgical techniques have improved survival in this disease. The appropriate therapy and timing of treatment should be individualized and determined by a multidisciplinary team of medical oncologists, radiation oncologists, interventional radiologists, and surgeons.

MEDICAL THERAPY

There are several different chemotherapeutic options for patients with liver metastases from CRC. These treatment approaches are discussed elsewhere.[72] *Adjuvant therapy* refers to systemic chemotherapy given after surgery to reduce the risk of recurrent disease. *Neoadjuvant therapy* refers to preoperative systemic chemotherapy to reduce the risk of recurrence and/or downstage the disease to allow for surgical resection. Often, systemic chemotherapy is administered both before and after surgery and is referred to as a *perioperative approach*.[72]

SURGICAL THERAPY

Surgical resection is considered the only curative option for patients with CRC metastases.[72] Before being considered for operation, it must be shown that the patient has little or no extrahepatic disease and has intrahepatic disease that can be safely resected. The goal of surgical resection is to remove all lesions with tumor-free margins.[89] For those patients who undergo resection for CRC metastases, the 5-year survival approaches 45% to 60%.[90,91] Combined modality approaches such as surgical resection and intraoperative ablation, staged bilobar surgical resection, and portal vein embolization with extended hepatectomy have all expanded the pool of surgical candidates with CRC.

CHEMOEMBOLIZATION

Historically, patients who had unresectable colorectal cancer metastases that progressed on chemotherapy were candidates for chemoembolization. A current area of research involves the use of irinotecan drug-eluting beads to treat patients with CRC liver metastases. *Irinotecan* is a chemotherapeutic agent that has been shown to increase survival and delay tumor progression when added to the treatment regimen for patients with metastatic colorectal cancer. Initial results of a phase II clinical trial reported an 80% response rate with reduction of contrast enhancement of treated tumors following treatment.[92] Other trials evaluating the safety and efficacy of irinotecan drug-eluting beads in liver metastases from CRC are ongoing.

RADIOEMBOLIZATION

Patients who have unresectable CRC metastases to the liver and are on systemic chemotherapy or have failed to respond to first- or second-line chemotherapeutic agents are considered candidates for radioembolization.[52] As mentioned previously, there are two commercially available agents (SIR-Sphere and TheraSphere). Currently, SIR-Sphere is FDA approved for patients with metastatic CRC (Fig. 24-10). In a metaanalysis of 19 studies and 792 patients with metastatic CRC treated with radioembolization (SIR-Sphere and TheraSphere), response rates of approximately 80% and 90% (as first-line treatment) were observed.[93] Two large randomized phase III clinical trials are currently enrolling patients to evaluate the benefit of adding radioembolization to standard first-line chemotherapy regimens.

PERCUTANEOUS ABLATION

Patient selection, technical aspects of the procedure, and complications associated with the percutaneous ablative therapies are discussed earlier. The published results of percutaneous RFA of small (≤5 cm) CRC metastases compares well with postresection survival data.[94] Also, emerging data concern the role of RFA in the palliation of CRC metastases. These data suggest a survival benefit over systemic chemotherapy, which was previously the sole mainstay of therapy in these patients.[95] Hepatic metastases from CRC are also amenable to cryoablation and microwave ablation, although there are fewer data to support their use. Many of the studies evaluating the efficacy of cryoablation therapy do not separate patient population by type of neoplasm, making it more difficult to ascertain whether cryoablation is more or less effective for specific tumor types.[96]

Neuroendocrine Liver Metastases

Etiology and Natural History

Neuroendocrine tumors are relatively rare entities with an estimated incidence of one or two cases per 100,000 persons per year in the United States.[97] They are a heterogenous group of neoplasms originating from endocrine cells. Thus, they can originate from anywhere that endocrine cells live (e.g., gastrointestinal tract, pituitary, pancreas). *Carcinoid, insulinoma,* and *glucagonoma* are just a few examples. Neuroendocrine tumors also have a strong predilection for developing liver metastases (up to 78% in some surgical series).[98] The tumors are generally slow growing and typically have a long, indolent disease course, particularly when the tumor is of the nonfunctional type. Still, metastatic neuroendocrine disease is associated with a 5-year survival rate of only 22%.[99]

Clinical Features

Patients' clinical presentations usually result from the tumor's biochemical activity or from local obstruction or infiltration of an adjacent anatomic structure.[100] For example, a patient with a carcinoid tumor may present with flushing, diarrhea, and weight loss.

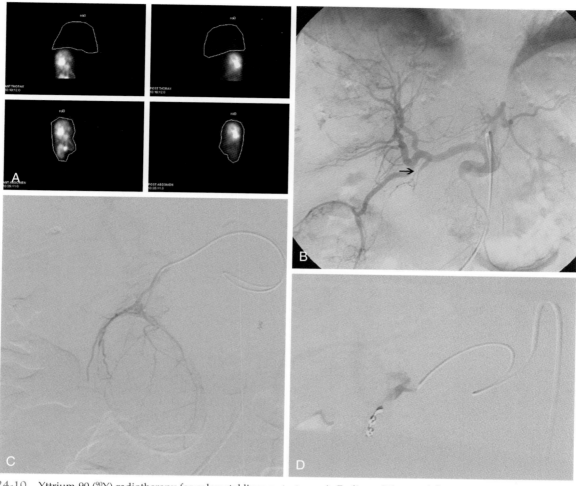

FIGURE 24-10 Yttrium-90 (^{90}Y) radiotherapy for colorectal liver metastases. **A,** Radionuclide scan following intraarterial injection of Tc-99m macroaggregated albumin excludes significant shunting to the lungs. **B,** Celiac arteriography shows multiple vascular masses in the liver. The cystic artery is identified *(arrow).* **C,** A coaxial microcatheter is used to select the artery, which is then embolized with coils. **D,** Inadvertent delivery of ^{90}Y to this site could lead to cholecystitis.

Imaging

Hepatic metastases from neuroendocrine tumors have variable appearance on cross-sectional imaging studies. Some metastases are hypervascular on early arterial imaging, whereas others are hypovascular. Octreotide scans as well as PET-CT can aid in the diagnosis and staging of these lesions. Usually, a combination of imaging modalities is used when evaluating patients with symptomatic neuroendocrine metastatic disease (Fig. 24-11).

Treatment

MEDICAL THERAPY

Somatostatin analogues (e.g., *octreotide*) are often initially effective in controlling symptoms because they interfere with the activity of hormones liberated by the tumors. The PROMID trial found that octreotide LAR (long-acting release) significantly lengthened the time to tumor progression compared with placebo in this population.[101] However, complete regression or prolonged response has yet to be proven.[102]

SURGICAL THERAPY

According to the latest National Comprehensive Cancer Network guidelines, patients with clinically significant progression of neuroendocrine metastases should undergo either cytoreductive surgery (if near complete resection can be achieved) or liver-directed therapy.[103] Symptomatic relief and survival benefit has been demonstrated in patients with metastatic neuroendocrine tumors.[104] One common theme in the current literature is that cytoreduction, regardless of whether complete surgical resection is achieved, has resulted in response of tumor markers and improvement in symptoms in patients with metastatic neuroendocrine

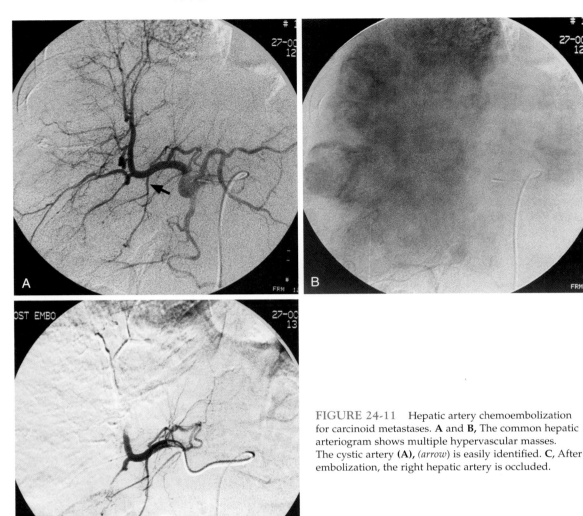

FIGURE 24-11   Hepatic artery chemoembolization for carcinoid metastases. **A** and **B,** The common hepatic arteriogram shows multiple hypervascular masses. The cystic artery **(A),** *(arrow)* is easily identified. **C,** After embolization, the right hepatic artery is occluded.

tumors.[105] Open or laparoscopic ablative therapies can be conducted at the time of surgical resection, allowing treatment of the primary and metastatic lesions in one setting.

LIVER DIRECTED THERAPY

Accepted indications for liver directed therapy are unresectable tumors with symptoms related to hormonal excess and tumor bulk. The techniques of chemoembolization and radioembolization are discussed previously in this chapter. An important adjunct to the preprocedure management of patients with neuroendocrine metastases is the administration of a somatostatin analogue before therapy whether the patient is currently receiving this therapy or not. This measure should limit

symptoms caused by hormonal release immediately following therapy.[106]

Several studies have reported the beneficial therapeutic effect of chemoembolization and bland hepatic embolization for patients with metastatic neuroendocrine tumors. In a study published in 2007 comparing TACE with bland embolization, patients treated with TACE demonstrated a trend toward improvement in time to progression, symptom control, and survival.[107] Likewise, published reports of radioembolization in patients with metastatic neuroendocrine tumors have been favorable. Prolonged response to treatment (i.e., >2 years) has been demonstrated.[108] Accordingly, the median survival was 70 months in a retrospective review of 148 patients with metastatic neuroendocrine tumors treated with radioembolization.[109]

The principles of percutaneous ablation for neuroendocrine metastases follow those mentioned previously in this chapter. Important factors include size, location, and number of lesions. As with embolotherapy, ablation of neuroendocrine metastases can be associated with release of hormonally active substances during the procedure and, in the case of carcinoid metastases, produce a tumor crisis.[110] Therefore, these patients should be pretreated with a somatostatin analogue. Heat-based ablation has shown benefit as an adjunctive treatment at the time of aggressive surgical resection and in palliation of symptoms in appropriately selected patients. Data regarding cryoablation and microwave ablation in this setting are sparse.

KIDNEY

Renal Cell Carcinoma

Etiology and Imaging

The American Cancer Society estimated 57,760 new cases of tumors of the kidney and renal pelvis with 12,980 deaths in the United States in 2009.[111] Most of these tumors will prove to be *renal cell carcinoma (RCC)*. The expanding role of cross-sectional imaging in daily medical practice continues to increase the detection of incidental small renal masses.[112] These tumors classically present as a heterogeneously enhancing mass that disturbs the renal contour. Multiphase contrast-enhanced imaging is typically used for staging purposes. Staging is performed with the TNM staging classifications system that includes anatomic factors such as tumor size, venous invasion, renal capsule invasion, adrenal involvement, and lymph node and distant metastasis.[113] A unique characteristic of this tumor is its tendency to spread in an intravascular manner, along with the development of distant metastatic lesions to the bone, brain, liver, and lungs. Even though the imaging diagnosis of RCC is sometimes straightforward by CT, problem-solving tools including MRI and ultrasound are often needed. The *Bosniak classification system* was developed as a means to separate cystic renal masses into surgical and nonsurgical categories based on specific features. Much effort has been invested in developing methods to distinguish RCCs from complex renal cysts, angiomyolipomas, oncocytomas, renal metastasis, and lymphoma.

At presentation, RCC is commonly asymptomatic and localized when detected. Whereas some studies advocate watchful waiting and active surveillance, many patients and physicians choose to treat these small, early stage tumors because there are less invasive options. Stage Ia (<4 cm) tumors represent the vast majority of lesions treated percutaneously or with nephron-sparing surgery.

Treatment

SURGICAL THERAPY

The gold standard for treatment of these small lesions is excision with a nephron-sparing approach.[114] This therapy is as effective as radical nephrectomy for tumors smaller than 4 cm.[115] Nephron-sparing surgery includes techniques such as laparoscopic ablation as well as partial resection. Resection requires access to the renal hilum and clamping of the renal vessels to achieve hemostasis while removing the mass. The propensity for intravascular spread and invasion of regional structures does not necessarily preclude nephrectomy based on current staging systems.

PERCUTANEOUS ABLATION

PATIENT SELECTION Thermal ablation has emerged as a treatment option for medically inoperable patients with RCC. The early success with thermal ablation in this population has provided an opportunity to treat patients who do not want to undergo surgery and those with underlying renal insufficiency, solitary kidney, transplanted kidney, or multifocal tumors (e.g., individuals with von Hippel Lindau syndrome.)[114] Biopsy of indeterminate renal masses may be obtained before or at the same setting as thermal ablation. Biopsy is often not performed at a separate preablation setting because controversy exists over its utility for characterizing small renal masses, thus limiting its value for clinical decision making. The timing and role of biopsy with regard to ablation is debated and more extensively reviewed elsewhere.[115]

TECHNIQUE RFA and cryoablation are the primary modalities used for percutaneous therapy of renal tumors.[116] There has been a recent trend favoring cryoablation in the kidney although both methods have certain advantages and disadvantages. A variety of imaging modalities can be used, including ultrasound, CT, and MRI, based largely on the interventionalist's experience, availability of equipment, and lesion location.[116] Tumors less than 4 cm in diameter (stage Ia) are most appropriate for these ablative techniques. Ablation of larger tumors is feasible, particularly if they are exophytic. Posterior exophytic lesions are the most favorable; central and hilar lesions are much more difficult. Extrarenal complications are uncommon but may occur with anterior tumors (bowel or visceral organ injury), central tumors (collecting system and main renal vessel injury), lower pole tumors (ureteral injury), or upper pole tumors (pleural effusion or pneumothorax).[116]

The procedure is most commonly performed under CT, CT fluoroscopy, or ultrasound/fluoroscopic guidance. Ultrasound has the advantage of real-time monitoring during the ablation, whereas CT provides more information about surrounding organs that must be avoided.[114] With the patient prone, scout CT images are obtained for planning purposes. The anticipated route may need to be altered due to differences in kidney position from the supine diagnostic scan or phases of respiration. "Hydrodissection" may be employed if there is need to displace nontarget structures. This technique entails needle placement and subsequent infusion of either sterile water or dextrose 5% in water to separate the target from nontarget structures. Saline solution should not be used for this purpose when performing RFA, because the conductive properties of saline may cause an unpredictable zone of ablation. A general guideline for probe placement is the "2 to 1 rule," in which probes should be placed no more than 2 cm apart from one another and within 1 cm of the tumor margin.[114] Once the probes are in satisfactory position, one may proceed with ablation according to the manufacturer's specifications and institutional protocol. With cryoablation, two freezing periods of 10 minutes are usually separated by an active thaw interval. Monitoring images are obtained every 5 minutes during the freeze periods. After the second freeze, a passive or active thaw is employed, the probes are removed, and final imaging is obtained. Patients are recovered according to the type of anesthesia/sedation they receive, observed overnight, and discharged the following morning.

RESULTS AND COMPLICATIONS Recovery is faster after percutaneous ablation than with the laparoscopic approach. Thumar and colleagues[114] recently summarized the results of RF ablation for RCC. At least 79% of tumors in all studies were treated in a single session. After complete necrosis was achieved by imaging criteria, the local progression rates ranged from 0% to 9.7%. Unfortunately, local progression was identified as late as 31 months after treatment, thus necessitating long-term surveillance. In the same review, initial success rates for cryoablation were reported as greater than 90% in all series.[114] The risk of local tumor progression appears lower than with RF ablation, but the series are smaller and the follow-up periods shorter.[114] For this reason, current follow-up strategies involve repeat CT or MRI with and without contrast at 1, 3, 6, 12, 18, and 24 months after ablation.[115]

LUNG

Lung Cancer

Etiology and Clinical Features

Lung cancer (bronchogenic carcinoma) refers to malignancies originating from the airway or pulmonary parenchyma. Primary lung cancer is the number one cause of cancer-related deaths in men and women in the United States. The American Cancer Society estimated 159,390 lung cancer deaths for 2009, or 28% of all cancer-related deaths, and 219,440 new cases of lung cancer, or 15% of cancer diagnoses.[111] The World Health Organization recognizes four major histologic subtypes: adenocarcinoma including bronchioalveolar carcinoma, squamous cell carcinoma, large cell carcinoma, and small cell carcinoma. Lung cancers are classified as either *small cell* (SCLC, 14% of cases) or *non–small cell* (NSCLC, 85% of cases). SCLC is the more aggressive of the two types.

Numerous environmental and lifestyle risk factors have been associated with lung cancer development, the most important being cigarette smoking, estimated to account for 90% of all lung cancers.[111] Other risk factors include radiation therapy, various environmental toxins, pulmonary fibrosis, infection with human immunodeficiency virus, genetic factors, and possibly dietary habits. Presenting symptoms depend on the extent of disease. Chest symptoms include cough, hemoptysis, chest pain, and dyspnea. Many patients present with lymph node or systemic involvement and are thus treated primarily with chemotherapy and irradiation.

Imaging

Because of the typically late presentation and dismal prognosis of most lung cancer, concerted efforts are underway in the United States and throughout the world to develop effective screening programs. Although many pulmonary neoplasms are still discovered on conventional chest radiographs, CT and PET-CT have emerged as the diagnostic workhorses in the diagnosis and staging of lung cancer. In addition, CT is now commonly used to guide percutaneous biopsy for tissue diagnosis.

Treatment

THERMAL ABLATION

PATIENT SELECTION Most published research in pulmonary tumor ablation is related to treatment of NSCLC. The primary scenario for percutaneous ablative therapy is the medically inoperable, high-risk patient with an early stage lung cancer.[117] This group typically includes patients who would normally qualify for surgical resection but will not tolerate an operation due to an inadequate pulmonary reserve or concomitant cardiopulmonary disease. Pulmonary ablation can also be used in individuals with small pulmonary metastases without hilar or mediastinal nodal involvement or extrathoracic disease.[117] Finally, palliative thermal ablation may be performed for patients experiencing tumor related symptoms (e.g., painful chest wall masses). RFA should be avoided in the lung apex and mediastinum due to the risk of mechanical and thermal injury.

TECHNIQUE RFA or microwave ablation may interfere with pacemaker or defibrillator function. Therefore, the interventionalist must consult with anesthesia or cardiology services regarding the need for external pacing or defibrillation.[117] Ablation may be done with midazolam and fentanyl, although some physicians prefer monitored anesthesia or a general anesthetic.

Although some chest wall or pleural masses may be ablated with ultrasound guidance, the vast majority are performed with CT guidance. A preprocedural CT should be reviewed for planning purposes. The overlying skin is prepped and local and extrapleural anesthesia is administered. A preliminary CT scan of the extrapleural needle is obtained to assess the potential trajectory of the probe or electrode. The size and depth of the lesion determine the length and active tip of the probe selected.[117] Treatment times vary by ablative technology and number of probes. After the lesion is treated, the probe is removed and a postprocedure CT scan is performed to evaluate for pneumothorax. Postprocedure observation is performed for 2 to 3 hours with a repeat chest radiograph to exclude pneumothorax.

Microwave ablation has many theoretical advantages over other ablation systems, including the ability to achieve higher intratumoral temperatures, larger ablation volumes, and faster ablation times.[118] In addition, microwave ablation does not rely on an electrical circuit; as such, multiple probes may be used simultaneously. The advantages of cryoablation over RFA include larger tumor ablation volumes, the ability to use multiple probes, and less procedural pain. The ability to see lower attenuation ice as it covers a soft tissue mass is also a consideration.

IMAGING FOLLOW-UP There is no consensus regarding the best imaging modality or surveillance protocol after lung ablation. A common strategy involves CT imaging at 1-, 3-, and then 6-month intervals. FDG PET-CT has been recently shown to depict a higher number of treatment failures earlier than chest CT.[119]. The initial postablation CT usually demonstrates a ground-glass opacity around the ablated mass which roughly equates to the ablation margin.[119] At 1 month, the lesion may have apparently increased in size and appear as a nodular consolidation. Diminished or absent activity on PET scans also suggests tumor necrosis without residual disease. Residual tumor is sometimes identified as uptake within the periphery of the lesion, although this finding is not entirely specific.[119]

RESULTS AND COMPLICATIONS The current literature regarding thermal ablation of the lung involves studies published with heterogenous groups with different follow-up periods and reporting standards.[120] There is currently greater experience with RFA in that the majority of studies involving pulmonary ablation involve this technology. A retrospective review was performed of 153 patients with 189 lesions who received RFA and a median 20.5-month follow-up. The Kaplan-Meier 1-, 2-, 3-, 4-, and 5-year survival rates for stage I non–small cell lung cancer were 78%, 57%, 36%, 27%, and 27%, respectively.[117] Another group followed 60 patients with five or fewer tumors per patient with a diameter of less than 4 cm. Overall survival rates at 18 months were 76% for primary lung tumors and 71% for metastatic disease.[117] Complications of percutaneous lung ablation include postablation syndrome (see earlier discussion), bleeding, cardiopulmonary collapse, pneumothorax, hemoptysis, pulmonary hemorrhage, reactive pleural effusion, bronchopleural fistula, infection or abscess formation, damage to adjacent anatomic structures, and skin burns during RFA secondary to incorrect grounding pad placement.[117]

BONE

Image-guided percutaneous treatment of bone tumors is another developing application of thermal ablation. In some patients, it is an effective alternative to surgery or external beam radiation. Percutaneous ablation is now the first line treatment for osteoid osteoma. It also has value in some other benign primary bone tumors and for palliation of painful bone metastases.[121] Thermal ablation can be combined with cementoplasty in metastases at risk for fracture to provide stability as well as pain control.

When considering a musculoskeletal lesion for potential ablation, a multidisciplinary approach should be used with involvement of the medical oncologist, musculoskeletal-trained radiologist, and orthopedic oncologist to verify tumor type and choose the most appropriate therapy. One should be familiar with the perilesional anatomy including adjacent nerves, blood vessels, and organs.[121] Additional tools such as motor-evoked potentials may be used when lesions are near the spinal cord or major motor nerves.[121] Preprocedure planning requires an understanding of the lesion being treated. CT is the most commonly used modality for skeletal ablation procedures because of the ability to rapidly and accurately place devices. Ultrasound may be used in the setting of soft tissue tumor treatment.

Osteoid Osteoma

Osteoid osteoma is a small, painful, benign bone tumor that typically occurs in children and young adults. The classic presentation is severe pain that is worse at night and is relieved with salicylates. Imaging demonstrates a radiolucent nidus composed of vascular osteoblastic tissue found primarily in the metaphysis and diaphysis of long bones.[121] Effective treatment requires destruction of the central nidus to achieve cure. Rosenthal and colleagues[122] first reported the use of RFA in osteoid osteoma and have since published additional series with longer follow-up. The standard treatment algorithm involves placement of a noncooled RF probe in the nidus of the lesion for 6 minutes at 90° C.[122]

Bone Metastases

Studies have demonstrated that up to 85% of patients with breast, prostate, and lung cancer have bone metastases at the time of death.[123] Palliation for skeletal metastases include local therapies (e.g., surgery, external beam radiation, thermal ablation), systemic therapies (e.g., chemotherapy, radiopharmaceuticals, bisphosphonates), and analgesics (e.g., nonsteroidal antiinflammatories, opioids).[121] Radiation therapy is currently the standard of care for management of localized painful metastases. However, data are mixed regarding the effectiveness and durability of this therapy. Surgery is typically reserved for recent or impending fracture. Recent publications have shown positive outcomes in the ablation of bone and soft tissue metastases with improved palliation with painful bone metastases. An American College of Radiology Imaging Network (ACRIN) single arm prospective trial evaluating the use of RFA in bone metastases showed decrease in pain severity at 1 and 3 months at follow-up.[124] When performing ablation for pain control, patient selection is crucial. Patients should have pain localized to one or two sites and at least moderate in severity (>4 on a 10-point scale for worst pain in a 24-hour period).[121]

Cementoplasty may be used alone or in combination with thermal ablation techniques to treat metastatic lesions. This technique involves percutaneous injection of polymethylmethacrylate cement to provide stability in the weight-bearing bones in the spine and pelvis in an effort to minimize the risk of pathologic fracture. Pain relief is believed to occur from a direct effect on nociceptors in addition to stabilization of microfractures. As with other applications of thermal ablation, further research is needed to define the role and outcomes of ablation with respect to bone tumors.

References

1. Parkin DM, Bray F, Ferlay J, et al. Global cancer statistics, 2002. *CA Cancer J Clin* 2005;**55**:74.
2. Jemal A, Bray F, Center MM, et al. Global cancer statistics 2011. *CA Cancer J Clin* 2011;**61**:69.
3. Bosch FX, Ribes J, Diaz M, et al. Primary liver cancer: worldwide incidence and trends. *Gastroenterology* 2004;**127**:S5.
4. Ries LAG, Eisner MP, Kosary CL, et al, editors. *SEER cancer statistics review, 1975–2002*. Bethesda (MD): National Cancer Institute; 2005.
5. Ananthakrishnan A, Gogineni V, Saeian K. Epidemiology of primary and secondary liver cancers. *Semin Interv Radiol* 2006;**23**:47.
6. Sherlock S. Viruses and hepatocellular carcinoma. *Gut* 1994;**35**:828.
7. Hassan MM, Hwang LY, Hatten CJ, et al. Risk factors for hepatocellular carcinoma: synergism of alcohol with viral hepatitis and diabetes mellitus. *Hepatology* 2002;**36**:1206.
8. Bralet MP, Regimbear JM, Pineau P, et al. Hepatocellular carcinoma occurring in nonfibrotic liver: epidemiologic and histopathologic analysis of 80 French cases. *Hepatology* 2000;**32**:200.
9. Llovet JM, Bustamante J, Castells A, et al. Natural history of untreated nonsurgical hepatocellular carcinoma: rationale for the design and evaluation of therapeutic trials. *Hepatology* 1999;**29**:62.
10. Bruix J, Sherman M. AASLD practice guideline: management of hepatocellular carcinoma. *Hepatology* 2005;**42**:1208.
11. Okuda K, Ohtsuki T, Obata H, et al. Natural history of hepatocellular carcinoma and prognosis in relation to treatment. *Cancer* 1985;**56**:918.
12. Levy I, Sherman M. Staging of hepatocellular carcinoma: assessment of the CLIP, Okuda, and Child-Pugh staging systems in a cohort of 257 patients in Toronto. *Gut* 2002;**50**:881.
13. Christiansen E. Prognostic models including the Child-Pugh, MELD and Mayo risk scores—where are we and where should we go? *J Hepatol* 2004;**41**:344.
14. Llovet JM, Bru C, Bruix J. Prognosis of hepatocellular carcinoma: the BCLC staging classification. *Semin Liver Dis* 1999;**19**:329.
15. Caturelli E, Pompili M, Bartolucci F, et al. Hemangioma-like lesions in chronic liver disease: diagnostic evaluation in patients. *Radiology* 2001;**220**:337.
16. Peterson MS, Baron RL. Radiologic diagnosis of hepatocellular carcinoma. *Clin Liver Dis* 2001;**5**:123.
17. Fielding, L. Current imaging strategies of primary and secondary neoplasms of the liver. *Semin Interv Radiol* 2006;**23**:3.
18. Hwang GJ, Kim MJ, Yoo HS, et al. Nodular hepatocellular carcinomas: detection with arterial-, portal-, and delayed phase images at spiral CT. *Radiology* 1997;**202**:383.
19. Colombo M. Screening and diagnosis of hepatocellular carcinoma. *Liver International* 2009;**29**:143.
20. Zech CJ, Reiser MF, Hermann KA. Imaging of hepatocellular carcinoma by computed tomography and magnetic resonance imaging: state of the art. *Dig Dis* 2009;**27**:114.
21. Burrel M, Llovet JM, Ayuso C, et al. MRI angiography is superior to helical CT for detection of HCC prior to liver transplantation: an explant correlation. *Hepatology* 2003;**38**:1034.
22. Llovet JM, Burroughs A, Bruix J. Hepatocellular carcinoma. *Lancet* 2003;**362**:1907.
23. Llovet JM, Bruix J. Systematic review of randomized trials for unresectable hepatocellular carcinoma: chemoembolization improves survival. *Hepatology* 2003;**37**:429.
24. Lopez PM, Villanueva A, Llovet JM. Systematic review: evidence-based management of hepatocellular carcinoma-an updated analysis of randomized controlled trials. *Aliment Pharmacol Ther* 2006;**23**:1535.
25. Llovet JM, Ricci S, Mazzafero V, et al. Sorafenib in advanced hepatocellular carcinoma. *N Engl J Med* 2008;**359**:378.
26. Song TJ, Wai Kit Ip E, Fong Y. Hepatocellular carcinoma: current surgical management. *Gastroenterology* 2004;**127**:S248.
27. Hemming AW, Reed AL, Howard RJ, et al. Preoperative portal vein embolization for extended hepatectomy. *Ann Surg* 2003;**237**:686.
28. Abulkhir A, Limongelli P, Healey AJ, et al. Preoperative portal vein embolization for major liver resection: a meta-analysis. *Ann Surg* 2008;**247**:49.
29. Patt CH, Thulvath PJ. Role of liver transplantation in the management of hepatocellular carcinoma. *J Vasc Interv Radiol* 2002;**13**:S205.
30. Shetty K, Timmins K, Brensinger C, et al. Liver transplantation for hepatocellular carcinoma: validation of the present selection criteria in predicting outcome. *Liver Transpl* 2004;**10**:911.

31. Breedis C, Young G. The blood supply of neoplasms in the liver. *Am J Pathol* 1954;**30**:969.

32. Shin SW. The current practice of transarterial chemoembolization for the treatment of hepatocellular carcinoma. *Korean J Radiol* 2009;**10**:425.

33. Yemane B, Weber S. Liver-directed treatment modalities for primary and secondary hepatic tumors. *Surg Clin N Am* 2009;**89**:97.

34. Tsochatzis EA, Germani G, Burroughs AK. Transarterial chemoembolization, transarterial chemotherapy, and intra-arterial chemotherapy for hepatocellular carcinoma treatment. *Semin Oncol* 2010; **37**:898.

35. Liapi E, Georgiades CC, Hong K, et al. Transcatheter arterial chemoembolization: current technique and future promise. *Tech Vasc Interv Radiol* 2007;**10**:2.

36. Dharancy S, Boitard J, Decaens T, et al. Comparison of two techniques of transarterial chemoembolization before liver transplantation for hepatocellular carcinoma: a case-control study. *Liver Transpl* 2007; **13**:665.

37. Kiely JM, Rilling WS, Touzios JG, et al. Chemoembolization in patients at high risk. *J Vasc Interv Radiol* 2003;**17**:47.

38. Georgiades CS, Hong K, D'Angelo M, et al. Safety and efficacy of transarterial chemoembolization in patients with unresectable hepatocellular carcinoma and portal vein thrombosis. *J Vasc Interv Radiol* 2005;**16**:1653.

39. Kim W, Clark T, Baum RA, et al. Risk factors for liver abscess formation after hepatic chemoembolization. *J Vasc Interv Radiol* 2001;**12**:965.

40. Geschwind JH, Kauchik S. Influence of new prophylactic antibiotic therapy on the incidence of liver abscesses after chemoembolization treatment of liver tumors. *J Vasc Interv Radiol* 2002;**13**:1163.

41. Okuda K, Mush H, Yamasaki T, et al. Angiographic demonstration of intrahepatic arterio-portal anastomoses in hepatocellular carcinoma. *Radiology* 1977;**122**:53.

42. Brown KT, Koh BY, Brody LA, et al. Particle embolization of hepatic neuroendocrine metastases for control of pain and hormonal symptoms. *J Vasc Interv Radiol* 1999;**10**:397.

43. Miyayama S, Matsui O, Taki K, et al. Extrahepatic blood supply to hepatocellular carcinoma: angiographic demonstration and transcatheter arterial chemoembolization. *Cardiovasc Interv Radiol* 2006; **29**:39.

44. Lo CM, Ngan H, Tso WK, et al. Randomized controlled trial of transarterial lipiodol chemoembolization for unresectable hepatocellular carcinoma. *Hepatology* 2002;**35**:1164.

45. Llovet J, Real MI, Montana X, et al. Arterial embolization or chemoembolization versus symptomatic treatment in patients with unresectable hepatocellular carcinoma: a randomized controlled trial. *Lancet* 2002;**359**:1734.

46. Leung DA, Goin JE, Sickles C, et al. Determinants of postembolization syndrome after hepatic chemoembolization. *J Vasc Interv Radiol* 2001;**12**:321.

47. Gonsalves CF, Brown DB. Chemoembolization of hepatic malignancy. *Abdom Imaging* 2009;**34**:557.

48. Brown DB, Cardella JF, Sacks D, et al. Quality improvement guidelines for transhepatic arterial chemoembolizawtion, embolization, and chemotherapeutic infusion for hepatic malignancy. *J Vasc Interv Radiol* 2006;**17**:225.

49. Sakamoto I, Aso N, Nagaoki K, et al. Complications associated with transcatheter arterial embolization for hepatic tumours. *Radiographics* 1998;**18**:605.

50. Geschwind JF, Salem R, Carr BI, et al. Yttrium-90 microspheres for the treatment of hepatocellular carcinoma. *Gastroenterology* 2004; **127**:S194.

51. Kennedy AS, Nag S, Salem R, et al. Recommendations for radioembolization of hepatic malignancies using yttrium-90 microsphere brachytherapy: a consensus panel report from the radioembolization brachytherapy oncology consortium. *Int J Radiat Oncol Biol Phys* 2007;**68**:13.

52. Kennedy AS, Salem R. Radioembolization (yttrium-90 microspheres) for primary and metastatic hepatic malignancies. *Cancer J* 2010;**16**:163.

53. *TheraSphere Yttruim-90 microspheres* [package insert]. Kanata (Canada): MDS Nordion; 2004.

54. Murthy R, Nunez R, Szklaruk J, et al. Yttrium-90 microsphere therapy for hepatic malignancy: devices, indications, technical considerations, and potential complications. *Radiographics* 2005; **25**:S41.

55. Salem R, Thruston KG. Radioembolization with 90Yttrium microspheres: a state-of-the-art brachytherapy treatment for primary and secondary liver malignancies: Part 1: technical and methodologic considerations. *J Vasc Interv Radiol* 2006;**17**:1251.

56. Salem R, Lewandowski RJ, Mulcahy MF, et al. Radioembolization for hepatocellular carcinoma using yttrium-90 microspheres: a comprehensive report of long-term outcomes. *Gastroenterology* 2010;**138**:52.

57. Sangro B, Bilbao JI, Boan J, et al. Radioembolization using 90Y-resin microspheres for patients with advanced hepatocellular carcinoma. *Int J Radiat Oncol Biol Phys* 2006;**66**:792.

58. Garin E, Rolland Y, Boucher E, et al. First experience of hepatic radioembolization using microspheres labeled with yttrium-90 (TheraSphere): practical aspects concerning its implementation. *Eur J Nucl Med Mol Imaging* 2010;**37**:453.

59. Geschwind JF, Salem R, Carr BI, et al. Yttrium-90 microspheres for the treatment of hepatocellular carcinoma. *Gastroenterology* 2004; **127**:S107.

60. Kooby DA, Egnatashvili V, Srinivasan S, et al. Comparison of yttrium-90 radioembolization and transcatheter arterial chemoembolization for the treatment of unresectable hepatocellular carcinoma. *J Vasc Interv Radiol* 2010;**21**:224.

61. Kulik LM, Atassi B, van Holsbeeck L, et al. Yttrium-90 microspheres (TheraSphere) treatment of unresectable hepatocellular carcinoma: downstaging to resection, RFA, and bridge to transplantation. *J Surg Oncol* 2006;**94**:572.

62. Salem R, Lewandowski RJ, Atassi B, et al. Treatment of unresectable hepatocellular carcinoma with use of 90Y microspheres (TheraSphere): safety, tumor response, and survival. *J Vasc Interv Radiol* 2005;**16**:1627.

63. Riaz A, Kulik LM, Mulcahy MF, et al. Yttrium-90 radioembolization in the management of liver malignancies. *Semin Oncol* 2010; **37**:94.

64. Kennedy AS, McNeillie P, Dezarn WA, et al. Treatment parameters and outcome in 680 treatments of internal radiation with resin 90Y-microspheres for unresectable hepatic tumors. *Int J Radiat Oncol Biol Phys* 2009;**74**:1494.

65. Saldanha DF, Khiatani VL, Carrillo TC, et al. Current tumor ablation technologies: basic science and device review. *Semin Interv Radiol* 2010;**27**:247.

66. Salloum C, Castaing D. Surgical margin status in hepatectomy for liver tumors. *Bull Cancer* 2008;**95**:1183.

67. Hong K, Georgiades C. Radiofrequency ablation: mechanism of action and devices. *J Vasc Interv Radiol* 2010;**21**:S179.

68. Erinjeri JP, Clark TW. Cryoablation: mechanism of action and devices. *J Vasc Interv Radiol* 2010;**21**:S187.

69. Hinshaw JL, Lee FT. Cryoablation for liver cancer. *Tech Vasc Interv Radiol* 2007;**10**:47.

70. Erinjeri JP, Clark TW. Cryoablation: Mechanism of action and devices. *J Vasc Interv Radiol* 2010;**21**:S187.

71. Lubner MG, Brace CL, Hinshaw JL, et al. Microwave tumor ablation: mechanisms of action, clinical results, and devices. *J Vasc Interv Radiol* 2010;**21**:S192.

72. Stone MJ, Wood BJ. Emerging local ablation techniques. *Semin Interv Rad* 2006;**23**:85.

73. Xu HX, Lu M, Xie X, et al. Prognostic factors for long-term outcome after percutaneous thermal ablation for hepatocellular carcinoma: a

survival analysis of 137 consecutive patients. *Clin Radiol* 2005; **60**:1018.

74. McWilliams JP, Yamamoto S, Raman SS, et al. Percutaneous ablation of hepatocellular carcinoma: current status. *J Vasc Interv Radiol* 2010;**21**:S204.

75. Tateishi R, Shiina S, Teratani T, et al. Percutaneous radiofrequency ablation for hepatocellular carcinoma: an analysis of 1000 cases. *Cancer* 2005;**103**:1201.

76. Lencioni R, Cioni D, Crocetti L, et al. Early stage hepatocellular carcinoma in patients with cirrhosis: long term results of percutaneous image-guided radiofrequency ablation. *Radiology* 2005;**234**:961.

77. N'Kontchou G, Mahamoudi A, Aout M, et al. Radiofrequency ablation of hepatocellular carcinoma: long-term results and prognostic factors in 235 Western patients with cirrhosis. *Hepatology* 2009;**50**:1475.

78. Chen MS, Li JQ, Zheng Y, et al. A prospective randomized trial comparing percutaneous ablative therapy and partial hepatectomy for small hepatocellular carcinoma. *Ann Surg* 2006;**243**:321.

79. Hinshaw JL, Lee FT. Cryoablation for liver cancer. *Tech Vasc Interv Rad* 2007;**10**:47.

80. Liang P, Dong B, Yu X, et al. Prognostic factors for survival in patients with hepatocellular carcinoma after percutaneous microwave ablation. *Radiology* 2005;**235**:299.

81. Mulier S, Mulier P, Ni Y, et al. Complications of radiofrequency coagulation of liver tumors. *Br J Surg* 2002;**89**:1206.

82. Siefert JK, Morris DL. World survey on the complications of hepatic and prostate cryotherapy. *World J Surg* 1999;**23**:109.

83. Lehner SG, Gould JE, Saad WE, et al. Tumor lysis syndrome after radiofrequency ablation of hepatocellular carcinoma. *AJR Am J Radiol* 2005;**185**:1307.

84. Jemal A, Siegel R, Ward E, et al. Cancer statistics, 2009. *CA Cancer J Clin* 2009;**59**:225.

85. Vogl TJ, Zangos S, Eichler K, et al. Colorectal liver metastases: regional chemotherapy via transarterial chemoembolization (TACE) and hepatic chemoperfusion: an update. *Eur Radiol* 2007; **17**:1025.

86. Alexander HR, Allegra CJ, Lawrence TS. Metastatic cancer to the liver. In: Devita VT, Hellman S, Rosenberg SA, editors. *Cancer: principles and practice of oncology* . 6th ed. Philadelphia: Lippincott Williams and Wilkins; 2001. p. 2690.

87. Stangl R, Altendorf-Hoffmann A, Charnley RM, et al. Factors influencing the natural history of colorectal liver metastases. *Lancet* 1994; **343**:1405.

88. Fielding L. Current imaging strategies of primary and secondary neoplasms of the liver. *Semin Interven Rad* 2006;**23**:3.

89. Garden OJ, Rees M, Poston GJ, et al. Guidelines for resection of colorectal cancer liver metastases. *Gut* 2006;**55**(suppl 3):iii1.

90. Abdalla EK, Vauthey JN, Ellis LM, et al. Recurrence and outcomes following hepatic resection, radiofrequency ablation, and combined resection/ablation for colorectal liver metastases. *Ann Surg* 2004; **239**:818.

91. Pawlik TM, Scoggins CR, Zorzi D, et al. Effect of surgical margin status on survival and site of recurrence after hepatic resection for colorectal metastases. *Ann Surg* 2005;**241**:715.

92. Fiorentini G, Aliberti C, Turrisi G, et al. Intraarterial hepatic chemoembolization of liver metastases from colorectal cancer adopting irinotecan-eluting beads: results of a phase II clinical study. *In Vivo* 2007;**21**:1085.

93. Vente MAD, Wondergem M, van der Tweel I, et al. Yttrium-90 microsphere radioembolization for the treatment of liver malignancies: a structured meta-analysis. *Eur Radiol* 2009;**19**:951.

94. Gillams AR, Lees WR. RFA of CRC in 167 patients. *Eur Radiol* 2004; **14**:2261.

95. Venkatesan AM, Gervais DA, Mueller PR. Percutaneous radiofrequency thermal ablation of primary and metastatic hepatic tumors: current concepts and review of the literature. *Semin Interv Radiol* 2006;**23**:73.

96. Smith MT, Ray CE. The treatment of primary and metastatic hepatic neoplasms using percutaneous cryotherapy. *Semin Interven Radiol* 2006;**23**:39.

97. Modlin IM, Lye KD, Kidd M. A 5-decade analysis of 13,715 carcinoid tumors. *Cancer* 2003;**97**:934.

98. Chu Q, Hill H, Douglass H, et al. Predictive factors associated with long-term survival in patients with neuroendocrine tumors of the pancreas. *Ann Surg Oncol* 2002;**9**:855.

99. Modlin IM, Sandor A. An analysis of 8305 cases of carcinoid tumors. *Cancer* 1997;**79**:813.

100. Liu DM, Kennedy A, Turner D, et al. Minimally invasive techniques in management of hepatic neuroendocrine metastatic disease. *Am J Clin Oncol* 2009;**32**:200.

101. Rinke A, Muller HH, Schade-Brittinger C, et al. Placebo-controlled, double-blind, prospective, randomized study on the effect of octreotide LAR in the Control of tumor growth in patients with metastatic neuroendocrine midgut tumors: a report from the PROMID Study Group. *J Clin Oncol* 2009;**27**:4656.

102. Modlin IM, Latich I, Kidd M, et al. Therapeutic options for gastrointestinal carcinoids. *Clin Gastroenterol Hepatol* 2006;**4**:526.

103. National Comprehensive Cancer Network. Available at www.nccn.org/professionals/physician_gls/pdf/neuroendocrine.pdf (by subscription).

104. Norton JA. Endocrine tumours of the gastrointestinal tract. Surgical treatment of neuroendocrine metastases. *Best Pract Res Clin Gastroenterol* 2005;**19**:577.

105. Boudreaux JP, Putty B, Frey DJ, et al. Surgical treatment of advanced-stage carcinoid tumors: lessons learned. *Ann Surg* 2005; **241**:839.

106. Gupta S, Yao JC, Ahrar K, et al. Hepatic artery embolization and chemoembolization for treatment of patients with metastatic carcinoid tumors: the M.D. Anderson experience. *Cancer J* 2003; **9**:261.

107. Ruutiainen AT, Soulen MC, Tuite CM, et al. Chemoembolization and bland embolization of neuroendocrine tumor metastases to the liver. *J Vasc Interv Radiol* 2007;**18**:847.

108. Rhee TK, Lewandowski RJ, Liu DM, et al. 90Y Radioembolization for metastatic neuroendocrine liver tumors: preliminary results from a multi-institutional experience. *Ann Surg* 2008;**247**:1029.

109. Kennedy AS, Dezarn WA, McNeillie P, et al. Radioembolization for unresectable neuroendocrine hepatic metastases using resin ^{90}Y-microspheres: early results in 148 patients. *Am J Clin Oncol* 2008;**31**:271.

110. Wettstein M, Vogt C, Cohnen M, et al. Serotonin release during percutaneous radiofrequency ablation in a patient with symptomatic liver metastases of a neuroendocrine tumor. *Hepatogastroenterology* 2004;**51**:830.

111. American Cancer Society. *Cancer statistics 2009*. Atlanta, American Cancer Society; 2009.

112. Parsons JK, Schoenberg MS, Carter HB. Incidental renal tumors: casting doubt on the efficacy of early intervention. *Urology* 2001; **57**:1013.

113. Greene F, Page D, Fleming I, et al. *AJCC cancer staging manual*. 6th ed. New York: Springer; 2002.

114. Thumar AB, Trabulsi EJ, Lallas CD, et al. Thermal ablation of renal cell carcinoma: triage, treatment, and follow-up. *J Vasc Interv Radiol* 2010;**21**:S233.

115. Fergany AF, Hafez KS, Novick AC. Long term results of nephron sparing surgery for localized renal cell carcinoma: 10-year follow up. *J Urol* 2000;**163**:442.

116. Maybody, M. An overview of image-guided percutaneous ablation of renal tumors. *Semin Interv Radiol* 2010;**27**:261.

117. Dupuy DE, Shulman M. Current status of thermal ablation treatments for lung malignancies. *Semin Intervent Radiol* 2010; **27**:268.

118. Lubner MG, Brace CL, Hinshaw JL, et al. Microwave tumor ablation: mechanism of action and devices. *J Vasc Interv Radiol* 2010; **21**:S179.

119. Deandrais D, Leboulleux S, Dromain C. Role of FDG PET/CT and chest CT in the follow-up of lung lesions treated with radiofrequency ablation. *Radiology* 2011;**258**:270.

120. McTaggart RA, Dupuy DE, Dipetrillo T. Image-guided ablation in the thorax. In: Geschwind J-F, Soulen MC, editors. *Interventional oncology: principles and practice*. New York: Cambridge University Press; 2008. p. 440.

121. Kurup AN, Callstrom MC. Image-guided percutaneous ablation of bone and soft tissue tumors. *Semin Interv Radiol* 2010;**27**:276.

122. Rosenthal DI, Alexander A, Rosenberg AE, et al. Ablation of osteoid osteomas with a percutaneously placed electrode: a new procedure. *Radiology* 1992;**183**:29.

123. Nielsen OS, Munro AJ, Tannock IF. Bone metastases: pathophysiology and management policy. *J Clin Oncol* 1991;**9**:509.

124. Dupuy DE, Liu D, Hartfeil D, et al. Percutaneous radiofrequency ablation of painful osseous metastases: a multicenter American College of Radiology Imaging Network trial. *Cancer* 2010;**116**:989.

Index

Note: Page numbers followed by b, f, and t indicate boxes, figures, and tables, respectively.